Fifth Edition

MEASUREMENT OF JOINT MOTION

A GUIDE TO GONIOMETRY

Cynthia C. Norkin, PT, EdD
Associate Professor Emerita
Division of Physical Therapy
College of Health Sciences and Professions
Ohio University
Athens, Ohio

D. Joyce White, PT, DSc
Associate Professor
Department of Physical Therapy
College of Health Sciences
University of Massachusetts Lowell
Lowell, Massachusetts

Photographs by Jason Torres, Jocelyn Greene Molleur, and Lucia Grochowska Littlefield
Illustrations by Timothy Wayne Malone and Graphic World Illustration Services

F. A. DAVIS COMPANY • Philadelphia

JAYPEE **The Health Sciences Publisher**
New Delhi | London | Panama

FIFTH INDIAN EDITION 2017

Measurement of Joint Motion

Printed in India

Published by
Jaypee Brothers Medical Publishers (P) Ltd

Corporate Office
4838/24, Ansari Road, Daryaganj, **New Delhi** 110002, India, Phone: +91-11-43574357

Registered Office
B-3, EMCA House, 23/23B, Ansari Road, Daryaganj, **New Delhi** 110002, India
Phones: +91-11-23272143, +91-91-23272703, +91-11-23282021, +91-11-23245672
Rel: +91-11-32558559, Fax: +91-11-23276490, +91-11-23245683
e-mail: jaypee@jaypebrothers.com, Website: www.jaypeebrothers.com

Branches
- **Ahmedabad** e-mail: ahmedabad@jaypeebrother.com
- **Bengaluru** e-mail: bangalore@jaypeebrothers.com
- **Chennai** e-mail: chennai@jaypeebrothers.com
- **Lucknow** e-mail: lucknow@jaypeebrothers.com
- **Hyderabad** e-mail: hyderabad@jaypeebrother.com
- **Kochi** e-mail: kochi@jaypeebrothers.com
- **Kolkata** e-mail: kolkata@jaypeebrothers.com
- **Mumbai** e-mail: mumabi@jaypeebrothers.com
- **Nagpur** e-mail: nagpur@jaypeebrothers.com

ISBN 978-93-5270-090-5

Preface

The measurement of joint motion is an important component of a thorough physical examination of the extremities and spine, one which helps health professionals determine function, identify impairments, and assess rehabilitative status. The need for a comprehensive text with sufficient written detail and photographs to allow for the standardization of goniometric measurement methods—both for the purposes of teaching and clinical practice—led to the development of the first edition of the *Measurement of Joint Motion: A Guide to Goniometry* in 1985. Our approach included a discussion and photographs of testing position, stabilization, end-feel, and goniometer alignment for each measurable joint in the body. The resulting text was extremely well received by a variety of health professional educational programs and was used as a reference in many clinical settings and research studies.

Subsequent editions were expanded to include muscle length testing at joints where muscle length is often a factor affecting range of motion. This addition integrated the measurement procedures used in this book with the American Physical Therapy Association's *Guide to Physical Therapy Practice*. Illustrations and anatomical descriptions were added so that the reader had a visual reminder of the joint structures and muscles involved in range of motion. Information on osteokinematics, arthrokinematics, and capsular and noncapsular patterns of limitation was included. Illustrations of bony anatomical landmarks and photographs of surface anatomy were added to help the reader align the goniometer accurately. Inclinometer techniques for measuring range of motion of the spine and some alternative positions and alignments for goniometric measurement of the range of motion of certain extremity joints were presented to coincide with current practice in some clinical settings.

In the years following initial publication, a considerable amount of research on the measurement of joint motion appeared in the literature. Consequently, later editions have included a chapter on the reliability and validity of joint measurement, as well as joint-specific research sections in each chapter that focus on measurement procedures. Research findings to establish normative range-of-motion values and the motion needed for a variety of functional tasks have been provided and updated with each edition. Current evidence of the effects on range of motion of an individual's characteristics such as age, gender, body mass, and recreational/occupational activities, as well as the effects of the testing process such as testing position and type of measuring instrument have been consistently included in each edition. In this manner, clinicians have been supported in their efforts to integrate evidence-based practice as they determine an individual's impairments and set rehabilitative goals.

We have made some changes in the fifth edition as part of our ongoing search for ways to present current information in an easily accessible format. New tables and text have been added that summarize up-to-date research findings on the reliability of the assessment of joint motion with universal goniometers and, where appropriate, inclinometers and smart phone applications. For the first time, these tables include absolute measures of reliability such as standard error of measurement (SEM) and minimal detectable change (MDC) that allow clinicians to estimate their measurement error to decide whether changes in range of motion values reflect real changes in their patients. Two exercises have been added to Chapter 3 that will help the reader understand and apply these statistical tests. Extensive new tables have been included that make it easy to find current research results on joint motions needed to perform a wide variety of functional tasks. Summary Guides for each joint that include essential information about testing positions, stabilization, and goniometer and/or inclinometer placement can be quickly located in a new Appendix B. In addition, readers will benefit from the more than 80 new photographs and illustrations that are included to better explain concepts and enhance learning.

In spite of the many changes over the years, this book continues to present goniometry logically and clearly. Chapter 1 discusses basic concepts regarding the use of goniometry to assess range of motion and muscle length in patient evaluation. Arthrokinematic and osteokinematic movements, elements of active and passive range of motion, hypomobility, hypermobility, and factors affecting joint motion are included. The inclusion of end-feels and capsular and noncapsular patterns of joint limitation introduces readers to current concepts in orthopedic manual therapy and encourages them to consider joint structure and muscle length while measuring joint motion.

Chapter 2 takes the reader through a step-by-step process to master the techniques of goniometric evaluation including positioning, stabilization, instruments used for measurement, goniometer alignment, and the recording of results. Exercises that help develop necessary psychomotor skills and demonstrate direct application of theoretical concepts facilitate learning.

Chapter 3 discusses the validity and reliability of measurement. The results of the most contemporary validity and reliability studies on the measurement of joint motion are summarized to help the reader focus on ways of improving and interpreting goniometric measurements. Mathematical methods of evaluating reliability are shown along with examples and exercises so that the reader can assess their reliability in taking measurements.

Chapters 4 through 13 present detailed information on goniometric testing procedures for the upper and lower extremities, spine, and temporomandibular joint. When appropriate, muscle length testing procedures are also included. In each chapter, a logical sequence progresses from an overview of joint structures, osteokinematic and arthrokinematic motions, and capsular patterns of limitation to specific measurement procedures. Information on anatomical landmarks, testing position, stabilization, testing motion, normal end-feel, and goniometer alignment for each joint and motion follows in a format that reinforces a consistent approach to evaluation. The extensive use of photographs, illustrations, and captions eliminates the need for repeated demonstrations by an instructor and provides the reader with a permanent reference for visualizing the procedures. At the end of each chapter there is a review of current literature regarding normal range of motion values; the effects of age, gender, and other factors on range of motion; functional range of motion; and the reliability and validity of measurement procedures. This structure makes it easy for readers who are focused on learning measurement techniques, as well as readers who are focused on reviewing the research literature for evidence-based practice, to find what they are seeking.

We believe that the fifth edition provides a comprehensive coverage of the clinical measurement of joint motion and muscle length that supports evidence-based practice. We hope that this book will make the teaching and learning of goniometry easier and improve the standardization and thus the reliability and validity of this examination tool. Readers are encouraged to provide us with feedback on our current efforts to bring you a high-quality, user-friendly text.

CCN
DJW

Contributing Authors

Erin Hartigan, PT, DPT, PhD, OCS, ATC
Associate Professor
Physical Therapy Department
University of New England
Portland, Maine

David A. Scalzitti, PT, PhD
Assistant Professor
Program in Physical Therapy
George Washington University
Washington, DC

Reviewers

Becca D. Jordre, PT, DPT, GCS
Associate Professor
Physical Therapy Department
The University of South Dakota
Vermillion, South Dakota

Heather MacKrell, PT, PhD
Physical Therapist Assistant Program Director
Health Sciences Department
Calhoun Community College
Tanner, Alabama

Jill Manners, MS, MPT, LAT, ATC, PT
Program Director and Professor
Athletic Training Education Program
Western Carolina University
Cullowhee, North Carolina

Mary T. Marchetti, PT, PhD, GCS
Assistant Professor
Physical Therapy Department
Duquesne University
Pittsburgh, Pennsylvania

Rebecca A Reisch, PT, PhD, DPT, OCS
Associate Professor
Physical Therapy Department
Pacific University
Hillsboro, Oregon

Kimberly Varnado, PT, DPT, OCS, FAAOMPT
Assistant Professor
Physical Therapy Department
Midwestern University
Glendale, Arizona

Acknowledgments

We are very grateful for the contributions of the many people who were involved in the development and production of *Measurement of Joint Motion*. We wish to thank David Scalzitti and Erin Hartigan who added their considerable expertise as researchers and educators to update Chapter 3: Validity and Reliability of Goniometric Measurement, and Chapter 8: The Hip, respectively. Photographer Jason Torres of J. Torres Photography in New York used his skills and experience to produce the new high-quality photographs that appear in this fifth edition. We are appreciative of the access provided by the University of Massachusetts Lowell to take these photographs in the teaching laboratories of the Department of Physical Therapy. The late Jocelyn Molleur, who assiduously took the photographs for the third and fourth editions, and Lucia Grochowska Littlefield, who produced the photographs for the first and second editions, are also responsible for this important feature of the book. Timothy Malone, an artist from Ohio, used his talents and knowledge of anatomy to create the excellent illustrations that appear in this as well as past editions. We also offer our thanks to colleagues Erika Lewis and Kyle Coffey, as well as Jessica LeBlanc, Conor Nordengren, Samantha Rollings, Rachel Blakeslee, Chris Fournier, Colleen DeCotret, Rebecca D'Amour, Alexander White, and Claudia Van Bibber, who graciously agreed to participate in the photographs or provided painstaking research support for the fifth edition.

We wish to express our appreciation to these dedicated professionals at F. A. Davis: Margaret Biblis, Editor in Chief, Melissa Duffield, Senior Acquisitions Editor, and Laura Horowitz, Developmental Editor, for their encouragement and commitment to excellence. Our thanks are also extended to George Lang, Director of Content Development; Jennifer Pine, Manager of Developmental Editing; Cindy Breuninger, Managing Editor; Sharon Lee, Production Manager; Carolyn O'Brien, Manager of Art and Design; Daniel Domzalski, Illustration Coordinator; Elizabeth Stepchin, Project Editor; Nichole Liccio, Administrative Assistant; and Marsha Hall, Project Manager, Progressive Publishing Services. We are very grateful to the numerous, faculty, students, and clinicians who over the years have used the book or formally reviewed portions of the manuscript and offered insightful comments and helpful suggestions that have improved this text.

Finally, we wish to thank our families: Cynthia's daughter, Alexandra, and her daughters, Taylor and Kimberly; and Joyce's husband, Jonathan, and sons, Alexander and Ethan, for their continuing encouragement and support. We will always be appreciative.

About the Authors

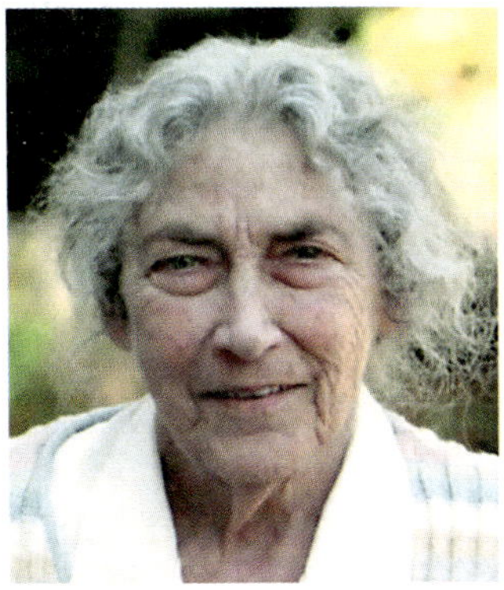

Dr. Cynthia C. Norkin is Associate Professor Emerita, School of Physical Therapy, Ohio University. She holds a Doctorate of Education degree and an Advanced Master of Science in Physical Therapy degree from Boston University, a Bachelor of Science degree from Tufts University, and Certificate in Physical Therapy from the Bouvé-Boston School. She founded the School of Physical Therapy at Ohio University and served as Director for 11 years. Previously, she spent 10 years at Boston University as an Assistant Professor of Physical Therapy, Sargent College, where she and Dr. White initially wrote *Measurement of Joint Motion: A Guide to Goniometry*. Dr. Norkin is the co-editor and contributing author of the book *Joint Structure and Function: A Comprehensive Analysis,* currently in its fifth edition.

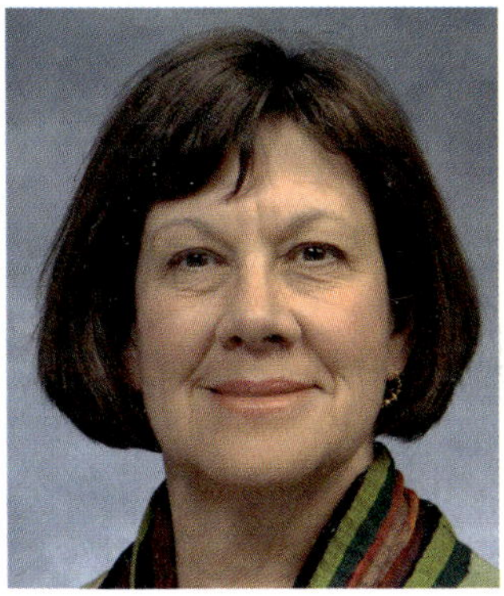

Dr. D. Joyce White is Associate Professor, Department of Physical Therapy, University of Massachusetts Lowell. She holds a Doctorate of Science degree in Epidemiology and an Advanced Master of Science degree in Physical Therapy from Boston University, and a Bachelor of Science degree in Physical Therapy from the University of Connecticut. Dr. White's research, teaching, and clinical experience have predominantly focused on the assessment, treatment, and contributing causes of musculoskeletal conditions of the upper and lower extremities. She has authored research articles and book chapters, and presented numerous conference papers in these areas. The American Physical Therapy Association has presented her with the Dorothy Briggs Memorial Scientific Inquiry Award. Dr. White is a recipient of the University of Massachusetts Lowell Award for Teaching Excellence where she has taught for over 25 years. She has also held academic appointments at Boston University, Sargent College.

Brief Contents

Contents

PART I

INTRODUCTION TO GONIOMETRY AND MUSCLE LENGTH TESTING

This book is designed to serve as a guide for learning how to assess range of motion and muscle length. Part I presents the background information on the principles and procedures necessary for understanding goniometry. Practice exercises are included at appropriate intervals to help the examiner apply this information and develop the psychomotor skills necessary for competency in measuring joint motion and muscle length. Different types of joint range-of-motion measuring instruments such as goniometers and inclinometers are introduced so that examiners become competent in their use. The validity and reliability of goniometric measurements are explored to encourage thoughtful and appropriate use of these techniques in clinical practice. Parts II through IV present the procedures for the examination of joint range of motion and muscle length testing of the upper and lower extremities, the spine, and temporomandibular joints.

OBJECTIVES

After completion of Part I, which includes chapters on *Basic Concepts*, *Procedures*, and *Validity and Reliability*, you will be able to:

1. Define:

goniometry
kinematics
arthrokinematics
osteokinematics
range of motion
end-feel
muscle length testing
reliability
validity

2. Identify the appropriate planes and axes for each of the following motions:

flexion–extension, abduction–adduction, and rotation

3. Compare:

active, active assistive, and passive ranges of motion
arthrokinematic and osteokinematic motions
soft, firm, and hard end-feels
hypomobility and hypermobility
capsular and noncapsular patterns of restricted motion
goniometer and inclinometer
reliability and validity
intratester and intertester reliability
face, content, criterion-related, and construct validity

4. Explain the importance of:

testing positions
stabilization
clinical estimates of range of motion
palpation of bony landmarks
recording starting and ending positions

5. Perform an evaluation of elbow joint motion, including:

a clear explanation of the procedure
proper placement of the individual in the recommended testing position
adequate stabilization of the proximal joint component

correct determination of the end of the range of motion
correct identification of the end-feel
palpation of the appropriate bony landmarks
accurate alignment of the goniometer
correct reading of both the goniometer and the inclinometer, and recording of the measurements

6. Give an example of a muscle length test.

7. Perform and interpret intratester and intertester reliability tests, including standard deviation, coefficient of variation, correlation coefficients, standard error of measurement, and minimal detectable change.

CHAPTER 1

Basic Concepts

D. Joyce White, PT, DSc
Cynthia C. Norkin, PT, EdD

Goniometry

The term **goniometry** is derived from two Greek words: *gonia,* meaning "angle," and *metron,* meaning "measure." Therefore, goniometry refers to the measurement of angles, in particular the measurement of angles created at human joints by the bones of the body. The examiner obtains these measurements by placing the parts of the measuring instrument, called a goniometer, along the bones immediately proximal and distal to the joint being evaluated. Goniometry may be used to determine both a particular joint position and the total amount of motion available at a joint.

Example: The elbow joint is evaluated by placing the parts of the measuring instrument on the humerus (proximal segment) and the forearm (distal segment) and measuring either a specific joint position or the total arc of motion (Fig. 1.1).

Goniometry is an important part of a comprehensive examination of joints and surrounding soft tissue. A comprehensive examination typically begins by interviewing the individual and reviewing records to obtain an accurate description of current symptoms; functional abilities and activities of daily living; occupational, social, and recreational activities; and medical history. Observation of the individual's body to assess bone and soft tissue contour, as well as skin and nail condition, usually follows the interview. Gentle palpation is used to determine skin temperature and the quality of soft tissue deformities and to locate pain symptoms in relation to anatomical structures. Anthropometric measurements such as leg length, leg circumference, and body volume may be indicated.

The performance of active joint motions by the individual during the examination allows the examiner to screen for abnormal movements and gain information about the individual's willingness to move. If abnormal active motions are found, the examiner performs passive joint motions in an attempt to determine reasons for joint limitation. Performing

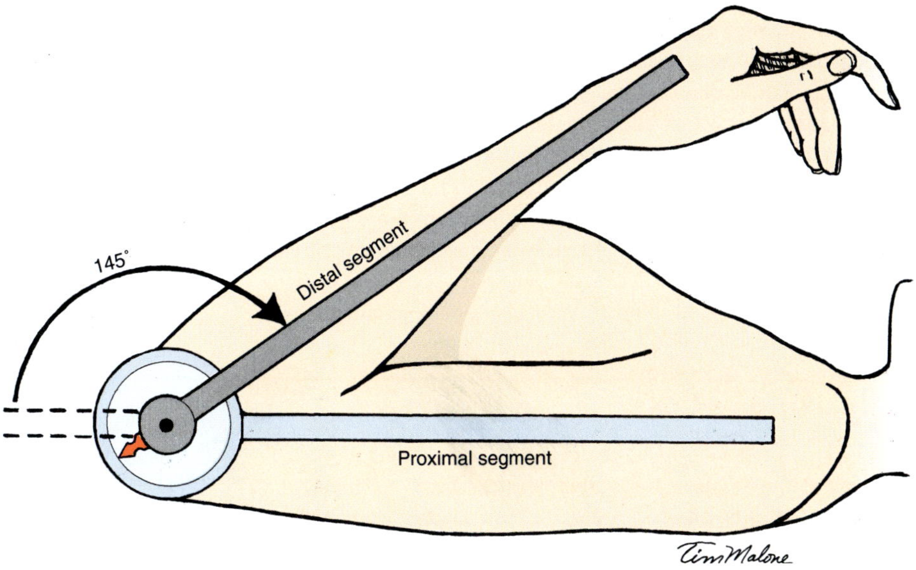

FIGURE 1.1 The left upper extremity of an individual in the supine position is shown. The parts of the measuring instrument have been placed along the proximal (humerus) and distal (radius) body segments and centered over the axis of the elbow joint. When the distal segment has been moved toward the proximal segment (elbow flexion), a measurement of the arc of motion can be obtained.

passive joint motions enables the examiner to assess the tissue that is limiting the motion, detect pain, and make an estimate of the amount of motion. Goniometry is used to measure and document the amount of active and passive joint motion as well as abnormal fixed joint positions.

Following the examination of active and passive range of motion, resisted isometric muscle contractions, joint integrity and mobility tests, and special tests for specific body regions are used in conjunction with goniometry to help identify the injured anatomical structures. Tests to assess muscle performance and neurological function are often included. Diagnostic imaging procedures and laboratory tests may be needed. Functional outcome measures are often required for Medicare, Medicaid, and health insurance documentation.

Goniometric data used in conjunction with other information can provide a basis for the following:

- Determining the presence, absence, or change in impairment[1]
- Establishing a diagnosis
- Developing a prognosis, treatment goals, and plan of care
- Evaluating progress or lack of progress toward rehabilitative goals
- Modifying treatment
- Motivating the individual
- Researching the effectiveness of therapeutic techniques or regimens (for example, measuring outcomes following exercises, medications, and surgical procedures)
- Fabricating orthotics and adaptive equipment

Kinematics

Kinematics is the study of motion without regard for the forces that are creating the motion. When referring to the human body, kinematics describes the motion of bony segments including the type, direction, and magnitude of motion; location of the bony segment in space; and the rate of change or velocity of the segment. The three types of motion that a bony segment can undergo are translatory (linear displacement), rotary (angular displacement), or more often a combination of translatory and rotary motion.[2] In translatory motion, all points on a segment move in the same direction at the same time. In rotary motion, the bone spins around a fixed point. These three types of motion will be explained in more detail in the following subdivisions of kinematics: arthrokinematics and osteokinematics. In arthrokinematics, the focus is on how joint surfaces move and interact, whereas in osteokinematics, the focus is on movements of the shafts of bones.

Arthrokinematics

Motion at a joint occurs as the result of movement of one joint surface in relation to another joint surface. **Arthrokinematics** is the term used to refer to the movement of joint surfaces.[3,4] The movements of joint surfaces are described as slides (or glides), spins, and rolls. A **slide (glide),** which is a translatory motion, is the sliding of one joint surface over another, as when a braked wheel skids (Fig. 1.2). A **spin** is a rotary motion, similar to the spinning of a toy top. All points on the moving joint surface rotate around a fixed axis of motion (Fig. 1.3). A **roll** is also a rotary motion, similar to the rolling of the bottom of a rocking chair on the floor or the rolling of a tire on the road (Fig. 1.4).

In the human body, slides, spins, and rolls usually occur in combination with one another and result in angular movement of the shafts of the bones. The combination of the sliding and rolling is referred to as roll-gliding or roll-sliding[4] and allows for increased motion at a joint by postponing the joint

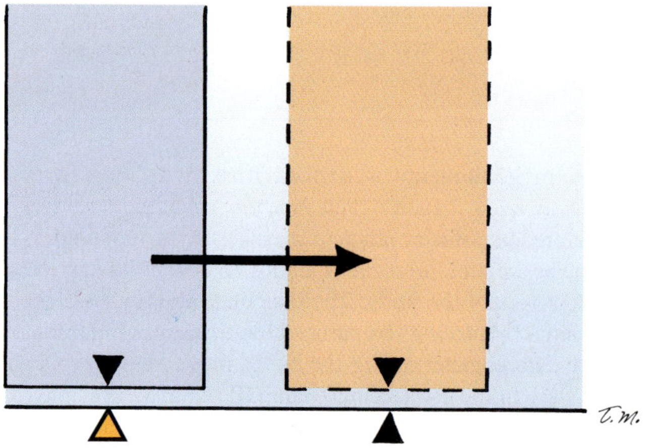

FIGURE 1.2 A slide (glide) is a translatory motion in which the same point on the moving joint surface comes in contact with new points on the opposing surface, and all the points on the moving surface travel the same amount of distance.

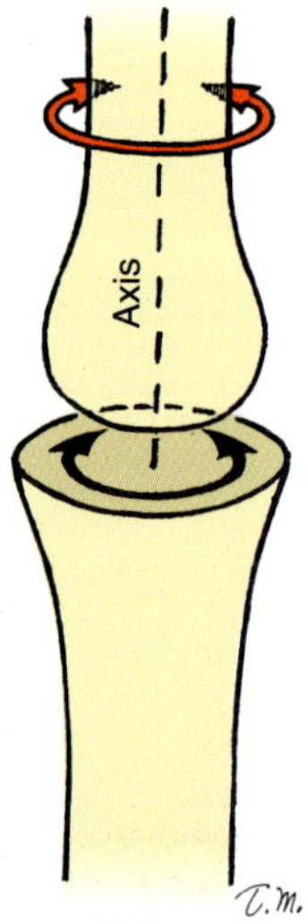

FIGURE 1.3 A spin is a rotary motion in which all the points on the moving surface rotate around a fixed central axis. The points on the moving joint surface that are closer to the axis of motion will travel a smaller distance than the points farther from the axis.

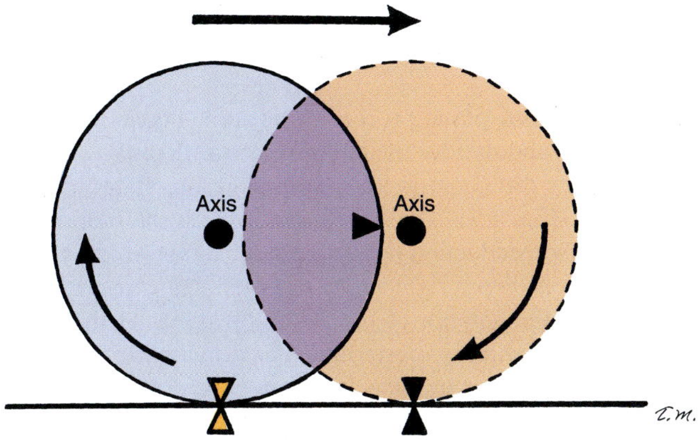

FIGURE 1.4 A roll is a rotary motion in which new points on the moving joint surface come in contact with new points on the opposing surface. The axis of rotation has also moved, in this case to the right.

TABLE 1.1 Arthrokinematic (Accessory/Joint Play) Joint Motion Grades

Grade	Joint Status
0	Ankylosed
1	Considerable hypomobility
2	Slight hypomobility
3	Normal
4	Slight hypermobility
5	Considerable hypermobility
6	Unstable

compression and separation that would occur at either side of the joint during a pure roll. The direction of the rolling and sliding components of a roll-slide will vary depending on the shape of the moving joint surface. If a convex joint surface is moving, the convex surface will roll in the same direction as the angular motion of the shaft of the bone but will slide in the opposite direction (Fig. 1.5A). If a concave joint surface is moving, the concave surface will roll and slide in the same direction as the angular motion of the shaft of the bone (Fig. 1.5B).

Arthrokinematic motions are examined for amount of motion, tissue resistance at the end of the motion, and effect on the individual's symptoms.[5] The ranges of arthrokinematic motions are very small and cannot be measured with a goniometer or standard ruler. Instead, arthrokinematic motions are subjectively compared with the same motion on the contralateral side of the body or with an examiner's past experience testing people of similar age and gender as the individual. An ordinal grading scale of 0 to 6 is often used to describe the amount of arthrokinematic motions[6] (Table 1.1). These motions are also called accessory or joint play motions.

Osteokinematics

Osteokinematics refers to the gross movement of the shafts of bony segments rather than the movement of joint surfaces. The movements of the shafts of bones are usually described in terms of the rotary or angular motion produced, as if the movement occurs around a fixed axis of motion. Goniometry measures the angles created by the rotary motion of the shafts of the bones. Some translatory shifting of the axis of motion usually occurs during movement; however, most clinicians find the description of osteokinematic movement in terms of

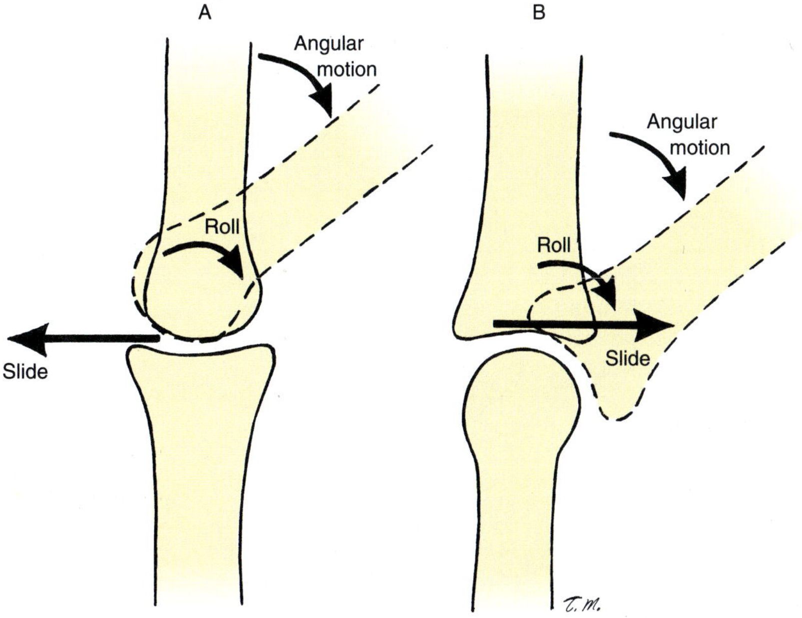

FIGURE 1.5 (A) If the joint surface of the moving bone is convex, sliding is in the opposite direction to the rolling and angular movement of the bone. (B) If the joint surface of the moving bone is concave, sliding is in the same direction as the rolling and angular movement of the bone.

just rotary motion to be sufficiently accurate and use goniometry to measure osteokinematic movements.

Planes and Axes

Osteokinematic motions are classically described as taking place in one of the three **cardinal planes** of the body (sagittal, frontal, transverse) around three corresponding **axes** (medial–lateral, anterior–posterior, vertical). The three planes lie at right angles to one another, whereas the three axes lie at right angles both to one another and to their corresponding planes.

The **sagittal plane** proceeds from the anterior to the posterior aspect of the body. The median sagittal plane divides the body into right and left halves.[7] The motions of flexion and extension occur in the sagittal plane (Fig. 1.6). The axis around which the motions of flexion and extension occur may be envisioned as a line that is perpendicular to the sagittal plane and proceeds from one side of the body to the other. This axis is called a **medial–lateral axis.** All motions in the sagittal plane take place around a medial–lateral axis.

The **frontal plane** proceeds from one side of the body to the other and divides the body into front and back halves. The motions that occur in the frontal plane are abduction and adduction (Fig. 1.7). The axis around which the motions of abduction and adduction take place is an **anterior–posterior axis.** This axis lies at right angles to the frontal plane and proceeds from the anterior to the posterior aspect of the body. Therefore, the anterior–posterior axis lies in the sagittal plane.

The **transverse plane** is horizontal and divides the body into upper and lower portions. The motion of rotation occurs in the transverse plane around a vertical axis (Fig. 1.8). The **vertical axis** lies at right angles to the transverse plane and proceeds in a cranial to caudal direction.

The osteokinematic motions described previously are considered to occur in a single plane around a single axis. Combination motions such as circumduction (flexion–abduction–extension–adduction) are possible at many joints, but because of the limitations imposed by the uniaxial design of the measuring instrument, only motion occurring in a single plane can be measured in goniometry.

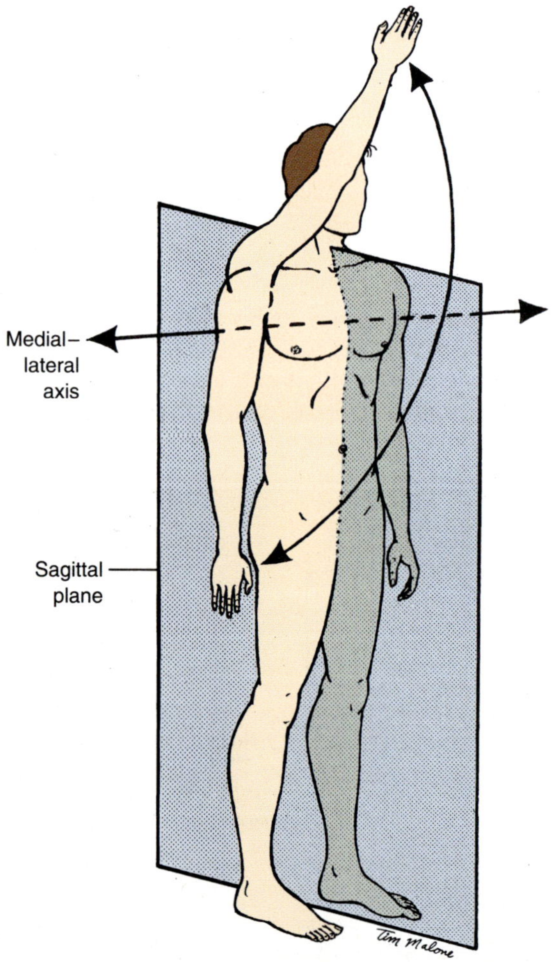

FIGURE 1.6 The shaded areas indicate the sagittal plane. This plane proceeds from the anterior aspect of the body to the posterior aspect. Motions in this plane, such as flexion and extension of the upper and lower extremities, take place around a medial–lateral axis.

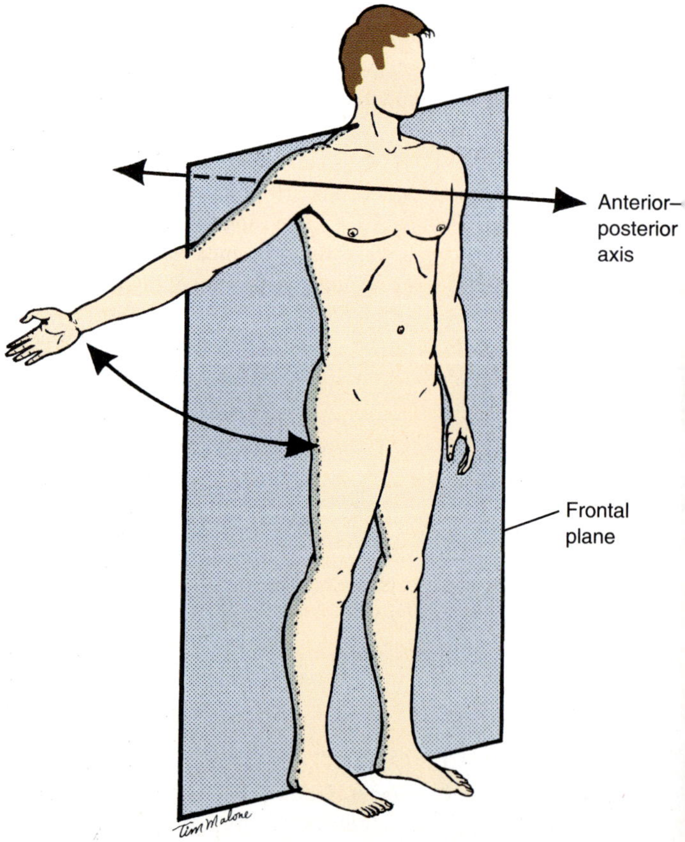

FIGURE 1.7 The frontal plane, indicated by the shaded area, proceeds from one side of the body to the other. Motions in this plane, such as abduction and adduction of the upper and lower extremities, take place around an anterior–posterior axis.

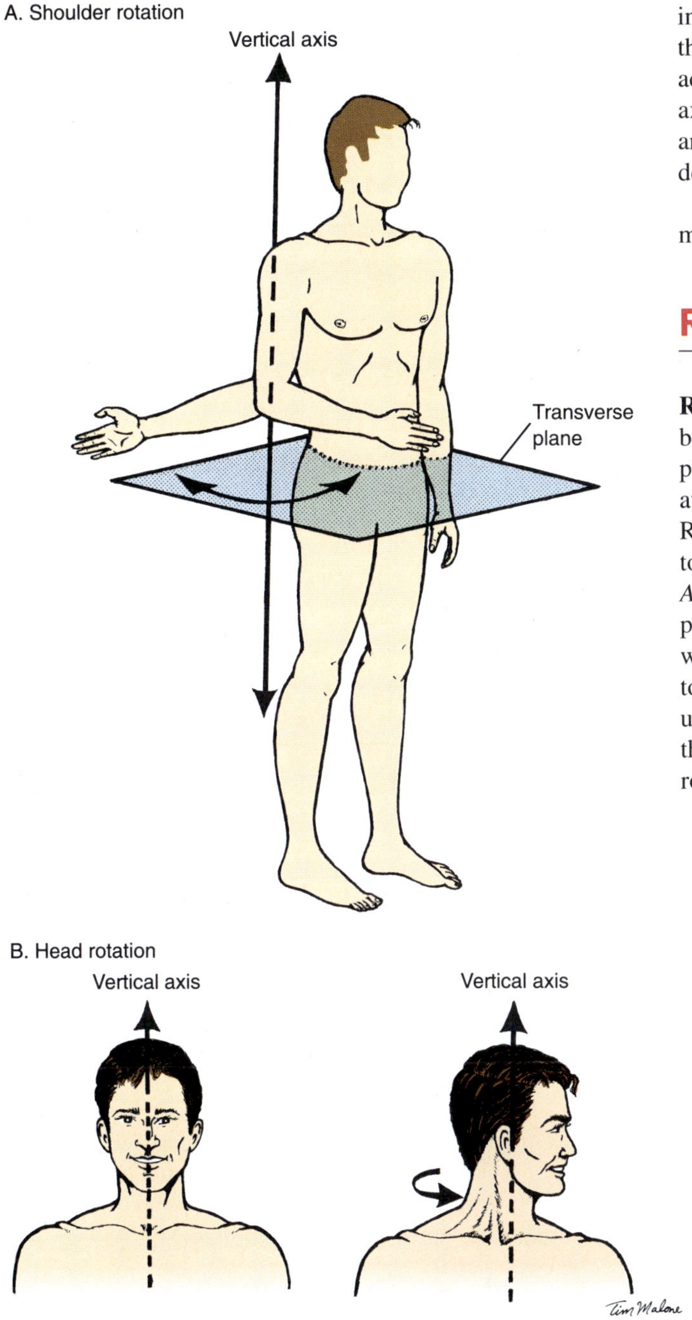

FIGURE 1.8 The transverse plane is indicated by the shaded area. Movements in this plane take place around a vertical axis. These motions include rotation of the shoulder (A), head (B), and hip, as well as pronation and supination of the forearm.

The type of motion that is available at a joint varies according to the structure of the joint. Some joints, such as the interphalangeal joints of the digits, permit a large amount of motion in only one plane around a single axis: flexion and extension in the sagittal plane around a medial–lateral axis. A joint that allows motion in only one plane is described as having one **degree of freedom of motion.** The interphalangeal joints of the digits have one degree of freedom of motion. Other joints, such as the glenohumeral joint, permit motion in three planes around three axes: flexion and extension in the sagittal plane around a medial–lateral axis, abduction and adduction in the frontal plane around an anterior–posterior axis, and medial and lateral rotation in the transverse plane around a vertical axis. The glenohumeral joint has three degrees of freedom of motion.

The planes and axes for each joint and joint motion to be measured are presented in Chapters 4 through 13.

Range of Motion

Range of motion (ROM) is the arc of motion in degrees between the beginning and the end of a motion in a specific plane.[1] The arc of motion may occur either at a single joint or at a series of joints.[5] The starting position for measuring all ROM is either the anatomical or neutral position. The anatomical position is described in the 41st edition of *Gray's Anatomy* as a posture in which the upper limbs are by the person's side and the palms of the hands are facing forward with the fingers extended[7] (Fig. 1.9A). The lower limbs are together and facing forward. The neutral position, which is used to measure rotation ROM in the transverse plane, places the upper extremity joints halfway between medial and lateral rotation, and supination and pronation (Fig. 1.9B).

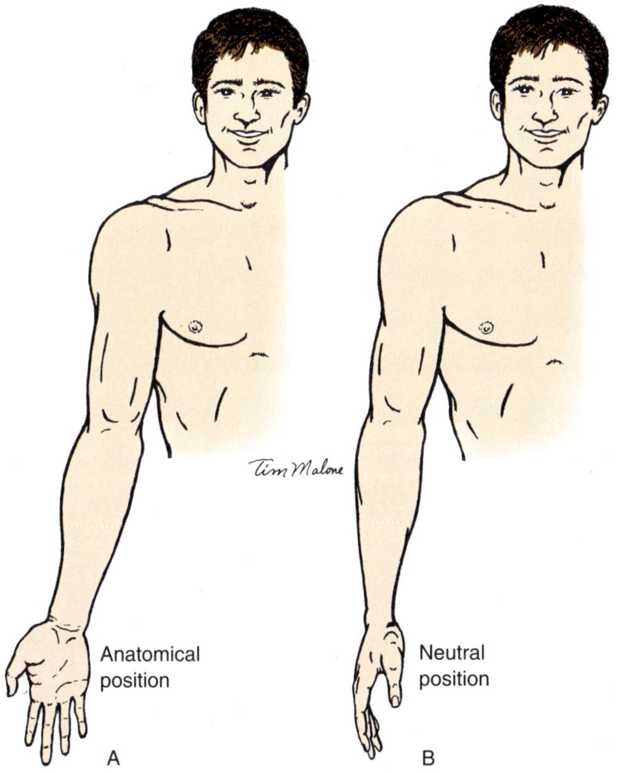

FIGURE 1.9 (A) In the anatomical position, the forearm is supinated so that the palms of the hands face anteriorly. (B) When the forearm is in a neutral position (with respect to rotation), the palm of the hand faces the side of the body.

The three notation systems used to define ROM are the 0- to 180-degree system, the 180- to 0-degree system, and the 360-degree system. In the **0- to 180-degree notation system,** the upper- and lower-extremity joints are at 0 degrees for flexion–extension and abduction–adduction when the body is in the anatomical position, and at 0 degrees for rotation when the body is in the neutral position (see Fig. 1.9). Normally, a ROM begins at 0 degrees and proceeds in an arc toward 180 degrees. This 0- to 180-degree system of notation, also called the **neutral zero method,** is widely used throughout the world. First described by Silver[8] in 1923, its use has been supported by many authorities, including Cave and Roberts,[9] Moore,[10] the American Academy of Orthopaedic Surgeons,[11,12] and the American Medical Association.[1]

Example: The ROM for shoulder flexion, which begins with the shoulder in the anatomical position (0 degrees) and ends with the arm overhead in full flexion (180 degrees), is expressed as 0 to 180 degrees.

In the preceding example, the portion of the extension ROM from full shoulder flexion back to the zero starting position does not need to be measured because this ROM represents the same arc of motion that was measured in flexion. However, the portion of the extension ROM that is available beyond the zero starting position must be measured (Fig. 1.10). Documentation of extension ROM usually incorporates only the extension that occurs beyond the zero starting position. The term **hyperextension** is used to describe a greater than normal extension ROM.

Two other systems of notation have been described. The **180- to 0-degree notation system,** first described by Clark, defines the anatomical position as 180 degrees.[13] The ROM begins at 180 degrees and proceeds in an arc toward 0 degrees. The **360-degree notation system,** first described by West, also defines the anatomical position as 180 degrees.[14] The motions of flexion and abduction begin at 180 degrees and proceed in an arc toward 0 degrees. The motions of extension and adduction begin at 180 degrees and proceed in an arc toward 360 degrees.[15] These two notation systems are more difficult to interpret than the 0- to 180-degree notation system and are infrequently used. Therefore, we have not included them in this text.

Active Range of Motion

Active ROM is the arc of motion produced by the individual's voluntary unassisted muscle contraction. Having an individual perform active ROM provides the examiner with information about the individual's willingness to move, coordination, muscle strength, and joint ROM. If pain occurs during active ROM, it may be due to contracting or stretching of "contractile" tissues, such as muscles, tendons, and their attachments to bone. Pain may also be due to stretching or pinching of noncontractile (inert) tissues, such as ligaments, joint capsules, bursa, fascia, and skin. Testing active ROM is a good screening technique to help focus a physical examination. If an individual can complete active ROM easily and painlessly,

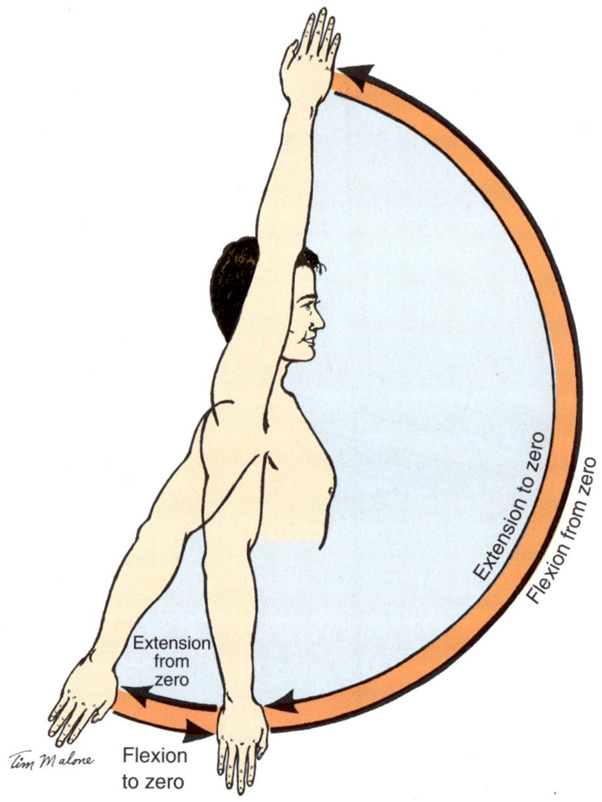

FIGURE 1.10 Flexion and extension of the shoulder begin with the shoulder in the anatomical position. The ROM in flexion proceeds anteriorly from the zero position through an arc toward 180 degrees. The long, bold arrow shows the ROM in flexion, which is measured in goniometry. The ROM in extension proceeds posteriorly from the zero position through an arc toward 180 degrees. The short, bold arrow shows the ROM in extension, which is measured in goniometry.

further testing of that motion probably is not needed. If, however, active ROM is limited, painful, or awkward, the physical examination should include an examination of passive ROM and additional testing to clarify the problem.

Active assistive ROM is the arc of motion produced by the individual's muscle contraction assisted by an external force. During the examination process the external force is provided by the examiner. In other instances the external force may be provided by an unimpaired region of the individual's body, or by a mechanical device.

Passive Range of Motion

Passive ROM is the arc of motion produced by the application of an external force by the examiner. The individual remains relaxed and plays no active role in producing the motion. Normally, passive ROM is slightly greater than active ROM[16–18] because each joint has a small amount of motion that is not under voluntary control. The additional passive ROM that is available at the end of the normal active ROM is due to the stretch of tissues surrounding the joint and the reduced bulk of relaxed muscles compared with contracting muscles. This additional passive ROM helps to protect joint structures because it allows the joint to absorb extrinsic forces.

Testing passive ROM provides the examiner with information about the integrity of the joint surfaces and the extensibility of the joint capsule and associated ligaments, muscles, fascia, and skin. Comparisons between passive ROM and active ROM provide information about the amount of motion permitted by the associated joint structures (passive ROM) relative to the individual's ability to produce motion at a joint (active ROM). In cases of impairment such as muscle weakness, passive ROM and active ROM may vary considerably.

Example: An examiner may find that an individual with a muscle paralysis has full passive ROM but no active ROM at the same joint. In this instance, the joint surfaces and the extensibility of the joint capsule, ligaments, muscles, tendons, fascia, and skin are sufficient to allow full passive ROM. The lack of muscle strength prevents active motion at the joint.

If pain occurs during passive ROM, it is often due to moving, stretching, or pinching of noncontractile (inert) structures. Pain occurring at the end of passive ROM may be due to stretching of contractile structures as well as noncontractile structures.[19] Pain during passive ROM is not due to active shortening (contracting) of contractile tissues. By comparing which motions (active versus passive) cause pain and noting the location of the pain, the examiner can begin to determine which injured tissues are involved. Careful consideration of the end-feel and location of tissue tension and pain during passive ROM also adds information about structures that are limiting ROM.

End-Feel

The amount of passive ROM is determined by the unique structure of the joint being tested. Some joints are structured so that the joint capsules limit the end of the ROM in a particular direction, whereas other joints are structured so that ligaments limit the end of a particular ROM. Other normal limitations to motion include passive tension in soft tissue such as muscles, fascia, and skin; soft tissue approximation; and contact of joint surfaces.

The type of structure that limits a ROM has a characteristic feel that may be detected by the examiner who is performing the passive ROM when slight overpressure is applied at the end of the motion. This feeling, which is experienced by an examiner as a barrier to further motion, is called the **end-feel.**[6,19,20] Developing the ability to determine the character of the end-feel requires practice and sensitivity. Determination of the end-feel must be carried out slowly and carefully to detect the end of the ROM and to distinguish among the various normal and abnormal end-feels. The ability to distinguish among the various end-feels helps the examiner identify the type of limiting structure. Cyriax,[19] Kaltenborn,[6] and Paris[20] have described a variety of types of normal (physiological) and abnormal (pathological) end-feels. Table 1.2, which describes normal end-feels, and Table 1.3, which describes abnormal end-feels, have been adapted from the works of these authors but are most similar to those presented by Kaltenborn.[6]

TABLE 1.2 Normal End-Feels

End-Feel	Description	Example
Soft	Soft tissue approximation	Knee flexion (contact between soft tissue of posterior leg and posterior thigh)
Firm	Muscular stretch	Hip flexion with the knee straight (passive tension of hamstring muscles)
	Capsular stretch	Extension of metacarpophalangeal joints of fingers (tension in the anterior capsule)
	Ligamentous stretch	Forearm supination (tension in the palmar radioulnar ligament of the inferior radioulnar joint, interosseous membrane, oblique cord)
Hard	Bone contacting bone	Elbow extension (contact between the olecranon process of the ulna and the olecranon fossa of the humerus)

Only recently have researchers begun to conduct studies to determine the validity and reliability of end-feels. Petersen and Hayes investigated Cyriax's theory that abnormal end-feels are significantly more painful than normal end-feels. The authors found partial confirmation of Cyriax's theory in that some abnormal end-feels were significantly more painful than normal end-feels at the two joints (knee and shoulder) included in their study.[21] Hayes and Petersen found that, generally, end-feel identification reliability was considered to be good when the same examiner made the identification of Cyriax's three normal and six abnormal end-feels at the knee and shoulder.[22] However, the ability of different examiners to agree on the same end-feels was poor. Manning et al[23] conducted a study to evaluate the reliability of end-feel identification, pain provocation, and hypomobility at each cervical joint from C2–C3 to C6–C7 in symptomatic individuals. Clinically acceptable reliability was found primarily for assessment of joint hypomobility and end-feel in the lower cervical disc segment of the less painful side but not in the more painful side.

TABLE 1.3 Abnormal End-Feels

End-Feel	Description	Example
Soft	Occurs sooner or later in the ROM than is usual or in a joint that normally has a firm or hard end-feel. Feels boggy.	Soft tissue edema Synovitis
Firm	Occurs sooner or later in the ROM than is usual or in a joint that normally has a soft or hard end-feel.	Increased muscular tonus Capsular, muscular, ligamentous, and fascial shortening
Hard	Occurs sooner or later in the ROM than is usual or in a joint that normally has a soft or firm end-feel. A bony grating or bony block is felt.	Chondromalacia Osteoarthritis Loose bone fragments in joint Myositis ossificans Fracture
Empty	No real end-feel because pain prevents reaching end of ROM. No resistance is felt except for individual's protective muscle splinting or muscle spasm.	Acute joint inflammation Bursitis Abscess Fracture Psychogenic disorder

In Chapters 4 through 11, we describe what we believe are the normal end-feels and the structures that limit the ROM for each joint and motion. Because of the paucity of specific literature in this area, these descriptions are based on our experience in evaluating joint motion and on information obtained from established anatomy[7,24–28] and biomechanics texts.[29,30] Controversy exists among experts concerning the structures that limit the ROM in some parts of the body. Normal individual variations in body structure may also cause instances in which the end-feel differs from our description. Examiners should practice trying to distinguish among the different types of end-feels. **Exercise 1 in Chapter 2** is included for this purpose.

Hypomobility

The term **hypomobility** refers to a decrease in ROM that is substantially less than normal values for that joint, given the individual's age and gender. For example, the end-feel occurs early in the ROM and may be different in quality from what is expected. This limitation in passive ROM may be due to a variety of causes, including abnormalities of the joint surfaces; passive shortening of joint capsules, ligaments, muscles, fascia, and skin; and inflammation of these structures.

Hypomobility has been associated with many orthopedic conditions such as osteoarthritis,[31] spinal disorders,[32] and metabolic disorders such as diabetes.[33,34] Decreased ROM is also a common consequence of immobilization after fractures and scar development after burns.[35,36] Neurological conditions such as stroke, head trauma, cerebral palsy, and complex regional pain syndrome can result in hypomobility owing to loss of voluntary movement, increased muscle tone, immobilization, and pain. Hypomobility also has been shown to impair function in the hand[37] and the ankle.[38]

Capsular Patterns of Restricted Motion

Cyriax[19] proposed that pathological conditions involving the entire joint capsule cause a particular pattern of restriction involving all or most of the passive motions of the joint. This pattern of restriction is called a **capsular pattern.** The restrictions do not involve a fixed number of degrees for each motion but rather a fixed proportion of one motion relative to another motion.

Example: The capsular pattern for the elbow joint is a greater limitation of flexion than of extension. The elbow joint normally has a passive flexion ROM of 0 to 150 degrees. If the capsular involvement is mild, the last 15 degrees of flexion and the last 5 degrees of extension might be restricted so that passive ROM is 5 to135 degrees. If the capsular involvement is more severe, the last 30 degrees of flexion and the last 10 degrees of extension might be restricted so that the passive ROM is 10 to120 degrees.

Capsular patterns vary from joint to joint (Table 1.4). The capsular patterns for each joint, as presented by Cyriax[19] and Kaltenborn,[6] are noted in the beginning of Chapters 4 through 10. Additional studies are needed to test the hypotheses regarding the cause of capsular patterns and to determine the capsular pattern for each joint. Several studies[21,39–41] have examined the construct validity of Cyriax's capsular pattern in individuals with arthritis or arthrosis of the knee. Although differing opinions exist, the findings seem to support the concept of a capsular pattern of restriction for the knee but with more liberal interpretation of the proportions of limitation than suggested by Cyriax.[19] Two studies[41,42] examining capsular patterns for the hip found decreases in all hip motions in osteoarthritic

TABLE 1.4 Capsular Pattern of Extremity Joints

Joint	Restricted Motions
Glenohumeral joint	Greatest loss of lateral rotation, moderate loss of abduction, minimal loss of medial rotation
Elbow complex (humeroulnar, humeroradial, proximal radioulnar joints)	Loss of flexion greater than loss of extension; rotations full and painless except in advanced cases
Forearm (proximal and distal radioulnar joints)	Equal loss of supination and pronation, only occurring if elbow has marked restrictions of flexion and extension
Wrist (radiocarpal and midcarpal joints)	Equal loss of flexion and extension, slight loss of ulnar and radial deviation (Cyriax) Equal loss of all motions (Kaltenborn)
Hand	
Carpometacarpal joint—digit 1	Loss of abduction (Cyriax); loss of abduction greater than extension (Kaltenborn)
Carpometacarpal joint—digits 2–5	Equal loss of all motions
Metacarpophalangeal and interphalangeal joints	Equal loss of flexion and extension (Cyriax) Restricted in all motions, but loss of flexion greater than loss of other motions (Kaltenborn)
Hip	Greatest loss of medial rotation and flexion, some loss of abduction, slight loss of extension; little or no loss of adduction and lateral rotation (Cyriax) Greatest loss of medial rotation, followed by less restriction of extension, abduction, flexion, and lateral rotation (Kaltenborn)
Knee (tibiofemoral joint)	Loss of flexion greater than extension
Ankle (talocrural joint)	Loss of plantarflexion greater than dorsiflexion
Subtalar joint	Loss of inversion (varus)
Midtarsal joint	Loss of inversion (adduction and medial rotation); other motions full
Foot	
Metatarsophalangeal joint—digit 1	Loss of extension greater than flexion
Metatarsophalangeal joint—digits 2–5	Loss of flexion greater than extension
Interphalangeal joints	Loss of extension greater than flexion

Adapted from Dyrek, DA: Assessment and Treatment Planning Strategies for Musculoskeletal Deficits. In O'Sullivan, SB, and Schmitz, TJ (eds): Physical Rehabilitation: Assessment and Treatment, ed 3. FA Davis, Philadelphia, 1994. Capsular patterns are from Cyriax[19] and Kaltenborn.[6]

hips as compared with nonosteoarthritic hips but raised questions concerning specific patterns of limitation proposed by Kaltenborn[6] and Cyriax.[19]

Hertling and Kessler[43] have extended Cyriax's concepts on causes of capsular patterns. They suggest that conditions resulting in a capsular pattern of restriction can be classified into two general categories:

1. Conditions in which there is considerable joint effusion or synovial inflammation
2. Conditions in which there is relative capsular fibrosis

Joint effusion and synovial inflammation accompany conditions such as traumatic arthritis, infectious arthritis, acute rheumatoid arthritis, and gout. In these conditions, the joint capsule is distended by excessive intra-articular synovial fluid, causing the joint to maintain a position that allows the greatest intra-articular joint volume. Pain triggered by stretching the capsule and muscle spasms that protect the capsule from further insult inhibit movement and cause a capsular pattern of restriction.

Relative capsular fibrosis often occurs during chronic low-grade capsular inflammation, immobilization of a joint, and resolution of acute capsular inflammation. These conditions increase the relative proportion of collagen compared with that of mucopolysaccharide in the joint capsule or they change the structure of the collagen. The resulting decrease in extensibility of the entire capsule causes a capsular pattern of restriction.

Noncapsular Patterns of Restricted Motion

A limitation of passive motion that is not proportioned similarly to a capsular pattern is called a **noncapsular pattern** of restricted motion.[19] A noncapsular pattern is usually caused by a condition involving structures other than the entire joint capsule. Internal joint derangement, adhesion of a part of a joint capsule, ligament shortening, muscle strains, and muscle contractures are examples of conditions that typically result in noncapsular patterns of restriction. Noncapsular patterns usually involve only one or two motions of a joint, in contrast to capsular patterns, which involve all or most motions of a joint.[6,19]

Example: A strain of the biceps muscle may result in pain and restriction at the end of the range of passive elbow extension. The passive motion of elbow flexion would not be affected.

Hypermobility

The term **hypermobility** refers to the ability of one or more joints to actively or passively move beyond normal limits given the individual's age and gender. For example, in adults the normal ROM for extension at the elbow joint is about 0 degrees.[11,12] A ROM measurement of 30 degrees or more of extension at the elbow is well beyond normal ROM and is indicative of a hypermobile joint in an adult. Children have some normally occurring specific instances of increased ROM compared with adults. For example, neonates 6 to 72 hours old have been found to have a mean ankle dorsiflexion passive ROM of 59 degrees,[44] which contrasts with mean adult ROM values of between 12 and 20 degrees.[11,12] The increased motion that is present in these children is normal for their age. If the increased motion persists beyond the expected age range, it would be considered abnormal and hypermobility would be present.

Hypermobility is due to the laxity of soft tissue structures such as ligaments, capsules, and muscles that normally prevent excessive motion at a joint. In some instances, the hypermobility may be due to abnormalities of the joint surfaces. A frequent cause of hypermobility is trauma to a joint. Hypermobility also occurs in serious hereditary disorders of connective tissue such as Marfan syndrome, rheumatic diseases, osteogenesis imperfecta, and Ehlers-Danlos syndrome. Research involving Ehlers-Danlos syndrome has found that in addition to joint hypermobility and widespread musculoskeletal pain, the syndrome involves all of the major systems of the body.[45]

Hypermobility syndrome (HMS) or benign joint hypermobility syndrome (BJHS) is used to describe otherwise healthy individuals who have generalized hypermobility accompanied by musculoskeletal symptoms.[46,47] An inherited abnormality in collagen and regular physical exercise are thought to be responsible for the joint laxity in these individuals.[48–50] Traditionally, the diagnosis of HMS involves the exclusion of other conditions, a score of at least 4 on the Beighton score (Table 1.5), and arthralgia for longer than 3 months in four or more joints.[51] Some researchers have noted that these criteria are inadequate for children because scores greater than 4 on the Beighton scale were found in 65% of a sample of 1,120 children aged 4 to 7 years in Brazil.[50] Jelsma and colleagues[53] also found an extremely high prevalence of hypermobility when they applied the cutoff score of 5 in children ages 3 to 9 years and a score of 4 in the 10 to 16 years age-group; they suggested that a cutoff of 7 would be more appropriate. The authors also stressed the need for international agreement on firm cutoff points and the use of standardized measurement for Beighton mobility tasks.[51] Other criteria have also been proposed, including additional joint motions and extra-articular signs.[52,53]

According to Grahame,[48] the following joint motions should also be considered: shoulder lateral rotation greater than 90 degrees, cervical spine lateral flexion greater than 60 degrees, distal interphalangeal joint hyperextension greater than 60 degrees, and first metatarsophalangeal joint extension greater than 90 degrees. In addition to Grahame's findings, Smith, Jermane, and Easton,[47] in a systematic review of studies involving BJHS, found evidence to suggest that people with the syndrome have significantly poor joint position sense compared with people without BJHS. Smits-Engelsman, Klerks, and Kirby[54] conducted a prospective study of 551 Dutch children aged 6 to 12 years to evaluate the validity of the Beighton score as a generalized measure of hypermobility. Qualified physical therapists assessed the children using goniometry to measure passive ROM. More

TABLE 1.5 Beighton Hypermobility Score

The Ability to	Points
Passively appose thumb to forearm	
Right	1
Left	1
Passively extend fifth MCP joint more than 90 degrees	
Right	1
Left	1
Hyperextend elbow more than 10 degrees	
Right	1
Left	1
Hyperextend knee more than 10 degrees	
Right	1
Left	1
Place palms on floor by flexing trunk with knees straight	1
Total Beighton Score = sum of points.	0–9

Adapted from Beighton, P, Solomon, L, and Soskolne, CL: Articular mobility in an African population. Ann Rheum Dis 32:23, 1973.

than 35% of children scored greater than 5/9 on the Beighton score. The authors concluded that when goniometry is used, the Beighton score is a valid instrument to measure generalized joint mobility in children aged 8 to 12 years and that additional items to improve the score, as suggested by Grahame,[48] are not needed.

Factors Affecting Range of Motion

Range of motion varies among individuals and is influenced by factors such as age, gender, and whether the motion is performed actively or passively. A fairly extensive amount of research on the effects of age and gender on ROM has been conducted for the upper and lower extremities as well as the spine. Other factors relating to characteristics such as body mass index, occupational activities, and recreational activities may affect ROM but have not been as extensively researched as age and gender. In addition, factors relating to the testing process, such as the testing position, type of instrument employed, experience of the examiner, and even time of day, have been identified as affecting ROM measurements. A brief summary of research findings that examine age and gender effects on ROM is presented in this introductory chapter. To assist the examiner, more detailed information about the effects of age and gender on the featured joints is presented at the end of Chapters 4 through 13. Information on the effects of characteristics and the testing process is included if available.

Ideally, to determine whether a ROM is impaired, the value of the ROM of the joint under consideration should be compared with ROM values from people of the same age and gender, and from studies that used the same method of measurement. Often such comparisons are not possible because age-related and gender-related norms have not been established for all groups. In such situations, the ROM of the joint should be compared with the same joint of the individual's contralateral extremity, providing that the contralateral extremity is not impaired or used selectively in athletic or occupational activities. Most studies have found little difference between the ROM of the right and left extremities.[54–57] A few studies[17,59,60] have found slightly less ROM in some joints of the upper extremity on the dominant or right side compared with the contralateral side, which Allender and coworkers[58] attribute to increased exposure to stress. If the contralateral extremity is inappropriate for comparison, the individual's ROM may be compared with average ROM values in handbooks of the American Academy of Orthopaedic Surgeons[11,12] and other standard texts.[1,3,7,60,61] However, in some of these texts, the populations from which the values were derived as well as the testing positions and type of measuring instruments used are not identified.

Mean ROM values published in several standard texts and research studies are summarized at the beginning of the Range of Motion Testing Procedures for each motion and in tables at the end of Chapters 4 through 13. The ROM values presented should serve as only a general guide to identifying normal versus impaired ROM. Considerable differences in mean ROM values are sometimes noted between the various references.

Age

Numerous studies have been conducted to determine the effects of age on ROM of the extremities and spine. General agreement exists among investigators regarding the age-related effects on the ROM of the extremity joints of newborns, infants, and young children up to about 2 years of age.[44,62–66] These age effects are joint and motion specific but do not seem to be affected by gender; both males and females are affected similarly. The youngest age-groups have more hip flexion, hip abduction, hip lateral rotation, ankle dorsiflexion, and elbow motion compared with adults. Limitations in hip extension, knee extension, and plantar flexion are considered to be normal for these youngest age-groups. Mean values for these age-groups differ by more than 2 standard deviations from mean values for adults published by the American Academy of Orthopaedic Surgeons,[12] and the American Medical Association.[1] Therefore, age-appropriate norms should be used whenever possible for newborns, infants, and young children up to 2 years of age.

Most investigators who have studied a wide range of age-groups have found that older adult groups have somewhat less ROM of the extremities than younger adult groups. These age-related changes in the ROM of older adults also are joint and motion specific and may affect males and females differently. Allender and associates[58] found that wrist flexion–extension, hip rotation, and shoulder rotation ROM decreased with increasing age, whereas flexion ROM in the metacarpophalangeal (MCP) joint of the thumb showed no consistent loss of motion. Roach and Miles[67] generally found a small decrease (3 to 5 degrees) in mean active hip and knee motions between the youngest age-group (25 to 39 years) and the oldest age-group (60 to 74 years). Except for hip extension ROM, these decreases represented less than 15% of the arc of motion. Stubbs, Fernandez, and Glenn[69] found a decrease of between 4% and 30% in 11 of 23 joints studied in men between the ages of 25 and 54 years. James and Parker[16] found systematic decreases in 10 active and passive lower-extremity motions in individuals who were between 70 and 92 years of age. Steinberg and associates[68] in a study of dancers and nondancers of the same ages (8 to 16 years) found that age differences not only occurred in different joints and motions but also varied with activity. For example, hip flexion and internal rotation and knee flexion ROM decreased with increasing age in both groups, but ankle plantar flexion and hip external rotation decreased with increasing age in nondancers and did not change in dancers.

As with the extremities, age-related effects on spinal ROM appear to be motion specific. Youdas and associates[75] found that with each decade, both females and males lose approximately 5 degrees of active motion in neck extension and 3 degrees in flexion, lateral flexion, and rotation. Chen and colleagues,[76] in a review of the literature regarding the effects of aging on cervical spine ROM, concluded that active cervical ROM decreased by 4 degrees per decade, which is similar to the findings of Youdas and associates. Salo and colleagues[77] in a study of 220 healthy women aged 20 to 59 years found that passive ROM of the cervical spine decreased with increasing age in all motions except forward flexion. Lansade and associates,[74] using the noninvasive infrared polaris system to investigate the effects of age on cervical ROM, found less of a decrease (only 0.55 to 0.79 degree) per decade between 20 and 93 years.

Investigators have reached varying conclusions regarding how large a decrease in ROM occurs with increasing age in the thoracolumbar spine. Loebl[78] found that thoracolumbar spinal mobility (flexion–extension) decreases with age an average of 8 degrees per decade. Fitzgerald and colleagues[79] found a systematic decrease in lateral flexion and extension of the lumbar spine at 20-year intervals but no differences in rotation and forward flexion. In contrast to Fitzgerald, Intolo and colleagues[80] in a systematic review and meta-analysis to determine the effect of age on lumbar range of motion found 16 studies with results that showed age-related reductions in flexion, extension, and lateral flexion occurred primarily from 40 to 50 years and after 60 years of age. There was little evidence of age effects on lumbar rotation. Trudelle-Jackson and associates[81] compared measurements of lumbar spine flexion and extension in a group of white and African American women between 20 and 83 years. Flexion and extension ROM in the young group (aged 20 to 39) was significantly greater than in the middle group (aged 40 to 59) and in the older group (aged 60 plus). In addition, the difference in extension ROM between the middle and older groups was also significant, but this difference was not significant for flexion ROM. Decreases in lumbar flexion ranged from 2.4 to 7.3 degrees, whereas differences in extension ranged from 4.9 degrees to 10.8 degrees. Extension and flexion showed a decreasing trend with increasing age in both racial groups.

Gender

The effects of gender on the ROM of the extremities and spine also appear to be joint and motion specific. If gender differences in the amount of ROM are found, females are more often reported to have slightly greater ROM than males. In general, gender differences appear to be more prevalent in adults than in young children.

Bell and Hoshizaki[71] found that females across an age range of 18 to 88 years had more flexibility than males in 14 of 17 joint motions tested. Beighton, Solomon, and Soskolne[51] in a study of an African population found that females between 0 and 80 years of age were more mobile than their male counterparts. Walker and coworkers[70] in a study of 28 joint motions in 60- to 84-year-olds reported that 8 motions were greater in females and 4 motions were greater in males, whereas the other motions showed little gender difference. Almquist and colleagues[73] found that women had 10% to 20% greater knee ROM than men in all age-groups between 15 and 60 plus years. Kalscheur and associates[72] measured 24 upper-extremity and cervical motions in men and women between the ages of 63 and 86 years. Gender differences were noted for 14 of the motions, and in all cases the older women had greater active ROM than the older men. Lansade[74] and associates found that gender had no significant influence on three-dimensional cervical range of motion except in the 70- to 79-year-old group.

Muscle Length Testing

Maximal **muscle length** is the greatest extensibility of a muscle-tendon unit.[5] It is the maximal distance between the proximal and the distal attachments of a muscle to bone. Clinically, muscle length is not measured directly; instead, it is measured indirectly by determining the maximal passive ROM of the joint(s) crossed by the muscle.[82–85] Muscle length, in addition to the integrity of the joint surfaces and the extensibility of the capsule, ligaments, fascia, and skin, affects the amount of passive ROM of a joint. The purpose of testing muscle length is to ascertain whether hypomobility or hypermobility is caused by the length of the inactive antagonist muscle or other structures. By ascertaining which structures are involved, the health professional can choose more specific and more effective treatment procedures.

Muscles can be categorized by the number of joints they cross from their proximal to their distal attachments. **One-joint muscles** cross and therefore influence the motion of only one joint. **Two-joint muscles** cross and influence the motion of two joints, whereas **multi-joint muscles** cross and influence multiple joints.

No difference exists between the measurement of the length of a one-joint muscle and the measurement of passive joint ROM in the direction opposite to the muscle's active motion. Usually, one-joint muscles have sufficient length to allow full passive ROM at the joint they cross. If a one-joint muscle is shorter than normal, passive ROM in the direction opposite to the muscle's action is decreased and the end-feel is firm owing to a muscular stretch. At the end of the ROM, the examiner may be able to palpate tension within the muscle-tendon unit if the structures are superficial. In addition, the individual may complain of pain in the region of the tight muscle and tendon. These signs and symptoms help to confirm muscle shortness as the cause of the joint limitation.

If a one-joint muscle is abnormally lax, passive tension in the capsule and ligaments may initially maintain a normal ROM. However, with time, these joint structures often lengthen as well and passive ROM at the joint increases. Because the indirect measurement of the length of one-joint muscles is the same as the measurement of passive joint ROM, we have not presented specific muscle length tests for one-joint muscles.

Example: The length of one-joint hip adductors such as the adductor longus, adductor magnus, and adductor brevis is assessed by measuring passive hip abduction ROM. The indirect measurement of the length of the hip adductor muscles is identical to the measurement of passive hip abduction ROM (Fig. 1.11).

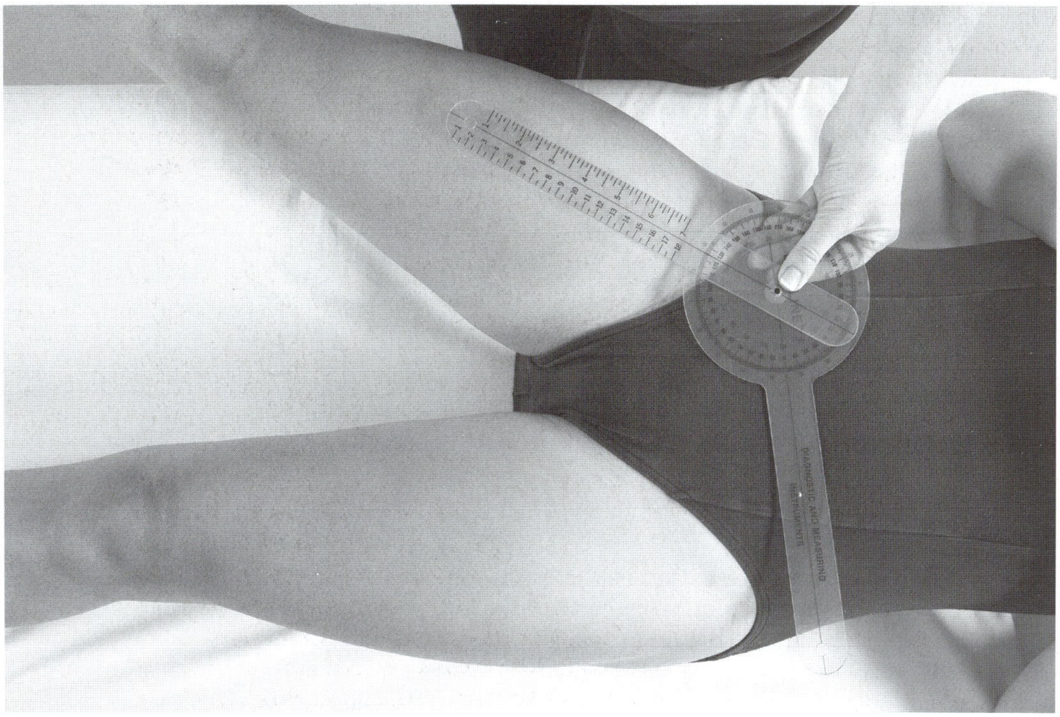

FIGURE 1.11 The indirect measurement of the muscle length of one-joint hip adductors is the same as measurement of passive hip abduction ROM.

In contrast to one-joint muscles, the length of two-joint and multi-joint muscles is usually not sufficient to allow full passive ROM to occur simultaneously at all joints crossed by these muscles. This inability of a muscle to lengthen and allow full ROM at all of the joints the muscle crosses is termed **passive insufficiency.** If a two-joint or multi-joint muscle crosses a joint that the examiner is assessing for ROM, the individual must be positioned so that passive tension in the muscle does not limit the joint's ROM. To allow full ROM at the joint under consideration and to ensure sufficient length in the muscle, the muscle must be put on slack at all of the joints the muscle crosses that are not being assessed. A muscle is put on slack by passively approximating the origin and insertion of the muscle.

Example: The triceps is a two-joint muscle that extends the elbow and shoulder. The triceps is passively insufficient during full shoulder flexion and full elbow flexion. When an examiner assesses elbow flexion ROM, the shoulder must be in a neutral position so there is sufficient length in the triceps to allow full flexion at the elbow (Fig. 1.12).

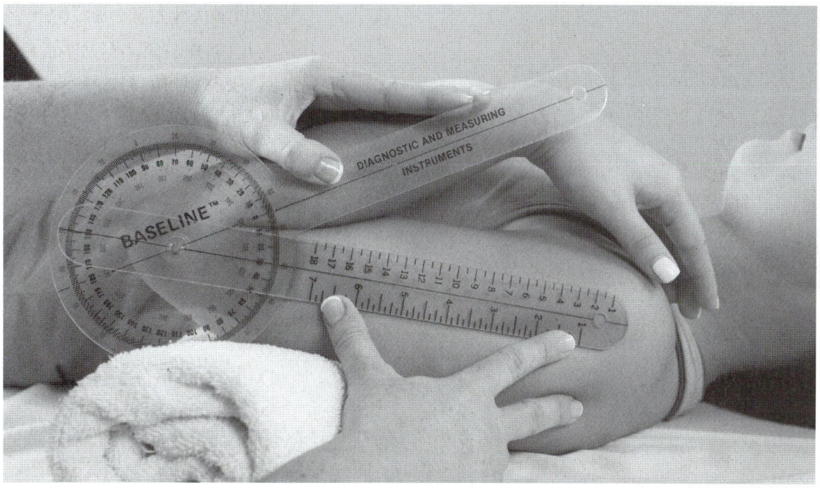

FIGURE 1.12 During the measurement of elbow flexion ROM, the shoulder must be in neutral to avoid passive insufficiency of the triceps, which would limit the ROM.

To assess the length of a two-joint muscle, the individual is positioned so that the muscle is lengthened over the proximal and distal joints that the muscle crosses. One joint is held in a full ROM position while the examiner attempts to further lengthen the muscle by moving the second joint through full ROM. The end-feel in this situation is firm owing to the development of passive tension in the stretched muscle. The length of the two-joint muscle is indirectly assessed by measuring the passive ROM in the direction opposite to the muscle's action at the second joint.

Example: To assess the length of a two-joint muscle such as the triceps, the shoulder is positioned and held in full flexion. The elbow is flexed until tension is felt in the triceps, creating a firm end-feel. The length of the triceps is determined by measuring passive ROM of elbow flexion with the shoulder in flexion (Fig. 1.13).

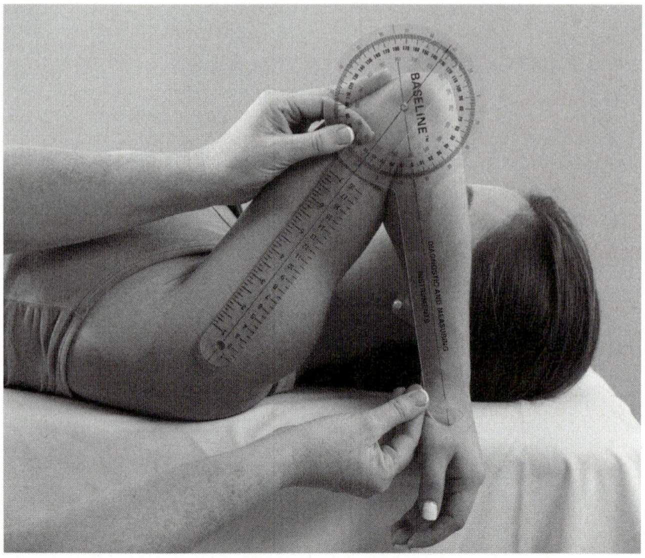

FIGURE 1.13 To assess the length of the two-joint triceps muscle, elbow flexion is measured while the shoulder is positioned in flexion.

The length of multi-joint muscles is assessed in a manner similar to that used in assessing the length of two-joint muscles. However, the individual is positioned and held so that the muscle is lengthened over all of the joints that the muscle crosses except for one last joint. The examiner attempts to further lengthen the muscle by moving the last joint through full ROM. Again, the end-feel is firm owing to tension in the stretched muscle. The length of the multi-joint muscle is determined by measuring passive ROM in the direction opposite to the muscle's action at the last joint to be moved. Commonly used muscle length tests that indirectly assess two-joint and multi-joint muscles have been included in Chapters 4 through 10 as appropriate. Normative values on joint angle at the end of the muscle length tests and information on the reliability and validity of these tests, if available, are presented as well.

In the next chapter, the examiner will have an opportunity to learn about the various instruments used to measure joint motion as well as participate in exercises designed to assist in identifying end-feels. Additional exercises are provided to assist the examiner in developing the skills that are necessary to use the instruments and record a ROM examination.

REFERENCES

1. Rondinelli, RD (ed): Guides to the Evaluation of Permanent Impairment, ed 6. American Medical Association Chicago, 2008.
2. Ward, SR: Biomechanical Applications to Joint Structure and Function. In Levangie, P, and Norkin, C (eds): Joint Structure and Function: A Comprehensive Analysis, ed 5. FA Davis, Philadelphia, 2011.
3. MacConaill, MA, and Basmajian, JV: Muscles and Movement: A Basis for Human Kinesiology, ed 2. Robert E. Krieger, New York, 1977.
4. Kisner, C, and Colby, LA: Therapeutic Exercise, ed 5. FA Davis, Philadelphia, 2007.
5. White, DJ: Musculoskeletal Examination. In O'Sullivan, SB, Schmitz, TJ, and Fulk, GD (eds): Physical Rehabilitation, ed 6. FA Davis, Philadelphia, 2014.
6. Kaltenborn, FM: Manual Mobilization of the Extremity Joints, ed 5. Olaf Norlis Bokhandel, Oslo, 1999.
7. Standring, S (ed): Gray's Anatomy, ed 41. Elsevier, New York, 2015.
8. Silver, D: Measurement of the range of motion in joints. J Bone Joint Surg 21:569, 1923.
9. Cave, EF, and Roberts, SM: A method for measuring and recording joint function. J Bone Joint Surg 18:455, 1936.
10. Moore, ML: The measurement of joint motion. Part II: The technic of goniometry. Phys Ther Rev 29:256, 1949.
11. American Academy of Orthopaedic Surgeons: Joint Motion: Methods of Measuring and Recording. AAOS, Chicago, 1965.
12. Greene, WB, and Heckman, JD (eds): The Clinical Measurement of Joint Motion. American Academy of Orthopaedic Surgeons, Rosemont, IL, 1994.
13. Clark, WA: A system of joint measurement. J Orthop Surg 2:687, 1920.
14. West, CC: Measurement of joint motion. Arch Phys Med Rehabil 26:414, 1945.
15. Cole, TM, and Tobis, JS: Measurement of Musculoskeletal Function. In Kottke, FJ, and Lehmann, JF (eds): Krusenn's Handbook of Physical Medicine and Rehabilitation, ed 4. WB Saunders, Philadelphia, 1990.
16. James, B, and Parker, AW: Active and passive mobility of lower limb joints in elderly men and women. Am J Phys Med Rehabil 68:162, 1989.
17. Gunal, I, et al: Normal range of motion of the joints of the upper extremity in male subjects, with special reference to side. J Bone Joint Surg Am 78(A):1401, 1996.
18. Smahel, Z, and Klimova, A: The influence of age and exercise on the mobility of hand joints: 1: Metacarpophalangeal joints of the three-phalangeal fingers. Acta Chirurgiae Plasricae 46:81, 2004.
19. Cyriax, J: Textbook of Orthopaedic Medicine: Diagnosis of Soft Tissue Lesions, ed 8. Bailliere Tindall, London, 1982.
20. Paris, SV: Extremity Dysfunction and Mobilization. Institute Press, Atlanta, 1980.
21. Petersen, CM, and Hayes, KW: Construct validity of Cyriax's selective tension examination. Association of end-feels with pain at the knee and shoulder. J Orthop Sports Phys Ther 30:512, 2000.
22. Hayes, KW, and Petersen, CM: Reliability of assessing end-feel and pain and resistance sequence in subjects with painful shoulders and knees. J Orthop Sports Phys Ther 31(8):432–445, 2001.
23. Manning, DM, et al: Reliability of a seated three-dimensional passive intervertebral motion test for mobility, end-feel, and pain provocation patients with cervicalgia. J Man Manip Ther 3:135, 2012.
24. Moore, KL, and Dalley, AF: Clinically Oriented Anatomy, ed 5. Lippincott, Williams & Wilkins, Baltimore, 2005.
25. Kapandji, IA: Physiology of the Joints, Vol 1, ed 2. Churchill Livingstone, London, 1970.
26. Kapandji, IA: Physiology of the Joints, Vol 2, ed 2. Williams & Wilkins, Baltimore, 1970.
27. Kapandji, IA: Physiology of the Joints, Vol 3, ed 2. Churchill Livingstone, London, 1970.
28. Steindler, A: Kinesiology of the Human Body. Charles C. Thomas, Springfield, IL, 1955.
29. Levangie, PL, and Norkin, CC: Joint Structure and Function: A Comprehensive Analysis, ed 5. FA Davis, Philadelphia, 2011.
30. Newmann, DA: Kinesiology of the Musculoskeletal System. Mosby, St. Louis, 2010.
31. Steultjens, MPM, et al: Range of joint motion and disability in patients with osteoarthritis of the knee or hip. Rheumatology 39:955, 2000.
32. Hermann, KM, and Reese, CS: Relationship among selected measures of impairment, functional limitation, and disability in patients with cervical spine disorders. Phys Ther 81:903, 2000.
33. Rao, SR, et al: Increased passive ankle stiffness and reduced dorsiflexion range of motion in individuals with diabetes mellitus. Foot Ankle Int 27:617, 2006.
34. Sauseng, S, Kastenbauer, T, and Irsigler, K: Limited joint mobility in selected hand and foot joints in patients with type 1 diabetes mellitus: A methodology comparison. Diabetes Nutr Metab 15:1, 2002.
35. Richard, RL, and Ward, RS: Burns. In O'Sullivan, SB, and Schmitz, TJ (eds): Physical Rehabilitation: Assessment and Treatment, ed 5. FA Davis, Philadelphia, 2014.
36. Johnson, J, and Silverberg, R: Serial casting of the lower extremity to correct contractures during the acute phase of burn care. Phys Ther 75:262, 1995.
37. deSouza Campos, C, Jr, Bracht, MA, and Dos Santos, MJ: The effect of joint hypomobility on precision grip force. J Hand Ther 26(4):323, 2013.
38. Beazell, JR, et al: Treatment of lateral knee pain in addressing tibiofibular hypomobility in a recreational runner. N Am J Sports Phys Ther 4(1):21, 2009.
39. Fritz, JM, et al: An examination of the selective tissue tension scheme, with evidence for the concept of a capsular pattern of the knee. Phys Ther 78:1046, 1998.
40. Hayes, KW, Petersen, C, and Falconer, J: An examination of Cyriax's passive motion tests with patients having osteoarthritis of the knee. Phys Ther 74:697, 1994.
41. Biji, D, et al: Validity of Cyriax's concept capsular pattern for the diagnosis of osteoarthritis of hip and/or knee. Scand J Rheumatol 27:347, 1998.
42. Klassbo, M, and Harms-Ringdahl, K: Examination of passive ROM and capsular pattern in the hip. Physiother Res Int 8:1, 2003.
43. Hertling, DH, and Kessler, RM: Management of Common Musculoskeletal Disorders, ed 4. Lippincott, Williams & Wilkins, Philadelphia, 2005.
44. Waugh, KG, et al: Measurement of selected hip, knee and ankle joint motions in newborns. Phys Ther 63:1616, 1983.
45. Castori, M: Ehler-Danlos syndrome, hypermobility type: An underdiagnosed hereditary connective tissue disorder with mucocutaneous, articular and systemic manifestations. G Ital Dermatol Venereol 1:13, 2013.
46. Everman, DB, and Robin, NH: Hypermobility syndrome. Pediatr Rev 19:111, 1998.
47. Smith, TO, et al.: Do people with benign joint hypermobility syndrome (BJHS) have reduced proprioception? A systematic review and meta-analysis. Rheumatol Int 33(11):2709, 2013.
48. Grahame, R: Hypermobility not a circus act. Int J Clin Pract 54:314, 2000.
49. Russek, LN: Hypermobility syndrome. Phys Ther 79:59, 1999.
50. Lamari, NM, Chueire, AG, and Cordeiro, JA: Analysis of joint mobility patterns among preschool children. Sao Paulo Med J 123:119, 2005.
51. Beighton, P, Solomon, L, and Soskolne, CL: Articular mobility in an African population. Ann Rheum Dis 32:23, 1973.
52. Remvig, L, Jensen, DV, and Ward, RC: Are diagnostic criteria for general joint hypermobility and benign joint hypermobility syndrome based on reproducible and valid tests? A review of the literature. J Rheumatol 34:798, 2007.
53. Jelsma, LD, et al: The relationship between joint mobility and motor performance in children with and without the diagnosis of developmental coordination disorder. BMC Pediatr 13:35, 2013.
54. Smits-Engelsman, B, Klerks, M, and Kirby, A: Beighton score: A valid measure for generalized hypermobility in children. J Pediatr 158(1):119, 2011.
55. Stefanyshyn, DJ, and Ensberg, JR: Right to left differences in the ankle joint complex range of motion. Med Sci Sports Exerc 26:551, 1993.
56. Mosley, AM, Crosbie, J, and Adams, R: Normative data for passive ankle plantar flexion-dorsiflexion flexibility. Clin Biomech 16:514, 2001.
57. Escalanate, A, et al: Determinants of hip and knee flexion range: Results from the San Antonio Longitudinal Study of Aging. Arthritis Care Res 12:8, 1999.
58. Allender, E, et al: Normal range of joint movements in shoulder, hip, wrist and thumb with special reference to side: A comparison between two populations. Int J Epidemiol 3:253, 1974.
59. Escalante, A, Lichtenstein, MJ, and Hazuda, HP: Determinants of shoulder and elbow flexion range: Results from the San Antonio Longitudinal Study of Aging. Arthritis Care Res 12:277, 1999.
60. Kendall, FP, et al: Muscles: Testing and Function With Posture and Pain, ed 5. Lippincott, Williams & Wilkins, Philadelphia, 2005.
61. Reese, NB, and Bandy, WD: Joint Range of Motion and Muscle Length Testing. WB Saunders, Philadelphia, 2010.

62. Drews, JE, Vraciu, JK, and Pellino, G: Range of motion of the joints of the lower extremities of newborns. Phys Occup Ther Pediatr 4:49, 1984.
63. Phelps, E, Smith, LJ, and Hallum, A: Normal range of hip motion of infants between nine and 24 months of age. Dev Med Child Neurol 27:785, 1985.
64. Wanatabe, H, et al: The range of joint motions of the extremities in healthy Japanese people: The differences according to age. Nippon Seikeigeka Gakkai Zasshi 53:275, 1979. Cited in Walker, JM: Musculoskeletal development: A review. Phys Ther 71:878, 1991.
65. Schwarze, DJ, and Denton, JR: Normal values of neonatal limbs: An evaluation of 1000 neonates. J Pediatr Orthop 13:758, 1993.
66. Broughton, NS, Wright, J, and Menelaus, MB: Range of knee motion in normal neonates. J Pediatr Orthop 13:263, 1993.
67. Roach, KE, and Miles, TP: Normal hip and knee active range of motion: The relationship to age. Phys Ther 71:656, 1991.
68. Steinberg, N, et al: Range of joint movement in female dancers and non-dancers aged 8–16 years: Anatomical and clinical implications. Am J Sports Med 34(5):814, 2006.
69. Stubbs, NB, Fernandez, JE, and Glenn, WM: Normative data on joint ranges of motion for 25- to 54-year-old males. Int J Ind Ergon 12:265, 1993.
70. Walker, JM, et al: Active mobility of the extremities in older subjects. Phys Ther 64:919, 1984.
71. Bell, RD, and Hoshizaki, TB: Relationship of age and sex with range of motion: Seventeen joint actions in humans. Can J Appl Sport Sci 6:202, 1981.
72. Kalscheur, JA, Costello, PS, and Emery, LJ: Gender differences in range of motion in older adults. Phys Occup Ther Geriatr 22:77, 2003.
73. Almquist, PO, et al: Knee motion in healthy individuals related to age and gender. J Orthop Res 31(1):23, 2013.
74. Lansade, C, et al: Three-dimensional analysis of the cervical spine kinematics: Effect of age and gender in healthy subjects. Spine 34(26):2900, 2009.
75. Youdas, JW, et al: Normal range of motion of the cervical spine: An initial goniometric study. Phys Ther 72:770, 1992.
76. Chen, J, et al: Meta-analysis of normative cervical motion. Spine 24:1571, 1999.
77. Salo, PK, et al: Quantifying the effect of age on passive range of motion of the cervical spine in healthy working-age women. J Orthop Sports Phys Ther 39:478, 2009.
78. Loebl, WY: Measurement of spinal posture and range of spinal movement. Ann Phys Med 9:103, 1967.
79. Fitzgerald, GK, et al: Objective assessment with establishment of normal values for lumbar spinal range of motion. Phys Ther 63:1776, 1983.
80. Intolo, P, et al: The effect of age on lumbar range of motion: A systematic review. Man Ther 14:596, 2009.
81. Trudelle-Jackson, E, et al: Lumbar spine flexion and extension extremes of motion in women of different age and racial groups. Spine 35(16):1539, 2010.
82. Gajdosik, RL, et al: Comparison of four clinical tests for assessing hamstring muscle length. J Orthop Sports Phys Ther 18:614, 1993.
83. Tardieu, G, Lespargot, A, and Tardieu, C: To what extent is the tibia-calcaneum angle a reliable measurement of the triceps surae length: Radiological correction of the torque-angle curve. Eur J Appl Physiol 37:163, 1977.
84. Gajdosik, RL: Passive extensibility of skeletal muscle: Review of the literature with clinical implications. Clin Biomech 16:87, 2001.
85. Gajdosik, RL, Hallett, JP, and Slaughter, LL: Passive insufficiency of two-joint shoulder muscles. Clin Biomech 9:377, 1994.

CHAPTER 2

Procedures

Cynthia C. Norkin, PT, EdD
D. Joyce White, PT, DSc

Competency in goniometry requires that the examiner learn the structure and function of each joint being measured. The examiner must also develop the necessary psychomotor skills for measuring range of motion and muscle length. This chapter contains exercises designed to assist the examiner in recognizing the end of the range of motion and identifying end-feels as well as exercises providing practice in reading the goniometer and other instruments employed in the measurement process. Positioning and stabilization are included in the chapter as initial parts of the 12-step examination sequence, which includes, among others, locating and palpating bony landmarks and methods of recording range of motion and muscle length.

Positioning

The **testing position** refers to the positions of the body recommended for obtaining both goniometric and muscle length measurements. Positioning is an important part of goniometry because it is used to place the joints in a zero starting position when measuring range of motion, and to lengthen a multi-joint muscle over all but the last joint crossed by the muscle when measuring muscle length. The last joint is moved to further stretch the muscle and determine the muscle length. In both goniometry and muscle length testing, positioning helps to stabilize the proximal joint segment. Positioning is important for the examiner, who should stand or sit close to the part of the individual's body being tested. If the examiner maintains a position close to the individual, it will improve the examiner's body mechanics and help prevent the examiner from incurring a back injury. Positioning is also important for the individual because choosing a comfortable and safe position relaxes the individual and may assist in reducing the amount of tension in soft tissue structures (capsule, ligaments, muscles) surrounding a joint. A testing position in which one or more of these soft tissues becomes taut results in a more limited range of motion (ROM) than a position in which the same structures become lax. However, when testing for muscle length, it is necessary to use an opposite position in which all of the tissues are stretched and taut. As can be seen in the following example, the use of different testing positions alters the ROM obtained for hip flexion.

Example: Consider the effects of muscle length on ROM. A testing position in which the knee is flexed relaxes the hamstring muscles and allows for greater hip flexion ROM (Fig. 2.1A) than a testing position in which the knee is extended (Fig. 2.1B). When the knee is extended, hip flexion is prematurely limited by the tension in the hamstring muscles. Muscles such as the hamstrings that cross two or more joints are not of sufficient length to allow a full ROM to occur simultaneously at all joints that they cross (in this instance, the knee and the hip joints). The tension developed in the hamstring muscles that are stretched over two joints prevents a full ROM of the hip. Knee flexion relaxes the hamstrings at the knee so that the muscle length is reduced to allow full ROM at the hip. In contrast to positioning for relaxation of opposing muscles in ROM testing, muscle length testing requires the stretching of muscles.

It is important for an examiner to use the same testing position and ideally conduct tests at the same time of day during successive measurements so that the relative amounts of tension in the soft tissue structures are the same as in previous measurements. A comparison of ROM measurements taken in the same position should yield similar results. When either different testing positions or different examiners are used for successive measurements of a joint ROM, more variability is added to the measurement, and less basis for comparison exists.[1–7] It becomes difficult to determine whether any differences in successive measurements are the result of a true change in joint ROM or the result of a different position or examiner.

Testing positions involve a variety of body positions such as supine, prone, sitting, and standing. When an examiner

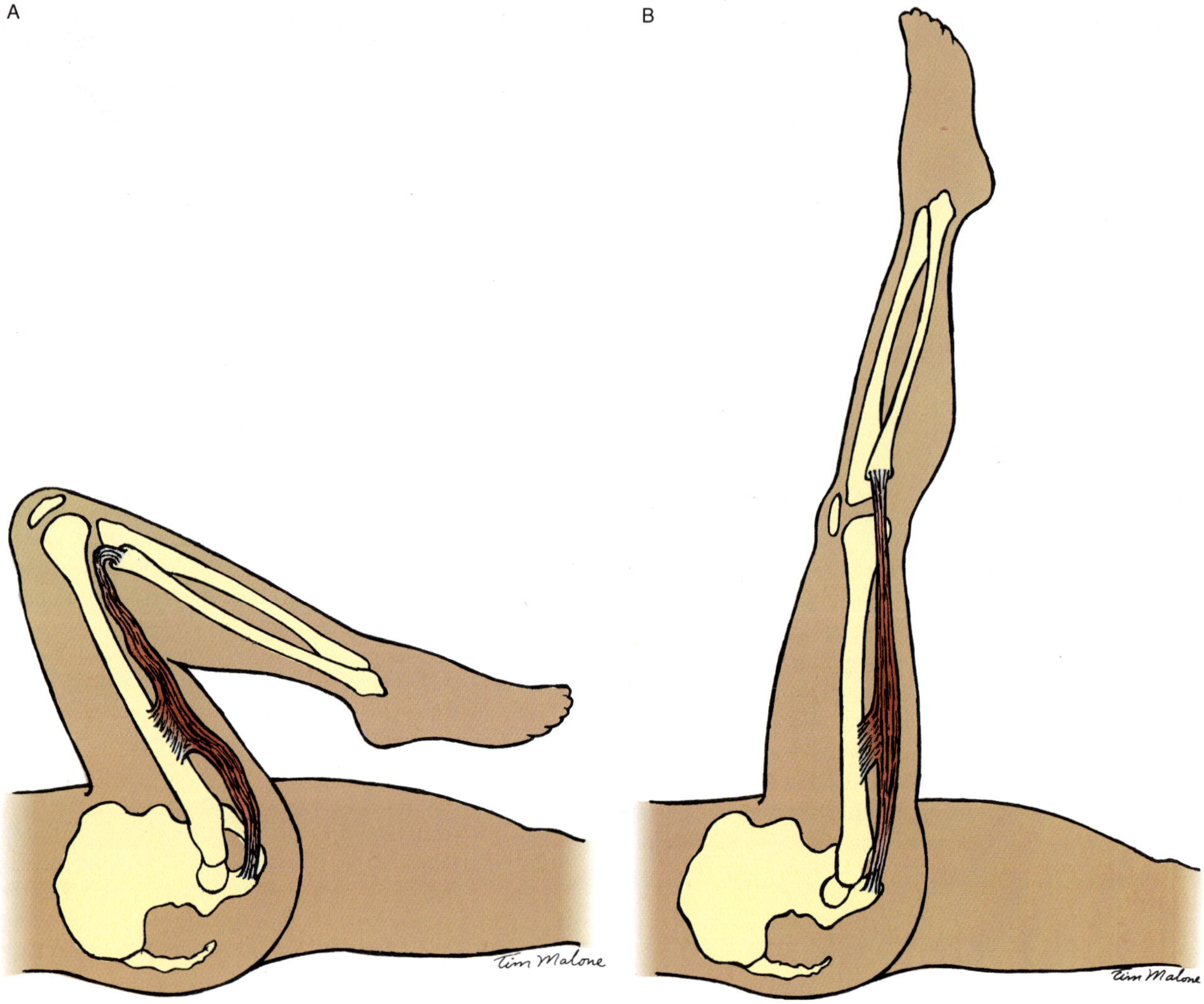

FIGURE 2.1 Positioning differs between ROM testing and muscle length testing. (A) Hip flexion ROM is tested with the knee flexed to relax the hamstring muscles, which will limit hip flexion ROM when the knee is extended. (B) To measure the muscle length of the hamstrings the knee must be extended and the hip flexed to ensure that the hamstring muscles are adequately lengthened.

intends to test several joints and motions during one testing session, the goniometric examination should be planned to avoid moving the individual unnecessarily. For example, if the individual is prone, all possible measurements in this position should be taken before the individual is moved into another position. Table 2.1, which lists joint measurements by body position, has been designed to help the examiner plan a goniometric examination.

The series of testing positions in this text are designed to follow the five guidelines discussed above. To summarize, the testing positions will do the following:

1. Ensure that the individual being tested is in a comfortable, safe, and stable position.
2. Place the joint being measured in a starting position of 0 degrees when testing for ROM.
3. Permit complete and unobstructed motion of the joint when testing for ROM.
4. Place the muscle in a lengthened position at all of the joints that the muscle crosses except for the one joint that will be measured for motion when testing for muscle length.
5. Provide stabilization for the proximal joint segment.

If a recommended testing position cannot be attained because of restrictions imposed by the environment or limitations of the individual, the examiner must use creativity to decide how to obtain a particular joint measurement. The alternative testing position that is created must serve the same five functions as the recommended testing position. In addition, the examiner must describe the position precisely in the individual's records so that the same position can be used for all subsequent measurements.

TABLE 2.1 Joint Measurements by Body Position

Joint/Body Region	Position			
	Prone	***Supine***	***Sitting***	***Standing***
Shoulder	Extension	Flexion Abduction Medial rotation Lateral rotation		
Elbow		Flexion		
Forearm			Pronation Supination	
Wrist			All motions	
Hand			All motions	
Hip	Extension Lateral rotation* Medial rotation*	Flexion Abduction Adduction	Medial rotation Lateral rotation	
Knee		Flexion		
Ankle and foot	Subtalar inversion Subtalar eversion	Dorsiflexion Plantar flexion Inversion Eversion Midtarsal inversion Midtarsal eversion	Dorsiflexion Plantar flexion Inversion Eversion Midtarsal inversion Midtarsal eversion	
Toes		All motions	All motions	
Cervical spine		Rotation†	Flexion Extension Lateral flexion Rotation	
Thoracolumbar spine			Rotation	Flexion Extension Lateral flexion Rotation†
Temporomandibular joint			All motions	

* = alternative position.

† = measured with inclinometer(s).

Stabilization

The testing position for ROM helps to stabilize the individual's body and proximal joint segment so that a motion can be isolated to the joint being examined. Isolating the motion to one joint helps to ensure that a true measurement of the motion is obtained, rather than a measurement of combined motions that occur at a series of joints. Positional stabilization may be supplemented by manual stabilization provided by the examiner.

Example: Measurement of medial rotation of the hip joint is performed with the individual in a sitting position (Fig. 2.2A). The pelvis (proximal segment) is partially stabilized by the body weight, but the individual is moving trunk and pelvis during hip rotation. Additional stabilization must be provided by the examiner and the individual (Fig. 2.2B). The examiner provides manual stabilization for the pelvis by exerting a downward pressure on the iliac crest of the side being tested. The individual shifts her body weight over the hip being tested to help keep the pelvis stabilized.

For most measurements, the amount of manual stabilization applied by an examiner must be sufficient to keep the proximal joint segment fixed during movement of the distal joint segment. If both the distal and the proximal joint segments are allowed to move during joint testing, the end of the ROM is difficult to determine. Learning how to stabilize requires practice because the examiner must stabilize with one hand while simultaneously moving the distal joint segment with the other hand. In the case of some hip joint motions, a second person may be necessary to help either by stabilizing the proximal joint segment or by supporting the distal joint segment after the end of the ROM has been determined. This assistance provided by the second person helps to ensure that the goniometer can be accurately aligned. The techniques of stabilizing the proximal joint segment and of determining the end of a ROM (end-feel) are basic to joint range-of-motion measurement and should be mastered prior to learning how to use either the goniometer or the inclinometer. **Exercise 1** is designed to help the examiner learn how to stabilize and determine the end of the ROM and end-feel.

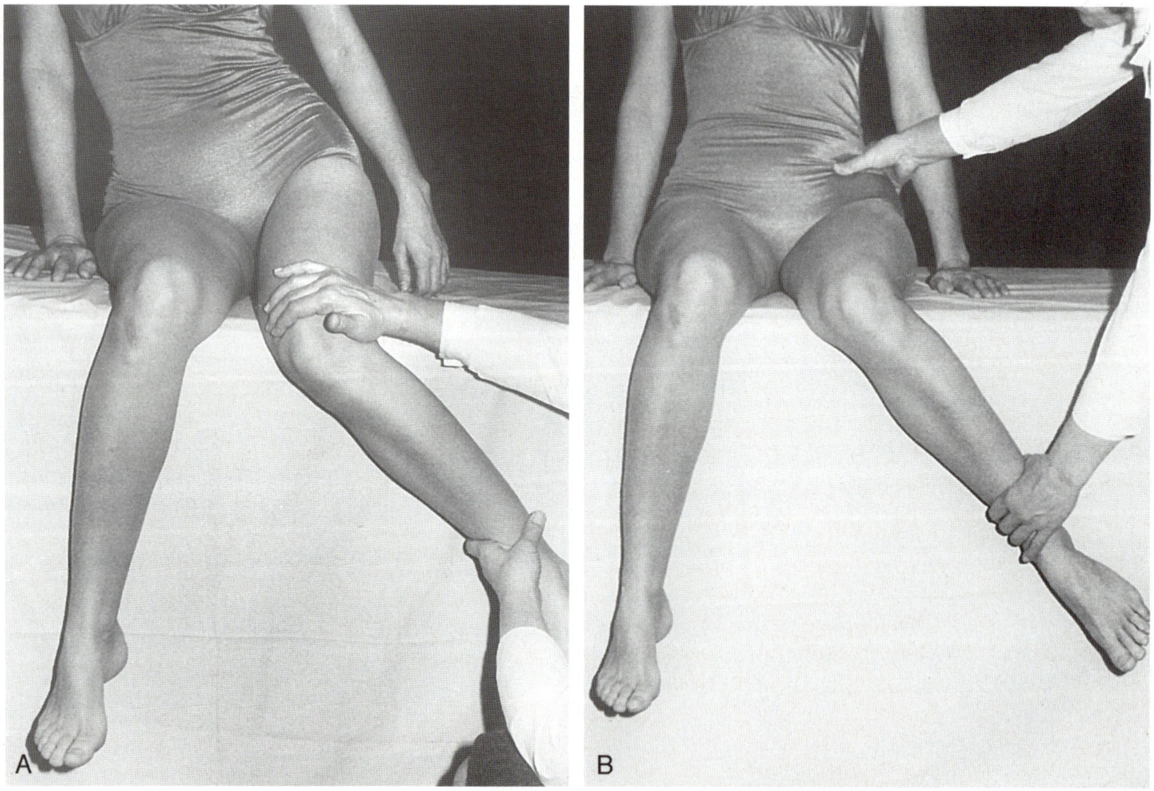

FIGURE 2.2 (A) The consequences of inadequate stabilization. The examiner has failed to stabilize the individual's pelvis and trunk; therefore, a lateral tilt of the pelvis and lateral flexion of the trunk accompany the motion of hip medial rotation. The range of medial rotation appears greater than it actually is because of the added motion from the pelvis and trunk. (B) The use of proper stabilization. The examiner uses her right hand to stabilize the pelvis (keeping the pelvis from rising off the table) during the passive range of motion (ROM). The individual assists in stabilizing the pelvis by placing her body weight on the left side. The individual keeps her trunk straight by placing both hands on the table.

Exercise 1

Determining the End of the Range of Motion and End-Feel

This exercise is designed to help the examiner determine the end of the ROM and to differentiate among the three normal end-feels: soft, firm, and hard.

ELBOW FLEXION: Soft End-Feel (Passive ROM)

Activities: See Figure 5.13 in Chapter 5.

1. Select an individual with whom to practice.
2. Position the individual supine with the arm placed close to the side of the body. A towel roll is placed under the distal end of the humerus to allow space for full elbow extension. The forearm is placed in full supination with the palm of the hand facing the ceiling.
3. With one hand, stabilize the distal end of the humerus (proximal joint segment) to prevent flexion of the shoulder.
4. With the other hand, slowly move the forearm through the full passive range of elbow flexion until you feel resistance limiting the motion.
5. Gently push against the resistance until no further flexion can be achieved. Carefully note the quality of the resistance. This soft end-feel is caused by compression of the muscle bulk of the anterior forearm with that of the anterior upper arm.
6. Compare this soft end-feel with the soft end-feel found in knee flexion (see ROM Testing Procedures: Knee and Fig. 9.6 in Chapter 9).

ANKLE DORSIFLEXION: Firm End-Feel (Passive ROM)

Activities: See Figure 10.11 in Chapter 10.

1. Select an individual with whom to practice.
2. Place the individual in a sitting position so that the lower leg is over the edge of the supporting surface and the knee is flexed at least 30 degrees.
3. With one hand, stabilize the distal end of the tibia and fibula to prevent knee extension and hip motions.
4. With the other hand on the plantar surface of the metatarsals, slowly move the foot through the full passive range of ankle dorsiflexion until you feel resistance limiting the motion.
5. Push against the resistance until no further dorsiflexion can be achieved. Carefully note the quality of the resistance. This firm end-feel is caused by tension in the Achilles tendon from the soleus muscle, the posterior portion of the deltoid ligament, the posterior talofibular ligament, the calcaneofibular ligament, the posterior joint capsule, and the wedging of the talus into the mortise formed by the tibia and fibula.
6. Compare this firm end-feel with the firm end-feel found in metacarpophalangeal (MCP) extension of the fingers (see ROM Testing Procedures for Fingers MCP Extension and Fig. 7.12 in Chapter 7).

ELBOW EXTENSION: Hard End-Feel (Passive ROM)

Activities: Select an individual with whom to practice.

1. Position the individual supine with the arm placed close to the side of the body. A small towel roll is placed under the distal end of the humerus to allow full elbow extension. The forearm is placed in full supination with the palm of the hand facing the ceiling.
2. With one hand resting on the towel roll and holding the posterior, distal end of the humerus, stabilize the humerus (proximal joint segment) to prevent extension of the shoulder.
3. With the other hand, slowly move the forearm through the full passive range of elbow extension until you feel resistance limiting the motion.
4. Gently push against the resistance until no further extension can be attained. Carefully note the quality of the resistance. When the end-feel is hard, it has no give to it. This hard end-feel is caused by contact between the olecranon process of the ulna and the olecranon fossa of the humerus.
5. Compare this hard end-feel with the hard end-feel usually found in radial deviation of the wrist (see ROM Testing Procedures for Radial Deviation and Fig. 6.18 in Chapter 6).

Measurement Instruments

A variety of instruments are available to measure joint motion and muscle length. These instruments range from tape measures to manual universal and digital goniometers,[8–10] manual and digital inclinometers,[9,11–13] cameras,[14–18] electrogoniometers,[19] gyroscopes,[20] motion analysis systems, and most recently goniometer and inclinometer applications (apps) for smartphones.[13,21,22] An examiner may choose to use a particular instrument based on the purpose of the measurement (clinical versus research); the motion being measured; and the instrument's accuracy, availability, cost, ease of use, size, and record of reliability and validity.

Universal Goniometer

The **universal goniometer** is the instrument most commonly used to measure ROM in the clinical setting. Moore designated this type of goniometer as "universal" because of its versatility.[23,24] It can be used to measure joint position and ROM at almost all joints of the body. The majority of measurement techniques presented in this book demonstrate the use of the universal goniometer. In the American Medical Association's sixth edition of the *Guides to the Evaluation of Permanent Impairment*,[25] the universal goniometer is the instrument recommended for obtaining ROM for the upper and lower extremities. In the fifth edition of the *Guides*,[26] the double inclinometer was the instrument recommended for measuring spinal ROM; however, the inclinometer was not included in the latest edition because there was insufficient evidence regarding its reliability/validity for measuring spinal motion. This change is one example of the need for more research to verify that the procedures and instruments used by physical therapists are thoroughly supported by evidence.

Goniometer Construction

Universal goniometers (UGs) may be constructed of plastic (Fig. 2.3) or metal (Fig. 2.4) and are produced in many sizes and shapes but adhere to the same basic design. Typically the

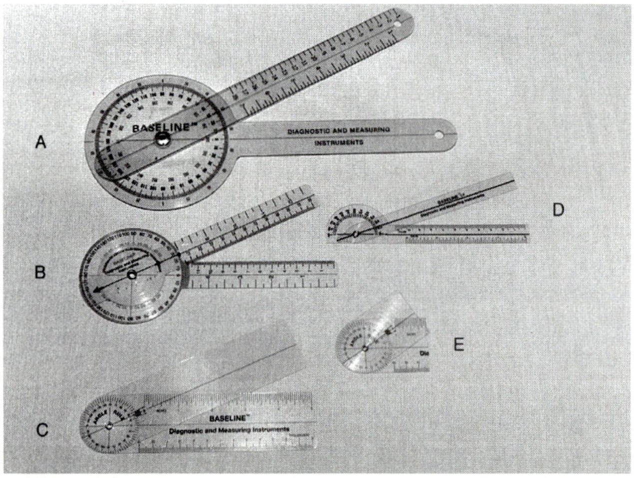

FIGURE 2.3 Plastic universal goniometers are available in different shapes and sizes. Some goniometers have full-circle bodies (A, B, C, E), whereas others have half-circle bodies (D). The 14-inch goniometer (A) is used to measure large joints such as the hip, knee, and shoulder. The level on one arm helps the examiner ensure that the arms are either horizontal or vertical. Six- to 8-inch goniometers (B, C, D) are used to assess midsized joints such as the wrist and ankle. The small goniometer (E) has been cut in length from a 6-inch goniometer (C) to make it easier to measure the fingers and toes.

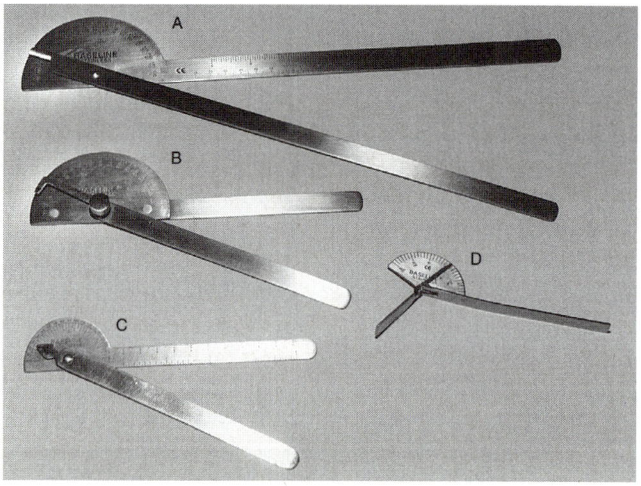

FIGURE 2.4 These metal goniometers are of different sizes but all have half-circle bodies. Metal goniometers with full-circle bodies are also available. The smallest goniometer (D) is specifically designed to lie on the dorsal or ventral surface of the fingers and toes while measuring joint motion. Goniometers A and B have a cut-out portion on the moving arm, whereas goniometers C and D have pointers on the moving arm to enable the reading of the scale on the bodies.

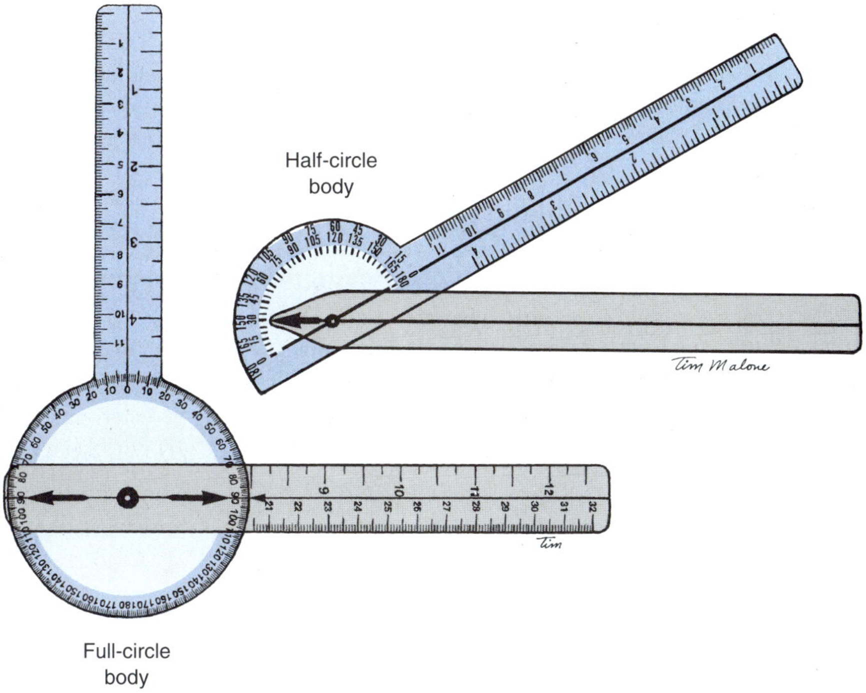

FIGURE 2.5 The body of the goniometer may be either a half circle (*top*) or a full circle (*bottom*). The scales on the body of the goniometer are usually in increments of 1 (*bottom*) or 5 degrees (*top*).

design includes a body and two thin extensions called arms—a stationary arm and a moving arm. A relatively new innovation is a gravitational level that can be slipped on to one arm of the goniometer. The level helps to ensure that the goniometer arm is either vertical or horizontal.

The *body* of a universal goniometer resembles a protractor and may form a half circle or a full circle (Fig. 2.5). The scales on a half-circle goniometer read from 0 to 180 degrees and from 180 to 0 degrees. The scales on a full-circle instrument may read either from 0 to 180 degrees and from 180 to 0 degrees, or from 0 to 360 degrees and from 360 to 0 degrees. Sometimes full-circle instruments have both 180-degree and 360-degree scales. Therefore, the examiner must pay close attention to avoid reading the wrong scale. The examiner should also check the increments on the scales, which may vary from 1 to 10 degrees, but 1- and 5-degree increments are the most common.

The *arms* of a universal goniometer are designated as moving or stationary according to how they are attached to the body of the goniometer (Fig. 2.6). The *stationary arm* is a structural part of the body of the goniometer and cannot be moved independently from the body. The *moving arm* is attached to the center of the body of most plastic goniometers by a rivet that permits the arm to move freely on the body. The moving arm may have one or more of the following features: a pointed end, a black or white line extending the length of the arm, or a cut-out portion (window). Goniometers that are used to measure ROM on radiographs have an opaque white line extending the length of the arms and opaque markings on the body. These features help the examiner to read the scales.

The length of the arms varies among instruments from approximately 1 to 14 inches. These variations in length represent an attempt on the part of the manufacturers to adapt the size of the instrument to the size of the joints. At least one manufacturer[9] has a goniometer with arms that can expand from 8 to 28 inches in length.

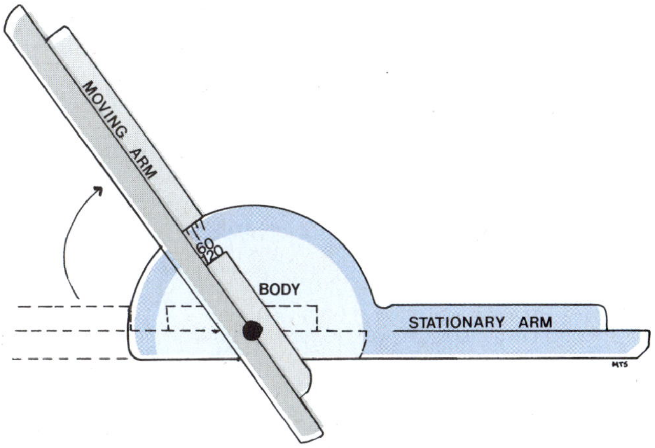

FIGURE 2.6 The body of this universal goniometer forms a half circle. The stationary arm (colored blue for emphasis) is an integral part of the body of the goniometer. The moving arm (colored gray for emphasis) is attached to the body by a rivet so that it can be moved independently from the body. In this example, a cut-out portion, sometimes referred to as a "window," is found in the center and at the end of the moving arm. The windows permit the examiner to read the scale on the body of the goniometer.

Example: A universal goniometer with 14-inch arms is appropriate for measuring motion at the knee joint because the arms are long enough to permit alignment with the greater trochanter of the femur and the lateral malleolus of the tibia (Fig. 2.7A). A goniometer with short arms would be difficult to use because the arms do not extend a sufficient distance along the femur and tibia to permit good alignment with the bony landmarks (see Fig. 2.7B). A goniometer with long arms would be awkward for measuring the MCP joints of the hand. Goniometers that are designed to measure the joints of the hand usually have arms that measure 4 to 6 inches in length and are well adapted to the small size of the fingers and thumb.

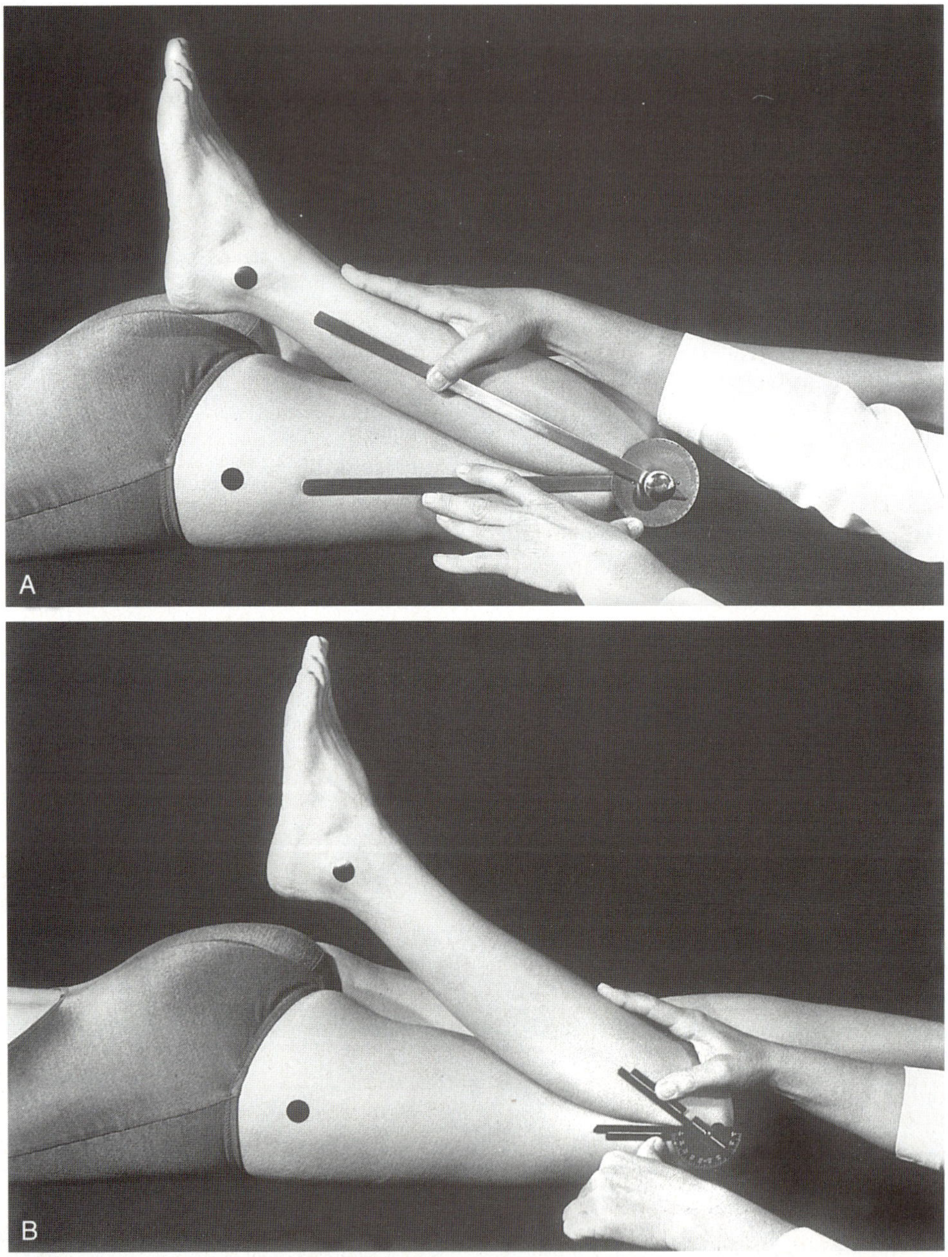

FIGURE 2.7 Selecting the right-sized goniometer makes it easier to measure joint motion. (A) The examiner is using a full-circle instrument with long arms to measure knee flexion ROM. The arms of the goniometer extend along the distal and proximal segments of the joint to within a few inches of the bony landmarks (black dots) that are used to align the arms. The proximity of the ends of the arms to the landmarks makes alignment easy and helps ensure that the arms are aligned accurately. (B) The small half-circle metal goniometer is a poor choice for measuring knee flexion ROM because the landmarks are so far from the ends of the goniometer's arms that accurate alignment is difficult.

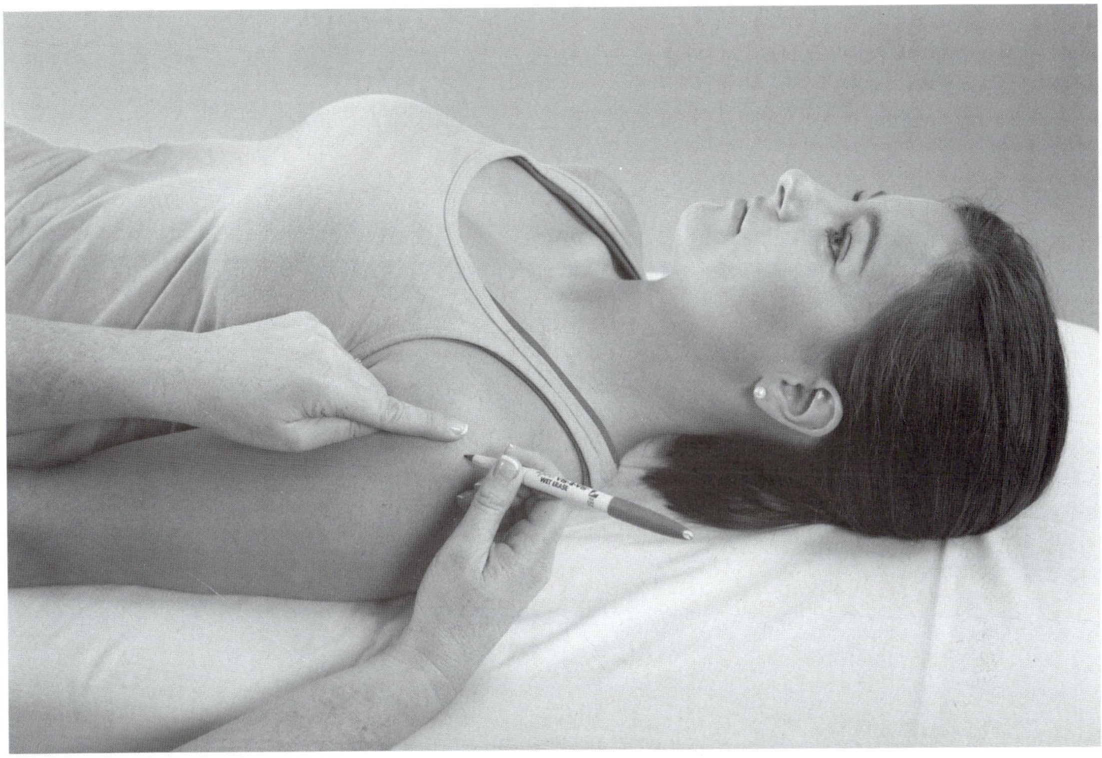

FIGURE 2.8 The examiner is using a washable ink pen to mark the location of the left acromion process. Note that the individual's clothing has been removed so that the bony landmark can be easily visualized. The examiner often uses the index and middle fingers to palpate the bony landmarks.

Alignment

Goniometer alignment refers to the alignment of the arms of the goniometer with the proximal and distal segments of the individual's joints. The examiner must learn and use the bony **anatomical landmarks** to more accurately visualize the joint segments. These landmarks, which have been identified for all joint measurements, should be exposed completely so that they may be easily located and palpated (Fig. 2.8). The careful visualization, palpation, and alignment of the arms of the goniometer with the landmarks improve the accuracy and consistency of the measurements.

Customarily, the stationary arm is aligned parallel to the longitudinal axis of the proximal segment of the joint and the moving arm is aligned parallel to the longitudinal axis of the distal segment of the joint (Fig. 2.9). In some situations, because of limitations imposed by either the goniometer or the individual, it may be necessary to reverse the alignment of the two arms so that the moving arm is aligned with the distal part and the stationary arm is aligned with the distal part (Fig. 2.10).

However, the angle measured by the goniometer will be the same regardless of which arms are aligned with the proximal or distal segments of the joint. Therefore, we use the term **proximal arm** to refer to the arm of the goniometer that is aligned with the proximal segment of the joint and the term **distal arm** to refer to the arm aligned with the distal segment

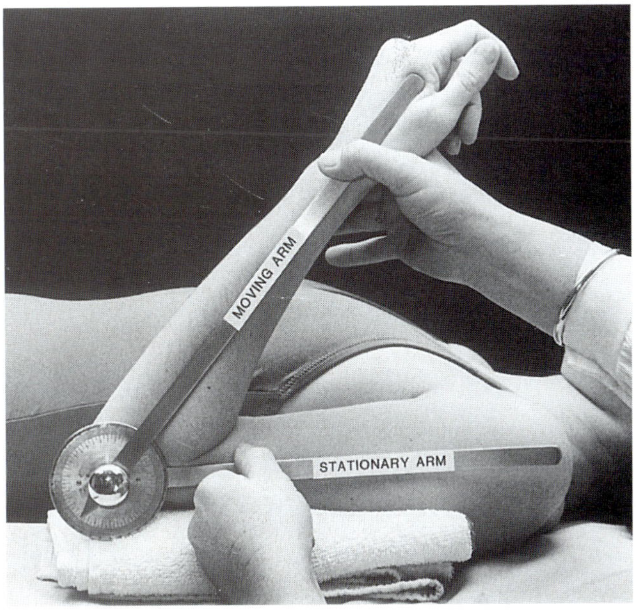

FIGURE 2.9 When using a full-circle goniometer to measure ROM of elbow flexion, the stationary arm is usually aligned parallel to the longitudinal axis of the proximal part (humerus) and the moving arm is aligned parallel to the longitudinal axis of the distal part (forearm). However, if the arms of the goniometer are reversed, the same angle will be measured.

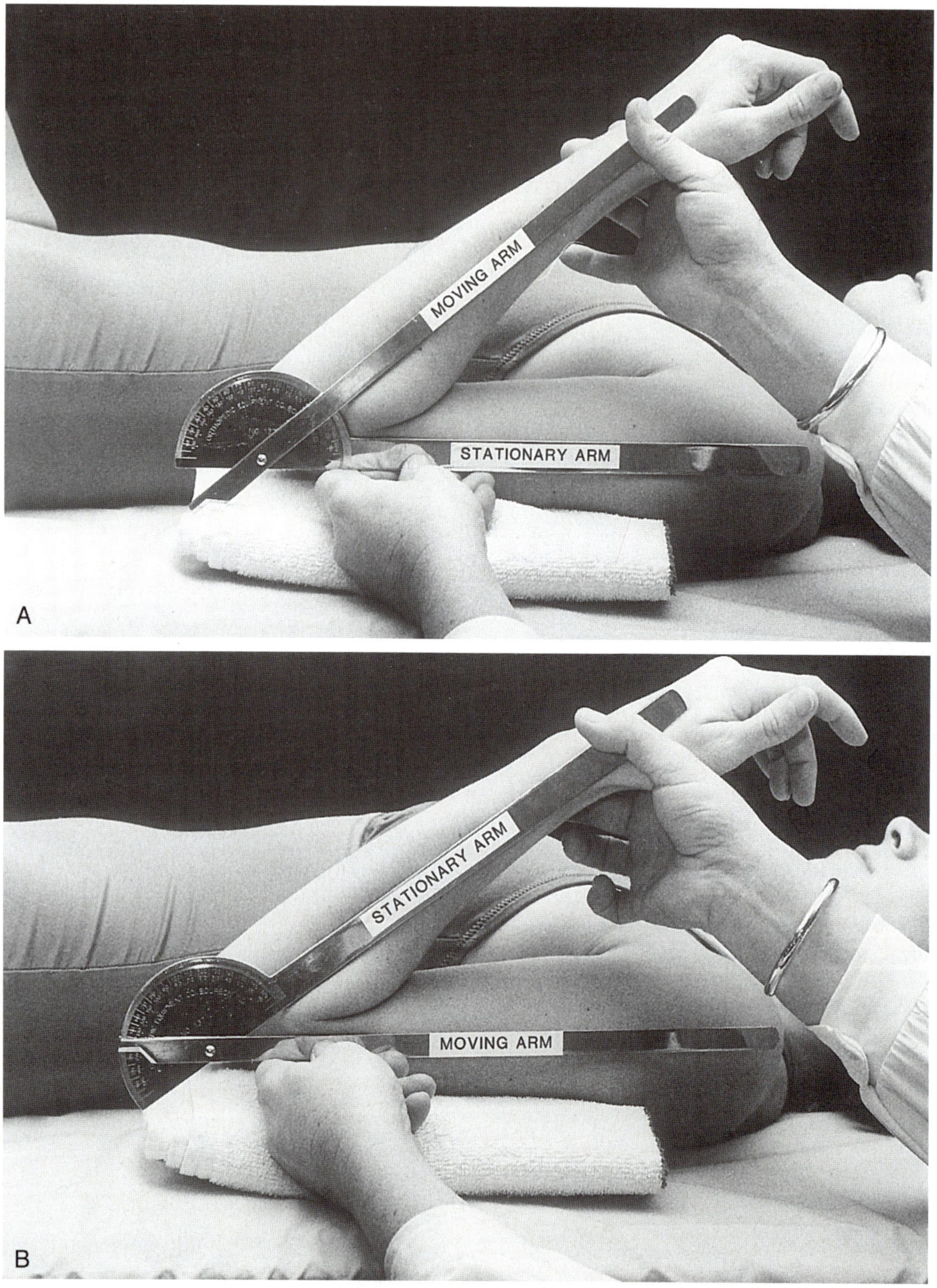

FIGURE 2.10 (A) When the examiner uses a half-circle goniometer to measure left elbow flexion, aligning the moving arm with the forearm causes the pointer to move beyond the goniometer body, which makes it impossible to read the scale. (B) Reversing the arms of the instrument so that the stationary arm is aligned parallel to the distal part and the moving arm is aligned parallel to the proximal part causes the pointer to remain on the body of the goniometer, enabling the examiner to read the scale along the pointer.

of the joint (Fig. 2.11). The anatomical landmarks provide reference points that help to ensure that the alignment of the arms is correct.

The **fulcrum** of the goniometer is usually placed over the approximate location of the axis of motion of the joint being measured. However, because the axis of motion changes during movement, the location of the fulcrum must be adjusted accordingly. Moore[23,24] suggested that careful alignment of the proximal and distal arms ensures that the fulcrum of the goniometer is located at the approximate axis of motion. Therefore, alignment of the arms of the goniometer with the proximal and distal joint segments should be emphasized more than placement of the fulcrum over the approximate axis of motion.

Errors in measuring joint position and motion with a goniometer can occur if the examiner is not careful. When aligning the arms and reading the scale of the goniometer, the examiner must be at eye level with the goniometer to avoid parallax. This situation occurs if the examiner is higher or lower than the goniometer; as a consequence, the alignment and scales are distorted. Often a goniometer will have several scales, one reading from 0 to 180 degrees and another reading from 180 to 0 degrees. Examiners must determine which scale is correct for the measurement. If a visual estimate is made before the measurement is taken, gross errors caused by reading the wrong scale will be obvious. Another source of error is misinterpretation of the intervals on the scale. For example, the smallest interval of a particular goniometer may be 5 degrees, but an examiner may believe the interval represents 1 degree. In this case, the examiner would incorrectly read 91 degrees instead of 95 degrees.

Cost

The cost of universal goniometers varies according to construction material (stainless steel or plastic), size, and special features for measuring particular joints. Universal goniometers range in cost from about $5.00 for a plastic goniometer with 6-inch arms to about $75.00 for a stainless steel goniometer with 14-inch arms. Goniometers specifically designed for measuring the finger joints cost anywhere from $20.00 to $100.00. Generally, universal goniometers are the least expensive and most cost–effective option for measuring joint motion and muscle length.

After the examiner has read this section on universal goniometer construction and alignment, **Exercises 2 and 3** should be completed.

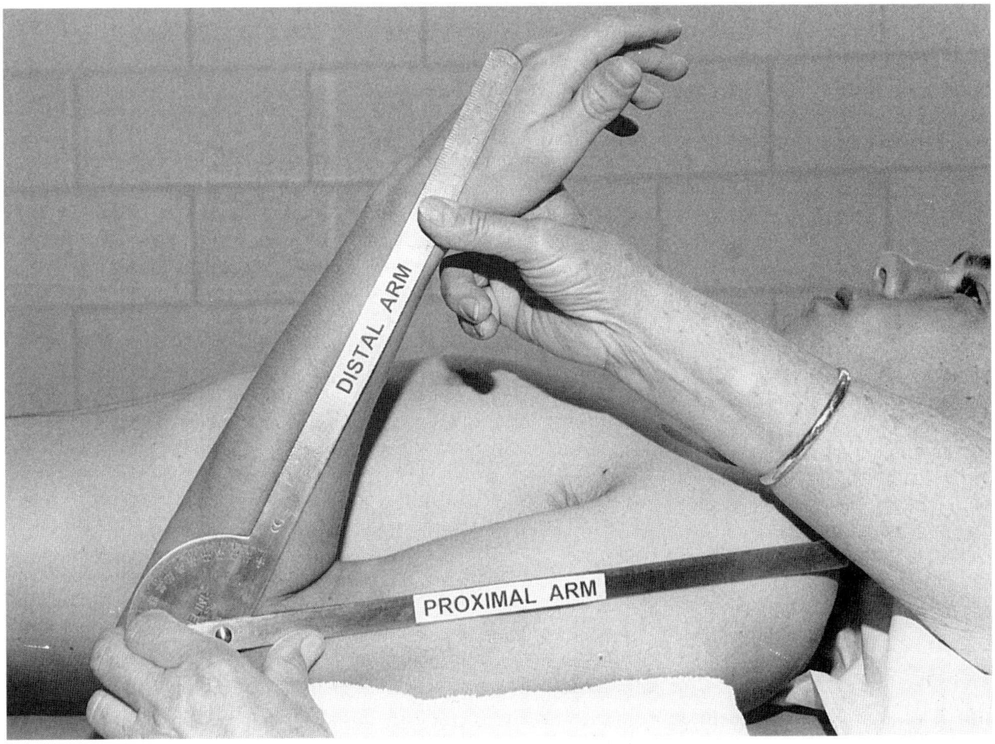

FIGURE 2.11 The term "proximal arm" indicates the arm of the goniometer that is aligned with the proximal segment of the joint being examined. The term "distal arm" is used to indicate the arm of the goniometer that is aligned with the distal segment of the joint. During the measurement of elbow flexion, the proximal arm is aligned with the humerus, and the distal arm is aligned with the forearm.

Exercise 2

The Universal Goniometer

The following activities are designed to help the examiner become familiar with the universal goniometer.

EQUIPMENT: Full-circle and half-circle universal goniometers made of plastic and metal.

Activities:

1. Select a goniometer.
2. Identify the type of goniometer selected (full-circle or half-circle) by noting the shape of the body.
3. Differentiate between the moving and the stationary arms of the goniometer. (Remember that the stationary arm is an integral part of the body of the goniometer.)
4. Observe the moving arm to see whether it has a cut-out portion or pointer.
5. Find the line in the middle of the moving arm and follow it to a number on the scale.
6. Study the body of the goniometer and answer the following questions:
   a. Is the scale located on one or both sides?
   b. Is it possible to read the scale through the body of the goniometer?
   c. What intervals are used?
   d. Does the body contain one, two, or more scales?
7. Hold the goniometer in both hands. Position the arms so that they form a continuous straight line. When the arms are in this position, find the scale that reads 0 degrees.
8. Keep the stationary arm fixed in place and shift the moving arm while watching the numbers on the scale, either at the tip of the moving arm or in the cut-out portion. Shift the moving arm from 0 to 45, 90, 150, and 180 degrees.
9. Keep the stationary arm fixed and shift the moving arm from 0 degrees through an estimated 45-degree arc of motion. Compare the visual estimate with the actual arc of motion by reading the scale on the goniometer. Try to estimate other arcs of motion and compare the estimates with the actual arc of motion.
10. Keep the moving arm fixed in place and move the stationary arm through different arcs of motion.
11. Repeat Steps 2 to 10 using different plastic and metal goniometers.

Exercise 3

Goniometer Alignment for Elbow Flexion

The following activities are designed to help the examiner learn how to align and read the universal goniometer.

EQUIPMENT: Full-circle and half-circle universal goniometers of plastic and metal in various sizes and a skin-marking pen or pencil.

Activities: See Figures 5.9 to 5.15 in Chapter 5.

1. Select a goniometer and an individual with whom to practice.
2. Position the individual supine. The individual's left arm should be positioned so that it is close to the side of the body with the forearm in supination (palm of hand faces the ceiling). A towel roll placed under the distal humerus helps to ensure that the elbow is fully extended. (See Fig. 5.14 in Chapter 5.)
3. Locate and mark each of the following landmarks: acromion process, lateral epicondyle of the humerus, radial head, and radial styloid process. (See Figs. 5.9 to 5.12 in Chapter 5.)
4. Align the proximal arm of the goniometer along the longitudinal axis of the humerus, using the acromion process and the lateral epicondyle as reference landmarks. To avoid parallax, make sure that you are positioned so that the goniometer is at eye level during the alignment process.
5. Align the distal arm of the goniometer along the longitudinal axis of the radius, using the radial head and the radial styloid process as reference landmarks. (See Fig. 5.14 in Chapter 5.)

6. The fulcrum should be close to the lateral epicondyle. Check to make sure that the body of the goniometer is not being deflected by the supporting surface.
7. Recheck the alignment of the arms and readjust the alignment as necessary.
8. Read the scale on the goniometer.
9. Remove the goniometer from the individual's arm and place it nearby so it is handy for measuring the next joint position.
10. Move the individual's forearm into various positions in the flexion ROM, including the end of the flexion ROM. At each joint position, align and read the goniometer. Remember that you must support the individual's forearm while aligning the goniometer. (See Fig. 5.15.)
11. Repeat Steps 3 to 10 on the individual's right upper extremity.
12. Repeat Steps 4 to 10 using goniometers of different sizes and shapes.
13. Answer the following questions:
    a. Did the length of the goniometer arms affect the accuracy of the alignment? Explain.
    b. What length goniometer arms would you recommend as being the most appropriate for this measurement? Why?
    c. Did the type of goniometer used (full-circle or half-circle) affect either joint alignment or the reading of the scale? Explain.
    d. Did the side of the body that you were testing make a difference in your ability to align the goniometer? Why?

Gravity-Dependent Goniometers (Inclinometers)

Although not as common as the universal goniometer, several other types of manual and digital goniometers may be found in the clinical setting. **Gravity-dependent goniometers** or **inclinometers** use gravity's effect on pointers and fluid levels to measure joint position and motion (Fig. 2.12). The **pendulum goniometer** consists of a 360-degree protractor with a weighted pointer hanging from the center of the protractor. This device was first described by Fox and Van Breemen[27] in 1934. The **fluid (bubble) goniometer,** which was developed by Schenkar[28] in 1956, has a fluid-filled circular chamber containing an air bubble. It is similar to a carpenter's level but being circular has a 360-degree scale motion.

Some inclinometers are either attached to or held on the distal segment of the joint being measured. The angle between the long axis of the distal segment and the line of gravity is noted. Inclinometers may be easier to use in certain situations than universal goniometers because they do not have to be aligned with two bony landmarks and centered over the axis of motion, but they do have to be put over particular landmarks for consistency. Misplacement over anatomical landmarks can give inaccurate readings. In addition, it is critical

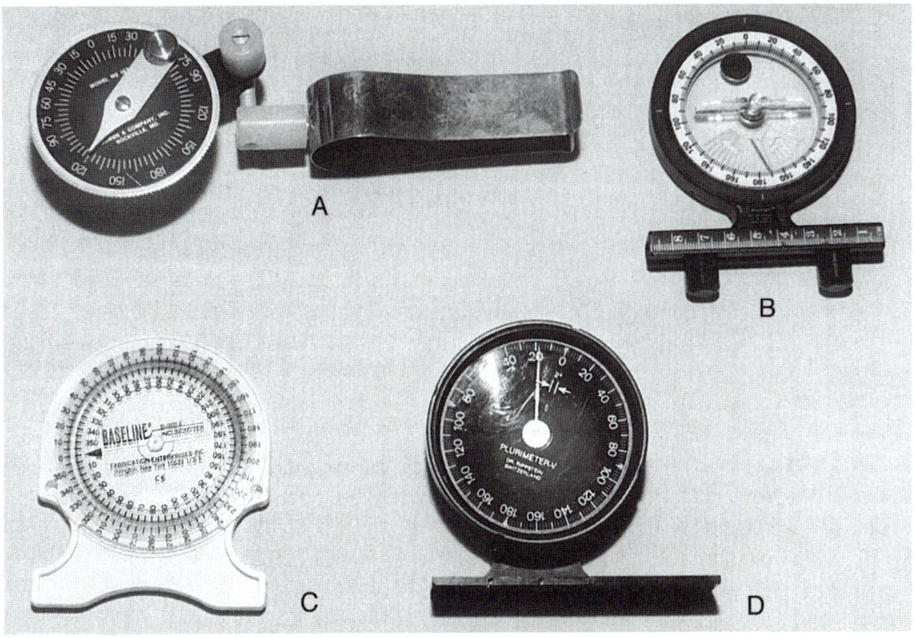

FIGURE 2.12 Each of these gravity-dependent goniometers uses a weighted pointer (A, B, D) or bubble (C) to indicate the position of the goniometer relative to the vertical pull of gravity. All of these inclinometers have a rotating dial so that the scale can be zeroed with the pointer or bubble in the starting position.

that the proximal segment of the joint being measured be positioned vertically or horizontally to obtain accurate measurements; otherwise, adjustments must be made in determining the measurement.[29] Inclinometers are also difficult to use on small joints and where there is soft tissue deformity or edema.

Some inclinometers are specifically used for measuring spinal motion. The cervical range of motion (CROM) device and back range of motion (BROM) device manufactured by Performance Attainment[30] are examples of inclinometers that are mounted on plastic frames. The CROM device (Fig. 2.13A) has three inclinometers fastened on a plastic frame that fits over the head. The inclinometer located on the frame on the lateral side of the head is used to measure lateral cervical flexion. The inclinometer on the front of the plastic frame is used to measure cervical flexion and extension. A compass inclinometer attached to the top of the headpiece is used to measure cervical rotation. The compass inclinometer reacts to the earth's magnetic field to measure motions in the horizontal plane and is used in conjunction with a magnetic yoke placed around the individual's shoulders. The BROM device (Fig. 2.13B) has similar arrangements for its inclinometers, with a compass inclinometer mounted horizontally to measure rotation in conjunction with a magnetic yoke fastened around the pelvis.

Although both universal and gravity-dependent goniometers may be available within a clinical setting, they should not be used interchangeably.[31–34] For example, an examiner should not use a universal goniometer on Tuesday and an inclinometer on Wednesday to measure the same individual's knee ROM. The two instruments may provide slightly different results, making comparisons for judging changes in ROM inappropriate. Given the adaptability and widespread use of the universal goniometer in the clinical setting, this book focuses primarily on teaching the measurement of the extremity joints using the universal goniometer. However, sections of the book that focus on the spine and temporomandibular joints use inclinometers and tape measures as well as the universal goniometer.

Cost

Generally, inclinometers are more expensive than universal goniometers.[9] The price of a bubble inclinometer ranges between $60.00 and $180.00, whereas the price of the Acumar Single Digital inclinometer is about $300.00.[9] Specialized inclinometers such as the CROM and the BROM cost about $380.00 to $400.00.[10]

After the examiner has read the preceding information about inclinometers, **Exercises 4 and 5** should be completed.

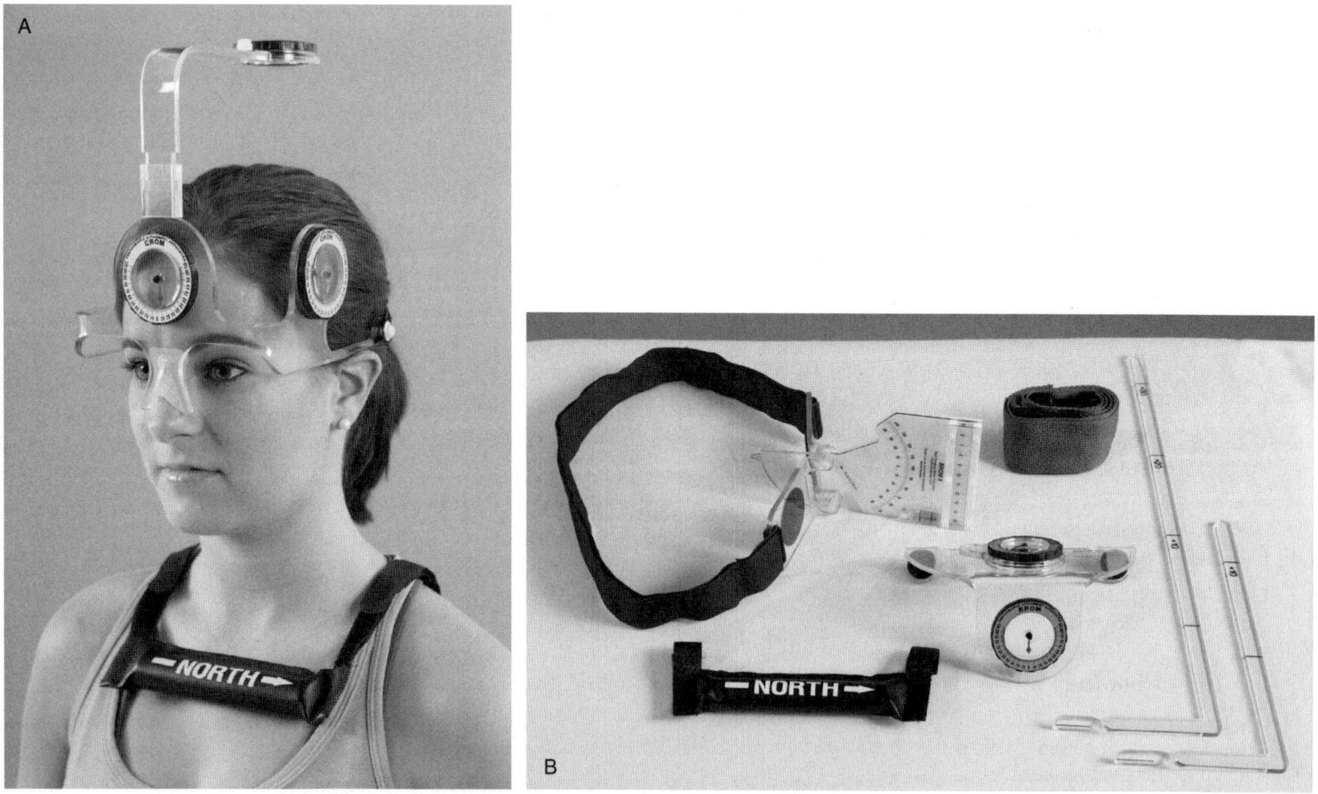

FIGURE 2.13 (A) The cervical range of motion (CROM) device has three inclinometers mounted on a plastic frame that fits over the head. One inclinometer is mounted on the side of the head to measure lateral motion of the head. A second inclinometer is located in front of the head in order to measure flexion and extension. A compass inclinometer mounted on top of the head is used in conjunction with a magnetic yoke placed around the individual's shoulder to measure rotation. (B) The back range of motion (BROM) device also has a compass inclinometer mounted horizontally that is used in conjunction with a magnetic yoke fastened around the pelvis to measure rotation.

Exercise 4

Inclinometers

The following activities are designed to help the examiner become familiar with inclinometers.

EQUIPMENT: Bubble inclinometer and pendulum inclinometer.

Activities

1. What does the face of the bubble inclinometer look like? The pendulum inclinometer? What do you see in the moveable clear plastic circle of the bubble inclinometer? What do you see in the face of the pendulum inclinometer? How are the two instruments alike and how are they different?
2. Stand the bubble inclinometer up vertically on its two legs. Note that there are inner and outer scales on the plastic circle. Does the pendulum inclinometer have the same arrangement?
   a. Are the increments the same on each instrument? The scales go from 0 to 350 on the bubble inclinometer and from 0 to 50 on the pendulum inclinometer.
   b. What happens to the inside scale on the bubble inclinometer if you set the outside scale to zero?
   c. On the bubble inclinometer, in which direction does the outside scale go—clockwise or counterclockwise?
   d. If you tilt the bubble inclinometer to the right, which scale should you use to take a measurement? If you tilt the pendulum inclinometer to the right, what happens? To the left?
3. If both the inside and outside scales on the bubble inclinometer are on zero, what does the scale directly across from the zero read? What does the scale directly across from zero read on the pendulum inclinometer?
4. Did you find it difficult to keep the liquid at zero in the bubble inclinometer? Did you have any difficulty maintaining a zero position on the pendulum inclinometer?
5. What happens to the liquid in the bubble inclinometer if you tilt it forward? Backward?
6. Which instrument appears to be the easiest to handle and read? Why?

Exercise 5

Inclinometer Alignment for Cervical Rotation

The following activities are designed to help the examiner learn how to align and read the bubble inclinometer.

Activities: Refer to Figures 11.42 and 11.43 in Chapter 11.

1. Select an inclinometer and an individual with whom to practice.
2. Position the individual in a supine position with arms at the side and head in a neutral position.
3. Stand or sit at the end of the table so that you are looking at the top of the individual's head.
4. Use your hands to roll the individual's head to the right and to the left, making sure that the end of the range of motion has been reached.
5. Ask the individual to repeat the motions until the motions are being performed correctly.
6. Reposition the individual's head in a neutral position.
7. Place the inclinometer on the individual's forehead, holding it firmly in contact with the skin while you zero the inclinometer.
8. Ask the individual to move her head to the right.
9. Hold the inclinometer firmly on the forehead throughout the motion, being careful not to tip it up or down.
10. Read the correct scale at the end of the ROM.
11. Record your findings.
12. Reposition the head in neutral and zero the inclinometer.
13. Repeat the activity by asking the individual to move her head to the left.
14. Hold the inclinometer firmly on the on the forehead throughout the motion.
15. Record your findings.
    a. Did you experience more or less difficulty holding the inclinometer to the right or the left?
    b. What things did you like about the inclinometer and what things did you dislike?

Electrogoniometers

Electrogoniometers, introduced by Karpovich and Karpovich[35] in 1959, are used primarily in research to obtain dynamic joint measurements. Most devices have two arms, similar to those of the universal goniometer, which are attached to the proximal and distal segments of the joint being measured.[34–39] A potentiometer is connected to the two arms. Changes in joint position cause the resistance in the potentiometer to vary. The resulting change in voltage can be used to indicate the amount of joint motion.

Some electrogoniometers resemble pendulum goniometers.[40,41] Changes in joint position cause a change in contact between the pendulum and the small resistors. Contact with the resistors produces a change in the electrical current, which is used to indicate the amount of joint motion.

Potentiometers measuring angular displacement have also been integrated with strain gauges and isokinetic dynamometers. Flexible electrogoniometers with two plastic end-blocks connected by a flexible strain gauge have been designed to measure angular displacement between the end-blocks in one or two planes of motion,[33,42] but cannot measure rotation. Torsiometers (single axis) are designed to measure rotations in one plane such as supination and pronation of the forearm. However, Shiratsu and Coury, in a study of torsiometers, found that the reliability and accuracy of the torsiometer sensors varied between sensors and movements. The authors concluded that electrogoniometers were more reliable and accurate than torsiometers.[43]

A systematic review of measurement tools (standard goniometers, fluid- and gravity-based inclinometers, photographs, and motion analysis systems) used to quantify knee joint motion found that for dynamic measurements, electrogoniometers and 3D motion analysis systems were the most reliable and had low measurement error. For quantifying static joint position, handheld goniometers and inclinometers followed sequential MRI and 2D motion analysis systems in having the least measurement error.[44] Perriman and colleagues[45] found that the flexible electrogoniometer demonstrated excellent accuracy and test-retest reliability when used to measure thoracic kyphosis.

Cost

Electrogoniometers are more expensive than most goniometers and inclinometers but less expensive than most motion analysis systems such as the magnetic motion capture system Flock of Birds, which costs about $40,000.00, and computer-assisted video motion analysis systems that cost about $150,000.00 to $200,000.00. Burnfield and Norkin[46] suggest that in comparison to motion analysis systems, electrogoniometers are an affordable means of measuring joint motion during walking.

Radiography

For many years, radiographs produced by x-ray imaging were the gold standard used to verify joint position measurements made with goniometers and inclinometers. However, this method had the major drawback of exposing the individual to radiation. Another problem was the length of time involved in developing the film. Digital radiography, which is a form of x-ray imaging using x-ray digital sensors instead of traditional photographic film, uses less radiation and gives instant images. This new technology is an important development and it is likely that in the future digital radiography may be used as the new gold standard.

Photography

The use of a goniometer to measure joint angles directly on photographs is another method of measuring joint motion and muscle length. This type of ROM measurement has received some reports of good to excellent reliability.[14,18] Photography has been used in the past to measure joint ROM, but it was considered to be a more time-consuming and expensive process than traditional goniometry. The ease of printing and transmitting photographs with small digital cameras and phones has made digital photography less expensive and time consuming than developing film, but according to Bennett and associates,[15] digital imaging is still relatively time consuming and a digital camera, computer, and angle measurement software are expensive and may be difficult to access. Another problem identified by Dunleavy, Cooney, and Gormley[16] is the perspective error that occurs when the photographed angle is rotated away from the camera's perpendicular view. Obviously, an examiner cannot operate a camera correctly if he or she is moving the individual's extremity throughout a ROM, and an examiner cannot determine an end-feel or palpate bony landmarks while using a camera.

Smartphones

Smartphones, such as the iPhone and phones with Android operating systems,[13,21,22] loaded with appropriate software applications (TiltMeter) can easily be turned into inclinometers by using their built-in tilt-sensitive systems. This capability increases the likelihood that they may be used in clinical settings in the future. In addition, some applications such as Dr. Goniometer enable a moveable angle to be superimposed over a digital photograph of body parts taken with a smartphone. However, there is an insufficient body of evidence regarding the reliability and validity of smartphone applications to support their use in the clinical setting at this time.[13,22]

A study by Anderson and associates[21] that compared the universal goniometer and the TiltMeter inclinometer's measurements of shoulder motion concluded that the two instruments were not interchangeable. The instruments were acceptable for clinical use only when the same examiner made the measurements using the same instruments. Kolber and Hanely[13] compared lumbar spine measurements made by a bubble inclinometer and an iPhone app. These authors found both instruments had good intra- and interrater reliability as well as concurrent validity when strict measurement procedures were followed. However, like Anderson and associates,[21] the authors cautioned clinicians about using these instruments interchangeably.

Visual Estimation

Although some examiners make visual estimates of joint position and motion rather than use a measuring instrument, we do not recommend this practice. The use of visual estimates in situations in which the individual has excessive soft tissue covering anatomical landmarks has been suggested,[47] but most authorities report more accurate and reliable measurements with a goniometer than with visual estimates.[48–52] Even when produced by a skilled examiner, visual estimates yield only subjective information in contrast to the objective information gotten from goniometric measurements. Visual estimates made prior to goniometric measurements may help to reduce errors attributable to incorrect reading of the goniometer. If the goniometric measurement is not made in the same quadrant as the estimate, the examiner is alerted to the possibility that the wrong scale is being read. However, there is a possibility that knowledge of the estimate may influence the results of the goniometric measurement.

Recording

Goniometric measurements are recorded in numerical tables, in pictorial charts, or within the written text of an evaluation. Regardless of which method is used, recordings should provide enough information to permit an accurate interpretation of the measurement. The following items are recommended to be included in the recording:

- Individual's name, age, and gender
- Examiner's name or initials
- Date and time of measurement
- Type of goniometer/inclinometer used
- Side of the body, joint, and motion being measured (for example, left knee flexion)
- For ROM, include the number of degrees at the beginning and end of the motion. For muscle length, include only the degrees at the end of the motion.
- Type of motion being measured (passive or active)
- Any subjective information, such as discomfort or pain, that is reported by the individual during the testing
- Any objective information obtained by the examiner during testing, such as a protective muscle spasm, crepitus, or capsular or noncapsular patterns of restriction
- A complete description of any deviation from the recommended testing positions

If an individual has normal pain-free ROM during active or passive motion, the ROM may be recorded as normal (N) or within normal limits (WNL). To determine whether the ROM is normal, the examiner should compare the ROM of the joint being tested with the tables that report normal values by age and gender and methods of measurement presented in the Research Findings sections in Chapters 4 through 13. A selection of normal ROM values for adults is usually presented at the beginning of testing procedures for each motion. The ROM of the joint being tested may be compared with the same joint of the individual's contralateral extremity, provided that the contralateral extremity is neither impaired nor used selectively in athletic or occupational activities.

Recordings of ROM values should include both the starting and the ending joint positions to completely define the ROM. A recording that includes only the total ROM, such as 50 degrees of flexion, gives no information as to where a motion begins and ends. Likewise, a recording that lists –20 degrees (minus 20 degrees) of flexion is open to misinterpretation because the lack of flexion could occur at either the end or the beginning of the ROM.

A motion such as flexion that begins at 0 degrees and ends at 50 degrees of flexion is recorded as 0–50 degrees of flexion (Fig. 2.14A). A motion that begins with the joint flexed at 20 degrees and ends at 70 degrees of flexion is recorded as 20–70 degrees of flexion (Fig. 2.14B). The total ROM is the same (50 degrees) in both instances, but the arcs of motion are different.

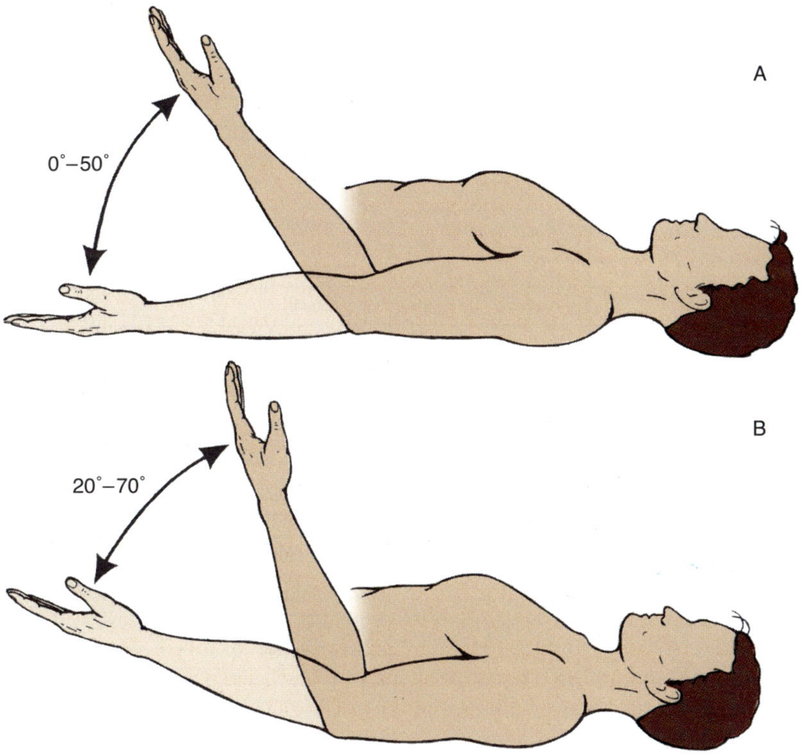

FIGURE 2.14 (A) Recording of ROM should include the beginning of the range as well as the end. In this illustration, the motion begins at 0 degrees and ends at 50 degrees so that the total ROM is 50 degrees. (B) In this illustration, the motion begins at 20 degrees of flexion and ends at 70 degrees, so that the total ROM is 50 degrees. For both individuals, the total ROM is the same, 50 degrees, even though the arcs of motion are different.

Because both the starting and the ending joint positions have been recorded, the measurement can be interpreted correctly. If we assume that the normal ROM for this movement is 0 to 140 degrees, the individual who has a flexion ROM of 0 to 50 degrees lacks motion at the end of the flexion ROM. The individual with a flexion ROM of 20 to 70 degrees lacks motion both at the beginning and at the end of the flexion ROM. The term **hypomobile** may be applied to both of these joints because both joints have a less-than-normal ROM.

Sometimes the opposite situation exists, in which a joint has a greater-than-normal range of motion and is **hypermobile.** If an elbow joint is hypermobile, the starting position for measuring elbow flexion may be in hyperextension rather than at 0 degrees. If the elbow was hyperextended 20 degrees in the starting position, the beginning of the flexion ROM would be recorded as 20 degrees of hyperextension (Fig. 2.15). To clarify that the 20 degrees represents hyperextension rather than limited flexion, a "0" representing the zero starting position, which is now within the ROM, is included. A ROM that begins at 20 degrees of hyperextension and ends at 140 degrees of flexion is recorded as 20–0–140 degrees of flexion.

A ROM that does not start with 0 degrees or ends prematurely indicates hypomobility. The addition of zero, representing the usual starting position within the ROM, indicates hypermobility.

Numerical Tables

Numerical tables typically list joint motions in a column down the center of the form (Fig. 2.16). Space to the left of the central column is reserved for measurements taken on the left side of the individual's body; space to the right is reserved for measurements taken on the right side of the body. The examiner's initials and the date of testing are noted at the top of the measurement columns. The instrument used is listed in the comment section along with any observations, such as the individual's pain or discomfort during the examination. Subsequent measurements are recorded on the same form and identified by the examiner's initials and the date at the top of the appropriate measurement column. The first set of measurements may be recorded in a column on either side of the central column, with subsequent measurements in the next

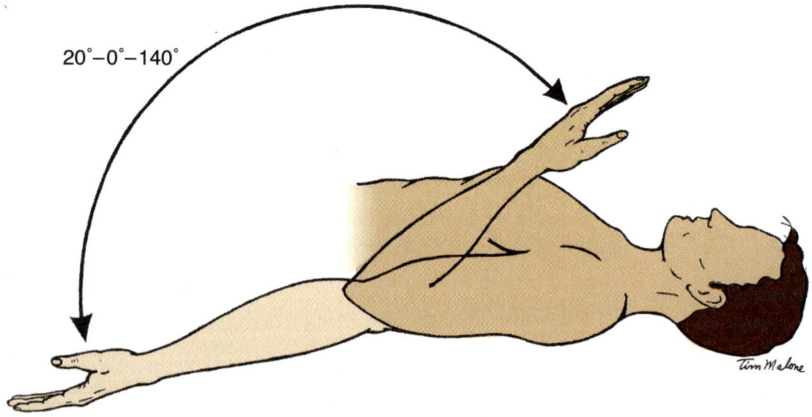

FIGURE 2.15 This individual has 20 degrees of hyperextension at his elbow. In this case, motion begins at 20 degrees of hyperextension and proceeds through the 0-degree position to 140 degrees of flexion.

Name Paul Jones Age 57 Gender M

Left					Right			
		JW	JW	**Examiner**	JW			
		4/1/16	3/18/16	**Date**	3/18/16			
				Hip				
		0-98	0-73	Flexion	0-118			
		0-5	0-5	Extension	0-12			
		0-28	0-18	Abduction	0-32			
		0-12	0-6	Adduction	0-15			
		0-35	0-24	Medial rotation	0-42			
		0-40	0-35	Lateral rotation	0-44			
				Comments: 14" universal goniometer				

FIGURE 2.16 This numerical table records the results of ROM measurements of an individual's left and right hips. The examiner has recorded her initials and the date of testing at the top of each column of ROM measurements. Note that the right hip was tested once, on March 18, 2016; and the left hip was tested twice, once on March 18, 2016, and again on April 1, 2016.

column toward the edges of the form (see Fig. 2.16). Alternately, the first set of measurements may be recorded in the left column, with subsequent measurements in the next column toward the right. Either format makes it easy to compare a series of measurements to identify problem motions and then to track rehabilitative response over time.

Pictorial Charts

Pictorial charts may be used in isolation or combined with numerical tables to record ROM measurements. Pictorial charts usually include a diagram of the normal starting and ending positions of the motion (Fig. 2.17).

Sagittal–Frontal–Transverse–Rotation (SFTR) Method of Recording

Although not commonly used in the United States, another recording method is the **sagittal–frontal–transverse–rotation (SFTR) method of recording**, developed by Gerhardt and Russe.[53,54] In the SFTR method, three numbers are used to describe all motions in a given plane. The first and last numbers indicate the ends of the ROM in that plane. The middle number indicates the starting position, which would be 0 in normal motion. The SFTR may be included in a written text or formatted into a table.

In the sagittal plane, represented by S, the first number indicates the end of the extension ROM, the middle number indicates the starting position, and the last number indicates the end of the opposite ROM in the same plane, that is, flexion. For example, if an individual has 50 degrees of shoulder extension and 170 degrees of shoulder flexion, these motions would be recorded: Shoulder S: 50–0–170 degrees. See Table 2.2 for information about recording motion in the other planes using this measurement system.

Limb position during measurement is noted if it varies from anatomical position. The notation (F90) would indicate that a measurement was taken with the limb positioned in 90 degrees of flexion. For example, if an individual has 45 degrees of lateral rotation and 35 degrees of medial rotation measured with the hip in 90 degrees of flexion, these ROM values would be recorded as: Hip R: (F90) 45–0–35 degrees.

Hypomobility is noted by the lack of 0 as the middle number or by less-than-normal values for the first and last numbers, which indicate the ends of the ROM. For example, if elbow flexion ROM was limited and could move only between 20 and 90 degrees of flexion, it would be recorded: Elbow S: 0–20–90 degrees. A fixed-joint limitation such as ankylosis is indicated by the use of only two numbers. The zero starting position is included to clarify in which motion the fixed position occurs. Therefore, a recording of Elbow S: 0–40 degrees would indicate that the elbow is fixed in 40 degrees of flexion.

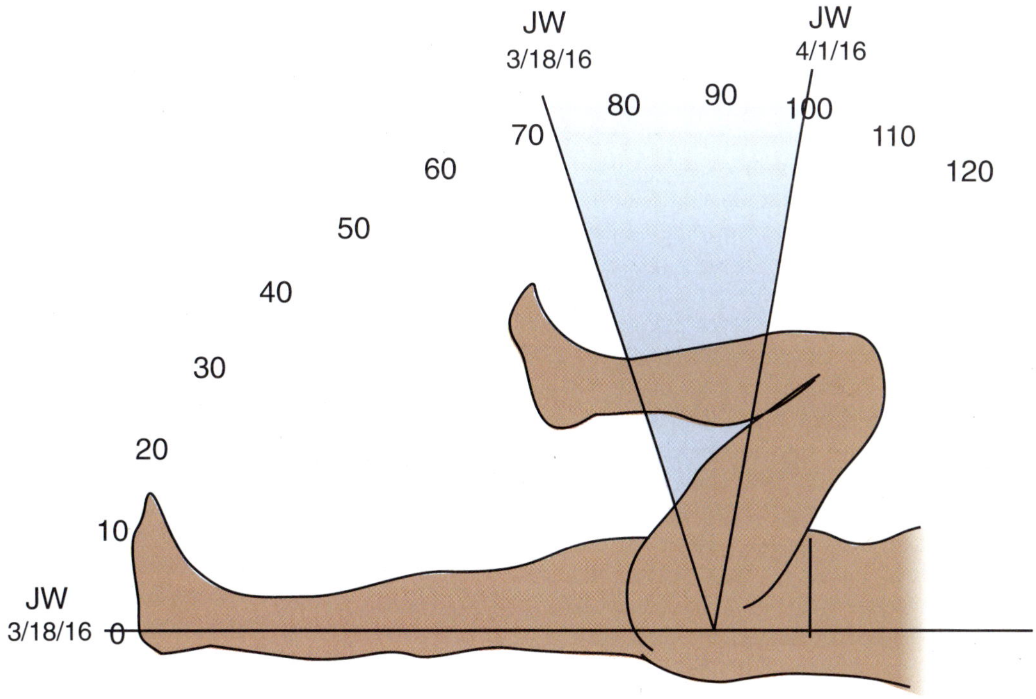

FIGURE 2.17 This pictorial chart records the results of flexion ROM measurements of an individual's left hip. For measurements taken on March 18, 2016, note the 0 to 73 degrees of left hip flexion; for measurements taken on April 1, 2016, note the 0 to 98 degrees of left hip flexion. Blue shading has been added to highlight the improvement in ROM values. (Adapted with permission from Range of Motion Test, New York University Medical Center, Rusk Institute of Rehabilitation Medicine.)

TABLE 2.2 Sagittal-Frontal-Transverse-Rotation Recording Method

Plane of Motion	First Number	Middle Number	Last Number
Sagittal	Extension	Start (0)	Flexion
	Dorsiflexion	Start (0)	Plantarflexion
Frontal	Abduction	Start (0)	Adduction
	Spinal lateral flexion Left	Start (0)	Spinal lateral flexion Right
Transverse	Horizontal abduction	Start (0)	Horizontal adduction
Rotation	Lateral rotation	Start (0)	Medial rotation
	Forearm supination	Start (0)	Forearm pronation
	Ankle eversion	Start (0)	Ankle inversion
	Spinal rotation Left	Start (0)	Spinal rotation Right

American Medical Association Guides to Evaluation of Permanent Impairment Method

The sixth edition of the American Medical Association's (AMA's) *Guides to the Evaluation of Permanent Impairment*[25] also uses the 0–180 degree system for recording ROM. The neutral starting position is recorded as 0 degrees with motions progressing toward 180 degrees. However, the recording system differs from the recording system used in this text. In the AMA book, extension that exceeds the neutral starting position even when normally found in the body is referred to as hyperextension and is expressed with the plus (+) symbol. The minus (–) symbol is used to indicate an extension limitation in which the neutral starting position cannot be attained. It should be noted that the American Academy of Orthopaedic Surgeons[51] does not use the minus (–) symbol to indicate an extension limitation or hypomobility. Likewise, we have avoided the use of plus (+) and minus (–) symbols in this text as we believe that these symbols can be interpreted in different ways and can create confusion.

Ratings of permanent impairment for all major body systems are provided in the AMA book, including three chapters on evaluation of the musculoskeletal system: upper extremities, lower extremities, and spine and pelvis. Restricted active motion, ankylosis, amputation, sensory loss, vascular changes, loss of strength, pain, joint crepitation, joint swelling, joint instability, and deformity are measured and converted to percentage of impairment for the body part. The total percentage of impairment for the body part is converted to the percentage of impairment for the extremity and, finally, to a percentage of impairment for the entire body. Often these permanent impairment ratings are used, along with other information, to determine the patient's level of disability and the amount of monetary compensation to be expected from the employer or the insurer. Physicians and therapists working with patients with permanent impairments who are seeking compensation for their disabilities should refer to the AMA's book for more detail.

Procedures

Precautions to Range of Motion and Muscle Length

Prior to conducting a goniometric evaluation, the examiner should review the individual's medical record and gather information during the interview process to determine whether any precautions to ROM and muscle length testing are present. Some precautions include suspected or confirmed: joint dislocation, joint subluxation, unstable bone fracture,[55] rupture of tendon or ligament, infectious or acute inflammatory process, and severe osteoporosis.[56] The examiner also should consider whether the ROM would disrupt the healing process and increase tissue damage following an acute injury or recent surgery. Measurement procedures may need to be modified or postponed if they increase an individual's pain or elicit an increase in muscle spasms.[57] Of course, ROM measurements are not possible if the joint to be tested is immobilized in a cast or external fixation device. Once these concerns have been addressed, the goniometric examination of ROM or muscle length can begin.

Preparation for Testing

This section includes exercises designed to prepare the examiner for carrying out goniometric testing procedures using the universal goniometer. Initially, examiners practice the testing procedures on classmates. Once examiners feel confident with the procedure, they proceed to the final exercise and perform an examination of elbow flexion ROM. The examiners follow the steps in the exercise while referencing Chapter 5 (The Elbow and Forearm).

Prior to beginning the measurement of joint ROM or muscle length the following information needs to be considered:

- Determine whether there are contraindications or precautions to ROM or muscle length testing
- Determine which joints and motions need to be tested
- Organize the testing sequence by body position

- Gather the necessary equipment, such as goniometers or inclinometers, towel rolls, and recording forms
- Prepare an explanation of the procedure for the individual

Explanation of Procedure

The listed steps and the example that follow provide the examiner with a suggested format for explaining the ROM testing procedure to an individual.

Steps

1. Introduce yourself and explain purpose of the visit.
2. Explain and demonstrate how the goniometer/inclinometer works and let the individual inspect the instrument.
3. Explain and demonstrate anatomical landmarks and why they need to be exposed.
4. Explain and demonstrate testing position and why positioning is important.
5. Explain and demonstrate the examiner's and the individual's roles.
6. Confirm the individual's understanding and willingness to participate.

During the explanation and testing procedure, common layperson terms rather than medical terms are used so that the individual can understand the procedure. The examiner should try to establish a good rapport and enlist the individual's participation in the evaluation process. After reading the example, the examiner should practice **Exercise 6**.

Example: Explanation of Goniometric Testing Procedure for Measuring Elbow Flexion ROM

1. Introduce Self and Explain Purpose

Introduction: My name is __________________. I am a (occupational title).

Explanation: I understand that you have been having some difficulty moving your elbow. I am going to measure the amount of motion that you have at your elbow joint to see if it differs from what is normally expected. I will use this information to plan a treatment program and assess its effectiveness.

Demonstration: The examiner flexes and extends his or her own elbow so that the individual is able to observe a joint motion.

2. Explain and Demonstrate Goniometer

Explanation: The instrument that I will use to take the measurements is called a goniometer. It is similar to a protractor, but it has two extensions called arms. It is placed on the outside of your body, next to your elbow.

Demonstration: The examiner presents the goniometer and encourages the individual to ask questions. The examiner shows the individual how the goniometer is used by holding it next to his or her own elbow.

3. Explain and Demonstrate Anatomical Landmarks

Explanation: To obtain accurate measurements, I need to identify some anatomical landmarks to help me to align the arms of the goniometer. To find these landmarks I may have to ask you to remove certain articles of clothing, such as your shirt. Also, to locate some of the landmarks, I may have to press my fingers against your skin.

Demonstration: The examiner shows the individual an easily identified anatomical landmark such as the radial styloid process.

4. Explain and Demonstrate Recommended Testing Positions

Explanation: Certain testing positions have been established to make joint measurements easier and more accurate. If you need some help in getting into a particular position, I will be happy to assist you. Please let me know if you need assistance.

Demonstration: The sitting or supine positions.

5A. Explain and Demonstrate Examiner's and Individual's Roles During Active Motion

Explanation: I will ask you to move your arm in exactly the same way that I move your arm.

Demonstration: The examiner takes the individual's arm through a passive ROM and then asks the individual to perform the same motion.

5B. Explain and Demonstrate Examiner's and Individual's Roles During Passive Motion

Explanation: I will move your arm and take a measurement. You should relax and let me do all of the work. These measurements should not cause discomfort so please let me know if you have any pain and I will stop moving your arm.

Demonstration: The examiner moves the individual's arm gently and slowly through the range of elbow flexion.

6. Confirm Individual's Understanding and Willingness to Participate.

Explanation: Do you have any questions? Are you ready to begin?

Testing Procedure

The testing procedure is initiated after the explanation has been given and the examiner is assured that the individual understands the nature of the testing process. The testing procedure consists of the following 12-step sequence of activities.

Steps

1. Position the individual in the recommended testing position and as close to the side of the bed or plinth as possible.
2. Stabilize the proximal joint segment.
3. Move the distal joint segment to the zero starting position. If the joint cannot be moved to the zero starting position, it should be moved as close as possible to the zero starting position. Slowly move the distal joint segment to the end of the passive ROM and determine the end-feel. Ask the individual whether there was any discomfort during the motion.
4. Make a visual estimate of the ROM.
5. Return the distal joint segment to the starting position.
6. Palpate the bony anatomical landmarks.
7. Align the goniometer.
8. Read and record the starting position. Remove the goniometer.
9. Stabilize the proximal joint segment.

10. Move the distal segment through the full ROM.
11. Replace and realign the goniometer. Palpate the anatomical landmarks again.
12. Read and record the ROM.

Exercise 6, which is based on the 12-step sequence, affords the examiner an opportunity to use the testing procedure for an evaluation of the elbow joint. This exercise should be practiced until the examiner is able to perform the activities sequentially without reference to the exercise.

Once these exercises have been completed, the examiner should be well prepared for conducting goniometric exercises on patients.

Exercise 6

Explanation of Goniometric Testing Procedure

EQUIPMENT: A universal goniometer.

Activities: Practice the following six steps with an individual.

1. Introduce yourself and explain the purpose of goniometric testing. Demonstrate a joint ROM on yourself.
2. Show the goniometer to the individual and demonstrate how it is used to measure a joint ROM. Let the individual inspect the instrument if he would like to do so.
3. Explain why bony landmarks must be located and palpated. Demonstrate how you would locate a bony landmark on yourself, and explain why clothing may have to be removed.
4. Explain and demonstrate why changes in position may be required.
5. Explain the individual's role in the procedure. Explain and demonstrate your role in the procedure.
6. Obtain confirmation of the individual's understanding of your explanation.

Exercise 7

Testing Procedure for Goniometric Measurement of Elbow Flexion ROM

EQUIPMENT: A universal goniometer, skin-marking pencil, recording form, and pencil.

Activities: See Figures 5.9 to 5.15 in Chapter 5.

1. Place the individual in a supine position, with the arm to be tested positioned close to the side of the body. Place a towel roll under the distal end of the humerus to allow full elbow extension. Position the forearm in full supination, with the palm of the hand facing the ceiling.
2. Stabilize the distal end of the humerus to prevent flexion of the shoulder.
3. Move the forearm to the zero starting position and determine whether there is any motion (extension) beyond zero. Move to the end of the passive range of flexion. Evaluate the end-feel. Usually the end-feel is soft because of compression of the muscle bulk on the anterior forearm in conjunction with that on the anterior humerus. Ask the individual whether there was any discomfort during the motion. (Refer to Fig. 5.13 in Chapter 5.)
4. Make a visual estimate of the beginning and end of the ROM.
5. Return the forearm to the starting position.
6. Palpate the bony anatomical landmarks (acromion process, lateral epicondyle of the humerus, radial head, and radial styloid process) and mark with a skin pencil. (Refer to Figs. 5.9 to 5.12 in Chapter 5.)
7. Align the arms and the fulcrum of the goniometer. Align the proximal arm with the lateral midline of the humerus, using the acromion process and lateral epicondyle for reference. Align the distal arm along the lateral midline of the radius, using the radial head and the radial styloid process for reference. The fulcrum should be close to the lateral epicondyle of the humerus.
8. Read the goniometer and record the starting position. (Refer to Fig. 5.14 in Chapter 5.) Remove the goniometer.
9. Stabilize the proximal joint segment (humerus).
10. Perform the passive ROM, making sure that you complete the available range.
11. When the end of the ROM has been attained, replace and realign the goniometer. Palpate the anatomical landmarks again, if necessary. (Refer to Fig. 5.15.)
12. Read the goniometer and record your reading. Compare your reading with your visual estimate to make sure that you are reading the correct scale on the goniometer.

REFERENCES

1. Sabari, JS, et al: Goniometric assessment of shoulder range of motion: Comparison of testing in supine and sitting positions. Arch Phys Med Rehabil 79:64, 1998.
2. Marshall, MM, Morzall, JR, and Shealy, JE: The effects of complex wrist and forearm posture on wrist range of motion. Hum Factors 41:205, 1999.
3. Werner, SL, and Plancher, KD: Biomechanics of wrist injuries in sports. Clin Sports Med 17:407, 1998.
4. Simoneau, GG, et al: Influence of hip position and gender on active hip internal and external rotation. J Orthop Sports Phys Ther 28:158, 1998.
5. Kebaetze, M, McClure, D, and Pratt, NA: Thoracic position effect on shoulder range of motion, strength, and three-dimensional scapular kinematics. Arch Phys Med Rehabil 80(8):945, 1999.
6. Van Dillen, LR, et al: Effect of knee and hip position on hip extension range of motion in individuals with and without low back pain. J Orthop Sports Phys Ther 30:307, 2000.
7. Gates, JJ, Gupta, A, and McGarry, MH: The effect of glenohumeral internal rotation deficit due to posterior capsular contracture on passive glenohumeral joint motion. Am J Sports Med 40(12):2794, 2012.
8. Carey, MA, et al: Reliability, validity and clinical usability of a digital goniometer. Work 36(1):55, 2010.
9. Lafayette Instrument Evaluation. 2016. Retrieved from www.lafayetteevaluation.com.
10. Halo Medical Devices. 2016. Retrieved from www.halomedicaldevices.com.
11. PT in Motion Magazine. Online Buyer's Guide. 5(7):58, 2013.
12. Kolber, MJ, et al: The reliability and concurrent validity of scapular plane shoulder elevation measurements using a digital inclinometer and goniometer. Physiother Theory Pract 28(2):161, 2012.
13. Kolber, MJ, and Hanley, WJ: The reliability and concurrent validity of measurements to quantify lumbar spine mobility: An analysis of an iPhone application and gravity based inclinometry. Int J Sports Phys Ther 7(3), 2012.
14. Blonna, D, et al: Validation of a photography-based goniometry method for measuring range of motion. J Shoulder Elbow Surg 21:29, 2012.
15. Bennett, D, et al: Measurement of knee joint motion using digital imaging. Int Orthop 33(6):1627, 2009.
16. Dunleavy, C, Cooney, M, and Gormley, J: Procedural considerations for photographic-based joint angle measurements. Physiother Res Int 10(4):190, 2005.
17. O'Neill, BJ, et al: Digital photography for assessment of shoulder range of motion: A novel clinical and research tool. Int J Shoulder Surg 7(1):23, 2013.
18. Naylor, JM, et al: Validity and reliability of using photography for measuring knee range of motion: A methodological study. BMC Musculoskelet Disord 12:77, 2012.
19. Tucker, WS, and Ingram, RL: Reliability and validity of measuring scapular elevation using an electrical inclinometer. J Electromyogr Kinesiol 22(3):419, 2012.
20. Penning, LI, et al: Reproducibility of a 3-dimensional gyroscope in measuring shoulder anteflexion and abduction. BMC Musculoskelet Disord 13:135, 2012.
21. Anderson, DS, et al: Reliability and validity of an iPhone inclinometer as compared to a universal goniometer as a tool for measuring joint motion of the shoulder in apparently healthy subjects. Orthop Pract 25(1):34–38, 2012.
22. Shin, SA, et al: Within-day reliability of range of motion measurement with a smart phone. Man Ther 17(4):298, 2012.
23. Moore, ML: The measurement of joint motion. Part II: The technic of goniometry. Phys Ther Rev 29:256, 1949.
24. Moore, ML: Clinical Assessment of Joint Motion. In Basmajian, JV (ed): Therapeutic Exercise, ed 4. Williams & Wilkins, Baltimore, 1984.
25. Rondinelli, RD (ed): Guides to the Evaluation of Permanent Impairment, ed 6. American Medical Association, Chicago, 2009.
26. Cocchiarella, L, and Anderson, GBJ (eds): Guides to the Evaluation of Permanent Impairment, ed 5. American Medical Association, Chicago, 2001.
27. Fox, RF, and Van Breemen, J: Chronic Rheumatism, Causation and Treatment. Churchill, London, 1934, p 327.
28. Schenkar, WW: Goniometry: An improved method of joint motion measurement. N Y State J Med 56:539, 1956.
29. Clarkson, HM: Musculoskeletal Assessment: Joint Motion and Muscle Testing, ed 3. Wolters Kluwer Lippincott Williams & Wilkins, Philadelphia, 2013.
30. Performance Attainment Associates. Product descriptions. 2016. Retrieved from http://www.spineproducts.com.
31. Petherick, M, et al: Concurrent validity and intertester reliability of universal and fluid-based goniometers for active elbow range of motion. Phys Ther 68:966, 1988.
32. Rheault, W, et al: Intertester reliability and concurrent validity of fluid-based and universal goniometers for active knee flexion. Phys Ther 68:1676, 1988.
33. Goodwin, J, et al: Clinical methods of goniometry: A comparative study. Disabil Rehabil 14:10, 1992.
34. Rome, K, and Cowieson, F: A reliability study of the universal goniometer, fluid goniometer, and electrogoniometer for the measurement of ankle dorsiflexion. Foot Ankle Int 17:28, 1996.
35. Karpovich, PV, and Karpovich, GP: Electrogoniometer: A new device for study of joints in action. Fed Proc 18:79, 1959.
36. Kettelkamp, DB, et al: An electrogoniometric study of knee motion in normal gait. J Bone Joint Surg Am 52:775, 1970.
37. Knutzen, KM, Bates, BT, and Hamill, J: Electrogoniometry of postsurgical knee bracing in running. Am J Phys Med Rehabil 62:172, 1983.
38. Carey, JR, Patterson, JR, and Hollenstein, PJ: Sensitivity and reliability of force tracking and joint-movement tracking scores in healthy subjects. Phys Ther 68:1087, 1988.
39. Torburn, L, Perry, J, and Gronley, JK: Assessment of rearfoot motion: Passive positioning, one-legged standing, gait. Foot Ankle Int 19:688, 1998.
40. Clapper, MP, and Wolf, SL: Comparison of the reliability of the Ortho-Ranger and the standard goniometer for assessing active lower extremity range of motion. Phys Ther 68:214, 1988.
41. Greene, BL, and Wolf, SL: Upper extremity joint movement: Comparison of two measurement devices. Arch Phys Med Rehabil 70:288, 1989.
42. Ball, P, and Johnson, GR: Reliability of hindfoot goniometry when using a flexible electrogoniometer. Clin Biomech 8:13, 1993.
43. Shiratsu, A, and Coury, HJ: Reliability and accuracy of different sensors of a flexible electrogoniometer. Clin Biomech 18(7):682, 2003.
44. Piriyaprasarth, P, and Morris, ME: Psychometric properties of measurement tools for quantifying knee joint position and movement: A systematic review. Knee 14(1):2, 2006.
45. Perriman, DM, et al: Validation of the flexible electrogoniometer for measuring thoracic kyphosis. Spine 15(14):35, 2010.
46. Burnfield, J, and Norkin, C: Examination of Gait. In O'Sullivan, S, Schmitz, TJ, and Fulk, GD (eds): Physical Rehabilitation, ed. 6. FA Davis, Philadelphia, 2014.
47. American Academy of Orthopaedic Surgeons: Joint Motion: Method of Measuring and Recording. AAOS, Chicago, 1965.
48. Youdas, JW, Bogard, CL, and Suman, VJ: Reliability of goniometric measurements and visual estimates of ankle joint range of motion obtained in a clinical setting. Arch Phys Med Rehabil 74:1113, 1993.
49. Watkins, MA, et al: Reliability of goniometric measurements and visual estimates of knee range of motion obtained in a clinical setting. Phys Ther 71:90, 1991.
50. Youdas, JW, Carey, JR, and Garrett, TR: Reliability of measurements of cervical spine range of motion: Comparison of three methods. Phys Ther 71:98, 1991.
51. Greene, WB, and Heckman, JD: The Clinical Measurement of Joint Motion. American Academy of Orthopaedic Surgeons, Rosemont, IL, 1994.
52. Van de Pol, RJ, van Triffel, E, and Lucas, C: Inter-rater reliability for measurement of passive physiological range of motion of upper extremity joints is better if instruments are used: A systematic review. J Physiother 56(1):7, 2010.
53. Gerhardt, JJ, and Russe, OA: International SFTR Method of Measuring and Recording Joint Motion. Hans Huber, Bern, 1975.
54. Gerhardt, JJ: Clinical measurement of joint motion and position in the neutral-zero method and SFTR: Basic principles. Int Rehabil Med 5:161, 1983.
55. Kisner, C, and Colby, LA: Therapeutic Exercise, ed. 5. FA Davis, Philadelphia, 2012.
56. Hertling, D, and Kessler, RM: Management of Common Musculoskeletal Disorders, ed 4. Lippincott Williams & Wilkins, Philadelphia, 2006.
57. Johansson, C, and Chinworth, SA: Mobility in Context: Principles of Patient Care Skills. FA Davis, Philadelphia, 2012.

CHAPTER 3

Validity and Reliability of Goniometric Measurement

David A. Scalzitti, PT, PhD
D. Joyce White, PT, DSc

Validity

For goniometry to provide meaningful information, measurements must be valid. **Validity** is "the degree to which a useful (meaningful) interpretation can be inferred from a measurement."[1] Stated in another way, the validity of a measurement refers to how well the measurement represents the true value of the variable of interest and how well this measurement can be used for a specific purpose. The purpose of goniometry is to measure the angle created at a joint by the adjacent bones of the body. Therefore, a valid goniometric measurement is one that represents the actual joint angle and one that can provide data for use in clinical decision-making. The joint angle obtained from a goniometric measurement is used to describe a specific joint position or, if a beginning and ending joint position are compared, a range of motion (ROM). In this section, the four main types of validity (face validity, content validity, criterion-related validity, and construct validity) are discussed as they relate to the measurement of joint motion.

Face Validity

Face validity indicates that the instrument generally appears to measure what it proposes to measure—that it is plausible to those using the test.[2–4] Much of the literature on goniometric measurement does not specifically address face validity because this type of validity is not generally tested. Rather, an assumption is made that the angle created by aligning the arms of a universal goniometer with bony landmarks truly represents the angle created by the proximal and distal bones composing the joint. One infers that changes in goniometer alignment reflect changes in joint angle and represent a range of joint motion. Portney and Watkins[3] report that face validity is easily established for some tests, such as the measurement of ROM, because the instrument measures the variable of interest through direct observation.

Content Validity

Content validity is determined by judging whether an instrument adequately measures and represents the domain of content—the substance—of the variable of interest.[1–4] Both content and face validity are based on opinion. However, face validity is the most basic and elementary form of validity, whereas content validity involves more rigorous and careful consideration of experts familiar with the content of interest. Gajdosik and Bohannon[5] state, "Physical therapists judge the validity of most ROM measurements based on their anatomical knowledge and their applied skills of visual inspection, palpation of bony landmarks, and accurate alignment of the goniometer. Generally, the accurate application of knowledge and skills, combined with interpreting the results as measurement of ROM only, provide sufficient evidence to ensure content validity."

Criterion-Related Validity

Criterion-related validity justifies the validity of the measuring instrument by comparing measurements made with the instrument to a well-established gold standard of measurement—the criterion.[1–4] If the measurements made with the instrument and criterion are taken at approximately the same time, **concurrent validity** is tested. Concurrent validity is a type of criterion-related validity and is the most frequent type of validity reported for goniometry. Criterion-related validity can be assessed using statistical methods such as correlation. In terms of goniometry, an examiner may question the construction of a particular goniometer on a very basic level and consider whether the degree units of the goniometer accurately represent the degree units of a circle. The angles of the goniometer can be compared with known angles of a protractor—the criterion. Usually the construction of goniometers is adequate, and concurrent validity may then focus on whether the measurement of joint position with a goniometer reflects the true joint angle. In this case, a measure of joint position obtained by radiography may serve as the criterion measure to represent the true joint angle.

Criterion-Related Validity Studies of Extremity Joints

Some of the classic studies that have examined the concurrent validity of goniometric and radiographic measurements for the extremity joints are summarized here. As appropriate, summaries of additional studies comparing goniometry to radiographs and/or photographs are included in the Research Findings sections of Chapters 4 through 13. Furthermore, recent systematic reviews have also reported strong concurrent validity between universal goniometers and radiographs for knee joint position[6] and between smartphone goniometer applications (apps) and radiographs.[7]

Gogia and associates[8] measured the knee position of 30 healthy individuals with radiography and with a universal goniometer. Knee positions ranged from 0 to 120 degrees. High correlation (correlation coefficient [*r*] = 0.97) and agreement (intraclass correlation coefficient [ICC] = 0.98) were found between the two types of measurements. These authors concluded that the measurement of knee joint position as obtained in their study was valid to reflect the actual joint position. Enwemeka[9] studied the validity of measuring knee ROM with a universal goniometer by comparing the goniometric measurements of 10 individuals with radiographs. No significant differences were found between the two types of measurements when ROM was within 30 to 90 degrees of flexion (mean difference between the two measurements ranged from 0.5 to 3.8 degrees). However, a significant difference was found when ROM was within 0 to 15 degrees of flexion (mean difference = 4.6 degrees). Ahlback and Lindahl[10] found that a joint-specific goniometer used to measure total hip flexion and extension of 14 hips closely agreed with radiographic measurements. Kato and coworkers[11] compared the accuracy of three types of goniometers aligned on the lateral and dorsal surfaces of the proximal interphalangeal joints of the 16 fixated fingers with radiographs. Mean differences between the goniometers and radiographs ranged from 0.5 to 3.3 degrees.

Criterion-Related Validity Studies of the Spine

Various instruments used to measure ROM of the spine have also been compared with a radiographic criterion, although some authors question the use of radiographs as the gold standard given the variability of total ROM measurements derived from summed segmental motions on spinal readiographs.[12] Three cross-sectional studies that contrasted cervical ROM measurements taken with gravity-dependent goniometers with those recorded on radiographs found concurrent validity to be high. Herrmann,[13] in a study of 11 adults, noted a high correlation (*r* = 0.97) and agreement (ICC = 0.98) between radiographic measures and pendulum goniometer measures of head and neck flexion–extension. Ordway and colleagues[14] simultaneously measured cervical flexion and extension in 20 healthy persons with a cervical ROM (CROM) device, a computerized tracking system, and radiographs. There were no significant differences between measurements taken with the CROM device and radiographic angles determined by an occipital line and a vertical line, although there were differences between the CROM device and the radiographic angles between the occiput and C7. Tousignant and coworkers[15] measured cervical flexion and extension in 31 volunteers with a CROM goniometer and radiographs that included cervical and upper thoracic motion. They found a high correlation between the two measurements for flexion (*r* = 0.97) and extension (*r* = 0.98). An additional study by Tousignant and colleagues[16] reported a high correlation for concurrent validity between cervical rotational and lateral flexion movements and an optoelectronic gold standard.

Studies that compared clinical ROM measurement methods for the lumbar spine with radiographic results have reported high to low values for validity. Macrae and Wright[17] measured lumbar flexion in 342 individuals by using a tape measure according to the Schober and modified Schober methods and compared these results with those shown in radiographs. Their findings support the validity of these measures: correlation coefficient values between the Schober method and the radiographic evidence were 0.90 (standard error = 6.2 degrees) and between the modified Schober and the radiographs were 0.97 (standard error = 3.3 degrees). Portek and associates,[18] in a study of 11 men, reported low correlations (0.42 to 0.57) for lumbar flexion and extension ROM measurements taken with a skin distraction method and with a single inclinometer as compared with radiographic evidence. Limitations of this study include the following: measurements were made sequentially rather than concurrently, and different test positions were used. Radiographs and skin distraction methods were performed with subjects standing, whereas inclinometer measurements were performed with subjects sitting for flexion and prone for extension.

Burdett, Brown, and Fall,[19] in a study of 27 healthy participants, found a fair correlation between measurements taken with a single inclinometer and radiographs for lumbar flexion (*r* = 0.73) and a very poor correlation for lumbar extension (*r* = 0.15). Mayer and coworkers[20] compared total lumbar flexion and extension motion in 12 persons with chronic low back pain as measured with a double inclinometer technique and radiographs. No significant difference in group means was observed between the two methods. Saur and colleagues,[21] in a study of 54 persons with chronic low back pain, found lumbar flexion ROM measurement taken with two inclinometers correlated highly with radiographs (*r* = 0.98). Extension ROM measurement correlated with radiographs to a fair degree (*r* = 0.75). Samo and associates[22] used double inclinometers and radiographs to measure 30 volunteers held in a position of flexion and extension. Radiographs resulted in flexion values that were 11 to 15 degrees greater than those found with inclinometers and extension values that were 4 to 5 degrees less than those found with inclinometers.

Construct Validity

Construct validity is the ability of an instrument to measure an abstract concept (construct) or to be used to make an inferred interpretation.[2,3] Rehabilitation professionals may use ROM measurements to make inferences about the function of a person. In Chapters 4 through 13 on measurement procedures, the results of research studies that report joint ROM observed during functional tasks are included. These findings begin to quantify the joint motion needed to avoid functional limitations. Several researchers have artificially restricted joint motion with splints or braces and examined the effect on function.[23–25] These studies have demonstrated that many functional tasks can be completed with severely restricted elbow or wrist ROM, provided other adjacent joints are able to compensate.

Some studies have measured the correlation between ROM values and the ability to perform functional tasks in patient populations. A study by Hermann and Reese[26] examined the relationship among impairments, functional limitations, and disability in 80 persons with cervical spine disorders. The highest correlation ($r = 0.82$) occurred between impairment measures and functional limitation measures, with ROM contributing more to the relationship than the other two impairment measures of cervical muscle force and pain. Triffitt[27] found significant correlations between the amount of shoulder ROM and the ability to perform nine functional activities in 125 persons with shoulder conditions. Wagner and colleagues[28] measured passive ROM of wrist flexion, extension, radial and ulnar deviation, and the strength of the wrist extensor and flexor muscles in 18 boys with Duchenne muscular dystrophy. A highly significant negative correlation was found between difficulty performing functional hand tasks and radial deviation ROM ($r = -0.76$ to -0.86) and between difficulty performing functional hand tasks and wrist extensor strength ($r = -0.61$ to -0.83). Other studies, however, have demonstrated weaker associations between ROM and function. For example, Waddell and colleagues[29] measured lumbosacral motion with inclinometers and compared the results with the Roland-Morris Low Back Pain Disability Questionnaire ($r = -0.47$ for lumbosacral flexion and $r = -0.33$ for lumbosacral extension). A less-than-perfect correlation between ROM and function is not surprising because function is a multidimensional construct and an impairment of one factor related to body functions and structure, such as joint motion, may be responsible only for a small component.[30,31]

Reliability

In order for a measurement to be valid, not only should the measurement represent the true variable of interest but the same value should be obtained when the measurement is repeated under the same conditions. **Reliability** refers to the amount of consistency between successive measurements of the same variable on the same individual under the same conditions.[1–3] A goniometric measurement is highly reliable if successive measurements of a joint angle or ROM on the same individual and under the same conditions yield the same results. A highly reliable measurement contains little measurement error. Assuming that a measurement is both highly reliable and valid, an examiner can confidently use its results to determine a true absence, presence, or change in dysfunction. For example, a highly reliable and valid goniometric measurement could be used to determine the presence of limited joint ROM, to evaluate progress toward rehabilitative goals, and to assess the effectiveness of therapeutic interventions.

Consistency is necessary for a measurement to be considered valid, although one can obtain a highly consistent measurement that is absent of meaning and therefore is still not valid. An unreliable measurement is inconsistent, does not produce the same results when the same variable is repeatedly measured on the same individual under the same conditions, and contains a large amount of measurement error. This lack of consistency and heightened error will make validity poor as well. A measurement that has poor reliability and validity is not dependable and should not be used to make clinical decisions.

Summary of Goniometric Reliability Studies

The reliability of goniometric measurement has been the focus of many research studies. Given the variety of study designs and measurement techniques, it is difficult to compare the results of many of these studies. However, some findings noted in several studies can be summarized. An overview of such findings is presented here. More information on reliability studies that pertain to the featured joint is reviewed in Chapters 4 through 13. Readers may also wish to refer to several review articles and book chapters on this topic.[32–37]

The measurement of joint position and ROM of the extremities with a universal goniometer has generally been found to have good-to-excellent reliability. Numerous reliability studies have been conducted on joints of the upper and lower extremities. Some studies have examined the reliability of measuring joints held in a fixed position, whereas others have examined the reliability of measuring passive or active ROM. Studies that measured a fixed joint position usually have reported higher reliability values than studies that measured ROM.[8,13,38,39] This finding is expected because more potential sources of error are present in measuring ROM than in measuring a fixed joint position. Additional sources of error in measuring ROM include movement of the joint axis, variations in manual force applied by the examiner during passive ROM, and variations in an individual's effort during active ROM.

The reliability of goniometric ROM measurements varies somewhat depending on the joint and motion. Range of motion measurements of upper-extremity joints have been found by several researchers to be more reliable than ROM measurements of lower-extremity joints,[36,37,40,41] although opposing results have also been reported.[42] Differences in reliability have also been reported for different joints and for different motions of the same joint. For example, Hellebrandt, Duvall, and Moore,[43] in a study of upper-extremity joints, noted that measurements of wrist flexion, medial rotation of the shoulder, and abduction of the shoulder were less reliable than measurements of other motions of the upper extremity. Low[44] found ROM measurements of wrist extension to be less reliable than measurements of elbow flexion. Greene and Wolf[45] reported ROM measurements of shoulder rotation and wrist motions to be more variable than elbow motion and other shoulder motions. Reliability studies on ROM measurement of the cervical and thoracic spine in which a universal goniometer was used have generally reported lower reliability values than studies of the extremity joints.[19,46–49] Many devices and techniques have been developed to try to improve the reliability of measuring spinal motions. Gajdosik and Bohannon[5] suggested that the reliability of measuring certain joints and motions might be adversely affected by the complexity of the joint. Measurement of motions that are influenced by movement of adjacent joints or multi-joint muscles may be less reliable than measurement of motions of simple hinge joints. Difficulty palpating bony landmarks and passively moving heavy body parts may also play a role in reducing the reliability of measuring ROM of the lower extremity and spine.[5,37,40]

Many studies of joint measurement methods have found intratester reliability to be higher than intertester reliability.[19,38–44,46,47,49–68] Reliability was higher when successive measurements were taken by the same examiner than when successive measurements were taken by different examiners. This is true for studies that measured joint position and ROM of the extremities and spine with universal goniometers and other devices such as joint-specific goniometers, inclinometers, tape measures, and flexible rulers. Only a few studies found intertester reliability to be higher than intratester reliability.[69–72] In most of these studies, the time interval between repeated measurements by the same examiner was considerably greater than the time interval between measurements by different examiners.

Boone et al[40] reported mean standard deviations of repeated measurements taken of six extremity joints by one examiner using a universal goniometer to range from 3.7 to 4.0 degrees, whereas Bovens et al[42] examined nine joint motions and reported mean standard deviations of repeated measurements of one examiner from 2.5 to 8.1 degrees. The mean of the mean standard deviations reported in these studies was 3.9 degrees and 4.8 degrees, respectively. One interpretation of these findings is that a difference of at least 5 degrees (1 standard deviation) to 10 degrees (2 standard deviations) may be necessary to show improvement or worsening of a joint motion measured by the same examiner. This is somewhat consistent with a recent study of 30 joint motions in 12 adult women that reported intratester standard error of measurement (SEM) values ranging from 1 to 7 degrees (mean SEM = 3.5 degrees), and minimal detectable change (MDC) values at the 95% confidence level ranging from 4 to 21 degrees (mean MDC_{95} = 9.6 degrees).[73] When more than one examiner took repeated goniometric measurements, the mean of the mean standard deviations increased to 4.7 degrees in the study by Boone et al[40] and to 5.9 degrees in the study by Bovens et al.[42] This implies a difference of at least 6 to 12 degrees (1 to 2 standard deviations) may be necessary to show true change when repeated measurements are taken by more than one examiner. These values should serve only as a very general guideline of the measurement error of goniometry of extremity joints. Readers are referred to the Research Findings sections of Chapters 4 through 13 for more joint-specific information on intratester and intertester reliability.

The reliability of goniometric measurements is affected by the measurement procedure. Several studies found that intertester reliability improved when all the examiners used consistent, well-defined testing positions and measurement methods.[51,53,54,74] Intertester reliability was lower if examiners used a variety of positions and measurement methods.

Several investigators have examined the reliability of using the mean of several goniometric measurements compared with using one measurement. Low[44] recommends using the mean of several measurements made with the goniometer to increase reliability over one measurement. Early studies by Cobe[75] and Hewitt[76] also used the mean of several measurements. However, Boone and associates[40] found no significant difference between repeated measurements made by the same examiner during one session and suggested that one measurement taken by an examiner is as reliable as the mean of repeated measurements. Rothstein, Miller, and Roettger,[54] in a study on knee and elbow ROM, found that intertester reliability determined from the means of two measurements improved only slightly from the intertester reliability determined from single measurements.

The authors of some texts on goniometric methods suggest the use of universal goniometers with longer arms to measure joints with large body segments such as the hip and shoulder.[33,77,78] Goniometers with shorter arms are recommended to measure joints with small body segments such as the wrist and fingers. Robson,[79] using a mathematical model, determined that goniometers with longer arms are more accurate in measuring an angle than goniometers with shorter arms. Goniometers with longer arms reduce the effects of errors in the placement of the goniometer axis. However, Rothstein, Miller, and Roettger[54] found no difference in reliability among large plastic, large metal, and small plastic universal goniometers used to measure knee and elbow ROM. Riddle, Rothstein, and Lamb[52] also reported no difference in reliability between large and small plastic universal goniometers used to measure shoulder ROM.

Numerous studies have compared the measurement values and reliability of different types of devices used to measure joint ROM. Universal and gravity-dependent (pendulum and fluid) goniometers; joint-specific devices; tape measures; and wire tracing are some of the devices that have been compared. Studies comparing clinical measurement devices have been conducted on the shoulder,[43,45,80] elbow,[38,43,44,62,81,82] wrist,[38,45] hand,[39,65,83,84] hip,[85,86] knee,[54,85,87] ankle,[87,88] cervical spine,[46,47,70] and thoracolumbar spine.[19,22,48,68,89–95] Many studies have found differences in values and reliability between measurement devices, whereas some studies have reported no differences. A recent systematic review reported that measurements of ROM of upper-extremity joints using instruments, including goniometers, were more reliable than measurements using visual estimation.[36]

In conclusion, on the basis of the literature and practical experience, several procedures are recommended to improve the reliability of goniometric measurements (Table 3.1). Examiners should use consistent, well-defined testing positions, stabilize the proximal body segment, and carefully palpate anatomical landmarks to align the arms of the goniometer. During successive measurements of passive ROM, examiners should strive to apply the same amount of manual force to move the limb segment. During successive measurements of active ROM, the individual should be urged to exert the same effort to perform a motion. To reduce measurement variability, it is prudent to take repeated measurements on an individual using the same type of measurement device. For example, an examiner should take all repeated measurements of a ROM with a universal goniometer, rather than taking the first measurement with a universal goniometer and the second measurement with an inclinometer. Most examiners should find it easier and more accurate to use a large universal goniometer when measuring joints with large body segments and a small goniometer when measuring joints with small body segments. Inexperienced examiners may wish to take several measurements and record the mean of those measurements to improve reliability, but one measurement is usually sufficient for more experienced examiners using good technique. Clinicians should also remember that successive measurements are more reliable if taken by the same examiner using the same methods than measurements obtained by different examiners. A final recommendation is to calibrate the device at regular intervals by checking the angles obtained with known standards. This recommendation is provided to ensure the measurements obtained reflect the true angle and is especially relevant for devices such as inclinometers and smartphone apps.

TABLE 3.1 Recommendations for Improving the Reliability of Goniometric Measurements

- Use consistent, well-defined testing positions.
- Stabilize the part of the body that is proximal to the joint being examined to prevent unwanted movements.
- Use consistent, well-defined, and carefully palpated anatomical landmarks to align the goniometer.
- Use the same amount of manual force to move the body part during successive measurements of passive ROM.
- Provide consistent direction, including asking that an individual exerts the same effort to move the body part during successive measurements of active ROM.
- Use the same device to take successive measurements.
- Use a goniometer that is suitable in size to the joint being measured.
- If the examiner is less experienced, record the mean of several measurements rather than a single measurement.
- Have the same examiner, rather than a different examiner, take successive measurements.
- Calibrate the measurement instrument at regular intervals.

Statistical Methods of Evaluating Measurement Reliability

Clinical measurements may be affected by three main sources of variation: (1) true biological variation, (2) temporal variation, and (3) measurement error.[96] **True biological variation** refers to variation in measurements from one individual to another, caused by factors such as age, sex, race, genetics, medical history, and condition. **Temporal variation** refers to variation in measurements made on the same individual at different times, caused by changes in factors such as a person's health status, activity level, emotional state, and circadian rhythms. **Measurement error** refers to variation in measurements made on the same individual under the same conditions at different times, caused by factors such as the examiners (testers), measuring instruments, and procedural methods. For example, the skill level and experience of the examiners, the accuracy of the measurement instruments, and the standardization of the measurement methods all may affect the amount of measurement error. Reliability reflects the degree to which a measurement is free of measurement error; therefore, highly reliable measurements have little measurement error.

Statistics can be used to assess variation in numerical data and hence to assess measurement reliability.[3,96] A brief digression into statistical methods of expressing reliability is included to assist the examiner in correctly interpreting goniometric measurements and in understanding the literature on joint measurement. This discussion starts with presenting measures of variability, including the standard deviation and the coefficient of variation. This is followed by a discussion of measures of relative reliability including the Pearson product-moment correlation coefficient and the intraclass correlation coefficient. Examples that show the calculation of these statistical tests are presented. This section finishes with a discussion of absolute measures of reliability that provide values for the amount of error associated with the measurement in the original units of the measurement. The measures discussed include the standard error of measurement and the minimal detectable change. For additional information, including the assumptions underlying the use of all of these statistical tests, the reader is referred to the cited references.

At the end of this chapter, four exercises are included for examiners to assess their consistency in obtaining goniometric measurements and performing the calculations for the measures presented. Clinicians are also encouraged to collect data from their staff and patient population to determine reliability of their own measurements. Miller[33] has presented a step-by-step procedure for conducting such studies.

Measures of Variation

Standard Deviation

In the biomedical literature, the statistic most frequently used to indicate variation in a sample is the standard deviation.[3,96,97] The **standard deviation** is the square root of the mean of the squares of the deviations from the mean. The standard deviation is symbolized in the literature as **SD, s,** or **sd.** The sample mean is generally denoted as $\bar{x}$, and is calculated by dividing the sum of each data observation (x) by the number of observations in the sample (n). The equation for the standard deviation of the distribution of the data around a mean is:

$$SD = \sqrt{\frac{\Sigma(x-\bar{x})^2}{n-1}}$$

The standard deviation is expressed in the same units as the original data observations. For example, in goniometry this will be in degrees. If the data observations have a normal (bell-shaped) distribution, one standard deviation above and below the mean includes about 68% of all the observations, and two standard deviations above and below the mean include about 95% of the observations. A large value for the standard deviation value indicates large variability in a series of measurements.

Several standard deviations may be determined from a single measurement study.[96] These standard deviations represent the dispersion of data around different means. Two of these standard deviations are discussed here. One standard deviation that can be determined represents mainly ***inter*****subject variation** around the mean of measurements taken of a group of individuals, indicating biological variation. This standard deviation may be of interest in deciding whether an individual has an abnormal ROM in comparison with other people of the same age and gender. Another standard deviation that can be determined represents ***intra*****subject variation** around the mean of repeated measurements taken of an individual, indicating measurement error. Assuming the individual's joint was in the same position for each measurement, this is the standard deviation of interest to indicate that the examiner was consistent in obtaining the measurement and was reliable.

An example of how to determine these two standard deviations is provided. Table 3.2 presents ROM measurements taken on five subjects.* Three repeated measurements (observations) were taken on each subject by the same examiner.

The **standard deviation indicating biological variation** (intersubject variation) is determined by first calculating the mean ROM measurement for each subject. The mean ROM measurement for each of the five subjects is found in the last column of Table 3.2. The grand mean of the mean ROM measurement for each of the five subjects equals 56 degrees. The grand mean is symbolized by $\bar{X}$. The standard deviation is determined by finding the differences between each of the five subjects' means and the grand mean. The differences are squared to ensure having positive numbers, and added together. The sum is used in the formula for the standard deviation. Calculation of the standard deviation indicating biological variation is found in Table 3.3.

In the example, the standard deviation indicating biological variation equals 13.6 degrees. This standard deviation denotes primarily intersubject variation. Knowledge of intersubject variation may be helpful in deciding whether a subject has an abnormal ROM in comparison with other people of the same age and gender. If a normal distribution of the measurements is assumed, one way of interpreting this standard deviation from the example is to predict that about 68% of all subjects' mean ROM measurements would fall between 42.4 degrees and 69.6 degrees (plus or minus 1 standard deviation around the grand mean of 56 degrees). One would expect that about 95% of all subjects' mean ROM measurements would fall between 28.8 degrees and 83.2 degrees (plus or minus 2 standard deviations around the grand mean of 56 degrees).

The **standard deviation indicating measurement error** (intrasubject variation) also is determined by first calculating the mean ROM measurement for each subject. However, this standard deviation is determined by finding the differences between each of the three repeated measurements taken on a subject and the mean of that subject's measurements. The differences are squared to ensure positive numbers and added together. The sum of these squared differences is then used in the formula for the standard deviation. Using the information on subject 1 in the example, the calculation of the standard deviation indicating measurement error is shown in Table 3.4.

Referring to Table 3.2 for information on each of the other subjects and using the same procedure as shown in Table 3.4, the standard deviation for subject 1 = 5.3 degrees, the standard deviation for subject 2 = 2.6 degrees, the standard deviation for subject 3 = 4.0 degrees, the standard deviation for subject 4 = 3.6 degrees, and the standard deviation for subject 5 = 3.0 degrees. The mean standard deviation for

* Five subjects are included in the example to illustrate the calculations. Ideally, a reliability study would include more than five individuals to ensure adequate statistical power.

TABLE 3.2 Three Repeated ROM Measurements in Degrees Taken on Five Subjects

Subject	First Measurement	Second Measurement	Third Measurement	Total	Mean of Three Measurements ($\bar{x}$)
1	57	55	65	177	59
2	66	65	70	201	67
3	66	70	74	210	70
4	35	40	42	117	39
5	45	48	42	135	45

$$\text{Grand mean } \left(\bar{X}\right) = \frac{(59+67+70+39+45)}{5} = 56 \text{ degrees}$$

TABLE 3.3 Calculation of the Standard Deviation Indicating Biological Variation in Degrees

Subject	Mean of Three Measurements ($\bar{x}$)	Grand Mean ($\bar{X}$)	($\bar{x} - \bar{X}$)	($\bar{x} - \bar{X}$)^2
1	59	56	3	9
2	67	56	11	121
3	70	56	14	196
4	39	56	−17	289
5	45	56	−11	121

$$\Sigma\left(\bar{x} - \bar{X}\right)^2 = 9 + 121 + 196 + 289 + 121 = 736 \text{ degrees; SD} = \sqrt{\frac{\Sigma(\bar{x} - \bar{X})^2}{(n-1)}} = \sqrt{\frac{736}{(5-1)}} = \sqrt{184} = 13.6 \text{ degrees}$$

TABLE 3.4 Calculation of the Standard Deviation Indicating Measurement Error in Degrees for Subject 1

Measurements (x)	Mean ($\bar{x}$)	($\bar{x} - \bar{X}$)	($\bar{x} - \bar{X}$)^2
57	59	−2	4
55	59	−4	16
65	59	6	36

$$(\bar{x}) = \frac{57+55+65}{3} = 59 \text{ degrees}$$

$$\text{SD} = \sqrt{\frac{\Sigma(x-\bar{x})^2}{(n-1)}} = \sqrt{\frac{56}{(3-1)}} = \sqrt{28} = 5.3 \text{ degrees}$$

all of the subjects combined is determined by summing the five subjects' standard deviations and dividing by the number of subjects:

$$\text{SD} = \frac{5.3+2.6+4.0+3.6+3.0}{5} = \frac{18.5}{5} = 3.7 \text{ degrees}$$

In the example, the standard deviation indicating intrasubject variation equals 3.7 degrees. This standard deviation is appropriate for indicating measurement error, especially if the repeated measurements on each subject were taken within a short period of time. Note that in this example the standard deviation indicating measurement error (3.7 degrees) is much smaller than the standard deviation indicating biological variation (13.6 degrees). One way of interpreting the standard deviation for measurement error is to predict that about 68% of the repeated measurements on a subject would fall within 3.7 degrees (1 standard deviation) above and below the mean of the repeated measurements of a subject because of measurement error (assuming a normal distribution). We would expect that about 95% of the repeated measurements on a subject would fall within 7.4 degrees (2 standard deviations) above and below the mean of the repeated measurements of a subject, again because of measurement error. A smaller value for the standard deviation of a series of measurements is indicative of less measurement error and therefore a more consistent and reliable measurement.

Coefficient of Variation

Sometimes it is helpful to consider the percentage of variation rather than the standard deviation, which is expressed in the units of the data observation (measurement). The **coefficient of variation (CV)** is a measure of variation that is relative to the mean and standardized so that the variations of different variables can be compared. The CV is the ratio of the standard deviation to the mean and is expressed as a percentage. The formula is:

$$CV = \frac{SD}{\bar{x}}(100\%)$$

For the example presented in Table 3.2, the coefficient of variation indicating biological variation uses the standard deviation for biological variation (standard deviation = 13.6 degrees).

$$CV = \frac{13.6}{56}(100\%) = 24.3\%$$

The coefficient of variation indicating measurement error uses the standard deviation for measurement error (standard deviation = 3.7 degrees).

$$CV = \frac{3.7}{56}(100\%) = 6.6\%$$

In this example the coefficient of variation for measurement error (6.6%) is less than the coefficient of variation for biological variation (24.3%).

A lower value for the coefficient of variation represents less measurement error and therefore a more consistent measurement. This statistic is especially useful in comparing the variability of two or more variables that have different units of measurement (for example, comparing ROM measurement methods recorded in inches versus degrees). However, the coefficient of variation is markedly influenced by the value of the mean. For example, a standard deviation indicating a measurement error of 5 degrees would result in a CV of about 3% if the mean ROM was 150 degrees, whereas the same standard deviation of 5 degrees would result in a CV of 25% if the mean ROM was 20 degrees.

Relative Measures of Reliability: Correlation Coefficients

Correlation coefficients are traditionally used to measure the relationship between two variables. They result in a number from –1.0 to +1.0, which indicates how closely one variable is related to another variable.[3,97,98] A value of +1.0 describes a perfect positive relationship between the two variables, whereas a value of –1.0 describes a perfect negative relationship. A correlation coefficient of 0 indicates that there is no relationship between the two variables. Correlation coefficients may be used to indicate measurement reliability because it is assumed that two repeated measurements should be highly correlated and approach +1.0. As discussed earlier in this chapter, correlation coefficients may also be used to demonstrate concurrent validity between two devices for measuring joint motion. Several different cut-off values to interpret reliability using correlation coefficients have been described.[3,97,98] For an example, Portney and Watkins[3] provide a general guideline in which coefficients below 0.50 represent poor reliability, 0.50 to 0.75 suggest moderate reliability, and values greater than 0.75 indicate good reliability. They caution, however, that these values should be interpreted in the context of the data and should not be used as strict cut-off points.

Pearson Product-Moment Correlation Coefficient

Because goniometric measurements produce ratio level data, and provided the other criteria for the use of parametric statistics are met, the **Pearson product-moment correlation coefficient** may be calculated to compare the association between pairs of goniometric measurements. The Pearson product-moment correlation coefficient is symbolized by the lowercase letter ***r***. The formula to calculate r is expressed in the following equation. In the case where r is used to indicate reliability of two measurements, x symbolizes the first measurement and y symbolizes the second measurement.

$$r = \frac{\Sigma(x-\bar{x})(y-\bar{y})}{\sqrt{\Sigma(x-\bar{x})^2}\sqrt{\Sigma(y-\bar{y})^2}}$$

Referring to the example in Table 3.2, the Pearson correlation coefficient can be used to determine the relationship between the first and the second ROM measurements on the five subjects. Calculation of the Pearson product-moment correlation coefficient for this example is found in Table 3.5. The resulting value of $r = 0.98$ indicates a highly positive linear relationship between the first and the second measurements. In other words, the two measurements are highly correlated.

The Pearson product-moment correlation coefficient indicates association between the pairs of measurements rather than agreement. Therefore, to decide whether the two measurements are identical, the equation of the straight line best representing the relationship should be determined. If the equation of the straight line representing the relationship includes a slope equal to 1 *and* an intercept equal to 0, then an r value that approaches +1.0 indicates that the two measurements are identical. However, in cases where the slope is not equal to 1 or the intercept is not equal to 0, the value of r only indicates association of the two measures and does not represent agreement.

Given the equation of a straight line $y = a + bx$, where x represents the first measurement, y the second measurement, a the intercept, and b the slope, the equation for the slope is:

$$b = \frac{\Sigma(x-\bar{x})(y-\bar{y})}{\Sigma(x-\bar{x})^2}$$

and the equation for the intercept is:

$$a = \bar{y} - b\bar{x}$$

TABLE 3.5 Calculation of the Pearson Product-Moment Correlation Coefficient for the First (x) and Second (y) ROM Measurements in Degrees

Subject	x	y	$(x-\bar{x})$	$(y-\bar{y})$	$(x-\bar{x})(y-\bar{y})$	$(\bar{x}-\bar{X})^2$	$(y-\bar{y})^2$
1	57	55	3.2	–0.6	–1.92	10.24	0.36
2	66	65	12.2	9.4	114.68	148.84	88.36
3	66	70	12.2	14.4	175.68	148.84	207.36
4	35	40	–18.8	–15.6	293.28	353.44	243.36
5	45	48	–8.8	–7.6	66.88	77.44	57.76
					$\Sigma = 648.60$	$\Sigma = 738.80$	$\Sigma = 597.20$

$$\bar{x} = \frac{57+66+66+35+45}{5} = 53.8 \text{ degrees; } \bar{y} = \frac{55+65+70+40+48}{5} = 55.6 \text{ degrees}$$

$$r = \frac{\Sigma(x-\bar{x})(y-\bar{y})}{\sqrt{\Sigma(x-\bar{x})^2}\sqrt{\Sigma(y-\bar{y})^2}} = \frac{648.6}{\sqrt{738.8}\sqrt{597.2}} = \frac{648.6}{(27.2)(24.4)} = 0.98$$

For the example using the data from Table 3.5, the calculation of the slope and intercept is:

$$b = \frac{648.6}{738.8} = 0.88$$

$$a = 55.6 - (0.88 \times 53.8) = 55.6 - 47.34 = 8.26 \text{ degrees}$$

The equation of the straight line best representing the relationship between the first and the second measurements in this example is $y = 8.26 + 0.88x$. Although the r value represents a high correlation, the two measurements are *not* identical given this linear equation.

One concern in interpreting correlation coefficients is that the value of the correlation coefficient is markedly influenced by the range of the measurements.[3,99] The greater the biological variation between individuals for the measurement is, the more extreme the r value will be, so that r is closer to –1.0 or +1.0. Another limitation is the fact that the Pearson product-moment correlation coefficient can evaluate the relationship between only two variables or two measurements at one time. An additional limitation to remember is that the value of r is a point-estimate of a population parameter and one should consider the confidence interval around r as an estimate of the true population value.

Intraclass Correlation Coefficient

To avoid the need for calculating and interpreting both the correlation coefficient and a linear equation, the **intraclass correlation coefficient (ICC)** is frequently used to evaluate reliability of goniometric measurements. The ICC also allows the comparison of two or more measurements at a time; one can think of it as an average correlation among all possible pairs of measurements.[99] This statistic is determined from an analysis of variance model, which compares different sources of variation. The ICC is conceptually expressed as the ratio of the variance associated with the subjects, divided by the sum of the variance associated with the subjects plus error variance.[100] The theoretical limits of the ICC are between 0.0 and +1.0; +1.0 indicates perfect agreement (no error variance), whereas 0.0 indicates no agreement (large amount of error variance).

There are six different formulas for determining ICC values based on the design of the study, the purpose of the study, and the type of measurement.[3,100–102] Three models have been described, each with two different forms. In Model 1, each subject is tested by a different set of testers (examiners), and the testers are considered representative of a larger population of testers—to allow the results to be generalized to other testers. In Model 2, each subject is tested by the same set of testers, and again the testers are considered representative of a larger population of testers. In Model 3, each subject is tested by the same set of testers, but the testers are the only testers of interest—the results are not intended to be generalized to other testers. The first form of all three models is used when single measurements (1) are compared, whereas the second form is used when the means of multiple measurements (k) are compared. The different formulas for the ICC are identified by two numbers enclosed by parentheses. The first number indicates the model, and the second number indicates the form. For further discussion, examples, and formulas, the reader is urged to refer to the referenced texts[3] and articles.[100–102]

In the example of the ROM measurements from five subjects (Table 3.2), a repeated measures analysis of variance was conducted and the ICC (3,1) was calculated as 0.94. This ICC model was selected because each measurement was taken by the same tester, there was only an interest in applying the results to this tester, and three separate single measurements were compared rather than the means of several measurements. This ICC value indicates high reliability between the three repeated measurements. However, this value is slightly lower than the Pearson product-moment correlation coefficient, as the calculation of the ICC is considering both association and agreement. This calculation of the ICC also differed from the calculation of the Pearson product-moment correlation coefficient as it incorporated the three repeated measurements as compared with a pair of repeated measurements. For recommendations to interpret ICC values, please refer to textbooks on clinical research.[3,98] Keep in mind that these values need to be interpreted in the context of the data and are not strict cut-offs.

Like the Pearson product-moment correlation coefficient, the ICC is also influenced by the range of measurements between the subjects. As the group of subjects becomes more homogeneous, the ability of the ICC to detect agreement is reduced and the ICC can erroneously indicate poor reliability.[3,100,102,103] Because correlation coefficients are sensitive to the range of the measurements and do not provide an index of reliability in the units of the measurement, some experts prefer the use of the standard deviation of the repeated measurements (intrasubject standard deviation) or the standard error of measurement to assess reliability.[102–105] Furthermore, like the correlation coefficient, the value of the ICC is a point-estimate of a population parameter and one should consider the confidence interval around this point-estimate.

Absolute Measures of Reliability

Earlier in this chapter, standard deviations were discussed as a measure of variability. A standard deviation is an absolute measure of reliability as it is reported in the same units as the original measurement. Absolute measures, such as the standard deviation, provide the clinician with a sense of the magnitude of the consistency of the measurement in units that are logical to understand and may be easily explained by the clinician to the person whose joint angle or ROM is being measured.

Standard Error of Measurement

The standard error of measurement is another absolute measure of measurement reliability that is expressed in the same units as the original measurement.[3,102,106,107] According to DuBois,[106] "The **standard error of measurement** is the likely standard deviation of the error made in predicting true scores when we have knowledge only of the obtained scores." The true scores are forever unknown, but several formulas have been developed to estimate this statistic. The standard error of measurement is generally symbolized as **SEM.**[†]

[†] Note that another statistic, the standard error of the mean, is often confused with the standard error of measurement.[3,96] The standard error of the mean may also be symbolized with the same abbreviation as the standard error of measurement, which may contribute to the confusion. These two statistics are not equivalent, nor do they have the same interpretation. The standard error of the mean is the standard deviation of a distribution of means taken from samples of a population.[3] The standard error of the mean describes how much variation can be expected in the means from future samples of the same size. Because we are interested in the variation of individual measurements when evaluating reliability rather than the variation of means, the standard deviation of the repeated measurements or the standard error of measurement are the appropriate statistical tests to use.[108]

One method to estimate the SEM considers the differences between the scores from two repeated measurements such as in a test-retest reliability study.[102,107] In other words, the difference between two repeated measurements of a joint motion is determined and a standard deviation from all of the difference scores is calculated. This standard deviation of the test-retest differences (SD_{diff}) is then divided by the square root of 2 to obtain the SEM.

$$\text{SEM} = \frac{SD_{diff}}{\sqrt{2}}$$

The SEM can also be estimated from a repeated measures analysis of variance (ANOVA) model.[107,109,110] This formula may be helpful when more than two repeated measurements are taken. In this case, the SEM is equivalent to the square root of the error variance. The error variance may also be referred to as the mean square error or within-subjects mean square. The value for the error variance is frequently available from the ANOVA summary table.

$$\text{SEM} = \sqrt{\text{error variance}}$$

A third method to estimate the SEM incorporates information from the variation of repeated measurements and the reliability coefficient. If the pooled standard deviation from a series of repeated measurements is denoted SD_p, a correlation coefficient such as the intraclass correlation coefficient is denoted ICC, and the Pearson product-moment correlation coefficient is denoted r, the formulas for the SEM are as follows:

$$\text{SEM} = SD_p\sqrt{1 - \text{ICC}}$$

or if the Pearson product-moment correlation is used for reliability

$$\text{SEM} = SD_p\sqrt{1 - r}$$

Returning to the example in Table 3.2, the SEM can be estimated using these three methods. First, the calculation of the SEM using the standard deviation of the differences of the first and second measurements is shown in Table 3.6. The resulting value for the SEM of 2.2 degrees is an indication of the stability of the observed scores. Because the SEM is a special case of the standard deviation, about 68% of the time the true measurement would be within 2.2 degrees of the observed measurement.

We can also use all three measurements from the five subjects in Table 3.2 and the results of a repeated measures analysis of variance to estimate the SEM. Given that the error variance in the ANOVA is equal to 10.9, the SEM is equal to the square root of the error variance or 3.3 degrees. Note in this case the value of the SEM is larger than when only the first two measurements were used because of the increased variation added by the third measurement in this example.

TABLE 3.6 Calculation of the Standard Error of Measurement (SEM) for the First (x) and Second (y) ROM Measurements in Degrees Using the Standard Deviation of the Differences (SD_{diff})

Subject	x	y	(x − y)	$(x - y) - (\bar{X}_{diff})$	$[(x - y) - (\bar{X}_{diff})]^2$
1	57	55	2	3.8	14.44
2	66	65	1	2.8	7.84
3	66	70	−4	−2.2	4.84
4	35	40	−5	−3.2	10.24
5	45	48	−3	−1.2	1.44
			Σ = −9		Σ = 38.80

$$\text{Mean of differences } (x-y) = \bar{X}_{diff} = \frac{\Sigma(x-y)}{n} = \frac{-9}{5} = -1.8 \text{ degrees}$$

$$\text{Standard deviation of differences } (SD_{diff}) = \sqrt{\frac{\Sigma[(x-y)-(\bar{X}_{diff})]^2}{(n-1)}} = \sqrt{\frac{38.80}{4}} = \sqrt{9.7} = 3.11 \text{ degrees}$$

$$\text{Standard error of measurement (SEM)} = \frac{SD_{diff}}{\sqrt{2}} = \frac{3.11}{\sqrt{2}} = \frac{3.11}{1.41} = 2.2 \text{ degrees}$$

Likewise, we can also use the value of the ICC, which was also obtained from a repeated measures ANOVA, to estimate the SEM. As you recall, in the example the value for the ICC is 0.94 and the value for the pooled standard deviation (SD_p) among the five subjects is 13.6 degrees (in this example the SD_p is also equal to the value of the standard deviation, indicating biological variation).

$$SEM = 13.6\sqrt{1-0.94} = 13.6\sqrt{0.06} = 3.3 \text{ degrees}$$

Both of these analyses using the three repeated measurements obtained a value of 3.3 degrees for the SEM, which informs us that 68% of the time the true measurement would be within 3.3 degrees of the observed measurement or 95% of the time the true measurement would be within 6.6 degrees of the observed measurement (i.e., within two SEM).

Minimal Detectable Change

A final absolute measure to discuss is the concept of **minimal detectable change (MDC),** which is the smallest amount of change in a measurement in excess of the measurement error.[3,97,107,111,112] The MDC uses information regarding the reliability of the measurement in order to provide a minimal value to determine whether a change has occurred. In the literature the MDC has also been referred to as the **minimal detectable difference (MDD),** the **minimal important difference,** and the **smallest detectable difference (SDD).**[3,112] The MDC at the 90% confidence level is calculated from the standard error of measurement using the following equation, with the value of 1.65 representing the z-score at the 90% confidence level.[‡] Like the SEM, the MDC is expressed in the same units as the original measurement.

$$MDC_{90} = SEM \times \sqrt{2} \times 1.65$$

Because the SEM may be calculated from the standard deviation of the test-retest differences divided by the square root of 2, the MDC may also be calculated as:

$$MDC_{90} = SD_{diff} \times 1.65$$

One may also see MDC values in the literature reported at other confidence levels. For example, equations for the MDC at the 95% confidence level are as follows and result in a larger value for the minimal change than the MDC_{90}.

$$MDC_{95} = SEM \times \sqrt{2} \times 1.96$$

or

$$MDC_{95} = SD_{diff} \times 1.96$$

Returning to our example of three repeated measurements of ROM and using a value for the SEM of 3.3 degrees, the MDC_{90} is calculated as 7.7 degrees.

$$MDC_{90} = 3.3 \times \sqrt{2} \times 1.65 = 7.7 \text{ degrees}$$

[‡] A z-score is the difference between an observation and the mean, divided by the standard deviation $[(x - \bar{x})/SD]$. The z-score, which is in standard deviation units and applied to a standard normal curve distribution in which the mean is 0 and the SD = 1, can be used to determine the probability of an observation.

The interpretation of this MDC is that 90% of individuals whose ROM has not changed will display random fluctuations of up to 7.7 degrees between measurements because of measurement error. Expressed another way, differences greater than 7.7 degrees between repeated measurements would likely represent a real change in ROM 90% of the time. Even though we had obtained a fairly high correlation coefficient in this example (ICC = 0.94), the variability within the data resulted in an MDC of 7.7 degrees. Please refer to the Research Findings sections of Chapters 4 through 13 for more joint-specific information on measures of absolute error. Please keep in mind these measures of absolute reliability will be specific for the population in which the measure was obtained and specific to the procedures used to obtain the measurement.

Exercises to Evaluate Reliability

Exercises 8 and 9 have been included to help examiners assess their reliability in obtaining goniometric measurements. Calculations of the standard deviation and coefficient of variation are included in the belief that understanding is reinforced by practical application. **Exercise 8** examines **intratester reliability.** Intratester reliability refers to the amount of agreement between repeated measurements of the same joint position or ROM by the same examiner (tester). An intratester reliability study answers the question: How accurately can an examiner reproduce his or her own measurements? **Exercise 9** examines **intertester reliability.** Intertester reliability refers to the amount of agreement between repeated measurements of the same joint position or ROM by different examiners (testers). An intertester reliability study answers the question: How accurately can one examiner reproduce measurements taken by other examiners? **Exercises 10 and 11** provide practice using different methods to obtain the **standard error of measurement** and the **minimal detectable change** from measurements repeated at two time points. In addition, Exercise 11 provides practice in calculating the Pearson product-moment correlation coefficient. Each of these four exercises provides instructions to calculate these values by hand, although the learner may also use calculators, spreadsheets, or computer applications to obtain the values for the different statistics.

Exercise 8

Intratester Reliability

1. Select a subject and a universal goniometer.
2. Measure elbow flexion ROM on your subject three times, following the steps outlined in Chapter 2, Exercise 7.
3. Record each measurement on the recording form (see opposite page) in the column labeled x.
4. Compare the measurements. If a discrepancy of more than 5 degrees exists between measurements, recheck each step in the procedure to make sure that you are performing the steps correctly, and then repeat this exercise.
5. Continue practicing until you have obtained three successive measurements that are within 5 degrees of each other.
6. To gain an understanding of several of the statistics used to evaluate intratester reliability, calculate the standard deviation and coefficient of variation by completing the following steps.
   a. Add the three measurements together to determine the sum of the measurements. The symbol for summation is Σ. Record the sum at the bottom of the column labeled x.
   b. To determine the **mean,** divide this sum by 3, which is the number of measurements. The number of measurements is denoted by n. The mean is denoted by $\bar{x}$. Space to calculate the mean is provided on the recording form.
   c. To continue the process of calculating the **standard deviation,** subtract the mean from each of the three measurements and record the results in the column labeled $(x - \bar{x})$. Space to calculate the standard deviation is provided on the recording form.
   d. Square each of the numbers in the column labeled $(x - \bar{x})$ and record the results in the column labeled $(x - \bar{x})^2$.
   e. Add the three numbers in column $(x - \bar{x})^2$ to determine the sum of the squares. Record the results at the bottom of the column labeled $(x - \bar{x})^2$.
   f. Divide this sum by 2, which is the number of measurements minus 1 $(n - 1)$. Then find the square root of this number. The units will be in degrees.
   g. To determine the **coefficient of variation,** divide the standard deviation by the mean. Multiply this number by 100%. Space to calculate the coefficient of variation is provided on the recording form.
7. Repeat this procedure with other joints and motions after you have learned the testing procedures.

RECORDING FORM FOR EXERCISE 8: INTRATESTER RELIABILITY

Follow the steps outlined in Exercise 8. Use this form to record your measurements and the result of your calculations.

Subject's Name ______________________ Date ____________________

Examiner's Name ______________________

Joint and Motion ______________________ Right or Left Side ____________

Passive or Active Motion ______________________ Type of Goniometer ____________

Measurement	x	$(x - \bar{x})$	$(x - \bar{x})^2$
1			
2			
3			
$n = 3$	$\Sigma x =$		$\Sigma(x - \bar{x})^2 =$

Mean of the three measurements $= \bar{x} = \dfrac{\Sigma x}{n} =$

Standard deviation $= \text{SD} = \sqrt{\dfrac{\Sigma(x-\bar{x})^2}{n-1}} =$

Coefficient of variation $= \text{CV} = \dfrac{\text{SD}}{\bar{x}}(100\%) =$

Exercise 9

Intertester Reliability

1. Select a subject and a universal goniometer.
2. Measure elbow flexion ROM on your subject once, following the steps outlined in Chapter 2, Exercise 7.
3. Ask two other examiners to measure the same elbow flexion ROM on your subject, using your goniometer and following the steps outlined in Chapter 2, Exercise 5.
4. Record each measurement on the recording form (see opposite page) in the column labeled *x*.
5. Compare the measurements. If a discrepancy of more than 5 degrees exists between measurements, repeat this exercise. The examiners should observe one another's measurements to discover differences in technique that might account for variability, such as faulty alignment, lack of stabilization, or reading the wrong scale.
6. To gain an understanding of several of the statistics used to evaluate intertester reliability, calculate the mean deviation, standard deviation, and coefficient of variation by completing the following steps.
   a. Add the three measurements together to determine the sum of the measurements. The symbol for summation is Σ. Record the sum at the bottom of the column labeled *x*.
   b. To determine the **mean,** divide this sum by 3, which is the number of measurements. The number of measurements is denoted by *n*. The mean is denoted by $\overline{x}$. Space to calculate the mean is provided on the recording form.
   c. To continue the process of calculating the **standard deviation,** subtract the mean from each of the three measurements and record the results in the column labeled $(x - \overline{x})$. Space to calculate the standard deviation is provided on the recording form.
   d. Square each of the numbers in the column labeled $(x - \overline{x})$ and record the results in the column labeled $(x - \overline{x})^2$.
   e. Add the three numbers in column $(x - \overline{x})^2$ to determine the sum of the squares. Record the results at the bottom of the column labeled $(x - \overline{x})^2$.
   f. Divide this sum by 2, which is the number of measurements minus 1 $(n - 1)$. Then find the square root of this number.
   g. To determine the **coefficient of variation,** divide the standard deviation by the mean. Multiply this number by 100%. Space to calculate the coefficient of variation is provided on the recording form.
7. Repeat this exercise with other joints and motions after you have learned the testing procedures.

RECORDING FORM FOR EXERCISE 9: INTERTESTER RELIABILITY

Follow the steps outlined in Exercise 9. Use this form to record your measurements and the results of your calculations.

Subject's Name ______________________ Date ______________________

Examiner 1. Name ______________________

Examiner 2. Name ______________________ Joint and Motion ______________________

Examiner 3. Name ______________________ Right or Left Side ______________________

Passive or Active Motion ______________________ Type of Goniometer ______________________

Measurement	x	$(x - \bar{x})$	$(x - \bar{x})^2$
1			
2			
3			
$n = 3$	$\Sigma x =$		$\Sigma(x - \bar{x})^2 =$

Mean of the three measurements $= \bar{x} = \dfrac{\Sigma x}{n} =$

Standard deviation $= \text{SD} = \sqrt{\dfrac{\Sigma(x - \bar{x})^2}{n - 1}} =$

Coefficient of variation $= \text{CV} = \dfrac{\text{SD}}{\bar{x}}(100\%) =$

Exercise 10

Calculation of the Standard Error of Measurement and Minimal Detectable Change

This exercise describes the calculation of the standard error of measurement (SEM) and minimal detectable change (MDC) from two repeated measurements of five subjects.

1. Select five subjects and a universal goniometer.
2. Measure elbow flexion ROM on each subject once, following the steps outlined in Chapter 2, Exercise 7.
3. After a short rest, repeat the measurement of the same elbow flexion ROM on the five subjects, using the same goniometer and following the steps outlined in Chapter 2, Exercise 7. Avoid referring to the value for the first measurement when obtaining the second measurement.
4. Record each measurement on the recording form (see opposite page) in the column labeled x for the first measurement with each subject, and in the column labeled y for the second measurement with each subject.
5. To gain an understanding of the statistics used to evaluate absolute reliability calculate the **SEM** and **MDC** by completing the following steps.
   a. To calculate the difference between the two measurements, subtract y from x for each of the five measurements, and record the results in the column labeled $(x - y)$. Add these differences together to determine the sum of the measurements in the $(x - y)$ column. The symbol for summation is Σ. Record the sum at the bottom of the column labeled $(x - y)$.
   b. To determine the **mean of the summed test-retest differences,** divide this sum by 5, which is the number of measurements. The number of measurements is denoted by n. The mean is denoted in the example by $\bar{X}_{\text{diff}}$. Record this value in the space provided on the recording form.
   c. Subtract the mean of the summed differences from each of the numbers in the column labeled $(x - y)$ and record the results in the column labeled $(x - y) - (\bar{X}_{\text{diff}})$.
   d. Square each of the numbers in the column labeled $(x - y) - (\bar{X}_{\text{diff}})$, and record the results in the column labeled $[(x - y) - (\bar{X}_{\text{diff}})]^2$.
   e. Add the five numbers in the column labeled $[(x - y) - (\bar{X}_{\text{diff}})]^2$ to determine their sum. Record the sum at the bottom of the column labeled $[(x - y) - (\bar{X}_{\text{diff}})]^2$.
   f. To determine the **standard deviation of the test-retest differences (SD_{diff}),** divide this sum by 4, which is the number of measurements minus 1 $(n - 1)$. Then find the square root of this number. Space to calculate and record the standard deviation of the differences is provided on the recording form.
   g. To determine the **standard error of measurement (SEM),** divide the standard deviation of the differences by the square root of 2. Record this value in the space provided. Remember to report the SEM in the same units as the original measurements (i.e., degrees).
   h. To determine the **minimal detectable change (MDC_{90}),** multiply the standard error of measurement by the square root of 2, and then multiply this value by 1.65. Space to calculate and record this value is provided on the recording form. Remember your result for the minimal detectable change will be in the units of the original measurement. You may also calculate the minimal detectable change by multiplying the standard deviation of the test-retest differences by 1.65.
6. Repeat this exercise with other joints and motions after you have learned the testing procedures.

RECORDING FORM FOR EXERCISE 10: CALCULATION OF THE STANDARD ERROR OF MEASUREMENT AND MINIMAL DETECTABLE CHANGE

Follow the steps outlined in Exercise 10. Use this form to record your measurements and the result of your calculations.

Subject 1. Name ______________________________ Date ____________________________

Subject 2. Name ______________________________

Subject 3. Name ______________________________ Joint and Motion ________________

Subject 4. Name ______________________________ Right or Left Side ______________

Subject 5. Name ______________________________ Passive or Active Motion ________

Examiner. Name ______________________________ Type of Goniometer ______________

Subject	x	y	(x – y)	$(x - y) - (\bar{X}_{diff})$	$[(x - y) - (\bar{X}_{diff})]^2$
1					
2					
3					
4					
5					
$n = 5$			$\Sigma(x - y) =$		$\Sigma[(x - y) - (\bar{X}_{diff})]^2 =$

Mean of summed test-retest differences $(x - y) = \bar{X}_{diff} = \dfrac{\Sigma(x-y)}{n} =$

Standard deviation of test-retest differences $(SD_{diff}) = \sqrt{\left(\dfrac{\Sigma[(x-y)-(\bar{x}_{diff})]^2}{(n-1)}\right)} =$

Standard error of measurement $(SEM) = \dfrac{SD_{diff}}{\sqrt{2}} =$

Minimal detectable change $= MDC_{90} = SEM \times \sqrt{2} \times 1.65 =$

Or use equation: $MDC_{90} = SD_{diff} \times 1.65 =$

Exercise 11

Calculation of the Pearson Product-Moment Correlation Coefficient, Standard Error of Measurement, and Minimal Detectable Change

This exercise describes the calculation of the Pearson product-moment correlation coefficient (r) from repeated measurements of five subjects. This correlation coefficient is then used to determine the standard error of measurement (SEM) and minimal detectable change (MDC). Alternatively, the learner may use the intraclass correlation coefficient (ICC) for the calculation of the SEM and MDC. Calculation of the ICC, however, is best obtained from statistical software instead of calculation by hand.

1. Select five subjects and a universal goniometer. (If you have completed Exercise 10, you may wish to use the same data. In this case, record the x and y values from Exercise 10 as described in Step 4 and then begin the calculations with Step 5.)
2. Measure elbow flexion ROM on each subject once, following the steps outlined in Chapter 2, Exercise 7.
3. After a short rest, repeat the measurement of the same elbow flexion ROM on the five subjects, using the same goniometer and following the steps outlined in Chapter 2, Exercise 7. Avoid referring to the value for the first measurement when obtaining the second measurement.
4. Record each measurement on the recording form (see opposite page) in the column labeled x for the first measurement with each subject, and in the column labeled y for the second measurement with each subject.
5. To gain an understanding of the statistics used to evaluate relative reliability calculate the **Pearson product-moment correlation coefficient** by completing the following steps.
   a. Add the measurements together to determine the sum of the measurements in the x and y columns. The symbol for summation is Σ. Record the sum at the bottom of the column labeled x and the column labeled y.
   b. To determine the **mean,** divide this sum by 5, which is the number of measurements. The number of measurements is denoted by n. The mean is denoted by $\overline{x}$ and $\overline{y}$. Space to calculate the means is provided on the recording form.
   c. To determine the **reliability correlation coefficient (Pearson's r),** first subtract the mean from each measurement for each subject and record the results in the appropriate columns [$(x-\overline{x})^2$ and $(y-\overline{y})^2$, respectively].
   d. Multiply each value for $(x-\overline{x})$ by $(y-\overline{y})$ and record the results in the column labeled $(x-\overline{x})\,(y-\overline{y})$.
   e. Square each of the numbers in the columns labeled $(x-\overline{x})$ and $(y-\overline{y})$ and record the results in the appropriate columns [$(x-\overline{x})^2$ and $(y-\overline{y})^2$, respectively].
   f. Add the five numbers in the columns $(x-\overline{x})\,(y-\overline{y})$, $(x-\overline{x})^2$, and $(y-\overline{y})^2$ to determine their sums. Record the sums in each respective column in the space provided beneath the five scores.
   g. Calculate the square roots of $\Sigma(x-\overline{x})^2$ and $\Sigma(y-\overline{y})^2$. Record these values in the space provided.
   h. Calculate the correlation coefficient (r) by dividing $\Sigma(x-\overline{x})\,(y-\overline{y})$ by the product of $\sqrt{\Sigma(x-\overline{x})^2}$ and $\sqrt{\Sigma(y-\overline{y})^2}$. Space to calculate and record this value is provided on the recording form.
6. To gain an understanding of statistics used to evaluate absolute reliability, calculate the standard error of measurement and minimal detectable change (MDC_{90}) by completing the following steps.
   a. To determine the **standard error of measurement,** next determine the **standard deviation for x (sd_x)** and the **standard deviation of y (sd_y).** Use $\Sigma(x-\overline{x})^2$ and $\Sigma(y-\overline{y})^2$, which were previously calculated. Divide these sums by 4, which is the number of measurements minus 1 (n – 1). Then find the square roots of these numbers. Record these values in the space provided.
   b. To obtain the **pooled standard deviation,** square the values for the standard deviation for x (sd_x) and the standard deviation of y (sd_y) and then add the square values together. Divide this sum by 2 (which is the number of times each subject was measured). Then obtain the square root of this value. Calculate and record this value in the space provided (SD_p).
   c. Multiply the pooled standard deviation by the square root of 1 minus the correlation coefficient (r). Space to calculate and record this value is provided on the recording form. Remember that your result for the standard error of measurement will be in the units of the original measurement, which in this case is in degrees.

d. To determine the **minimal detectable change** (MDC_{90}), multiply the standard error of measurement by the square root of 2 and then multiply this value by 1.65. Space to calculate and record this value is provided on the recording form. Remember that your result for the minimal detectable change will be in the units of the original measurement.

7. Repeat this exercise with other joints and motions after you have learned the testing procedures.

RECORDING FORM FOR EXERCISE 11: CALCULATION OF THE PEARSON PRODUCT-MOMENT CORRELATION COEFFICIENT, STANDARD ERROR OF MEASUREMENT, AND MINIMAL DETECTABLE CHANGE

Follow the steps outlined in Exercise 11. Use this form to record your measurements and the result of your calculations.

Subject 1. Name ______________________ Date ______________________

Subject 2. Name ______________________

Subject 3. Name ______________________ Joint and Motion ______________________

Subject 4. Name ______________________ Right or Left Side ______________________

Subject 5. Name ______________________ Passive or Active Motion ______________________

Examiner. Name ______________________ Type of Goniometer ______________________

Subject	x	y	$(x-\bar{x})$	$(y-\bar{y})$	$(x-\bar{x})(y-\bar{y})$	$(x-\bar{x})^2$	$(y-\bar{y})^2$
1							
2							
3							
4							
5							
n = 5	$\Sigma x =$	$\Sigma y =$			$\Sigma(x-\bar{x})(y-\bar{y}) =$	$\Sigma(x-\bar{x})^2 =$	$\Sigma(y-\bar{y})^2 =$
						$\sqrt{\Sigma(x-\bar{x})^2} =$	$\sqrt{\Sigma(y-\bar{y})^2} =$

Mean of first 3 measurements $(x) = \bar{x} = \dfrac{\Sigma x}{n} =$

Mean of second 3 measurements $(y) = \bar{y} = \dfrac{\Sigma y}{n} =$

Pearson product-moment correlation coefficient $= r = \dfrac{\Sigma(x-\bar{x})(y-\bar{y})}{\sqrt{\Sigma(x-\bar{x})^2}\sqrt{\Sigma(y-\bar{y})^2}} =$

Standard deviation of x = $\mathbf{sd}_x = \sqrt{\dfrac{\Sigma(x-\bar{x})^2}{(n-1)}} =$

Standard deviation of y = $\mathbf{sd}_y = \sqrt{\dfrac{\Sigma(y-\bar{y})^2}{(n-1)}} =$

Pooled standard deviation $= SD_p = \sqrt{\dfrac{sd_x^2 + sd_y^2}{2}} =$

Standard error of the measurement $= SEM = SD_p\sqrt{1-r} =$

Minimal detectable change $= MDC_{90} = SEM \times \sqrt{2} \times 1.65 =$

REFERENCES

1. Rothstein, JM, and Echternach, JL: Primer on Measurement: An Introductory Guide to Measurement Issues. American Physical Therapy Association, Alexandria, VA, 1993.
2. Guide to Physical Therapist Practice 3.0. Alexandria, VA, American Physical Therapy Association, 2014. Available at: http://guidetopractice.apta.org.
3. Portney, LG, and Watkins, MP: Foundations of Clinical Research: Applications to Practice, ed 3. FA Davis, Philadelphia, PA, 2015.
4. Sim, J, and Arnell, P: Measurement validity in physical therapy research. Phys Ther 73:102, 1993.
5. Gajdosik, RL, and Bohannon, RW: Clinical measurement of range of motion: Review of goniometry emphasizing reliability and validity. Phys Ther 67:1867, 1987.
6. Piriyaprasarth, P, and Morris ME: Psychometric properties of measurement tools for quantifying knee joint position and movement: A systematic review. Knee 14:2, 2007.
7. Milani, P, et al: Mobile smartphone applications for body position measurement in rehabilitation: A review of goniometric tools. PM&R 6: 1038, 2014.
8. Gogia, PP, et al: Reliability and validity of goniometric measurements at the knee. Phys Ther 67:192, 1987.
9. Enwemeka, CS: Radiographic verification of knee goniometry. Scand J Rehabil Med 18:47, 1986.
10. Ahlback, SO, and Lindahl, O: Sagittal mobility of the hip-joint. Acta Orthop Scand 34:310, 1964.
11. Kato, M, et al: The accuracy of goniometric measurements of proximal interphalangeal joints in fresh cadavers: Comparison between methods of measurement, types of goniometers, and fingers. J Hand Ther 20:12, 2007.
12. Chen, J, et al: Meta-analysis of normative cervical motion. Spine 24:1571, 1999.
13. Herrmann, DB: Validity study of head and neck flexion-extension motion comparing measurements of a pendulum goniometer and roentgenograms. J Orthop Sports Phys Ther 11:414, 1990.
14. Ordway, NR, et al: Cervical sagittal range-of-motion analysis using three methods: Cervical range-of-motion device, space, and radiography. Spine 22:501, 1997.
15. Tousignant, M, et al: Criterion validity of the cervical range of motion (CROM) goniometer for cervical flexion and extension. Spine 25:324, 2000.
16. Tousignant, M, et al: Criterion validity of the cervical range of motion (CROM) device for rotational range of motion on healthy adults. J Orthop Sports Phys Ther 35:242, 2006.
17. Macrae, JF, and Wright, V: Measurement of back movement. Ann Rheum Dis 28:584, 1969.
18. Portek, I, et al: Correlation between radiographic and clinical measurement of lumbar spine movement. Br J Rheumatol 22:197, 1983.
19. Burdett, RG, Brown, KE, and Fall, MP: Reliability and validity of four instruments for measuring lumbar spine and pelvic positions. Phys Ther 66:677, 1986.
20. Mayer, TG, et al: Use of noninvasive techniques for quantification of spinal range-of-motion in normal subjects and chronic low-back dysfunction patients. Spine 9:588, 1984.
21. Saur, PM, et al: Lumbar range of motion: Reliability and validity of the inclinometer technique in the clinical measurement of trunk flexibility. Spine 21:1332, 1996.
22. Samo, DG, et al: Validity of three lumbar sagittal motion measurement methods: Surface inclinometers compared with radiographs. J Occup Environ Med 39:209, 1997.
23. Vasen, AP, et al: Functional range of motion of the elbow. J Hand Surg Br 20A:288, 1995.
24. Cooper, JE, et al: Elbow joint restriction: Effect on functional upper limb motion during performance of three feeding activities. Arch Phys Med Rehabil 74:805, 1993.
25. Nelson, DL: Functional wrist motion. Hand Clin 13:83, 1997.
26. Hermann, KM, and Reese, CS: Relationships among selected measures of impairment, functional limitation, and disability in patients with cervical spine disorder. Phys Ther 81:903, 2001.
27. Triffitt, PD: The relationship between motion of the shoulder and the stated ability to perform activities of daily living. J Bone Joint Surg 80:41, 1998.
28. Wagner, MB, et al: Assessment of hand function in Duchenne muscular dystrophy. Arch Phys Med Rehabil 74:801, 1993.
29. Waddell, G, et al: Objective clinical evaluation of physical impairment in chronic low back pain. Spine 17:617, 1992.
30. World Health Organization: International Classification of Functioning, Disability and Health: ICF. World Health Organization, Geneva, 2001.
31. Scalzitti, DA: Examination of Function. In O'Sullivan, SB, Schmitz, TJ, and Fulk, GD (eds): Physical Rehabilitation, ed 6. FA Davis, Philadelphia, 2014.
32. Moore, ML: Clinical Assessment of Joint Motion. In Basmajian, JV (ed): Therapeutic Exercise, ed 3. Williams & Wilkins, Baltimore, 1978.
33. Miller, PJ: Assessment of Joint Motion. In Rothstein, JM (ed): Measurement in Physical Therapy. Churchill Livingstone, New York, 1985.
34. Lea, RD, and Gerhardt, JJ: Current concepts review: Range-of-motion measurements. J Bone Joint Surg Am 77:784, 1995.
35. Williams, MA, et al: A systematic review of reliability and validity studies of methods for measuring active and passive cervical range of motion. J Manipulative Physiol Ther 33:138, 2010.
36. van de Pol R, et al: Inter-rater reliability for measurement of passive physiological range of motion of upper extremity joints is better if instruments are used: A systematic review. J Physiother 56:7, 2010.
37. van Trijffel E, et al: Inter-rater reliability for measurement of passive physiological movements in lower extremity joints is generally low: A systematic review. J Physiother 56:223, 2010.
38. Grohmann, JE: Comparison of two methods of goniometry. Phys Ther 63:922, 1983.
39. Hamilton, GF, and Lachenbruch, PA: Reliability of goniometers in assessing finger joint angle. Phys Ther 49:465, 1969.
40. Boone, DC, et al: Reliability of goniometric measurements. Phys Ther 58:1355, 1978.
41. Pandya, S, et al: Reliability of goniometric measurements in patients with Duchenne muscular dystrophy. Phys Ther 65:1339, 1985.
42. Bovens, AM, et al: Variability and reliability of joint measurements. Am J Sport Med 18:58, 1990.
43. Hellebrandt, FA, Duvall, EN, and Moore, ML: The measurement of joint motion. Part III: Reliability of goniometry. Phys Ther Rev 29:302, 1949.
44. Low, JL: The reliability of joint measurement. Physiotherapy 62:227, 1976.
45. Greene, BL, and Wolf, SL: Upper extremity joint movement: Comparison of two measurement devices. Arch Phys Med Rehabil 70:299, 1989.
46. Tucci, SM, et al: Cervical motion assessment: A new, simple and accurate method. Arch Phys Med Rehabil 67:225, 1986.
47. Youdas, JW, Carey, JR, and Garrett, TR: Reliability of measurements of cervical spine range of motion: Comparison of three methods. Phys Ther 71:2, 1991.
48. Fitzgerald, GK, et al: Objective assessment with establishment of normal values for lumbar spine range of motion. Phys Ther 63:1776, 1983.
49. Nitschke, JE, et al: Reliability of the American Medical Association Guides' model for measuring spinal range of motion. Spine 24:262, 1999.
50. Mayerson, NH, and Milano, RA: Goniometric measurement reliability in physical medicine. Arch Phys Med Rehabil 65:92, 1984.
51. Watkins, MA, et al: Reliability of goniometric measurements and visual estimates of knee range of motion obtained in a clinical setting. Phys Ther 71:90, 1991.
52. Riddle, DL, Rothstein, JM, and Lamb, RL: Goniometric reliability in a clinical setting: Shoulder measurements. Phys Ther 67:668, 1987.
53. Ekstrand, J, et al: Lower extremity goniometric measurements: A study to determine their reliability. Arch Phys Med Rehabil 63:171, 1982.
54. Rothstein, JM, Miller, PJ, and Roettger, RF: Goniometric reliability in a clinical setting: Elbow and knee measurements. Phys Ther 63:1611, 1983.
55. Solgaard, S, et al: Reproducibility of goniometry of the wrist. Scand J Rehabil Med 18:5, 1986.
56. Lovell, FW, Rothstein, JM, and Personius, WJ: Reliability of clinical measurements of lumbar lordosis taken with a flexible rule. Phys Ther 69:96, 1989.
57. Bartlett, JD, et al: Hip flexion contractures: A comparison of measurement methods. Arch Phys Med Rehabil 66:620, 1985.
58. Jonson, SR, and Gross, MT: Intraexaminer reliability, interexaminer reliability, and mean values for nine lower extremity skeletal measures in healthy naval midshipmen. J Orthop Sports Phys Ther 25:253, 1997
59. Elveru, RA, Rothstein, JM, and Lamb, RL: Goniometric reliability in a clinical setting. Phys Ther 68:672, 1988.
60. Diamond, JE, et al: Reliability of a diabetic foot evaluation. Phys Ther 69:797, 1989.
61. MacDermid, JC, et al: Intratester and intertester reliability of goniometric measurement of passive lateral shoulder rotation. J Hand Ther 12:187, 1999.

62. Armstrong, AD, et al: Reliability of range-of-motion measurement in the elbow and forearm. J Shoulder Elbow Surg 7:573, 1998.
63. Boon, AJ, and Smith, J: Manual scapular stabilization: Its effect on shoulder rotational range of motion. Arch Phys Med Rehabil 81:978, 2000.
64. Horger, MM: The reliability of goniometric measurements of active and passive wrist motions. Am J Occup Ther 44:342, 1990.
65. Ellis, B, Bruton, A, and Goddard, JR: Joint angle measurement: A comparative study of the reliability of goniometry and wire tracing for the hand. Clin Rehabil 11:314, 1997.
66. Pellecchia, GL, and Bohannon, RW: Active lateral neck flexion range of motion measurements obtained with a modified goniometer. Reliability and estimates of normal. J Manipulative Physiol Ther 21:443, 1998.
67. Nilsson, N: Measuring passive cervical motion: A study of reliability. J Manipulative Physiol Ther 18:293, 1995.
68. Williams, R, et al: Reliability of the modified-modified Schober and double inclinometer methods for measuring lumbar flexion and extension. Phys Ther 73:26, 1993.
69. Defibaugh, JJ: Measurement of head motion. Part II: An experimental study of head motion in adult males. Phys Ther 44:163, 1964.
70. Balogun, JA, et al: Inter- and intratester reliability of measuring neck motions with tape measure and Myrin Gravity-Reference Goniometer. J Orthop Sports Phys Ther 10:248, 1989.
71. Capuano-Pucci, D, et al: Intratester and intertester reliability of the cervical range of motion. Arch Phys Med Rehabil 72:338, 1991.
72. LaStayo, PC, and Wheeler, DL: Reliability of passive wrist flexion and extension goniometric measurements: A multicenter study. Phys Ther 74:162, 1994.
73. Macedo, LG, and Magee DJ: Effects of age on passive range of motion of selected peripheral joints in healthy adult females. Physiother Theory Pract 25:145, 2009.
74. Mayer, TG, et al: Spinal range of motion. Spine 22:1976, 1997.
75. Cobe, HM: The range of active motion at the wrist of white adults. J Bone Joint Surg Br 10:763, 1928.
76. Hewitt, D: The range of active motion at the wrist of women. J Bone Joint Surg Br 10:775, 1928.
77. Palmer, ML, and Epler, M: Clinical Assessment Procedures in Physical Therapy, ed 2. JB Lippincott, Philadelphia, 1998.
78. Clarkson, HM: Musculoskeletal Assessment: Joint Range of Motion and Manual Muscle Strength, ed 2. Williams & Wilkins, Baltimore, 2000.
79. Robson, P: A method to reduce the variable error in joint range measurement. Ann Phys Med 8:262, 1966.
80. Mullaney, MJ, et al: Reliability of shoulder range of motion comparing a goniometer to a digital level. Physiother Theory Pract 26:327, 2010.
81. Goodwin, J, et al: Clinical methods of goniometry: A comparative study. Disabil Rehabil 14:10, 1992.
82. Petherick, M, et al: Concurrent validity and intertester reliability of universal and fluid-based goniometers for active elbow range of motion. Phys Ther 68:966, 1988.
83. Brown, A, et al: Validity and reliability of the Dexter hand evaluation and therapy system in hand-injured patients. J Hand Ther 13:37, 2000.
84. Weiss, PL, et al: Using the Exos Handmaster to measure digital range of motion: Reliability and validity. Med Eng Phys 16:323, 1994.
85. Clapper, MP, and Wolf, SL: Comparison of the reliability of the Ortho Ranger and the standard goniometer for assessing active lower extremity range of motion. Phys Ther 68:214, 1988.
86. Ellison, JB, Rose, SJ, and Sahrman, SA: Patterns of hip rotation: A comparison between healthy subjects and patients with low back pain. Phys Ther 70:537, 1990.
87. Rheault, W, et al: Intertester reliability and concurrent validity of fluid-based and universal goniometers for active knee flexion. Phys Ther 68:1676, 1988.
88. Rome, K, and Cowieson, F: A reliability study of the universal goniometer, fluid goniometer, and electrogoniometer for the measurement of ankle dorsiflexion. Foot Ankle Int 17:28, 1996.
89. Reynolds, PM: Measurement of spinal mobility: A comparison of three methods. Rheumatol Rehabil 14:180, 1975.
90. Miller, MH, et al: Measurement of spinal mobility in the sagittal plane: New skin distraction technique compared with established methods. Br J Rheumatol 11:4, 1984.
91. Gill, K, et al: Repeatability of four clinical methods for assessment of lumbar spinal motion. Spine 13:50, 1988.
92. Lindahl, O: Determination of the sagittal mobility of the lumbar spine. Acta Orthop Scand 37:241, 1966.
93. Mayer, RS, et al: Variance in the measurement of sagittal lumbar range of motion among examiners, subjects, and instruments. Spine 20:1489, 1995.
94. Chen, SP, et al: Reliability of the lumbar sagittal motion measurement methods: Surface inclinometers. J Occup Environ Med 39:217, 1997.
95. Breum, J, Wilberg, J, and Bolton, JE: Reliability and concurrent validity of the BROM II for measuring lumbar mobility. J Manipulative Physiol Ther 18:497, 1995.
96. Colton, T: Statistics in Medicine. Little, Brown, Boston, 1974.
97. Fetters, L, and Tilson, J. Evidence Based Physical Therapy. FA Davis, Philadelphia, 2013.
98. Di Fabio, RD. Essentials of Rehabilitation Research: A Statistical Guide to Clinical Practice. FA Davis, Philadelphia, 2013.
99. Bland, JM, and Altman, DG: Measurement error and correlation coefficients [statistics notes]. BMJ 313:41, 1996.
100. Lahey, MA, Downey, RG, and Saal, FE: Intraclass correlations: There's more there than meets the eye. Psychol Bull 93:586, 1983.
101. Shrout, PE, and Fleiss, JL: Intraclass correlations: Uses in assessing rater reliability. Psychol Bull 86:420, 1979.
102. Weir, JP: Quantifying test-retest reliability using the intraclass correlation coefficient and the SEM. J Strength Cond Res 19:231, 2005.
103. Stratford, P: Reliability: Consistency or differentiating among subjects? [letters to the editor]. Phys Ther 69:299, 1989.
104. Bland, JM, and Altman, DG: Measurement error [statistics notes]. BMJ 312:1654, 1996.
105. Rothstein, JM: Measurement and Clinical Practice: Theory and Application. In Rothstein, JM (ed): Measurement in Physical Therapy. Churchill Livingstone, New York, 1985, p 41.
106. DuBois, PH: An Introduction to Psychological Statistics. Harper & Row, New York, 1965, p 401.
107. Riddle, DL, and Stratford, PW: Is This Change Real? Interpreting Patient Outcomes in Physical Therapy. FA Davis, Philadelphia, 2013.
108. Bartko, JJ: Rationale for reporting standard deviations rather than standard errors of the mean. Am J Psychiatry 142:1060, 1985.
109. Stratford, P: Use of the standard error as a reliability index of interest: An applied example using elbow flexor strength data. Phys Ther 77:745, 1997.
110. Eliasziw, M, et al: Statistical methodology for the concurrent assessment of interrater and intrarater reliability: Using goniometric measurement as an example. Phys Ther 74:777, 1994.
111. Stratford, PW, and Riddle, DL: When minimal detectable change exceeds a diagnostic test-based threshold change value for an outcome measure: Resolving the conflict. Phys Ther 92:1338, 2012.
112. Haley, SM, and Fragala-Pinkham, MA: Interpreting change scores of tests and measures used in physical therapy. Phys Ther 86:735, 2006.

PART II

UPPER-EXTREMITY TESTING

OBJECTIVES

On completion of Part II, you will be able to:

1. Identify:

appropriate planes and axes for each upper-extremity joint motion
normal ranges of motion for each upper-extremity joint
structures that limit the end of the range of motion (ROM)
expected normal end-feels

2. Describe:

testing positions used for each upper-extremity joint motion and muscle length test
goniometer alignment for each motion and muscle length test
capsular pattern of restricted motion
range of motion necessary for selected functional activities at each major upper-extremity joint

3. Explain:

how age, gender, and other factors can affect the range of motion
how sources of error in measurement can affect testing results

4. Perform goniometric measurement of joint ROM and muscle length testing for the shoulder, elbow, wrist, and hand that includes:

a clear explanation of the testing procedure
proper placement of the individual in the testing position
adequate stabilization
correct determination of the end of the motion
correct identification of the end-feel
palpation of the appropriate bony landmarks
accurate alignment of the goniometer and correct reading and recording of goniometric measurements

5. Plan goniometric measurements of the shoulder, elbow, wrist, and hand that are organized by body position.

6. Assess intratester and intertester reliability of the reader's goniometric measurements of the upper-extremity joints using the statistical methods described in Chapter 3.

CHAPTER 4

The Shoulder

D. Joyce White, PT, DSc

Structure and Function

Shoulder Complex

The shoulder complex is composed of four joints: the glenohumeral (GH), sternoclavicular (SC), acromioclavicular (AC), and scapulothoracic joints. Full range of motion (ROM) of the shoulder requires coordinated motion at all four of these joints. Although there is some individual and motion-specific variability, about two-thirds of shoulder ROM occurs at the glenohumeral joint and one-third occurs at the remaining joints.[1–3] The distribution of shoulder complex motion across these multiple joints enables greater ROM and stability than if all motion were restricted to a single joint. The congruency between the head of the humerus and glenoid fossa of the scapula is improved, which reduces bone shearing forces. In addition, the muscles acting across the glenohumeral joint are maintained in a more optimal length-tension relationship, which reduces the potential problem of active insufficiency.[2]

The motions that occur at these joints must be coordinated to enable full, pain-free shoulder motions. For example, to achieve active flexion of the shoulder, the humerus undergoes flexion and some lateral rotation at the GH joint; the clavicle typically undergoes posterior rotation, retraction, and elevation at the SC joint; and the scapula undergoes posterior tilting, upward rotation, and protraction relative to the clavicle at the AC joint.[4] The combination of retraction of the clavicle and protraction of the scapula results in some retraction of the scapula relative to the thorax. Specific information about the GH, SC, AC, and scapulothoracic joints that comprise the shoulder complex is presented in the following sections.

Glenohumeral Joint

The glenohumeral (GH) joint is a synovial ball-and-socket joint. The ball is the convex head of the humerus, which faces medially, superiorly, and posteriorly with respect to the shaft of the humerus (Fig. 4.1).[1,2] The socket is formed by the concave glenoid fossa of the scapula and faces laterally, superiorly, and anteriorly. The socket is shallow and smaller than the humeral head but is deepened and enlarged by the fibrocartilaginous glenoid labrum. The joint capsule is thin and lax, blends with the glenoid labrum, and is reinforced by the glenohumeral (superior, middle, inferior) and coracohumeral ligaments (Fig. 4.2), as well as the tendons of the rotator cuff muscles (subscapularis, supraspinatus, infraspinatus, and teres minor) and long head of the biceps brachii muscle.

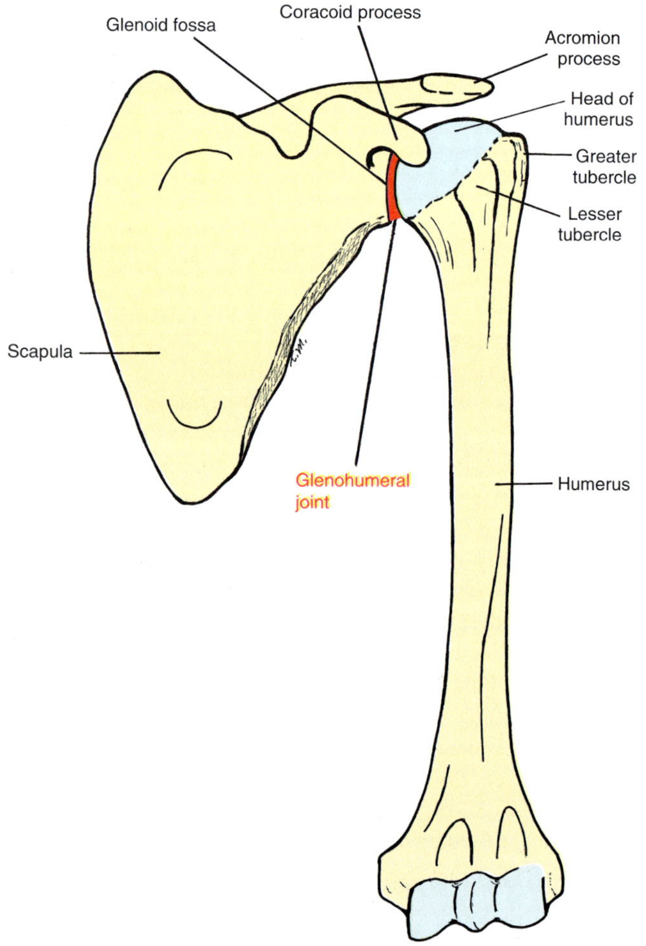

FIGURE 4.1 An anterior view of the left glenohumeral joint.

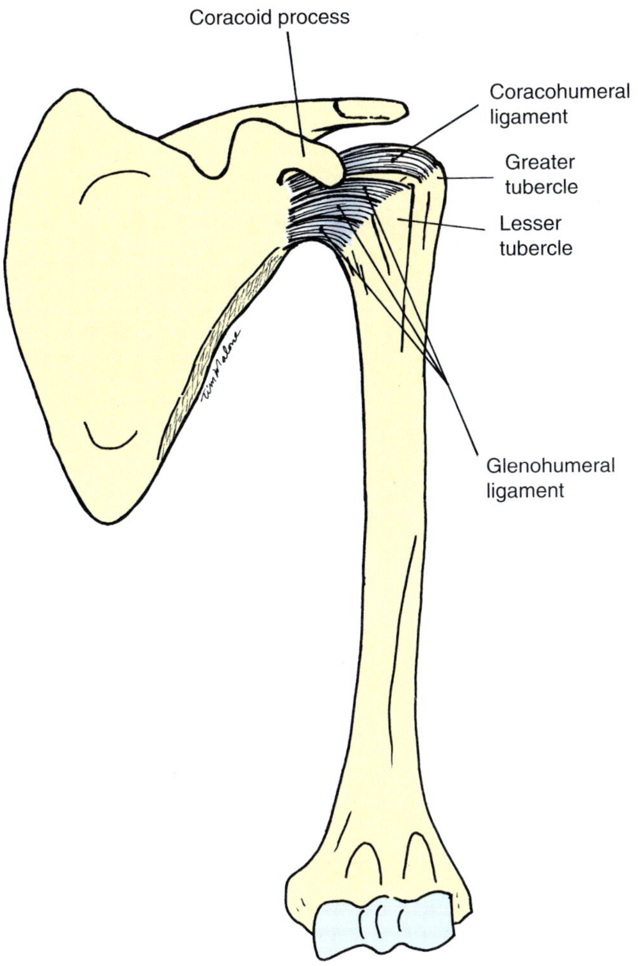

FIGURE 4.2 An anterior view of the left glenohumeral joint showing the coracohumeral and glenohumeral ligaments.

Osteokinematics

The GH joint has 3 degrees of freedom. The motions permitted at the joint are flexion–extension, abduction–adduction, and medial–lateral rotation that lie in the sagittal, frontal, and transverse cardinal planes, respectively.[2,3] Normative ROM values for these glenohumeral motions are presented in the Testing Procedures and Research Findings sections of this chapter.

In addition, horizontal abduction and horizontal adduction are functional motions performed at the level of the shoulder: Horizontal abduction is created by combining abduction and extension, and horizontal adduction is created by combining adduction and flexion. Another functional motion, often referred to as scapular plane abduction or scaption, is elevation of the humerus in a plane of motion that is 30 to 45 degrees anterior to the frontal plane of the body.[2,3,5] This plane of movement more closely matches the plane of the scapula and the anterior lateral orientation of the glenoid fossa than it does pure abduction in the frontal plane.

Arthrokinematics

Motion at the GH joint occurs as a rolling and sliding of the head of the humerus on the glenoid fossa. The convex joint surface of the head of the humerus slides in the opposite direction and rolls in the same direction as the osteokinematic movements of the shaft of the humerus.[2,3,6,7] The sliding motions help to maintain contact between the head of the humerus and the glenoid fossa of the scapular during the rolling motions and reduce translational movement of the axis of rotation in the humerus. During abduction, the surface of the humeral head slides inferiorly while rolling superiorly. The opposite motions occur during adduction. In medial rotation and flexion, the surface of the humeral head slides posteriorly and rolls anteriorly. In lateral rotation and extension, the surface of the humeral head slides anteriorly and rolls posteriorly on the glenoid fossa. Arthrokinematic motions during flexion and extension have also been described as a spin.[3]

Capsular Pattern

The greatest restriction of passive motion is in lateral rotation, followed by some restriction in abduction and less restriction in medial rotation.[7,8]

Sternoclavicular Joint

The sternoclavicular (SC) joint is a synovial joint linking the medial end of the clavicle with the sternum and the cartilage of the first rib (Fig. 4.3A). The joint surfaces are saddle-shaped.[1–3] The clavicular joint surface is convex cephalocaudally and concave anteroposteriorly. The opposing joint surface, located at the notch formed by the manubrium of the sternum and the first costal cartilage, is concave cephalocaudally and convex anteroposteriorly. An articular disc divides the joint into two separate compartments.

The associated joint capsule is strong and is reinforced by anterior and posterior sternoclavicular ligaments (Fig. 4.3B).[2,3] These ligaments limit anterior–posterior movement of the medial end of the clavicle. The costoclavicular ligament, which extends from the inferior surface of the medial end of the clavicle to the first rib, limits clavicular elevation and protraction.[2] The interclavicular ligament extends from one clavicle to another and limits excessive inferior movement of the clavicle.[2,3]

Osteokinematics

The SC joint has 3 degrees of freedom, and motion consists of movement of the clavicle on the sternum. These motions are described by the movement at the lateral end of the clavicle. Clavicular motions include elevation–depression in the frontal plane, protraction–retraction in the horizontal plane, and anterior–posterior rotation around the longitudinal axis through the length of the clavicle.[2,3,5]

Arthrokinematics

During clavicular elevation and depression, the convex portion of the joint surface of the clavicle slides on the concave manubrium in the opposite direction and rolls in the same direction as movement of the lateral end of the clavicle.[2,3,6,7] In protraction and retraction, the concave portion of the clavicular joint surface slides and rolls on the convex surface of the manubrium in the same direction as the lateral end of the clavicle. In rotation, the clavicular joint surface spins on the opposing joint surface. In summary, the clavicle slides inferiorly in

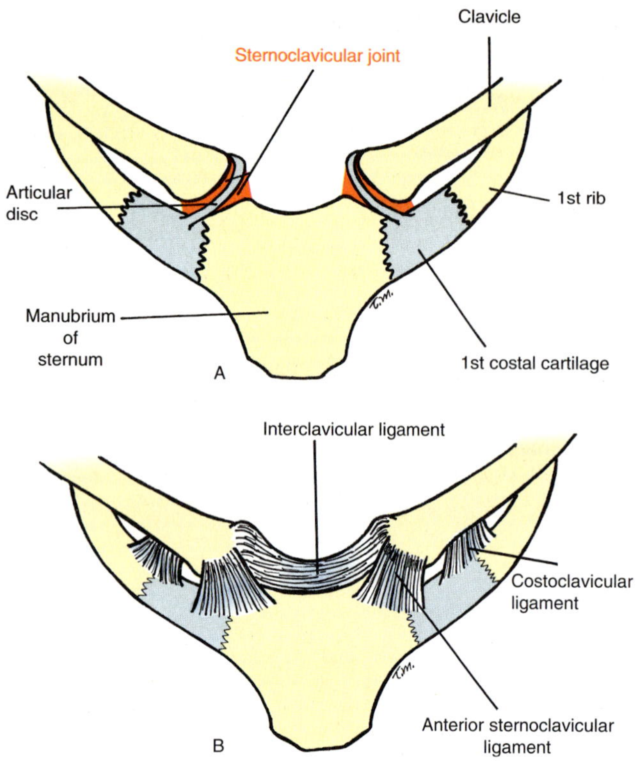

FIGURE 4.3 (A) An anterior view of the sternoclavicular joint showing the bone structures and articular disc. (B) An anterior view of the sternoclavicular joint showing the interclavicular, sternoclavicular, and costoclavicular ligaments.

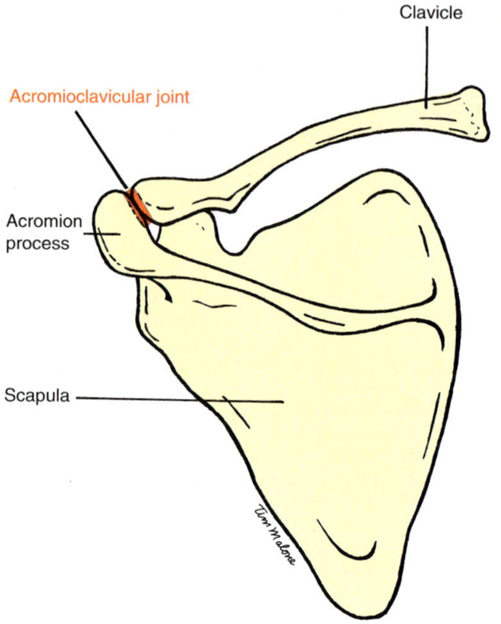

FIGURE 4.4 A posterior–superior view of the left acromioclavicular joint.

elevation, superiorly in depression, anteriorly in protraction, and posteriorly in retraction.

Acromioclavicular Joint

The acromioclavicular (AC) joint is a synovial joint linking the scapula to the clavicle. The scapular joint surface is a shallow concave facet located on the medial aspect of the acromion of the scapula (Fig. 4.4).[2,3] The clavicular joint surface is a slightly convex facet located on the lateral end of the clavicle. However, in some individuals the joint surfaces may be flat or the reverse pattern of convex–concave shapes.[1] The joint contains a fibrocartilaginous disc and is surrounded by a weak joint capsule. The superior and inferior acromioclavicular ligaments reinforce the capsule (Fig. 4.5). The coracoclavicular ligament, which extends between the clavicle and the scapular coracoid process, provides additional stability.

Osteokinematics

The AC joint has 3 degrees of freedom and permits angular movement of the scapula on the clavicle in three planes.[2,3] Tilting (tipping) is movement of the scapula in the sagittal plane around a coronal axis. During anterior tilting the superior border of the scapula and glenoid fossa move anteriorly, whereas the inferior angle moves posteriorly. During posterior tilting (tipping) the superior border of the scapula and glenoid fossa move posteriorly, whereas the inferior angle moves anteriorly.

Upward and downward rotations of the scapula occur in the frontal plane around an anterior–posterior axis. During upward rotation the glenoid fossa moves cranially, whereas during downward rotation the glenoid fossa moves caudally.

Protraction and retraction of the scapula occur in the transverse plane around a vertical axis. During protraction (also termed winging) the glenoid fossa moves medially and anteriorly, whereas the vertebral border of the scapula moves away from the spine. During retraction the glenoid fossa moves laterally and posteriorly, whereas the vertebral border of the scapula moves toward the spine.

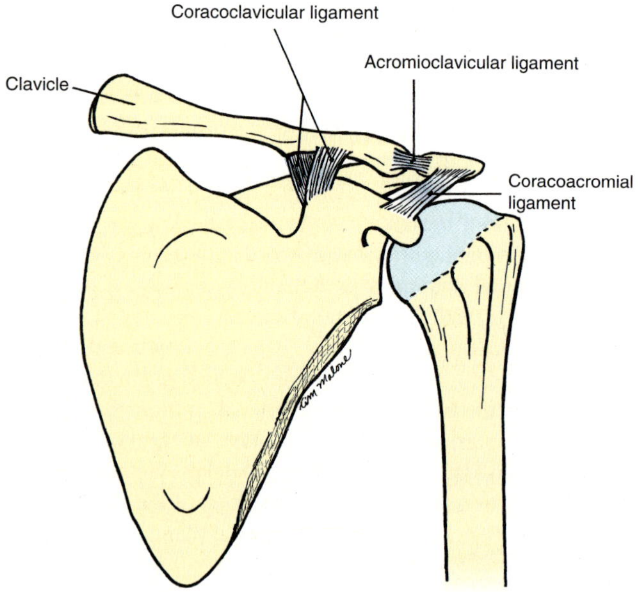

FIGURE 4.5 An anterior view of the left acromioclavicular joint showing the coracoclavicular, acromioclavicular, and coracoacromial ligaments.

Numerous terms have been used to describe AC motions, but we find the terms described above to be most easily understood. Some sources have used the terms "medial rotation" and "lateral rotation" to describe protraction and retraction. However, depending on whether the glenoid fossa or vertebral border of the scapula is referenced, protraction has been described as either medial rotation[2–4] or lateral rotation,[1,7] respectively. Similar issues arise with the use of rotation to describe retraction. We have also avoided the use of abduction–adduction to describe scapula motion because these terms have been used to indicate the motions of upward rotation–downward rotation as well as protraction–retraction.[5]

Arthrokinematics

If the acromial facet is concave in shape, it will slide and roll on the lateral end of the clavicle in the same direction as the osteokinematic movement of the scapula.[6,7]

Scapulothoracic Joint

The scapulothoracic joint is considered to be a functional rather than an anatomical joint. The joint surfaces are the anterior surface of the scapula and the posterior surface of the thorax.

Osteokinematics

The motions that occur at the scapulothoracic joint are caused by the independent or combined motions of the sternoclavicular and acromioclavicular joints. These motions are described in many ways and include scapular elevation–depression, upward–downward rotation, anterior–posterior tilting, and protraction–retraction.

Arthrokinematics

Motion consists of a sliding of the scapula on the thorax.

RANGE OF MOTION TESTING PROCEDURES: Shoulder

To make measurements more informative for the clinician, we suggest using two methods of measuring the ROM of the shoulder. One method measures passive motion primarily at the glenohumeral joint. The other method measures passive or active ROM at all the joints included in the shoulder complex.

We have found the method that measures primarily glenohumeral motion is helpful in identifying glenohumeral joint problems within the shoulder complex. The ability to differentiate and quantify ROM at the glenohumeral joint from other joints in the shoulder complex is important in diagnosing and treating many shoulder conditions. This method of measuring glenohumeral motion requires the use of passive motion and careful stabilization of the scapula. Active motion is avoided because it results in synchronous motion throughout the shoulder complex, making isolation of glenohumeral motion difficult. Some studies have begun establishing normative values and assessing the reliability of this glenohumeral measurement method.[9–15]

The second method measures full motion of the shoulder complex and is useful in evaluating the functional ROM of the shoulder. This more traditional method of assessing shoulder motion incorporates the stabilization of the thoracic spine and rib cage. Both methods of measuring the ROM of the shoulder are presented in the following discussions of stabilization techniques and end-feels. However, the alignment of the goniometer is the same for measuring glenohumeral and shoulder complex motions.

Landmarks for Testing Procedures

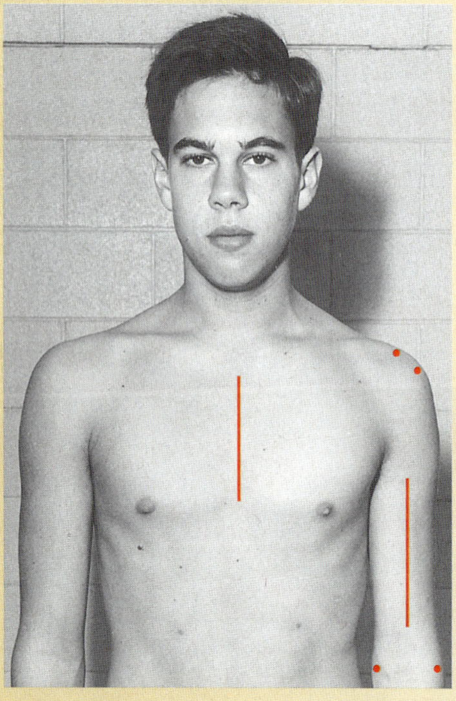

FIGURE 4.6 An anterior view of the humerus, clavicle, sternum, and scapula showing surface anatomy landmarks for aligning the goniometer.

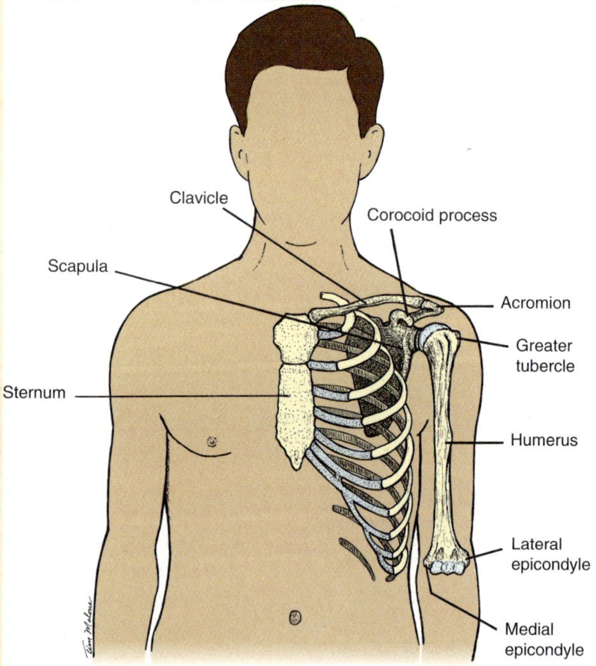

FIGURE 4.7 An anterior view of the humerus, clavicle, sternum, and scapula showing bony anatomical landmarks for aligning the goniometer.

Landmarks for Testing Procedures (continued)

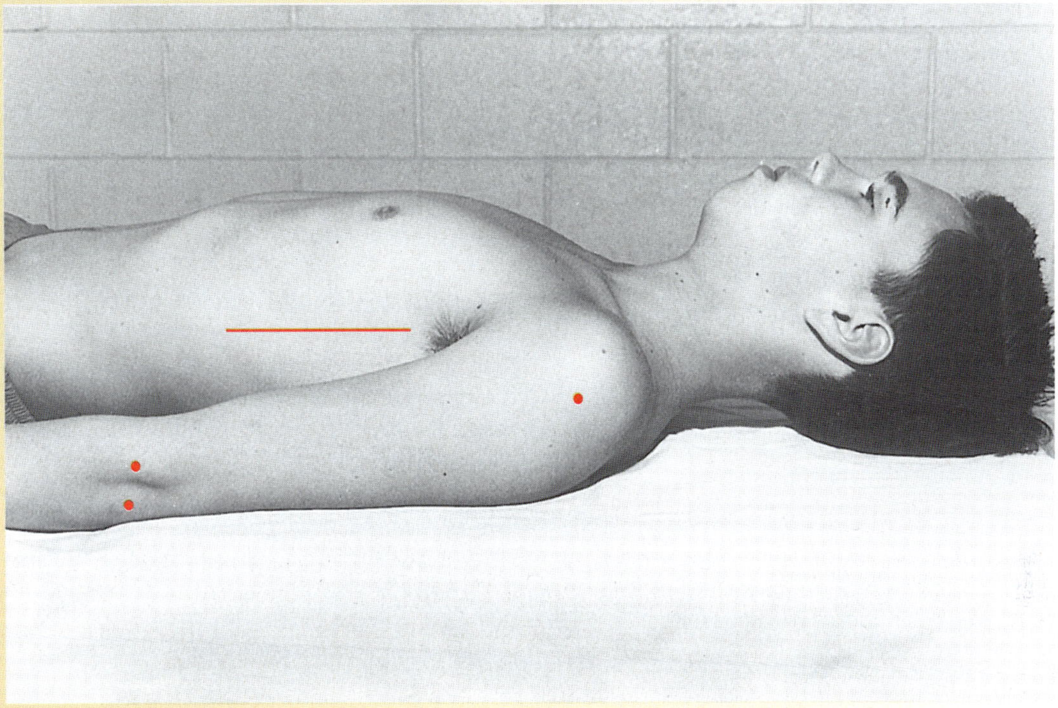

FIGURE 4.8 A lateral view of the upper arm showing surface anatomy landmarks for aligning the goniometer.

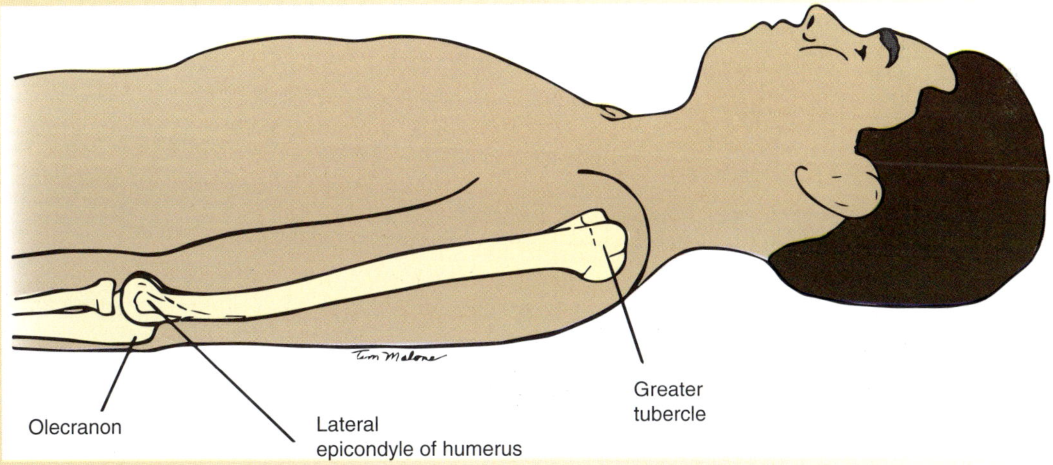

FIGURE 4.9 A lateral view of the upper arm showing bony anatomical landmarks for aligning the goniometer.

FLEXION

Motion occurs in the sagittal plane around a medial–lateral axis. Normal *shoulder complex* flexion ROM values for adults vary from about 165 to 180 degrees. Normal *glenohumeral* flexion ROM values for adults vary from about 100 to 115 degrees. See Research Findings and Tables 4.1 to 4.4 for more detailed normal ROM values by age and joint.

Testing Position

Place the individual supine with the knees flexed to flatten the lumbar spine. Position the shoulder in 0 degrees of abduction, adduction, and rotation. Place the elbow in extension so that tension in the long head of the triceps muscle does not limit the motion. Position the forearm in 0 degrees of supination and pronation so that the palm of the hand faces the body.

Stabilization

Glenohumeral Flexion

Stabilize the scapula to prevent posterior tilting, upward rotation, and elevation of the scapula.

Shoulder Complex Flexion

Stabilize the thorax to prevent extension of the spine and movement of the ribs. The weight of the trunk may assist stabilization.

Testing Motion

Flex the shoulder by lifting the humerus off the examining table, bringing the hand up over the individual's head. Maintain the extremity in neutral abduction and adduction during the motion. Slight rotation is allowed to occur as needed to attain maximal flexion.

Glenohumeral Flexion

The end of glenohumeral flexion ROM occurs when resistance to further motion is felt and attempts to overcome the resistance cause upward rotation, posterior tilting, or elevation of the scapula (Fig. 4.10).

Shoulder Complex Flexion

The end of shoulder complex flexion ROM occurs when resistance to further motion is felt and attempts to overcome the resistance cause extension of the spine or motion of the ribs (Fig. 4.11).

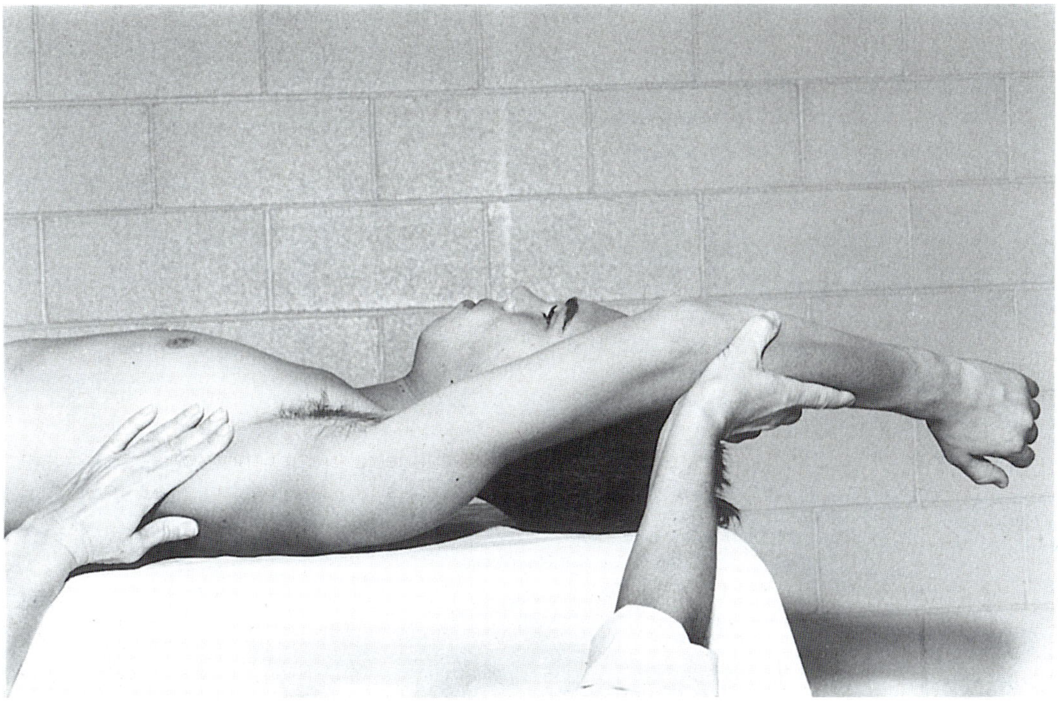

FIGURE 4.10 The end of glenohumeral flexion ROM. The examiner stabilizes the lateral border of the scapula with her hand. The examiner is able to determine that the end of the ROM has been reached because any attempt to move the extremity into additional flexion causes the lateral border of the scapula to move anteriorly and laterally.

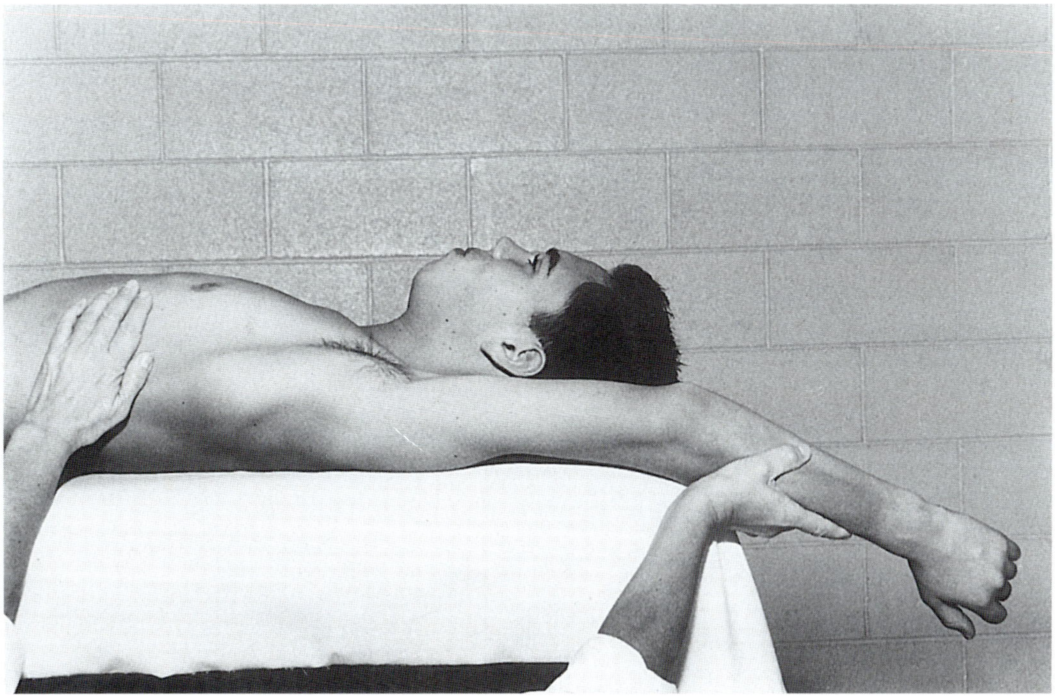

FIGURE 4.11 The end of shoulder complex flexion ROM. The examiner stabilizes the individual's trunk and ribs with her hand. The examiner is able to determine that the end of the ROM has been reached because any attempt to move the extremity into additional flexion causes extension of the spine and movement of the ribs.

Normal End-Feel

Glenohumeral Flexion

The end-feel is firm because of tension in the posterior band of the coracohumeral ligament; the posterior joint capsule; and the posterior deltoid, teres minor, teres major, and infraspinatus muscles.

Shoulder Complex Flexion

The end-feel is firm because of tension in the costoclavicular ligament and SC capsule and ligaments, and the latissimus dorsi, sternocostal fibers of the pectoralis major and pectoralis minor, and rhomboid major and minor muscles.

Goniometer Alignment

This goniometer alignment is used for measuring glenohumeral and shoulder complex flexion (Figs. 4.12 through 4.14).

1. Center **fulcrum** of the goniometer over the lateral aspect of the greater tubercle.
2. Align **proximal arm** parallel to the midaxillary line of the thorax.
3. Align **distal arm** with the lateral midline of the humerus. Depending on how much flexion and rotation occur, the lateral epicondyle of the humerus or the olecranon process of the ulnar may be helpful references.

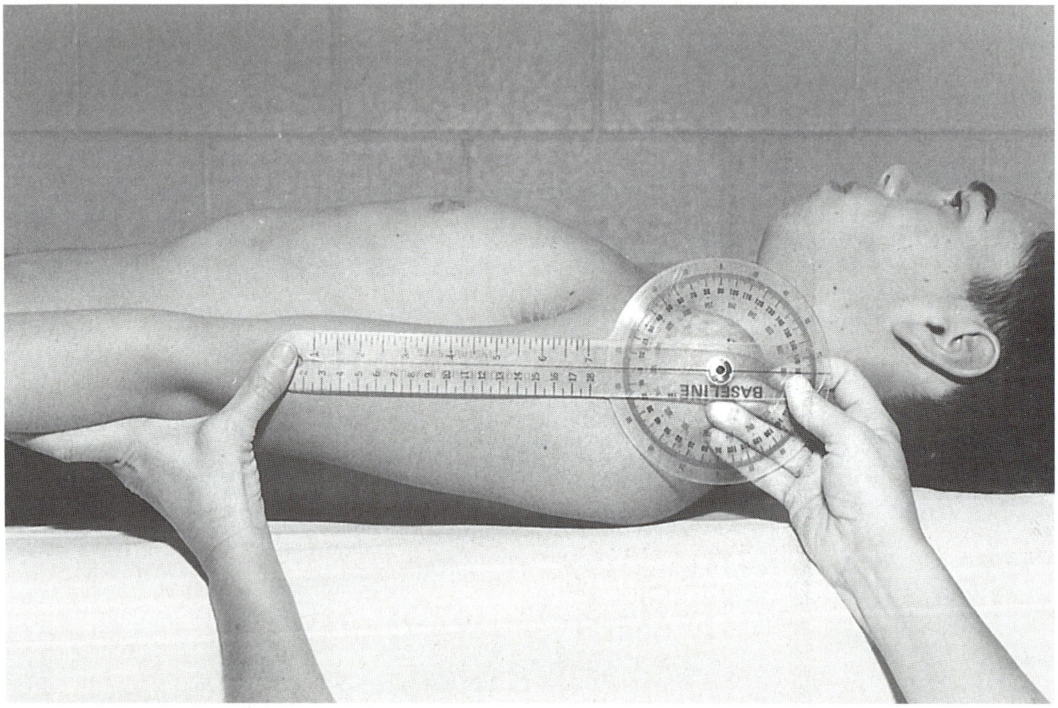

FIGURE 4.12 The alignment of the goniometer at the beginning of glenohumeral and shoulder complex flexion ROM.

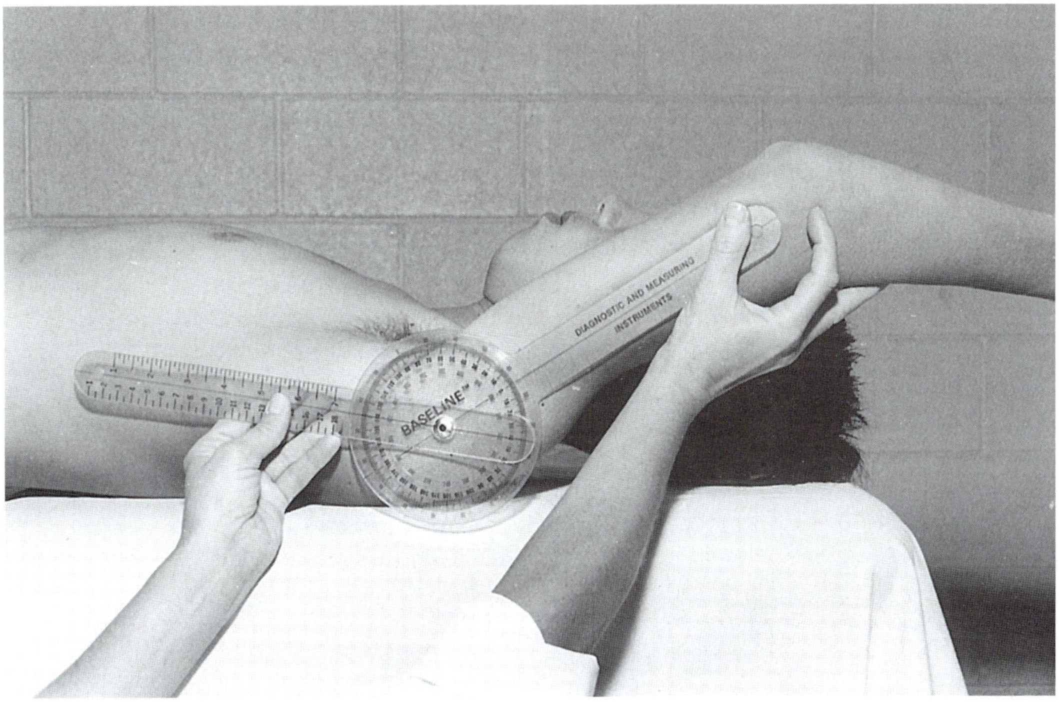

FIGURE 4.13 The alignment of the goniometer at the end of glenohumeral flexion ROM. The examiner's hand supports the individual's extremity and maintains the goniometer's distal arm in correct alignment over the lateral epicondyle. The examiner's other hand releases its stabilization and aligns the goniometer's proximal arm with the lateral midline of the thorax.

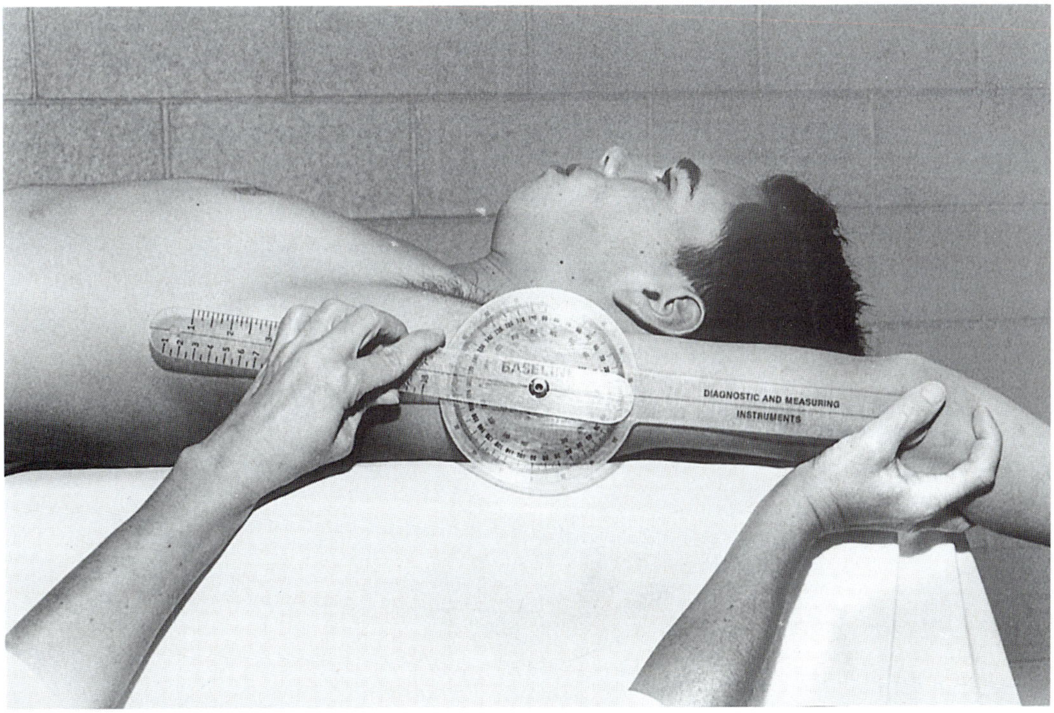

FIGURE 4.14 The alignment of the goniometer at the end of shoulder complex flexion ROM. More motion is noted during shoulder complex flexion than in glenohumeral flexion.

EXTENSION

Motion occurs in the sagittal plane around a medial–lateral axis. Normal *shoulder complex* extension ROM values for adults vary from about 50 to 60 degrees. Normal *glenohumeral* extension ROM values for adults vary from about 20 to 25 degrees. See Research Findings and Tables 4.1 to 4.4 for more detailed normal ROM values by age and joint.

Testing Position

Position the individual prone, with the face turned away from the shoulder being tested. A pillow is not used under the head. Place the shoulder in 0 degrees of abduction, adduction, and rotation. Position the elbow in slight flexion so that tension in the long head of the biceps brachii muscle will not restrict the motion. Place the forearm in 0 degrees of supination and pronation so that the palm of the hand faces the body.

Stabilization

Glenohumeral Extension

Stabilize the scapula at the inferior angle or at the acromion and coracoid processes to prevent elevation and anterior tilting (inferior angle moves posteriorly) of the scapula.

Shoulder Complex Extension

The examining table and the weight of the trunk stabilize the thorax to prevent forward flexion of the spine. The examiner can also stabilize the trunk to prevent rotation of the spine.

Testing Motion

Extend the shoulder by lifting the humerus off the examining table. Maintain the extremity in neutral abduction and adduction during the motion.

Glenohumeral Extension

The end of ROM occurs when resistance to further motion is felt and attempts to overcome the resistance cause anterior tilting or elevation of the scapula (Fig. 4.15).

Shoulder Complex Extension

The end of ROM occurs when resistance to further motion is felt and attempts to overcome the resistance cause forward flexion or rotation of the spine (Fig. 4.16).

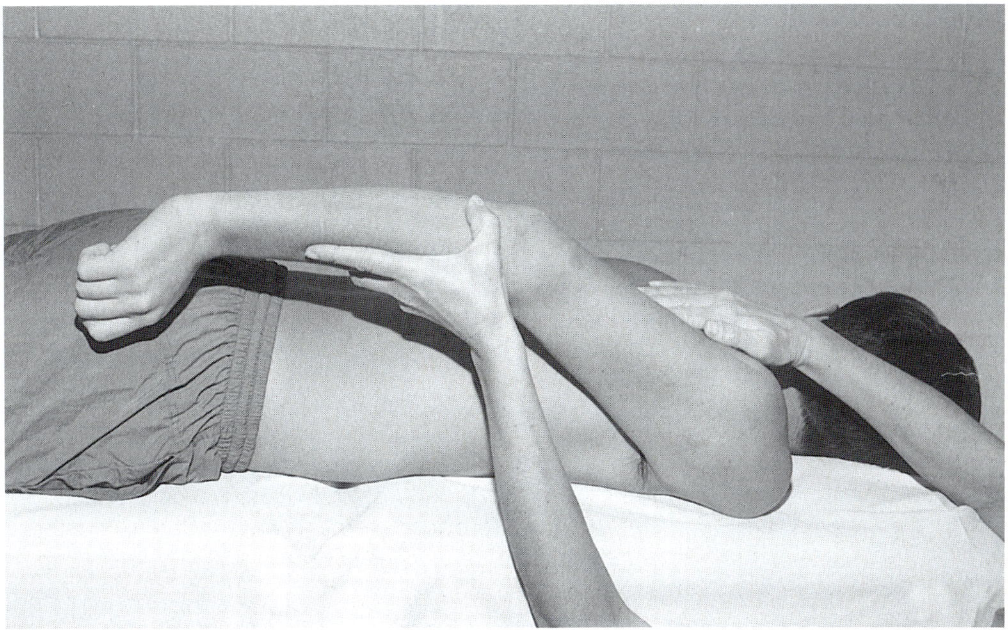

FIGURE 4.15 The end of glenohumeral extension ROM. The examiner is stabilizing the inferior angle of the scapula with her hand. The examiner is able to determine that the end of the ROM in extension has been reached because any attempt to move the humerus into additional extension causes the scapula to tilt anteriorly and to elevate, causing the inferior angle of the scapula to move posteriorly. Alternatively, the examiner may stabilize the acromion and coracoid processes of the scapula.

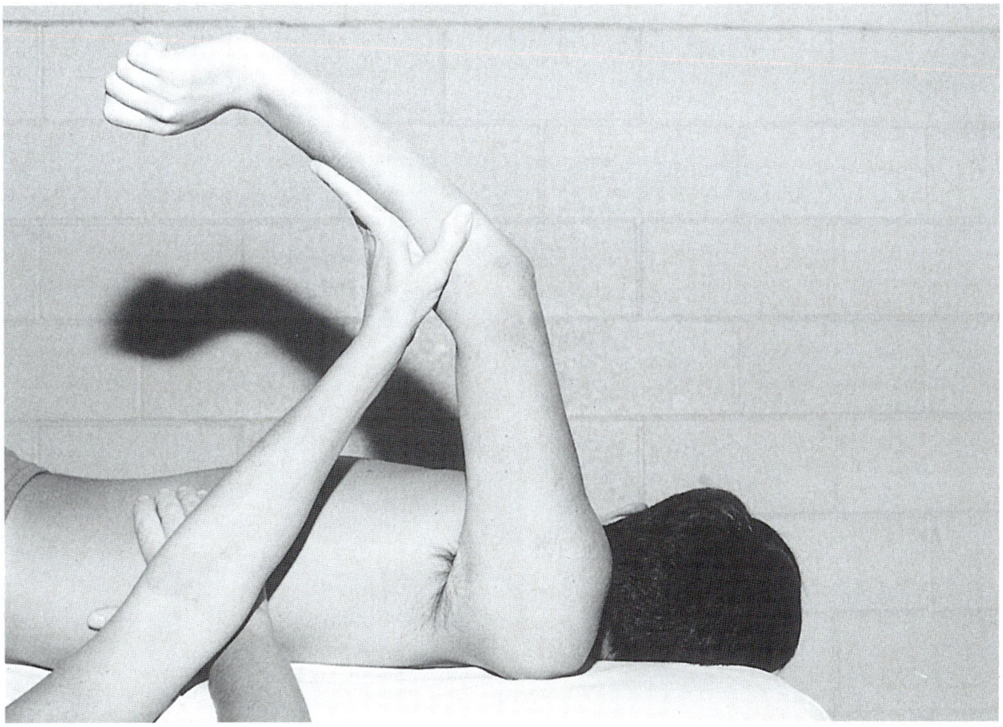

FIGURE 4.16 The end shoulder complex extension ROM. The examiner stabilizes the individual's trunk and ribs with her hand. The examiner is able to determine that the end of the ROM has been reached because any attempt to move the extremity into additional extension causes flexion and rotation of the spine.

Normal End-Feel

Glenohumeral Extension

The end-feel is firm because of tension in the anterior band of the coracohumeral ligament; anterior joint capsule; and clavicular fibers of the pectoralis major, coracobrachialis, and anterior deltoid muscles.

Shoulder Complex Extension

The end-feel is firm because of tension in the SC capsule and ligaments and in the serratus anterior muscle.

Goniometer Alignment

This goniometer alignment is used for measuring glenohumeral and shoulder complex extension (Figs. 4.17 to 4.19).

1. Center **fulcrum** of the goniometer over the lateral aspect of the greater tubercle.
2. Align **proximal arm** parallel to the midaxillary line of the thorax.
3. Align **distal arm** with the lateral midline of the humerus, using the lateral epicondyle of the humerus for reference.

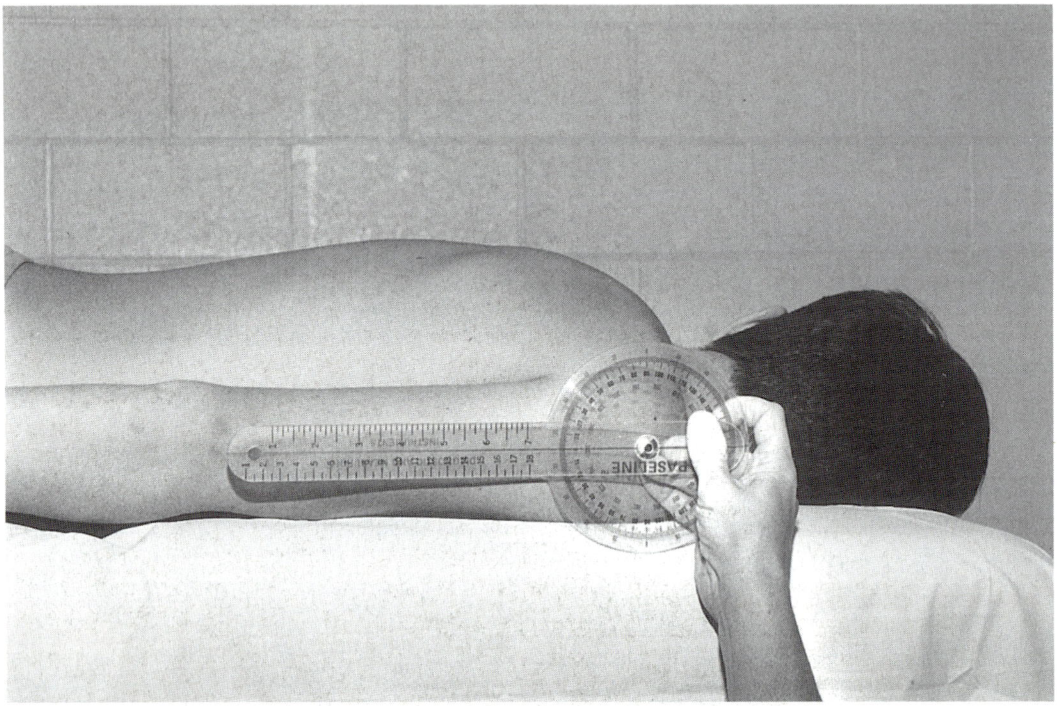

FIGURE 4.17 The alignment of the goniometer at the beginning of glenohumeral and shoulder complex extension ROM.

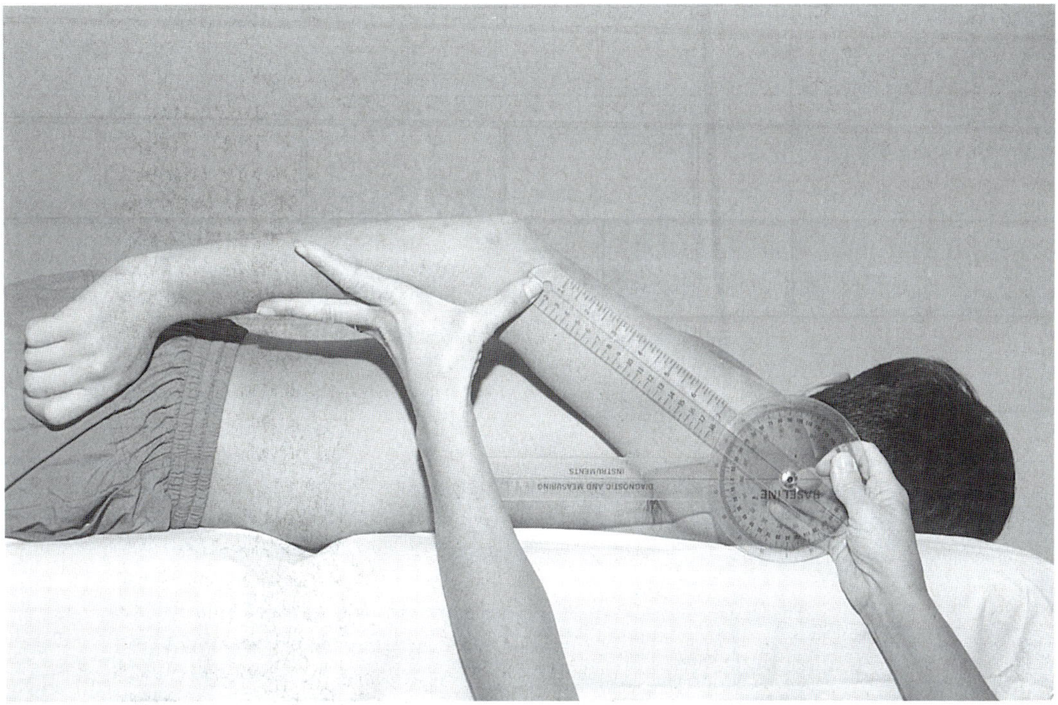

FIGURE 4.18 The alignment of the goniometer at the end of glenohumeral extension ROM. The examiner's left hand supports the individual's extremity and holds the distal arm of the goniometer in correct alignment over the lateral epicondyle of the humerus.

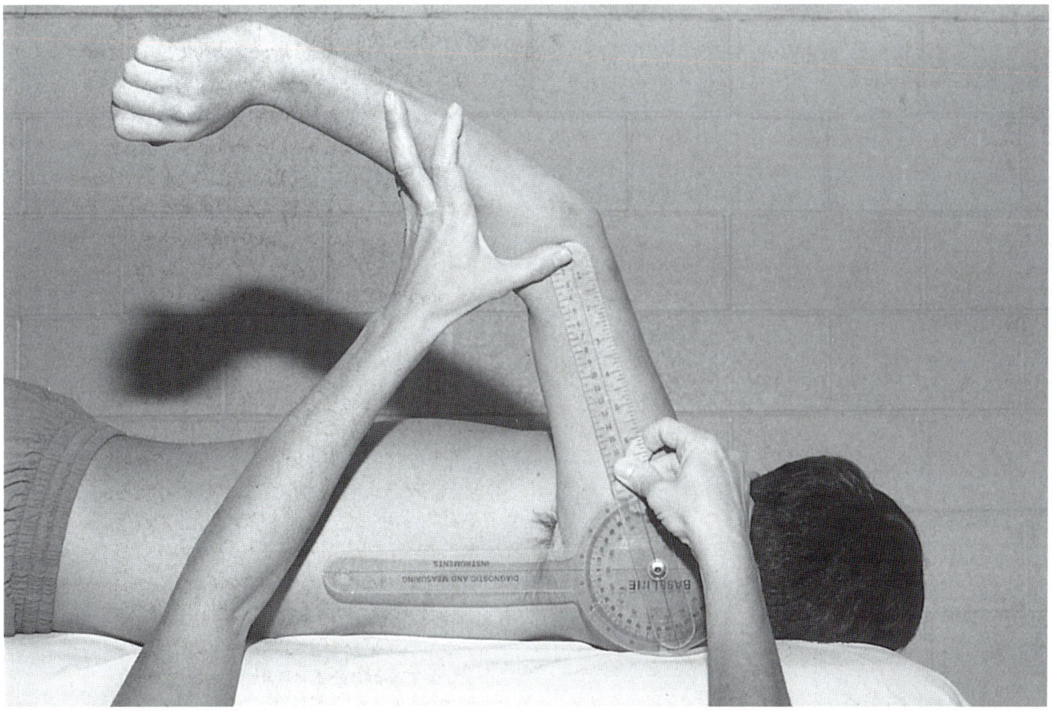

FIGURE 4.19 The alignment of the goniometer at the end of shoulder complex extension ROM. The examiner's hand that formerly stabilized the individual's trunk now positions the goniometer.

ABDUCTION

Motion occurs in the frontal plane around an anterior–posterior axis. Normal *shoulder complex* abduction ROM values for adults vary from about 170 to 180 degrees. Normal *glenohumeral* abduction ROM values for adults vary from about 90 to 125 degrees. See Research Findings and Tables 4.1 to 4.4 for more detailed normal ROM values by age and joint.

Testing Position

Position the individual supine, with the shoulder in lateral rotation and 0 degrees of flexion and extension so that the palm of the hand faces anteriorly. If the humerus is not laterally rotated, contact between the greater tubercle of the humerus and the upper portion of the glenoid fossa or the acromion process will restrict the motion. The elbow should be extended so that tension in the long head of the triceps does not restrict the motion.

Stabilization

Glenohumeral Abduction

Stabilize the scapula to prevent upward rotation and elevation of the scapula.

Shoulder Complex Abduction

Stabilize the thorax to prevent lateral flexion of the spine. The weight of the trunk may assist stabilization.

Testing Motion

Abduct the shoulder by moving the humerus laterally away from the individual's trunk. Maintain the upper extremity in lateral rotation and neutral flexion and extension during the motion.

Glenohumeral Abduction

The end of ROM occurs when resistance to further motion is felt and attempts to overcome the resistance cause upward rotation or elevation of the scapula (Fig. 4.20).

Shoulder Complex Abduction

The end of ROM occurs when resistance to further motion is felt and attempts to overcome the resistance cause lateral flexion of the spine (Fig. 4.21).

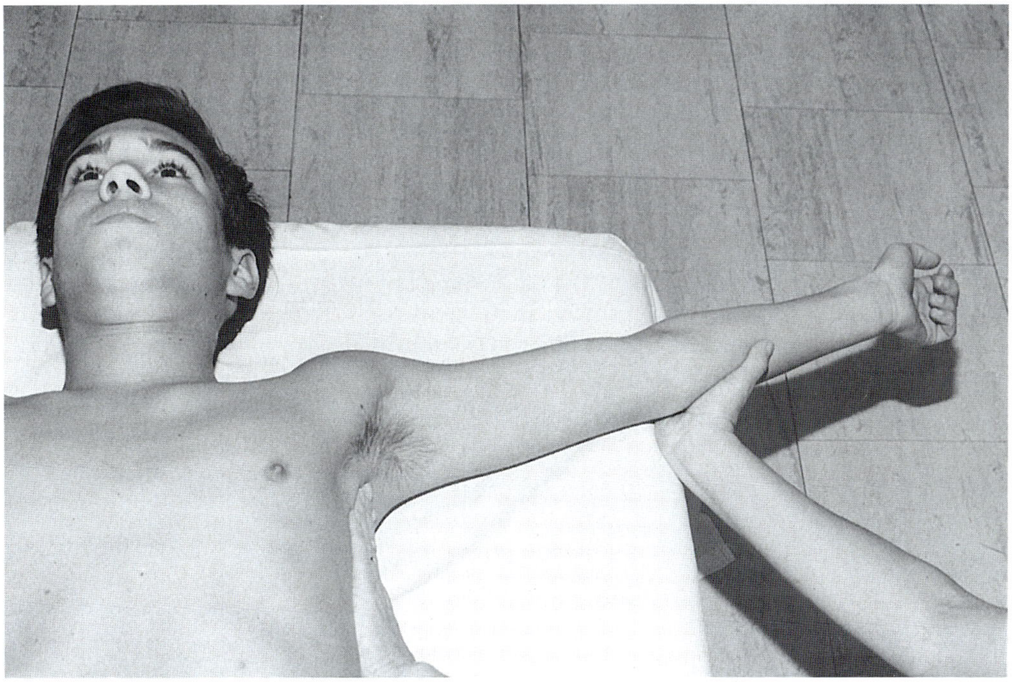

FIGURE 4.20 The end of the ROM of glenohumeral abduction. The examiner stabilizes the lateral border of the scapula with her hand to detect upward rotation of the scapula. Alternatively, the examiner may stabilize the acromion and coracoid processes of the scapula to detect elevation of the scapula.

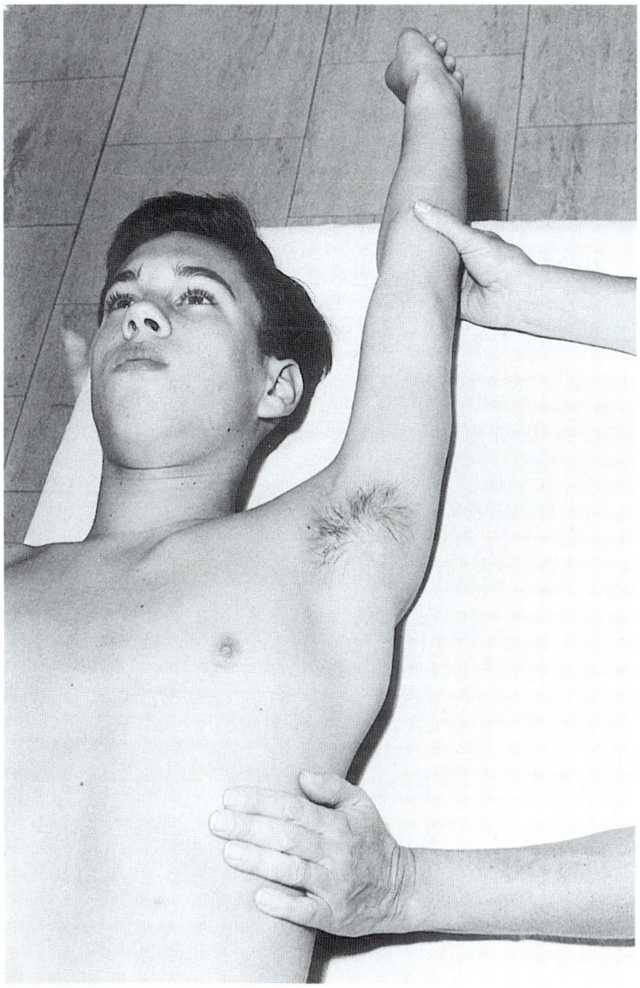

FIGURE 4.21 The end of the ROM of shoulder complex abduction. The examiner stabilizes the individual's trunk and ribs with her hand to detect lateral flexion of the spine and movement of the ribs.

Normal End-Feel

Glenohumeral Abduction

The end-feel is usually firm because of tension in the middle and inferior bands of the glenohumeral ligament, inferior joint capsule, and the teres major and clavicular fibers of the pectoralis major muscles.

Shoulder Complex Abduction

The end-feel is firm because of tension in the costoclavicular ligament; sternoclavicular capsule and ligaments; and latissimus dorsi, sternocostal fibers of the pectoralis major, and major and minor rhomboid muscles.

Goniometer Alignment

This goniometer alignment is used for measuring glenohumeral and shoulder complex abduction (Figs. 4.22 to 4.24).

1. Center **fulcrum** of the goniometer close to the anterior aspect of the acromial process.
2. Align **proximal arm** so that it is parallel to the midline of the anterior aspect of the sternum.
3. Align **distal arm** with the anterior midline of the humerus. Depending on the amount of abduction and lateral rotation that has occurred, the medial epicondyle may be a helpful reference.

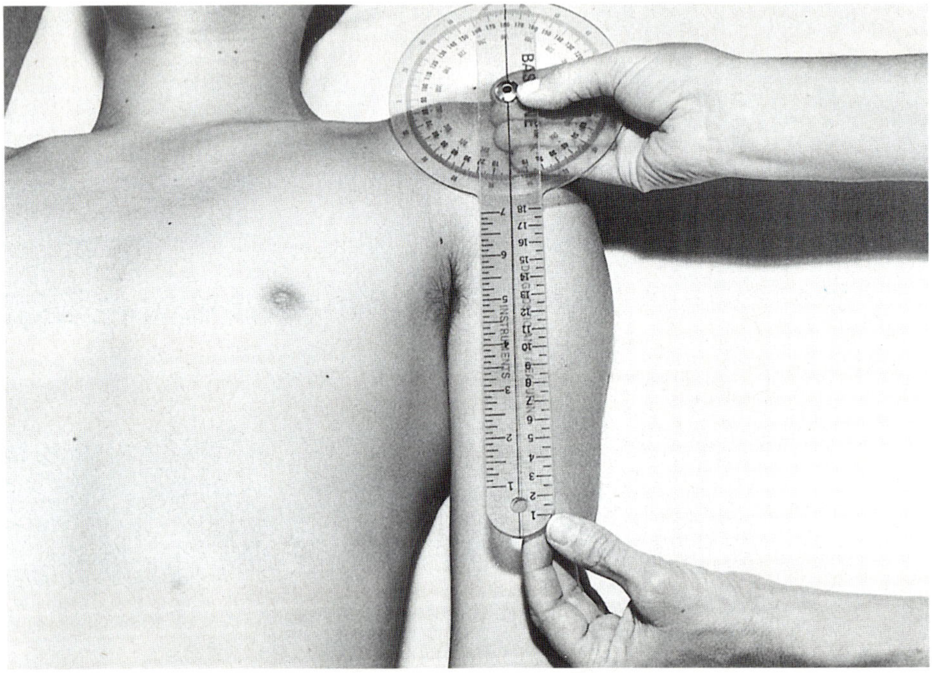

FIGURE 4.22 The alignment of the goniometer at the beginning of glenohumeral and shoulder complex abduction ROM.

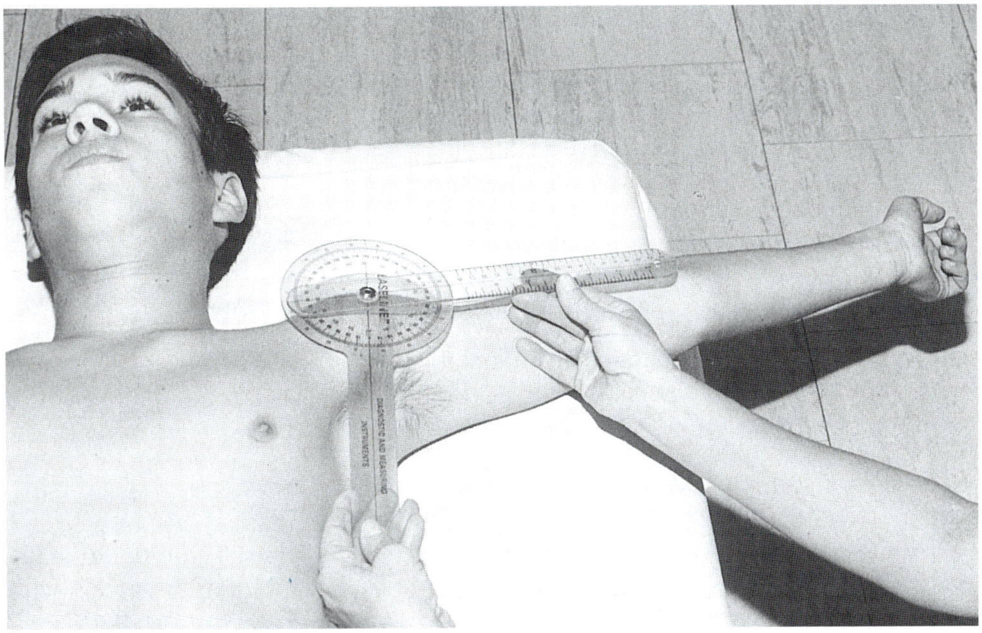

FIGURE 4.23 The alignment of the goniometer at the end of glenohumeral abduction ROM. The examining table or the examiner's hand can support the individual's extremity and align the goniometer's distal arm with the anterior midline of the humerus. The examiner's other hand has released its stabilization of the scapula and is holding the proximal arm of the goniometer parallel to the sternum.

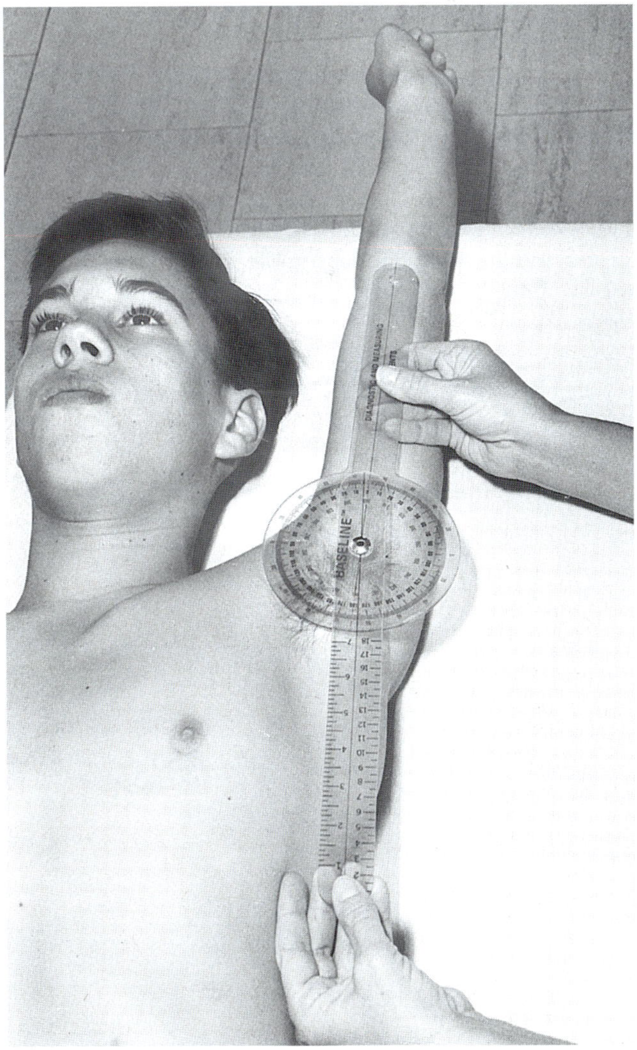

FIGURE 4.24 The alignment of the goniometer at the end of shoulder complex abduction ROM. The humerus has laterally rotated, and the medial epicondyle is now a helpful anatomical landmark for aligning the distal arm of the goniometer. Note that the placement of the stationary and moving arms of the goniometer with the proximal and distal joint segments have inadvertently been switched from that in Figure 4.23, but both placements will give an accurate measurement of the angle at the end of motion.

ADDUCTION

Motion occurs in the frontal plane around an anterior–posterior axis. Adduction in the frontal plane is not usually measured and recorded because it is the return to the zero starting position from full abduction. Further adduction can occur if the arm is positioned anterior to the body so that contact is avoided, but in that case adduction is combined with shoulder flexion.

MEDIAL (INTERNAL) ROTATION

When the individual is in anatomical position, the motion occurs in the transverse plane around a vertical axis. When the individual is in the testing position, the motion occurs in the sagittal plane around a medial–lateral (coronal) axis. Normal *shoulder complex* medial rotation ROM values for adults vary from about 70 to 90 degrees. Normal *glenohumeral* medial rotation ROM values for adults vary from about 50 to 60 degrees. See Research Findings and Tables 4.1 to 4.4 for more detailed normal ROM values by age and joint.

Testing Position

Position the individual supine, with the arm being tested in 90 degrees of shoulder abduction. Place the forearm perpendicular to the supporting surface and in 0 degrees of supination and pronation so that the palm of the hand faces the feet. Rest the full length of the humerus on the examining table. The elbow is not supported by the examining table. Place a pad under the humerus so that the humerus is level with the acromion process.

Stabilization

Glenohumeral Medial Rotation

In the beginning of the ROM, stabilization is often needed at the distal end of the humerus to keep the shoulder in 90 degrees of abduction. Toward the end of the ROM, the clavicle and coracoid and acromion processes of the scapula are stabilized to prevent anterior tilting and **protraction of the scapula.**

Shoulder Complex Medial Rotation

Stabilization is often needed at the distal end of the humerus to keep the shoulder in 90 degrees of abduction. The thorax may be stabilized by the weight of the individual's trunk or with the examiner's hand to prevent flexion or rotation of the spine.

Testing Motion

Medially rotate the shoulder by moving the forearm anteriorly, bringing the palm of the hand toward the floor. Maintain the shoulder in 90 degrees of abduction and the elbow in 90 degrees of flexion during the motion.

Glenohumeral Medial Rotation

The end of ROM occurs when resistance to further motion is felt and attempts to overcome the resistance cause an anterior tilt or protraction of the scapula (Fig. 4.25).

Shoulder Complex Medial Rotation

The end of ROM occurs when resistance to further motion is felt and attempts to overcome the resistance cause flexion or rotation of the spine (Fig. 4.26).

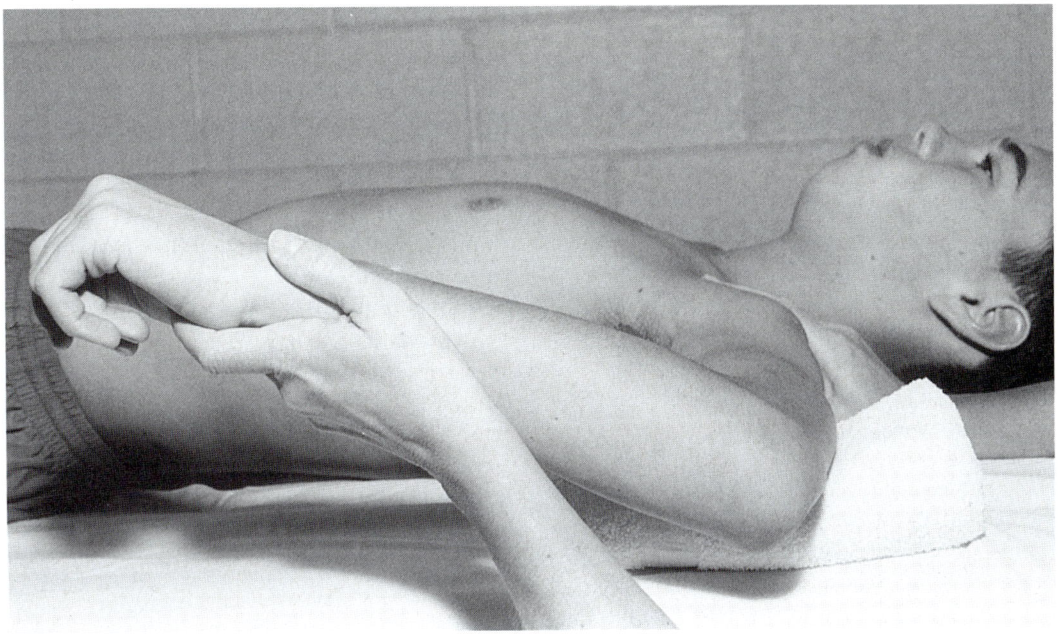

FIGURE 4.25 The end of glenohumeral medial (internal) rotation ROM. The examiner stabilizes the acromion and coracoid processes of the scapula. The examiner is able to determine that the end of the ROM has been reached because any attempt to move the extremity into additional medial rotation causes the scapula to tilt anteriorly or protract. The examiner should also maintain the shoulder in 90 degrees of abduction and the elbow in 90 degrees of flexion during the motion. A towel roll is placed under the distal humerus to keep the humerus horizontal to the ground.

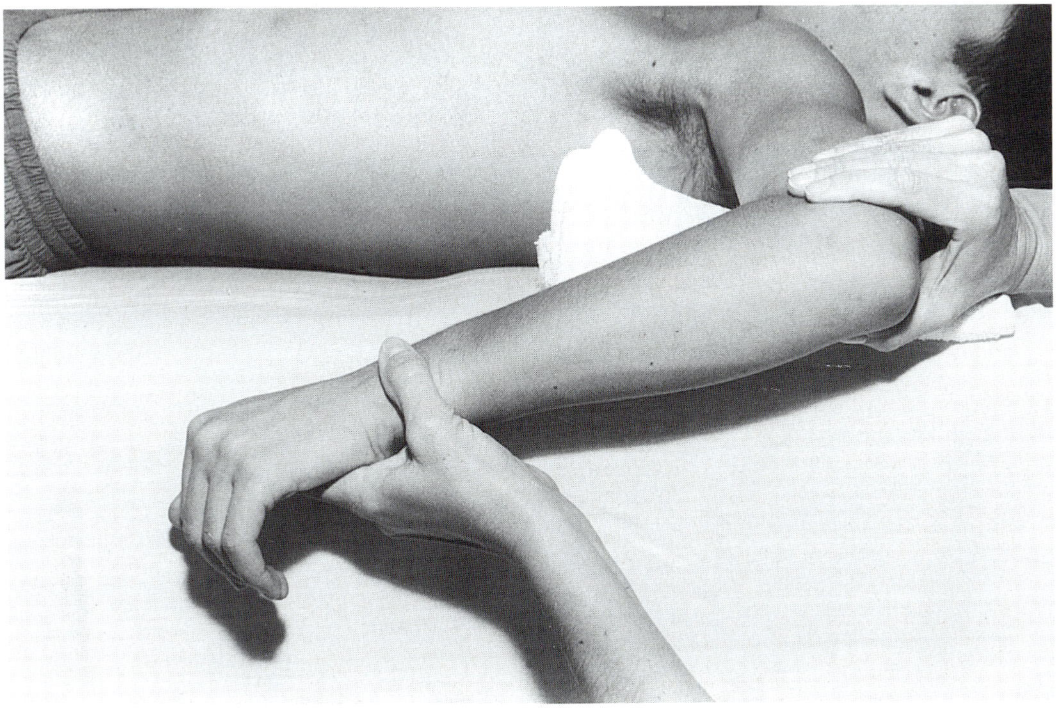

FIGURE 4.26 The end of shoulder complex medial (internal) rotation ROM. The examiner stabilizes the distal end of the humerus to maintain the shoulder in 90 degrees of abduction and the elbow in 90 degrees of flexion during the motion. Resistance is noted at the end of medial rotation of the shoulder complex because attempts to move the extremity into further motion cause the spine to flex or rotate. The clavicle and scapula are allowed to move as they participate in shoulder complex motions.

Normal End-Feel

Glenohumeral Medial Rotation

The end-feel is firm because of tension in the posterior joint capsule and the infraspinatus and teres minor muscles.

Shoulder Complex Medial Rotation

The end-feel is firm because of tension in the sterno-clavicular capsule and ligaments, the costoclavicular ligament, and the major and minor rhomboid and trapezius muscles.

Goniometer Alignment

This goniometer alignment is used for measuring glenohumeral and shoulder complex medial rotation (Figs. 4.27 to 4.29).

1. Center **fulcrum** of the goniometer over the olecranon process.
2. Align **proximal arm** so that it is either perpendicular to or parallel with the floor.
3. Align **distal arm** with the ulna, using the olecranon process and ulnar styloid for reference.

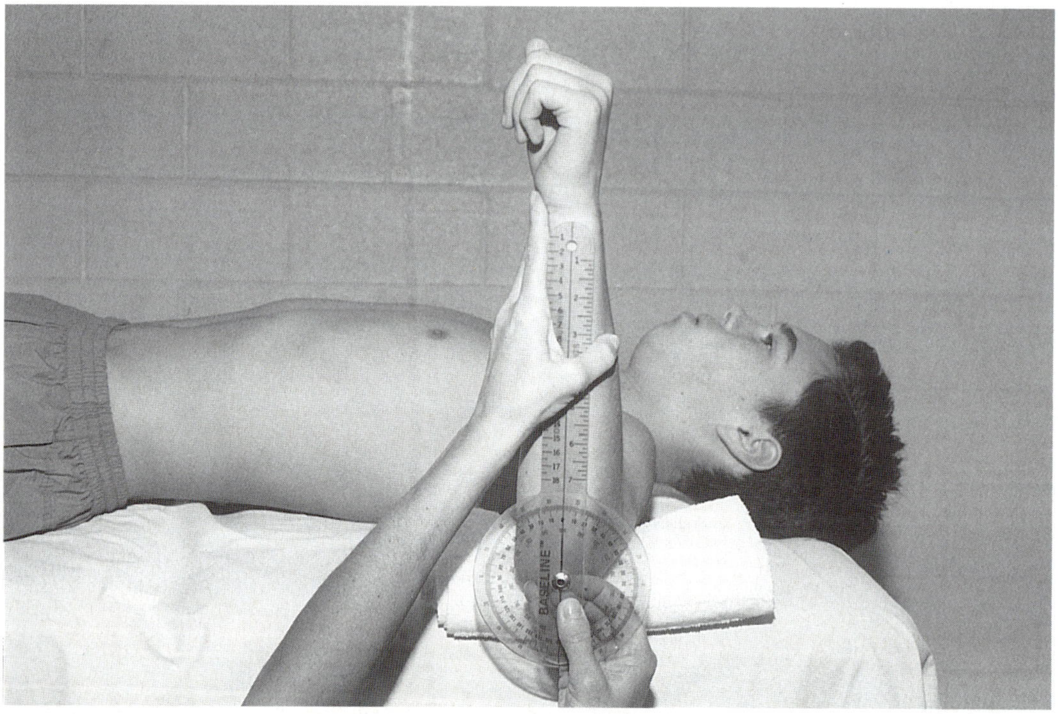

FIGURE 4.27 The alignment of the goniometer at the beginning of medial rotation ROM of the glenohumeral and shoulder complex.

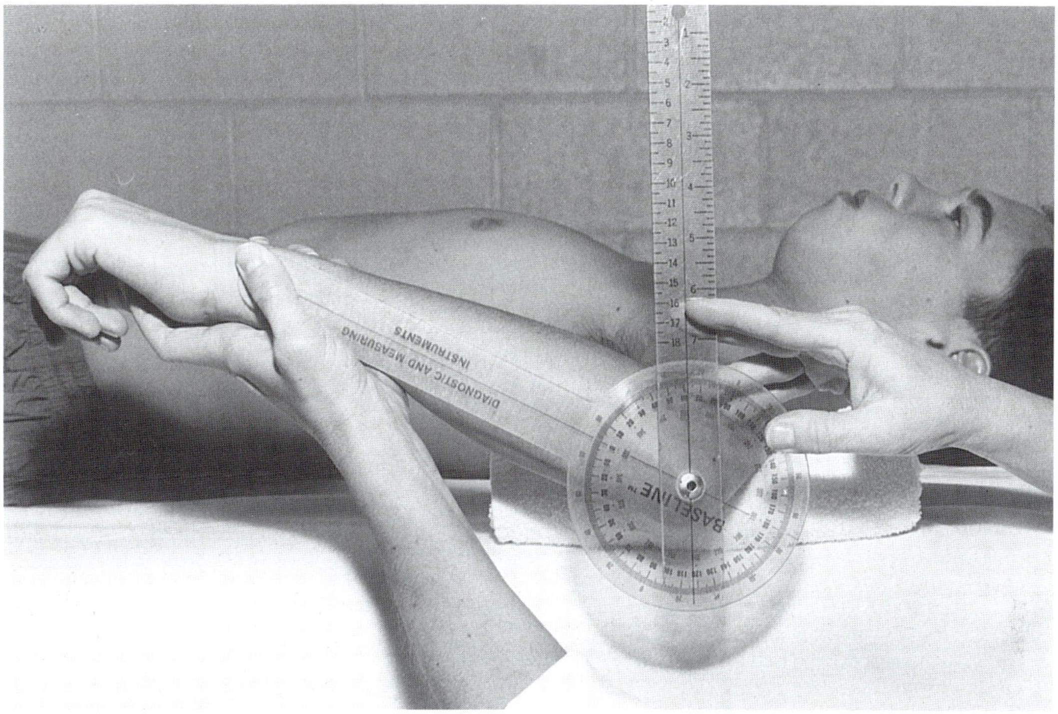

FIGURE 4.28 The alignment of the goniometer at the end of medial rotation ROM of the glenohumeral joint. The examiner uses one hand to support the individual's forearm and the distal arm of the goniometer. The examiner's other hand holds the body and the proximal arm of the goniometer.

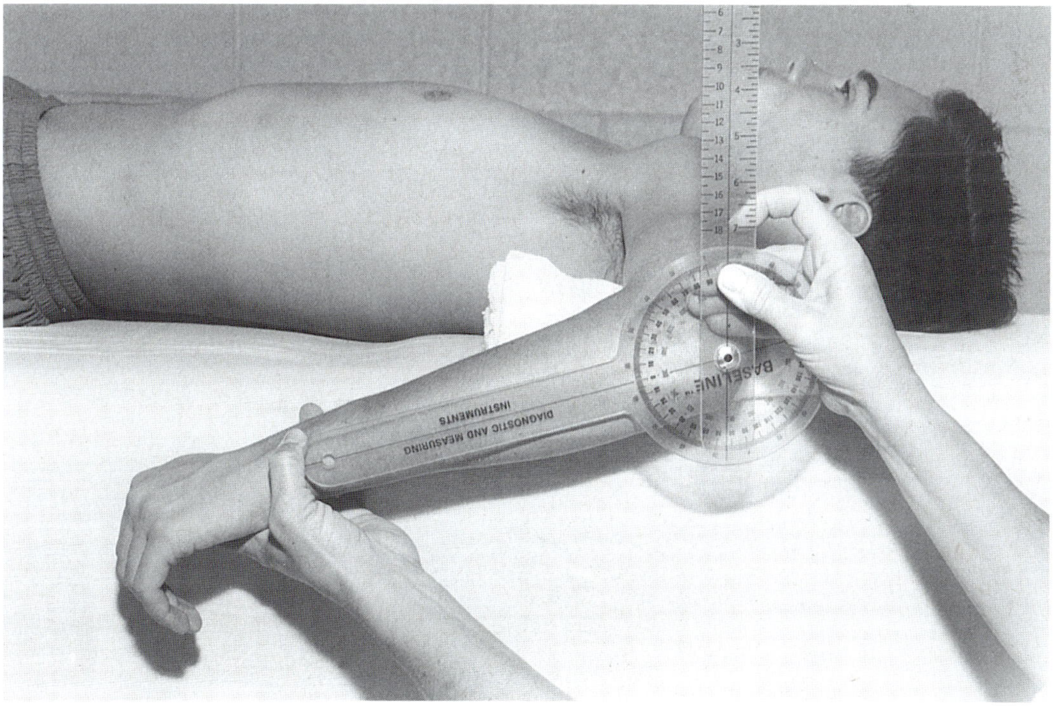

FIGURE 4.29 The alignment of the goniometer at the end medial rotation ROM of the shoulder complex.

LATERAL (EXTERNAL) ROTATION

When the individual is in anatomical position, the motion occurs in the transverse plane around a vertical axis. When the individual is in the testing position, the motion occurs in the sagittal plane around a medial–lateral (coronal) axis. Normal *shoulder complex* lateral rotation ROM values for adults vary from about 90 to 100 degrees. Normal *glenohumeral* lateral rotation ROM values for adults vary from about 80 to 90 degrees. Generally, these values for shoulder complex and glenohumeral lateral rotation ROM values were obtained with individuals in supine and the scapula resting on the examining table while the shoulder was abducted to 90 degrees. This stabilization of the scapula by the examining table for both types of measurements likely contributed to the relatively similar results. See Research Findings and Tables 4.1 to 4.4 for more detailed normal ROM values by age and joint.

Testing Position

Position the individual supine, with the arm being tested in 90 degrees of shoulder abduction. Place the forearm perpendicular to the supporting surface and in 0 degrees of supination and pronation so that the palm of the hand faces the feet. Rest the full length of the humerus on the examining table. The elbow is not supported by the examining table. Place a pad under the humerus so that the humerus is level with the acromion process.

Stabilization

Glenohumeral Lateral Rotation

At the beginning of the ROM, stabilization is often needed at the distal end of the humerus to keep the shoulder in 90 degrees of abduction. Toward the end of the ROM, the spine of the scapula is stabilized to prevent posterior tilting and retraction.

Shoulder Complex Lateral Rotation

Stabilization is often needed at the distal end of the humerus to keep the shoulder in 90 degrees of abduction. To prevent extension or rotation of the spine, the thorax may be stabilized by the weight of the individual's trunk or by the examiner's hand.

Testing Motion

Rotate the shoulder laterally by moving the forearm posteriorly, bringing the dorsal surface of the palm of the hand toward the floor. Maintain the shoulder in 90 degrees of abduction and the elbow in 90 degrees of flexion during the motion.

Glenohumeral Lateral Rotation

The end of ROM occurs when resistance to further motion is felt and attempts to overcome the resistance cause a posterior tilt or retraction of the scapula (Fig. 4.30).

Shoulder Complex Lateral Rotation

The end of ROM occurs when resistance to further motion is felt and attempts to overcome the resistance cause extension or rotation of the spine (Fig. 4.31).

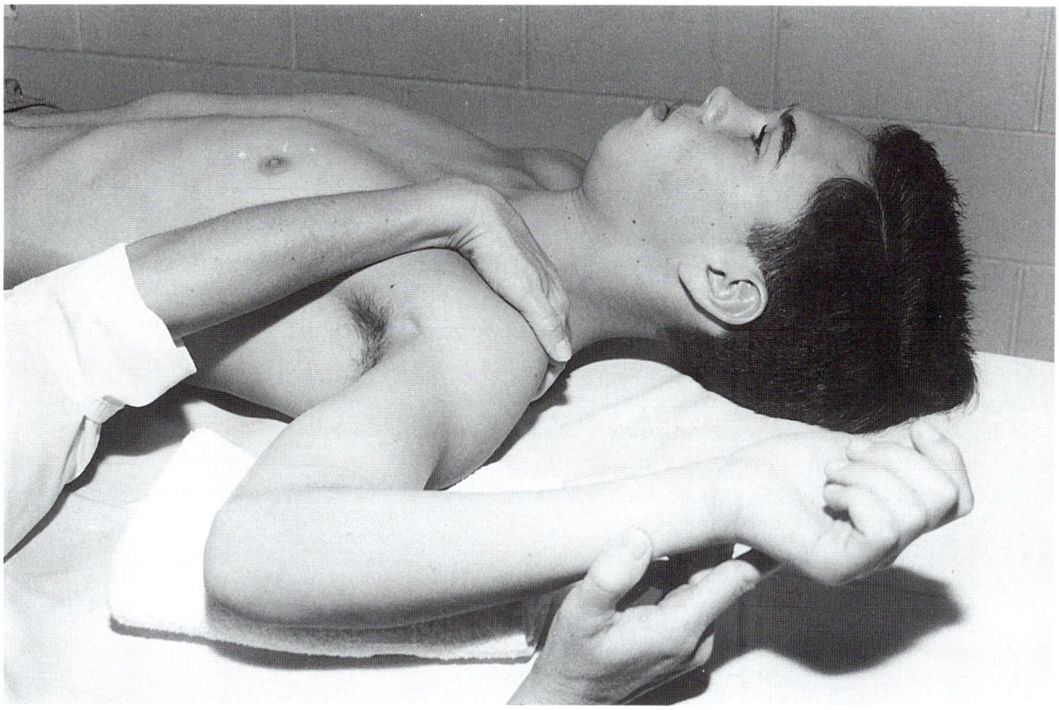

FIGURE 4.30 The end of lateral rotation ROM of the glenohumeral joint. The examiner's hand stabilizes the spine of the scapula. The end of the ROM is reached when additional motion causes the scapula to posteriorly tilt or retract and push against the examiner's hand.

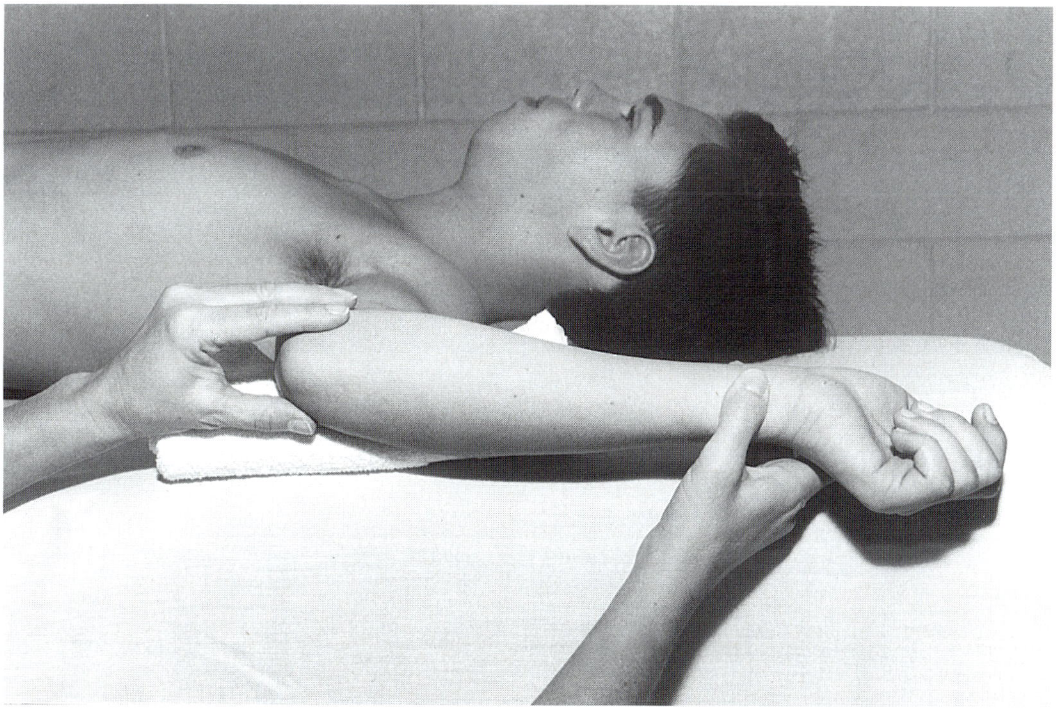

FIGURE 4.31 The end of lateral rotation ROM of the shoulder complex. The examiner stabilizes the distal humerus to prevent shoulder abduction beyond 90 degrees, while the elbow is maintained in 90 degrees of flexion. The clavicle and scapular are allowed to move as they participate in shoulder complex motions.

Normal End-Feel

Glenohumeral Lateral Rotation

The end-feel is firm because of tension in the anterior joint capsule; the three bands of the glenohumeral ligament; the coracohumeral ligament; and the subscapularis, the teres major, and the clavicular fibers of the pectoralis major muscles.

Shoulder Complex Lateral Rotation

The end-feel is firm because of tension in the SC capsule and ligaments and in the latissimus dorsi, sternocostal fibers of the pectoralis major, pectoralis minor, and serratus anterior muscles.

Goniometer Alignment

This goniometer alignment is used for measuring glenohumeral and shoulder complex lateral rotation (Figs. 4.32 to 4.34).

1. Center **fulcrum** of the goniometer over the olecranon process.
2. Align **proximal arm** so that it is either parallel to or perpendicular to the floor.
3. Align **distal arm** with the ulna, using the olecranon process and ulnar styloid for reference.

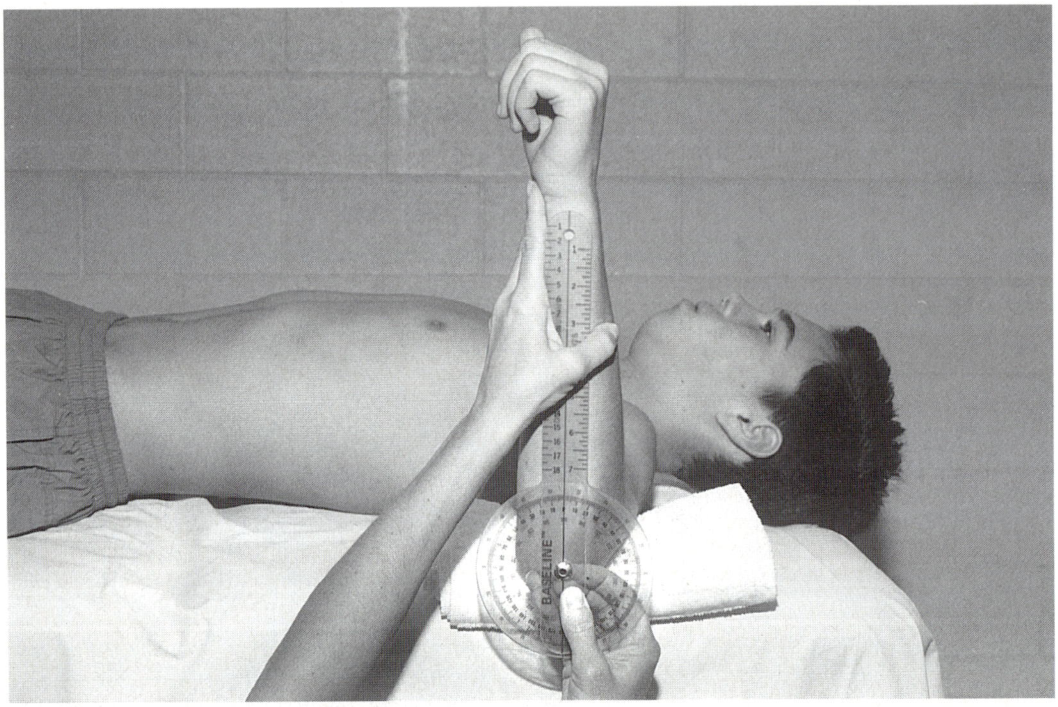

FIGURE 4.32 The alignment of the goniometer at the beginning of lateral rotation ROM of the glenohumeral joint and shoulder complex.

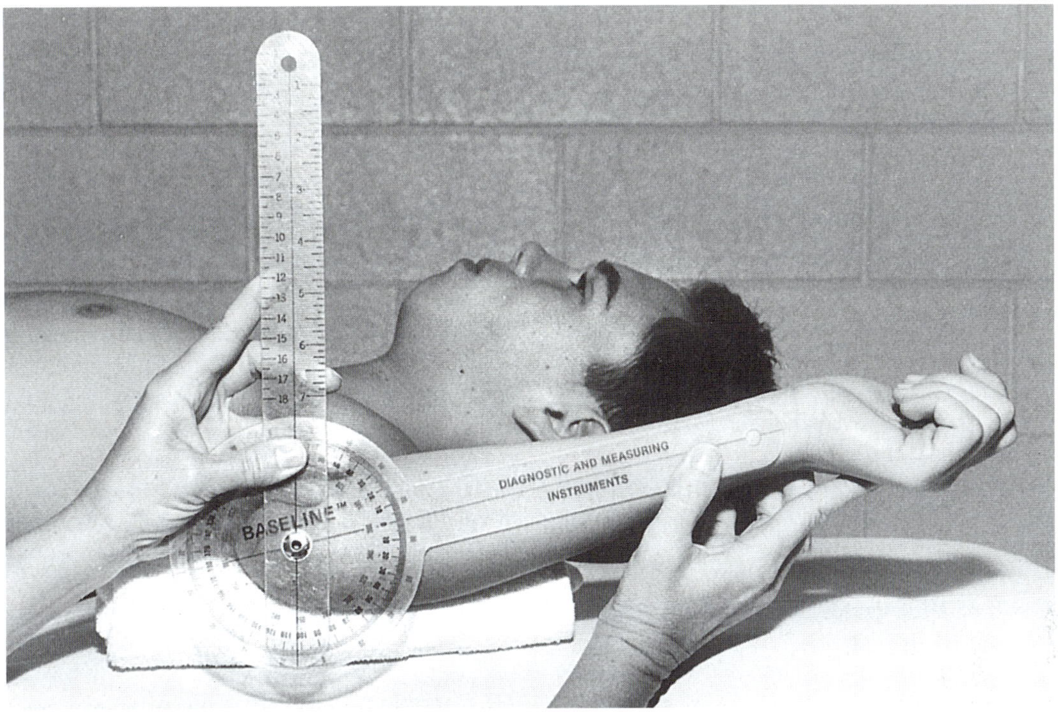

FIGURE 4.33 The alignment of the goniometer at the end of lateral rotation ROM of the glenohumeral joint. The examiner's hand supports the individual's forearm and the distal arm of the goniometer. The examiner's other hand holds the body and proximal arm of the goniometer. The placement of the examiner's hands would be reversed if the right shoulder was being tested.

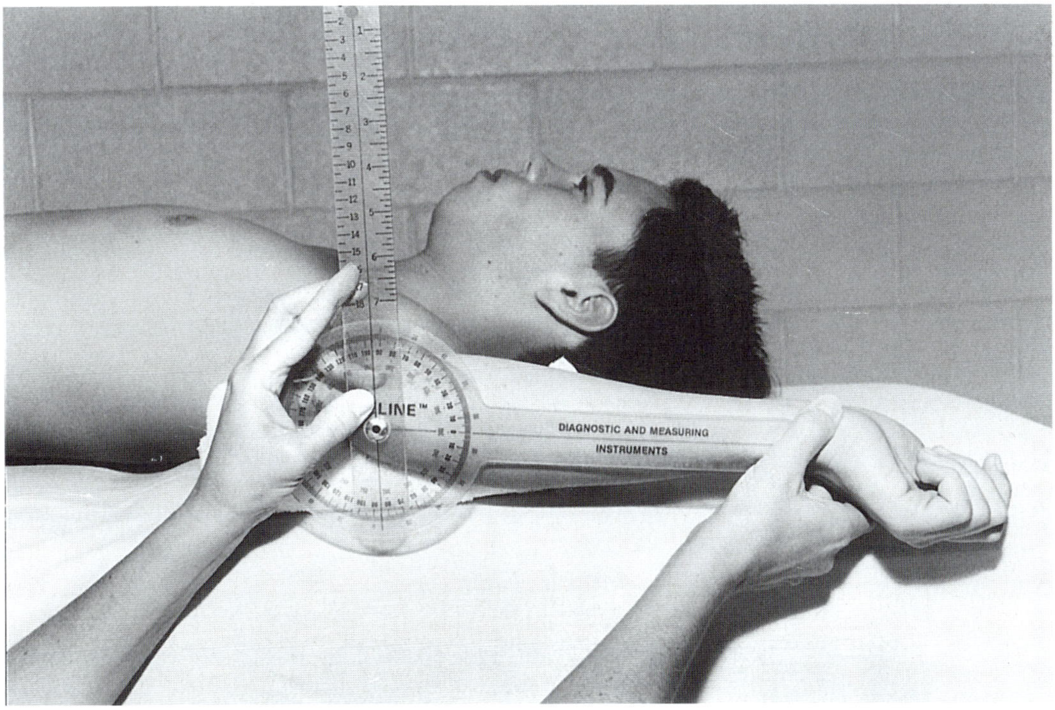

FIGURE 4.34 The alignment of the goniometer at the end of lateral rotation ROM of the shoulder complex.

Research Findings

Effects of Age, Gender, and Other Factors

Table 4.1 shows normal values of shoulder complex ROM for healthy adults from five sources.[10,15,17–19] In general, these mean values range from 155 to 185 degrees for shoulder complex flexion, 50 to 70 degrees for extension, 165 to 185 degrees for abduction, 50 to 90 degrees for medial rotation, and 85 to 105 degrees for lateral rotation. There is some variation in these values possibly due to differences in measurement methods (active versus passive ROM) and study populations (exclusively male, exclusively female, or both genders). The data on age, gender, and number of subjects that were measured to obtain the values reported for the AAOS[15,16] and AMA[17] were not specified; however, the other sources used universal goniometers and included similarly aged adults. Other researchers have also reported normative shoulder complex ROM values for healthy adults.[14,19–21] Unless otherwise noted in this section, Research Findings, the reader should assume that shoulder ROM refers to shoulder complex ROM.

Some studies have specifically measured glenohumeral ROM using clinical tools such as a universal goniometer. Table 4.2 shows normal values of glenohumeral ROM for healthy adults and adolescents obtained from four sources.[9–12] These studies used manual stabilization of the scapula and universal goniometers to obtain passive glenohumeral measurements but included different-aged subjects and genders. Although variations are noted in glenohumeral flexion and abduction ROM values, some motions seem to be more consistent: extension ranging from about 20 to 25 degrees, medial rotation from 50 to 60 degrees, and lateral rotation from about 90 to 100 degrees in adults. In addition to the sources included in Table 4.2, Boon and Smith[13] reported a mean of 62.8 degrees of medial rotation and 108.1 degrees of lateral rotation in 50 high school athletes (18 males and 32 females) aged 12 to 18 years. In a similar population of 32 healthy male and 24 female adolescent athletes, Awan, Smith, and Boon[14] found mean glenohumeral medial rotation to be between 63.2 and 70.2 degrees with the scapula manually stabilized, and between 60.6 and 70.7 degrees using visualized movement of the scapula to determine end range. Rundquist and coworkers[22] also provide some glenohumeral and shoulder complex ROM data measured with electromagnetic tracking sensors on the humerus and scapula in 10 asymptomatic adults with a mean age of 51 years. These investigators reported 97 degrees of GH flexion during 148 degrees of shoulder complex flexion, and 100 degrees of GH abduction during 151 degrees of shoulder complex abduction. Pearl and associates[23] noted a mean of 10 degrees of GH extension during 58 degrees of maximal shoulder complex extension in a study of 15 normal subjects using a scapular locating device and a goniometer. More studies are needed to establish normative values for glenohumeral ROM using clinical methods, especially in older adults.

The measurement of osteokinematic motions isolated to the sternoclavicular (SC) and acromioclavicular (AC) joints using clinical tools has not been widely practiced or studied. However, up to about 45 degrees of clavicular elevation at the SC joint, 10 to 15 degrees of depression, 15 to 30 degrees of protraction, 15 to 30 degrees of retraction, 50 degrees of posterior rotation, and less than 10 degrees of anterior rotation have been reported using research methods that typically involve electromagnetic or visual markers with 3-dimensional motion analysis equipment.[2–4,24] Acromioclavicular motions are generally reported to be between 10 and 30 degrees in vivo using research methods.[2–4,24] Nadeau and associates[25] in a study of 30 healthy subjects reported elevation to be about 28 degrees (standard deviation [SD] = 5.2) using a goniometer and 9.4 centimeters (SD = 2.2) using a tape measure.

Several clinical methods of measuring scapulothoracic motion, which incorporates SC and AC joint motion, have undergone preliminary study. Some researchers have

TABLE 4.1 Normal Shoulder Complex ROM Values for Adults in Degrees From Selected Sources

	AAOS[15]	AMA[17]	Boone and Azen[18]		Greene and Wolf[19]	Macedo and Magee[10]	
			20–54 yr *n* = 56 Males AROM		18–55 yr *n* = 20 Males and Females AROM	18–59 yr *n* = 90 Females PROM	
Motion			***Mean***	***(SD)***	***Mean***	***Mean***	***(SD)***
Flexion	180	180	165.0	(5.0)	155.8	189	(14)
Extension	60	50	57.3	(8.1)	—	70	(12)
Abduction	180	170	182.7	(9.0)	167.6	188	(10)
Medial rotation	70	80	67.1	(4.1)	48.7	94	(14)
Lateral rotation	90	60	99.6	(7.6)	83.6	109	(11)

AROM = Active range of motion; PROM = Passive range of motion; SD = Standard deviation.

TABLE 4.2 Normal Passive Glenohumeral ROM Values in Degrees From Selected Sources

	Lannan et al[9]		Macedo and Magee[10]		Goddu et al[11]		Ellenbecker et al[12]			
	21–40 yr n = 20 Males and 40 Females		18–59 yr n = 90 Females		18–90 yr n = 45 Males and 45 Females		11–17 yr n = 113 Males		11–17 yr n = 90 Females	
Motion	**Mean**	**(SD)**	**Mean**	**(SD)**	**Mean**	**(SD)**	**Mean**	**(SD)**	**Mean**	**(SD)**
Flexion	106.2	(10.2)	41	(14)	117.7	(14.1)	—	—	—	—
Extension	20.1	(5.8)	27	(9)	26.1	(6.5)	—	—	—	—
Abduction	128.9	(9.1)	85	(19)	123.3	(8.8)	—	—	—	—
Medial rotation	49.2	(9.0)	64	(14)	50.4	(12.7)	50.9	(12.6)	56.3	(10.3)
Lateral rotation	94.2	(12.2)	94	(12)	80.9	(13.8)	102.8	(10.9)	104.6	(10.3)

SD = Standard deviation.

proposed measuring linear distances between the spine and anatomical landmarks on the scapula,[25–27] linear movement of the metacarpals in an outstretched arm,[28] universal and specialized goniometers aligned with the acromion or clavicle,[25] inclinometers on the spine of the scapula,[26] or the use of specialized scapular-locating devices[23,29] to quantify scapular position and movement. A research summit meeting on the scapula, held in 2009,[30] identified the need for testing the reliability, validity, and clinical utilization of inclinometer measures of scapular position. We await more research in this area before including specific clinical methods of measuring scapulothoracic ROM in future editions of this textbook

Age

Very minimal differences have been noted in shoulder complex ROM values among children from birth through adolescence (see Table 4.3). Although the values obtained from Wanatabe and coworkers[31] for infants are greater than those obtained from Boone[32] for children aged 1 to 19 years and from Vairo and associates[33] for military cadets with a mean age of 18 years, it is difficult to compare values across studies. Within one study, Boone[32] and Boone and Azen[18] found that shoulder ROM varied little in males between 1 and 19 years of age.

There is some indication that children have greater values than adults for certain shoulder complex motions. Wanatabe and coworkers[31] found that the passive ROM in shoulder extension and lateral rotation was greater in Japanese infants than the average values typically reported for adults. Boone and Azen[18] found significantly greater active ROM in all shoulder motions except for abduction in male children between 1 and 19 years of age compared with male adults between 20 and 54 years of age.

TABLE 4.3 Effects of Age and Gender on Shoulder Complex ROM: Normal Values in Degrees for Newborns, Children, and Adolescents

	Wanatabe et al[31]	Boone[32]						Vairo[33]	
	2 wk–2 yr* n = 45 Males & Females	18 mo–5 yr† n = 19 Males		6–12 yr† n = 17 Males		13–19 yr† n = 17 Males		x̄ = 19 yr* n = 548 Males	
Motion	**Range of Means**	**Mean**	**(SD)**	**Mean**	**(SD)**	**Mean**	**(SD)**	**Mean**	**(SD)**
Flexion	172–180	168.8	(3.7)	169.0	(3.5)	167.4	(3.9)	170.6	(7.7)
Extension	79–89	68.9	(6.6)	69.6	(7.0)	64.0	(9.3)	—	—
Abduction	177–187	186.3	(2.6)	184.7	(3.8)	185.1	(4.3)	—	—
Medial rotation	72–90	71.2	(3.6)	70.0	(4.7)	70.3	(5.3)	58.9	(14.0)
Lateral rotation	118–134	110.0	—	107.4	(3.6)	106.3	(6.1)	104.6	(10.8)

SD = Standard deviation.

* Values are for passive ROM measured with a universal goniometer. Vairo et al values are for the dominant arm.

† Values are for active ROM measured with a universal goniometer.

Table 4.4 summarizes the effects of age on shoulder complex ROM in adults. There appears to be a trend for older adults (over age 60) to have lower values than younger adults for the motions of extension, lateral rotation, and abduction. There seems to be less of a reduction in medial rotation ROM with increased age. In any case, the ROM values for adults over 60 years of age in all of these studies[34–36] were less than the normal values listed by the AAOS[15,16] and AMA[17] (Table 4.1). Kalscheur, Costello, and Emery[36] in their study of older adults aged 63 to 86 years, developed mathematical models that predicted an annual decrease ranging from 0.1 degrees for medial rotation to 1.1 degrees for lateral rotation and 1.3 degrees for abduction. It is interesting to note that the standard deviations for the older groups in Table 4.4 are much larger than the values reported for the younger groups. The larger standard deviations appear to indicate that ROM is more variable in the older groups than in the younger groups. However, the fact that the measurements were obtained by different investigators should be considered when drawing conclusions from this information.

In addition to the evidence for age-related changes presented in Tables 4.3 and 4.4, other investigators have identified age-related trends. West[37] found that older subjects had between 15 and 20 degrees less shoulder complex flexion ROM and 10 degrees less extension ROM than younger subjects. Subjects ranged in age from the first decade to the eighth decade. Soucie et al[21] in a study of 674 persons reported a decrease in shoulder complex flexion of about 14 degrees in males and 10 degrees in females between the age-group of 2- to 8-year-olds and the age-group of 45- to 69-year-olds. Clarke and coworkers[38] found significant decreases with age in passive glenohumeral lateral rotation, total rotation, and abduction in a study that included 60 normal males and females ranging in age from 21 to 80 years. Mean reduction in these three glenohumeral ROMs ranged from 7 to 29 degrees in those aged 71 to 80 years compared with those aged 21 to 30 years. Stathokostas and coworkers[39] also found a decline in shoulder abduction ROM averaging 5 degrees per decade in 205 males and 6 degrees per decade in 231 females between the ages of 55 and 86 years. Linear regression showed an accelerated decline of 0.8 degrees per year starting at age 71 years in males and a decline of 0.7 degrees per year starting at age 63 years in females.

Age-related changes in shoulder rotation have been noted in the following studies. Macedo and Magee,[10] in a study of 90 females aged 18 to 59 years, found a statistically significant decrease in passive shoulder complex and GH lateral rotation, and shoulder complex abduction and extension. However, only lateral rotation of the shoulder complex and GH joint decreased more than 10 degrees over the 40-year age range of the subjects. Mathematical models predicting a change in motion in people from 18 to 59 years ranged from +0.01 degrees annually for GH medial rotation to –0.42 per year for GH lateral rotation. Roy and coworkers[20] in a study of 121 males and 173 females also found the greatest decrease in lateral rotation of the shoulder in the over-60 age category compared to the 18 to 39 age category. The mean reduction was about 7 degrees on the dominant side and 5 degrees on the nondominant side when measured in supine. A significant decrease in passive total shoulder rotation was associated with increasing age especially on the right side in a study by Allander and associates[40] of 517 females and 203 males aged 33 to 70 years. Barnes, Van Steyn, and Fischer,[41] in a study of 140 males and 140 females ranging in age from 7 to 70, found a decrease in all shoulder motions with increasing age except for medial rotation, which increased.

Gender

Several studies have reported that females have greater shoulder complex ROM than males, especially in older populations.

TABLE 4.4 Effects of Age and Gender on Active Shoulder Complex ROM: Normal Values in Degrees for Adults 20 to 93 Years of Age

	Boone[32]						Walker et al[34]		Downey et al[35]		Kalscheur et al[36]			
	20–29 yr n = 19 Males		30–39 yr n = 18 Males		40–54 yr n = 19 Males		60–85 yr* n = 30 Males		61–93 yr n = 140 Females & Males		63–85 yr* n = 61 Females		66–86 yr* n = 25 Males	
Motion	**Mean**	**(SD)**	**Mean**	**(SD)**	**Mean**	**(SD)**	**Mean**	**(SD)**	**Mean**	**(SD)**	**Mean**	**(SD)**	**Mean**	**(SD)**
Flexion	164.5	(5.9)	165.4	(3.8)	165.1	(5.2)	160	(11)	165.0	(10.7)	158.2	(19.6)	151.8	(16.5)
Extension	58.3	(8.3)	57.5	(8.5)	56.1	(7.9)	38	(11)	—	—	—	—	—	—
Abduction	182.6	(9.8)	182.8	(7.7)	182.6	(9.8)	155	(22)	157.9	(17.4)	154.6	(21.4)	130.5	(35.3)
Medial rotation	65.9	(4.0)	67.1	(4.2)	68.3	(3.8)	59	(16)	65.0	(11.7)	52.9	(9.0)	45.6	(9.5)
Lateral rotation	100.0	(7.2)	101.5	(6.9)	97.5	(8.5)	76	(13)	80.6	(11.0)	76.1	(16.3)	66.4	(12.6)

SD = Standard deviation.

* For right shoulder.

Walker and coworkers[34] in a study of 30 men and 30 women between 60 and 84 years of age found that women had statistically significant greater ROM than their male counterparts in all shoulder motions studied except for medial rotation. The mean differences for women were 20 degrees greater than those of males for shoulder abduction, 11 degrees greater for shoulder extension, and 9 degrees greater for shoulder flexion and lateral rotation. Escalante, Lichenstein, and Hazuda[42] studied shoulder flexion in 687 community-dwelling adults aged 65 to 74 years and found that women had 3 degrees more flexion than men. In a study of older adults aged 63 to 86 years conducted by Kalscheur and associates,[36] females were found to have more shoulder abduction, flexion, and medial and lateral rotation than males, with differences ranging from about 24 degrees for abduction to 6 degrees for flexion and medial rotation. In a study of 208 male and female subjects between the ages of 4 and 70 years, Barnes and coworkers[41] found that females had greater ROM for all active and passive shoulder complex motions that were measured: forward elevation, extension, abduction, and medial and lateral rotation. Allander and associates,[40] in a study of passive shoulder rotation in 208 Swedish women and 203 men aged 45 to 70 years, found that women had a greater ROM in total shoulder rotation than men. Although women generally appeared to have greater lateral and medial rotation in sitting and supine than men, only lateral rotation of the nondominant side measured in sitting rose to the level of the significance in a study by Roy et al[20] of 294 adults aged 18 to 60 years; overall mean difference was 7.6 degrees with a maximal difference of 15.2 degrees in the 40- to 59-year age category. In contrast to the aforementioned studies, Stathokostas and associates[39] found no differences in shoulder abduction ROM between males and females in their study population of 436 individuals aged 55 to 86 years.

Gender differences have also been noted in most glenohumeral motions with females having more motion than males. Clarke and associates[38] in a study that included 60 males and 60 females between the ages of 20 and 40 years found that females had greater glenohumeral ROM for shoulder abduction as well as lateral and total rotation for all age-groups. Males had, on average, 92% of the ROM of their female counterparts, the difference being most marked in abduction. Lannan, Lehman, and Toland[9] in a study of 40 women and 20 men aged 21 to 40 years found that women had statistically significant greater amounts of glenohumeral flexion, extension, abduction, and medial and lateral rotation than men. The mean differences typically varied between 3 and 8 degrees. Boon and Smith,[13] in a study of 32 females and 18 males aged 12 to 18 years, reported that females had significantly more lateral and total rotation than males. The mean difference in lateral and total rotation was 4.5 and 9.1 degrees, respectively. Ellenbecker and colleagues[12] studied 113 male and 90 female elite tennis players aged 11 to 17 years (see Table 4.2). Their data seem to indicate that the females had greater ROM than males for glenohumeral medial and lateral rotation, although no statistical tests focused on the effect of gender on ROM.

Body Mass Index

The influence of body mass index (BMI) on shoulder ROM measurements is not well defined and results of research studies vary as to whether or not there is an effect. Obesity, defined as a BMI greater than 30 kg/m^2, was associated with a decrease in shoulder complex extension and adduction ROM in a small study by Park and colleagues[43] that included 20 obese and 20 nonobese young adult males. Obesity-associated reductions in mean ROM ranged from 21% to 22% for extension, and 36% to 39% for adduction. Other shoulder complex motions of flexion, abduction, and medial and lateral rotation were examined but showed no effect.

Increasing BMI was associated with decreasing ROM for shoulder complex and GH extension, shoulder complex abduction, and GH external rotation in a study of 90 females aged 18 to 59 years by Macedo and Magee.[10] However, increasing BMI was associated with increasing shoulder complex medial rotation and glenohumeral abduction. The authors state that although changes were statistically significant, changes per BMI categories were minimal and considered insignificant. Similarly, a study by Escalante, Lichenstein, and Hazuda[42] found no relationship between shoulder flexion and body mass index in 695 community-dwelling subjects aged 65 to 74 years who participated in the San Antonio Longitudinal Study of Aging.

Testing Position

An individual's posture and testing position have been shown to affect the shoulder complex motions of abduction and lateral rotation. These findings support the use of consistent, well-defined positions to enable an examiner to compare shoulder measurements with normative values and accurately assess rehabilitative progress. Kebaetse, McClure, and Pratt[44] in a study of 34 healthy adults measured active shoulder abduction and scapula ROM while subjects were sitting in both erect and slouched trunk postures. There was significantly less active shoulder abduction ROM in the slouched than in the erect postures (mean difference = 23.6 degrees). The slouched posture also resulted in more scapula elevation during 0 to 90 degrees of abduction and less scapula posterior tilting in the interval between 90-degree and maximal abduction.

Sabari and associates[45] studied 30 adult subjects and noted greater amounts of active and passive shoulder abduction measured in the supine position than in the sitting position. The mean differences in abduction ranged from 3.0 to 7.1 degrees. On visual inspection of the data there were also greater amounts of shoulder flexion in the supine versus the sitting position; however, these differences did not attain significance. A supine position with the shoulder at 90 degrees of abduction also resulted in greater lateral rotation ROM than the sitting position with the shoulder in 0 degrees of abduction in 294 subjects in a study by Roy and associates.[20] Mean difference ranged from about 16 to 24 degrees. However, passive ROM was measured in supine position whereas active ROM was measured in sitting position, which may have influenced the results.

Right Versus Left Side

In a general population that does not engage in upper-extremity-intense sports or manual labor, most research findings support the use of the opposite side of the body in unilateral shoulder conditions as an indicator of pre-injury or normal ROM. If differences between sides are noted, studies seem to indicate that the left/nondominant shoulder has slightly more motion than the right/dominant shoulder especially for medial rotation and extension. However, these differences may be of questionable clinical importance because most were reported to be between 2 to 5 degrees and in almost all cases were less than 10 degrees. Only one study suggested using side-specific values for medial and lateral rotation.[41]

Several studies have found no or minimal differences in shoulder ROM between sides. Boone and Azen[18] studied 109 males between the ages of 18 months and 54 years and found no statistical differences between the right and left shoulders for flexion, extension, abduction, medial and lateral rotation, horizontal flexion, and horizontal extension in almost all age-groups. Soucie and coworkers[21] found a statistically significant but small difference of less than 1 degree between sides for shoulder flexion in a study of 674 male and female subjects aged 8 to 69. Likewise, several studies on older adults have found no or small differences of 2 to 3 degrees based on side. Kalscheur, Emery, and Costello[46] in a study of 61 older women aged 63 to 83 years found no significant differences between the right and left sides for shoulder complex flexion, abduction, medial or lateral rotation, with all mean differences less than 3.5 degrees. A larger study of 695 community-dwelling male and female adults aged 65 to 74 years found a statistically significant but small increase of 2 degrees in left shoulder flexion as compared with the right.[42]

A few studies have reported slightly larger differences due to side or hand dominance in particular shoulder motions. Gunal and coworkers[47] found most active and passive shoulder motions had statistically greater motion on the left or nondominant side in a large study of 1,000 right-handed healthy Turkish males 18 to 21 years of age. Most mean differences were small and between 2.5 to 4 degrees, except for active horizontal flexion, active medial rotation, and active glenohumeral abduction, which had mean differences of between 6.2 to 9.5 degrees. Macedo and Magee[48] included 90 female subjects aged 18 to 59 years in a study that measured 60 active and passive motions of the upper and lower extremities. Shoulder complex and glenohumeral ROM for flexion and abduction were generally found to be similar between sides, whereas extension and medial rotation had more motion on the nondominant side with mean differences of about 2 to 4 degrees and 5 to 7.5 degrees, respectively. Lateral rotation was greater on the dominant side with mean differences ranging from 2.5 to 6 degrees. These authors generally considered these differences, especially those less than 5 degrees, to be relatively small in consideration of the minimal detectible differences that are needed to identify clinically important change. Barnes and associates[41] reported a similar pattern of greater active and passive medial rotation and extension on the nondominant side and greater active and passive lateral rotation on the dominant side in 280 healthy male and female subjects aged 4 to 70 years. However, because they found mean differences between sides of 8 to 15 degrees for medial and lateral rotation ROM they suggested that using the uninjured contralateral side for comparison may be misleading for rotation. No differences were found for shoulder abduction and forward elevation. All passive motions were greater than active motions.

Sports

In contrast to studies of the general population, numerous studies of professional, collegiate, and high school baseball players have consistently found mean increases in lateral rotation of between 5 to 12 degrees, and mean decreases in medial rotation shoulder ROM of 8 to 15 degrees in the dominant (throwing) arm as compared with the nondominant (nonthrowing arm).[49–55] Measurements of rotation were taken with the shoulder in 90 degrees of abduction as opposed to 0 degrees of abduction. Total shoulder rotation, which combines medial and lateral ROM, remained relatively stable and symmetrical between sides. These findings have been noted in position players as well as in pitchers. Variation from these usual differences such as the loss of more than 20 degrees of GH medial rotation, less than 5 degrees of increase of GH lateral rotation, or a loss of greater than 5 degrees (10%) of total shoulder rotation in the dominant arm as compared with the nondominant shoulder have been suggested as risk factors for increased shoulder injury and pathology.[56–59]

Decreases in shoulder medial rotation ROM and total rotation ROM have also been noted in the dominant (playing) compared with the nondominant (nonplaying) arms of male and female professional[60,61] and elite junior tennis players.[12] Decreases in medial rotation ranged from about 7 to 12 degrees. These differences in medial rotation ROM increased with age and years of tournament play in a study by Kibler and colleagues[61] of 39 members of the U.S. Tennis Association National Tennis Team and touring professional program. Some studies also reported an increase in lateral glenohumeral rotation on the dominant arm in professional adult players,[60,61] whereas others found no significant difference in lateral rotation between sides in young elite players.[12]

Studies of overhead athletes who play sports that use both upper extremities such as swimming generally reported no differences in shoulder ROM between sides.[62,63] Studies that include direct comparisons of athletes with nonathletes are lacking, but ROM values in swimmers appear greater than normative values for most shoulder complex movements, especially abduction, flexion, and lateral rotation. However, medial rotation in swimmers appears to be less than normal. Beech and coauthors,[62] in a small study of 28 Division I collegiate swimmers and 4 club swimmers, found mean abduction of the left and right sides to be 196 and 195 degrees, flexion to be 188 and 187 degrees, lateral rotation to be 100 and 101 degrees, and medial rotation to be 49 and 45 degrees, respectively. These typical increases in forward flexion and abduction allow the arms and body to achieve a more horizontal plane to the water surface to reduce drag and to allow for a greater stroke length.[64] However, the increases in ROM may reduce shoulder stability and contribute to shoulder pathology. Water polo players, whose sport requires swimming and throwing a ball, were found by Witwer and Sauers[65] to have more passive glenohumeral lateral rotation ROM and total rotation on the dominant (throwing arm) than on the nondominant arm. No differences in passive GH medial rotation, scapular upward rotation, and posterior shoulder tightness between sides were found in this study of 31 Division I water polo athletes.

Power lifters were found to have decreased ROM in shoulder complex flexion, extension, and medial and lateral rotation compared with nonlifters in a study by Chang, Buschbacker, and Edlich.[66] Ten male power lifters and 10 age-matched male nonlifters were included in the study. The authors suggest that athletic training programs that emphasize muscle-strengthening exercise without stretching exercise may cause progressive loss of ROM.

General physical activity level was not found to effect shoulder complex abduction or hip flexion in a study of 436 individuals aged 55 to 86 years in a study by Stathokostas and associates.[39] Activity level was measured by the Minnesota Leisure-Time Physical Activity Questionnaire.

Functional Range of Motion

Numerous activities of daily living require adequate shoulder ROM. Tiffitt[67] in a study of 125 patients found a significant correlation between the amount of specific shoulder complex motions and a patient's reported ability to perform activities such as combing the hair, putting on a coat, washing the back, washing the contralateral axilla, using the toilet, reaching a high shelf, lifting above the shoulder level, pulling, and sleeping on the affected side. Flexion and adduction ROM correlated best with the ability to comb the hair, whereas medial and lateral rotation ROM correlated best with the ability to wash the back.

If patients have difficulty performing certain functional activities, evaluation and treatment procedures need to focus on the shoulder motions necessary for the activity. Likewise, if patients have known limitations in shoulder ROM, therapists and physicians should anticipate patient difficulty in performing these activities and adaptations should be suggested. To assist in this process, studies have examined the ROM that occurs in healthy adults and children during certain functional activities.

Table 4.5 presents shoulder ROM findings for selected feeding, reaching, and common tasks from some of these studies. A global system proposed by the International Society of Biomechanics (ISB)[68] is used to describe shoulder motion in terms of three planes: (1) elevation, which is movement in a vertical plane around any horizontal axis through the shoulder and is similar to latitude; (2) plane of elevation, which is movement in a horizontal plane around a vertical axis through the shoulder and is similar to longitude; and (3) medial–lateral rotation around the long axis of the upper arm. For example, 70 degrees of flexion in the sagittal plane would be described as 70 degrees of elevation in a 90-degree plane of elevation. One hundred degrees of abduction in the frontal plane would be described as 100 degrees of elevation in a 0-degree plane of elevation. The plane of elevation that is closest to abduction (Abd), flexion (F), extension (E), and scaption (S) is indicated in Table 4.5 to assist with interpretation. This system seems most successful and consistent in describing elevation motions such as flexion, abduction, and extension but has more difficulty describing shoulder rotation.[69] Some researchers used traditional methods of describing shoulder motion, so we have translated their values into the global ISB system for ease of comparison. In any case, there are variations in the ROM values as differences exist in motion analysis methods, anatomical landmarks used for attaching tracking markers, soft tissue artifact due to movement of skin and markers, and subject selection. In addition, there may be different upper-extremity movement strategies employed by individuals for performing the same functional tasks. Most studies presented in Table 4.5 describe humeral motion relative to the thorax (shoulder complex motion) but several describe humeral motion relative to the scapula (glenohumeral motion). In spite of these many differences, some ROM trends for functional tasks are evident.[84]

The greatest amount of shoulder flexion (about 120 degrees in adults, 140 degrees in children) is needed to reach a high shelf (Fig. 4.35), whereas less flexion (about 35 to 80 degrees) is needed for self-feeding and face-washing tasks (Fig. 4.36). A large amount of abduction in the frontal plane or scapular plane (about 100 to 120 degrees) and lateral rotation (40 to 80 degrees) is required to reach behind the head for activities such as grooming the hair (Fig. 4.37), fastening a necklace, and washing the neck and upper back. To reach behind the mid- and lower back for tasks such as fastening a bra (Fig. 4.38), tucking in a shirt, and reaching the perineum to perform hygiene activities, large amounts of shoulder extension (about 35 to 50 degrees) and medial rotation (100 degrees) are necessary. Some horizontal adduction is needed for activities performed in front of the body such as washing the contralateral axilla and eating. Varying amounts of shoulder motions have been noted during wheelchair propulsion at different speeds; however, it seemed most relevant to include ROM values during self-selected speeds in Table 4.5.[81–83,85]

TABLE 4.5 Shoulder Motion During Functional Activities: Mean Maximal Values in Degrees

Activity	Study			Motion			
	First author	N	Measurement	Elevation	Plane of Elevation*	Medial Rotation	Lateral Rotation
Feeding Tasks							
Drink with glass/cup	Aizawa[69]	20	3D electromagnetic (EM) system	87	80 (F)		62, 60†
	Cooper[§70]	19	3D optical video system	34 26	90 (F) 0 (Abd)	25	
	Safaee-Rad[71]	10	3D optical video system	43 31	90 (F) 0 (Abd)	23	
	Van Andel[72]	10	3D optical system	64	62 (S)	59	
Eat with spoon	Magermans[73]	24	3D EM system, GH motion	74	60 (S)		49
	Safaee-Rad[71]	10	3D optical video system	36 22	90 (F) 0 (Abd)	17	
Eat with fork	May-Lisowski[74]	20	3D EM system	58 47	90 (F) 0 (Abd)		7
	Safaee-Rad[71]	10	3D optical video system	35 19	90 (F) 0 (Abd)	18	
Eat meal	Hermi[75]	5	3D optical system	43	90 (F)		
Pour from pitcher	O'Neill[76]	10	3D EM system	74	42 (S)		
Reaching Tasks for Personal Care							
Hand to occiput/ back of head	Namdari[77]	20	3D EM system	127	0 (Abd)		61
	O'Neill[76]	10	3D EM system	127	57 (S)		
	Sheikhzadeh[78]	8	3D EM system	110	47 (S)		42
Put on necklace	Aizawa[69]	20	3D EM system	106	65 (S)		58, 77†
Hand to back of neck	Sheikhzadeh[78]	8	3D EM system	124	47 (S)		42
Comb hair/hand to top of head	Aizawa[69]	20	3D EM system	110	60 (S)		57, 79†
	Magermans[73]	24	3D EM system, GH motion	90	59 (S)		70
	Namdari[77]	20	3D EM system	108	86 (F)		
	Petuskey[79]	28	3D optical system	85 36	90 (F) 0 (Abd)		
	Van Andel[72]	10	3D optical system	98	64 (S)		81
Wash face	Aizawa[69]	20	3D EM system	44	111 (F)	17 NSAR	57 ISBAR
	Hermi[75]	5	3D optical system	50	90 (F)		
Hand to forehead	Mackey[80]	10‡	3D optical system	105 49	90 (F) 0 (Abd)		
	Sheikhzadeh[78]	8	3D EM system	64	80 (F)		39
Hand to mouth	Mackey[80]	10‡	3D optical system	70 46	90 (F) 0 (Abd)		
	O'Neill[76]	10	3D EM system	87	77 (F)		
Hand to chin	Sheikhzadeh[78]	8	3D EM system	38	77 (F)		32
Hand to axilla (ipsilateral)	Aizawa[69]	20	3D EM system	51	−27(E)	53, 31†	
Hand to axilla (contralateral)	Aizawa[69]	20	3D EM system	42	109 (F)	65 NSAR	11 ISBAR
	Magermans[73]	24	3D EM system, GH motion	53	100 (F)		15

TABLE 4.5 Shoulder Motion During Functional Activities: Mean Maximal Values in Degrees (continued)

Activity	Study			Motion			
	First author	N	Measurement	Elevation	Plane of Elevation*	Medial Rotation	Lateral Rotation
Hand to shoulder (contralateral)	Van Andel[72]	10	3D optical system	53	102 (F)	27	
	O'Neill[76]	10	3D EM system	69	124 (F)		
	Sheikhzadeh[78]	8	3D EM system	54	111 (F)		37
Wash back of opposite shoulder	Namdari[77]	20	3D EM system	95	116 (F)		116
Hand to midback/ unhook bra	Namdari[77]	20	3D EM system	47	−90 (E)	99	
Hand to back pocket	Van Andel[72]	10	3D optical system	48	−53 (E)	102	
	Petuskey[79]	28[‡]	3D optical system	47	−88 (E)	27	
Hand to sacrum/ perineum	Aizawa[69]	20	3D EM system	41	−86 (E)	135, 66[†]	
	Magermans[73]	24	3D EM system, GH motion	35	−67 (E)	105	
	O'Neill[76]	10	3D EM system	31	−77 (E)		
Hand to shoe	O'Neill[76]	10	3D EM system	72	88 (F)		
Common Tasks							
Reach over head	Magermans[73]	24	3D EM system, GH motion	121	73 (F)		61
	Petuskey[79]	28[‡]	3D optical system	142 34	90 (F) 0 (Abd)		
Reach high shelf	Namdari[77]	20	3D EM system	121	90 (F)		38
	O'Neill[76]	10	3D EM system	105	61 (S)		
Reach midshelf/ shoulder height	Mackey[80]	10[‡]	3D optical system	94 58	90 (F) 0 (Abd)		
	Namdari[77]	20	3D EM system	105	90 (F)		34
	O'Neill[76]	10	3D EM system	62	66 (S)		
Turn steering wheel	O'Neill[76]	10	3D EM system	70	90 (F)		
Propel wheel chair	Collinger[81]	61**	3D optical systems, self-selected speed	24 52 47	90 (F) 0 (Abd) −90 (E)	84	
	Rao[82]	16**	3D optical system, self-selected speed	57 23	23 (Abd) −57 (E)	86	
	Koontz[83]	27**	3D optical system, 0.9 m/s speed	19 42 43	90 (F) 0 (Abd) −90 (E)	52	

* Plane of Elevation indicates the horizontal positioning of the humerus during elevation: 0 degrees = elevation in the frontal plane, which is equivalent to abduction; 90 degrees = elevation in the sagittal plane anterior to body, which is equivalent to flexion; −90 = elevation in the sagittal plane posterior to the body, which is equivalent to extension; and 45 degrees = elevation 45 degrees anterior to the frontal plane, which is commonly termed scaption. Plane of elevation that is closest to Abduction (Abd), Flexion (F), Extension (E), and Scaption (S) is indicated in the table to assist with interpretation.

† First number used is the International Society of Biomechanics definition for axial rotation (ISBAR) method, second number used is the nonsingular axial rotation (NSAR) method. The zero position of rotation differs in the two definitions.

‡ Subjects were healthy male and female children aged 9 to 12 years.

** Subjects were adults with paraplegia due to a spinal cord injury below T1.

§ Cooper studied three feeding tasks with cup, spoon, fork, but drink with cup provided maximal ROM values. Values were averaged from males and females.

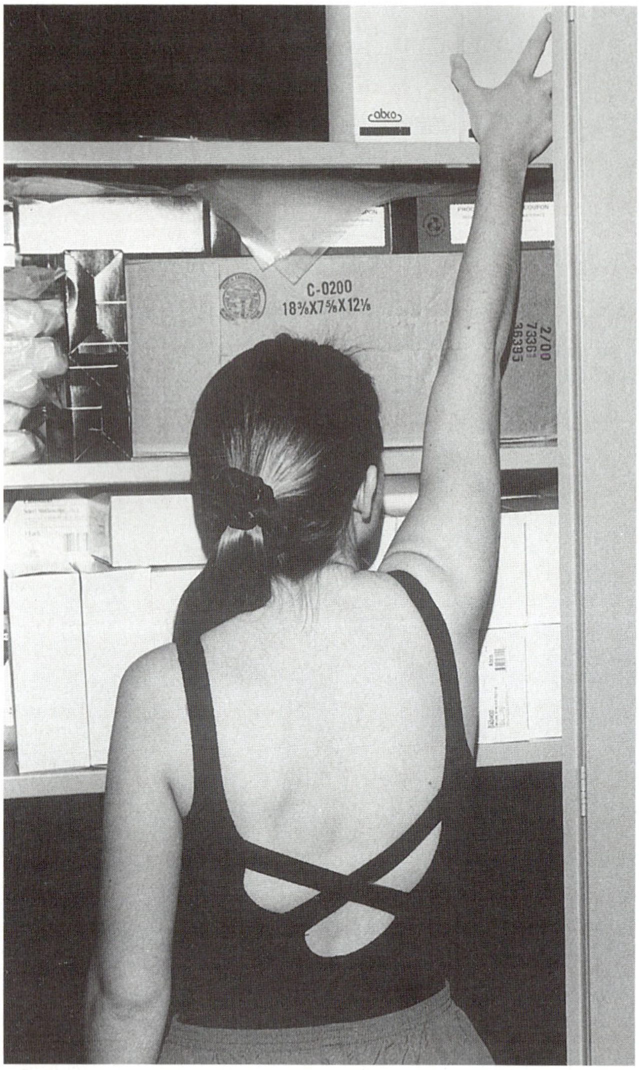

FIGURE 4.35 Reaching objects on a high shelf requires about 120 degrees of shoulder flexion in adults[77] and about 140 degrees in children.[79] The amount of motion depending on the height of the shelf and height of the individual.

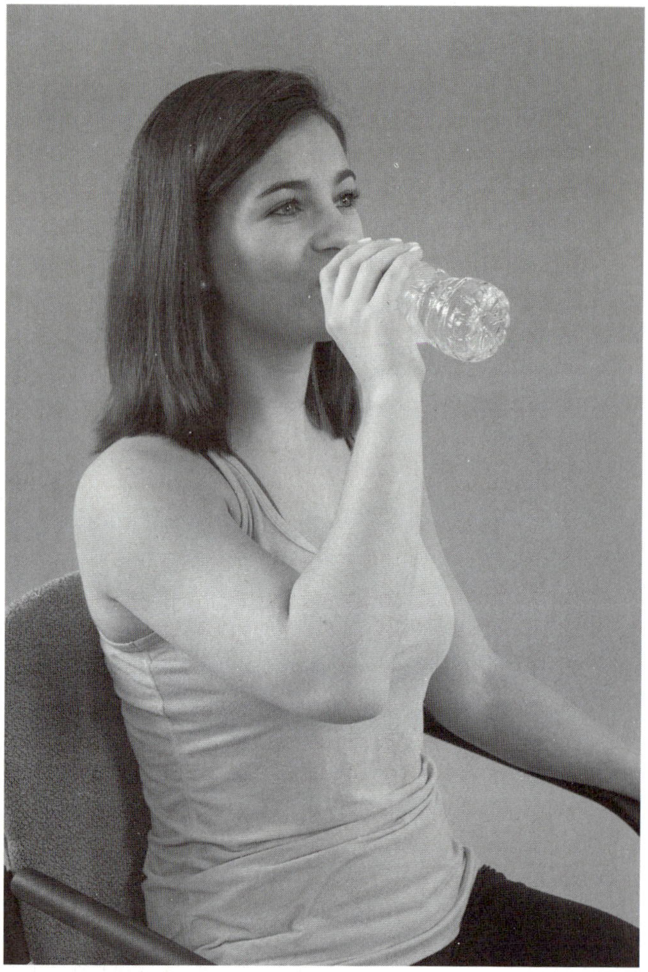

FIGURE 4.36 Feeding tasks such as eating with a fork and spoon, and drinking from a cup or in this case a water bottle, require about 35 to 85 degrees of shoulder flexion.[69,71]

Namdari and associates,[77] in a study of 20 healthy adults performing 10 activities of daily living, found that subjects required 57% to 76% of full shoulder motion to successfully complete a task. To complete all 10 tasks required approximately 120 degrees of flexion, 45 degrees of extension, 130 degrees of abduction, 115 degrees of cross-body (horizontal) adduction, and 60 degrees of lateral rotation with the arm abducted to 90 degrees. The 10 tasks were taken from functional assessment sections of three commonly used standardized outcome tools.

Reliability and Validity

Reliability of Universal Goniometers

The intratester and intertester reliability of measurements of shoulder motions with a universal goniometer have been studied by many researchers. The results of some of these studies are presented in Tables 4.6 and 4.7 and are briefly summarized in this section. Reliability varies according to the motion being measured, but no shoulder motions were consistently found to be less reliable than other motions across multiple studies. Most studies presented evidence that measurements taken by the same tester (intratester reliability) are more consistent and have less measurement error than measurements taken by different testers (intertester reliability). It is suggested that the same tester take repeated measurements of patient ROM whenever possible so that differences in measurement values more likely reflect change in patient status than measurement error. Some studies indicate that adding consistent stabilization through positioning (supine versus standing or sitting) or manual contact is helpful. Likewise, testers who are more familiar and experienced with goniometry usually have better reliability than novice users.

Healthy Populations

Many studies have focused on the reliability of shoulder ROM measurement taken with a universal goniometer in healthy populations. Boone and coworkers[86] examined the reliability

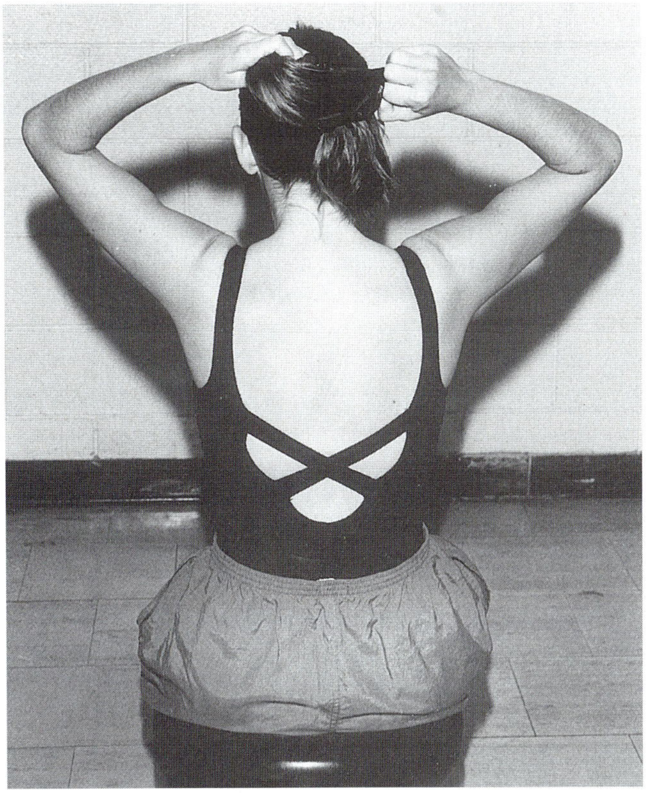

FIGURE 4.37 Reaching behind the head requires 110 to 125 degrees of abduction/scaption and 40 to 60 degrees of lateral rotation of the shoulder.[76–78]

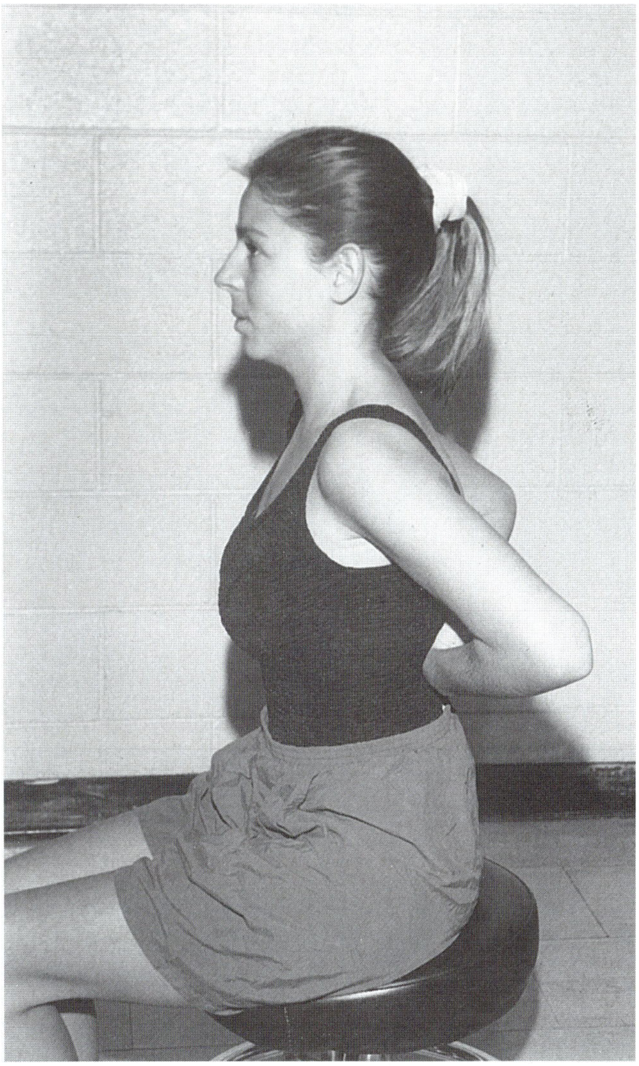

FIGURE 4.38 Reaching behind the back to fasten a bra or bathing suit requires about 50 degrees of extension and a large amount of medial rotation of the shoulder.[77]

of measuring active ROM for lateral rotation of the shoulder complex, elbow extension–flexion, wrist ulnar deviation, hip abduction, knee extension–flexion, and foot inversion. Four physical therapists used universal goniometers to measure these motions in 12 healthy males once a week for 4 weeks. Measurement of lateral rotation of the shoulder was more reliable than that of the other motions tested. For all motions except lateral rotation of the shoulder, intratester reliability was noted to be greater than intertester reliability. Intratester and intertester reliability for lateral rotation ROM were excellent and similar with Pearson's correlation coefficient (r) of 0.96 and 0.97, respectively.

Boon and Smith[13] studied 50 high school athletes to determine the reliability of measuring passive shoulder rotation ROM with and without manual stabilization of the scapula. Four experienced physical therapists working in pairs took goniometric measurements with the shoulder in 90 degrees of abduction and repeated those measurements 5 days later. Scapular stabilization, which resulted in more isolated glenohumeral motion, produced significantly smaller ROM values than when the scapula was not stabilized. According to the authors, intratester reliability for medial rotation was poor for nonstabilized motion (intraclass correlation coefficient [ICC] = 0.23, standard error of measurement [SEM] = 20.2 degrees) and good for stabilized motion (ICC = 0.60, SEM = 8.0 degrees). The authors state that intratester reliability for lateral rotation was good for both nonstabilized (ICC = 0.79, SEM = 5.6) and stabilized motion (ICC = 0.53, SEM = 9.1). Intertester reliability for medial rotation improved from nonstabilized motion (ICC = 0.13, SEM = 21.5) to stabilized motion (ICC = 0.38, SEM = 10.0), and was similar for both nonstabilized and stabilized lateral rotation (ICC = 0.84, SEM = 4.9 and ICC = 0.78, SEM = 6.6, respectively).

Bovens and associates,[87] in a study of the variability and reliability of nine joint motions throughout the body, used a universal goniometer to examine active lateral rotation ROM of the shoulder complex with the arm at the side. Three physician testers and eight healthy subjects participated in the study. Intratester reliability coefficients for lateral rotation of the shoulder ranged from 0.76 to 0.83, whereas the intertester reliability coefficient was 0.63. Mean intratester standard deviations for the measurements taken on each subject ranged from 5.0 to 6.6 degrees, whereas the mean intertester

Text continued on page 109

TABLE 4.6 Intratester Reliability of Shoulder ROM Measurements With Universal Goniometers and Other Devices for Healthy and Patient Populations

Study	N	Sample	Methods	Motion	r	ICC	Absolute Measures (degrees)
Healthy Populations							
Boone et al[86]	12	Healthy males	AROM, 4 testers (PT) universal goniometer	Lateral rotation	.96		Intra SD = 0.6 Total SD = 3.8
Boone and Smith[13]	50	Healthy high school athletes	PROM, 4 testers (PT), universal goniometer with and without scapula stabilized				SEM:
				GH Medial rotation		.60	8.0
				GH Lateral rotation		.58	9.1
				Medial rotation		.23	20.2
				Lateral rotation		.79	5.6
Bovens et al[87]	8	Healthy adults	AROM, 3 testers (physicians), universal goniometer, with arm at side, elbows flexed 90°	Lateral rotation	.76, .80, .83		Repeated measures SD: 5.0 6.6 5.6
Carey et al[88]	18	Healthy adults	AROM, PROM, 5 testers (PT). universal goniometer, new prototype digital inclinometer	Universal goniometer:			
				Medial rotation			
				PROM	.73–.90		
				AROM	.66–.80		
				Lateral rotation			
				PROM	.41–.81		
				AROM	.34–.80		
				Digital inclinometer:			
				Medial rotation			
				PROM	.75–.91		
				AROM	.81–.86		
				Lateral rotation			
				PROM	.85–.92		
				AROM	.64–.94		
Greene and Wolf[19]	20	Healthy adults	AROM, 1 tester (PT), universal goniometer and Ortho Ranger inclinometer	Universal goniometer:			Repeated measures SD:
				Flexion		.96	1.4
				Extension		.98	1.1
				Abduction		.96	1.8
				Adduction		.97	1.7
				Medial rotation		.93	2.8
				Lateral rotation		.91	3.0

				Inclinometer:		
				Flexion	.94	3.1
				Extension	.97	2.2
				Abduction	.94	3.7
				Adduction	.94	4.0
				Medial rotation	.91	3.5
				Lateral rotation	.87	3.8
Kolber and Hanney[89]	30	Healthy adults	AROM, 2 testers (PT students), universal goniometer and digital inclinometer	Universal goniometer:		SEM:
				Flexion	.95	2
				Abduction	.97	2
				Medial rotation	.95	2
				Lateral rotation	.94	3
				Digital inclinometer:		
				Flexion	.95	2
				Abduction	.97	2
				Medial rotation	.97	2
				Lateral rotation	.98	2
Macedo and Magee[10]	12	Healthy females	PROM, 2 testers (PT) 1 measured, 1 read universal goniometer	Glenohumeral:		SEM; MDC:
				Flexion	.98	6.3; 17.4
				Extension	.78	4.9; 13.5
				Abduction	.84	5.8; 16.0
				Medial rotation	.97	2.8; 7.6
				Lateral rotation	.84	5.5; 15.3
				Shoulder complex:		
				Flexion	.98	1.9; 5.2
				Extension	.94	5.1; 14.2
				Abduction	.95	3.4; 9.5
				Medial rotation	.97	2.5; 6.8
				Lateral rotation	.96	2.8; 7.8
Sabari et al[45]	30	19 healthy adults and 11 adult rehabilitation patients	AROM, PROM, 1 tester (OT), universal goniometer, supine and sitting	Flexion:		
				AROM supine	.95	
				AROM sitting	.97	
				PROM supine	.94	
				PROM sitting	.95	
				Abduction:		
				AROM supine	.99	
				AROM sitting	.97	
				PROM supine	.98	
				PROM sitting	.95	

(table continues on page 104)

TABLE 4.6 Intratester Reliability of Shoulder ROM Measurements With Universal Goniometers and Other Devices for Healthy and Patient Populations (continued)

Study	*N*	Sample	Methods	Motion	*r*	ICC	Absolute Measures (degrees)
Patient Populations							
Hayes et al[90]	9	Adult patients with shoulder complaint seen by orthopedic surgeon	AROM, PROM, 1 tester (orthopedic surgeon) Rotation in sitting with arm at side and elbow flexed 90° for UG and visual; in supine for photograph. Flexion and abduction in sitting or standing.	Universal goniometer and AROM:			SEM:
				Flexion		.53	17
				Abduction		.58	23
				External rotation		.65	14
				Visual estimate PROM:			
				Flexion		.59	13
				Abduction		.60	21
				External rotation		.67	11
				Photography AROM:			
				Flexion		.56	19
				Abduction		.61	22
				External rotation		.60	13
Hellebrandt et al[91]	77	Adult patients seen at arthritic or orthopedic clinic	AROM, 1 tester (experienced PT), universal goniometer				Mean differences:
				Flexion			0.3
				Extension			0.5
				Abduction			1.5
				Medial rotation			1.0
				Lateral rotation			0.2
MacDermid et al[92]	30	Adult patients with variety of shoulder pathologies	PROM, 2 experienced testers (PT), universal goniometer, in 20°–30° shoulder abduction and 90° elbow flexion	Lateral rotation:			SEM:
				trial 1		.89	7.0
				trial 2		.94	4.9
Mullaney et al[93]	20	Adult patients with unilateral shoulder pathology, 9 males, 11 females	AROM, 2 testers (PT), 2 devices: universal goniometer, construction grade digital level (inclinometer)	Universal goniometer			95% LOA:
				Involved shoulder:			
				Flexion		.96, .97	7, 8
				Lateral rotation		.99, .99	6, 7
				Medial rotation		.97, .98	9, 8
				Noninvolved shoulder:			
				Flexion		.97, .91	3, 5
				Lateral rotation		.97, .98	6, 5
				Medial rotation		.94, .95	7, 8
				Digital level			
				Involved shoulder:			
				Flexion		.97, .98	6, 6
				Lateral rotation		.99, .98	6, 9
				Medial rotation		.97, .91	6, 9

				Noninvolved shoulder:		
				Flexion	.94, .96	5, 3
				Lateral rotation	.99, .98	5, 5
				Medial rotation	.98, .92	5, 7
Pandya et al[94]	150	Children and teen patients with Duchenne muscular dystrophy, aged 1 to 20 years	PROM, 5 testers (PT), universal goniometer	Abduction	.84	
Riddle et al[95]	50	Adult patients who required shoulder examinations	PROM, 16 testers (PT), universal goniometer in 2 sizes: large (10-inch) and small (5-inch) goniometers, positions varied	Large goniometer:		
				Flexion	.98	
				Extension	.94	
				Abduction	.98	
				Medial rotation	.94	
				Lateral rotation	.99	
				Horz. abduction	.90	
				Horz. adduction	.95	
				Small goniometer:		
				Flexion	.98	
				Extension	.94	
				Abduction	.98	
				Medial rotation	.93	
				Lateral rotation	.98	
				Horz. abduction	.93	
				Horz. adduction	.96	
Shin et al[96]	41	Adult patients with shoulder symptoms	AROM (included here), AROM with passive overpressure, 3 testers (2 orthopedic residents, 1 orthopedic surgeon), 2 devices: universal goniometer, smartphone inclinometer			SEM least experienced tester:
				Universal goniometer:		
				Flexion	.80, .92, .96	6.3
				Abduction	.99, .98, .94	14.7
				Lateral rot. (0° Abd)	.98, .96, .96	7.6
				Lateral rot. (90° Abd)	.99, .97, .96	7.0
				Medial rot. (90° Abd)	.98, .94, .96	4.3
				Smartphone inclinometer:		
				Flexion	.99, .97, .97	2.7
				Abduction	.96, .99, .97	6.3
				Lateral rot. (0° Abd)	.97, .97, .95	3.3
				Lateral rot. (90° Abd)	.98, .97, .96	3.0
				Medial rot. (90° Abd)	.99, .79, .97	1.9

All measurements of medial and lateral rotation are with shoulder abducted and elbow flexed 90° unless otherwise noted. AROM = Active range of motion; PROM = Passive range of motion; r = Pearson's product moment correlation coefficient; ICC = Interclass correlation coefficient; SD = Standard deviation; SEM = Standard error of measurement; MDC = Minimal detectible change with 95% confidence; 95% LOA = 95% limits of agreement; Abd = Abduction; rot. = rotation; Horz. = horizontal; PT = physical therapist; OT = occupational therapist.

TABLE 4.7 Intertester Reliability of Shoulder ROM Measurements With Universal Goniometers and Other Devices for Healthy and Patient Populations

Study	N	Sample	Methods	Motion	r	ICC	Absolute Measures (degrees)
Healthy Populations							
Boone et al[86]	12	Healthy males	AROM, 4 physical therapist (PT) testers, universal goniometer	Lateral rotation	.97		Intra SD = 1.5 Total SD = 4.0
Boone and Smith[13]	50	Healthy high school athletes; 18 males, 32 females	PROM, 4 testers (PT), universal goniometer with and without scapula stabilized				SEM:
				GH Medial rotation		.38	10.0
				GH Lateral rotation		.78	6.6
				Medial rotation		.13	21.5
				Lateral rotation		.84	4.9
Bovens et al[87]	8	Healthy adults	AROM, 3 testers (physicians), universal goniometer, with arm at side and elbow flexed 90°	Lateral rotation	.63		Repeated measures SD: 7.4
Carey et al[88]	18	Healthy adults	AROM, PROM, 5 testers (PT). universal goniometer, and new prototype digital inclinometer	Universal goniometer:			
				Medial rotation			
				PROM		.60	
				AROM		.60	
				Lateral rotation			
				PROM		.46	
				AROM		.46	
				Digital inclinometer:			
				Medial rotation			
				PROM		.62	
				AROM		.61	
				Lateral rotation			
				PROM		.53	
				AROM		.48	
Patient Populations							
Hayes et al[90]	8	Adult patients with shoulder complaint seen by orthopedic surgeon	AROM, PROM, 4 testers (orthopedic surgeon, sport physician trainee, 2 PTs). Rotation in sitting with arm at side and elbow flexed 90° for UG and visual; in supine for photography. Flexion and abduction in sitting or standing.	Universal goniometer AROM:			SEM:
				Flexion		.69	25
				Abduction		.69	21
				Lateral rotation		.64	14
				Visual estimate PROM:			
				Flexion		.57	19
				Abduction		.66	19
				Lateral rotation		.57	14

				Photography AROM:		
				Flexion	.73	23
				Abduction	.73	23
				Lateral rotation	.62	15
Hellebrandt et al[91]	77	Adult patients seen at arthritic or orthopedic clinics	AROM, 9 testers (PT) universal goniometer	Flexion Extension Abduction Medial rotation Lateral rotation		Mean differences = 2.8
MacDermid et al[92]	30	Adult patients with variety of shoulder pathologies	PROM, 2 experienced testers (PT), universal goniometer, in 20–30° shoulder abduction and 90° elbow flexion	Lateral rotation		SEM:
				trial 1	.86	7.5
				trial 2	.85	8.0
Mullaney et al[93]	20	Adult patients with unilateral shoulder pathology, 9 males, 11 females	AROM, 2 testers (PT), 2 devices: universal goniometer, construction grade digital level (inclinometer)	Universal goniometer		95% LOA:
				Involved shoulder:		
				Flexion	.88, .93	14, 10
				Lateral rotation	.95, .92	13, 17
				Medial rotation	.87, .82	14, 16
				Noninvolved shoulder:		
				Flexion	.79, .74	7, 9
				Lateral rotation	.76, .79	17, 16
				Medial rotation	.63, .62	20, 23
				Digital level		
				Involved shoulder:		
				Flexion	.91, .91	11, 11
				Lateral rotation	.91, .93	20, 17
				Medial rotation	.82, .84	14, 13
				Noninvolved shoulder:		
				Flexion	.87, .86	6, 7
				Lateral rotation	.82, .85	18, 16
				Medial rotation	.47, .31	20, 25
Pandya[94]	21	Children and young adult patients with Duchenne muscular dystrophy, aged 1 to 20 years	PROM, 5 testers (PT), universal goniometer	Abduction	.67	

(table continues on page 108)

TABLE 4.7 Intertester Reliability of Shoulder ROM Measurements With Universal Goniometers and Other Devices for Healthy and Patient Populations (continued)

Study	*N*	Sample	Methods	Motion	*r*	ICC	Absolute Measures (degrees)
Riddle et al[95]	50	Adult patients who required shoulder examination	PROM, 16 testers (PT), universal goniometer in 2 sizes: large (10-inch) and small (5-inch) goniometers, positioned varied	Large goniometer:			
				Flexion		.89	
				Extension		.27	
				Abduction		.87	
				Medial rotation		.55	
				Lateral rotation		.88	
				Horz. abduction		.30	
				Horz. adduction		.41	
				Small goniometer:			
				Flexion		.87	
				Extension		.26	
				Abduction		.84	
				Medial rotation		.43	
				Lateral rotation		.90	
				Horz. abduction		.28	
				Horz. adduction		.35	
Shin et al[96]	41	Adult patients with shoulder symptoms	AROM (included here), AROM with passive overpressure, 3 testers (2 orthopedic residents, 1 orthopedic surgeon), 2 devices: universal goniometer, smartphone inclinometer	Universal goniometer:			SEM:
				Flexion		.77, .86	12.0, 8.8
				Abduction		.85, .89	11.9, 10.0
				Lateral rot. (0° Abd)		.81, .80	8.4, 8.3
				Lateral rot. (90° Abd)		.91, .87	6.3, 7.5
				Medial rot. (90° Abd)		.67, .67	10.9, 11.4
				Smartphone inclinometer:			
				Flexion			
				Abduction		.83, .84	10.0, 9.6
				Lateral rot. (0° Abd)		.78, .79	13.8, 13.2
				Lateral rot. (90° Abd)		.77, .76	9.4, 9.7
				Medial rot. (90° Abd)		.87, .87	7.8, 7.8
						.76, .66	10.3, 10.6

All measurements of medial and lateral rotation are with shoulder abducted and elbow flexed 90° unless otherwise noted. AROM = Active range of motion; PROM = Passive range of motion; *r* = Pearson's product moment correlation coefficient; ICC = Interclass correlation coefficient; SD = Standard deviation; SEM = Standard error of measurement; MDC = Minimal detectible change with 95% confidence; 95% LOA = 95% limits of agreement; Abd = Abduction.

standard deviation was 7.4 degrees. The measurement of lateral rotation ROM of the shoulder was more reliable than were ROM measurements of the forearm and wrist. Mean standard deviations between repeated measurements of shoulder lateral rotation ROM were similar to those of the forearm and larger than those of the wrist.

Carey and coworkers[88] examined the reliability of measuring active and passive shoulder rotations with a universal goniometer and new prototype digital inclinometer in 18 healthy subjects. Five physical therapists measured each motion twice with each device. Intratester reliability for measuring passive medial rotation ROM was similar for both devices ($r = 0.73$ to 0.91), but active medial rotation and active and passive lateral rotation measurements were more reliable with the prototype digital inclinometer (see Tables 4.6 and 4.7). Intertester reliability as indicated by Pearson's correlation coefficient was generally low for both devices and motions ($r = 0.46$ to 0.62). Passive ROM measurements had better reliability than active ROM measurements using both devices, as did medial rotation as compared with lateral rotation ROM measurements. In this small study population, no statistically significant differences in measurement values were noted between devices; however, mean values for each device were not provided for comparison.

Greene and Wolf[19] compared the reliability of the Ortho Ranger, an electronic pendulum inclinometer, with that of a standard universal goniometer for active upper-extremity motions in 20 healthy adults. Shoulder complex motions were measured by one physical therapist three times with each instrument during three sessions that occurred over a 2-week period. Both instruments demonstrated high intrasession correlations (ICCs ranged from 0.98 to 0.87), but correlations were higher and 95% confidence intervals about the mean on the same subjects were considerably lower for the universal goniometer (3.9 to 17.2 degrees) versus the inclinometer (9.8 to 31.1 degrees). Measurements of medial rotation and lateral rotation ROM were less reliable than were measurements of flexion, extension, abduction, and adduction. There were significant differences between measurements taken with the Ortho Ranger and the universal goniometer. Interestingly, there were significant differences in measurements between sessions for both instruments. The authors noted that the daily variations that were found might have been caused by normal fluctuation in ROM, as suggested by Boone and colleagues,[86] or by daily differences in subjects' efforts while performing active ROM.

Kolber and Hanney[89] likewise compared the reliability of shoulder ROM measurements taken with a 12-inch universal goniometer and a digital inclinometer (Acumar) in 30 healthy adults. One physical therapy student took two measurements for each motion with the goniometer and another took two measurements for each motion with the inclinometer. Intratester reliability for both devices was excellent with all ICC values greater than 0.94 and SEM values ranging from 2 to 3 degrees. Concurrent validity between the two devices was good with ICC values of greater than 0.85. There appeared to be some differences in mean values taken with the two devices and testers: 1 degree for abduction, 5 degrees for medial rotation, and 8 degrees for flexion and lateral rotation. The 95% limits of agreement (LOA) between the two devices ranged from 2 to 20 degrees.

Macedo and Magee,[10] in a preliminary study of 12 healthy females aged 18 to 59 years, found the intratester reliability of measuring passive glenohumeral and shoulder complex ROM to be good to excellent with ICC values ranging from 0.78 to 0.98. Standard error of measurement (SEM) values ranged from about 3 to 6 degrees for glenohumeral motions and from 2 to 5 degrees for shoulder complex motions. On visual inspection of the results, intratester reliability appeared to be slightly better for shoulder complex versus glenohumeral ROM measurements. Measurements were taken with a universal goniometer by two physical therapists using methods described in the 2003 edition of this textbook.

Sabari and associates[45] examined intrarater reliability in the measurement of active and passive shoulder complex flexion and abduction ROM when 30 adults were positioned in supine and sitting positions. The ICCs between two trials by the same tester for each procedure ranged in value from 0.94 to 0.99, indicating high intratester reliability regardless of whether the measurements were active or passive or whether they were taken with the subject in the supine or the sitting position. There were no significant differences between comparable flexion measurements taken in supine and sitting positions. However, significantly greater abduction ROM was found in the supine than in the sitting position with mean differences ranging from 3 to 7.1 degrees.

Patient Populations

The reliability of using a universal goniometer to take measurements on patients with shoulder conditions has also been studied. Hayes and coworkers[90] measured the intratester reliability of shoulder flexion, abduction, and lateral rotation in nine patients with shoulder complaints using one tester who was an orthopedic surgeon. They also measured the intertester reliability of shoulder motion in eight patients using four testers of varying backgrounds. A universal goniometer was aligned with the humerus and various planes of motion with the patients in sitting position. Intratester reliability ICC values for the universal goniometer ranged from 0.53 to 0.65, and intertester values ranged from 0.64 to 0.69. The reliability of using visual estimation and still photography with labeled landmarks was also studied and produced similar results. The use of a tape measure to note distance between T1 and the thumb during reaching behind the back produced the worst ICC values of 0.39 and SEM values of 6 centimeters.

Hellebrandt, Duvall, and Moore[91] in a study of 77 patients found the intratester reliability of goniometric measurements of active ROM of shoulder complex abduction and medial rotation to be less than the reliability of measurements of shoulder flexion, extension, and lateral rotation. Mean differences between the repeated measurements taken by one experienced therapist ranged from 0.2 to 1.5 degrees. Mean differences between goniometric measurements taken by eight therapists averaged 2.8 degrees. Measurements were also taken with devices designed by the U.S. Army for specific joints. For most ROM measurements taken throughout the body, the universal goniometer was a more dependable tool than were the special devices.

In a study by MacDermid and colleagues,[92] two experienced physical therapists measured passive shoulder complex rotation ROM in 34 patients with a variety of shoulder pathologies. A universal goniometer was used to measure lateral rotation with the shoulder in 20 to 30 degrees of abduction. Intratester ICCs (0.88 and 0.93) and intertester ICCs (0.85 and 0.80) were high. Intratester standard errors of measurement (SEM; 4.9 and 7.0 degrees) and intertester SEM (7.5 and 8.0 degrees) also indicated good reliability. The SEMs indicate that differences of 5 to 7 degrees could be attributed to measurement error when the same tester repeats a measurement and about 8 degrees could be attributed to measurement error when different testers take a measurement.

Mullaney and coworkers[93] examined active ROM of the involved and noninvolved shoulders of 20 patients with unilateral shoulder pathology. Two physical therapists used a 12-inch universal goniometer and a construction-grade digital level (inclinometer) to take two repeated ROM measurements with each device of shoulder flexion, lateral rotation, and medial rotation in supine. Intratester reliability was excellent for both devices, with ICC values ranging from 0.91 to 0.99 and 95% LOA ranging from 3 to 9 degrees. Intertester reliability for both devices was lower, with ICC between 0.31 and 0.98 and 95% LOA values from 6 to 25 degrees. Measurements of flexion were the most reliable, whereas measurements of medial rotation were the least reliable in this particular study. Based on average LOA values in the involved shoulder, the authors suggest that a change of 6 to 11 degrees is needed for clinicians to be 95% certain that a true change has occurred when measurements are taken by the same tester, and a change of 15 degrees is needed if measurements are taken by different testers. Measurements taken with the two devices were not interchangeable because the level (inclinometer) consistently resulted in 3 to 5 degrees of greater lateral and medial rotation ROM values than occurred using the goniometer.

Pandya and associates,[94] in a study in which five physical therapists measured the passive ROM of shoulder complex abduction of 150 children and young adults with Duchenne muscular dystrophy, found that intratester reliability was good, with mean intraclass correlation coefficient (ICC) values of 0.84. The intertester reliability for measuring shoulder abduction in 21 patients was lower (ICC = 0.67). The researchers suggest that the same examiner be used for long-term follow-up and to assess results of treatment interventions in patient populations.

Riddle, Rothstein, and Lamb[95] conducted a study to determine intratester and intertester reliability for passive ROM measurements of the shoulder complex of 50 patients. Sixteen physical therapists, assessing in pairs, used two different-sized universal goniometers (large and small) for their measurements. Patient position and goniometer placement during measurements were not controlled. Intratester reliability for all motions was excellent, as indicated by ICC values ranging from 0.87 to 0.99. Intertester reliability for flexion, abduction, and lateral rotation was good, with ICC values ranging from 0.84 to 0.90. Intertester reliability was considerably lower for measurements of horizontal abduction, horizontal adduction, extension, and medial rotation, with ICC values ranging from 0.26 to 0.55. The authors concluded that passive ROM measurements for all shoulder motions can be reliable when taken by the same physical therapist regardless of whether large or small goniometers are used. Measurements of flexion, abduction, and lateral rotation can be reliable when assessed by different therapists. However, because repeated measurements of horizontal abduction, horizontal adduction, extension, and medial rotation were unreliable when taken by more than one tester, the same therapist should take these measurements.

The reliability of measuring active ROM and passive overpressure of five shoulder complex motions using an 18-centimeter universal goniometer and a smartphone were studied by Shin and coworkers[96] in 41 adult patients with shoulder symptoms. A smartphone, equipped with a gyrosensor system and inclinometer application, was attached to the forearm. The goniometer was aligned with the humerus and either a vertical or horizontal axis. Flexion and abduction were measured standing and rotations were measured in supine. In almost all motions, for all three testers (two orthopedic residents and one orthopedic surgeon) and both devices intratester reliability was excellent, with ICC values greater than 0.92. Intertester reliability for all motions and both devices was considered satisfactory, with ICC values greater than 0.70, except for medial rotation, which was 0.63 to 0.68 in both devices. Varying amounts of scapula motion control during medial rotation was believed to contribute to these differences. There was a fairly high positive correlation (ICC 0.72 to 0.97) between the measurements taken with both devices, but the 95% LOA ranged from 10 to 40 degrees. Lower correlation values and greater differences for flexion and abduction ROM might have been affected by carrying angle and elbow flexion because the smartphone was attached to the distal forearm, as opposed to the goniometer, which was aligned with the humerus. In addition, these motions were measured in standing rather than supine so that movement of the trunk may have contributed to inconsistencies.

Reliability of Inclinometers and Other Clinical Devices

The reliability of measurement devices other than a universal goniometer for assessing shoulder ROM has also been studied and is briefly mentioned here. Readers are encouraged to seek out the original articles for details if they are considering using inclinometers or other devices. Because the reliability of measuring shoulder motion using an inclinometer was usually similar to or less than the reliability using a universal goniometer and universal goniometers are less expensive to purchase, we continue to recommend the use of the universal goniometer for shoulder ROM measurements. Some examiners may find the placement of an inclinometer on the body to be easier than the alignment of two arms of a goniometer. However, inclinometer measurements are sensitive to slight changes in body positioning that affect the relationship of the trunk and upper extremity to gravity, as well as to inclinometer location, body contour, and to the carrying angle and amount of elbow flexion if the inclinometer is positioned on the forearm. Similar to reliability studies using goniometers, reliability studies using inclinometers also have found intratester reliability to be better than intertester reliability. The same device, method procedures, and ideally the same tester should be used for repeated measurements on a patient to reduce measurement error.

Some studies have examined the reliability of using various manual inclinometers to measure shoulder ROM. Clarke and coworkers[97] and Bower[98] examined the reliability of measuring passive glenohumeral motions with a hydrogoniometer strapped to the arms of 5 and 10 subjects, respectively. More recently, de Jong and associates[99,100] used a hydrogoniometer to measure the interrater reliability of three passive shoulder motions in two studies of patients after stroke. Overall, ICC values were between 0.84 and 0.99, SEM values between 2 and 7 degrees, and smallest detectible difference (SDD) between 6 and 22 degrees. The reliability of measuring active shoulder complex ROM with a Plurimeter-V inclinometer in six patients with shoulder pain and stiffness was investigated by Green and associates.[101] Tiffitt, Wildin, and Hajioff[102] studied the reliability of using an inclinometer to measure active shoulder complex motions in 36 patients with shoulder disorders. Valentine and Lewis[103] included 45 subjects with and 45 subjects without shoulder symptoms in a study of the intratester reliability of shoulder flexion and abduction using a manual inclinometer, lateral rotation using a tape measure, and medial rotation using visual estimation. Mullaney and associates[93] studied the reliability of using a construction-grade digital level and a universal goniometer to measure active shoulder motion in 20 patients with shoulder pathology (see Tables 4.6 and 4.7 for more details).

Several researchers have investigated the reliability of electronic or digital inclinometers in measuring shoulder ROM. Greene and Wolf[19] examined the intratester reliability of using the Ortho Ranger, an electronic device based on a pendulum inclinometer, and a universal goniometer to measure active ROM in upper-extremity joints including the shoulder of 20 healthy adults (see Table 4.6). De Winter and coworkers[104] examined the intertester reliability of an electronic digital inclinometer (Cybex EDI-320) to measure glenohumeral flexion and shoulder lateral rotation in 155 patients with shoulder pain. The reliability of the Acumar digital inclinometer to measure active shoulder ROM in two groups of 30 asymptomatic subjects was studied by Kolber and associates[105] and Kolber and Hanney[89] (see Table 4.6). As mentioned, Shin and colleagues[96] examined the reliability of using a smartphone attached to the forearm and equipped with a gyro-sensor system and inclinometer application to measure shoulder ROM in 41 adult patients with shoulder symptoms (Tables 4.6 and 4.7)

In an unusual study, Croft and colleagues[106] reported the reliability of observing shoulder complex flexion and lateral rotation and sketching the ROMs onto diagrams that were then measured with a protractor. The reliability of visual estimates and photography of shoulder ROM has also been reported by Hayes et al[90] and Valentine and Lewis.[103]

Validity of Universal Goniometers and Inclinometers

We are unaware of any research studies that examined the concurrent validity of shoulder ROM measurements taken with a universal goniometer or an inclinometer to the gold standard of radiographs. However, the face and content validity of using the universal goniometer that measures angles to determine the angle between the humerus and thorax seems logical.

Establishing the face and content validity of inclinometers that measure the angle of the soft tissue of the upper arm or forearm to the vertical pull of gravity may be more of a challenge. The careful placement and stabilization of the trunk in vertical, zeroing the inclinometer at the start of the motion, and aligning the inclinometer with the long axis of a bony lever such as the humerus may improve the validity.

Some researchers have studied the concurrent validity of manual inclinometers,[93] digital inclinometers,[19,88,89,93] and smartphone inclinometer applications[96] to universal goniometers. Green and Wolf[19] reported poor correlations (r = 0.52 to 0.59) between measurements taken with the Ortho Ranger and universal goniometer for shoulder flexion, extension, abduction, and adduction, and high correlations (r = 0.90, 0.92) for medial and lateral rotation. Differences between the measurement means ranged from 9.6 degrees for abduction to 2.2 degrees for medial rotation. Kolber and Hanney[89] found measurements with a digital inclinometer and universal goniometer to have good correlation for flexion and abduction (ICC = 0.86, 0.85) and excellent correlation for medial and lateral rotation (ICC = 0.95, 0.97). Mean differences between devices ranged from 1 to 8 degrees and 95% LOA ranged from 2 to 20 degrees. Shin et al[96] noted acceptable correlations between shoulder ROM measurements using a smartphone inclinometer application and a universal goniometer (ICC = 0.72 to 0.97), but 95% LOA ranged from 10 to 40 degrees. The differences found in these studies may be due to the placement of inclinometers on the skin surfaces of the upper or lower arm as compared with the usual alignment of universal goniometers with the long axes of the humerus and thorax. Differences between devices were generally smaller for measurements of shoulder rotation in which the arms of the universal goniometer were also aligned vertically and with the forearm. Given these findings, different ROM measuring devices are not interchangeable. Repeated measurement should be taken with the same device, measurement procedure, and tester to reduce measurement error. Clinicians should keep in mind that normative ROM values established using universal goniometers may differ from values measured with other devices.

REFERENCES

1. Standring, S (ed): Gray's Anatomy, ed 41. Elsevier, New York, 2016.
2. Ludewig, PM, and Borstead, JD: The Shoulder Complex. In Levangie, P, and Norkin, C (eds): Joint Structure and Function: A Comprehensive Analysis, ed 5. FA Davis, Philadelphia, 2011.
3. Neumann, DA: Kinesiology of the Musculoskeletal System, ed 2. Mosby, St. Louis, 2009.
4. Ludewig, PM, et al: Motion of the shoulder complex during multiplanar humeral elevation. J Bone Joint Surg Am 91:378, 2009.
5. Culham, E, and Peat, M: Functional anatomy of the shoulder complex. J Orthop Sports Phys Ther 18:342, 1993.
6. Kisner, C, and Colby, LA: Therapeutic Exercise, ed 6. FA Davis, Philadelphia, 2012.
7. Kaltenborn, FM: Manual Mobilization of the Extremity Joints, ed 7. Olaf Norlis Bokhandel, Oslo, 2011.
8. Cyriax, JH, and Cyriax, PJ: Illustrated Manual of Orthopaedic Medicine. Butterworths, London, 1983.
9. Lannan, D, Lehman, T, and Toland, M: Establishment of normative data for the range of motion of the glenohumeral joint. Master of Science Thesis, University of Massachusetts, Lowell, MA, 1996.
10. Macedo, LG, and Magee, DJ: Effects of age on passive range of motion of selected peripheral joints in healthy adult females. Physiother Theory Pract 25:145, 2009.
11. Goddu, R, Iby, C, and Poirier, S: Establishment of normative data for the range of motion of the glenohumeral joint with respect to age and gender. Doctorate of Physical Therapy Thesis, University of Massachusetts, Lowell, MA, 2009.
12. Ellenbecker, TS, et al: Glenohumeral joint internal and external rotation range of motion in elite junior tennis players. J Orthop Sports Phys Ther 24:336, 1996.
13. Boon, AJ, and Smith, J: Manual scapular stabilization: Its effect on shoulder rotational range of motion. Arch Phys Med Rehabil 81:978, 2000.
14. Awan, R, Smith, J, and Boon, AJ: Measuring shoulder internal rotation range of motion: A comparison of 3 techniques. Arch Phys Med Rehabil 83:1229, 2002.
15. American Academy of Orthopaedic Surgeons: Joint Motion: Method of Measuring and Recording. AAOS, Chicago, 1965.
16. Greene, WB, and Heckman, JD: The Clinical Measurement of Joint Motion. American Academy of Orthopaedic Surgeons, Rosemont, IL, 1994.
17. Rondinelli, RD (ed): American Medical Association: Guides to the Evaluation of Permanent Impairment, ed 6. AMA, Chicago, 2008.
18. Boone, DC, and Azen, SP: Normal range of motion in male subjects. J Bone Joint Surg Am 61:756, 1979.
19. Greene, BL, and Wolf, SL: Upper extremity joint movement: Comparison of two measurement devices. Arch Phys Med Rehabil 70:288, 1989.
20. Roy, JS, et al: Rotational strength, range of motion, and function in people with unaffected shoulders from various stages of life. Sports Med Arthrosc Rehabil Ther Technol 1:4, 2009.
21. Soucie, JW, et al: Range of motion measurements: Reference values and a database for comparison studies. Haemophilia 17:500, 2011.
22. Rundquist, PJ, et al: Shoulder kinematics in subjects with frozen shoulder. Arch Phys Med Rehabil 84:1473, 2003.
23. Pearl, ML, et al: Humeroscapular positions in a shoulder range-of-motion examination. J Shoulder Elbow Surg 1:296, 1992.
24. Sahara, W, et al: Three-dimensional clavicular and acromioclavicular rotations during arm abduction using vertically open MRI. J Orthop Res 25:1243, 2007.
25. Nadeau, S, et al: Active movement measurements of the shoulder girdle in healthy subjects with goniometer and tape measure techniques: A study on reliability and validity. Physiother Theory Pract 23:179, 2007.
26. T'Jonck, L, Lysens, R, and Grasses, G: Measurements of scapular position and rotation: A reliability study. Physiother Res Int 1:148, 1996.
27. Thomas, SJ, et al: Glenohumeral rotation and scapular position after a single high school female sports season. J Athl Train 44:230, 2009.
28. Schenkman, M, et al: Measures of shoulder protraction and thorocolumbar rotation. J Orthop Sports Phys Ther 25:329, 1997.
29. Plafcan, DM, et al: An objective measurement technique for posterior scapular displacement. J Orthop Sports Phys Ther 25:336, 1997.
30. Kibler, WB, et al: Scapular Summit 20009: Introduction. J Orthop Sports Phys Ther 39:A1, 2009.
31. Wanatabe, H, et al: The range of joint motions of the extremities in healthy Japanese people: The difference according to age. Nippon Seikeigeka Gakkai Zasshi 53:275, 1979. Cited by Walker, JM: Musculoskeletal development: A review. Phys Ther 71:878, 1991.
32. Boone, DC: Techniques of measurement of joint motion. (Unpublished supplement to Boone, DC, and Azen, SP: Normal range of motion in male subjects. J Bone Joint Surg Am 61:756, 1979.)
33. Vairo, GL, et al: Clinical descriptive measures of shoulder range of motion for a healthy, young and physically active cohort. Sports Med Arthrosc Rehabil Ther Technol 4:33, 2012.
34. Walker, JM, et al: Active mobility of the extremities in older subjects. Phys Ther 64:919, 1984.
35. Downey, PA, Fiebert, I, and Stackpole-Brown, JB: Shoulder range of motion in persons aged sixty and older [abstract]. Phys Ther 71:S75, 1991.
36. Kalscheur, JA, Costello, PS, and Emery, LJ: Gender differences in range of motion in older adults. Phys Occup Ther Geriatr 22:77, 2003.
37. West, CC: Measurement of joint motion. Arch Phys Med Rehabil 26:414, 1945.
38. Clarke, GR, et al: Preliminary studies in measuring range of motion in normal and painful stiff shoulders. Rheumatol Rehabil 14:39, 1975.
39. Stathokostas, L, et al: Flexibility of older adults aged 55–86 years and the influence of physical activity. J Aging Res, article ID 743843, 2013.
40. Allander, E, et al: Normal range of joint movement in shoulder, hip, wrist and thumb with special reference to side: A comparison between two populations. Int J Epidemiol 3:253, 1974.
41. Barnes, CJ, Van Steyn, SJ, and Fischer, RA: The effect of age, sex, and shoulder dominance on range of motion of the shoulder. J Shoulder Elbow Surg 10:242, 2001.
42. Escalante, A, Lichenstein, MJ, and Hazuda, HP: Determinants of shoulder and elbow flexion range: Results from the San Antonio longitudinal study of aging. Arthritis Care Res 12:277, 1999.
43. Park, W, et al: Obesity effect of male active joint range of motion. Ergonomics 53:102, 2010.
44. Kebaetse, M, McClure, P, and Pratt, NA: Thoracic position effect on shoulder range of motion, strength, and three-dimensional scapular kinematics. Arch Phys Med Rehabil 80:945, 1999.
45. Sabari, JS, et al: Goniometric assessment of shoulder range of motion: Comparison of testing in supine and sitting positions. Arch Phys Med Rehabil 79:64, 1998.
46. Kalscheur, JA, Emery, LJ, and Costello, PS: Range of motion in older women. Phys Occup Ther Geriatr 16:77, 1999.
47. Gunal, I, et al: Normal range of motion of the joints of the upper extremity in male subjects, with special reference to side. J Bone Joint Surg 78A:1401, 1996.
48. Macedo, LG, and Magee, DJ: Differences in range of motion between dominant and nondominant sides of upper and lower extremities. J Manipulative Physiol Ther 31:577, 2008.
49. Bigliani, LU, et al: Shoulder motion and laxity in the professional baseball player. Am J Sports Med 25:609, 1997.
50. Baltaci, G, Johnson, R, and Kohl, H: Shoulder range of motion characteristics in collegiate baseball players. J Sports Med Phys Fitness 41:236, 2001.
51. Downar, JM, and Sauers, EL: Clinical measures of shoulder mobility in the professional baseball player. J Athl Train 40:23, 2005.
52. Borsa, PA, Laudner, KG, and Sauers, EL: Mobility and stability adaptations in the shoulder of the overhead athlete: A theoretical and evidence-based perspective. Sports Med 38:17, 2008.
53. Hurd, WJ, et al: A profile of glenohumeral internal and external rotation motion in the uninjured high school baseball pitcher: Part I: Motion. J Athl Train 46:282, 2011.
54. Shanley, E, et al: Shoulder range of motion measures as risk factors for shoulder and elbow injuries in high school softball and baseball players. Am J Sports Med 39:1997, 2011.
55. Wilk, KE, Macrina, LC, and Arrigo, C: Passive range of motion characteristics in the overhead baseball pitcher and their implications for rehabilitation. Clin Orthop Relat Res 470:1586, 2012.
56. Meyers, JP, et al: Glenohumeral range of motion deficits and posterior shoulder tightness in throwers with pathologic internal impingement. Am J Sports Med 34:385, 2006.
57. Manske, R, and Ellenbecker, T: Current concepts in shoulder examination of the overhead athlete. Int J Sport Phys Ther 8:554, 2013.
58. Manske, R, et al: Glenohumeral motion deficits: Friend or foe? Int J Sport Phys Ther 8:537, 2013
59. Kibler, WB, et al: The disabled throwing shoulder: Spectrum of pathology: 10 year update. Arthroscopy 29:141, 2013.
60. Chinn, CJ, Priest, JD, and Kent, BA: Upper extremity range of motion, grip strength and girth in highly skilled tennis players. Phys Ther 54:474, 1974.

61. Kibler, WB, et al: Shoulder range of motion in elite tennis players: Effect of age and years of tournament play. Am J Sports Med 24:279, 1996.
62. Beech, ML, Whitney, SL, and Dickoff-Hoffman, SA: Relationship of shoulder flexibility, strength, and endurance to shoulder pain in competitive swimmers. J Orthop Sports Phys Ther 16:262, 1992.
63. Bak, K, and Magnusson, SP: Shoulder strength and range of motion in symptomatic and pain-free elite swimmers. Am J Sports Med 25:454, 1997.
64. Weldon, EJ, III, and Richardson, AB: Upper extremity overuse injuries in swimming: A discussion of swimmer's shoulder. Clin Sports Med 20:423, 2001.
65. Witwer, A, and Sauers, E: Clinical measures of shoulder mobility in college water-polo players. J Sports Rehabil 15:45, 2006.
66. Chang, DE, Buschbacker, LP, and Edlich, RF: Limited joint mobility in power lifters. Am J Sports Med 16:280, 1988.
67. Tiffitt, PD: The relationship between motion of the shoulder and the stated ability to perform activities of daily living. J Bone Joint Surg 80:41, 1998.
68. Wu, G, et al: ISB recommendation on definitions of joint coordinate systems of various joints for the reporting of human joint motion. Part II: Shoulder, elbow, wrist and hand. J Biomech 38:981, 2005.
69. Aizawa, J, et al: Three-dimensional motion of the upper extremity joints during various activities of daily living. J Biomech 43:2915, 2010.
70. Cooper, JE, et al: Elbow joint restriction: Effect on functional upper limb motion during performance of three feeding activities. Arch Phys Med Rehabil 74:805, 1993.
71. Safaee-Rad, R, et al: Normal functional range of motion of upper limb joints during performance of three feeding activities. Arch Phys Med Rehabil 71:505, 1990.
72. Van Andel, CJ, et al: Complete 3D kinematics of upper extremity functional tasks. Gait Posture 27:120, 2007.
73. Mangermans, DJ, et al: Requirements for upper extremity motions during activities of daily living. Clin Biomech 20:591, 2005.
74. May-Lisowski, TL, and Kine, PM: Effect of wearing a static wrist orthosis on shoulder movement during feeding. Am J Occup Ther 62:438, 2008.
75. Henmi, S, et al: A biomechanical study of activities of daily living using neck and upper limbs with an optical three-dimensional motion analysis system. Mod Rheumatol 16:289, 2006.
76. O'Neill, OR, et al: Compensatory motion in the upper extremity after elbow arthrodesis. Clin Orthop Relat Res 281:89, 1992.
77. Namdari, S, et al: Defining functional shoulder range of motion for activities of daily living. J Shoulder Elbow Surg 21:1177, 2012.
78. Sheikhzadeh, A, et al: Three-dimensional motion of the scapula and shoulder during activities of daily living. J Shoulder Elbow Surg 17:936, 2008.
79. Petuskey, K, et al: Upper extremity kinematics during functional activities: Three-dimensional studies in a normal pediatric population. Gait Posture 25:573, 2007.
80. Mackey, AH, Walt, SE, and Stott, NS: Deficits in upper-limb task performance in children with hemiplegic cerebral palsy as defined by 3-dimensional kinematics. Arch Phys Med Rehabil 87:207, 2006.
81. Collinger, JL, et al: Shoulder biomechanics during the push phase of wheelchair propulsion: A multisite study of persons with paraplegia. Arch Phys Med Rehabil 89:667, 2008.
82. Rao, SS, Bontrager, EL, and Gronley, JK: Three-dimensional kinematics of wheelchair propulsion. IEEE Trans Rehabil Eng 4:152, 1996.
83. Koontz, AM, et al: Shoulder kinematics and kinetics during two speeds of wheelchair propulsion. J Rehabil Res Dev 39:635, 2002.
84. Buckley, MA, et al: Dynamics of upper limb during performance of the task of everyday living: A review of the current knowledge base. Proc Inst Mech Eng H 210:242, 1996.
85. Morrow, MMB, et al: Upper extremity joint kinetics expression during wheelchair propulsion. J Rehabil Res Dev 46:939, 2009.
86. Boone, DC, et al: Reliability of goniometric measurements. Phys Ther 58:1355, 1978.
87. Bovens, AMP, et al: Variability and reliability of joint measurements. Am J Sports Med 18:58, 1990.
88. Carey, MA, et al: Reliability, validity, and clinical usability of a digital goniometer. Work 36:55, 2010.
89. Kolber, MJ, and Hanney, WJ: The reliability and concurrent validity of shoulder mobility measurements using a digital inclinometer and goniometer: A technical report. Int J Sports Phys Ther 7:306, 2012.
90. Hayes, K, et al: Reliability of five methods for assessing shoulder range of motion. Aust J Physiother 47:289, 2001.
91. Hellebrandt, FA, Duvall, EN, and Moore, ML: The measurement of joint motion. Part III: Reliability of goniometry. Phys Ther Rev 29:302, 1949.
92. MacDermid, JC, et al: Intratester and intertester reliability of goniometric measurement of passive lateral shoulder rotation. J Hand Ther 12:187, 1999.
93. Mullaney, MJ, et al: Reliability of shoulder range of motion comparing a goniometer to a digital level. Physiother Theory Pract 26:327, 2010.
94. Pandya, S, et al: Reliability of goniometric measurements in patients with Duchenne muscular dystrophy. Phys Ther 65:1339, 1985.
95. Riddle, DL, Rothstein, JM, and Lamb, RL: Goniometric reliability in a clinical setting: Shoulder measurements. Phys Ther 67:668, 1987.
96. Shin, SH, et al: With-in day reliability of shoulder range of motion measurement with a smartphone. Man Ther 17:298, 2012.
97. Clarke, GR, et al: Assessment of movement at the gleno-humeral joint. Orthopaedics 2:55, 1974.
98. Bower, KD: The hydrogoniometer and assessment of glenohumeral joint motion. Aust J Physiother 28:12, 1982
99. de Jong, LD, Nieuwboer, A, and Aufdemkampe, G: The hemiplegic arm: Interrater reliability and concurrent validity of passive range of motion measurements. Disabil Rehabil 29:1442, 2007.
100. de Jong, LD, et al: Repeated measurements of arm joint passive range of motion after stroke: Interobserver reliability and sources of variation. Phys Ther 92:1027, 2012.
101. Green, A, et al: A standardized protocol for measurement of range of movement of the shoulder using the Plurimeter-V inclinometer and assessment of its intrarater and interrater reliability. Arthritis Care Res 11:43, 1998.
102. Tiffitt, PD, Wildin, C, and Hajioff, D: The reproducibility of measurement of shoulder movement. Acta Orthop Scand 70:322, 1999.
103. Valentine, RE, and Lewis, JS: Intraobserver reliability of 4 physiologic movements of the shoulder in subjects with and without symptoms. Arch Phys Med Rehabil 87:1242, 2006.
104. de Winter, AF, et al: Inter-observer reproducibility of measurements of range of motion in patients with shoulder pain using a digital inclinometer. BMC Musculoskelet Disord 5:18, 2004. doi:10 1186/1471-2474-5-18.
105. Kolber, MJ, et al: The reliability and minimal detectable change of shoulder mobility measurements using a digital inclinometer. Physiother Theory Pract 27:176, 2011.
106. Croft, P, et al: Observer variability in measuring elevation and external rotation of the shoulder. Br J Rheumatol 33:942, 1994.

CHAPTER 5

The Elbow and Forearm

D. Joyce White, PT, DSc
Cynthia C. Norkin, PT, EdD

Structure and Function

Humeroulnar and Humeroradial Joints

The humeroulnar and humeroradial joints, which make up the medial and lateral sides of the elbow joint, are considered to be a modified-hinge compound synovial joint (Figs. 5.1 and 5.2). The proximal joint surface of the humeroulnar joint consists of the convex, hourglass-shaped trochlea located on the anterior medial surface of the distal humerus. The distal joint surface is the concave trochlear notch on the proximal ulna.

The proximal joint surface of the humeroradial joint is the convex capitulum located on the anterior lateral surface of the distal humerus. The concave, shallow, cup-shaped surface of the proximal end of the radial head is the opposing joint surface.

The joints are enclosed in a large, loose, weak joint capsule that also encloses the superior radioulnar joint. Medial and lateral collateral ligaments reinforce the sides of the capsule and help to provide medial–lateral stability (Figs. 5.3 and 5.4).[1]

When the arm is in the anatomical position of full elbow extension and supination, the long axes of the humerus and the forearm form an acute angle at the elbow in the frontal plane. This angle, which is called the "carrying angle" (Fig. 5.5), is the result of the slightly more distal projection of the medial epicondyle and trochlear, than the lateral epicondyle. The carrying angle is approximately 10 to 12 degrees in men and 13 to 17 degrees in women.[2,3] However, large interindividual variations are present so that some men have greater carrying angles than do some women.[3] Children usually have a smaller carrying angle than adults, with the angle gradually increasing with age until puberty when adult values are attained.[4,5] The carrying angle of the dominant arm has been reported to be about 1 to 2 degrees greater than the nondominant arm,[6] but others have found no differences[3] or

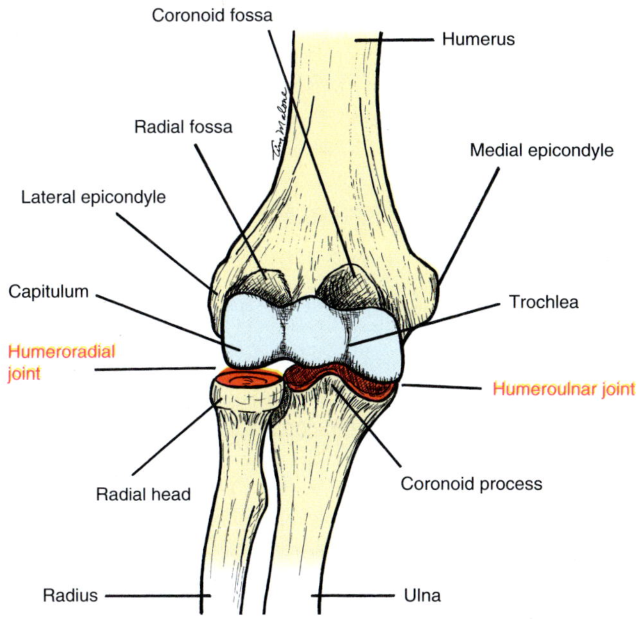

FIGURE 5.1 An anterior view of the right elbow showing the humeroulnar and humeroradial joints.

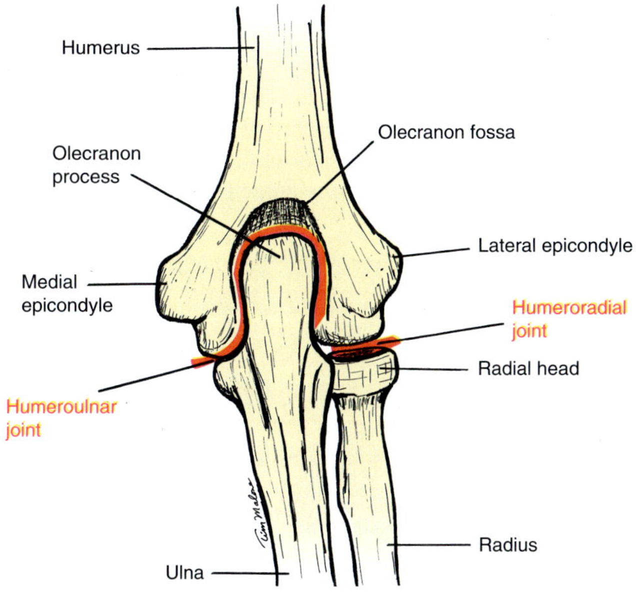

FIGURE 5.2 A posterior view of the right elbow showing the humeroulnar and humeroradial joints.

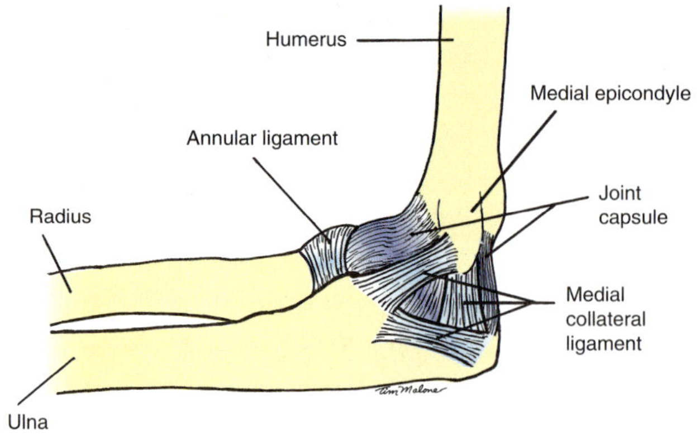

FIGURE 5.3 A medial view of the right elbow showing the medial (ulnar) collateral ligament, annular ligament, and joint capsule.

have found the angle of the left arm to be slightly greater than that of the right.[5] A carrying angle that is greater (more acute) than average is called "excessive cubitus valgus," whereas an angle that is less than average is called "cubitus varus."[7]

Osteokinematics

The humeroulnar and humeroradial joints have 1 degree of freedom; flexion–extension occurs in the sagittal plane around a medial–lateral (coronal) axis. In elbow flexion and extension, the axis of motion lies approximately through the center of the trochlea.[3] There is a slight amount of axial rotation and side-to-side motion of the ulnar during flexion and extension; therefore, the term *modified* hinge is best used to describe the elbow joint.[1,8,9]

Arthrokinematics

At the humeroulnar joint, posterior sliding of the concave trochlear notch of the ulna on the convex trochlea of the humerus continues during extension until the ulnar olecranon process enters the humeral olecranon fossa. In flexion, the ulna slides anteriorly along the humerus until the coronoid process of the ulna reaches the floor of the coronoid fossa of the humerus or until soft tissue in the anterior aspect of the elbow blocks further flexion.

At the humeroradial joint, the concave radial head slides posteriorly on the convex surface of the capitulum during extension. In flexion, the radial head slides anteriorly until the rim of the radial head enters the radial fossa of the humerus.

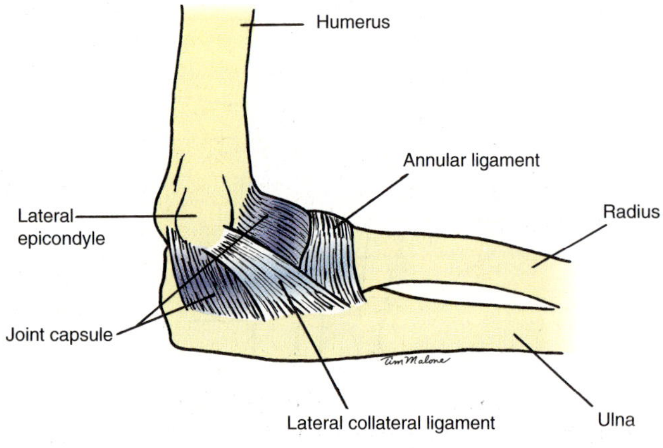

FIGURE 5.4 A lateral view of the right elbow showing the lateral (radial) collateral ligament, annular ligament, and joint capsule.

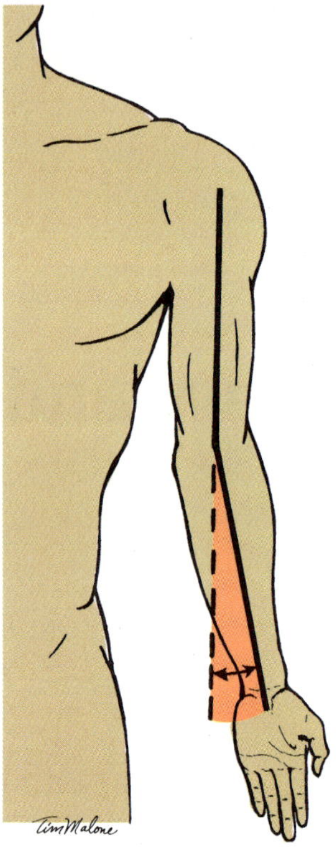

FIGURE 5.5 An anterior view of the right upper extremity showing the carrying angle between the longitudinal midline of the humerus and forearm.

Capsular Pattern

Most authorities agree that the range of motion (ROM) in flexion is more limited than it is in extension.[10–12] Only in severe cases would supination and pronation be slightly limited.[10] The literature varies as to the proportions of limitation in the capsular pattern for the elbow. For example, according to Cyriax 30 degrees of limitation in flexion would typically correspond to about 10 degrees of limitation in extension.[10] Kaltenborn notes that "with flexion limited to 90 degrees (60-degree limitation) there is only 10 degrees of limited extension."[11]

Superior and Inferior Radioulnar Joints

The ulnar portion of the superior radioulnar joint includes both the radial notch located on the lateral aspect of the proximal ulna and the annular ligament (Fig. 5.6). The radial notch and the annular ligament form a concave joint surface. The radial aspect of the joint is the convex head of the radius.

The ulnar component of the inferior radioulnar joint is the convex ulnar head (see Fig. 5.6). The opposing articular surface is the ulnar notch of the radius.

The interosseous membrane, a broad sheet of collagenous tissue linking the radius and ulna, provides stability for both joints (Fig. 5.7). The following three structures provide stability for the superior radioulnar joint: the annular ligament, quadrate ligament, and oblique cord. Stability of the inferior radioulnar joint is provided by the articular disc and the anterior and posterior radioulnar ligaments (Fig. 5.8).[1]

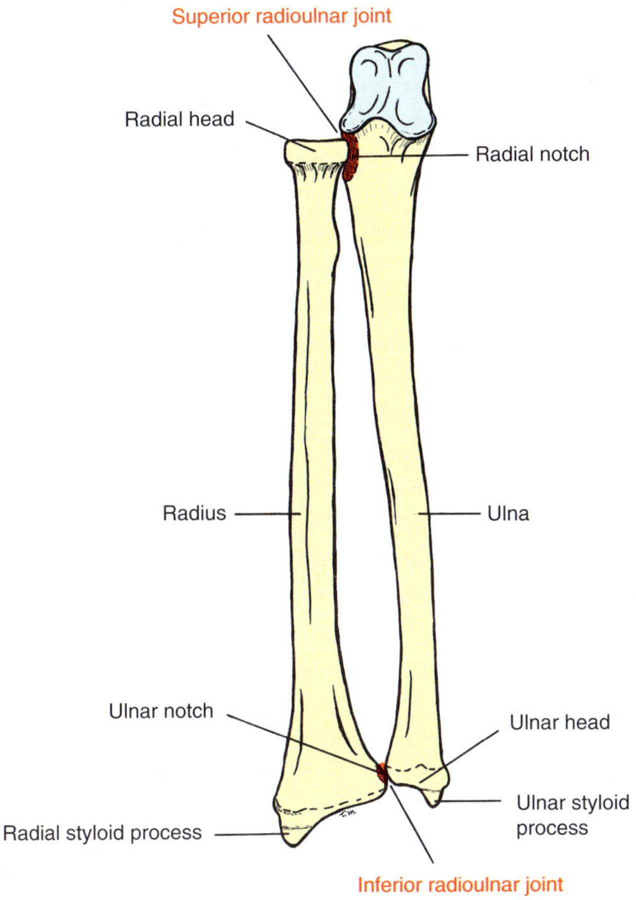

FIGURE 5.6 Anterior view of the superior and inferior radioulnar joints of the right forearm.

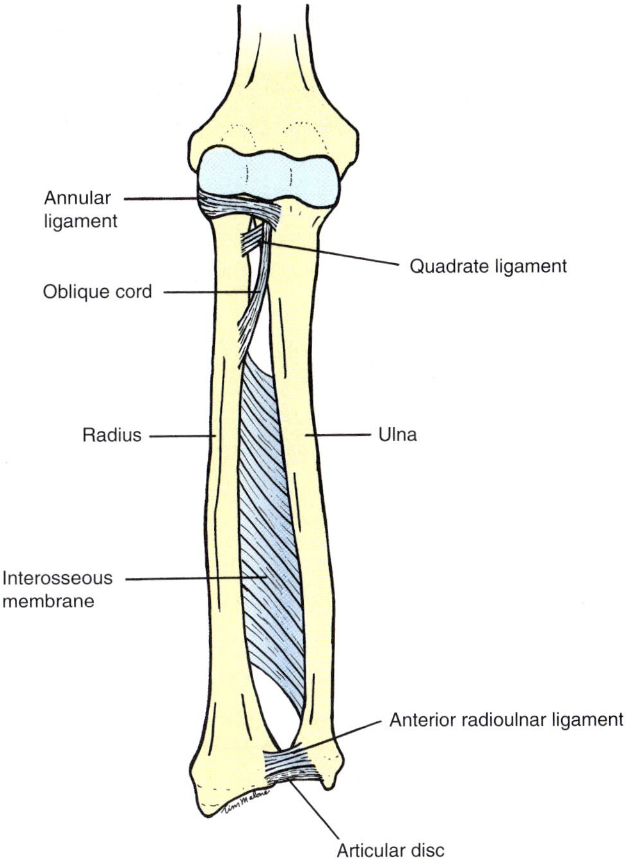

FIGURE 5.7 Anterior view of the superior and inferior radioulnar joints showing the annular ligament, quadrate ligament, oblique cord, interosseous membrane, anterior radioulnar ligament, and articular disc.

Osteokinematics

The superior and inferior radioulnar joints are mechanically linked. Therefore, motion at one joint is always accompanied by motion at the other joint. The axis for motion is a longitudinal axis extending from the radial head to the ulnar head. The mechanically linked synovial joints have 1 degree of freedom, permitting the motions of pronation and supination in the transverse plane when the individual is standing in anatomical position. However, pronation and supination are usually measured with the elbow flexed to 90 degrees to isolate the motions at the forearm and prevent rotation from also occurring at the glenohumeral joint. When the elbow is flexed to 90 degrees, pronation and supination occur in the frontal plane around an anterior–posterior axis. In pronation, the radius crosses over the ulna, whereas in supination the radius and ulna lie parallel to each other.

Arthrokinematics

At the superior radioulnar joint, the convex rim of the radial head spins within the annular ligament and the concave radial notch of the ulna during pronation and supination. The articular surface on the radial head spins posteriorly during pronation and anteriorly during supination.

At the inferior radioulnar joint, the concave surface of the ulnar notch on the radius slides over the ulnar head. The concave articular surface of the radius slides anteriorly (in the same direction as the hand) during pronation and slides posteriorly (in the same direction as the hand) during supination.

Capsular Pattern

The capsular pattern is an equal limitation of supination and pronation according to Cyriax and Cyriax[10] and Kaltenborn.[11]

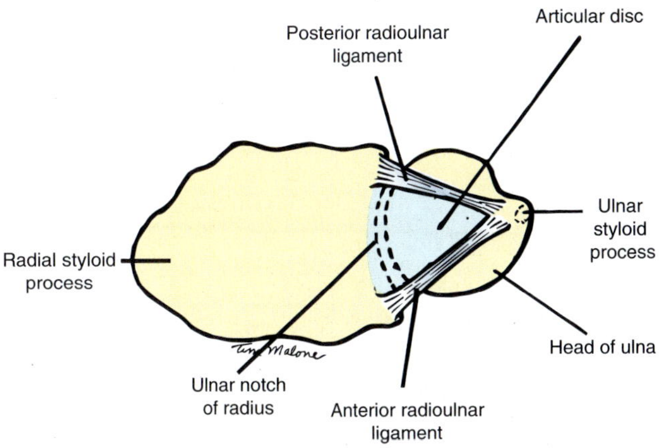

FIGURE 5.8 Distal aspect of the inferior radioulnar joint showing the articular disc (also called the triangular fibrocartilage) and radioulnar ligaments.

RANGE OF MOTION TESTING PROCEDURES: Elbow and Forearm

Landmarks for Testing Procedures

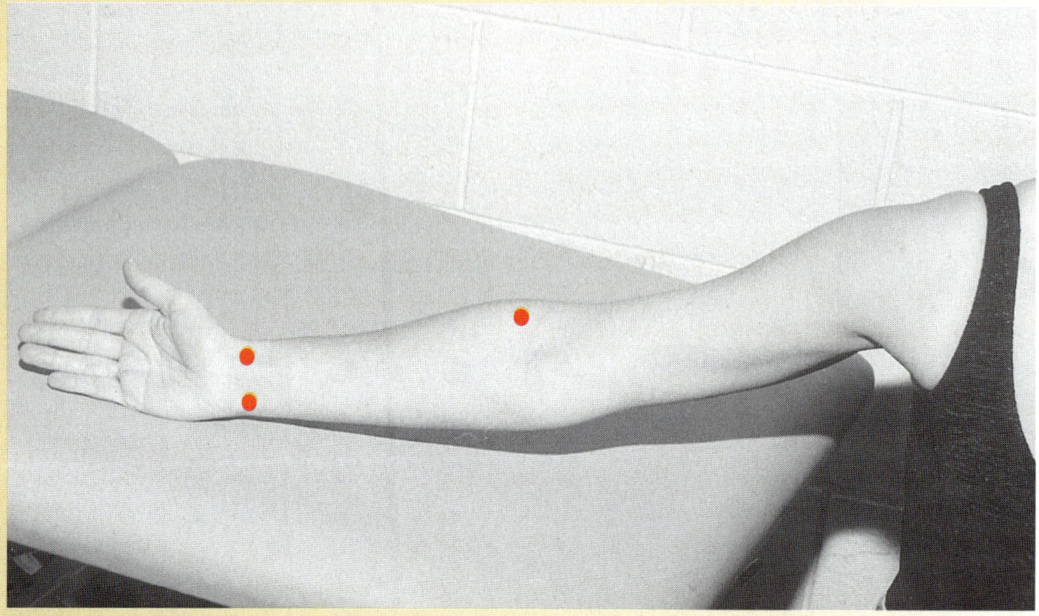

FIGURE 5.9 Anterior view of the right upper extremity showing surface anatomy landmarks for goniometer alignment during the measurement of elbow and forearm ROM.

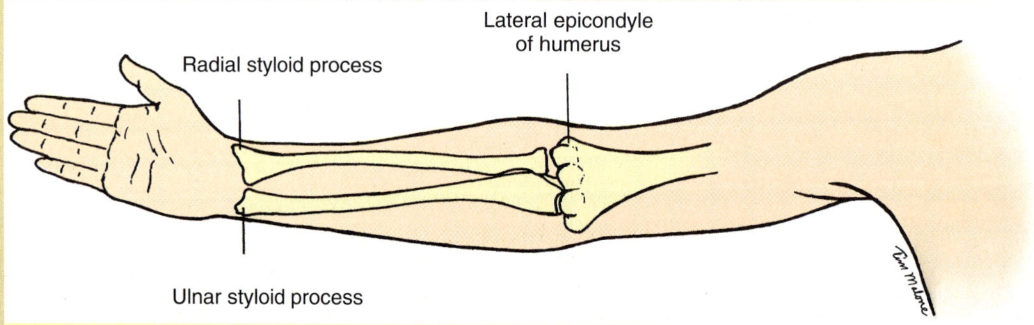

FIGURE 5.10 Anterior view of the right upper extremity showing bony anatomical landmarks for goniometer alignment during the measurement of elbow and forearm ROM.

Landmarks for Testing Procedures (continued)

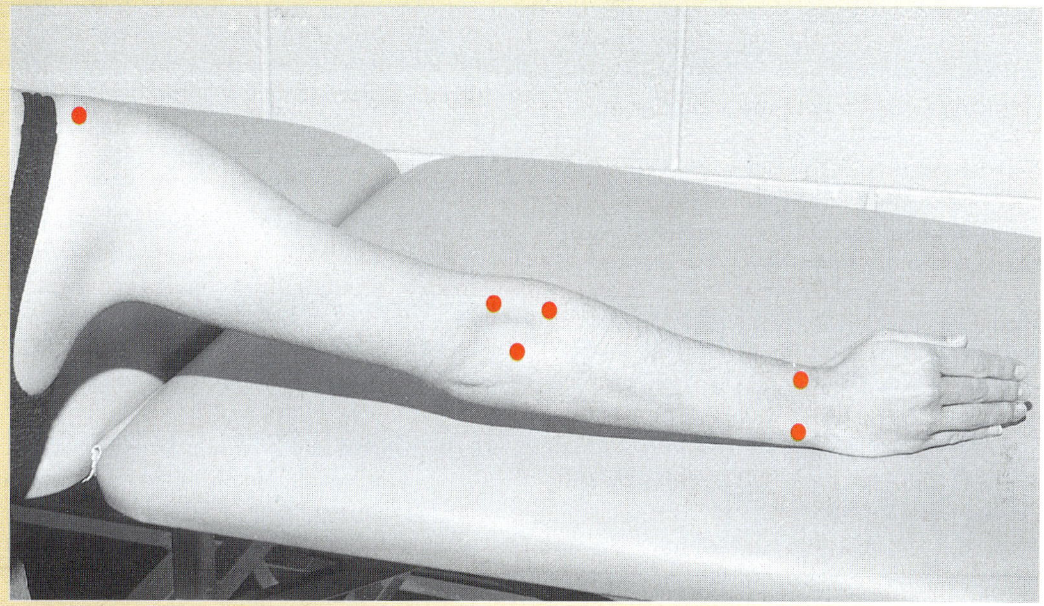

FIGURE 5.11 Posterior view of the right upper extremity showing surface anatomy landmarks for goniometer alignment during the measurement of elbow and forearm ROM.

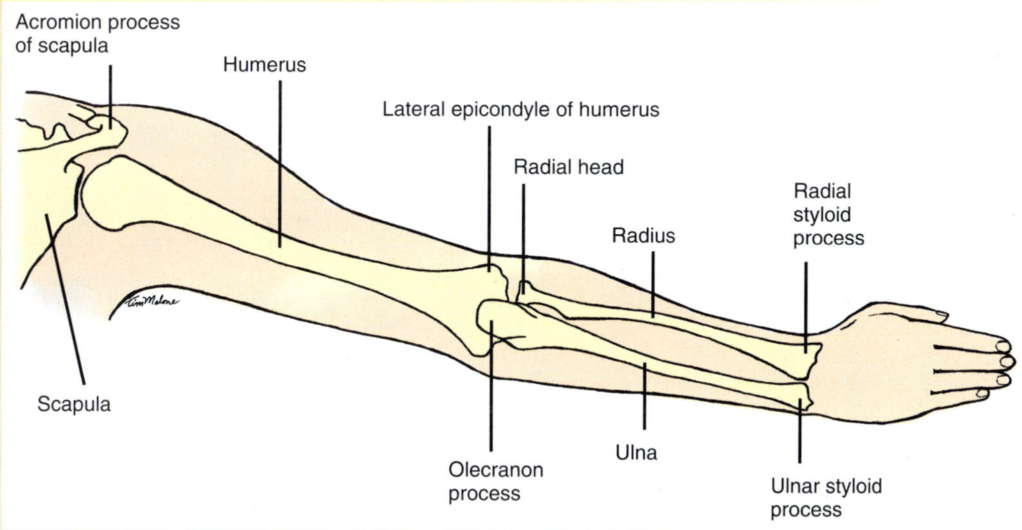

FIGURE 5.12 Posterior view of the right upper extremity showing anatomical landmarks for goniometer alignment during the measurement of elbow and forearm ROM.

ELBOW FLEXION

Motion occurs in the sagittal plane around a medial–lateral axis. Normal flexion ROM values for adults range from about 140 to 150 degrees. See Research Findings and Tables 5.1 to 5.3 for normal ROM values by age and gender.

Testing Position

Position the individual supine with the shoulder in 0 degrees of flexion, extension, and abduction so that the arm is close to the side of the body. Place a pad or towel roll under the distal end of the humerus to allow full elbow extension. Position the forearm in full supination with the palm of the hand facing the ceiling.

Stabilization

Stabilize the humerus to prevent flexion of the shoulder. The pad under the distal humerus and the examining table prevents extension of the shoulder.

Testing Motion

Flex the elbow by moving the hand toward the shoulder. Maintain the forearm in supination during the motion (Fig. 5.13). The end of flexion ROM occurs when resistance to further motion is felt and attempts to overcome the resistance cause flexion of the shoulder.

Normal End-Feel

Usually the end-feel is soft because of compression of the muscle bulk of the anterior forearm with that of the anterior upper arm. If the muscle bulk is small, the end-feel may be hard because of contact between the coronoid process of the ulna and the coronoid fossa of the humerus, and because of contact between the head of the radius and the radial fossa of the humerus. The end-feel may be firm because of tension in the posterior joint capsule, the lateral and medial heads of the triceps muscle, and the anconeus muscle.

Goniometer Alignment

See Figures 5.14 and 5.15.

1. Center **fulcrum** of the goniometer over the lateral epicondyle of the humerus.
2. Align **proximal arm** with the lateral midline of the humerus, using the center of the acromion process for reference.
3. Align **distal arm** with the lateral midline of the radius, using the radial head and radial styloid process for reference.

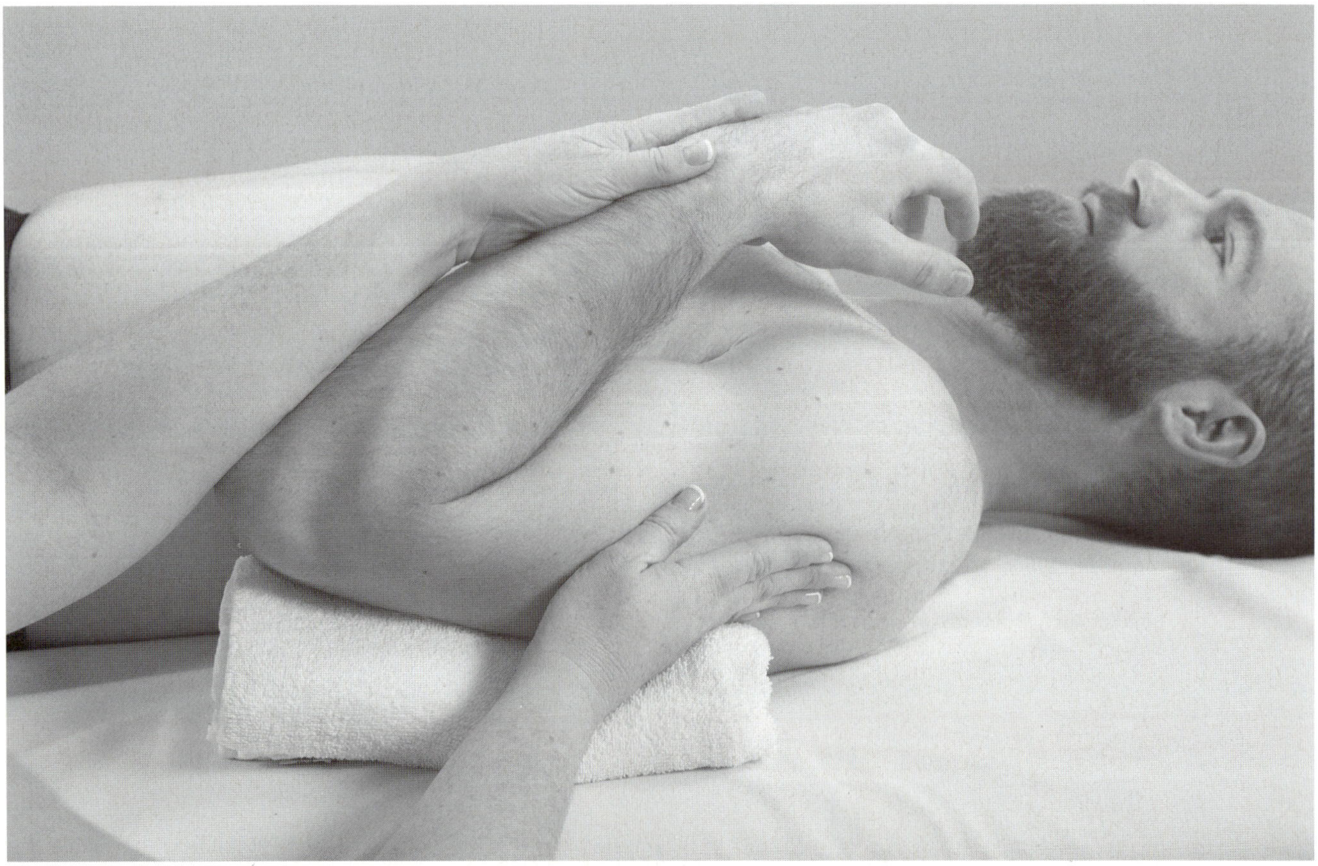

FIGURE 5.13 End of elbow flexion ROM. The examiner's hand stabilizes the humerus, but it must be positioned so it does not limit the motion.

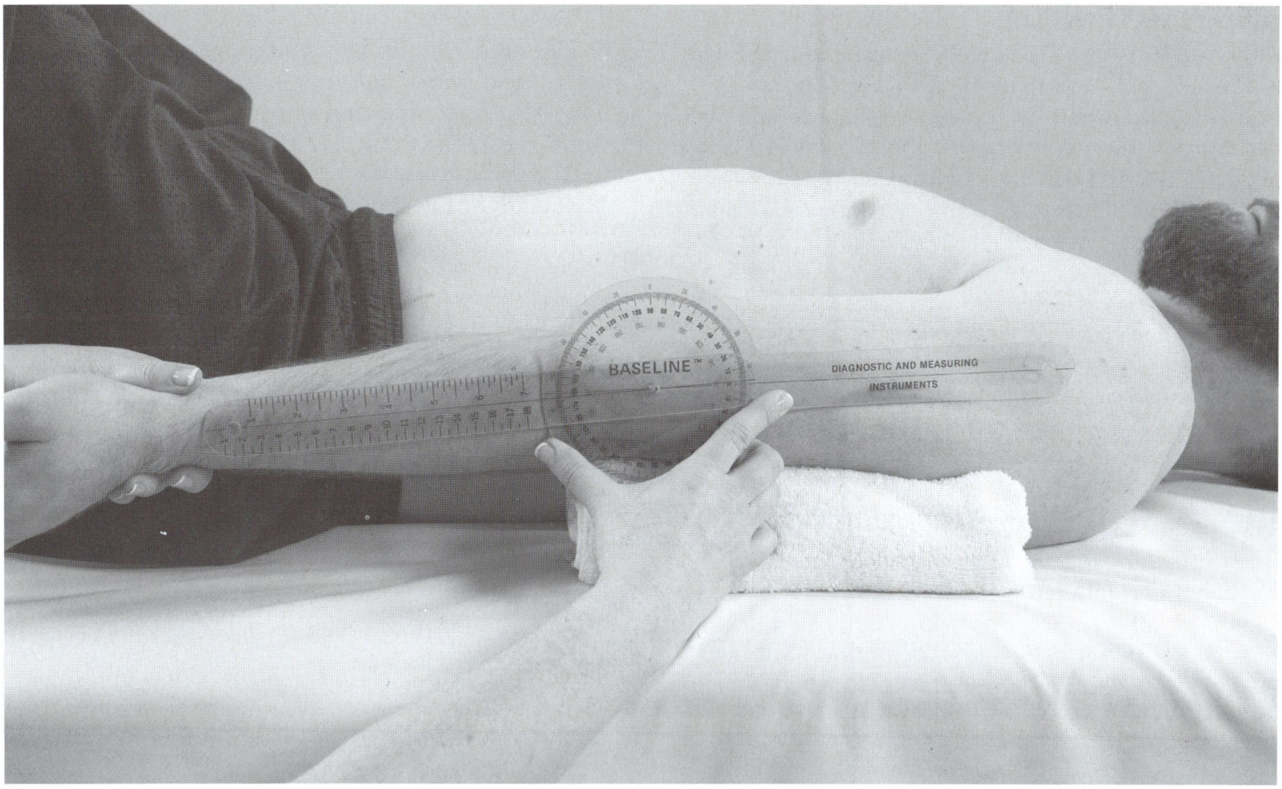

FIGURE 5.14 Alignment of the goniometer at the beginning of elbow flexion ROM. A towel is placed under the distal humerus to ensure that the supporting surface does not prevent full elbow extension.

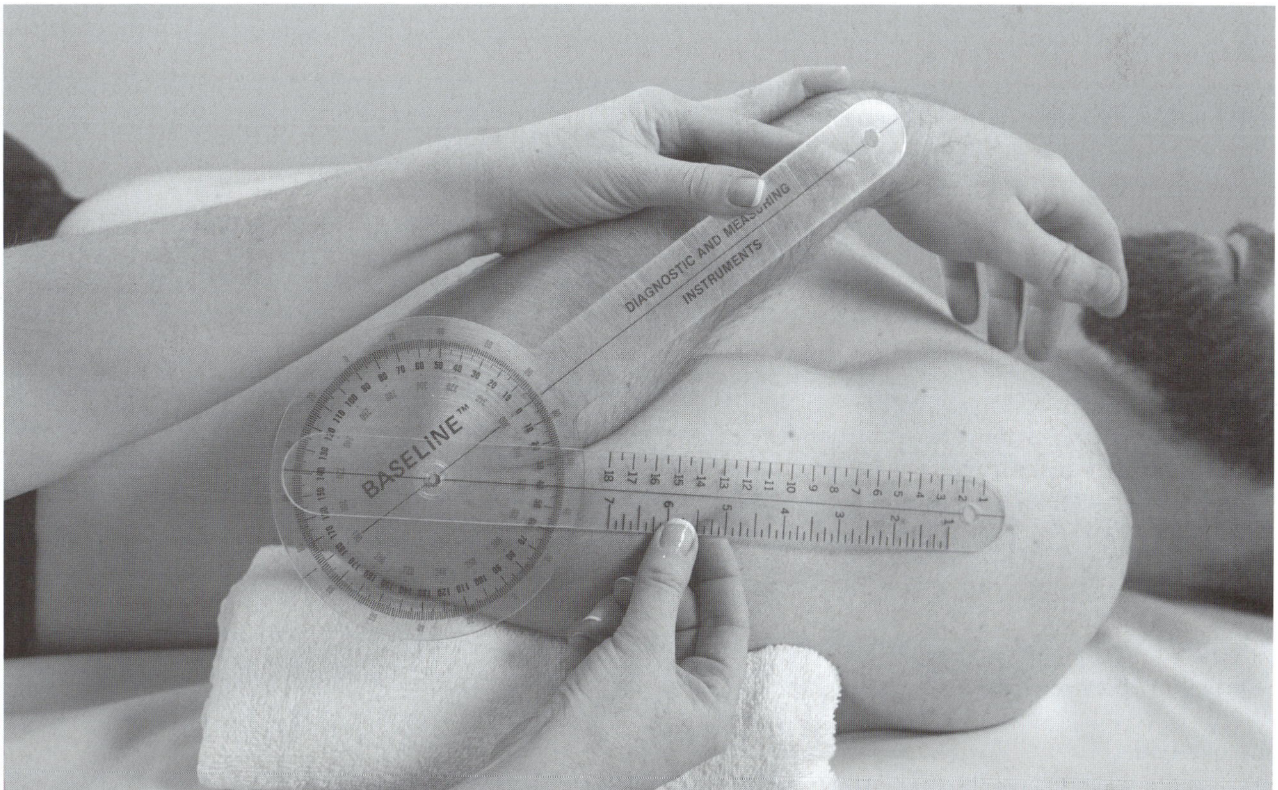

FIGURE 5.15 Alignment of the goniometer at the end of elbow flexion ROM. The forearm is kept in full supination so that the greatest amount of elbow flexion can occur.

ELBOW EXTENSION

Motion occurs in the sagittal plane around a medial–lateral axis. Elbow extension ROM is not usually measured and recorded separately because it is the starting position for measuring and recording elbow flexion ROM. The normal extension ROM value for adults is about 0 degrees. See Research Findings and Tables 5.1 to 5.3 for normal ROM values by age and gender.

Testing Position, Stabilization, and Goniometer Alignment

The testing position, stabilization, and alignment are the same as those used for elbow flexion. Refer to Figure 5.14.

Testing Motion

Extend the elbow by moving the hand dorsally toward the examining table. Maintain the forearm in supination during the motion. The end of extension ROM occurs when resistance to further motion is felt and attempts to overcome the resistance cause extension of the shoulder.

Normal End-Feel

Usually the end-feel is hard because of contact between the olecranon process of the ulna and the olecranon fossa of the humerus. Sometimes the end-feel is firm because of tension in the anterior joint capsule, the collateral ligaments, and the brachialis muscle.

FOREARM PRONATION

When the individual is in the testing position with the elbow flexed to 90 degrees, the motion occurs in the frontal plane around an anterior–posterior axis. Normal ROM values for adults range from about 75 to 85 degrees. See Research Findings and Tables 5.1 to 5.3 for normal ROM values by age and gender.

Testing Position

Position the individual sitting with the shoulder in 0 degrees of flexion, extension, abduction, adduction, and rotation so that the upper arm is close to the side of the body. Flex the elbow to 90 degrees and support the forearm. This testing position helps to isolate the motion to the forearm and prevent glenohumeral rotation. Initially position the forearm midway between supination and pronation so that the thumb is aligned with the humerus; in most individuals the thumb will be pointing up toward the ceiling.

Stabilization

Stabilize the distal end of the humerus to prevent medial rotation and abduction of the shoulder.

Testing Motion

Pronate the forearm by moving the distal radius in a volar direction so that the palm of the hand faces the floor (Fig. 5.16). The end of pronation ROM occurs when resistance to further motion is felt and attempts to overcome the resistance cause medial rotation and abduction of the shoulder.

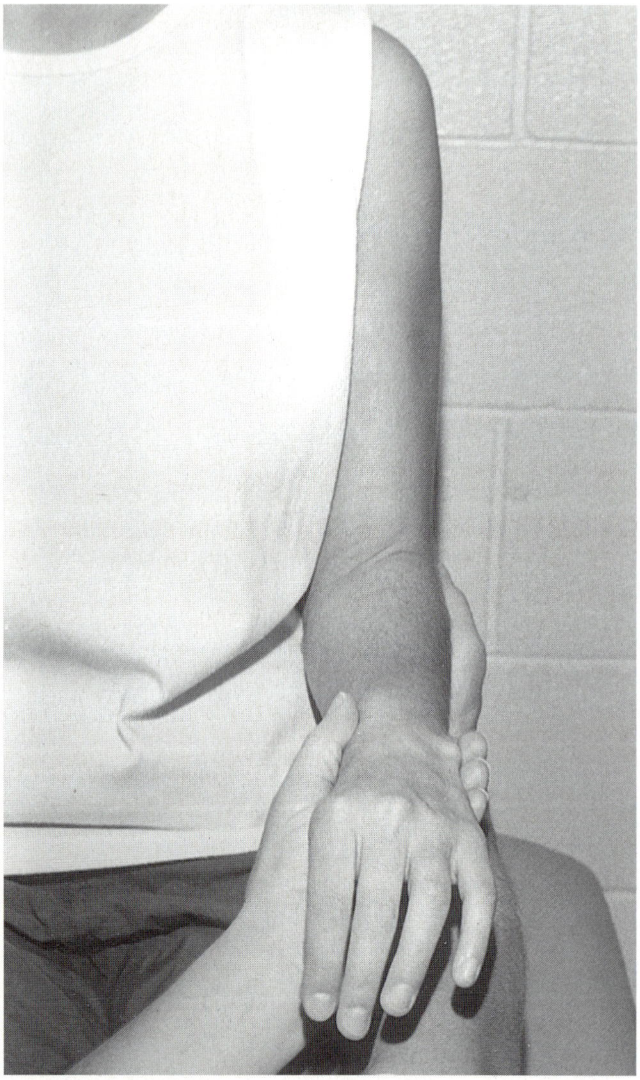

FIGURE 5.16 End of pronation ROM. The individual is sitting on the edge of a table, and the examiner is standing facing the arm that will be tested. The examiner uses one hand to hold the elbow close to the individual's body and in 90 degrees of elbow flexion to help prevent both medial rotation and abduction of the shoulder. The examiner's other hand pushes on the radius rather than on the hand. If the examiner pushes on the individual's hand, movement of the wrist may be mistaken for movement at the radioulnar joints.

Normal End-Feel

The end-feel may be hard because of contact between the ulna and the radius, or it may be firm because of tension in the dorsal radioulnar ligament of the inferior radioulnar joint, the interosseous membrane, and the supinator muscle.

Goniometer Alignment

See Figures 5.17 and 5.18.

1. Center **fulcrum** of the goniometer laterally and proximally to the ulnar styloid process.
2. Align **proximal arm** parallel to the anterior midline of the humerus.
3. Place **distal arm** across the dorsal surface of the forearm, just proximal to the styloid processes of the radius and ulna, where the forearm is most level and free of muscle bulk. The distal arm of the goniometer should be parallel to the styloid processes of the radius and ulna.

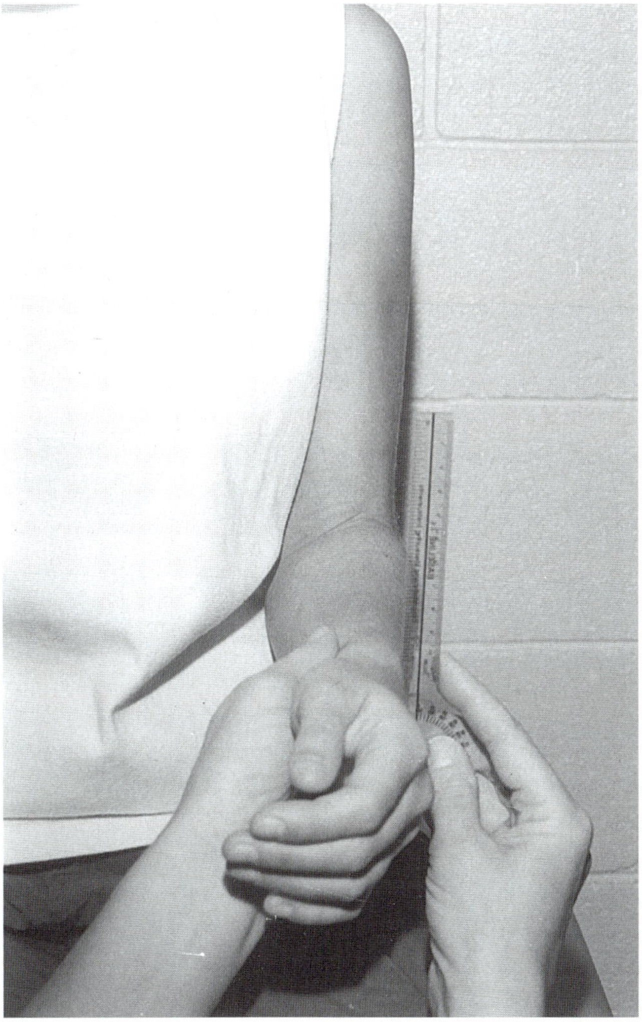

FIGURE 5.17 Alignment of the goniometer in the beginning of pronation ROM. The goniometer is placed laterally to the distal radioulnar joint. The arms of the goniometer are aligned parallel to the anterior midline of the humerus.

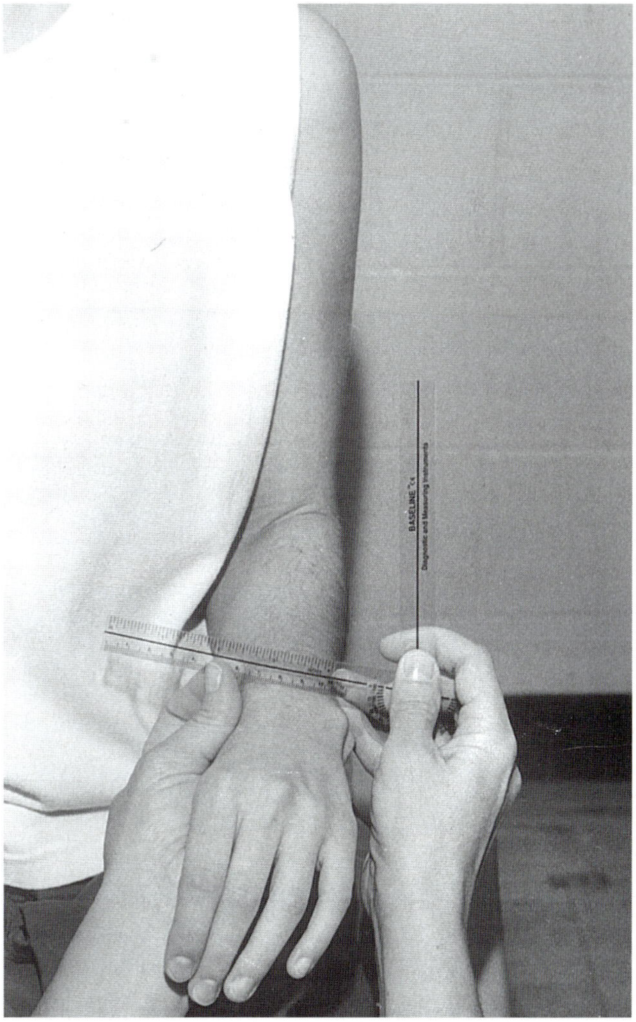

FIGURE 5.18 Alignment of the goniometer at the end of pronation ROM. The examiner uses one hand to hold the proximal arm of the goniometer parallel to the anterior midline of the humerus. The examiner's other hand supports the forearm and assists in placing the distal arm of the goniometer across the dorsum of the forearm just proximal to the radial and ulnar styloid process. The fulcrum of the goniometer is proximal and lateral to the ulnar styloid process.

FOREARM SUPINATION

When the individual is in the testing position with the elbow flexed to 90 degrees, the motion occurs in the frontal plane around an anterior–posterior axis. Normal ROM values for adults range from about 80 to 90 degrees. See Research Findings and Tables 5.1 to 5.3 for normal ROM values by age and gender.

Testing Position

Position the individual sitting with the shoulder in 0 degrees of flexion, extension, abduction, adduction, and rotation so that the upper arm is close to the side of the body. Flex the elbow to 90 degrees and support the forearm. This testing position helps to isolate the motion to the forearm and prevent glenohumeral rotation. Initially position the forearm midway between supination and pronation so that the thumb is aligned with the humerus; in most individuals the thumb will be pointing up toward the ceiling.

Stabilization

Stabilize the distal end of the humerus to prevent lateral rotation and adduction of the shoulder.

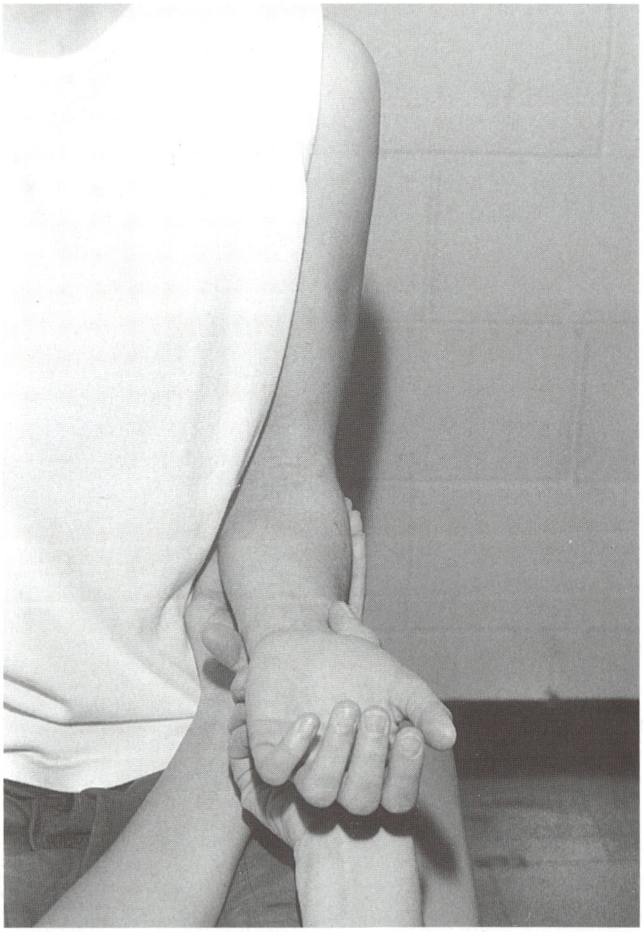

FIGURE 5.19 End of supination ROM. The examiner uses one hand to hold the elbow close to the individual's body and in 90 degrees of elbow flexion, preventing lateral rotation and adduction of the shoulder. The examiner's other hand pushes on the distal radius while supporting the forearm.

Testing Motion

Supinate the forearm by moving the distal radius in a dorsal direction so that the palm of the hand faces the ceiling. See Figure 5.19. The end of supination ROM occurs when resistance to further motion is felt and attempts to overcome the resistance cause lateral rotation and adduction of the shoulder.

Normal End-Feel

The end-feel is firm because of tension in the palmar radioulnar ligament of the inferior radioulnar joint, oblique cord, interosseous membrane, and pronator teres and pronator quadratus muscles.

Goniometer Alignment

See Figures 5.20 and 5.21.

1. Place **fulcrum** of the goniometer medially and just proximally to the ulnar styloid process.
2. Align **proximal arm** parallel to the anterior midline of the humerus.
3. Place **distal arm** across the ventral surface of the forearm, just proximal to the styloid processes, where the forearm is most level and free of muscle bulk. The distal arm of the goniometer should be parallel to the styloid processes of the radius and ulna.

Refer to Appendix B for a summary of measuring elbow and forearm ROM.

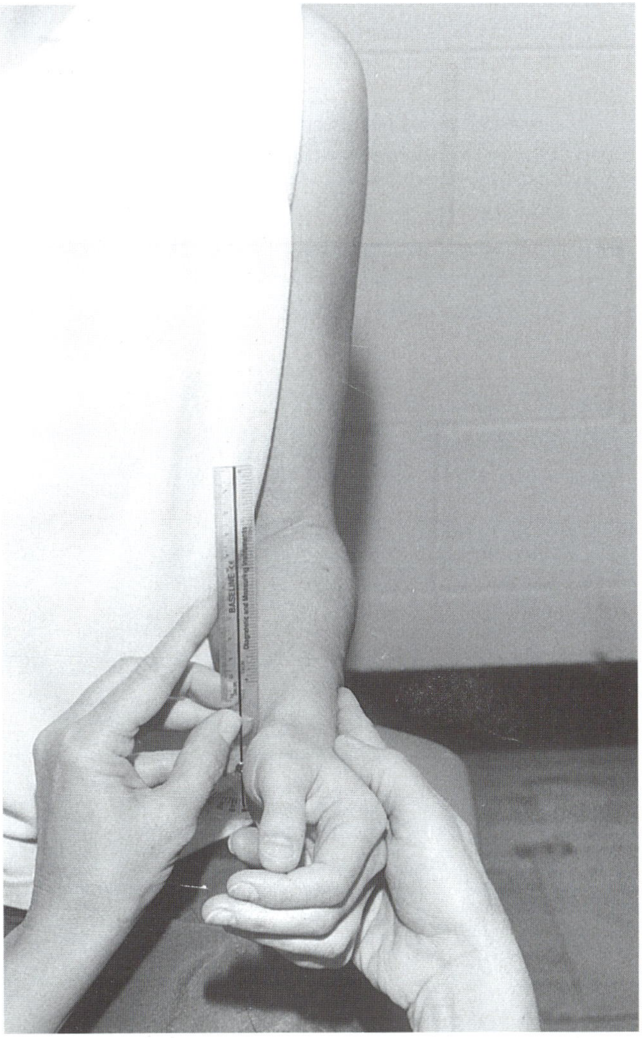

FIGURE 5.20 Alignment of the goniometer at the beginning of supination ROM. The body of the goniometer is medial to the distal radioulnar joint and the arms of the goniometer are parallel to the anterior midline of the humerus.

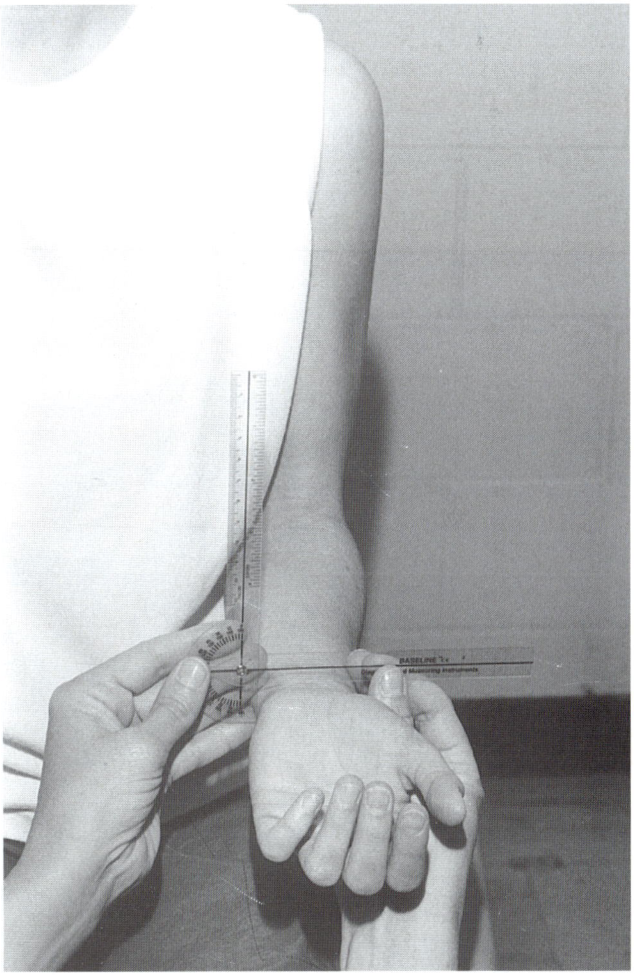

FIGURE 5.21 Alignment of the goniometer at the end of supination ROM. The examiner uses one hand to hold the proximal arm of the goniometer parallel to the anterior midline of the humerus. The examiner's other hand supports the forearm while holding the distal arm of the goniometer across the volar surface of the forearm just proximal to the radial and ulnar styloid process. The fulcrum of the goniometer is proximal and medial to the ulnar styloid process.

MUSCLE LENGTH TESTING PROCEDURES: Elbow and Forearm

Landmarks for Testing Procedures

Refer to Figures 5.9 through 5.12.

ELBOW FLEXORS

Several muscles flex the elbow and will limit elbow extension if they are short in length. The **biceps brachii** crosses multiple joints in the shoulder and elbow regions: the glenohumeral, humeroulnar, humeroradial, and superior radioulnar joints. The short head of the biceps brachii originates proximally from the coracoid process of the scapula (Fig. 5.22). The long head originates from the supraglenoid tubercle of the scapula. The biceps brachii attaches distally to the radial tuberosity. When the biceps brachii contracts, it flexes the elbow and shoulder and supinates the forearm. The muscle is passively lengthened by placing the shoulder and elbow in full extension and the forearm in full pronation.

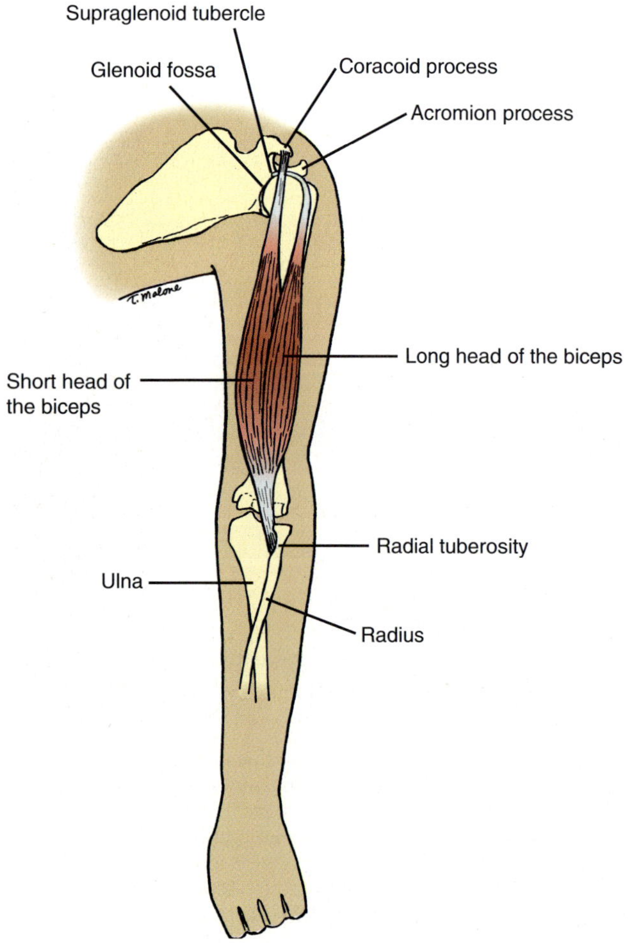

FIGURE 5.22 A lateral view of the left upper extremity showing the origins and insertion of the biceps brachii while being stretched over the glenohumeral, elbow, and superior radioulnar joints.

In contrast to the biceps brachialis, the brachialis and brachioradialis each cross only one joint, the humeroulnar and humeroradial joints, respectively. The **brachialis** originates proximally from the distal half of the anterior humerus and medial and lateral intermuscular septa. The brachialis attaches distally to the tuberosity and coronoid process of the ulna. The **brachioradialis** originates from the upper two-thirds of the lateral supracondylar ridge of the humerus and lateral intermuscular septa. The brachioradialis attaches distally to the styloid process of the radius. Both the brachialis and the brachioradialis are passively lengthened by elbow extension, regardless of the position of the shoulder or forearm. The length of these two muscles is automatically tested along with other joint structures during the measurement of elbow extension ROM (in which the shoulder is in neutral and the forearm is in supination); therefore, we do not include a separate test of the length of these muscles here.

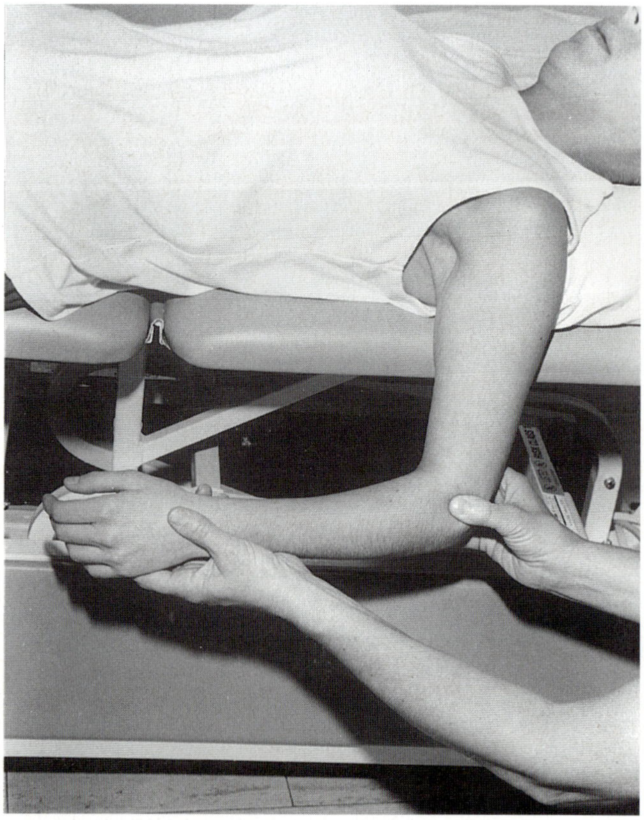

FIGURE 5.23 Starting position for testing the length of the biceps brachii.

BICEPS BRACHII MUSCLE LENGTH TEST

The length of the biceps brachii is evaluated by carefully positioning the shoulder in extension and the forearm in pronation and then extending the elbow.

Testing Position

Position the individual supine at the edge of the examining table (Fig. 5.23). Flex the elbow and position the shoulder in full extension and 0 degrees of abduction, adduction, and rotation.

Stabilization

Stabilize the humerus to maintain shoulder extension. The examining table helps to stabilize the scapula.

Testing Motion

Extend the elbow while holding the forearm in pronation (Fig. 5.24). The end of the testing motion occurs when resistance is felt and additional elbow extension causes shoulder flexion.

Normal End-Feel

The end-feel is firm because of tension in the biceps brachii muscle.

Goniometer Alignment

See Figure 5.25.

1. Center **fulcrum** of the goniometer over the lateral epicondyle of the humerus.
2. Align **proximal arm** with the lateral midline of the humerus, using the center of the acromion process for reference.
3. Align **distal arm** with the lateral midline of the ulna, using the ulna styloid process for reference.

Interpretation

If the biceps brachii is short, it limits elbow extension when the shoulder is positioned in full extension and the forearm is in full pronation. If elbow extension is limited regardless of shoulder and forearm position, the limitation is due to abnormalities of the elbow joint surfaces, to shortening of the anterior joint capsule and collateral ligaments, or to muscles that cross only the elbow region such as the brachialis and brachioradialis. We are unaware of any published normative values for the muscle length test of the biceps brachii.

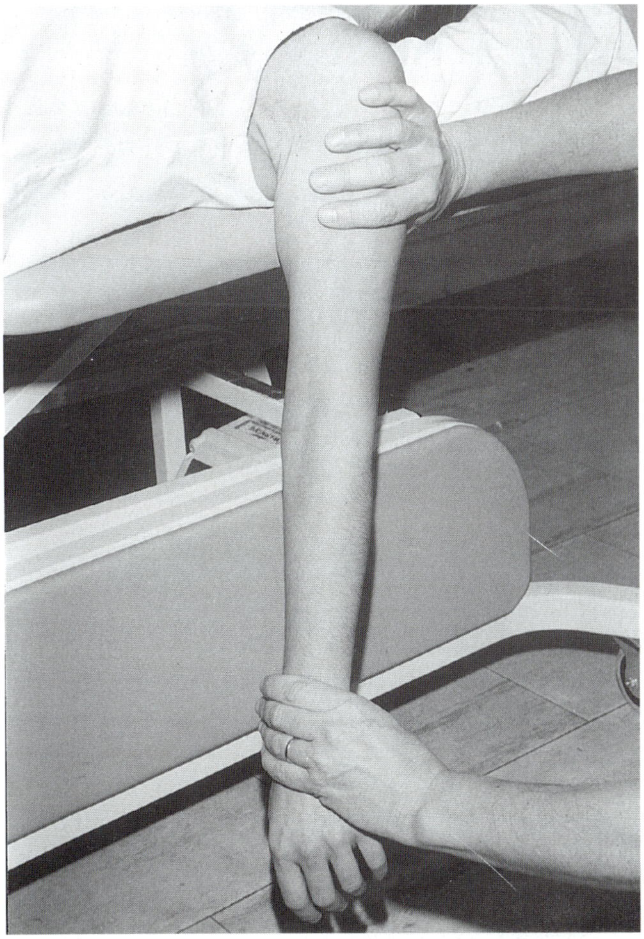

FIGURE 5.24 End of the testing motion for the length of the biceps brachii. The examiner uses one hand to stabilize the humerus in full shoulder extension while the other hand holds the forearm in pronation and moves the elbow into extension.

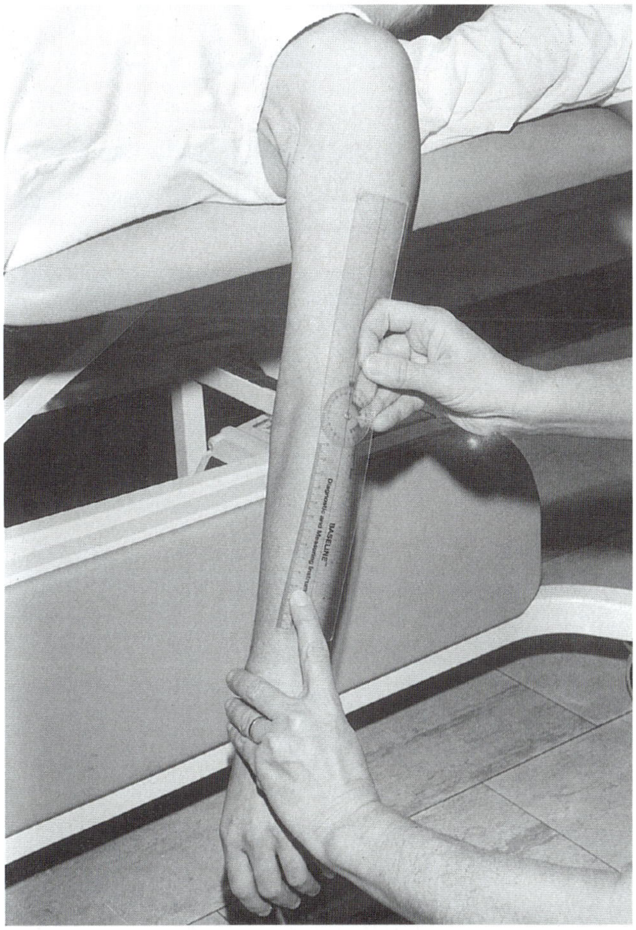

FIGURE 5.25 Alignment of the goniometer at the end of testing the length of the biceps brachii. The examiner releases the stabilization of the humerus and now uses her hand to position the goniometer.

ELBOW EXTENSORS

The triceps brachii and anconeus extend the elbow and they will limit elbow flexion if they are short in length. The **triceps brachii** muscle crosses the glenohumeral and humeroulnar joints. The long head of the triceps brachii muscle originates proximally from the infraglenoid tubercle of the scapula (Fig. 5.26). The lateral head of the triceps brachii originates from the posterior and lateral surfaces of the humerus, whereas the medial head originates from the posterior and medial surfaces of the humerus. All parts of the triceps brachii insert distally on the olecranon process of the ulna. When this muscle contracts it extends the shoulder and elbow. The long head of the triceps brachii is passively lengthened by placing the shoulder and elbow in full flexion.

The **anconeus** crosses only the humeroulnar joint. The anconeus originates proximally from the lateral epicondyle of the humerus and inserts distally on the lateral surface of the olecranon and posterior superior aspect of the ulna. The anconeus is passively lengthened by flexing the elbow, regardless of the position of the shoulder or forearm. The length of the anconeus is automatically tested along with other joint structures during the measurement of elbow flexion ROM (in which the shoulder is in neutral); therefore, we do not include a separate test of the length of the anconeus here.

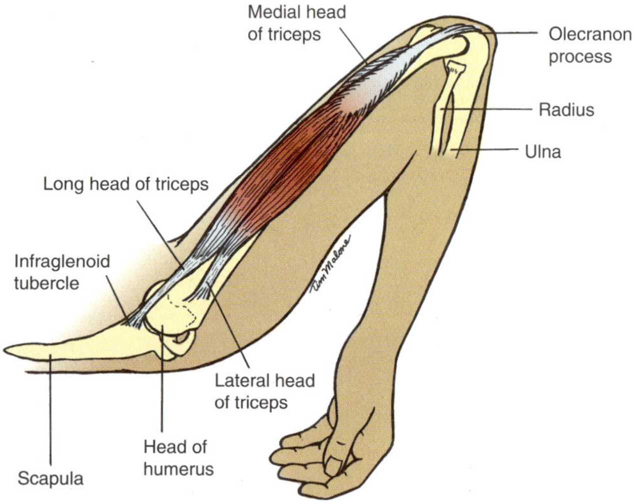

FIGURE 5.26 A lateral view of the left upper extremity showing the origins and insertions of the triceps brachii while being stretched over the glenohumeral and elbow joints.

LONG HEAD OF THE TRICEPS BRACHII MUSCLE LENGTH TEST

The length of the long head of the triceps brachii is evaluated by carefully positioning the shoulder in flexion and then flexing the elbow.

Testing Position

Position the individual supine close to the edge of the examining table. Extend the elbow and position the shoulder in full flexion and 0 degrees of abduction, adduction, and rotation. Supinate the forearm (Fig. 5.27).

Stabilization

Stabilize the humerus to maintain shoulder flexion. The weight of the trunk on the examining table and the passive tension in the latissimus dorsi, pectoralis minor, and rhomboid major and minor muscles help to stabilize the scapula.

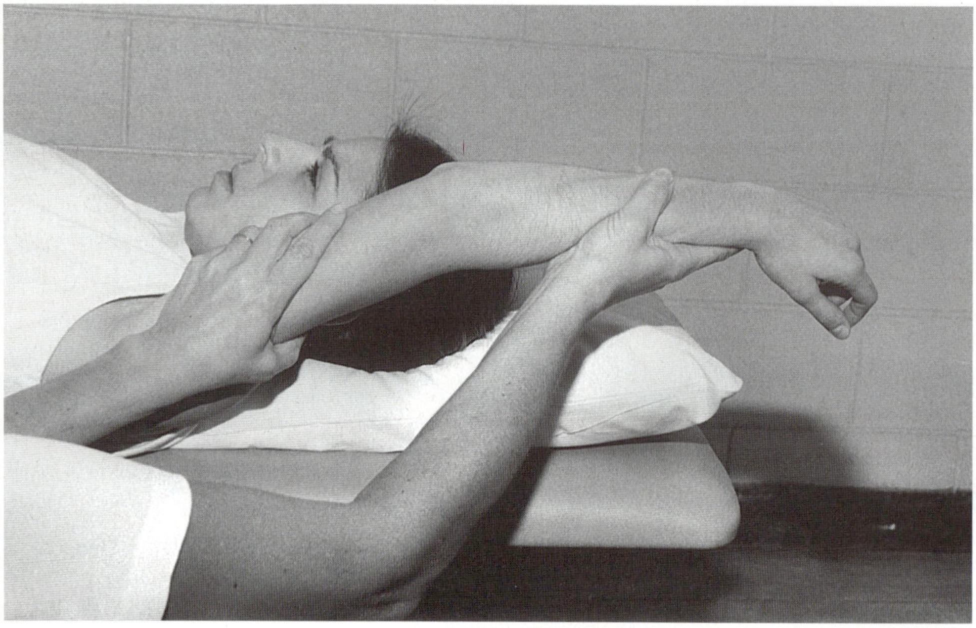

FIGURE 5.27 Starting position for testing the length of the triceps brachii.

Testing Motion

Flex the elbow by moving the hand closer to the shoulder (Fig. 5.28). The end of the testing motion occurs when resistance is felt and additional elbow flexion causes shoulder extension.

Normal End-Feel

The end-feel is firm because of tension in the long head of the triceps brachii muscle.

Goniometer Alignment

See Figure 5.29.

1. Center **fulcrum** of the goniometer over the lateral epicondyle of the humerus.
2. Align **proximal arm** with the lateral midline of the humerus, using the center of the acromion process for reference.
3. Align **distal arm** with the lateral midline of the radius, using the radial styloid process for reference.

Interpretation

If the long head of the triceps brachii is short in length, it will limit elbow flexion when the shoulder is positioned in full flexion. If elbow flexion is limited regardless of shoulder position, the limitation is due to abnormalities of the joint surfaces, to shortening of the posterior capsule, or to muscles that cross only the elbow, such as the anconeus and the lateral and medial heads of the triceps brachii. We are unaware of any published normative values for the muscle length test of the triceps brachii.

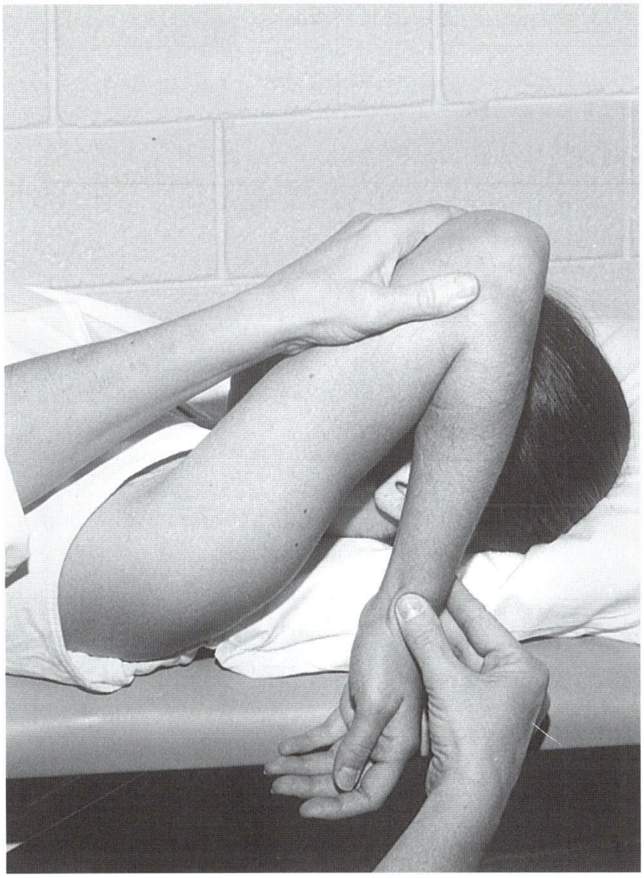

FIGURE 5.28 End of the testing motion for the length of the triceps brachii. The examiner uses one hand to stabilize the humerus in full shoulder flexion and the other hand to move the elbow into flexion.

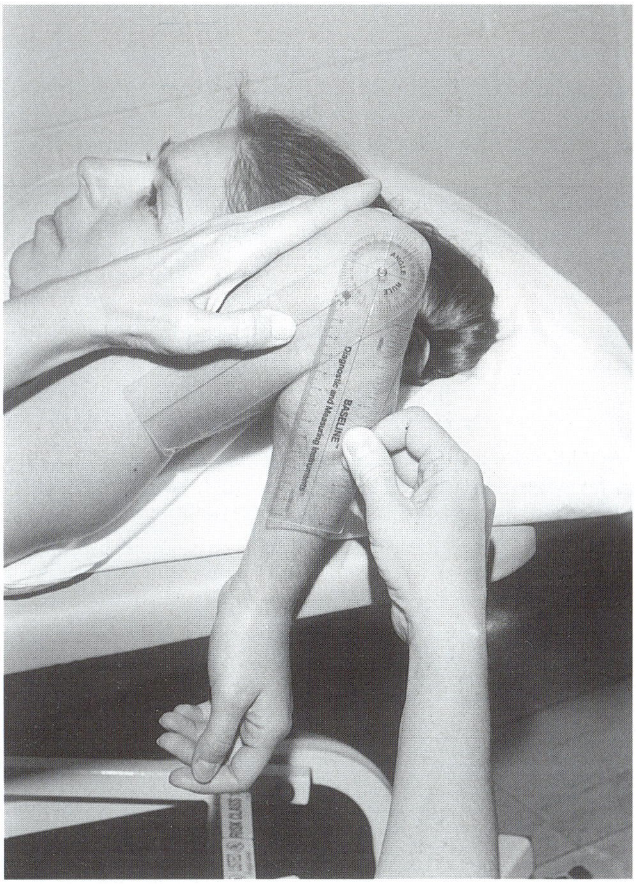

FIGURE 5.29 Alignment of the goniometer at the end of testing the length of the triceps brachii. The examiner uses one hand to continue to stabilize the humerus and align the proximal arm of the goniometer. The examiner's other hand holds the elbow in flexion and aligns the distal arm of the goniometer with the radius.

Research Findings

Effects of Age, Gender, and Other Factors

Table 5.1 provides normal elbow and forearm ROM values for healthy adults.[13–18] Other sources in addition to those listed in Table 5.1 report similar values. Greene and Wolf[19] in a study of 10 males and 10 females between the ages of 18 and 55 years found active flexion to be 145.3 degrees, pronation 84.4 degrees, and supination 76.9 degrees. Goodwin and colleagues[20] reported mean active elbow flexion to be 148.9 degrees in 23 females between 18 and 31 years of age. Petherick and associates[21] found mean active elbow flexion to be 145.8 degrees in 10 males and 20 females with a mean age of 24.0 years. Sanya and Chinyelu[22] studied 50 healthy adults (27 females and 23 males) between 20 and 71 years of age and found mean active elbow flexion to be 137.8 degrees. All of these sources used universal goniometers to obtain measurements.

Age

Cross-sectional studies of normal ROM values for various age-groups suggest that elbow and forearm ROM decreases slightly with increasing age. The elbow and forearm ROM values in infants reported by Wanatabe and colleagues,[23] as noted in Table 5.2, and the mean elbow flexion of 151.4 degrees in young male children aged 1 to 7 years reported by Hacker, Funk, and Manco-Johnson[24] are generally greater than the normal values for adult males found in Tables 5.1 and 5.3.

Other researchers have reported mean ROM values for elbow flexion in children that are not greater but are similar to published values for adults. Golden et al,[5] in a study of 300 children between the ages of 4 months and 18 years, found mean elbow flexion to be 143.8 degrees for males and 145.3 degrees for females. Barad and associates[25] found a mean of 142 degrees of flexion and 11 degrees of extension beyond 0 degrees in 747 male and 614 female children between the ages of 1 and 16 years (mean age 4.9 years). Flexion values in these children were similar to those in adults, but extension values were somewhat greater. Females had 1 to 2 degrees more extension and flexion ROM than males, which the researchers did not consider to be clinically significant. In any case, it can be difficult to compare values obtained from various studies because subject selection and measurement methods can differ.

Within one study of 109 males ranging in age from 18 months to 54 years, Boone and Azen[16] noted a significant difference in elbow flexion and supination between subjects younger and older than 19 years of age. Further analyses found that the group between 6 and 12 years of age had more elbow flexion and extension than other age-groups. The youngest group (between 18 months and 5 years) had a significantly greater amount of pronation and supination than other age-groups. However, the greatest differences between the age-groups were relatively small: 6.8 degrees of flexion, 4.4 degrees of supination, 3.9 degrees of pronation, and 2.5 degrees of extension.[26]

Likewise, Soucie and colleagues,[18] in a normative study of 674 subjects between the ages of 2 and 69 years, found that joint mobility was the greatest in the youngest age-group and lowest in the oldest age-group, but the differences in ROM at the elbow and forearm were less than 10 degrees. This trend of decreasing ROM with advancing age occurred in both males and females. Chapleau and associates[27] reported a negative correlation between age and elbow flexion and total ROM, in which elbow motion decreased with increasing age in 51 healthy male and female subjects between the ages of 19 and 50 years. Interestingly, Macedo and Magee[28] did not find a statistically significant decrease in elbow flexion or forearm ROM but did find a decrease in elbow extension (1.3 degrees)

TABLE 5.1 Normal Elbow and Forearm ROM Values for Adults in Degrees From Selected Sources

	AAOS[13,14]	AMA[15]	Boone and Azen[16]	Gunal et al[17]	Soucie et al[18]			
			20–54 yr* n = 56 Males	18–22 yr† n = 1000 Males	20–44 yr† n = 114 Males	20–44 yr† n = 143 Females	45–69 yr† n = 96 Males	45–69 yr† n = 123 Females
Motion			**Mean (SD)**	**Mean (SD)**	**Mean (SD)**	**Mean (SD)**	**Mean (SD)**	**Mean (SD)**
Flexion	150	140	140.5 (4.9)	144.2 (5.8)	144.6 (5.5)	150.0 (5.5)	143.5 (6.0)	148.3 (5.6)
Extension	0	0	0.3 (2.7)	4.9 (11.1)	0.8 (3.8)	4.7 (4.8)	–0.7 (3.9)	3.6 (5.5)
Pronation	80	80	75.0 (5.3)		76.9 (7.0)	82.0 (5.8)	77.7 (6.0)	80.8 (6.3)
Supination	80	80	81.1 (4.0)	91.7 (9.6)	85.0 (6.6)	90.6 (8.5)	82.4 (7.5)	87.2 (6.9)

SD = Standard deviation.

* Values are for active ROM measured with a universal goniometer.

† Values are for passive ROM measured with a universal goniometer.

– Minus sign indicates flexion.

TABLE 5.2 Effects of Age and Gender on Elbow and Forearm Motion: Normal Values in Degrees for Newborns, Children, and Adolescents

	Wanatabe et al[23]	Boone[26]			Soucie et al[18]			
	2 wk–2 yr* n = 45 Males and Females	18 mo–5 yr† n = 19 Males	6–12 yr† n = 17 Males	13–19 yr† n = 17 Males	2–8 yr* n = 55 Males	2–8 yr* n = 39 Females	9–19 yr* n = 48 Males	9–19 yr* n = 56 Females
Motion	**Range of Means**	**Mean (SD)**	**Mean (SD)**	**Mean (SD)**	**Mean (SD)**	**Mean (SD)**	**Mean (SD)**	**Mean (SD)**
Flexion	148–158	144.9 (5.7)	146.5 (4.0)	144.9 (6.0)	151.4 (2.4)	152.9 (4.4)	148.3 (5.2)	149.7 (4.7)
Extension		0.4 (3.4)	2.1 (3.2)	0.1 (3.8)	2.2 (5.0)	6.8 (5.2)	5.3 (6.0)	6.4 (6.3)
Pronation	90–96	78.9 (4.4)	76.9 (3.6)	74.1 (5.3)	79.6 (3.0)	84.6 (5.8)	79.8 (7.2)	81.2 (6.0)
Supination	81–93	84.5 (3.8)	82.9 (2.7)	81.8 (3.2)	86.4 (4.2)	93.7 (7.3)	87.8 (7.3)	90.0 (7.5)

SD = Standard deviation.

* Values are for passive ROM measured with a universal goniometer.

† Values are for active ROM measured with a universal goniometer.

with increasing age in the sample of 90 healthy females aged 18 to 59 years. The authors believed these differences to be small (0.5–1.5 degrees) between the youngest and oldest age-groups and well within the margin of error associated with goniometric measurements. A linear regression model projected a change in passive motions at the elbow and forearm to be between 0.01 and 0.10 degrees per year during this 40-year period.

Older persons appear to have difficulty fully extending their elbows to 0 degrees. Walker and associates[29] found that the older men and women (60–84 years of age) in their study were unable to extend their elbows to 0 degrees to attain a neutral starting position for flexion. The mean value for the starting position was 6 degrees in men and 1 degree in women. Boone and Azen[16] also found that the oldest subjects in their study (40–54 years of age) lost elbow extension and began flexion from a slightly flexed position. Bergstrom and colleagues[30] performed a study of 52 women and 37 men aged 79 years and found that 11% had flexion contractures of the right elbow greater than 5 degrees and 7% had bilateral flexion contractures. Fiebert, Fuhri, and New[31] measured elbow extension with a universal goniometer and elbow flexion and forearm motions with an electronic inclinometer in 124 men and women, 60 to 99 years of age. They also found that these older adults were unable to fully extend their elbows (mean extension −1 degree). Elbow flexion was 147 degrees, pronation 84 degrees, and supination 85 degrees, which are greater than reported values for this aged population measured with a goniometer.

Kalscheur, Emery, and Costello examined the effect of age in 61 older women and 25 older men aged 63 to 86 years.[32,33] Depending on the linear regression models used, they found that elbow flexion declined about 0.1 to 0.2 degrees per year from age 65 to 85 years, pronation declined about

TABLE 5.3 Effects of Age and Gender on Active Elbow and Forearm Motion: Normal Values in Degrees for Adults 20 to 85 Years of Age

	Boone[26]			Walker et al[29]		Kalscheur et al[33]	
	20–29 yr n = 19 Males	30–39 yr n = 18 Males	40–54 yr n = 19 Males	60–85 yr n = 30 Males	60–85 yr n = 30 Females	66–86 yr n = 25 Males	63–85 yr n = 61 Females
Motion	**Mean (SD)**	**Mean (SD)**	**Mean (SD)**	**Mean (SD)**	**Mean (SD)**	**Mean (SD)**	**Mean (SD)**
Flexion	140.1 (5.2)	141.7 (3.2)	139.7 (5.8)	139.0 (14)	148.0 (5)	142.9 (6.8)	149.0 (5.2)
Extension	0.7 (3.2)	0.7 (1.7)	−0.4 (3.0)	−6 (5)	−1 (5)		
Pronation	76.2 (3.9)	73.6 (4.3)	75.0 (7.0)	68 (9)	73 (12)	82.9 (9.2)	87.8 (6.7)
Supination	80.1 (3.7)	81.7 (4.2)	81.4 (4.0)	83 (11)	65 (11)	87.4 (12.1)	88.3 (6.4)

SD = Standard deviation.

– Minus sign indicates flexion.

0.1 to 0.4 degrees per year, and supination declined about 0.0 to 1.0 degrees per year. It was projected that over a 20-year period elbow flexion could be expected to decline approximately 3 degrees, pronation 5 degrees, and right supination 6 degrees.[33] Only declines in right supination and pronation ROM were statistically significant.

Gender

Studies that include a wide range of age-groups seem to concur that females have slightly more elbow flexion and extension ROM than males. Most studies support similar gender differences in forearm supination and pronation ROM, but some exceptions have been reported.

Female children and adolescents have been found to have greater ROM than males of a similar age. Golden and colleagues,[5] using a universal goniometer to measure bilateral elbow ROM in 300 healthy children aged 4 months to 18 years, found that females had statistically significantly more motion than males. However, mean differences were small: 1.5 degrees for flexion and 0.9 degrees for extension.

Females had greater mobility than males in all four age-groups from 2 to 69 years that were studied by Soucie and associates[18] (see Tables 5.1 and 5.2). Gender difference ranged from 1.4 to 5.4 degrees for elbow flexion, 1.1 to 4.6 degrees for elbow extension, 1.4 to 5.0 degrees for pronation, and 2.2 to 7.3 degrees for supination. Likewise, Chapleau and colleagues[27] reported that females had on average 4.0 degrees greater elbow ROM than males as measured by radiographs in a study of 31 females and 20 males ranging in age from 19 to 50 years. In another study that included a wide range of ages, Bell and Hoshizaki,[34] using a Leighton Flexometer, studied the ROM of 124 females and 66 males between the ages of 18 and 88 years. Females had significantly more elbow flexion than males, with mean differences ranging from about 2 to 14 degrees depending on the age-group. Although females had greater supination–pronation ROM than males, this increase was not statistically significant. Salter and Darcus,[35] measuring forearm supination–pronation with a specialized arthrometer in 20 males and 5 females between the ages of 16 and 29 years, found that the females had an average of 8 degrees more forearm rotation than males, although the difference was not statistically significant in this small sample.

Studies of older adults also found that females have greater elbow flexion–extension and pronation ROM than males (see Table 5.3). However, study results vary concerning supination: Studies have found that older males have more or the same amount of supination as older females. In a study of 695 community-dwelling older subjects between 65 and 74 years of age, Escalante, Lichenstein, and Hazuda[36] found that females had an average of 4 degrees more elbow flexion than males. Thirty older females and 30 older males, aged 60 to 84 years, were included in a study by Walker and associates.[29] Older females had significantly more flexion ROM (1–148 degrees) than older males (5–139 degrees), but males had significantly more supination (83 degrees) than females (65 degrees). Females had more pronation ROM than males, but the difference was not significant. Kalscheru and colleagues found that older women had more elbow and forearm ROM than older men in a study of 61 women and 25 men ranging in age from 63 to 86 years.[34,35] These gender differences were statistically significant for elbow flexion and pronation, with mean differences of 6.2 and 4.9 degrees, respectively. There was no significant difference in supination ROM between the men and women.

Ethnicity

Although some normative ROM studies have noted the race and nationality of their subjects in demographic summaries, only a few research studies have specifically examined the effect of ethnic background on ROM values at the elbow and forearm. Generally, ethnic differences, if evident, have been only about 2 to 3 degrees. Escalante, Lichenstein, and Hazuda,[36] in a study of 695 community-dwelling older adults living in San Antonio, Texas, found that Mexican Americans had an average of 2 to 3 degrees less elbow ROM than European Americans. However, this difference became nonsignificant in multivariate models. Golden and colleagues[5] studied 300 healthy children aged 4 months to 18 years of various ethnicities. The 110 Caucasian children had statistically significantly greater range of elbow flexion than the 100 African American and 77 Hispanic children who were included, with differences being 2.1 degrees and 3.2 degrees, respectively. The Caucasian children had significantly greater elbow extension ROM than African American subjects as well (mean difference = 2.6 degrees).

Body Mass Index

Increases in body mass index (BMI) have been associated with decreases in elbow flexion ROM in children as well as in older adults. This decrease in elbow motion may be due to an increase in soft tissue around the elbow joint that provides a mechanical block to full flexion.[27,37] Hacker and colleagues[24] found an association between increased BMI and decreased elbow ROM in 72 healthy boys aged 1 to 7 years. These findings were also supported in a study by Golden and colleagues[37] of 113 healthy children 2 to 18 years of age. Body mass index was negatively correlated with right and left elbow ROM. Likewise, Chapleau and associates,[27] in a study of 51 healthy adults aged 19 to 51, reported a similar correlation of increased BMI and midbrachial and forearm circumference with decreased elbow flexion. Escalante, Lichenstein, and Hazuda[36] also found BMI to be inversely associated with elbow flexion in 695 older subjects. Each unit increase in BMI (kg/m^2) was significantly associated with a 0.22 decrease in degrees of elbow flexion. Park and colleagues[38] found a reduction of about 3 degrees in elbow flexion in adult males whose BMI was greater than 30 kg/m^2 compared with nonobese males, but this difference was not significant in a study of 40 subjects.

Right Versus Left Side

Studies comparing ROM between the right and left sides or between the dominant and nondominant limbs have generally found no clinically relevant differences in elbow and forearm

ROM. Studies that included large numbers of subjects had the statistical power to find differences of 2 to 3 degrees to be significant. If differences were found, the left or nondominant side had more motion. For all practical purposes, ROM values taken from the healthy contralateral limb can be used for comparison in evaluation and treatment planning.

Boone and Azen[16] studied 109 males between the ages of 18 months and 54 years who were subdivided into six age-groups. They found no significant differences between right and left elbow flexion, extension, supination, and pronation, except for the age-group of subjects between 20 and 29 years of age whose elbow flexion ROM was greater on the left than on the right. This one significant finding was attributed to chance. Hacker and colleagues[24] found no significant difference between sides for elbow ROM in 72 healthy boys aged 1 to 7 years. Likewise, Chapleau and colleagues[27] reported no differences in elbow ROM between dominant and nondominant sides in 51 healthy adults.

Several studies have noted small but statistically significant differences between sides for certain elbow and forearm motions that are of questionable clinical importance. Soucie and associates,[18] in a study of 674 subjects aged 2 to 69 years, found statistically significant differences between the right and left sides for elbow flexion and supination ROM; however, the absolute differences were less than 1 degree in all cases and were considered inconsequential. Macedo and Magee[39] reported a greater amount of supination on the nondominant forearm of 90 females aged 19 to 59 years, but the mean difference was only 3.6 degrees. No significant differences were noted for elbow flexion, extension, and pronation. Gunal and colleagues,[17] in a study of 1,000 males between 18 to 22 years of age, found significantly greater elbow flexion, extension, and supination ROM on the left compared with the right; mean differences were 2.6 degrees, 2.0 degrees, and 2.2 degrees, respectively.

Studies on older subjects have noted similar results. Escalante, Lichenstein, and Hazudal,[36] in a study of 695 older subjects, found significantly greater elbow flexion on the left than on the right, but the difference averaged only 2 degrees. Kalscheur and colleagues[32] reported no significant differences between sides for elbow flexion and pronation ROM in a study of 61 older women. A statistically significant difference between sides was noted for supination ROM, with the left side being an average of 3.0 degrees greater than the right.

Testing Position

Elbow position has been shown to affect the range of forearm supination and pronation. Usually supination and pronation ROM are measured with the elbow in 90 degrees of flexion, but normative values may vary if the elbow is positioned in different amounts of flexion and extension. A study of 50 healthy adults (25 men and 25 women) found that supination ROM significantly increased to a maximum of 115.3 degrees with the elbow in full flexion and decreased to 47.4 degrees in full extension.[40] Likewise, there was a reciprocal decrease in pronation to a minimum of 55.4 degrees with the elbow in full flexion and increase to a maximum of 111.9 degrees in full extension. Although the authors propose that these differences are due to the trapezoidal shape of the radial notch of the ulnar and intra-articular movement of the radius at the proximal radioulnar joint, these measurement differences may also be related to the slightly diagonal orientation of the axis of rotation in the humeroulnar joint that brings the hand closer to the midline of the body and into slight supination with elbow flexion, and brings the hand laterally away from the midline of the body and into slight pronation with elbow extension. Maximum total forearm rotation (supination and pronation combined) was noted between 45 and 90 degrees of flexion, which is the most functional part of elbow ROM. Passive ROM resulted in approximately 11 degrees more supination and pronation each than active motion.

Sports

It appears that the frequent use of the upper extremities in sport activities may reduce elbow and forearm ROM. Possible causes for this association include muscle hypertrophy, muscle tightness, and joint trauma from overuse.

Chinn, Priest, and Kent,[41] in a study of 53 male and 30 female national and international tennis players, found significantly less active ROM in pronation (mean difference = 5.8 degrees) and supination (4.6 degrees) in the playing arms of all subjects. Male players also demonstrated a significant decrease (4.1 degrees) in elbow extension in the playing arm versus the nonplaying arm. Chang, Buschbacher, and Edlich[42] studied 10 power lifters and 10 age-matched nonlifters and found less active elbow flexion in the power lifters than in the nonlifters. No significant differences were found between the two groups for supination and pronation ROM. Wright and colleagues[43] noted an average decrease of 7.9 degrees for elbow extension ROM and 5.5 degrees for elbow flexion ROM in the dominant versus the nondominant arm of 33 professional pitchers. No significant differences were noted between the dominant and nondominant sides for supination and pronation ROM.

Functional Range of Motion

The elbow joint is critical for performing upper-extremity functional tasks as it is the only joint capable of substantially increasing and decreasing the length of the arm, thus allowing the hand to reach for objects and also touch the face and body for eating and personal care. It appears that almost the full range of elbow flexion (about 140 degrees), within 20 degrees of full elbow extension, 50 degrees of pronation, and 60 degrees of supination is needed to complete most common tasks without compensatory shoulder, wrist, and neck movements.

The amount of elbow and forearm motion that occurs during activities of daily living has been studied by researchers using electrogoniometers,[44–46] as well as three-dimensional optical[47–57] and electromagnetic motion analysis systems.[58–60] The research predominantly focused on adults but children were also studied.[61,62] Table 5.4 presents detailed results of

TABLE 5.4 Elbow and Forearm Motion During Functional Activities: Mean Values in Degrees

Activity	Study			Flexion		Pronation		Supination	
	First Author	N	Method	Min	Max	Min	Max	Min	Max
Feeding Tasks									
Drink from cup	Aizawa[59]	20	3D electromagnetic (EM) system		115				
	Morrey[44]	33	Triaxial electrogoniometer	45	130		10		13
	Safaee-Rad[47]	10 M	3D video system	72	129			3	31
Eat with fork	Morrey[44]	33	Triaxial electrogoniometer	85	128		10		52
	Safaee-Rad[47]	10 M	3D video system	94	122		38		59
Eat with spoon	Aizawa[59]	20	3D EM system		123				
	Magermans[58]	24 F	EM tracking system		132				
	Sanz[46]	10	Electrogoniometric system						55
	Packer[45]	5	Uniaxial electrogoniometer	70	115				
	Safaee-Rad[47]	10 M	3D video system	101	123		23		59
Take meal	Henmi[54]	5	3D optical system		146				
Hand to mouth	Mackey[61]	10 (6–12 yr)	8-camera video system	53	153		5		79
Cut with knife	Morrey[44]	33	Triaxial electrogoniometer	89	107	27	42		
Pour from pitcher	Aizawa[59]	20	3D EM system		93				
	Morrey[44]	33	Triaxial electrogoniometer	36	58		43		22
	Raiss[49]	7	Infrared light-reflecting system				55		
Reaching Tasks for Personal Care and Hygiene									
Hand to forehead	Aizawa[59]	20	3-D EM system		124				
	Morrey[44]	33	Triaxial electrogoniometer		119				47
Hand to forehead with palm	Mackey[61]	10 (6–12 yr)	8-camera video system	108	166		12		77
Wash face	Aizawa[59]	20	3D EM system		128				
	Henmi[54]	5	3D optical system		140		20		
	Romilly[52]	6	Biplanar video system						86
Hand to occiput	Morrey[44]	33	Triaxial electrogoniometer		144				2
	Sardelli[51]	25	3D optical system		143				
Hand to top of head	Petuskey[62]	28	3D imaging system		110				43
Comb hair	Aizawa[59]	20	3D EM system		119				
	de Groot[60]	10	6D EM system		145				
	Magermans[58]	24 F	EM tracking system		136				
	Van Andel[56]	10	3D optical system		139				
Shampoo hair	Henmi[54]	5	3D optical system		151				
Hand to neck	Aizawa[59]	20	3D EM system		134				
	Sardelli[51]	25	3D optical system		144				
Hand to axilla (contralateral)	Aizawa[59]	20	3D EM system		100				
	Magermans[58]	16	EM system		118				
Hand to axilla (ipsilateral)	Aizawa[59]	20	3D EM system		137				
Hand to sacrum	Morrey[44]	33	Triaxial electrogoniometer		70				56
Hand to perineum	Aizawa[59]	20	3D EM system		56				
	Magermans[58]	16	EM system		61				
	Raiss[49]	7	Infrared light-reflecting system						72

TABLE 5.4 Elbow and Forearm Motion During Functional Activities: Mean Values in Degrees (continued)

Activity	Study			Flexion		Pronation		Supination	
	First Author	N	Method	Min	Max	Min	Max	Min	Max
Hand to back pocket	Petuskey[62]	28 (9–12 yr)	3D imaging system		63				61
	Van Andel[56]	10	3D optical system		85				
Hand to shoe	de Groot[60]	10	6D EM system		39				
	Morrey[44]	33	Triaxial electrogoniometer		16		19		
	Sardelli[51]	25	3D optical system		27				
Common Tasks									
Use telephone	Morrey[44]	33	Triaxial electrogoniometer	43	136		41		23
	Packer[45]	5	Uniaxial electrogoniometer	75	140				
Use cell phone	Sardelli[51]	25	3D optical system		147				
	Romilly[52]	6	Biplanar video system		151				
Rise from chair	Morrey[44]	33	Triaxial electrogoniometer	20	95	10	34		
	Packer[34]	5	Uniaxial electrogoniometer	15	100				
Open door-turn door knob	Morrey[44]	33	Triaxial electrogoniometer	24	57		35		23
	Sardelli[51]	25	3D optical system						77
	Romilly[52]	6	Biplanar video system		42				
Read newspaper	Morrey[44]	33	Triaxial electrogoniometer	78	104	7	49		
Turn page	Romilly[52]	6	Biplanar video system				61		
Use keyboard	Sardelli[51]	25	3D optical system				65		
Reach above/to shoulder height	Magermans[58]	8			39				
	Mackey[61]	10 (6–12 yr)	8-camera video system	3	140		13		66
Reach overhead	Petuskey[62]	28 (9–12 yr)	3D imaging system	18			79		
Propel wheelchair	Rudins[57]	10	3D video system	5	61				

M = male; F = female

some of these studies and clusters the motions into three general categories: (1) feeding tasks, (2) reaching tasks that are necessary for personal care and hygiene, and (3) common activity tasks. Range of motion values reported by the studies vary because of differences in the type of equipment and placement of skin markers used to collect data, the tasks that are included, the starting position of the upper extremity (arm at side versus arm resting on tabletop), which often affects the minimum motion and arc, and joint axes definitions.[53] Assessment of the forearm pronation–supination presents more of a methodological challenge than assessing elbow flexion–extension because of variations in defining the zero position and difficulty in isolating forearm rotation from glenohumeral rotation. In addition, it appears that people perform upper-extremity tasks using a variety of movement strategies—much more so than the more consistent strategies used in the lower extremities for gait and transfers. However, some conclusions can be drawn about the arc of motion and average maximum values that occur while performing activities of daily living. These values can assist health-care providers in setting patient treatment goals to enable the completion of functional tasks.

In an oft-cited study, Morrey, Askew, and Chao[44] used a triaxial electrogoniometer attached to the upper extremity to measure elbow and forearm motion in 33 normal subjects. They concluded that most of the 15 activities of daily living that were studied required a total arc of about 100 degrees of elbow flexion (30–130 degrees) and 100 degrees of rotation (50 degrees of supination to 50 degrees of pronation). More elbow flexion was required to reach the back of the head (144 degrees), whereas more extension was needed to rise from a chair (20 degrees). The inclusion of these activities would require a total arc of elbow flexion of about 120 degrees (20–140 degrees). Packer and colleagues[45] found that a relatively similar range of 15 to 140 degrees of flexion (arc of 125 degrees) was needed to complete the three activities (using a telephone, rising from a chair to standing, and eating with a spoon) included in their study using a uniaxial electrogoniometer of five healthy adults. Sanz and associates,[46] using an electrogoniometric system, found that an arc of 130 degrees of flexion (10–141 degrees) and an arc of 100 degrees of pronation–supination (45 degrees pronation to 55 degrees supination) were required to complete 19 of the 20 activities performed by the 10 healthy adults in their study.

Other studies have used optical-based video cameras and electromagnetic systems to determine the maximal values and arc of motion at the elbow during certain tasks. These systems, which record and analyze the position of multiple markers attached to body parts, generally have noted similar or slightly greater values than those measured with electrogoniometers during the same activities. Safaee-Rad and colleagues[47] measured the ROM of 10 healthy males during three feeding activities: eating with a spoon, eating with a fork, and drinking from a handled cup (Fig. 5.30). The feeding activities required approximately 70 to 130 degrees of elbow flexion (arc of 60 degrees), 40 degrees of pronation, and 60 degrees of supination (arc of 100 degrees). Cooper et al[48] also studied three feeding tasks in 19 healthy adults with unrestricted upper extremities and found relatively similar results. Combining the results from both males and females, 82 to 130 degrees of elbow flexion (arc of 49 degrees), 42 degrees of pronation, and 52 degrees of supination (arc of 94 degrees) were required to complete the feeding tasks.

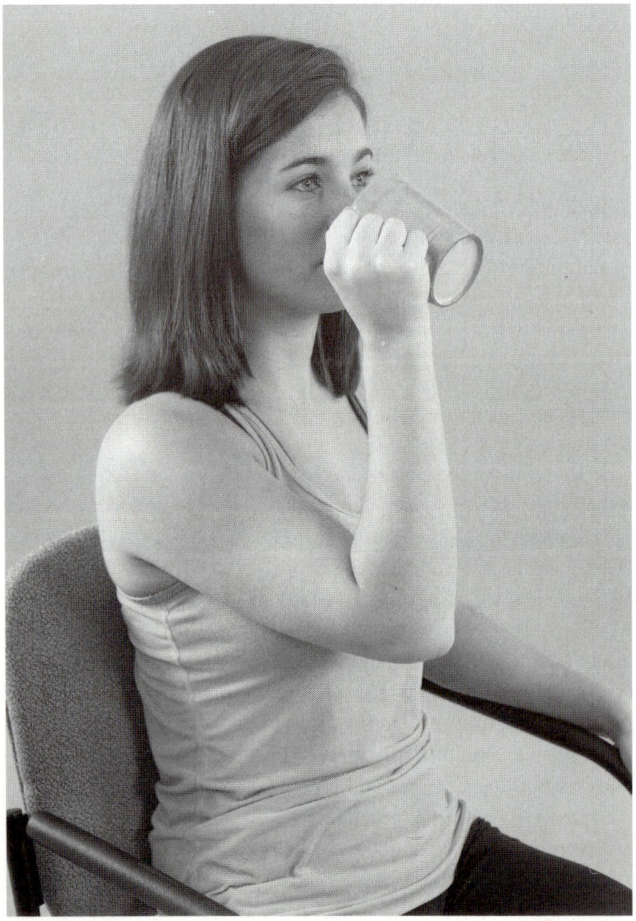

FIGURE 5.30 Drinking from a cup requires about 130 degrees of elbow flexion.

The inclusion of activities in addition to feeding tasks increases the required arc of motion. Raiss et al,[49] in a study of seven adults, found that a mean arc of 110 degrees of elbow flexion (36–146 degrees) and mean arc of 127 degrees of pronation–supination (55 pronation to 72 degrees supination) were required to complete 10 activities of daily living. The 10 activities included combing hair, genital hygiene, using a telephone, typing on a keyboard, turning a key, turning a page, and drawing in addition to eating tasks. Murray and Johnson,[50] in a study of 10 male adults, found that a slightly greater arc of 149 degrees of elbow flexion (16–165 degrees) and an arc of 119 degrees of pronation–supination (65 degrees of pronation to 54 degrees of supination) were needed to perform all of the 10 tasks related to eating, hygiene, and lifting objects. Extrapolating from the maximal values measured by Sardelli, Tashjian, and MacWilliams[51] during 6 positional and 11 functional tasks, an arc of 126 degrees of flexion (23–149 degrees) and an arc of 142 degrees of pronation–supination (65 pronation to 77 supination) were necessary to complete all of these 17 tasks.

In general, it appears that feeding activities required the least amount of elbow motion, instrument use such as writing and telephoning demanded a moderate amount of motion, and reaching needed for hygiene and dressing activities required the greatest motion. A number of studies indicated that maximal amounts of elbow flexion are needed for touching the forehead, back and side of the head (for washing and combing the hair, putting on a necklace), and ipsilateral axilla. Reaching for shoes on the floor or an object placed overhead and rising from a chair required the greatest amount of elbow extension (Fig. 5.31). The greatest arc of flexion–extension occurred using a phone.

Reaching activities and instrument use, such as reading a newspaper (Fig. 5.32), cutting with a knife, and pouring from a pitcher, required the most pronation. Eating with a spoon required the most supination. Eating with a fork (continental style), using a corkscrew, and turning a doorknob required the greatest arcs of pronation–supination.

Several investigators have taken a different approach in determining the amount of elbow and forearm motion needed for activities of daily living by immobilizing the arm and then determining what functional tasks are possible. Vasen and associates[63] studied the ability of 50 healthy adults to comfortably complete 12 activities of daily living while their elbows were restricted in an adjustable Bledsoe brace. Forty-nine subjects were able to complete all of the tasks with the elbow limited to motion between 75 and 120 degrees of flexion. Subjects used compensatory motions at adjacent normal joints to complete the activities.

Cooper and colleagues[48] studied upper-extremity motion in subjects during three feeding tasks with the elbow unrestricted and then fixed in 110 degrees of flexion with a splint. The 19 subjects were assessed with a video-based, three-dimensional motion analysis system while they were drinking with a handled cup, eating with a fork, and eating with a spoon. Compensatory motions to accommodate the fixed

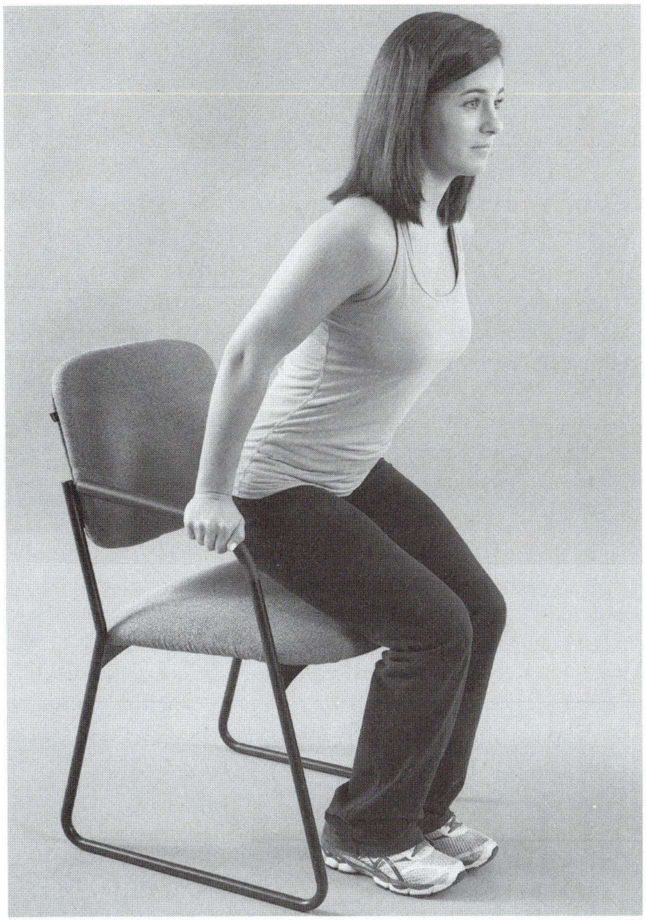

FIGURE 5.31 Studies report that rising from a chair using the upper extremities requires a large amount of elbow and wrist extension.

elbow occurred to a large extent at the shoulder and to a lesser extent at the wrist.

De Groot and associates[60] studied the elbow motion of 10 healthy adults with an electromagnetic tracking device during five activities of daily living (hand to occiput to represent combing hair, hand to sacrum to represent perineal care, hand to contralateral axilla for washing, hand to ipsilateral

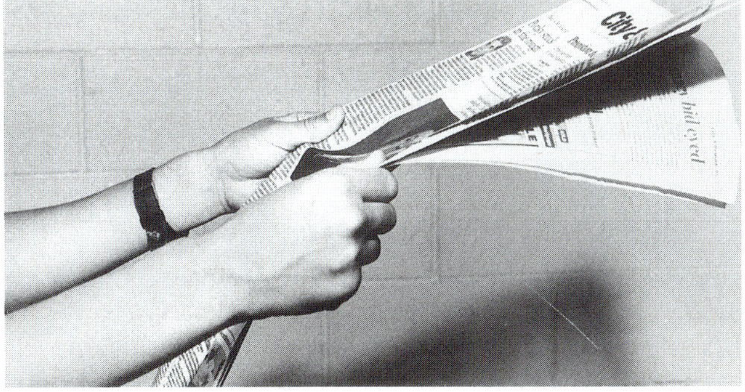

FIGURE 5.32 Approximately 50 degrees of pronation occur during the action of reading a newspaper.

shoe, and cup to mouth for drinking). Activities were performed with elbow flexion and extension unrestricted and then progressively restricted by an adjustable brace in increments of 30 degrees until the five activities could not be performed. A minimum average angle of 86 degrees of flexion and an additional range of 36 degrees of flexion (to 122 degrees) were required to complete the five tasks, as well as large compensatory motions at the shoulder and wrist. No one fixed elbow position allowed the performance of all five tasks, and none of the tasks could be performed with the elbow fixed between 97 and 110 degrees. These findings should be kept in mind if patients are immobilized in casts or splints, or the elbow joint is fused.

Reliability and Validity

Numerous studies have examined the reliability of the measuring elbow and forearm ROM. Most investigators have found the intratester and intertester reliability of measuring ROM with a universal goniometer at these joints to be good to excellent. However, studies indicate that larger differences in repeated measurements are needed to detect meaningful change when examining forearm supination and pronation as compared with elbow flexion and extension. Comparisons between ROM measurements taken with different devices have also been conducted, giving some indication of the concurrent validity of these devices with the universal goniometer. It is recommended that clinicians use the same device and alignment method to improve reliability because the measurement devices are not interchangeable.

Reliability of Universal Goniometers and Inclinometers

Tables 5.5 and 5.6 provide an overview of studies that assessed the intratester and intertester reliability of ROM measurements at the elbow and forearm using a universal goniometer and inclinometer. A brief summary of many of these studies is also included in this section, beginning with studies that were conducted with healthy adults and followed by studies with patient populations.

Healthy Population

Boone and colleagues[64] examined the reliability of measuring six passive motions including elbow extension–flexion. Four physical therapists used universal goniometers to measure these motions in 12 healthy males weekly for 4 weeks. They found that intratester reliability for elbow motion (Pearson product-moment correlation $r = 0.94$) was slightly higher than intertester reliability ($r = 0.88$).

Grohmann[65] found that in a study involving 40 testers and one subject, no significant differences existed between elbow measurements obtained by an over-the-joint method for goniometer alignment and the traditional lateral method. Differences between the means of the measurements were less than 2 degrees. The elbow was held in two fixed positions (an acute and an obtuse angle) by a plywood stabilizing device.

Text continued on page 142

TABLE 5.5 Intratester Reliability of Elbow and Forearm ROM Measurements With Goniometers and Inclinometers for Healthy and Patient Populations

Study	N	Sample	Methods	Motion	r	ICC	Absolute Measures (degrees)
Boone et al[64]	12	Healthy males	AROM, 4 testers, supine, universal goniometer	Extension–flexion	.94		Intra SD = .2 Total SD = 3.7
Carey et al[68]	18	Healthy adults	AROM, 5 testers				
			Digital goniometer	Flexion	.60 to .87		
			Universal goniometer	Flexion	.66 to .90		
Chapleau et al[80]	51	Healthy adults, right and left sides	AROM, 1 tester, sitting with shoulder in anterior flexion, forearm neutral, universal goniometer	Flexion		0.95	
				Extension		0.97	
Gajdosik[67]	31	Healthy adults	AROM, 1 tester, sitting, universal goniometer, 3 alignment methods	Pronation		.81 to .97	
				Supination		.81 to .97	
Goodwin et al[20]	23	Healthy females	AROM, supine, forearm supinated				
			Universal goniometer	Flexion		.56 to .91	
			Fluid inclinometer	Flexion		.50 to .84	
			Electrogoniometer	Flexion		.00 to .43	
Greene and Wolf[19]	20	Healthy adults	AROM, 1 tester,				Within-session SD =
			Universal goniometer	Flexion		.94	1.2
				Extension		.95	1.0
				Pronation		.90	2.2
			Ortho Ranger (electroinclinometer)	Supination		.98	2.1
				Flexion		.84	3.6
				Extension		.86	3.7
				Pronation		.89	3.8
				Supination		.94	3.5
Solveborn and Olerud[66]	16	Healthy adults, right and left sides	1 tester, universal goniometer, alignment for supination and pronation with handheld pencil, right, left sides	Flexion AROM			SD of error = 2, 2
				Extension AROM			SD of error = 1, 2
				Pronation			
				AROM			SD of error = 6, 5
				PROM			SD of error = 6, 5
				Supination			
				AROM			SD of error = 5, 6
				PROM			SD of error = 5, 5
Walker et al[29]	4	Healthy adults	AROM, 4 testers, universal goniometer	Flexion	>.81		Mean error = 5 ± 1
Armstrong et al[73]	38	Adult patients	AROM, sitting, 5 testers, 3 devices, universal goniometer	Flexion		.55 to .98	Mean difference = 3.2 95% CI of diff = 5.9
				Extension		.45 to .98	Mean difference = 3.5 95% CI of diff = 6.6
				Pronation		.96 to .99	Mean difference = 4.2 95% CI of diff = 7.7
				Supination		.96 to .99	Mean difference = 4.0 95% CI of diff = 7.7

de Jong et al[78]	48	Adult patients with subacute stroke	PROM, 2 testers, hydrogoniometer (gravity based)	Extension	.92		SEM = 1.0 SDD= 2.7
				Supination	.89		SEM = 2.2 SDD = 6.2
Flower et al[75]	30	Adult orthopedic patients	PROM, 3 testers, sitting,				
			Universal goniometer	Pronation		.79	SEM = 7.0
				Supination		.95	SEM = 3.7
			Handheld plumbline goniometer	Pronation		.87	SEM = 6.2
				Supination		.95	SEM = 3.7
Geertzen et al[74]	29	Adult patients with reflex sympathetic dystrophy (affected and nonaffected sides)	AROM, 2 testers, standing,				
			Universal goniometer	Flexion			
				Affected	.84, 84		
				Nonaffected	.66, .84		
				Extension			
				Affected	.90, .92		
				Nonaffected	.88, .88		
			Inclinometer	Supination			
				Affected	.92, .93		
				Nonaffected	.94, .92		
Hellebrandt et al[69]	77	Arthritic and orthopedic patients	AROM, 1 expert tester, positions not defined, universal goniometer	Flexion			Mean difference = 1.0
				Extension			Mean difference = .1
				Pronation			Mean difference = .6
				Supination			Mean difference = 1.5
Karagiannopoulos et al[76]	20	Adult orthopedic patients	AROM, 2 testers				
	20	Healthy adults	Universal goniometer aligned with handheld pencil	Pronation			
				injured		.95, .97	SEM = 2.0, 2.2
				healthy		.86, .98	SEM = 1.4, 2.8
				Supination			
				injured		.98, .98	SEM = 2.0, 2.2
				healthy		.96, .96	SEM = 2.0, 2.2
				Pronation			
				injured		.96, .98	SEM = 1.8, 2.1
				healthy		.95, .97	SEM = 1.8, 2.0
			Handheld plumbline goniometer	Supination			
				injured		.98, .98	SEM = 1.4, 2.1
				healthy		.94, .98	SEM = 1.5, 2.6
Pandya et al[72]	150	1- to 20-yr-olds with Duchenne muscular dystrophy	PROM, 5 testers, universal goniometer	Extension		.94	
Rothstein et al[70]	12	Adult patients	PROM, 12 therapists (2 per patient), 3 types of universal goniometers	Flexion	.95 to .98	.94 to .97	
				Extension	.95 to .99	.86 to .99	

r = Pearson correlation coefficient; ICC = Intraclass correlation coefficient; SD = Standard deviation; 95% CI of diff = 95% confidence interval for the difference between measurements; SEM = Standard error of the measurement; SDD = Smallest detectible difference.; AROM = active range of motion; PROM = passive range of motion.

TABLE 5.6 Intertester Reliability of Elbow and Forearm ROM Measurements With Goniometers and Inclinometers for Healthy and Patient Populations

Study	n	Sample	Methods	Motion	r	ICC	Absolute Measures (degrees)
Boone et al[64]	12	Healthy males	AROM, 4 testers, supine, universal goniometer	Extension–flexion	.88		Intra SD = 2.6 Total SD = 4.5
Carey et al[68]	18	Healthy adults	AROM, 5 testers				
			Universal goniometer	Flexion		.63	
			Digital goniometer	Flexion		.69	
Escalante et al[36]	24	Healthy older adults (65–80 yr)	PROM, 4 testers, supine, universal goniometer	Flexion		.84	
Petherick et al[21]	30	Healthy adults	AROM, 2 testers, supine				
			Universal goniometer Fluid inclinometer	Extension–flexion		.53 .92	
Walker et al[29]	4	Healthy adults	AROM, 2 testers, universal goniometer	Flexion			Mean difference = 6±5
Armstrong et al[73]	38	Orthopedic patients	AROM, 5 testers, sitting, 3 devices, universal goniometer	Flexion		.58, .62	Mean difference = 6.4 95% CI of diff = 9.2
				Extension		.58, .87	Mean difference = 7.0 95% CI of diff = 9.0
				Pronation		.83, .86	Mean difference = 7.9 95% CI of diff = 8.9
				Supination		.90, .93	Mean difference = 8.2 95% CI of diff = 9.5
Blonna et al[79]	50	Patients with elbow contractures	AROM, 4 testers (3 experienced, 1 inexperienced), standing with shoulder actively flexed 90°, universal goniometer				
			Experienced testers	Flexion		.96 to .98	Mean difference = −1 to 1 95% LOA = 5 to 7
				Extension		.94 to .98	Mean difference = −1 to 1 95% LOA = 7 to 12
			Inexperienced tester	Flexion		.81 to .86	Mean difference = 4 to 5 95% LOA = 14 to 16
				Extension		.76 to .78	Mean difference = 9 to 10 95% LOA = 17 to 18

Geertzen et al[74]	29	Patients with reflex sympathetic dystrophy (affected and nonaffected sides)	AROM, 2 testers, standing, universal goniometer for flexion and extension, inclinometer for supination	Flexion			
				Affected	.57 to .72		SDD = 9.6
				Nonaffected	.63 to .75		SDD = 7.1
				Extension			
				Affected	.66 to .80		SDD = 12.1
				Nonaffected	.66 to .80		SDD = 12.1
				Supination			
				Affected	.89 to .93		SDD = 19.3
				Nonaffected	.89 to .92		SDD = 16.5
Karagiannopoulos et al[76]	20	Orthopedic patients	AROM, 2 testers				
	20	Healthy adults	Universal goniometer aligned with handheld pencil	Pronation			
				injured		.95	SEM = 2.4
				healthy		.92	SEM = 3.0
				Supination			
				injured		.96	SEM = 2.9
				healthy		.94	SEM = 3.9
			Handheld plumbline goniometer	Pronation			
				injured		.92	SEM = 3.6
				healthy		.91	SEM = 3.0
				Supination			
				injured		.96	SEM = 3.0
				healthy		.96	SEM = 2.2
Pandya et al[72]	150	1- to 20-yr-olds with Duchenne muscular dystrophy	PROM, 5 testers, universal goniometer	Extension		.91	
Rothstein et al[70]	12	Adult patients	PROM, 12 therapists (2 per patient), 3 types of universal goniometers	Flexion	.91 to .97	.85 to .97	
				Extension	.92 to .96	.92 to .96	

r = Pearson correlation coefficient; ICC = Intraclass correlation coefficient; SD = Standard deviation; 95% CI of diff = 95% confidence interval for the difference between measurements; 95% LOA = 95% limits of agreement based on mean and standard deviation of the difference; SEM = Standard error of the measurement; SDD = Smallest detectible difference; AROM = active range of motion; PROM = passive range of motion.

The reliability of ROM measurements taken with a universal goniometer at the elbow and forearm were studied by Solveborn and Olerud[66] in 16 healthy adults as a preliminary part of a more extensive study of patients with tennis elbow. The standard deviation of the random error of the mean ranged from 1 to 2 degrees for elbow flexion and extension, up to 5 to 6 degrees for pronation and supination. During measurements of forearm rotation the goniometer was aligned with a pencil that was held in the hand. The goniometer alignment during elbow flexion and extension was parallel to the lateral aspect of the upper arm and forearm.

A study by Gajdosik[67] of 31 healthy subjects compared three methods of measuring active ROM for supination and pronation. All three methods aligned the stationary arm of a universal goniometer parallel to the humerus. However, Method I aligned the moveable arm of the goniometer with a pencil held in the hand. Method II placed the moveable arm of the goniometer over the anterior or posterior surface of the distal forearm. Method III aligned the moveable arm of the goniometer parallel to a visualized line connecting the styloid processes of the radius and ulna. There was a significant difference in values between the three methods, with Method I having the greatest amount of supination and the least amount of pronation. All methods were highly reliable with intraclass correlation coefficient (ICC) values ranging from 0.81 to 0.97 for three trials by one tester in one session and from 0.86 to 0.96 for two sessions conducted 30 minutes apart. The author noted that Method I was the most reliable but was confounded during supination by movement of the fourth and fifth metacarpals. Methods II and III were recommended as reliable and more valid for clinical use but should not be used interchangeably.

Researchers have conducted a number of studies comparing measurements of elbow and forearm motions using a universal goniometer with other devices. Petherick and associates,[21] in a study in which two testers measured 30 healthy young adults found that intertester reliability for measuring active elbow ROM with a fluid-based goniometer was higher than with a universal goniometer. The Pearson product-moment correlation between the two devices was 0.83, which is considered good; however, there was a significant difference between the two devices (145.8 degrees for the goniometer versus 149.4 for the inclinometer). The authors concluded that the fluid-based and the universal goniometers could not be used interchangeably.

Greene and Wolf[19] compared the reliability of the Ortho Ranger, an electronic pendulum goniometer, with the intratester reliability of a universal goniometer for active upper-extremity motions in 20 healthy adults. Elbow flexion, extension, pronation, and supination were measured three times for each instrument during each session. The three sessions were conducted by one physical therapist during a 2-week period. Within-session reliability was higher for the universal goniometer. Measurements taken with the Ortho Ranger correlated poorly with those taken with the universal goniometer for flexion (r = 0.21), extension (r = 0.11), and slightly better for pronation (r = 0.65), and supination (r = 0.81). There were significant differences in mean measurements taken with the two devices ranging from 10.4 to 18.1 degrees.

Goodwin and colleagues[20] evaluated the reliability of a universal goniometer, a fluid goniometer, and an electrogoniometer for measuring active elbow ROM in 23 healthy women. Three testers took three consecutive readings using each type of goniometer on two occasions that were 4 weeks apart. Significant differences were found between types of goniometers, testers, and replications. Measurements taken with the universal and fluid goniometers correlated the best (r = 0.90), whereas the electrogoniometer correlated poorly with the universal goniometer (r = 0.51) and fluid goniometer (r = 0.33). Intratester reliability within each occasion and between occasions was highest for the universal goniometer. Similar to other researchers, the authors do not advise the interchangeable use of different types of goniometers in the clinical setting.

Carey and colleagues[68] compared the reliability of a digital goniometer prototype with the universal goniometer during active elbow flexion ROM in 18 healthy subjects using five physical therapists to take the measurements. Both devices had similar intratester reliability for measuring elbow flexion, with the digital prototype having ICC values ranging from 0.66 to 0.90 and the universal goniometer from 0.60 to 0.87. Likewise, there was no significant difference in intertester reliability between the two devices (Pearson correlation coefficient r values ranged from 0.46 to 0.69).

Patient Population

In a study published in 1949 by Hellebrandt, Duvall, and Moore,[69] one therapist repeatedly measured 13 active upper-extremity motions, including elbow flexion and extension and forearm pronation and supination, in 77 patients. The differences between the means of two trials ranged from 0.1 degrees for elbow extension to 1.5 degrees for supination. A significant difference between the measurements was noted for elbow flexion, although the difference between the means was only 1.0 degrees. Significant differences were also noted between measurements taken with a universal goniometer and those obtained with specialized devices, leading the author to conclude that different measuring devices could not be used interchangeably. The universal goniometer was generally found to be the more reliable device.

Rothstein, Miller, and Roettger[70] found high intratester and intertester reliability for passive ROM of elbow flexion and extension. Their study involved 12 testers who used three different commonly used universal goniometers (large plastic, small plastic, and large metal) to measure 12 patients with elbow conditions. Intratester and intertester reliability was high (0.85–0.97) for both elbow extension and flexion as measured by all three types of universal goniometers. The use of the means of two measurements rather than one measurement did not improve intertester reliability at this joint. This was the only elbow ROM study that met all inclusion criteria in a review conducted in 2009 by van de Pol and colleagues[71] on interrater reliability for passive ROM of upper-extremity joints; however, not all of the criteria for external and internal validity were fulfilled.

Pandya and colleagues[72] studied the reliability of elbow extension measured with a universal goniometer in 150 children aged 1 to 20 years with Duchenne muscular dystrophy. Five experienced physical therapists took measurements on each patient on admission, at 1 week, and at 4 weeks. Intratester and intertester reliability was excellent with ICC values of 0.94 and 0.91, respectively.

Armstrong and associates[73] examined the intratester, intertester, and interdevice reliability of active ROM measurements of the elbow and forearm in 38 surgical patients. Five testers measured each motion twice with each of the three devices: a universal goniometer, an electrogoniometer, and a mechanical rotation-measuring device. Intratester reliability was high (r values generally greater than 0.90) for all three devices and all motions. Intertester reliability was high for pronation and supination with all three devices. Intertester reliability for elbow flexion and extension was high for the electrogoniometer and moderate for the universal goniometer. Measurements taken with different devices varied widely. The authors concluded that meaningful changes in intratester ROM taken with a universal goniometer occur with 95% confidence if they are greater than 6 degrees for flexion, 7 degrees for extension, and 8 degrees for pronation and supination. Meaningful changes in intertester ROM taken with a universal goniometer occur if they are greater than 10 degrees for flexion, extension, and pronation and greater than 11 degrees for supination.

Two examiners who used either an inclinometer or universal goniometer measured the active ROM of several upper-extremity joints in 29 patients with reflex sympathetic dystrophy in a study by Geertzen and colleagues.[74] Each examiner measured the motions of each patient once per session, and the session was repeated 30 minutes later. The smallest detectable difference (SDD), defined as the smallest amount of change in a variable that can be measured with statistical significance, for elbow flexion and extension with a universal goniometer was 9.6 and 12.1 degrees on the affected side and 7.1 and 12.1 degrees on the nonaffected side, respectively. The smallest detectable difference for supination measured with an inclinometer was 19.3 degrees on the affected side and 16.5 degrees on the nonaffected side. It was unclear whether the SDD referred to repeated measurements made by the same tester or different testers. All correlation coefficients between repeated measurements ranged from 0.57 to 0.84 for flexion, 0.66 to 0.92 for elbow extension, and 0.85 to 0.94 for supination.

Flower and associates[75] measured passive supination and pronation ROM in 30 orthopedic patients (31 wrists) with a traditional 6-inch universal goniometer aligned with the humerus and placed on the distal forearm and a new offset goniometer with a tubular handle and plumbline design. Three therapists measured each motion with each device once per session and repeated the session 20 minutes later. Intratester reliability was excellent (ICC = 0.95) for supination with both the universal and new goniometer and good for pronation with the universal (ICC = 0.79) and new goniometer (ICC = 0.87). Average standard error of the measurement for supination was 3.7 degrees for both the universal and new goniometer, and 7.0 and 6.2 degrees for pronation with the universal and new goniometer, respectively. The authors stated that the difference in reliability between the two methods is probably not clinically significant.

Karagiannopoulos, Sitler, and Michlovitz[76] assessed the reliability of two methods of measuring a functional combination of active forearm and wrist rotation in 20 injured and 20 noninjured subjects. One method placed the stationary arm of a universal goniometer vertically and aligned the moveable arm with a pencil held in the hand. The second method utilized an investigator-constructed tubular handle attached to a single-arm plumbline goniometer. Measurements were taken three times with each method by the two examiners during one session. Reliability was high and error was low for both methods and subject groups. Intratester and intertester ICC values ranged from 0.86 to 0.98 and from 0.91 to 0.96, respectively. Intratester standard error of the measurement (SEM) values ranged from 1.4 to 2.1 degrees, whereas intertester SEM values ranged from 2.2 to 3.9 degrees. To assess functional supination and pronation, the authors recommended the clinical use of the handheld pencil method over the slightly more reliable plumbline method because of the simplicity and greater availability of the equipment for the handheld pencil method.

The reliability of electronic digital inclinometer in measuring elbow flexion and extension was studied in 42 healthy adults by Cleffken and associates.[77] A variety of shoulder positions and stabilizations were studied with the inclinometer placed 3 centimeters distal to the olecranon and 3 centimeters proximal to the epicondyles. Pearson correlation r values ranged from 0.85 to 0.89, indicating good intratester reliability, and ranged from 0.66 to 0.82, indicating poor to good intertester reliability, using one measurement. Intertester reliability improved when the means of three measurements were used in the analyses (r ranging from 0.77 to 0.89). Reliability also improved with the addition of stabilization. The SDD at a 95% confidence limit were also reported: Intratester values ranged from 6 to 9 degrees and intertester values ranged from 4 to 17 degrees.

De Jong and colleagues[78] studied 48 patients with subacute stroke at four measurement sessions over a 20-week period. Seven upper-extremity motions were measured by two therapists within each session using a hydrogoniometer (inclinometer). Averaged interobserver reliability coefficients for elbow extension and forearm supination within sessions were 0.92 and 0.89, respectively, indicating very good reliability. The standard error of measurement and SDD at 95% confidence level were 1.0 and 2.7 degrees for elbow extension and 2.2 and 6.2 degrees for supination.

Blonna and associates[79] had four testers with different levels of expertise measure active elbow flexion and extension in 50 patients with elbow contractures. Measurements were taken with a universal goniometer placed directly on each patient once and with a goniometer placed on a previously taken digital photograph of the patient twice. Measurements were made with the patients in standing and the shoulder actively flexed forward to horizontal. Intertester reliability was high (ICC = 0.91–0.98) for both the clinical use of the universal goniometer and photography-based goniometry between the three experienced testers (surgeon, physician assistant, clinical fellow), but was only high for the study coordinator (who had no experience examining elbows) using the photograph-based goniometry. The average error (difference) between experienced testers for elbow motions using the goniometer was generally −1 to 1 degrees, and 95% limits of agreement (1.96 × standard deviation [SD]) were ±5 to 7 degrees, but results were worse for the inexperienced tester.

Validity of Universal Goniometric Measurements

Only one published study was found that reported the validity of elbow ROM measurements taken with a universal goniometer compared with the gold standard of measurement taken by radiographs. Chapleau and colleagues[80] studied the intratester reliability and concurrent validity of measuring active elbow motions and carrying angles with a universal goniometer and radiographs in 51 healthy adults (102 elbows). One tester took three goniometric measurements and two testers each took one measurement of the same radiographs for each motion of flexion and extension. Radiographic measurements were slightly (but statistically) lower than goniometric measurements with mean differences of 2.4 degrees for flexion, 1.1 degrees for extension, and 1.3 degrees for total ROM. Ninety-five percent of the goniometric measurements for flexion, extension, and total ROM were less than 7.0, 10.3, and 11.5 degrees different from the radiographs, respectively. Pearson correlation coefficients between the goniometric and radiographic measurements were 0.65 for flexion, 0.69 for extension, and 0.73 for total ROM. Some difference may have been due to variations in aligning the goniometer with external landmarks of the acromion process, lateral epicondyle, and midwrist, whereas the radiographs utilized the midshaft of the humerus and ulna. Both measurement methods were highly reliable: mean intratester ICCs for goniometry ranged from 0.95 to 0.97, whereas mean intertester ICCs for radiographs ranged from 0.98 to 0.99.

Reliability of Photography and Smartphone Applications Based on Photography

Several studies have examined the reliability of photography-based goniometric measurements of the elbow joint. The studies generally report high repeatability of measuring joint angles with a goniometer from a photograph and agreement with goniometric measurements taken directly on a person. However, the photographs were not taken by each tester on each study subject and then measured, as would be expected in a clinical setting. More research is needed to establish the reliability and validity of measuring joint motion using digital photographs from cameras and cell phones in a more realistic manner.

As reported previously, Blonna and associates[79] had four testers with different levels of expertise measure active elbow flexion and extension in 50 patients with elbow contractures. Measurements were taken with a universal goniometer placed directly on each patient once and with a goniometer placed on a previously taken digital photograph of the patient twice. Intratester and intertester reliability for elbow flexion and extension was high (ICC = 0.89–0.99) for the photography-based goniometry for all four testers regardless of their level of expertise. The average error (difference) between testers for the photography-based motions was −4 to 4 degrees, with 95% limits of agreement (LOA = 1.96 × SD) ranging from ±6 to 11 degrees. Eighty-nine percent of the photography-based goniometry measurements made by the expert surgeon were within 5 degrees of the values determined directly by goniometer, and the surgeon's interdevice validity was excellent (ICC = 0.96–0.98).

In a study by Fish and Wingate,[81] 46 physical therapy students used plastic and metal universal goniometers to measure the angle of an elbow fixed in approximately 50 and 135 degrees of flexion by a splint. In some cases the landmarks were prelabeled, whereas in others the testers had to palpate and identify the landmarks for goniometer alignment. Measurements were also determined from photographs of the prelabeled fixed elbow. In addition, passive elbow flexion ROM was measured in the unsplinted elbow. Except for one case, there were small but significant differences (ranging from 0.6 to 5.1 degrees) between the means of the goniometric measurements as compared with the photographic measurements. The standard deviation of the measurements increased from a low of 0.7 to 1.1 degrees with photographic measurements to a high of 3.4 to 4.2 degrees with passive ROM measured with goniometers. The authors proposed that small systematic errors in alignment of the goniometer, identification of bony landmarks, and variations in the amount of torque applied by the tester may account for these differences.

One study by Ferriero and associates[82] examined the reliability of measuring elbow ROM using the DrGoniometer application (C.D.M., Srl, Milano, Italy) on an iPhone (Apple Inc., Cupertino, CA). This application superimposes a virtual goniometer on a digital photograph previously taken with the smartphone. Seven experienced raters measured 28 previously taken photographs of healthy elbows once with a universal goniometer and with the smartphone. Measurements were repeated after 1 week. Intratester and intertester reliability was excellent with ICC values above 0.99. The width of the 95% LOA between the two devices was about 10 degrees (LOA = +4.5, −5.8). The practicality, reliability, and validity of using a smartphone with goniometer application to measure range of elbow motion directly from a patient still needs to be evaluated in future studies. The ability to store the measurement data for later analysis and download to a computer for written reports appears to be beneficial.

Reliability and Validity of Visual Estimates

A study by Blonna and colleagues[83] compared the reliability of previously reported data on goniometric measurements[79] with visual estimates of active elbow flexion and extension in 50 patients with elbow contractures. Patients were asked to stand with shoulder forward and flexed to horizontal and then to extend and flex their elbows. Three experienced testers (surgeon, physician assistant, clinical fellow) and one inexperienced tester (study coordinator) visually estimated and then measured each patient once. Intertester reliability for visual estimates was good to excellent between experienced testers (ICC = 0.87–0.96), but poor between the inexperienced tester and the others (ICC = 0.38–0.53). Experienced testers were capable of relatively accurate measurements with the average error (difference) of −3 to 1 degrees and 95% limits of agreement between ±10 to 15 degrees; however, there were very large systematic errors of 8 to 18 degrees and 95% limits of agreement from ±32 to 40 degrees between the inexperienced tester and the other testers.

REFERENCES

1. Levangie, PK, and Norkin, CC: Joint Structure and Function: A Comprehensive Analysis, ed 5. FA Davis, Philadelphia, 2011.
2. Amis, AA, and Miller, JH: The elbow. Clin Rheum Dis 8:571, 1982.
3. Van Roy, P, et al: Arthro-kinematics of the elbow: Study of the carrying angle. Ergonomics 48:11, 2005.
4. Balasubramanian, P, Madhuri, V, and Muliyil, J: Carrying angle in children: A normative study. J Pediatr Orthop B 15:37, 2006.
5. Golden, DW, et al: Elbow range of motion and clinical carrying angle in a healthy pediatric population. J Pediatr Orthop B 16:144, 2007.
6. Yilmaz, E, et al: Variation of carrying angle with age, sex, and special reference to side. Orthopedics 28:1360, 2005.
7. Hoppenfeld, S: Physical Examination of the Spine and Extremities. Appleton-Century-Crofts, New York, 1977.
8. Morrey, BF, and Chao, EYS: Passive motion of the elbow joint. J Bone Joint Surg Am 58:50, 1976.
9. Neumann, DA: Kinesiology of the Musculoskeletal System: Foundations for Physical Rehabilitation, ed 2. Mosby, St Louis, MO, 2009.
10. Cyriax, JH, and Cyriax, PJ: Illustrated Manual of Orthopaedic Medicine. Butterworths, London, 1983.
11. Kaltenborn, FM: Manual Mobilization of the Extremity Joints, ed 7. Olaf Norlis Bokhandel, Oslo, 2011.
12. Magee, DJ: Orthopedic Physical Assessment, ed 5. WB Saunders, Philadelphia, 2007.
13. American Academy of Orthopaedic Surgeons: Joint Motion: Methods of Measuring and Recording. AAOS, Chicago, 1965.
14. Green, WB, and Heckman, JD (eds): The Clinical Measurement of Joint Motion. American Academy of Orthopaedic Surgeons, Rosemont, IL, 1994.
15. American Medical Association: Guides to the Evaluation of Permanent Impairment, ed 5. Cocchiarella, L, and Andersson, GBJ (eds). AMA, Chicago, 2001.
16. Boone, DC, and Azen, SP: Normal range of motion in male subjects. J Bone Joint Surg Am 61:756, 1979.
17. Gunal, I, et al: Normal range of motion of the joints of the upper extremity in male subjects, with special reference to side. J Bone Joint Surg Am 78(A):1401, 1996.
18. Soucie, JM, et al: Range of motion measurements: Reference values and a database for comparison studies. Haemophilia 17:500, 2011.
19. Greene, BL, and Wolf, SL: Upper extremity joint movement: Comparison of two measurement devices. Arch Phys Med Rehabil 70:288, 1989.
20. Goodwin, J, et al: Clinical methods of goniometry: A comparative study. Disabil Rehabil 14:10, 1992.
21. Petherick, M, et al: Concurrent validity and intertester reliability of universal and fluid-based goniometers for active elbow range of motion. Phys Ther 68:966, 1988.
22. Sanya, AO, and Chinyelu SO: Range of motion in selected joints of diabetic and non-diabetic subjects. Afr J Health Sci 6:17, 1999.
23. Wanatabe, H, et al: The range of joint motions of the extremities in healthy Japanese people: The difference according to age. Nippon Seikeigeka Gakkai Zasshi 53:275, 1979. (Cited in Walker, JM: Musculoskeletal development: A review. Phys Ther 71:878, 1991.)
24. Hacker, MR, Funk, SM, and Manco-Johnson, MJ: The Colorado Hemophilia Paediatric Joint Physical Examination Scale: Normal values and interrater reliability. Haemophilia 13:71, 2007.
25. Barad, JH, et al: Range of motion of the healthy pediatric elbow: Cross-sectional study of a large population. J Pediatr Orthop B 22:117, 2013.
26. Boone, DC: Techniques of measurement of joint motion. Unpublished supplement to Boone, DC, and Azen, SP: Normal range of motion in male subjects. J Bone Joint Surg Am 61:756, 1979.
27. Chapleau, J, et al: Demographic and anthropometric factors affecting elbow range of motion in healthy adults. J Shoulder Elbow Surg 22:88, 2013.
28. Macedo, LG, and Magee, DJ: Effects of age on passive range of motion of selected peripheral joints in healthy adult females. Physiother Theory Pract 25:145, 2009.
29. Walker, JM, et al: Active mobility of the extremities in older subjects. Phys Ther 64:919, 1984.
30. Bergstrom, G, et al: Prevalence of symptoms and signs of joint impairment. Scand J Rehabil Med 17:173, 1985.
31. Fiebert, I, Fuhri, JR, and New, MD: Elbow, forearm and wrist passive range of motion in persons aged sixty and older. Phys Occup Ther Geriatr 10:17, 1992.
32. Kalscheur, JA, Emery, LJ, and Costello, PS: Range of motion in older women. Phys Occup Ther Geriatr 16:77, 1999.
33. Kalscheur, JA, Costello, PS, and Emery, LJ: Gender differences in range of motion in older adults. Phys Occup Ther Geriatr 22:77, 2003.
34. Bell, RD, and Hoshizaki, TB: Relationships of age and sex with range of motion of seventeen joint actions in humans. Can J Appl Sport Sci 6:202, 1981.
35. Salter, N, and Darcus, HD: The amplitude of forearm and of humeral rotation. J Anat 87:407, 1953.
36. Escalante, A, Lichenstein, MJ, and Hazuda, HP: Determinants of shoulder and elbow flexion range: Results from the San Antonio Longitudinal Study of Aging. Arthritis Care Res 12:277, 1999.
37. Golden, DW, et al: Body mass index and elbow range of motion in a healthy pediatric population: A possible mechanism of overweight in children. J Pediatr Gastroenterol Nutr 46:196, 2008. doi:10.1097/MPG.0b013e31812f568b.
38. Park, W, et al: Obesity effect on male active joint range of motion. Ergonomics 53:102, 2010.
39. Macedo, LG, and Magee, DJ: Differences in range of motion between dominant and nondominant sides of upper and lower extremities. J Manipulative Physiol Ther 31:577, 2008.
40. Shaaban, H, et al: The effect of elbow position on the range of supination and pronation of the forearm. J Hand Surg Eur 33E:3, 2008.
41. Chinn, CJ, Priest, JD, and Kent, BA: Upper extremity range of motion, grip strength and girth in highly skilled tennis players, Phys Ther 54:474, 1974.
42. Chang, DE, Buschbacher, LP, and Edlich, RF: Limited joint mobility in power lifters. Am J Sports Med 16:280, 1988.
43. Wright, RW, et al: Elbow range of motion in professional baseball pitchers. Am J Sports Med 34:190, 2006.
44. Morrey, BF, Askew, KN, and Chao, EYS: A biomechanical study of normal functional elbow motion. J Bone Joint Surg Am 63:872, 1981.
45. Packer, TL, et al: Examining the elbow during functional activities. Occup Ther J Res 10:323, 1990.
46. Sanz, MC, et al: Kinematic analysis of the elbow in the activities. Rehabilitacion 33:293, 1999.
47. Safaee-Rad, R, et al: Normal functional range of motion of upper limb joints during performance of three feeding activities. Arch Phys Med Rehabil 71:505, 1990.
48. Cooper, JE, et al: Elbow joint restriction: Effect on functional upper limb motion during performance of three feeding activities. Arch Phys Med Rehabil 74:805, 1993.
49. Raiss, G, et al: Range of motion of shoulder and elbow in activities of daily life in 3D motion. Z Orthop Unfall 145:493, 2007.
50. Murray, IA, and Johnson, GR: A study of the external forces and moments at the shoulder and elbow while performing everyday tasks. Clin Biomech 19:586, 2004.
51. Sardelli, M, Tashjian, RZ, and MacWilliams, BA: Functional elbow range of motion for contemporary tasks. J Bone Joint Surg Am 93:471, 2011.
52. Romilly, DP, et al: A functional task analysis and motion simulation for the development of a powered upper-limb orthosis. IEEE Trans Neural Syst Rehabil Eng 2:119, 1994.
53. Buckley, MA, et al: Dynamics of the upper limb during performance of the tasks of everyday living: A review of the current knowledge base. Proc Inst Mech Eng 210:241, 1996.
54. Henmi, S, et al: A biomechanical study of activities of daily living using neck and upper limbs with an optical three-dimensional motion analysis system. Mod Rheumatol 16:289, 2006.
55. Pieniazek, M, et al: Upper limb joint mobility ranges during activities of daily living determined by three-dimensional motion analysis—preliminary report. Ortop Traumatol Rehabil 9:413, 2007.
56. Van Andel, CJ, et al: Complete 3D kinematics of upper extremity functional tasks. Gait Posture 27:120, 2007. doi:10.1016/j.gaitpost.2007.03.002.
57. Rudins, A, et al: Kinematics of the elbow during wheelchair propulsion: A comparison of two wheelchairs and two stoking techniques. Arch Phys Med Rehabil 78:1204, 1997
58. Magerman, DJ, et al: Requirements for upper extremity motions during activities of daily living. Clin Biomech 20:591, 2005
59. Aizawa, J, et al: Three-dimensional motion of the upper extremity joints during various activities of daily living. J Biomech 43:2915, 2010.
60. de Groot, JH, et al: Reduced elbow mobility affects the flexion or extension domain in activities of daily living. Clin Biomech 26:713, 2011.
61. Mackey, AH, Walt, SE, and Stott, S: Deficits in upper-limb task performance in children with hemiplegic cerebral palsy as defined by 3-dimensional kinematics. Arch Phys Med Rehabil 87:207, 2006.

62. Petuskey, K, et al: Upper extremity kinematics during functional activities: Three-dimensional studies in a normal pediatric population. Gait Posture 25:573, 2007.
63. Vasen, AP, et al: Functional range of motion of the elbow. J Hand Surg 20A:288, 1995.
64. Boone, DC, et al: Reliability of goniometric measurements. Phys Ther 58:1355, 1978.
65. Grohmann, JEL: Comparison of two methods of goniometry. Phys Ther 63:922, 1983.
66. Solveborn, SA, and Olerud, C: Radial epicondylalgia (tennis elbow): Measurement of range of motion of the wrist and the elbow. J Orthop Sports Phys Ther 23:251, 1996.
67. Gajdosik, RL: Comparison and reliability of three goniometric methods for measuring forearm supination and pronation. Percept Mot Skills 93:353, 2001.
68. Carey, MA, et al: Reliability, validity, and clinical usability of a digital goniometer. Work 36:55, 2010.
69. Hellebrandt, FA, Duvall, EN, and Moore, ML: The measurement of joint motion. Part III: Reliability of goniometry. Phys Ther Rev 29:302, 1949.
70. Rothstein, JM, Miller, PJ, and Roettger, RF: Goniometric reliability in a clinical setting: Elbow and knee measurements. Phys Ther 63:1611, 1983.
71. van de Pol, RJ, van Triffel, E, and Lucas, C: Inter-rater reliability for measurement of passive physiological range of motion of upper extremity joints is better if instruments are used: A systematic review. J Physiother (Australian) 56(1):7, 2010.
72. Pandya, S, et al: Reliability of goniometric measurements in patients with Duchenne muscular dystrophy. Phys Ther 65:1339, 1985.
73. Armstrong, AD, et al: Reliability of range-of-motion measurement in the elbow and forearm. J Shoulder Elbow Surg 7:573, 1998.
74. Geertzen, JHB, et al: Variation in measurements of range of motion: A study in reflex sympathetic dystrophy patients. Clin Rehabil 12:254, 1998.
75. Flower, KR, et al: Intrarater reliability of a new method and instrumentation for measuring passive supination and pronation: A preliminary study. J Hand Ther 14:30, 2001.
76. Karagiannopoulos, C, Sitler, M, and Michlovitz, S: Reliability of 2 functional goniometric methods for measuring forearm pronation and supination active range of motion. J Orthop Sports Phys Ther 33:523, 2003.
77. Cleffken, B, et al: Test-retest reproducibility of elbow goniometric measurements in a rigid double-blinded protocol: Intervals for distinguishing between measurement error and clinical change. J Shoulder Elbow Surg16:788, 2007.
78. de Jong, LD, et al: Repeated measurements of arm joint passive range of motion after stroke: Interobserver reliability and sources of variation. Phys Ther 92:1027, 2012.
79. Blonna, D, et al: Validation of a photography-based goniometry method for measuring joint range of motion. J Shoulder Elbow Surg 21:29, 2012.
80. Chapleau, J, et al: Validity of goniometric elbow measurements: Comparative study with a radiographic method. Clin Orthop Relat Res 469:3134, 2011.
81. Fish, DR, and Wingate, L: Sources of goniometric error at the elbow. Phys Ther 65:1666, 1985.
82. Ferriero, G, et al: Reliability of a new application for smartphones (DrGoniometer) for elbow angle measurement. PM R 3:1153, 2011.
83. Blonna, D, et al: Accuracy and inter-observer reliability of visual estimation compared to clinical goniometry of the elbow. Knee Surg Sports Traumatol Arthrosc 20:1378, 2012.

CHAPTER 6

The Wrist

D. Joyce White, PT, DSc

Structure and Function

Radiocarpal and Midcarpal Joints

The wrist is composed of two joints, the radiocarpal and midcarpal joints, both of which are important to function. The radiocarpal joint lies closer to the forearm, whereas the midcarpal joint is closer to the hand. The proximal joint surface of the radiocarpal joint consists of the distal radius and radioulnar articular disc (Fig. 6.1; see also Fig. 5.8).[1] The disc connects the medial aspect of the distal radius to the distal ulna. The distal radius and the disc form a continuous concave surface.[2,3] The distal joint surface includes three bones from the proximal carpal row—the scaphoid, lunate, and triquetrum—which are connected by interosseous ligaments to form a convex surface (Fig. 6.1). The radius articulates with the scaphoid and lunate, whereas the radioulnar disc articulates with the triquetrum and, to a lesser extent, the lunate. The pisiform, although found in the proximal row of carpal bones, does not participate in the radiocarpal joint. The joint is enclosed by a strong capsule and is reinforced by the palmar radiocarpal, ulnocarpal, dorsal radiocarpal, ulnar collateral, and radial collateral ligaments and numerous intercarpal ligaments (Figs. 6.2 and 6.3).

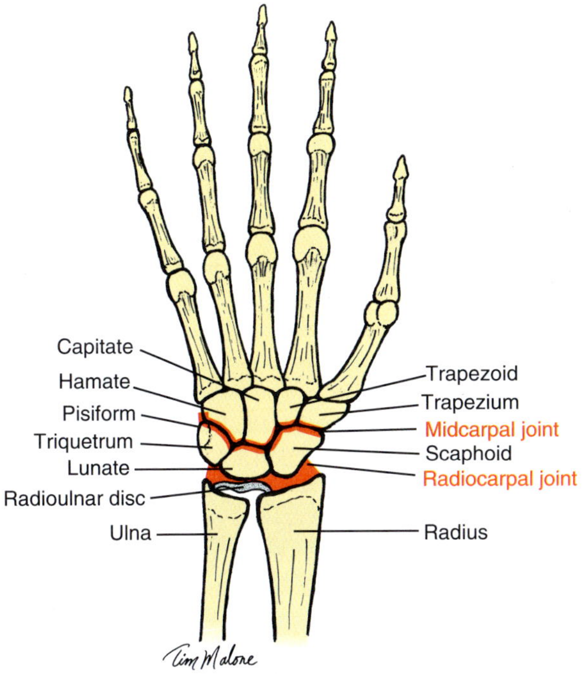

FIGURE 6.1 An anterior (palmar) view of the right wrist showing the radiocarpal and midcarpal joints.

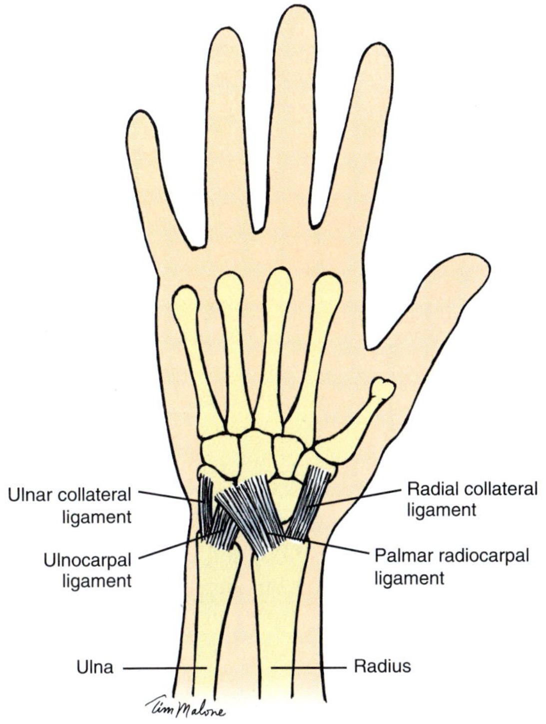

FIGURE 6.2 An anterior (palmar) view of the right wrist showing the palmar radiocarpal, ulnocarpal, and collateral ligaments.

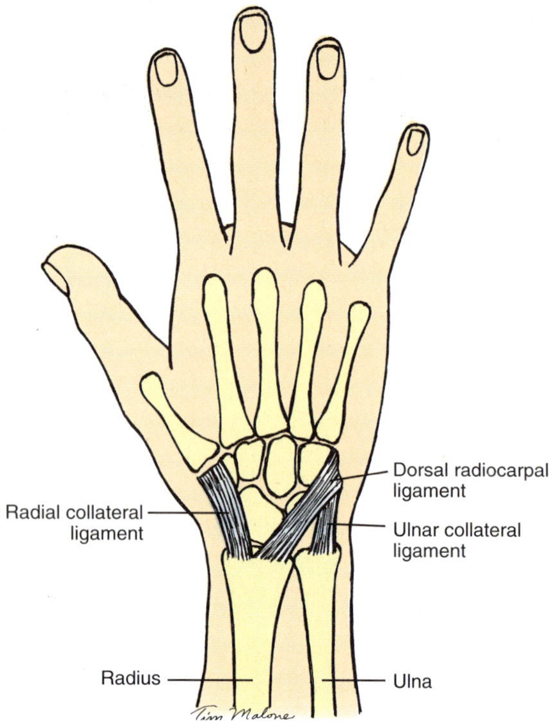

FIGURE 6.3 A posterior view of the right wrist showing the dorsal radiocarpal and collateral ligaments.

The midcarpal joint is distal to the radiocarpal joint. The predominant central and ulnar side of the midcarpal joint consists of the concave surfaces of the scaphoid, lunate, and triquetrum proximally and the convex surfaces of the capitate and hamate distally (Fig. 6.1).[1] On the radial side of the midcarpal joint, a smaller convex surface of the scaphoid contacts the concave surfaces of the trapezium and trapezoid. The midcarpal joint has a joint capsule that is continuous with each intercarpal joint and some carpometacarpal and intermetacarpal joints. Many of the ligaments that reinforce the radiocarpal joint also support the midcarpal joint (Figs. 6.2 and 6.3).

Osteokinematics

The radiocarpal and midcarpal joints are of the condyloid type, with 2 degrees of freedom.[2] The wrist complex (radiocarpal and midcarpal joints) permits flexion–extension in the sagittal plane around a medial–lateral axis, and radial–ulnar deviation in the frontal plane around an anterior–posterior axis. Both joints contribute to these motions.[4–7] The distal end of the radius is angled about 25 degrees toward the ulnar and results in more range of motion (ROM) in ulnar deviation than radial deviation.[4] Also, the distal end of the radius is angled about 10 degrees in the palmar direction contributing to a slightly greater range of wrist flexion than extension. Some sources report that a small amount of supination–pronation occurs at the wrist complex,[8,9] but this rotation is not usually measured in the clinical setting. Circumduction, a combination of flexion, extension, and radial and ulnar deviation in an egg-shaped asymmetrical pattern, is also possible; its measurement has begun to be quantified in the research setting.[10,11]

Arthrokinematics

Motion at the radiocarpal joint occurs because the convex surfaces of the proximal row of carpals roll and slide on the concave surfaces of the radius and radioulnar disc. The proximal row of carpals rolls in the same direction but slides in the opposite direction to movement of the hand.[3,4,12] The carpals slide dorsally on the radius and disc during wrist flexion, and ventrally toward the palm during wrist extension. During ulnar deviation, the carpals roll in an ulnar direction and slide in a radial direction. During radial deviation, the proximal row of carpals rolls in a radial direction and slide in an ulnar direction.

Motion at the midcarpal joint occurs because the distal row of carpals rolls and slides on the proximal row of carpals. Similar to the radiocarpal joint, the distal joint surface of the midcarpal joint is predominantly convex and rolls in the same direction and slides in the opposite direction to the osteokinematic movements of the wrist. During flexion, the large and markedly convex surfaces of the capitate and hamate roll ventrally and slide dorsally on the concave surfaces of the scaphoid, lunate, and triquetrum.[3,4,12] However, there is more complexity at the midcarpal joint than at the radiocarpal joint. On the lateral side of the midcarpal joint, the smaller, shallow surfaces of the trapezium and trapezoid are slightly concave, and roll and slide ventrally on the convex surface of the scaphoid with flexion creating slight pronation.[9] The movements during extension are opposite to that of flexion.

During radial deviation at the midcarpal joint, the convex surfaces of the predominant carpal bones, the capitate and hamate, roll in a radial direction and slide in an ulnar direction on the concave surfaces of the scaphoid, lunate, and triquetrum. However, the concave surfaces of the smaller trapezium and trapezoid roll and slide slightly dorsally into extension on the scaphoid during radial deviation.[3,9,11–14] With ulnar deviation, the surfaces on the capitate and hamate roll in an ulnar direction and slide in a radial direction. The joint surfaces of the trapezium and trapezoid roll and slide slightly ventrally into flexion.

Several studies using serial radiographs and CT scanning have also noted minimal amounts of flexion of the scaphoid and lunate on the radius during radial deviation, as well as minimal amounts of extension of the scaphoid and lunate on the radius during ulnar deviation. These slight motions at the radiocarpal joint compensate for the small motions occurring in the distal row of carpal bones at the midcarpal joint during radial and ulnar deviation. These small compensatory motions help to keep the hand in the frontal plane during radial and ulnar deviation[9] and perhaps allow a little more range of motion to occur.[4]

Capsular Pattern

Cyriax and Cyriax[15] report that the capsular pattern at the wrist is an equal limitation of flexion and extension and a slight limitation of radial and ulnar deviation. Kaltenborn[3] notes that the capsular pattern is an equal restriction in all motions.

RANGE OF MOTION TESTING PROCEDURES: Wrist

Landmarks for Testing Procedures

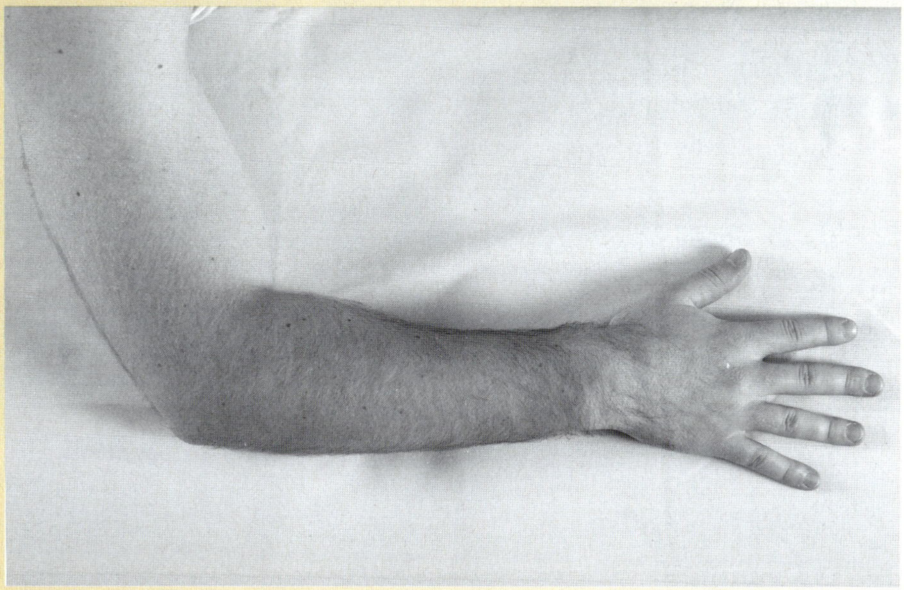

FIGURE 6.4 Posterior view of the right upper extremity showing surface anatomy landmarks for goniometer alignment during the measurement of wrist ROM.

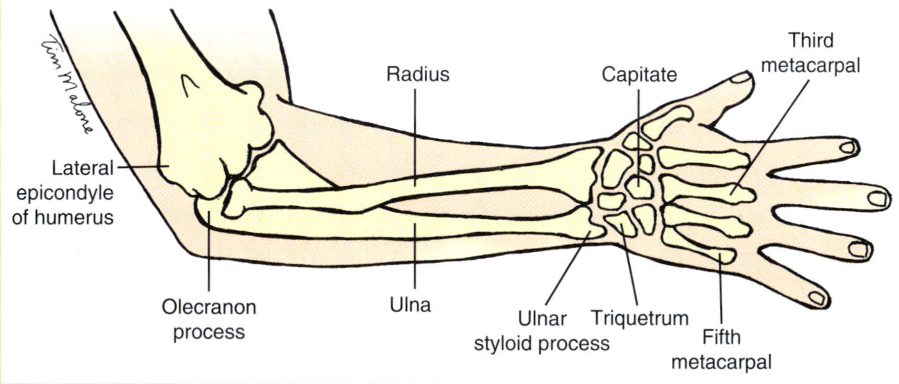

FIGURE 6.5 Posterior view of the right upper extremity showing bony anatomical landmarks for goniometer alignment during the measurement of wrist ROM.

Landmarks for Testing Procedures (continued)

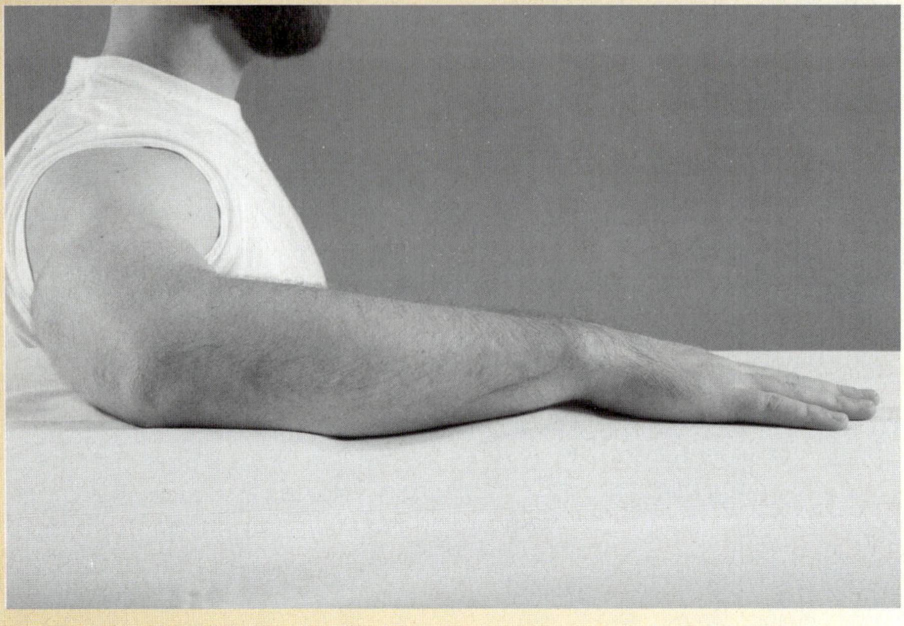

FIGURE 6.6 Lateral view of the right upper extremity showing surface anatomy landmarks for goniometer alignment during the measurement of wrist flexion and extension ROM.

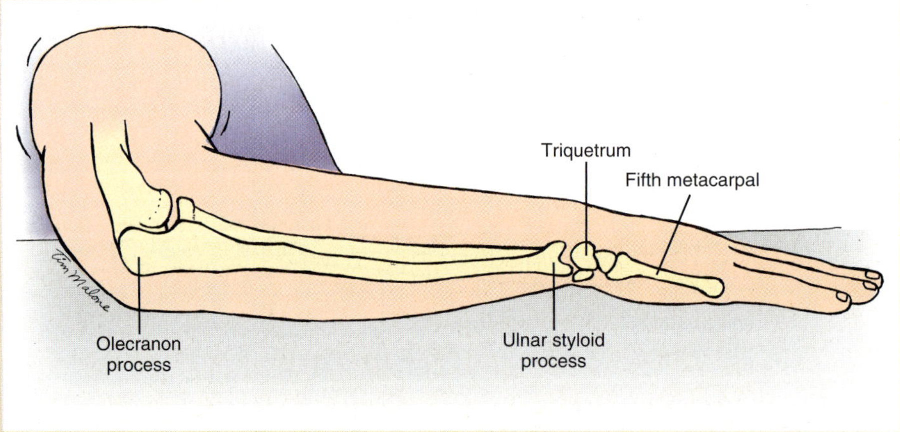

FIGURE 6.7 Lateral view of the right upper extremity showing bony anatomical landmarks for goniometer alignment during the measurement of wrist flexion and extension ROM.

WRIST FLEXION

This motion occurs in the sagittal plane around a medial–lateral axis. Wrist flexion is sometimes referred to as volar or palmar flexion. Normal ROM values for adults vary from about 60 to 80 degrees. Refer to Research Findings and Tables 6.1 through 6.4 for normal ROM values by age and gender.

Testing Position

Position the individual sitting next to a supporting surface with the shoulder abducted to 90 degrees, the elbow flexed to 90 degrees, and the palm of the hand facing the ground. In this position the forearm will be midway between supination and pronation. Rest the forearm on the supporting surface, but leave the hand free to move. Avoid radial or ulnar deviation of the wrist and flexion of the fingers. If the fingers are flexed, tension in the extensor digitorum communis, extensor indicis, and extensor digiti minimi muscles will restrict the motion.

If the individual cannot be positioned in 90 degrees of shoulder abduction, a more adducted shoulder position may be used, but the forearm will be in some pronation when the palm is facing the floor.

Stabilization

Stabilize the radius and ulna to prevent supination or pronation of the forearm and motion of the elbow.

Testing Motion

Flex the wrist by pushing on the dorsal surface of the third metacarpal, moving the hand toward the floor (Fig. 6.8). Maintain the wrist in 0 degrees of radial and ulnar deviation, being careful not to twist the hand. The end of flexion ROM occurs when resistance to further motion is felt and attempts to overcome the resistance cause the forearm to lift off the supporting surface.

Normal End-Feel

The end-feel is firm because of tension in the dorsal radiocarpal ligament and the dorsal joint capsule. Tension in the extensor carpi radialis brevis and longus and extensor carpi ulnaris muscles may also contribute to the firm end-feel.

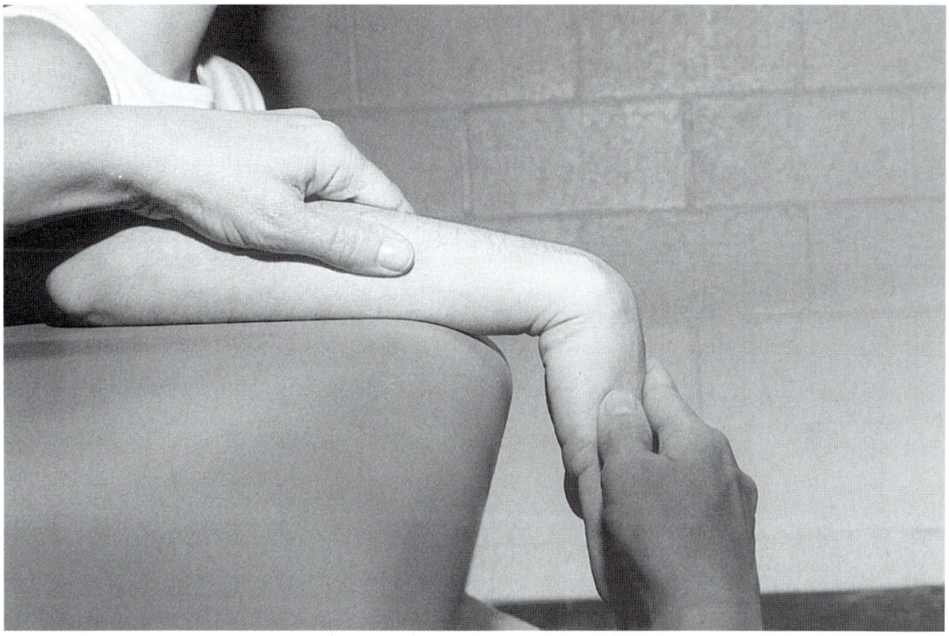

FIGURE 6.8 The end of wrist flexion ROM. Only about three-quarters of the forearm is supported by the examining table so that there is sufficient space for the hand to complete the motion.

Goniometer Alignment

See Figures 6.9 and 6.10.

1. Center **fulcrum** on the lateral aspect of the wrist over the triquetrum.
2. Align **proximal arm** with the lateral midline of the ulna, using the olecranon and ulnar styloid processes for reference.
3. Align **distal arm** with the lateral midline of the fifth metacarpal. Do not use the soft tissue of the hypothenar eminence for reference.

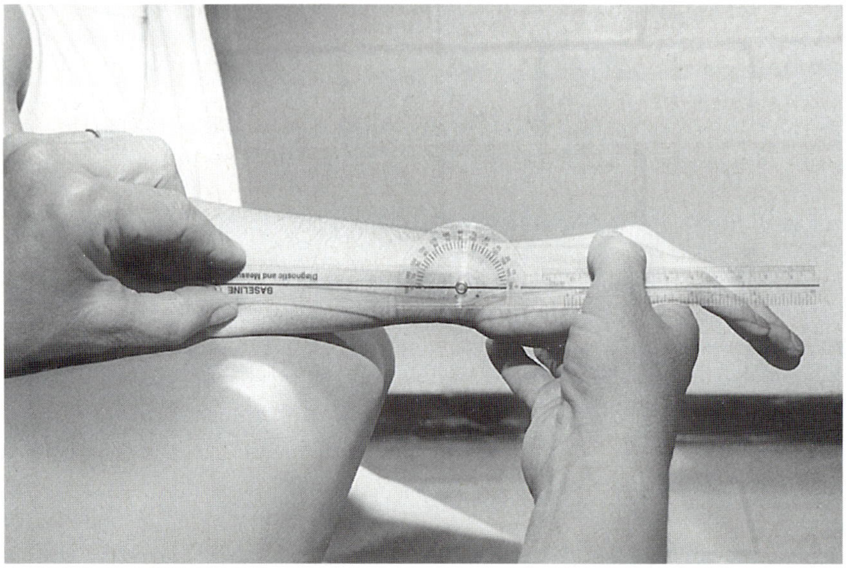

FIGURE 6.9 The alignment of the goniometer at the beginning of wrist flexion ROM.

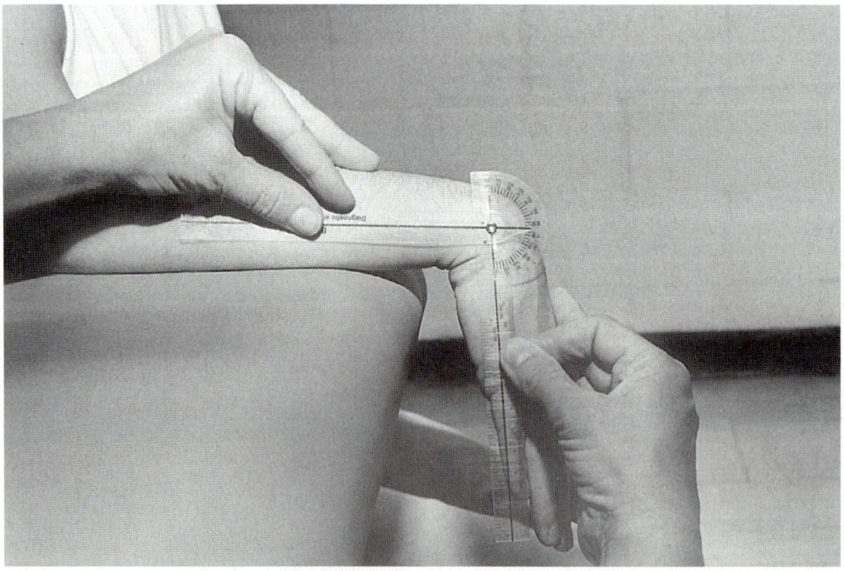

FIGURE 6.10 At the end of wrist flexion ROM the examiner uses one hand to align the distal arm of the goniometer with the fifth metacarpal while maintaining the wrist in flexion. The examiner exerts pressure on the middle of the dorsum of the individual's hand and avoids exerting pressure directly on the fifth metacarpal because such pressure will distort the goniometer alignment.

Alternative Goniometer Alignment: Dorsal Aspect

See Figures 6.11 and 6.12.

This alternative goniometer alignment is recommended by several authors providing that edema, bony deformity, or other topography aberrance is not present in the forearm and hand.[16,17] The dorsal alignment technique will likely result in lower wrist flexion ROM values than the lateral alignment technique (mean differences of 3 to 10 degrees reported).[16] This difference should be taken into account when comparing an individual's results with normative data that use a lateral alignment. Most important, the same alignment techniques should be used in repetitive measurements to evaluate change in wrist flexion ROM.

1. Center **fulcrum** dorsal to the wrist joint near the capitate.
2. Align **proximal arm** with the dorsal midline of the forearm.
3. Align **distal arm** with the dorsal aspect of the third metacarpal.

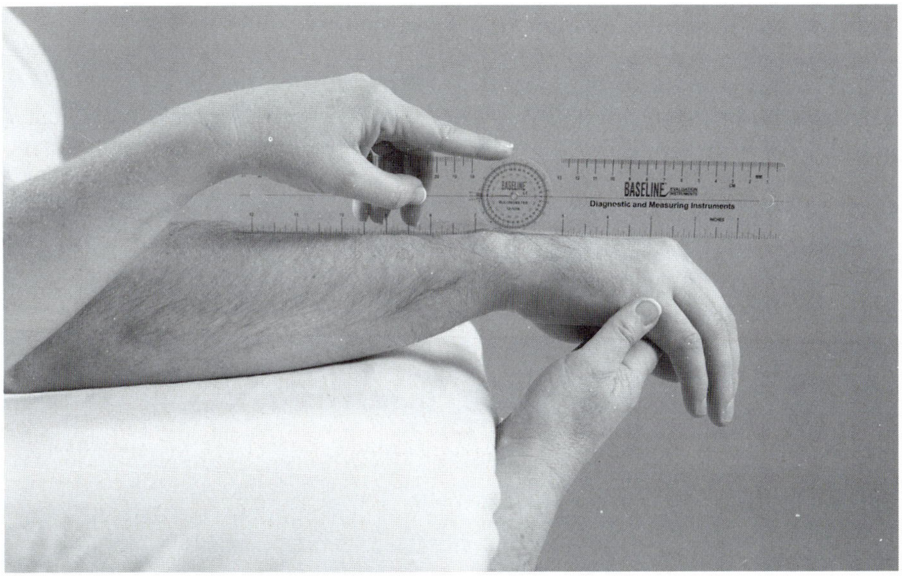

FIGURE 6.11 The alternative dorsal alignment of the goniometer at the beginning of wrist flexion ROM.

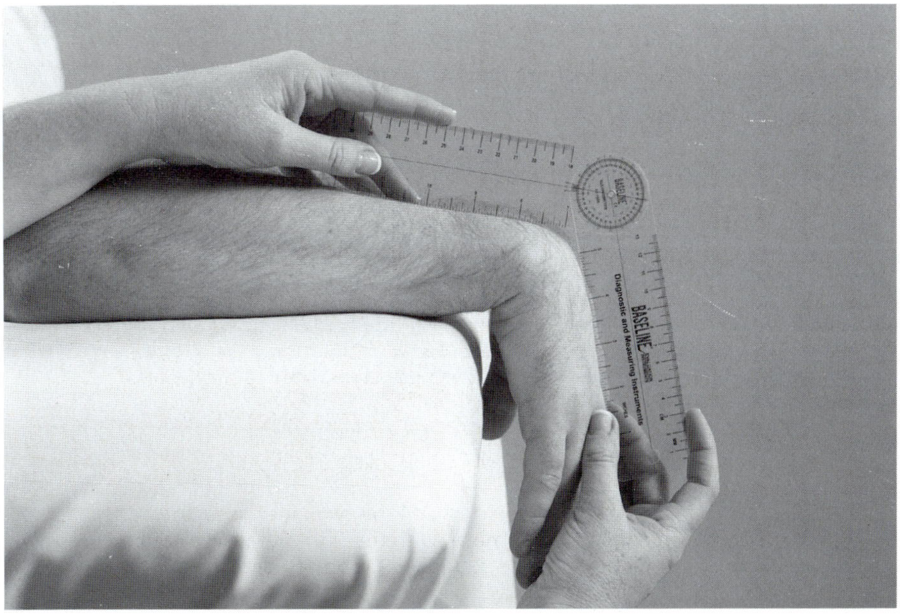

FIGURE 6.12 At the end of wrist flexion ROM using the alternative dorsal alignment, the arms of the goniometer are placed in firm contact with the dorsal surfaces of the forearm and third metacarpal. The axis of the goniometer will lie outside of the body in the region of the capitate.

WRIST EXTENSION

Motion occurs in the sagittal plane around a medial–lateral axis. Wrist extension is sometimes referred to as dorsal flexion. Normal ROM values for adults vary from about 60 to 75 degrees. See Research Findings and Tables 6.1 through 6.4 for normal ROM values by age and gender.

Testing Position

Position the individual sitting next to a supporting surface with the shoulder abducted to 90 degrees, the elbow flexed to 90 degrees, and the palm of the hand facing the ground. In this position the forearm will be midway between supination and pronation. Rest the forearm on the supporting surface, but leave the hand free to move. Avoid radial or ulnar deviation of the wrist and extension of the fingers. If the fingers are held in extension, tension in the flexor digitorum superficialis and profundus muscles will restrict the motion.

If the individual cannot be positioned in 90 degrees of shoulder abduction, a more adducted shoulder position may be used, but the forearm will be in some pronation when the palm is facing the floor.

Stabilization

Stabilize the radius and ulna to prevent supination or pronation of the forearm and motion of the elbow.

Testing Motion

Extend the wrist by pushing evenly across the palmar surface of the metacarpals, moving the hand in a dorsal direction toward the ceiling (Fig. 6.13). Maintain the wrist in 0 degrees of radial and ulnar deviation. The end of extension ROM occurs when resistance to further motion is felt and attempts to overcome the resistance cause the forearm to lift off the supporting surface.

Normal End-Feel

Usually the end-feel is firm because of tension in the palmar radiocarpal ligament, ulnocarpal ligament, and palmar joint capsule. Tension in the palmaris longus, flexor carpi radialis, and flexor carpi ulnaris muscles may also contribute to the firm end-feel. Sometimes the end-feel is hard because of contact between the radius and the carpal bones.

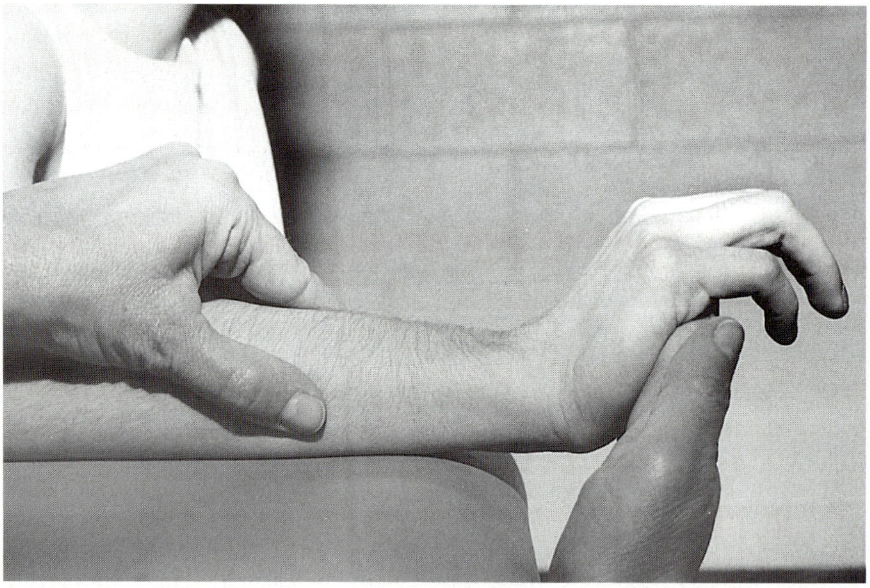

FIGURE 6.13 At the end of the wrist extension ROM, the examiner stabilizes the forearm with one hand and uses her other hand to hold the wrist in extension. The examiner is careful to distribute pressure equally across the metacarpals.

Goniometer Alignment

See Figures 6.14 and 6.15.

1. Center **fulcrum** on the lateral aspect of the wrist over the triquetrum.
2. Align **proximal arm** with the lateral midline of the ulna, using the olecranon and ulnar styloid process for reference.
3. Align **distal arm** with the lateral midline of the fifth metacarpal. Do not use the soft tissue of the hypothenar eminence for reference.

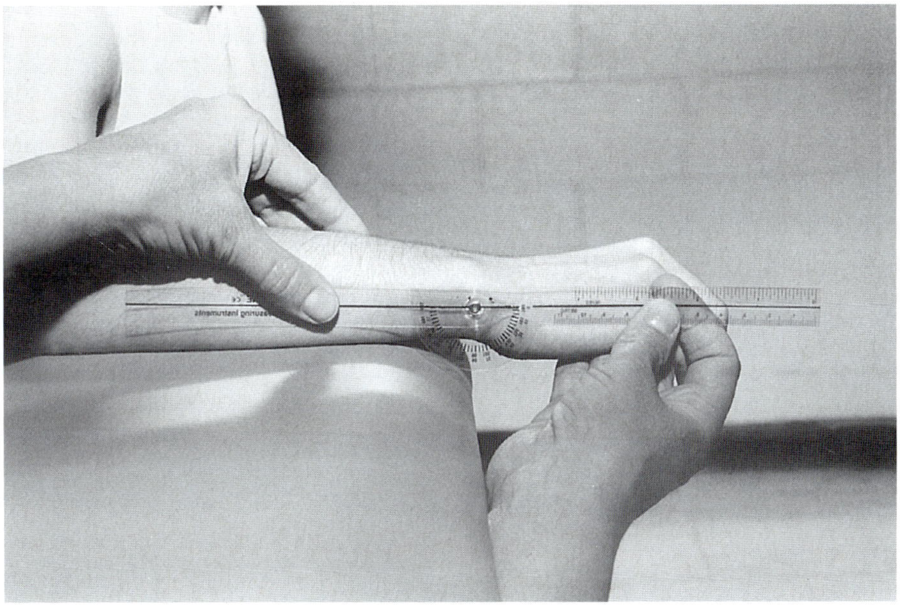

FIGURE 6.14 The alignment of the goniometer at the beginning of wrist extension ROM.

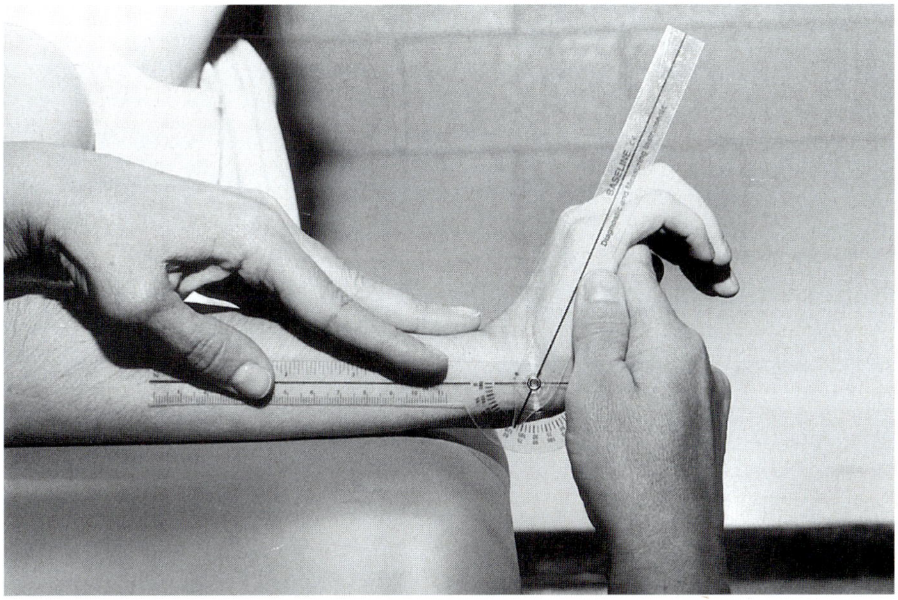

FIGURE 6.15 At the end of the ROM of wrist extension, the examiner aligns the distal goniometer arm with the fifth metacarpal while holding the wrist in extension. The examiner avoids exerting excessive pressure on the fifth metacarpal.

Alternative Goniometer Alignment: Palmar Aspect

See Figures 6.16 and 6.17.

This alternative goniometer alignment is recommended by several authors,[16,17] although edema and bony deformities in the forearm or hand may make accurate alignment over the palmar surfaces difficult. This alternative palmar technique requires a change in the testing position so that the forearm is supinated and the elbow extended. The palmar alignment technique will likely result in lower wrist extension ROM values than the lateral alignment technique (mean differences of 0–7 degrees reported[16]). This difference should be taken into account when comparing an individual's results with normative data using a lateral alignment. Most important, the same alignment techniques should be used in repetitive measurements to evaluate change in wrist extension ROM.

1. Center **fulcrum** palmar to the wrist joint near the capitate.
2. Align **proximal arm** with the palmar midline of the forearm.
3. Align **distal arm** with the palmar midline of the third metacarpal.

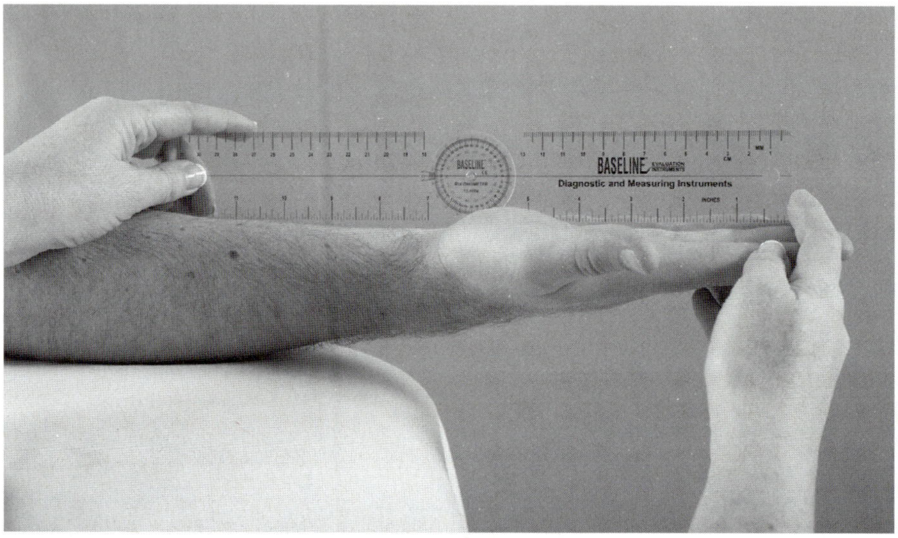

FIGURE 6.16 The alternative palmar alignment of the goniometer at the beginning of wrist extension ROM.

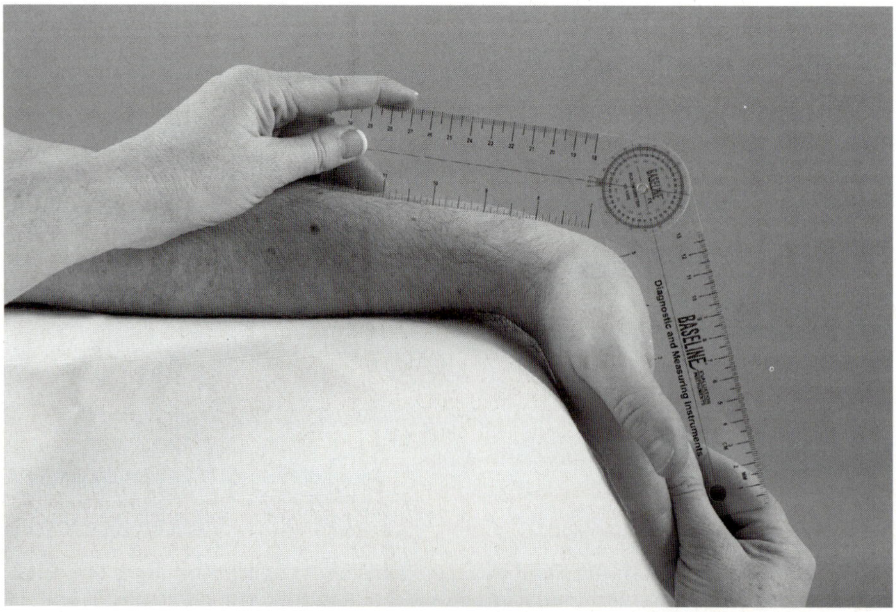

FIGURE 6.17 At the end of wrist extension ROM using the alternative palmar alignment, the arms of the goniometer are placed in firm contact with the palmar surfaces of the forearm and third metacarpal. The axis of the goniometer will lie outside of the body in the region of the capitate.

WRIST RADIAL DEVIATION

Motion occurs in the frontal plane around an anterior–posterior axis. Radial deviation is sometimes referred to as radial flexion or abduction. Normal ROM values for adults vary from about 20 to 25 degrees. See Research Findings and Tables 6.1 through 6.4 for normal ROM values by age and gender.

Testing Position

Position the individual sitting next to a supporting surface with the shoulder abducted to 90 degrees, the elbow flexed to 90 degrees, and the palm of the hand facing the ground. In this position the forearm will be midway between supination and pronation. Rest the forearm and hand on the supporting surface.

If the individual cannot be positioned in 90 degrees of shoulder abduction, a more adducted shoulder position may be used. However, the bony landmark of the lateral epicondyle of the humerus will not be accurate for aligning the proximal arm of the goniometer. In this case the proximal arm of the goniometer should be centered over the dorsal midline of the forearm.

Stabilization

Stabilize the radius and ulna to prevent pronation or supination of the forearm and elbow flexion beyond 90 degrees.

Testing Motion

Radially deviate the wrist by moving the hand toward the thumb (Fig. 6.18). Maintain the wrist in 0 degrees of flexion and extension, and avoid rotating the hand. The end of radial deviation ROM occurs when resistance to further motion is felt and attempts to overcome the resistance cause the elbow to flex.

Normal End-Feel

Usually the end-feel is hard because of contact between the radial styloid process and the scaphoid or trapezium, but it may be firm because of tension in the ulnar collateral ligament, the ulnocarpal ligament, and the ulnar portion of the joint capsule. Tension in the extensor carpi ulnaris and flexor carpi ulnaris muscles may also contribute to the firm end-feel.

Goniometer Alignment

See Figures 6.19 and 6.20.

1. Center **fulcrum** on the dorsal aspect of the wrist over the capitate.
2. Align **proximal arm** with the dorsal midline of the forearm. If the shoulder is in 90 degrees of abduction and the elbow is in 90 degrees of flexion, the lateral epicondyle of the humerus can be used for reference.
3. Align **distal arm** with the dorsal midline of the third metacarpal. Do not use the third phalanx for reference.

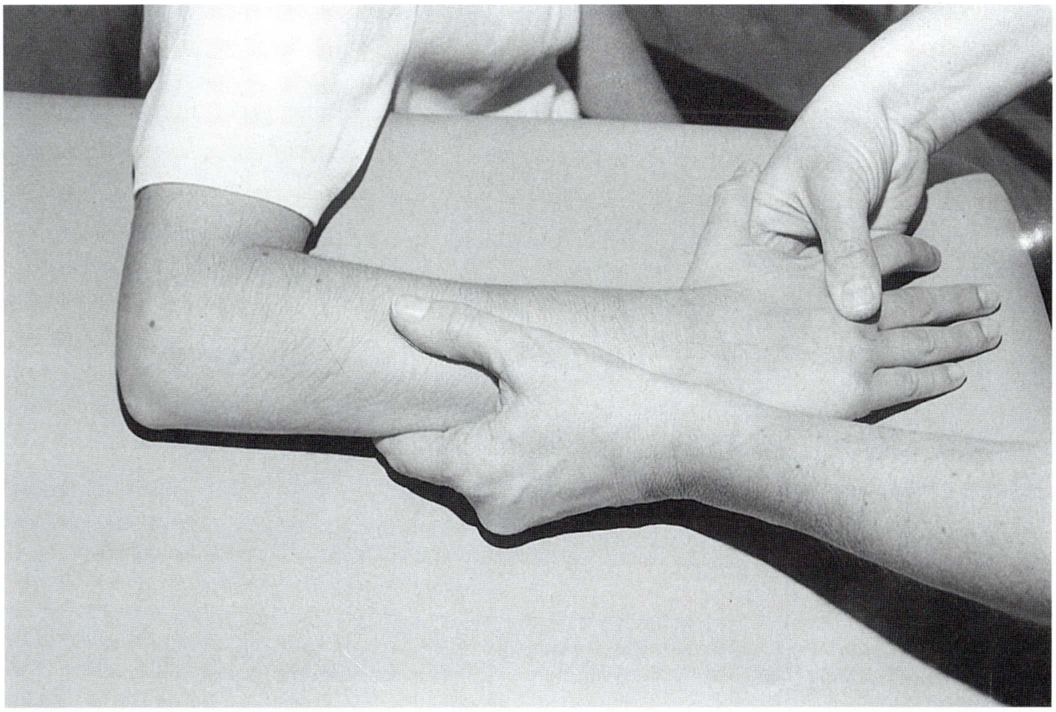

FIGURE 6.18 The examiner stabilizes the forearm to prevent flexion of the elbow beyond 90 degrees when the wrist is moved into radial deviation. The examiner avoids moving the wrist into either flexion or extension.

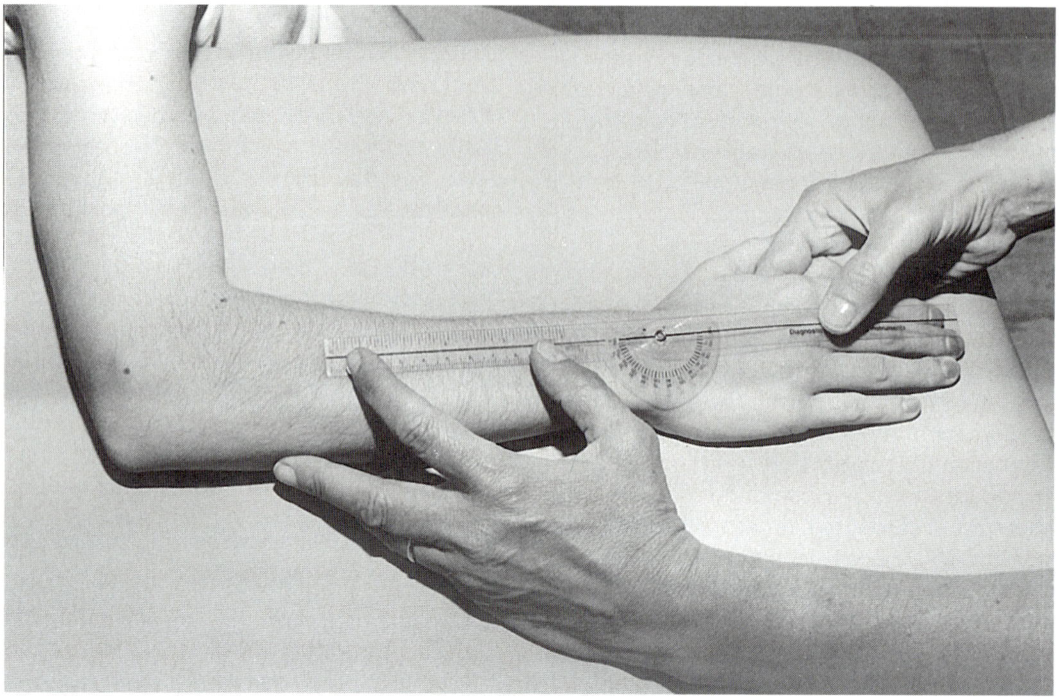

FIGURE 6.19 The alignment of the goniometer at the beginning of radial deviation ROM. The examining table can be used to support the hand.

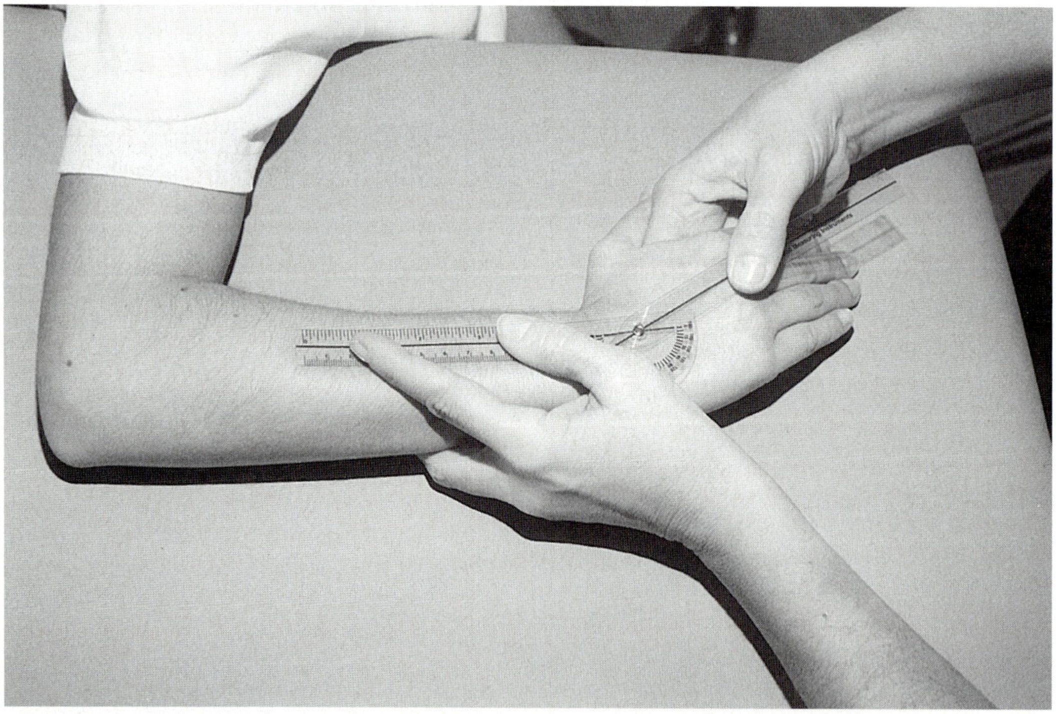

FIGURE 6.20 The alignment of the goniometer at the end of radial deviation ROM. The examiner must center the fulcrum over the dorsal surface of the capitate. If the fulcrum shifts to the ulnar side of the wrist, there will be an incorrect measurement of excessive radial deviation.

WRIST ULNAR DEVIATION

Motion occurs in the frontal plane around an anterior–posterior axis. Ulnar deviation is sometimes referred to as ulnar flexion or adduction. Normal ROM values for adults vary from about 30 to 40 degrees. See Research Findings and Tables 6.1 to 6.4 for normal ROM values by age and gender.

Testing Position

Position the individual sitting next to a supporting surface with the shoulder abducted to 90 degrees, the elbow flexed to 90 degrees, and the palm of the hand facing the ground. In this position the forearm will be midway between supination and pronation. Rest the forearm and hand on the supporting surface.

If the individual cannot be positioned in 90 degrees of shoulder abduction, a more adducted shoulder position may be used. However, the bony landmark of the lateral epicondyle of the humerus will not be accurate for aligning the proximal arm of the goniometer. In this case the proximal arm of the goniometer should be centered over the dorsal midline of the forearm.

Stabilization

Stabilize the radius and ulna to prevent pronation or supination of the forearm and less than 90 degrees of elbow flexion.

Testing Motion

Deviate the wrist in the ulnar direction by moving the hand toward the little finger (Fig. 6.21). Maintain the wrist in 0 degrees of flexion and extension, and avoid rotating the hand. The end of ulnar deviation ROM occurs when resistance to further motion is felt and attempts to overcome the resistance cause the elbow to extend.

Normal End-Feel

The end-feel is firm because of tension in the radial collateral ligament and the radial portion of the joint capsule. Tension in the extensor pollicis brevis and abductor pollicis longus muscles may contribute to the firm end-feel.

Goniometer Alignment

See Figures 6.22 and 6.23.

1. Center **fulcrum** on the dorsal aspect of the wrist over the capitate.
2. Align **proximal arm** with the dorsal midline of the forearm. If the shoulder is in 90 degrees of abduction and the elbow is in 90 degrees of flexion, the lateral epicondyle of the humerus can be used for reference.
3. Align **distal arm** with the dorsal midline of the third metacarpal. Do not use the third phalanx for reference.

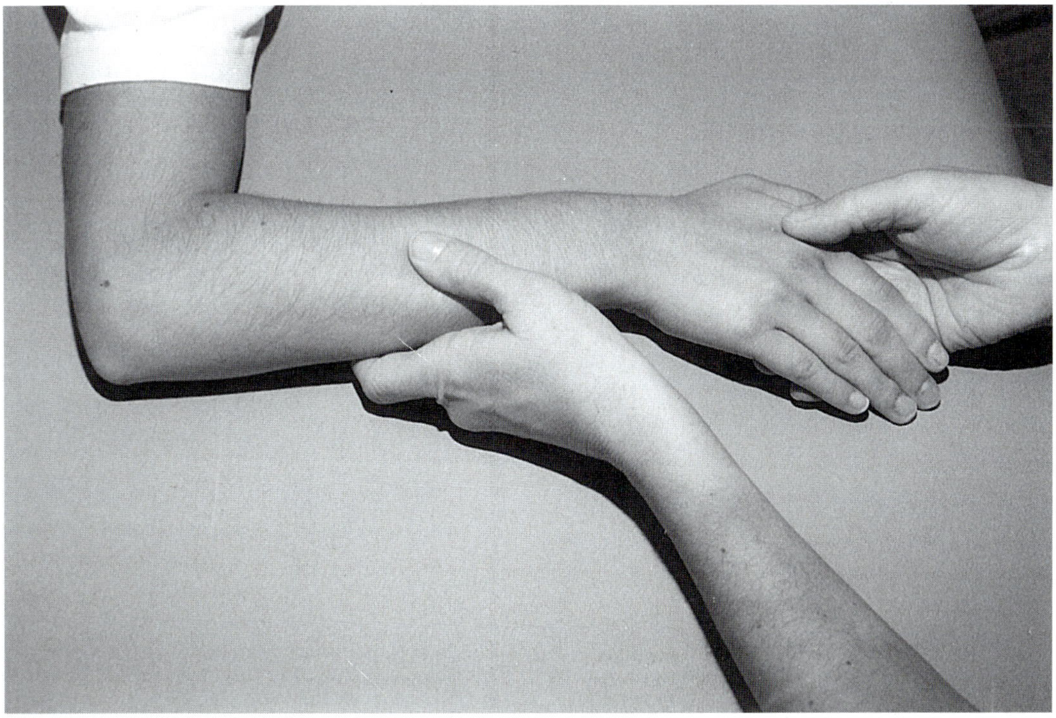

FIGURE 6.21 The examiner uses one hand to stabilize the forearm and maintain the elbow in 90 degrees of flexion. The examiner's other hand moves the wrist into ulnar deviation, being careful not to flex or extend the wrist.

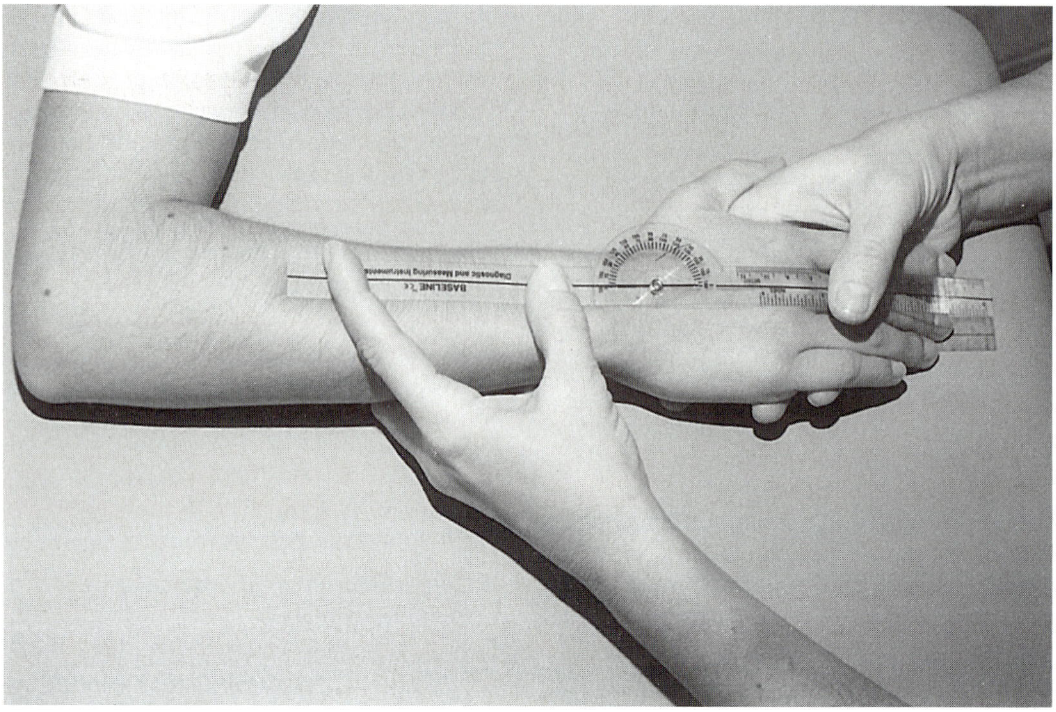

FIGURE 6.22 The alignment of the goniometer at the beginning of ulnar deviation ROM. Sometimes if a half-circle goniometer is used, the proximal and distal arms of the goniometer will have to be reversed so that the pointer remains on the body of the goniometer at the end of the ROM.

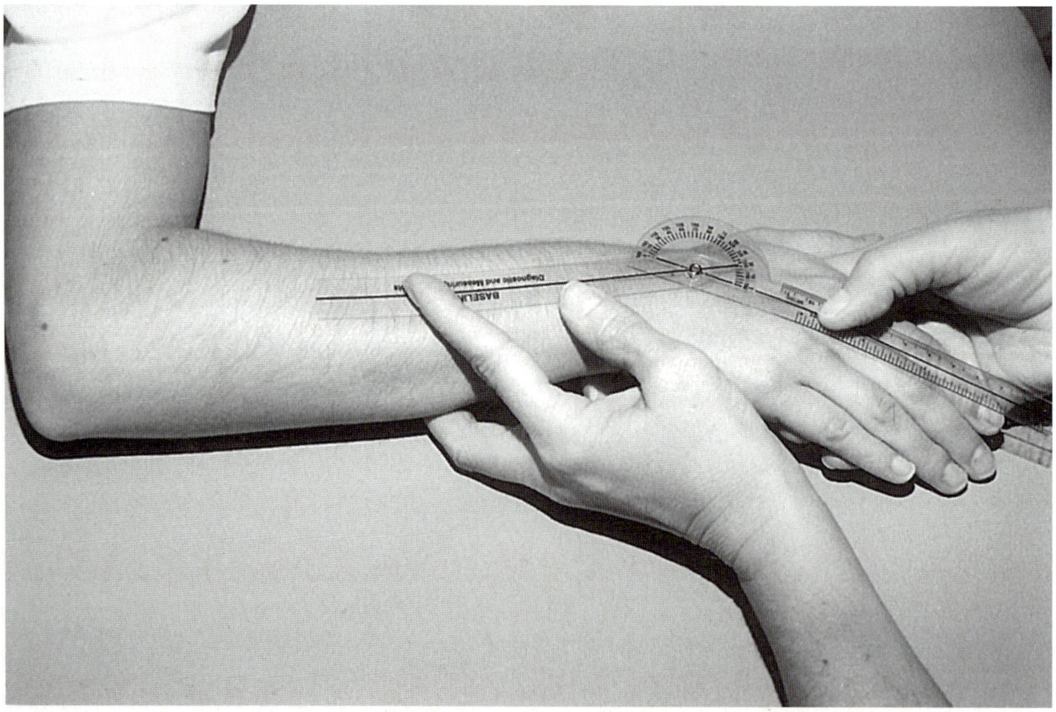

FIGURE 6.23 The alignment of the goniometer at the end of the ulnar deviation ROM. The examiner must center the fulcrum over the dorsal surface of the capitate. If the fulcrum shifts to the radial side of the wrist, there will be an incorrect measurement of excessive ulnar deviation.

MUSCLE LENGTH TESTING PROCEDURES: Wrist

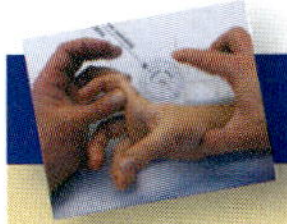

Landmarks for Testing Procedures

Refer to Figures 6.4 through 6.7 for landmarks for testing procedures of the wrist.

WRIST FLEXORS

A number of muscles perform wrist flexion and will limit wrist extension if they are short in length. The flexor digitorum profundus and the flexor digitorum superficialis cross the elbow, wrist, metacarpophalangeal (MCP), proximal interphalangeal (PIP), and distal interphalangeal (DIP) joints.[1] The **flexor digitorum profundus** originates proximally from the upper three-fourths of the ulna, the coronoid process of the ulna, and the interosseus membrane (Fig. 6.24). This muscle inserts distally on to the palmar surface of the bases of the distal phalanges of the fingers. The humeroulnar head of the **flexor digitorum superficialis** muscle originates proximally from the medial epicondyle of the humerus, the ulnar collateral ligament, and the coronoid process of the ulna (Fig. 6.25). The radial head of the flexor digitorum superficialis muscle originates proximally from the anterior surface of the radius. This muscle inserts distally via two slips into the sides of the bases of the middle phalanges of the fingers. When the flexor digitorum profundus and superficialis contract, they flex the MCP and IP joints of the fingers and flex the wrist. These muscles are passively lengthened by placing the elbow, wrist, MCP, and IP joints in extension. If the flexor digitorum profundus and flexor digitorum superficialis muscles are short, they will limit wrist extension when the elbow, MCP, PIP, and DIP joints are positioned in extension.

The flexor carpi radialis, flexor carpi ulnaris, and palmaris longus also flex the wrist, but do not cross the MCP and IP joints of the fingers.[1] The **flexor carpi radialis** originates proximally from the medial epicondyle of the humerus, and inserts distally into the base of the second and third metacarpals. The **flexor carpi ulnaris** originates proximally from the medial epicondyle of the humerus and from the proximal two-thirds of the ulna. It inserts distally into the pisiform, and eventually into the hamate and base of the fifth metacarpal via the pisohamate and pisometacarpal ligaments, respectively. The **palmaris longus** muscle originates proximally from the medial epicondyle of the humerus, and distally inserts into the palmar aponeurosis. The length of the flexor carpi radialis, carpi radialis ulnaris, and palmaris longus is automatically tested along with other joint structures during the measurement of wrist extension ROM (in which the elbow is flexed and the fingers are relaxed in flexion); therefore, we do not include a separate test of the length of these muscles.

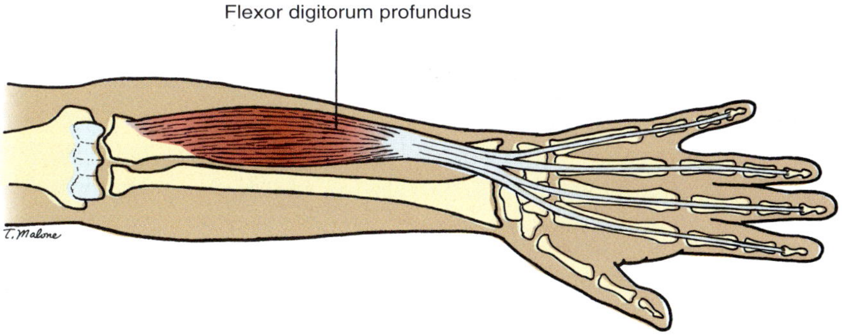

FIGURE 6.24 An anterior view of the right forearm showing the attachments of the flexor digitorum profundus muscle.

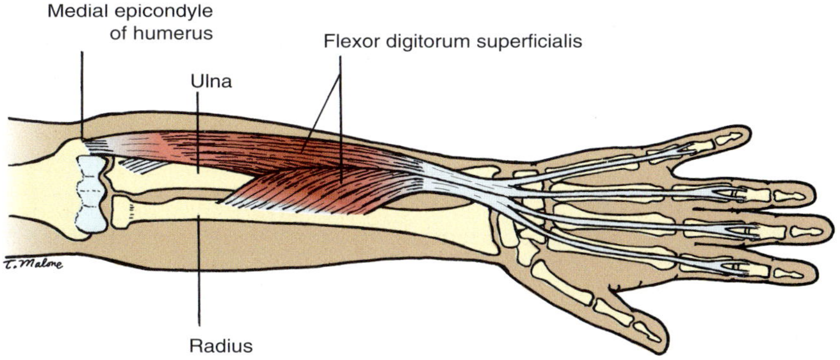

FIGURE 6.25 An anterior view of the right forearm and hand showing the attachments of the flexor digitorum superficialis muscle.

THE FLEXOR DIGITORUM PROFUNDUS AND FLEXOR DIGITORUM SUPERFICIALIS MUSCLE LENGTH TEST

This test is used to evaluate the length of the flexor digitorum profundus and flexor digitorum superficialis by carefully positioning the elbow in extension and the MCP, PIP, and DIP joints in extension, and then extending the wrist.

Testing Position

Position the individual sitting next to a supporting surface with the upper extremity resting on the surface. Place the elbow, MCP, PIP, and DIP joints in extension (Fig. 6.26). Pronate the forearm and place the wrist in neutral.

Stabilization

Stabilize the forearm to prevent elbow flexion.

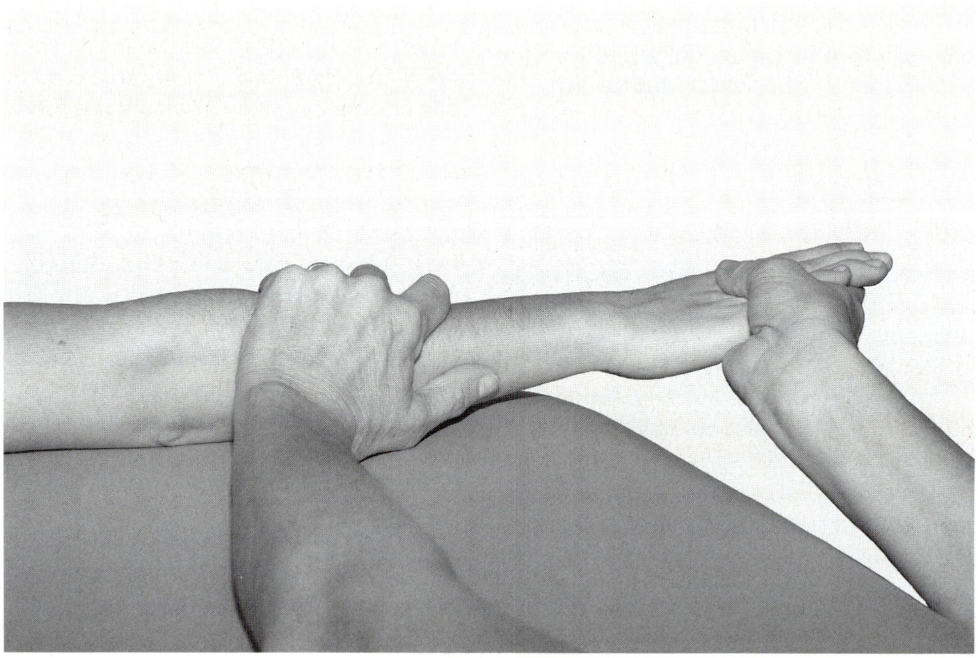

FIGURE 6.26 The starting position for testing the length of the flexor digitorum profundus and flexor digitorum superficialis muscles.

Testing Motion

Hold the MCP, PIP, and DIP joints in extension while extending the wrist (Figs. 6.27 and 6.28). The end of the testing motion occurs when resistance is felt and additional wrist extension causes the fingers or elbow to flex.

End-Feel

The end-feel is firm because of tension in the flexor digitorum profundus and flexor digitorum superficialis muscles.

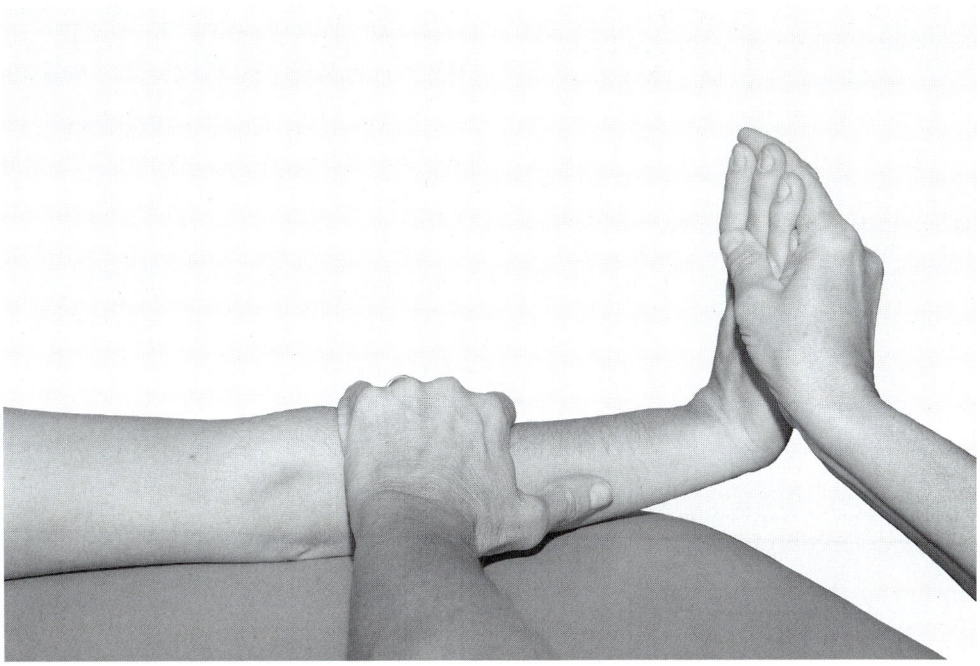

FIGURE 6.27 The end of the testing motion for the length of the flexor digitorum profundus and flexor digitorum superficialis muscles. The examiner uses one hand to stabilize the forearm, while the other hand holds the fingers in extension and moves the wrist into extension. The examiner has moved her right thumb from the dorsal surface of the fingers to allow a clearer photograph, but keeping the thumb placed on the dorsal surface would help to prevent the fingers from flexing at the PIP joints.

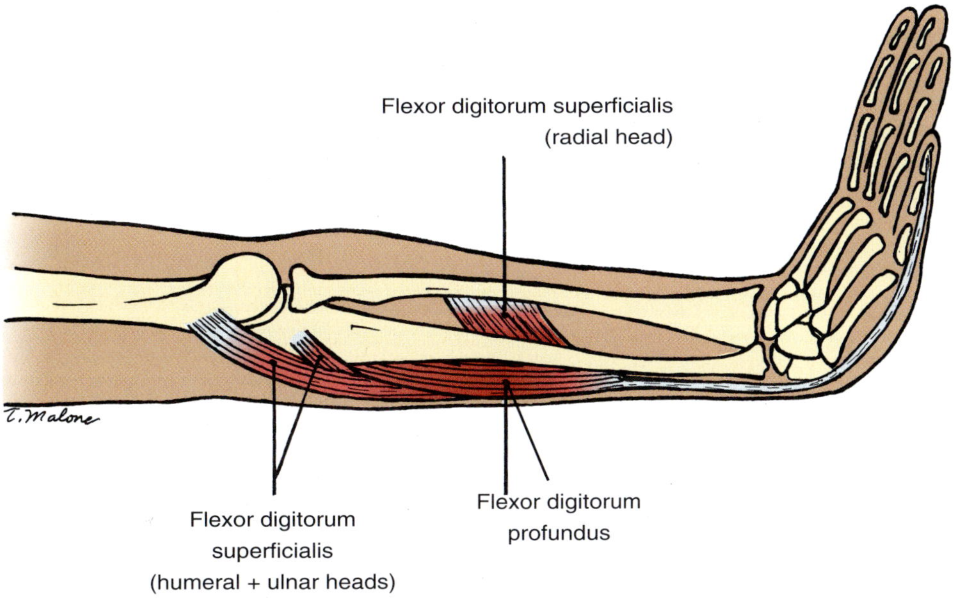

FIGURE 6.28 A lateral view of the right forearm and hand showing the flexor digitorum profundus and flexor digitorum superficialis being stretched over the elbow, wrist, MCP, PIP, and DIP joints.

Goniometer Alignment

See Figure 6.29.

1. Center **fulcrum** on the lateral aspect of the wrist over the triquetrum.
2. Align **proximal arm** with the lateral midline of the ulna, using the olecranon and ulnar styloid process for reference.
3. Align **distal arm** with the lateral midline of the fifth metacarpal. Do not use the soft tissue of the hypothenar eminence for reference.

Interpretation

If the flexor digitorum profundus and flexor digitorum superficialis are short in length, they will limit wrist extension when the elbow, MCP, and IP joints are held in extension. We are unaware of any published normative values for this test, but suggest that normally wrist extension will be about 10 to 15 degrees less than wrist extension ROM with the elbow, MCP, and IP joints in a relaxed flexed position.

If passive wrist extension is limited regardless of the position of the MCP, PIP, and DIP joints, the limitation is due to abnormalities of wrist joint surfaces or shortening of the palmar joint capsule, palmar radiocarpal ligament, ulnocarpal ligament, flexor carpi radialis, flexor carpi ulnaris, or palmaris longus muscles.

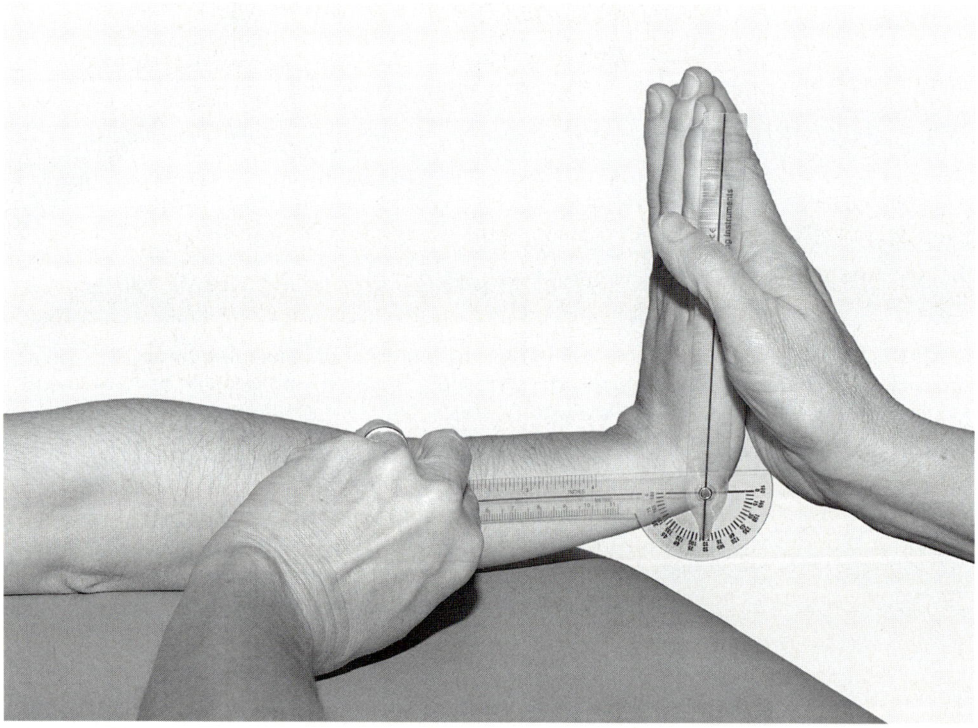

FIGURE 6.29 The alignment of the goniometer at the end of testing the length of the flexor digitorum profundus and flexor digitorum superficialis muscles.

WRIST EXTENSORS

A number of muscles assist in performing wrist extension and will limit wrist flexion if they are short in length. The extensor digitorum, extensor indicis, and extensor digiti minimi muscles all cross the elbow; wrist; and MCP, PIP, and DIP joints.[1] The **extensor digitorum** originates proximally from the lateral epicondyle of the humerus, and inserts distally on to the middle and distal phalanges of the fingers via the extensor hood (Figs. 6.30 and 6.33). The **extensor indicis** originates proximally from the posterior surface of the ulna and the interosseous membrane. This muscle inserts distally on to the extensor hood of the index finger. The **extensor digiti minimi** also originates proximally from the lateral epicondyle of the humerus, but inserts distally on to the extensor hood of the little finger. If the extensor digitorum, extensor indicis, and extensor digiti minimi muscles are short, they will limit wrist flexion when the elbow is positioned in extension and the MCP, PIP, and DIP joints are positioned in full flexion.

The extensor carpi radialis longus and brevis and extensor carpi ulnaris are considered prime movers for performing wrist extension, but do not cross the MCP, PIP, and DIP joints of the fingers. The extensor **carpi radialis longus** originates proximally from the lateral supracondylar ridge of the humerus and inserts distally on to the base of the second metacarpal. The extensor **carpi radialis brevis** originates proximally from the lateral condyle of the humerus and radial collateral ligament of the elbow. It inserts distally on to the base of the third metacarpal. The **extensor carpi ulnaris** originates proximally from the lateral epicondyle of the humerus and inserts distally on to the base of the fifth metacarpal. The length of these three muscles is automatically tested along with other joint structures during the measurement of wrist flexion ROM (in which the elbow is flexed and the fingers are relaxed in extension); therefore, we do not include a separate test of the length of these three muscles.

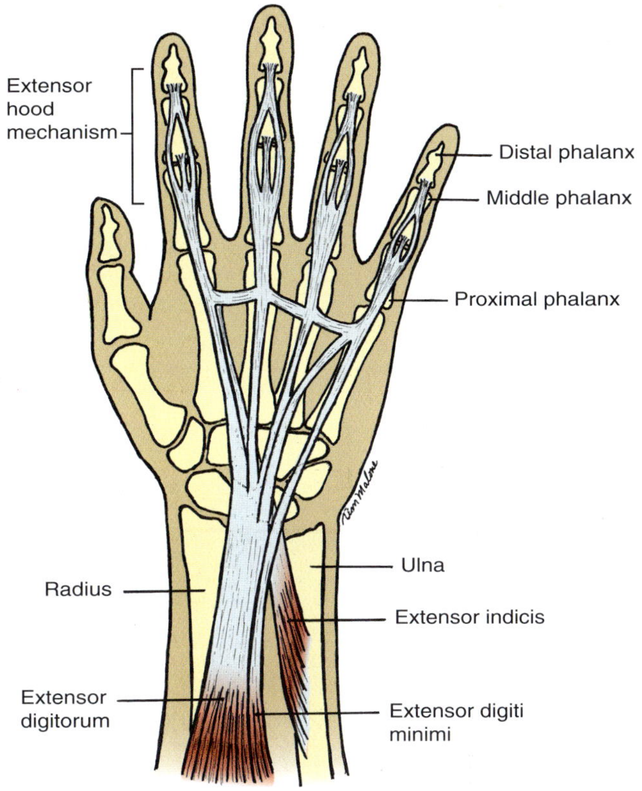

FIGURE 6.30 A posterior view of the right forearm and hand showing the distal attachments of the extensor digitorum, extensor indicis, and extensor digiti minimi muscles.

THE EXTENSOR DIGITORUM, EXTENSOR INDICIS, AND EXTENSOR DIGITI MINIMI MUSCLE LENGTH TEST

This test is used to evaluate the length of the extensor digitorum, extensor indicis, and extensor digiti minimi by carefully positioning the elbow in extension and the MCP, PIP, and DIP joints in flexion, and then flexing the wrist.

Testing Position

Position the individual sitting next to a supporting surface. The upper arm and the forearm should rest on the supporting surface, but the hand should be free to move into flexion. Place the elbow in full extension and the MCP, PIP, and DIP joints in full flexion (Fig. 6.31). Place the forearm in pronation and the wrist in neutral.

Stabilization

Stabilize the forearm to prevent elbow flexion.

Testing Motion

Hold the MCP, PIP, and DIP joints in full flexion while flexing the wrist (Figs. 6.32 and 6.33). The end of the testing motion occurs when resistance is felt and additional wrist flexion causes the fingers to extend or the elbow to flex.

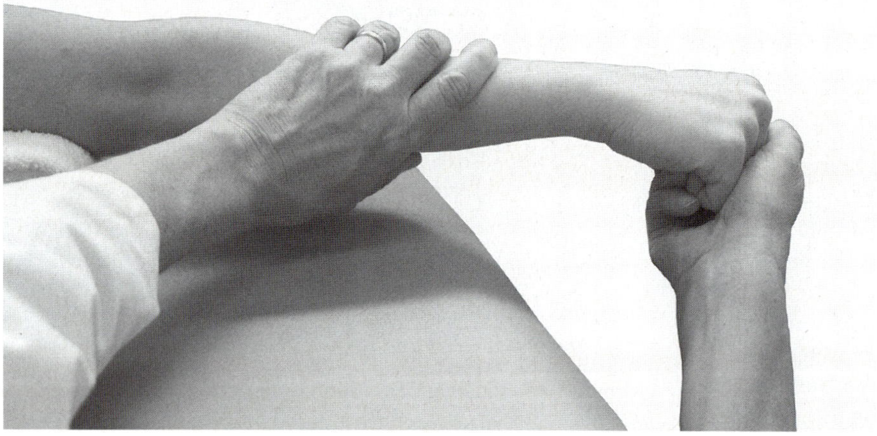

FIGURE 6.31 The starting position for testing the length of the extensor digitorum, extensor indicis, and extensor digiti minimi muscles. The hand is positioned off the end of the examining table to allow room for finger and wrist flexion.

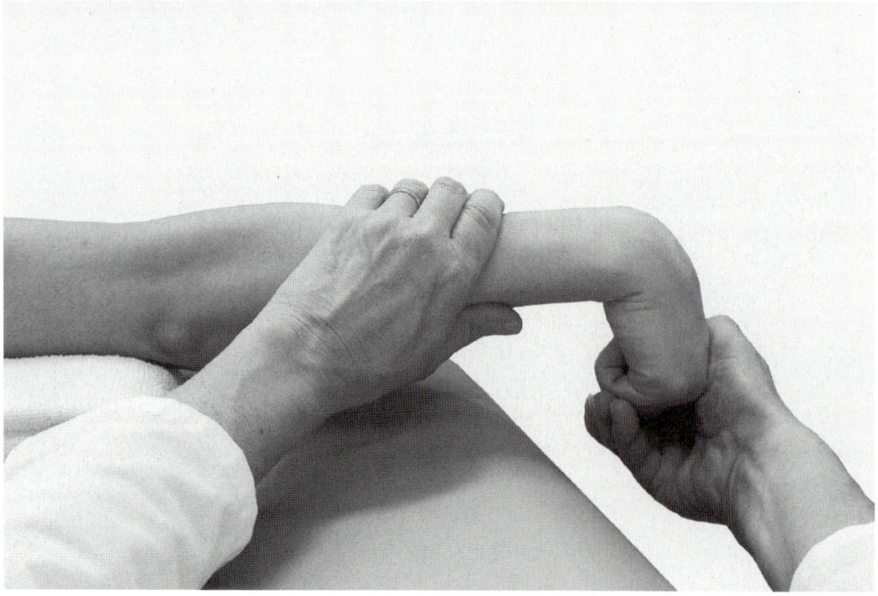

FIGURE 6.32 The end of the testing motion for the length of the extensor digitorum, extensor indicis, and extensor digiti minimi muscles. One of the examiner's hands stabilizes the forearm, while the other hand holds the fingers in full flexion and moves the wrist into flexion.

Normal End-Feel

The end-feel is firm because of tension in the extensor digitorum, extensor indicis, and extensor digiti minimi muscles.

Goniometer Alignment

See Figure 6.34.

1. Center **fulcrum** on the lateral aspect of the wrist over the triquetrum.
2. Align **proximal arm** with the lateral midline of the ulna, using the olecranon and ulnar styloid process for reference.
3. Align **distal arm** with the lateral midline of the fifth metacarpal. Do not use the soft tissue of the hypothenar eminence for reference.

Interpretation

If the extensor digitorum, extensor indicis, and extensor digiti minimi muscles are short, they will limit wrist flexion when the elbow is positioned in extension and the MCP, PIP, and DIP joints of the fingers are positioned in full flexion. We are unaware of any published normative values for this test, but suggest that normally wrist flexion will be about 10 to 15 degrees less than wrist flexion ROM with the elbow, MCP, PIP, and DIP joints in a relaxed extended position.

If wrist flexion is limited regardless of the position of the MCP, PIP, and DIP joints, the limitation is due to abnormalities of joint surfaces of the wrist or shortening of the dorsal joint capsule, dorsal radiocarpal ligament, extensor carpi radialis longus, extensor carpi radialis brevis, or extensor carpi ulnaris muscles.

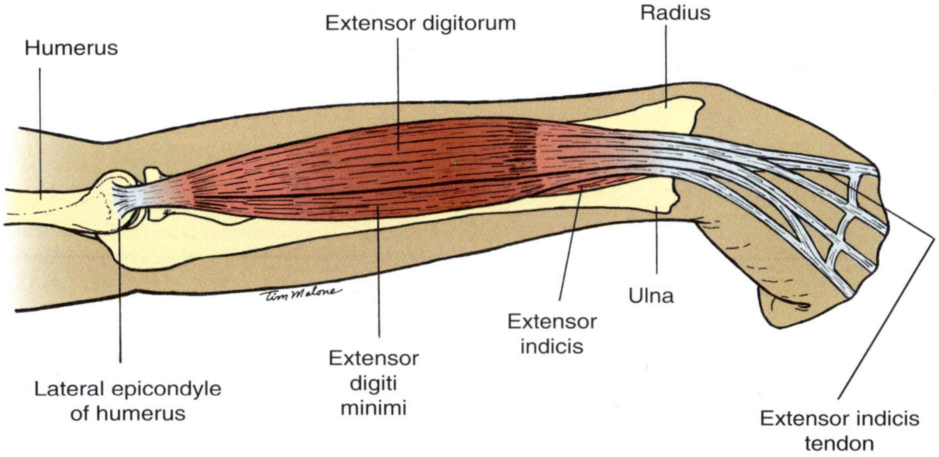

FIGURE 6.33 A posterior view of the right forearm and hand showing the extensor digitorum, extensor indicis, and extensor digiti minimi muscles stretched over the elbow, wrist, MCP, PIP, and DIP joints.

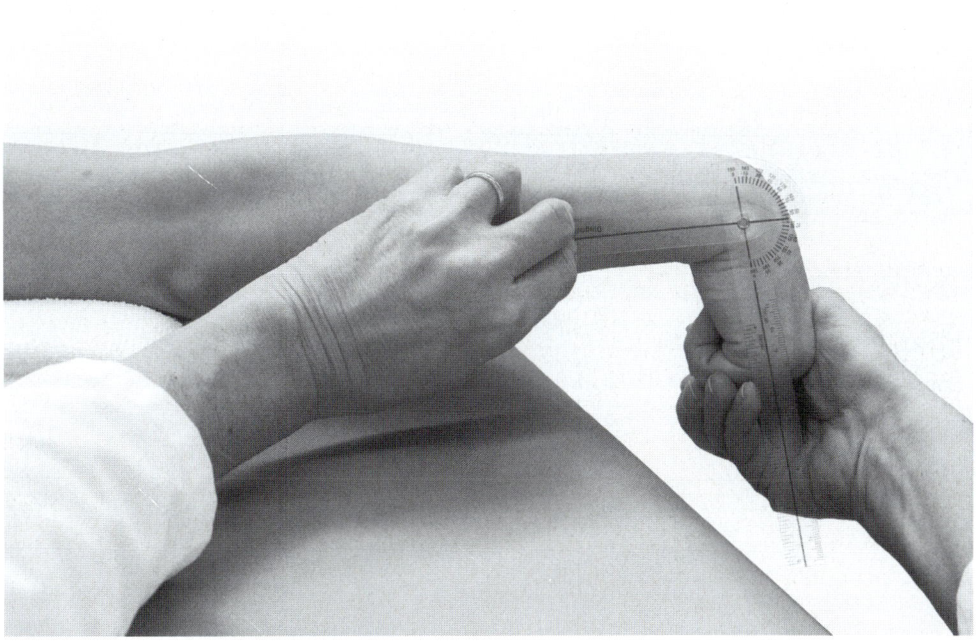

FIGURE 6.34 The alignment of the goniometer at the end of testing the length of the extensor digitorum, extensor indicis, and extensor digiti minimi muscles.

Research Findings

Effects of Age, Gender, and Other Factors

Table 6.1 provides normal wrist ROM values for healthy adults from five sources.[18–23] In general, these values range from 70 to 80 degrees for flexion, 60 to 75 degrees for extension, 20 to 25 degrees for radial deviation, and 30 to 40 degrees for ulnar deviation. Other studies that provide wrist ROM data for adults between the ages of 18 to 60 years include Solgaard and colleagues,[24] Solveborn and Olerud,[25] Stubbs, Fernandez, and Glenn,[26] Gunal et al,[27] Macedo and Magee,[28] and Klum and associates.[29]

Age

Most studies support a small, gradual decrease in the amount of wrist motion with increasing age. Age-related ROM changes appear to be most marked in young children and seniors, whereas changes in young and middle-aged adults seem minimal.

Normative wrist ROM values for newborns and children are provided in Table 6.2. Although caution must be used in drawing conclusions from comparisons between values obtained by different researchers, the mean flexion and extension values for infants from Wanatabe and coworkers[30] are larger than values for males aged 18 months to 19 years reported by Boone and Azen.[21,31] Within one study by Boone and Azen, wrist flexion and ulnar and radial deviation motions for the youngest age-group (18 months to 5 years) were significantly larger than the values for other age-groups (see Tables 6.2 and 6.3). Wrist extension values were significantly larger for males aged 6 to 12 years than for those in the other age-groups.

Table 6.3 provides wrist ROM values in men aged 18 to 54 years. The effect of age on wrist motion among this age range of adults appears to be small. Boone and Azen[21,31] found a statistically significant difference in wrist flexion and extension ROM between males younger than or equal to 19 years of age and those who were older. However, the effects of age on wrist flexion and extension in adults aged 20 to 54 years appear to be very slight with changes of about

TABLE 6.1 Normal Wrist ROM Values for Adults in Degrees From Selected Sources

	AAOS[18,19]	AMA[2]	Boone and Azen[21]	Greene and Wolf[22]	Ryu et al[23]
			20–54 yr *n* = 56 Males	18–55 yr *n* = 20 Males and Females	*n* = 40 Males and Females
Motion			***Mean (SD)***	***Mean***	***Mean***
Flexion	80	60	74.8 (6.6)	73.3	79.1
Extension	70	60	74.0 (6.6)	64.9	59.3
Radial deviation	20	20	21.1 (4.0)	25.4	21.1
Ulnar deviation	30	30	35.3 (3.8)	39.2	37.7

AAOS = Academy of Orthopaedic Surgeons; AMA = American Medical Association; SD = Standard deviation.

TABLE 6.2 Effects of Age on Wrist ROM in Newborns, Children, and Adolescents: Normal Values in Degrees

	Wanatabe et al[30]	Boone and Azen[21,31]		
	2 wk–2 yr *n* = 45 Males and Females	18 mo–5 yr *n* = 19 Males	6–12 yr *n* = 17 Males	13–19 yr *n* = 17 Males
Motion	***Range of Means***	***Mean (SD)***	***Mean (SD)***	***Mean (SD)***
Flexion	88–96	82.2 (3.8)	76.3 (5.6)	75.4 (4.5)
Extension	82–89	76.1 (4.9)	78.4 (5.9)	72.9 (6.4)
Radial deviation		24.2 (3.7)	21.3 (4.1)	19.7 (3.0)
Ulnar deviation		38.7 (3.6)	35.4 (2.4)	35.7 (4.2)

SD = Standard deviation.

TABLE 6.3 Effects of Age on Wrist ROM in Adult Males 18 to 54 Years Old: Normal Values in Degrees

	Boone and Azen[21,31]			Stubbs et al[26]		
	20–29 yr *n* = 19	30–39 yr *n* = 18	40–54 yr *n* = 19	25–34 yr *n* = 15	35–44 yr *n* = 20	45–54 yr *n* = 20
Motion	*Mean (SD)*	*Mean (SD)*	*Mean (SD)*	*Mean (SD)*	*Mean (SD)*	*Mean (SD)*
Flexion	76.8 (5.5)	74.9 (4.0)	72.8 (8.9)	70.6 (9.3)	73.5 (10.4)	68.9 (8.4)
Extension	77.5 (5.1)	72.8 (6.9)	71.6 (6.3)	78.3 (11.8)	76.4 (10.4)	76.7 (11.7)
Radial deviation	21.4 (3.6)	20.3 (3.1)	21.6 (5.1)	23.8 (9.5)	22.5 (7.9)	18.9 (7.9)
Ulnar deviation	35.1 (3.8)	36.1 (2.9)	34.7 (4.5)	51.1 (9.0)	49.9 (7.0)	44.1 (4.3)

SD = Standard deviation.

4 to 6 degrees. Decreases in ulnar and radial deviation were less than 1 degree. Stubbs and associates[26] placed 55 male subjects between the ages of 25 and 54 years into three age-groups, and found no significant difference among the age-groups for wrist flexion, extension, and radial deviation ROM. However, a significant difference in ulnar deviation (7 degrees) was found between the oldest and the youngest age-groups, with the oldest group having less motion.

Wrist ROM values in males 60 years of age and older are presented in Table 6.4. Flexion and extension ROM in these older adults, as presented by Walker and associates,[32] Chaparro and colleagues,[33] and Kalscheur and coworkers[34] are less than the values for the younger adult age-groups presented in Table 6.3. Chaparro and colleagues[33] further subdivided the 62 male subjects in their study into four age-groups: 60 to 69 years of age, 70 to 79 years of age, 80 to 89 years of age, and 90 years of age and older. They found a trend of decreasing ROM with increasing age, with the oldest group having significantly lower wrist flexion and ulnar deviation values than the two youngest groups.

TABLE 6.4 Effects of Age on Wrist ROM in Men Older Than 60 Years: Normal Values in Degrees

	Walker et al[32]	Chaparro et al[33]	Kalscheur et al[34]
	60–85 yr *n* = 30	60–90+ yr *n* = 62	66–86 yr *n* = 25
Motion	*Mean (SD)*	*Mean (SD)*	*Mean (SD)*
Flexion	62.0 (12.0)	50.8 (13.8)	64.9 (8.7)
Extension	61.0 (6.0)	44.0 (9.9)	58.2 (10.9)
Radial deviation	20.0 (6.0)		
Ulnar deviation	28.0 (7.0)	35.0 (9.5)	

SD = Standard deviation.

Other studies aside from those cited in Tables 6.1 through 6.4 offer additional information on the effects of age on wrist motion and generally support a decrease in wrist motion with increasing age. Hewitt,[35] in a study of 112 females between 11 and 45 years of age, found slight differences in the average amount of active motion in various age-groups, but no statistical analyses were performed. Allander and coworkers,[36] in a study of 309 Icelandic females, 208 Swedish females, and 203 Swedish males ranging in age from 33 to 70 years, found that with increasing age there was a decrease in flexion and extension ROM at both wrists. Males lost an average of 2.2 degrees of motion every 5 years. Bell and Hoshizaki[37] studied 124 females and 66 males ranging in age from 18 to 88 years. A significant negative correlation was noted between ROM and age for wrist flexion–extension and radial–ulnar deviation in females and for wrist flexion–extension in males. As age increased, wrist motions generally decreased. There was a significant difference among the five age-groups of females for all wrist motions, although the difference was not significant for males. Kalscheur and associates,[38] in a study of 61 women between the ages of 63 and 85 years, found a significant inverse linear relationship between age and right wrist flexion and extension, with ROM decreasing an average of 0.4 to 0.5 degrees per year in these older women. The relationships between age and left wrist motions were not statistically significant. Macedo and Magee[28] included 90 Caucasian women between the ages of 18 and 59 years in a study that examined the effect of age on passive ROM at the wrist as well as the ankle, knee, hip, shoulder, and elbow. Although many joints showed a decrease in ROM with increasing age, age effects on ROM at the wrist joint were not statistically significant. A large study by Klum and associates[29] of 387 men and 365 women between 18 and 65 years reported age to be inversely correlated (Pearson correlation coefficient $r = -0.4$) with wrist ROM in both sexes, with the greatest wrist motion in the young adult group ranging from 18 and 29 years.

Gender

The following six studies offer evidence of gender effects on the wrist joint, with most supporting the belief that women have slightly more wrist ROM than men. Cobe,[39] in a study of 100 college men and 15 women ranging in age from 20 to 30 years, found that women had a greater active ROM in all motions at the wrist than men. Allander and coworkers[36] compared wrist flexion and extension ROM in 203 Swedish men and 208 Swedish women aged 45 to older than 70 years and noted that women had significantly greater motion than men. Klum and coworkers[29] studied 387 German men and 363 German women between the ages of 18 and 65 years for wrist and hand function taking into account age, gender, body mass index (BMI), left versus right side, and whether their work involved low or high manual strain. They found that women had significantly greater wrist flexion–extension and ulnar–radial ROM than men, with most mean differences ranging from about 1 to 3 degrees for flexion–extension and from 1 to 2 degrees for ulnar–radial deviation in low manual strain workers.

Among older men and women aged 60 to 84 years, Walker and associates[32] found that the 30 women included in the study had more active wrist extension and flexion than the 30 men; however, the men had more ulnar and radial deviation than the women. These differences were statistically significant for wrist extension (4 degrees) and ulnar deviation (5 degrees). Chaparro and colleagues[33] examined wrist flexion, extension, and ulnar deviation ROM in 62 men and 85 women aged 60 to older than 90 years. Women had significantly greater wrist extension (6.4 degrees) and ulnar deviation (3.0 degrees) than men. Kalscheur and coworkers[34] found that women had more wrist flexion and extension ROM than men in a study of 61 women and 25 men between the ages of 63 and 86 years. These differences ranged from 1.7 to 5.3 degrees and were statistically significant for right wrist flexion (5.0 degrees) and left wrist extension (5.3 degrees).

Body Mass Index

Although a number of investigators have examined the effect of body mass on ROM at various joints, we are aware of only one study that focused on the wrist. Klum and coworkers,[29] in a study of 750 German subjects between the ages of 18 and 65 years, found a reduction in wrist extension ROM in those with high BMI. No mention was made of the effects of BMI on wrist flexion or deviations. Measurements were taken with a full-circle plastic goniometer on the dorsal surface of the wrist and third metacarpal

Right Versus Left Sides

Study results vary as to whether there is a difference between left and right wrist ROM. Some studies have found no differences based on side or handedness, whereas others have reported slightly greater range in the left or nondominant wrist. Generally, it appears that a patient's uninjured contralateral wrist can be used for normative comparisons in the clinical setting, perhaps taking into account that the left wrist may have slightly greater ROM than the right wrist, especially in individuals who perform heavy manual labor.

Among studies that reported no effect of handedness, Boone and Azen[21] found no significant difference in wrist flexion, extension, and radial and ulnar deviation between sides in 109 normal males between 18 months and 54 years of age. Likewise, Chang, Buschbacher, and Edlich[40] found no significant difference between right and left wrist flexion and extension in the 10 power lifters and 10 nonlifters who were their subjects. Solgaard and coworkers[24] studied 8 males and 23 females aged 24 to 65 years. Right and left wrist extension and radial deviation differed significantly, but the differences were small and not significant when the total range (i.e., flexion and extension) was assessed. The authors stated that the opposite wrist could be satisfactorily used as a reference. A study by Gunal and coworkers[27] of 1,000 healthy Turkish males between the ages of 18 to 22 years likewise found no significant difference between sides for wrist flexion and ulnar deviation. However, a greater amount of left wrist extension (average 10 degrees) and radial deviation (average 4 degrees active, 6 degrees passive) ROM was reported.

Several other studies have found the left wrist to have slightly greater ROM than the right or dominant wrist. These differences may be related to the greater strain put on the dominant wrist. Cobe[39] measured wrist motions in the positions of pronation and supination in 100 men and 15 women. He found that men had greater ROM in their left wrist than in their right for all motions except ulnar deviation measured in pronation. However, he reported that the women had greater wrist motion on the right except for extension in pronation and radial deviation in supination. No statistical tests were conducted in Cobe's 1928 study, but Allander and associates[36] reported that a recalculation of the original data collected by Cobe found a significantly greater ROM on the left in men. Cobe[39] suggests that the heavy work that men performed using their right extremities may account for the decrease in right-side motion in comparison with left-side motion.

In support of these findings, a study by Klum and coworkers[29] of 750 German workers found significantly lower wrist flexion and extension ROM values for those employed in high manual stress jobs compared with low manual stress jobs for both sexes. Among high manual stress workers, there was less wrist flexion and extension motion in the dominant hand (usually the right hand). Regardless of manual stress exposure, women had more flexion, extension, and radial deviation on the left and ulnar deviation on the right. Likewise, men showed greater extension on the left and ulnar deviation on the right.

Allander and associates,[36] in a study subgroup of 309 Icelandic women aged 34 to 61 years, found no significant difference between the right and the left wrists. However, a subgroup of 208 women and 203 Swedish men in the study showed significantly smaller ranges of wrist flexion and extension on the right than on the left, independent of gender. The authors state that these differences may be due to a higher level of exposure to trauma of the right hand in a predominantly right-handed society.

Solveborn and Olerud[25] measured wrist ROM in 16 healthy subjects in addition to 123 patients with unilateral tennis elbow. Among the healthy subjects, a significantly greater ROM was found for wrist flexion and extension on the left compared with the right. However, mean differences between sides were only 2 degrees. Given these small differences, the authors concurred with Boone and Azen[21] that a patient's healthy limb can be used to establish a norm for comparing with the affected side.

Macedo and Magee[41] included 90 Caucasian women between the ages of 18 and 59 years in a study that examined dominant versus nondominant sides on passive and active ROM at the wrist, ankle, knee, hip, shoulder, and elbow. Active wrist motions of flexion, extension, radial and ulnar deviation, and passive motions of extension and radial deviation were significantly different between sides. Most wrist motions had a greater range on the nondominant side; however, the differences were small, appearing to be 5 degrees or less in the diagrams.

Testing Position

Several studies have reported differences in wrist ROM depending on the testing position of the forearm during measurement. Generally, a greater amount of ulnar deviation has been noted with the forearm in supination, and greater amounts of wrist flexion, extension, and radial deviation with the forearm in pronation. These findings support the use of consistent forearm positions during wrist ROM measurements.

Cobe,[39] in a study of 100 men and 15 women, found that ulnar deviation ROM was greater in supination, whereas radial deviation was greater in pronation. It is interesting that the total amount of ulnar and radial deviation combined was similar between the two positions. Hewitt[35] measured wrist ROM in 112 females in supination and pronation and likewise found that ulnar deviation was greater in supination, whereas radial deviation, flexion, and extension were greater in pronation. Werner and Plancher,[7] in a review article, also stated that ulnar deviation has a greater ROM when the forearm is supinated than when the forearm is pronated. They noted that radial and ulnar deviation ROMs become minimal when the wrist is fully flexed or extended. No specific references for these observations were cited.

Spilman and Pinkston[42] examined the effect of three frequently used goniometric testing positions on active wrist radial and ulnar deviation ROM in 100 subjects (63 males, 37 females). In Position One, the subject's arm was at the side, with the elbow flexed to 90 degrees and the forearm fully pronated. In Position Two, the shoulder was in 90 degrees of flexion, with the elbow extended and the hand prone. In Position Three, the subject's shoulder was in 90 degrees of abduction, with the elbow in 90 degrees of flexion and the hand prone (in this position, the forearm is in neutral pronation). Ulnar deviation and the total range of radial and ulnar deviation were significantly greater when measured in Position Three. Radial deviation was significantly greater when the subject was in Position Three or Position Two than in Position One. The differences between the means for the three positions were small—approximately 3 degrees.

Wrist position during testing has also been found to affect ROM values. It appears that the greatest ROM values are obtained with the wrist in a neutral position. For example, it is recommended that radial and ulnar deviations be measured with the wrist in 0 degrees of flexion and extension. Flexion and extension of the wrist should be measured with the wrist in 0 degrees of radial and ulnar deviation.

Marshall, Morzall, and Shealy[43] evaluated 35 men and 19 women for wrist ROM in one plane of motion while the subjects were fixed in secondary wrist and forearm positions. For example, during the measurement of radial and ulnar deviation, the wrist was alternatively positioned in 0 degrees, 40 degrees of flexion, and 40 degrees of extension. During the measurement of flexion and extension, the wrist was positioned in 0 degrees, 15 degrees radial deviation, and 25 degrees ulnar deviation. The effects of the secondary wrist and forearm postures, although statistically significant, were generally small (less than 5 degrees), with most motions having the greatest range with the wrist in neutral. However, radial deviation ROM was greatest when performed in wrist extension. The authors believed that the changes that occur in wrist ROM with positional alterations might have been the result of changes in contact between articular surfaces and tautness of ligaments that span the wrist region.

In a study of 10 subjects performing active circumduction, Li and associates[44] found that maximum ROM in flexion and extension occurred with the wrist near 0 degrees of radial and ulnar deviation. Likewise, maximum ROM in radial and ulnar deviation occurred with the wrist near 0 degrees of flexion and extension. Wrist deviation from the neutral position in one plane of motion reduced wrist ROM in other planes of motions.

Functional Range of Motion

Several investigators have examined the ROM that occurs at the wrist during activities of daily living (ADLs), during the placement of the hand on the body areas necessary for personal care, and during common tasks. Table 6.5 presents findings from nine of these studies. Differences in ROM values reported for certain functional tasks were most likely the result of variations in task definitions, measurement methods, and subject selection. However, in spite of the range of values reported, certain trends are evident.

A review of Table 6.5 shows that the majority of ADLs and common tasks required wrist extension and ulnar deviation. Using a conventional telephone, turning a steering wheel or a doorknob, brushing teeth, washing the face, and rising from a chair (see Fig. 5.31) required the greatest amounts of extension (generally 40 to 63 degrees). The greatest amounts of ulnar deviation (32 to 48 degrees) were noted while pouring from a pitcher, combing hair, tying/untying shoes,

TABLE 6.5 Wrist ROM During Functional Activities: Mean Values in Degrees

Activity	Study			Flexion		Extension		Radial Deviation		Ulnar Deviation	
	First Author	Subjects (healthy adults)	Measurement Method	Min	Max	Min	Max	Min	Max	Min	Max
Feeding Tasks											
Drink from glass	Brumfield[45]	19	Uniaxial electrogoniometer			11	24				
	Ryu[23]	40	Biaxial electrogoniometer			3	22			6	20
	Romilly[50]	6	3D video system		16		24		8		11
	Aizawa[49]	20	3D electromagnetic system				15		3		
Drink from handled cup	Safee-Rad[47]	10	3D video system		8		6			8	16
Eat with fork	Brumfield[45]	19	Uniaxial electrogoniometer			9	37				
	Safee-Rad[47]	10	3D video system			3	18		5		3
Eat with spoon	Aizawa[49]	20	3D electromagnetic system				21				11
Use fork, spoon, cup	Cooper[48]	19	3D video system		7		21		2		19
Cut with knife	Brumfield[45]	19	Uniaxial electrogoniometer		4		20				
	Ryu[23]	40	Biaxial electrogoniometer	5	31					13	27
Pour from pitcher	Brumfield[45]	19	Uniaxial electrogoniometer			9	30				
	Ryu[23]	40	Biaxial electrogoniometer		20		22			12	32
	Aziawa[49]	20	3D electromagnetic system				10				3
Reaching Tasks for Personal Care											
Brush teeth (inside)	Ryu[23]	40	Biaxial electrogoniometer		30		42		10		24
	Romilly[50]	6	3D video system		39		32		17		22
Comb hair	Ryu[23]	40	Biaxial electrogoniometer		36		32		3		38
	Aizawa[49]	20	3D electromagnetic system				3				9
	Romilly[50]	6	3D video system		36		35		24		18
Wash face	Aizawa[49]	20	3D electromagnetic system				29		7		
	Romilly[50]	6	3D video system		14		42		15		19
Hand to top of head	Brumfield[45]	19	Uniaxial electrogoniometer		2						
	Ryu[23]	40	Biaxial electrogoniometer		21						16
Hand to occiput	Brumfield[45]	19					13				
	Ryu[23]	40	Biaxial electrogoniometer		1						
Hand to chest	Brumfield[45]	19	Uniaxial electrogoniometer		19						
	Ryu[23]	40	Biaxial electrogoniometer		25				5		

Tie/untie necktie or scarf	Ryu[23]	40		Biaxial electrogoniometer		51		41		15		40
Hand to axilla (ipsilateral)	Aizawa[49]	20		3D electromagnetic system		76						33
Hand to axilla (opposite)	Aizawa[49]	20		3D electromagnetic system		32						18
Hand to perineum	Aizawa[49]	20		3D electromagnetic system		1				5		
Perineal care	Ryu[23]	40		Biaxial electrogoniometer	16	54				5		21
Hand to sacrum	Brumfield[45]	19		Uniaxial electrogoniometer		1						
	Ryu[23]	40		Biaxial electrogoniometer		20						48
Hand to back	Aizawa[49]	20		3D electromagnetic system		45						20
Hand to foot/shoe	Brumfield[45]	19		Uniaxial electrogoniometer				14				
	Ryu[23]	40		Biaxial electrogoniometer				1				9
Tie/untie shoes	Ryu[23]	40		Biaxial electrogoniometer		30		36		10		32
Common Tasks												
Open/close jar lid	Ryu[23]	40		Biaxial electrogoniometer		35		6		12		36
Turn doorknob	Ryu[23]	40		Biaxial electrogoniometer		40		45		12		32
Use telephone	Brumfield[45]	19		Uniaxial electrogoniometer				43				
	Ryu[23]	40		Biaxial electrogoniometer		15		42		10		12
	Romilly[50]	6		3D video system		9		32		11		14
Writing	Ryu[23]	40		Biaxial electrogoniometer			16	30			5	17
Turn steering wheel	Ryu[23]	40		Biaxial electrogoniometer		15		45		17		28
Rise from chair	Brumfield[45]	19		Uniaxial electrogoniometer			1	63				
	Ryu[23]	40		Biaxial electrogoniometer		10		60		4		30
Propel wheelchair	Boninger[53]		9 paralympic athletes	3D camera system, 1.3 m/sec speed		7		39		25		20
	Veeger[52]		5 nonimpaired; 4 wheelchair users	3D optical-electronic system		14		34		13		24
	Wei[54]		11 wheelchair users	2D electrogoniometer, low seat, midposition backrest			1	37		22		19
	Wei[54]		11 wheelchair users	2D electrogoniometers, high seat, midposition backrest		9		35		17		26

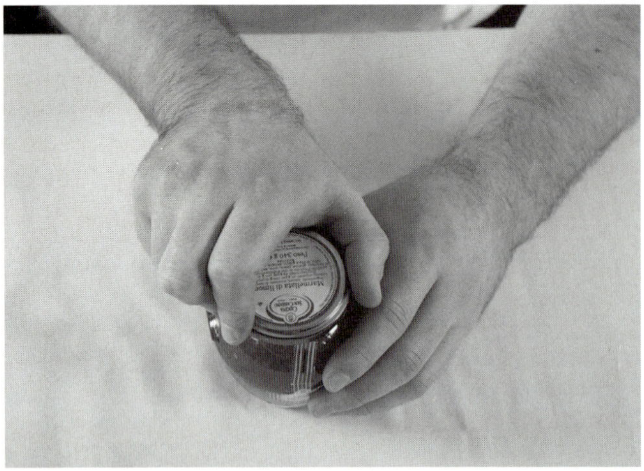

FIGURE 6.35 Opening the lid of a jar requires about 36 degrees of ulnar deviation and 12 degrees of radial deviation.[23]

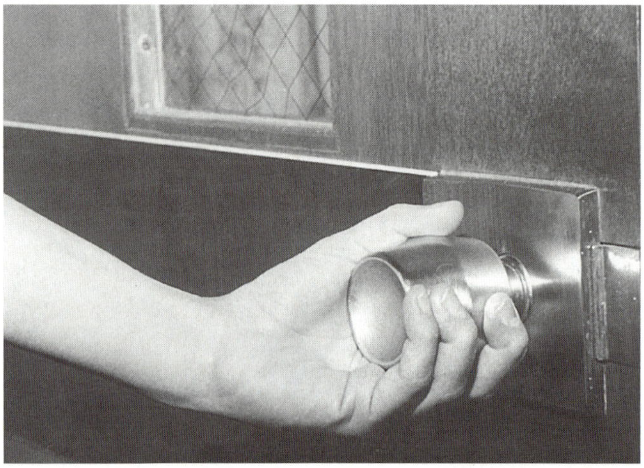

FIGURE 6.36 Turning a doorknob requires about 40 degrees of wrist flexion and 45 degrees of wrist extension.[23]

opening/closing jar lid (Fig. 6.35), and placing a hand on the sacrum. As seen in Table 6.5, wrist flexion more frequently occurred during the placement of a hand on body areas commonly touched during personal care. The greatest amounts of flexion were reported while brushing teeth, combing hair, performing perineum care, and placing the hand on the back and to the ipsilateral axilla as might occur during dressing and bathing (42 to 76 degrees). Among common tasks, turning a doorknob (Fig. 6.36) involved the greatest amount of flexion (40 degrees). Reaching the neck to tie/untie a necktie or scarf was particularly challenging, requiring large amounts of flexion, extension, and ulnar deviation (51, 41, and 40 degrees, respectively).

Brief summaries of some of the studies that have examined wrist ROM during ADLs, personal care, and common tasks are presented here. Brumfield and Champoux[45] used a uniaxial electrogoniometer to determine the range of wrist flexion and extension during 14 ADLs performed by 12 men and 7 women. They determined that ADLs such as eating and drinking were accomplished with 5 degrees of flexion to 35 degrees of extension. Personal care activities that involved placing the hand on the body required 20 degrees of flexion to 15 degrees of extension. The authors concluded that an arc of wrist motion of 45 degrees (10 degrees of flexion to 35 degrees of extension) is sufficient to perform most of the activities studied.

Palmer and coworkers[46] used a triaxial electrogoniometer to study 10 normal subjects while they performed 52 tasks. A range of 33 degrees of flexion, 59 degrees of extension, 23 degrees of radial deviation, and 22 degrees of ulnar deviation was used in performing ADLs and personal hygiene. During these tasks the average amount of motion was about 5 degrees of flexion, 30 degrees of extension, 10 degrees of radial deviation, and 15 degrees of ulnar deviation. Range-of-motion values for individual tasks were not presented in the study and therefore are not included in Table 6.5.

Ryu and associates[23] found that 31 examined tasks could be performed with 54 degrees of flexion, 60 degrees of extension, 17 degrees of radial deviation, and 40 degrees of ulnar deviation. The 20 men and 20 women were evaluated with a biaxial electrogoniometer during performance of palm placement activities, personal care and hygiene, diet and food preparation, and miscellaneous ADLs. Most tasks could be performed with about 70% of maximal wrist ROM. The authors agreed with other researchers that ulnar deviation and wrist extension are the most important positions for wrist activities.

Studies by Safaee-Rad and coworkers[47] and Cooper and coworkers[48] examined wrist ROM with a video-based three-dimensional motion-analysis system during three feeding tasks: drinking from a cup, eating with a fork, and eating with a spoon. The 10 males studied by Safaee-Rad and coworkers used from 10 degrees of wrist flexion to 25 degrees of extension and from 20 degrees of ulnar deviation to 5 degrees of radial deviation during the tasks. Cooper and coworkers examined 10 males and 9 females during feeding tasks, with the elbow unrestricted and then fixed in 110 degrees of flexion. With the elbow unrestricted, males used from 7 degrees of wrist flexion to 21 degrees of extension and from 19 degrees of ulnar deviation to 2 degrees of radial deviation. Females had similar values for flexion and extension but used from 3 degrees of ulnar deviation to 18 degrees of radial deviation. Both studies found that drinking from a cup required less of an arc of wrist motion than eating with a fork or spoon.

Aizawa and coworkers[49] studied the joint angles of upper-extremity joints of 20 healthy adults at the completion of 16 ADL tasks using a three-dimensional electromagnetic tracking system. Wrist extension was needed for many of the tasks, but less ulnar deviation was noted as compared with previous studies. This difference in ROM values between studies was attributed by the authors to differences in task instructions; for example, the current study asked subjects to drink until the glass was empty (rather than a sip), which required more radial deviation as the tasked was completed. The difference may also be related to reporting the joint angle at the completion of the tasks rather than the maximal values that occurred during the tasks. Washing the face (29 degrees) and the ipsilateral ear (25 degrees) required large amounts of wrist extension, whereas touching the ipsilateral axilla (76 degrees) and the back (45 degrees) required a large amount of flexion. The authors pointed out that these ipsilateral tasks are important motions for patients who cannot use one upper extremity because of conditions such as hemiplegia or amputation.

Romilly and colleagues[50] examined upper-extremity motions needed by six able-bodied subjects to perform 22 tasks that included eating and drinking, reaching, personal hygiene, and ADL tasks such as turning a doorknob, turning a page, and flipping a light switch. A three-dimensional video-based motion-analysis system was employed. The greatest amount of wrist extension occurred during face washing (42 degrees), whereas the greatest amount of wrist flexion (53 degrees) occurred during eating with a spoon using an overhand cylindrical grasp. However, the authors noted that many tasks centered on 10 degrees of wrist extension, so that if the wrist were immobilized in that position and other upper-extremity joints were free to move, many tasks could still be performed.

Van Andel et al[51] studied the wrist, elbow, and shoulder joints during four tasks in 10 healthy adults with a three-dimensional video-based motion-analysis system. Tasks included hand to the opposite shoulder, hand to mouth with a cup for a sip, combing hair, and hand to back pocket to represent back and perineal care. Peak wrist flexion was 66 degrees and peak wrist extension was 64 degrees during the four tasks. Large variations in motions were noted between the subjects with some using more forearm rotation in place of wrist extension and flexion during the tasks. Values for radial and ulnar deviations were not reported.

Wrist ROM during handrim wheelchair propulsion has been investigated under a variety of speeds and slopes, as well as seat height and horizontal positions. The results of several of these studies are presented in Table 6.5. A mix of wheelchair and nonwheelchair users was studied by Veeger and associates[52] at three wheelchair velocities and three incline slopes. The push phase started in a combination of radial deviation and extension, and changed into ulnar deviation and flexion. Maximum values for ulnar and radial deviation during wheelchair use were close to normal ROM values found in the literature, whereas maximal wrist extension was about 50% of normal ROM. The authors propose that the repetitive extremes of wrist ulnar deviation and extension, especially during wrist and finger muscle flexor activity, and pressure on the wrist region from contact with the rim may contribute to carpal tunnel syndrome in wheelchair users. Boninger and coworkers,[53] in a study of six manual wheelchair users, found stable ROM values for wrist flexion and ulnar deviation for the two propulsion speeds. Maximal wrist radial deviation and extension was greater by 4 degrees during the slower speed; however, only the difference in radial deviation was statistically significant. Eleven wheelchair users were included in a study by Wei and associates[54] that examined the effect of two seat heights and horizontal backrest position on wrist angle and muscle activity. The lower seat height significantly decreased maximal wrist flexion and forced the wrist to be in constantly maintained extension. The lower seat position also resulted in an increase in maximal radial deviation and decrease in ulnar deviation. Changes in horizontal seatback positions did not affect wrist motions. An ideal seat height was not indicated.

Repetitive trauma disorders such as carpal tunnel syndrome and wrist/hand tendinitis have been found to occur more frequently with certain types of work, sports, and artistic endeavours. To elucidate the cause of these higher incidences of injury, studies have been conducted on the wrist positions used and the amount and frequency of wrist motions required during grocery bagging,[55] grocery scanning,[56] piano playing,[57] computer use,[58–60] office and industrial work,[61–63] and in playing sports such as basketball, baseball pitching, and golf.[7,64] The reader is advised to refer directly to these studies to gain information about the amount of wrist ROM that occurs during these activities. In general, an association has been noted between activities that require extreme wrist postures and the prevalence of hand/wrist tendinitis.[65] Tasks that involve repeated wrist flexion and extreme wrist extension, repetitive work with the hands, and repeated force applied to the base of the palm and wrist have been associated with carpal tunnel syndrome.[66]

In contrast to the studies that reported on the amount of wrist motion that occurs during or at the completion of functional and occupational tasks, other investigators have limited wrist motion with splints in healthy adults to see the effect on upper-extremity function. Nelson[67] evaluated the ability of 9 males and 3 females to perform 123 ADLs with a splint on the dominant wrist that limited motion to 5 degrees of flexion, 6 degrees of extension, 7 degrees of radial deviation, and 6 degrees of ulnar deviation. All 123 activities could be completed with the splint in place, with 9 activities having a mean difficulty rating of greater than or equal to 2 (could be done with minimal difficulty or frustration and with satisfactory outcome). The most difficult activities included putting on/taking off a bra (Fig. 6.37), washing legs/back, writing, dusting low surfaces, cutting vegetables, handling a sharp knife, cutting meat, using a can opener, and using a manual egg-beater. It should be noted that these subjects were pain free and had normal shoulders and elbows to compensate for the restricted wrist motions. The ability to generalize these results to patient populations with pain and multiple involved joints may be limited. Compensatory motions of increased shoulder elevation, lateral and medial rotation, and abduction have been documented in patients with a history of distal radial fractures that reduced active wrist ROM and forearm rotation during the functional task of page turning.[68]

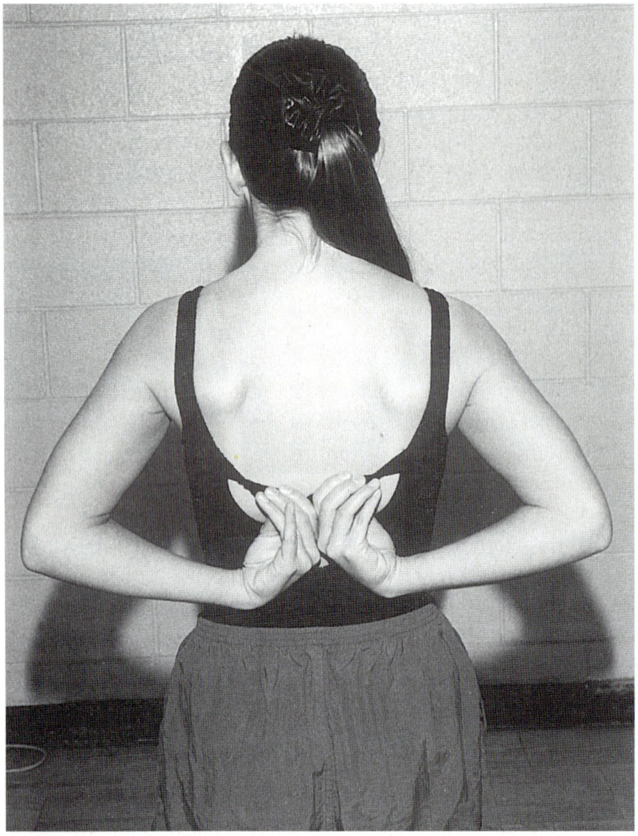

FIGURE 6.37 A large amount of wrist flexion is needed to fasten a bra or bathing suit. This is one of the most difficult activities to perform if wrist motion is limited.

Franko, Zurakowshi, and Day[69] found a strong association between wrist ROM and functional disability outcome measures in 42 healthy adults restricted with low-profile wrist splints for 24 hours. Subjects completed four functional disability tests: Disabilities of the Arm, Shoulder and Hand (DASH), Patient-Rated Wrist Evaluation (PRWE), Modern Activity Subjective Survey (MASS), and Modern Activity Timed Test (MATT) at baseline and in a partially and highly restricted splint. At baseline the median arc of wrist flexion–extension was 138 degrees and radial–ulnar deviation was 63 degrees. In a partially restricted splint the arc of flexion–extension was 58 degrees and radial–ulnar deviation was 41 degrees, whereas in a highly restricted splint the arc of flexion–extension was 20 degrees and radial–ulnar deviation was 21 degrees. A dose response was noted with greater reductions in functional disability scores reported as wrist motion became more restricted. This study also supports the construct validity of wrist ROM values to measure the abstract concept of functional limitation and disability (see end of this chapter).

Reliability and Validity

The following sections focus on the reliability and validity of wrist ROM measurements. At this time, no studies have been found that examined the reliability and validity of muscle length tests measured at the wrist.

Reliability of Universal Goniometer and Inclinometer Measurements

Healthy Populations

Studies of intratester and intertester reliability of wrist ROM measurements have been conducted by many researchers on healthy people using universal goniometers and, in a few cases, inclinometers. Reliability varied according to the motions being measured with no consistent motion being the most or least reliably measured. Universal goniometers were generally found to have good to excellent intratester reliability, with the majority of intraclass correlation coefficient (ICC) values ranging from 0.80 to 0.95, and the standard deviations (SDs) or standard errors of the repeated measurements (SEMs) ranging from about 3 to 5 degrees. The majority of these investigators found that intratester reliability was slightly better than intertester reliability, thus supporting having the same examiner take follow-up measurements on an individual whenever possible. In addition, repeated measurements should be taken with the same device and alignment methods to improve reliability, as different devices and methods were sometimes found to result in different measurements.

Tables 6.6 and 6.7 provide an overview of studies that assessed the intratester and intertester reliability of ROM measurements at the wrist using a universal goniometer or an inclinometer. The tables begin with studies that were conducted with healthy adults, followed by studies with patient populations. A brief written summary of many of these studies is also included below. One review article on the interrater reliability of ROM measurements (published in 2010) included five of these studies on the wrist.[70] Bird and Stowe[71] conducted a study in which two observers repeatedly measured active and passive wrist ROM with a universal goniometer in three subjects. Flexion and extension were measured from the lateral aspect of the ulna and fifth metacarpal, whereas radial and ulnar deviation was taken over the dorsal surface of the forearm and third metacarpal. They concluded that interobserver error was greatest for extension (±8 degrees) and least for radial and ulnar deviation (±2–3 degrees). Error during passive ROM measurements was slightly greater than error during active ROM measurements in these healthy subjects.

In a study by Boone et al,[72] four physical therapists, using a universal goniometer aligned on the dorsal surface of the forearm and third metacarpal, measured ulnar deviation on 12 healthy male volunteers. Measurements were repeated over a period of 4 weeks. Intratester reliability was found to be slightly better than intertester reliability. Total standard deviations of the repeated measurements that included intratester or intertester variation as well as goniometer error variation were about 4 degrees for wrist ulnar deviation. The authors generally concluded that to determine true change when more than one tester measures the same motion, differences in motion should exceed 5 degrees.

TABLE 6.6 Intratester Reliability of Wrist ROM Measurements With Goniometers and Inclinometers for Healthy and Patient Populations

Study	*N*	Sample	Methods	Motion	*r*	ICC	Absolute Measures (degrees)
Healthy Populations							
Boone et al[72]	12	Healthy males	AROM, 4 testers, supine, universal goniometer on dorsal surface	Ulnar dev	.76		Intra SD = 1.3 Total SD = 3.9
Bovens et al[73]	8	Healthy adults	PROM, 3 testers, universal goniometer, lateral alignment (ulnar and fifth metacarpal)	Flexion Extension	.27, .62, .87 .09, .28, .40		SD within tester = 4.3, 4.8, 3.9 SD = 3.2, 4.3, 2.8
Greene and Wolf[22]	20	Healthy adults	AROM, 1 tester, Universal goniometer:	Flexion Extension Radial dev Ulnar dev		.96 .94 .91 .94	Within-session SD = 2.1 2.2 2.0 2.1
			Ortho Ranger: (electroinclinometer)	Flexion Extension Radial dev Ulnar dev		.92 .90 .88 .89	3.4 3.6 3.1 3.1
Low[74]	1	Healthy adults	AROM, 50 testers, universal goniometer, any alignment allowed	Extension			Mean error ranged from 3.5 to 5.0
Macedo and Magee[28]	12	Healthy adults	PROM, 1 tester, universal goniometer, Norkin and White method	Flexion Extension Radial dev Ulnar dev		.83 .85 .81 .86	SEM = 3.9 MDC = 10.7 SEM = 2.9 MDC = 8.1 SEM = 3.0 MDC = 8.3 SEM = 7.4 MDC = 20.6
Solgaard et al[24]	31	Healthy adults	4 testers, universal goniometer, lateral alignment for flexion and extension, dorsal for deviations	Flexion Extension Radial dev Ulnar dev			SD within observer = 5.2 SD = 5.8 SD = 5.2 SD = 6.4
Solveborn and Olerud[25]	16	Healthy adults, right and left sides	1 tester, AROM, PROM, universal goniometer, dorsal alignment for flexion and deviations, lateral alignment for extension	AROM Flexion Extension Radial dev Ulnar dev PROM Flexion Extension			 SD of error = 2.5 SD of error = 4.5 SD of error = 4.5 SD of error = 4.0 SD of error = 2.5 SD of error = 3.0
Walker et al[32]	4	Healthy adults	AROM, 4 testers, universal goniometer	Flexion Extension Radial dev Ulnar dev	all >.81		Mean error = 5 ± 1
Patient Populations							
Hellebrandt et al[77]	77	Arthritic and orthopedic patients	AROM, 1 skilled tester, universal goniometer, undefined alignment	Flexion Extension Radial dev Ulnar dev			Mean difference between trials = 1.1 Mean difference = .9 Mean difference = .3 Mean difference = .3

(table continues on page 180)

TABLE 6.6 Intratester Reliability of Wrist ROM Measurements With Goniometers and Inclinometers for Healthy and Patient Populations (continued)

Study	*N*	Sample	Methods	Motion	*r*	ICC	Absolute Measures (degrees)
Horger[76]	48	Patients with wrist injury and/or surgery	AROM, PROM, 13 testers, universal goniometer, any alignment	AROM			
				Flexion		.96	SEM = 3.5
				Extension		.96	SEM = 3.7
				Radial dev		.90	SEM = 2.6
				Ulnar dev		.92	SEM = 3.5
				PROM			
				Flexion		.96	SEM = 4.4
				Extension		.96	SEM = 3.5
				Radial dev		.91	SEM = 2.7
				Ulnar dev		.94	SEM = 3.0
LaStayo et al[16]	120	Patients with wrist conditions	PROM, 32 testers, universal goniometer, 3 different goniometer alignments	Flexion			
				Radial align		.86	SEM = 7.2
				Ulnar align		.87	SEM = 7.4
				Dorsal align		.92	SEM = 5.7
				Extension			
				Radial align		.80	SEM = 7.8
				Ulnar align		.80	SEM = 8.1
				Dorsal align		.84	SEM = 5.6
Pandya et al[79]	150	Children with Duchene muscular dystrophy	PROM, 5 testers, universal goniometer, AAOS method	Extension		.87	

r = Pearson correlation coefficient; ICC = Intraclass correlation coefficient; Ulnar dev = Ulnar deviation; Radial dev = Radial deviation; SD = Standard deviation (of the repeated measurements); SEM = Standard error of the repeated measurements; MDC = Minimal detectable change; SDD = smallest detectable difference; 95% CI = 95 percent confidence interval; AROM = active range of motion; PROM = passive range of motion

Bovens and coworkers[73] measured nine motions at the wrist, forearm, shoulder, and ankle with a universal goniometer in eight healthy adults for intratester and intertester reliability, and in another group of 48 healthy athletic adults for intertester reliability. The three physicians who performed the measurements initially had little experience measuring joint ROM but were taught a set measurement protocol. Passive wrist motions were measured aligning the goniometer with the lateral ulnar and fifth metacarpal. The standard deviations of the repeated measurements taken by each of testers on the initial eight subjects ranged from 4 to 5 degrees for wrist flexion and 3 to 4 degrees for wrist extension. The standard deviations of the repeated measurements between the testers increased to 6 degrees for wrist flexion and 5 degrees for wrist extension. The authors suggest that it is difficult to demonstrate an improvement or worsening of a joint motion if the difference between the measurements is less than 5 to 10 degrees for most joints (2 × SD). Reliability coefficients were also provided, but the authors noted that the low reliability coefficients were explained by the relatively small interindividual variations. Intertester reliability coefficients from the last three sessions in 28 of the athletic subjects were 0.74 for flexion and 0.58 for extension.

Greene and Wolf[22] compared the reliability of the Ortho Ranger, an electronic pendulum goniometer, with a universal goniometer for active upper-extremity motions in 20 healthy adults. Wrist ROM was measured by one therapist three times with each instrument during each of three sessions over a 2-week period. There was a significant difference between instruments for wrist extension and ulnar deviation. Within-session reliability was slightly higher for the universal goniometer (ICC = 0.91–0.96) than for the Ortho Ranger (ICC = 0.88–0.92). The 95% confidence level, which represents the variability around the mean, ranged from 7.6 to 9.3 degrees for the goniometer and from 18.2 to 25.6 degrees for the Ortho Ranger. The authors concluded that the Ortho Ranger provided no advantages over the universal goniometer.

In a study by Low,[74] 50 testers visually estimated and then measured the author's active wrist extension and elbow flexion using a universal goniometer. Five testers also took 10 repeated measurements over the course of 5 to 10 days. Intraobserver error was less than interobserver error. Intertester mean error improved from 12.8 degrees for visual estimates to 7.8 degrees for goniometric measurement. The measurement of wrist extension was less reliable than the measurement of elbow flexion, with intertester mean errors

TABLE 6.7 Intertester Reliability of Wrist ROM Measurements With Goniometers and Inclinometers for Healthy and Patient Populations

Study	*N*	Sample	Methods	Motion	*r*	ICC	Absolute Measures (degrees)
Healthy Populations							
Bird and Stowe[71]	3	Healthy adults	AROM, 2 testers, universal goniometer	Flexion Extension Radial dev Ulnar dev			Error = ± 4 Error = ± 8 Error = ± 2 Error = ± 3
Boone et al[72]	12	Healthy males	AROM, 4 testers, supine, universal goniometer	Ulnar dev	.73		Intra SD = 1.6 Total SD = 4.0
Bovens et al[73]	8	Healthy adults	PROM, 3 testers, universal goniometer, aligned with ulnar and fifth metacarpal	Flexion Extension	.59, .74* .09, .58*		SD between testers = 5.7 SD = 5.1
Solgaard et al[24]	31	Healthy adults	4 testers, universal goniometer aligned with ulna and fifth metacarpal for flexion and extension, or dorsal aspect of forearm and third metacarpal for deviations	Flexion Extension Radial dev Ulnar dev			SD between testers = 6.0 SD = 6.2 SD = 5.4 SD = 8.8
Walker et al[32]	4	Healthy adults	AROM, 2 testers, universal goniometer	Flexion Extension Radial dev Ulnar dev			Mean error = 6 ± 5
Patient Populations							
Edgar et al[75]	45	Burn survivors 22 pairs of wrist measures	AROM, 4 testers, universal goniometer, aligned with ulnar and fifth metacarpal	Flexion–extension		.96	MDD = 7.7
Horger[76]	48	Patients with wrist injury and/or surgery	AROM, PROM, 13 testers, universal goniometer, any alignment allowed	AROM Flexion Extension Radial dev Ulnar dev PROM Flexion Extension Radial dev Ulnar dev		 .91 .85 .86 .78 .86 .84 .66 .83	 SEM = 6.6 SEM = 7.0 SEM = 3.0 SEM = 5.8 SEM = 8.2 SEM = 7.0 SEM = 5.3 SEM = 4.8
LaStayo et al[16]	120	Patients with wrist condition	PROM, 32 testers, universal goniometer, 3 different goniometer alignments	Flexion Radial align Ulnar align Dorsal align Extension Radial align Ulnar align Dorsal align		 .88 .89 .93 .80 .80 .84	 SEM = 6.6 SEM = 6.8 SEM = 5.5 SEM = 7.7 SEM = 7.9 SEM = 6.0

(table continues on page 182)

TABLE 6.7 Intertester Reliability of Wrist ROM Measurements With Goniometers and Inclinometers for Healthy and Patient Populations (continued)

Study	N	Sample	Methods	Motion	r	ICC	Absolute Measures (degrees)
Pandya et al[79]	21	Children with Duchenne muscular dystrophy	PROM, 5 testers, universal goniometer, AAOS method	Extension		.83	
de Jong et al[80]	48	Patients with subacute stroke	PROM, 2 testers, hydrogoniometer	Extension: fingers flexed			SEM = 1.0 SDD = 2.6
				Extension: fingers extended			SEM = 1.7 SDD = 4.7

ICC = Intraclass correlation coefficient; *r* = Pearson correlation coefficient; Ulnar dev = Ulnar deviation; Radial dev = Radial deviation; SD = Standard deviation (of the repeated measurements); SEM = Standard error of the repeated measurements; MDC = Minimal detectable change; MDD = Minimal detectable difference; SDD = Smallest detectable difference; AROM = active range of motion; PROM = passive range of motion.

* Values from an additional group of 28 healthy athletic subjects and measured when testers had acquired more experience.

of 7.8 and 5.0 degrees, respectively. Testers were allowed to align the goniometer using any method.

Macedo and Magee[28] included a preliminary study of intratester reliability in a larger study of 90 Caucasian women that examined the effect of age on passive ROM at the wrist, the ankle, knee, hip, shoulder, and elbow. One physical therapist took measurements with a universal goniometer using methods described by Norkin and White (third edition). The reliability coefficients for all wrist motions ranged from 0.81 to 0.86, indicating good reliability. Standard errors of the repeated measurement were similar (3–4 degrees) for flexion, extension, and radial deviation, but were higher (7 degrees) for ulnar deviation.

Solgaard and coworkers[24] found intratester standard deviations of 5 to 6 degrees and intertester standard deviations of 6 to 9 degrees in a study of wrist motions involving 31 healthy subjects. Measurements were taken with a universal goniometer by four testers on three different occasions. The goniometer was aligned on the lateral surface of the ulna and fifth metacarpal for flexion and extension, and on the dorsal surface of the forearm and third metacarpal for radial and ulnar deviations. Normative ROM values were also provided.

Solveborn and Olerud[25] examined the intratester reliability of measuring bilateral wrist motions with a universal goniometer in 16 healthy adults as a preliminary part of a study of patients with radial epicondylalgia. Wrist flexion was measured on the dorsal surface of the forearm and third metacarpal, whereas extension was measured parallel to the lateral aspect of the ulnar and third metacarpal. Radial and ulnar deviations were assessed on the dorsal surface of the radius and third finger. Wrist flexion was the most reliable measurement with standard deviations of the repeated measurements ranging from 2 to 3 degrees, whereas extension was the least with SD ranging from 3 to 5 degrees.

Walker and associates[32] conducted a small reliability study as part of a larger study determining normative ROM data on older men and women. Four healthy adult subjects were evaluated by four testers five times for each of 24 joint motions including wrist flexion, extension, and radial and ulnar deviation. All correlations for intratester reliability were greater than 0.81 and the mean error between the repeated measurements was 5 ± 1 degree. Two testers took all the measurements in the larger study and the mean error between the testers, indicating intertester reliability was 6 ± 5 degrees.

Patient Populations

A review of studies that assessed wrist ROM in patient populations provides evidence similar to studies on healthy populations: Universal goniometers can be reliably used to take wrist ROM measurements. Although both intratester reliability and intertester reliability are generally good to excellent, intratester reliability is higher than intertester reliability. Therefore, it is better to have the same tester take repeated measurements on an individual to assess change. Similarly, the same alignment method and measurement device should be used during repeated measurements to reduce measurement error.

Edgar and coworkers[75] examined the reliability of using a universal goniometer to measure active ROM in burn-affected joints of 45 patients. One physical therapist took two repeated measurements to assess intratester reliability, while four physical therapists took one measurement of each motion to assess intertester reliability. All measurements were made the same day using the lateral ulnar and fifth metacarpal for goniometer alignment. Intratester and intertester reliability was found to be excellent, with ICC values greater than 0.96 for the wrist. There were only enough data points to calculate minimal detectable differences (MDD) between the four testers for intertester reliability at the wrist, which was 7.7 degrees. According to the authors, the study demonstrated that clinically relevant, accurate, objective measures can be made in burn populations.

Horger[76] conducted a study in which 13 randomly paired therapists performed repeated measurements of active and passive wrist motions on 48 patients. Therapists were free to select their own method of measurement with a universal goniometer. The six specialized hand therapists used an ulnar alignment for flexion and extension, whereas the nonspecialized therapists used a radial goniometer alignment. Intratester reliability of both active and passive wrist motions was highly reliable (all ICCs higher than 0.90) for all motions. Intratester reliability was consistently higher than intertester reliability (ICC = 0.66–0.91). Standard errors of measurements ranged from 2.6 to 4.4 degrees for intratester values and from 3.0 to 8.2 degrees for intertester values. Agreement between measures was better for flexion and extension than it was for radial and ulnar deviation. Intertester reliability coefficients for measurements of active motion (ICC = 0.78–0.91) were slightly higher than were coefficients for passive motion (ICC = 0.66–0.86) except for radial deviation, and were similar to intratester reliability. Generally, reliability was higher for the specialized therapists than for the nonspecialized therapists. The author determined that the presence of pain reduced the reliability of both active and passive measurements, but active measurements were affected more than passive measurements.

Hellebrandt, Duvall, and Moore[77] found that wrist motions measured with a universal goniometer were more reliable than those measured with a joint-specific device in 30 patients at a clinic for arthritic and orthopedic conditions. Measurements of wrist flexion and extension were less reliable than measurements of radial and ulnar deviation, although mean differences between successive measurements taken with a universal goniometer by a skilled tester were small (1.1 degrees for flexion, 0.9 degrees for extension, and 0.3 degrees for radial and ulnar deviations). The mean differences between successive measurements increased to 5.4 degrees for flexion, 5.7 degrees for extension, 2.8 degrees for radial deviation, and 1.6 degrees for ulnar deviation when successive measurements were taken with different instruments.

LaStayo and Wheeler[16] studied the intratester and intertester reliability of passive ROM measurements of wrist flexion and extension in 120 patients as measured by 32 randomly paired therapists, who used three goniometric alignments (ulnar, radial, and dorsal–volar). The reliability of measuring wrist flexion ROM was consistently higher than that of measuring extension ROM. Mean intratester ICCs for wrist flexion were 0.86 for radial, 0.87 for ulnar, and 0.92 for dorsal alignment. Mean intratester ICCs for wrist extension were 0.80 for radial, 0.80 for ulnar, and 0.84 for volar alignment. The authors recommended that these three alignments, although generally having good reliability, should not be used interchangeably because there were some significant differences between the measurements taken with the three alignments. The authors suggested that the dorsal–volar alignment should be the technique of choice for measuring passive wrist flexion and extension, given its higher reliability. In an invited commentary on this study, Flower[78] suggested using the fifth metacarpal, which is easier to visualize and align with the distal arm of the goniometer in the ulnar technique, rather than the third metacarpal, which was used in the study. Flower noted that the presence and fluctuation of edema on the dorsal surface of the hand may reduce the reliability of the dorsal alignment and necessitate the use of the ulnar (fifth metacarpal) alignment in the clinical setting.

Pandya and coworkers[79] studied the reliability of wrist extension measured with a universal goniometer in 150 children aged 1 to 20 years with Duchenne muscular dystrophy. Five experienced physical therapists took measurements on each patient on admission, at 1 week, and at 4 weeks. Twenty-five patients were included in the part of the study that focused on intertester reliability. Intratester and intertester reliability was good, with ICC values of 0.87 and 0.83, respectively.

In addition to the universal goniometer, the reliability of wrist ROM measurements taken with other devices on patient populations has been studied. De Jong and associates,[80] using a gravity-based hydrogoniometer, investigated the reliability of two trained physical therapists to measure seven passive arm motions, four times over 20 weeks in 48 patients with subacute strokes. Wrist extension with the fingers flexed as compared with fingers extended resulted in slightly less variability and higher reliability. As one would expect, reliability was better during a single measurement session as compared with sessions spaced over 20 weeks. For example, the intertester SEM for wrist extension with the fingers flexed went from 1.0 degree during one session to 3.3 degrees over the 20-week study period, whereas the smallest detectible difference (SDD) was 2.6 during one session and increased to 9.1 degrees over the 20-week study period.

In a study by Geertzen and coworkers,[81] two examiners measured the active wrist ROM with an inclinometer in 29 patients with reflex sympathetic dystrophy as part of a larger study. Each examiner measured the motions of each patient in the affected and unaffected sides once per session, and the session was repeated 30 minutes later. All correlation coefficients between repeated measurements ranged from 0.66 to 0.94 for wrist flexion, 0.57 to 0.96 for wrist extension, 0.60 to 0.89 for ulnar deviation, and 0.55 to 0.73 for radial deviation. The SDD, defined as the smallest amount of change in a variable that can be measured with statistical significance, for wrist flexion, extension, and ulnar deviation ranged from 14 to 16 degrees. The SDD for radial deviation was higher, from 20 to 22 degrees, with the authors noting that the patients had difficulty performing this isolated motion. It was unclear whether the SDD referred to repeated measurements made by the same tester or different testers, and appears to include biological variation between patients, which would inflate these values.

Validity of Goniometric Measurements

We are unaware of any published studies that report criterion-related validity of wrist ROM measurements taken with a goniometer to the gold standard radiographs. However, the universal goniometer has been used to try to validate other measurement tools.[22,39,77,82] Kim et al,[82] in a study of 53 healthy adults, had one examiner measure wrist motions with a universal goniometer that was aligned with the forearm and fingers, and with an iPhone attached to the dorsum of the hand that used a gyroscope application. Differences between mean values varied from 0.2 to 0.4 degrees and were not statistically significant. An electronic pendulum inclinometer, the Ortho Ranger, was compared with the universal goniometer with mixed results. Greene and Wolf[22] found a significant difference between instruments for wrist extension and ulnar deviation.

Several studies have examined construct validity between impairment measures, such as wrist ROM, and ratings of functional limitation or disability. A review of 32 published wrist outcome instruments noted that ROM was the most frequently included variable, present in 82% of the outcome instruments.[83] Several studies that examined a relationship between reduced wrist ROM and functional outcome scores are discussed below.

The effect of reduced wrist motion in the plane of flexion and extension on Disabilities of the Arm, Shoulder and Hand (DASH) scores was studied by De Smet[84] in 205 patients who had undergone various wrist operations. This functional outcome measure had a significant but weak correlation ($r = 0.24$) with wrist flexion–extension arcs of motion (expressed as percentages of the unaffected side) when the cohort of patients with wrist arthrodeses was removed; however, the strength of the relationship increased to $r = 0.45$ when this cohort was included. The author stated that this finding showed the functional impact of complete loss of wrist motion versus restricted motion.

The relationship between wrist ROM and activity limitation, pain, and disability following wrist fractures has been examined. Tremayne and associates,[85] in a study of 20 patients with distal radius fractures, found strong, significant correlations ($r = -0.51$ to -0.76) between grip strength and tasks limitations measured with the Jebsen Test of Hand Function (JTHF) test, and weaker correlations ($r = -0.17$ to -0.55) between wrist extension ROM and task limitations in the JTHF. In a subset of 11 patients with Colles type fractures, there were significant correlations ($r = -0.74$ to -0.84) between wrist extension ROM and limitation during three of seven tasks (turning cards, stimulated feeding, and lifting large light objects) included in the JTHF.

In a study of 120 patients with distal radius fractures, MacDermid and coworkers[86] found that higher patient-rated pain and disability scores 6 months postinjury (6-month Patient-Rated Wrist Evaluation [PRWE] scores) were moderately associated ($r = -0.41$) with lower composite ROM scores. Composite ROM scores were based on wrist flexion, extension, ulnar and radial deviation, supination, pronation, and finger flexion.

Karnezis and Fragkiadakis,[87] in a study of 25 patients recovering from distal radial fractures, reported correlations between the "Function Score" of the PRWE score and grip strength ($r = 0.80$), wrist extension ROM ($r = 0.78$), pronation ($r = 0.70$), supination ($r = 0.63$), and wrist flexion ROM ($r = 0.62$). They concluded that grip strength, followed by wrist extension and forearm pronation were the most sensitive clinical indicators of return of wrist function. In another report of 31 patients recovering from distal radial fracture, the same authors noted that flexion–extension and pronation–supination arcs of motion (expressed as percentages of the unaffected side) were not significantly associated with total PRWE scores in a multiple regression model that included grip strength, age, gender, presence of high-energy injury, and intra-articular fracture.[88] The possibility that some of the variables included in the regression model may be inadvertent markers for diminished ROM values may have affected the findings.

REFERENCES

1. Standring, S (ed): Gray's Anatomy, ed 41. Elsevier Churchill Livingston, Philadelphia, 2016
2. Austin, NM: The Wrist and Hand Complex. In Levangie, PK, and Norkin, CC (eds): Joint Structure and Function: A Comprehensive Analysis, ed 5. FA Davis, Philadelphia, 2011.
3. Kaltenborn, FM: Manual Mobilization of the Extremity Joints, ed 7. Olaf Norlis Bokhandel, Oslo, 2011.
4. Neumann, DA: Kinesiology of the Musculoskeletal System: Foundations for Physical Rehabilitation, ed 2. Mosby, St Louis, 2009.
5. Sarrafian, SH, Melamed, JL, and Goshgarian, GM: Study of wrist motion in flexion and extension. Clin Orthop 126:153, 1977.
6. Youm, Y, et al: Kinematics of the wrist: I. An experimental study of radial-ulnar deviation and flexion-extension. J Bone Joint Surg Am 60:423, 1978.
7. Werner, SL, and Plancher, KD: Biomechanics of wrist injuries in sports. Clin Sports Med 17:407, 1998.
8. Ritt, M, et al: Rotational stability of the carpus relative to the forearm. J Hand Surg Am 20:305, 1995.
9. Camus, EJ, et al: Kinematics of the wrist using 2D and 3D analysis: Biomechanical and clinical deductions. Surg Radiol Anat 26:399, 2004.
10. Franko, OI, et al: Validation of an objective device for assessing circumductive wrist motion. J Hand Surg Am 33(8):1293, 2008.
11. Li, ZM, et al: Coupling between wrist flexion-extension and radial-ulnar deviation. Clin Biomech 20:177, 2005.
12. Kisner, C, and Colby, LA: Therapeutic Exercise: Foundations and Techniques, ed 6. FA Davis, Philadelphia, 2012.
13. Kapandji, IA, and Kandel, MJ: The Physiology of the Joints, Vol 1, ed 5. Churchill-Livingstone, Edinburgh, 1997
14. Kobayashi, M, et al: Normal kinematics of carpal bones: A three-dimensional analysis of carpal bones relative to the radius. J Biomech 30:787, 1997.
15. Cyriax, JH, and Cyriax, PJ: Illustrated Manual of Orthopaedic Medicine. Butterworths, London, 1983.
16. LaStayo, PC, and Wheeler, DL: Reliability of passive wrist flexion and extension measurements: A multicenter study. Phys Ther 74:162, 1994
17. Carter, TI, et al: Accuracy and reliability of three different techniques for manual goniometry for wrist motion: A cadaveric study. J Hand Surg Am 34:1422, 2009.
18. American Academy of Orthopaedic Surgeons: Joint Motion: Methods of Measuring and Recording. AAOS, Chicago, 1965.
19. Greene, WB, and Heckman, JD (eds): The Clinical Measurement of Joint Motion. American Academy of Orthopaedic Surgeons, Rosemont, IL, 1994.
20. Cocchiarella, L, and Andersson, GBJ (eds): American Medical Association: Guides to the Evaluation of Permanent Impairment, ed 5. AMA, Chicago, 2001.
21. Boone, DC, and Azen, SP: Normal range of motion in male subjects. J Bone Joint Surg Am 61:756, 1979.
22. Greene, BL, and Wolf, SL: Upper extremity joint movement: Comparison of two measurement devices. Arch Phys Med Rehabil 70:288, 1989.
23. Ryu, J, et al: Functional ranges of motion of the wrist joint. J Hand Surg Am 16:409, 1991.
24. Solgaard, S, et al: Reproducibility of goniometry of the wrist. Scand J Rehabil Med 18:5, 1986.
25. Solveborn, SA, and Olerud, C: Radial epicondylalgia (tennis elbow): Measurement of range of motion of the wrist and the elbow. J Orthop Sports Phys Ther 23:251, 1996.
26. Stubbs, NB, Fernandez, JE, and Glenn, WM: Normative data on joint ranges of motion of 25- to 54-year-old males. Int J Ind Ergon 12:265, 1993.
27. Gunal, I, et al: Normal range of motion of the joints of the upper extremity in male subjects, with special reference to side. J Bone Joint Surg Am 78:1401, 1996.
28. Macedo, LG, and Magee, DJ: Effects of age on passive range of motion of selected peripheral joints in healthy adult females. Physiother Theory Pract 25:145, 2009.
29. Klum, M, et al: Normative data on wrist function. J Hand Surg Am 37:2050, 2012.
30. Wanatabe, H, et al: The range of joint motions of the extremities in healthy Japanese people: The difference according to age. Nippon Seikeigeka Gakkai Zasshi 53:275, 1979. (Cited in Walker, JM: Musculoskeletal development: A review. Phys Ther 71:878, 1991.)
31. Boone, DC: Techniques of measurement of joint motion. (Unpublished supplement to Boone, DC, and Azen, SP: Normal range of motion in male subjects. J Bone Joint Surg Am 61:756, 1979.)
32. Walker, JM, et al: Active mobility of the extremities in older subjects. Phys Ther 64:919, 1984.
33. Chaparro, A, et al: Range of motion of the wrist: Implications for designing computer input devices for the elderly. Disabil Rehabil 22:633, 2000.
34. Kalscheur, JA, et al: Gender differences in range of motion in older adults. Phys Occup Ther Geriatr 22:77, 2003.
35. Hewitt, D: The range of active motion at the wrist of women. J Bone Joint Surg Br 26:775, 1928.
36. Allander, E, et al: Normal range of joint movements in shoulder, hip, wrist and thumb with special reference to side: A comparison between two populations. Int J Epidemiol 3:253, 1974.
37. Bell, RD, and Hoshizaki, TB: Relationships of age and sex with range of motion of seventeen joint actions in humans. Can J Appl Sport Sci 6:202, 1981.
38. Kalscheur, JA, et al: Range of motion in older women. Phys Occup Ther Geriatr 16:77, 1999
39. Cobe, HM: The range of active motion of the wrist of white adults. J Bone Joint Surg Br 26:763, 1928.
40. Chang, DE, Buschbacher, LP, and Edlich, RF: Limited joint mobility in power lifters. Am J Sports Med 16:280, 1988.
41. Macedo, LG, and Magee, DJ: Differences in range of motion between dominant and nondominant sides of upper and lower extremities. J Manipulative Physiol Ther 31:577, 2008.
42. Spilman, HW, and Pinkston, D: Relation of test positions to radial and ulnar deviation. Phys Ther 49:837, 1969.
43. Marshall, MM, Morzall, JR, and Shealy, JE: The effects of complex wrist and forearm posture on wrist range of motion. Hum Factors 41:205, 1999.
44. Li, ZM, et al: Coupling between wrist flexion–extension and radial–ulnar deviation. Clin Biomech 20:177, 2005.
45. Brumfield, RH, and Champoux, JA: A biomechanical study of normal functional wrist motion. Clin Orthop 187:23, 1984.
46. Palmer, AK, et al: Functional wrist motion: A biomechanical study. J Hand Surg Am 10:39, 1985.
47. Safaee-Rad, R, et al: Normal functional range of motion of upper limb joints during performance of three feeding tasks. Arch Phys Med Rehabil 71:505, 1990.
48. Cooper, JE, et al: Elbow joint restriction: Effect on functional upper limb motion during performance of three feeding tasks. Arch Phys Med Rehabil 74:805, 1993.
49. Aizawa, J, et al: Three-dimensional motion of the upper extremity joints during various activities of daily living. J Biomech 43:2915, 2010.
50. Romilly, DP, et al: A functional task analysis and motion simulation for the development of a powered upper-limb orthosis. IEEE Trans Neural Syst Rehabil Eng 2:119, 1994.
51. van Andel, DJ, et al: Complete 3D kinematics of upper extremity functional tasks. Gait Posture 27:120, 2007. doi:10.1016/j.goitpost.2007.03.002.
52. Veeger, DHEJ, et al: Wrist motion in handrim wheelchair propulsion. J Rehabil Res Dev 35:305, 1998
53. Boninger, ML, et al: Wrist biomechanics during two speeds of wheelchair propulsion: An analysis using a local coordinate system. Arch Phys Med Rehabil 78:364, 1997.
54. Wei, S, et al: Wrist kinematic characterization of wheelchair propulsion in various seating positions: Implication to wrist pain. Clin Biomech 18:S46, 2003.
55. Estill, CF, and Kroemer, KH: Evaluation of supermarket bagging using a wrist motion monitor. Hum Factors 40:624, 1998.
56. Marras, WS, et al: Quantification of wrist motion during scanning. Hum Factors 37:412, 1995.
57. Wagner, CH: The pianist's hand: Anthropometry and biomechanics. Ergonomics 31:97, 1988.
58. Burgess-Limerick, R, et al: Wrist posture during computer pointing device use. Clin Biomech 14:280, 1999.
59. Marras, WS, and Schoenmarklin, RW: Wrist motions in industry. Ergonomics 36:341, 1995.
60. Simoneau, GG, Marklin, RW, and Monroe, JF: Wrist and forearm postures of users of conventional computer keyboards. Hum Factors 41:413, 1999.
61. Simoneau, GG, Marklin, RW, and Berman, JE: Effect of computer keyboard slope on wrist position and forearm electromyography of typist without musculoskeletal disorders. Phys Ther 83:816, 2003.
62. Hansson, GA, et al: Physical workload in various types of work: Part I. Wrist and forearm. Int J Ind Ergon 39:221, 2009.

63. Balogh, I, et al: Precision of measurements of physical workload during standardized manual handling part III: Goniometry of the wrists. J Electromyogr Kinesiol 19:1005, 2009.
64. Ohinishi, N, et al: Analysis of Wrist Motion During Basketball Shooting. In Nakamura, RL, Linscheid, RL, and Miura, T (eds): Wrist Disorder: Current Concepts and Challenges. New York, Springer-Verlag, 1992.
65. Bernard, BP (ed): Musculoskeletal Disorders and Workplace Factors. National Institute of Occupational Safety and Health, Cincinnati, 1997.
66. Armstrong, TJ, et al: Ergonomic considerations in hand and wrist tendinitis. J Hand Surg Am 12:830, 1982.
67. Nelson, DL: Functional wrist motion. Hand Clin 13:83, 1997.
68. Murgia, A, Kyberd, P, and Barnhill, T: The use of kinematic and parametric information to highlight lack of movement and compensation in the upper extremities during activities of daily living. Gait Posture 31:300, 2010.
69. Franko, OI, Zurakowshi, D, and Day, CS: Functional disability of the wrist: Direct correlation with decreased wrist motion. J Hand Surg Am 33:485, 2008.
70. Van de Pol, van Trijffel, E, and Lucas, C: Inter-rater reliability for measurement of passive physiological range of motion of upper extremity joints is better if instruments are used: A systematic review. Aust J Physiother 56:7, 2010.
71. Bird, HA, and Stowe, J: The wrist. Clin Rheum Dis 8:559, 1982.
72. Boone, DC, et al: Reliability of goniometric measurements. Phys Ther 58:1355, 1978
73. Bovens, AMPM, et al: Variability and reliability of joint measurements. Am J Sports Med 18:58, 1990.
74. Low, JL: The reliability of joint measurement. Physiotherapy 62:227, 1976.
75. Edgar, D, et al: Goniometry and linear assessment to monitor movement outcomes: Are they reliable tools in burn survivors? Burns 35:58, 2008.
76. Horger, MM: The reliability of goniometric measurements of active and passive wrist motions. Am J Occup Ther 44:342, 1990.
77. Hellebrandt, FA, Duvall, EN, and Moore, ML: The measurement of joint motion. Part III: Reliability of goniometry. Phys Ther Rev 29:302, 1949.
78. Flower, KR: Invited commentary. Phys Ther 74:174, 1994.
79. Pandya, S, et al: Reliability of goniometric measurements in patients with Duchenne muscular dystrophy. Phys Ther 65:1339, 1985.
80. de Jong, LD, et al: Repeated measurements of arm joint passive range of motion after stroke: Interobserver reliability and sources of variation. Phys Ther 92:1027, 2012
81. Geertzen, JHB, et al: Variation in measurements of range of motion: A study in reflex sympathetic dystrophy patients. Clin Rehabil 12:254, 1998.
82. Kim, TS, et al: A study on the measurement of wrist motion range using the iPhone 4 gyroscope application. Ann Plast Surg 0:1, 2013.
83. Bialocerkowski, AE, et al: A systematic review of the content and quality of wrist outcome instruments. Int J Qual Health Care 12:149, 2000.
84. De Smet, L: Does restricted wrist motion influence the disability of the upper limb? Acta Orthop Belg 73:446, 2007.
85. Tremayne, A, et al: Correlation of impairment and activity limitation after wrist fracture. Physiother Res Int 7:90, 2002.
86. MacDermid, JC, et al: Patient versus injury factors as predictors of pain and disability six months after a distal radius fracture. J Clin Epidemiol 55:849, 2002.
87. Karnezis, IA, and Fragkiadakis, EG: Objective clinical parameters and patient-rated wrist function. J Bone Joint Surg Br 85 (Suppl 1):7, 2003.
88. Karnezis, IA, and Fragkiadakis, EG: Association between objective clinical variables and patient-rated disability of the wrist. J Bone Joint Surg Br 84:967, 2002.

CHAPTER 7

The Hand

D. Joyce White, PT, DSc

Structure and Function

Fingers: Metacarpophalangeal Joints

The metacarpophalangeal (MCP) joints of the fingers are composed of the convex distal end of each metacarpal and the concave base of each proximal phalanx (Fig. 7.1). The joints are enclosed in fibrous capsules (Fig. 7.2).

Ligamentous support of the MCP joints is provided by the palmar, collateral, and deep transverse metacarpal ligaments. The anterior portion of each capsule has a fibrocartilaginous thickening called the palmar plate or palmar ligament, which is firmly attached to the proximal phalanx and loosely attached to the metacarpals.[1,2] The palmar ligaments also blend with the deep transverse metacarpal ligament that connects the MCP joints of the second through fifth digits (Fig. 7.2). The two collateral ligaments on either side of each MCP joint have a strong, cord-like part that attaches between the metacarpal and proximal phalange, running in a distal and slightly palmar direction (Fig. 7.3). A fan-shaped accessory part of the collateral ligaments connects with the palmar ligaments.[1–3]

Osteokinematics

The MCP joints are biaxial condyloid joints that have 2 degrees of freedom, allowing flexion–extension in the sagittal plane and abduction–adduction in the frontal plane. Abduction–adduction is possible with the MCP joints positioned in extension, but it is limited with the MCP joints in flexion because of

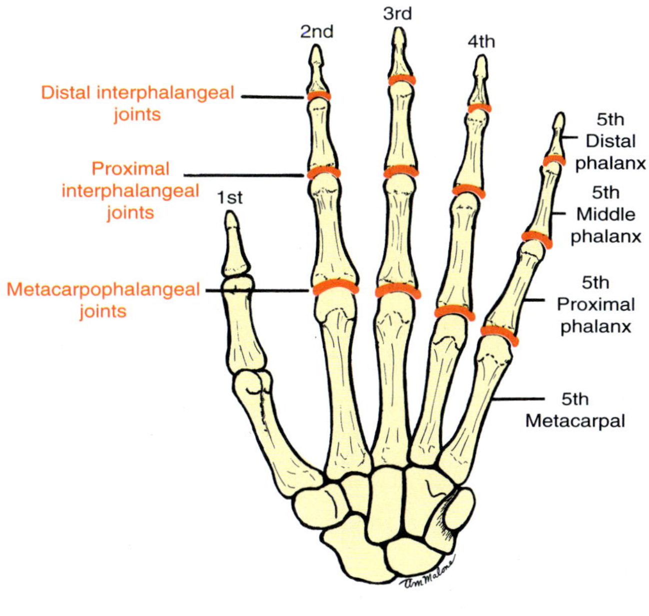

FIGURE 7.1 An anterior (palmar) view of the hand showing metacarpophalangeal, proximal interphalangeal, and distal interphalangeal joints.

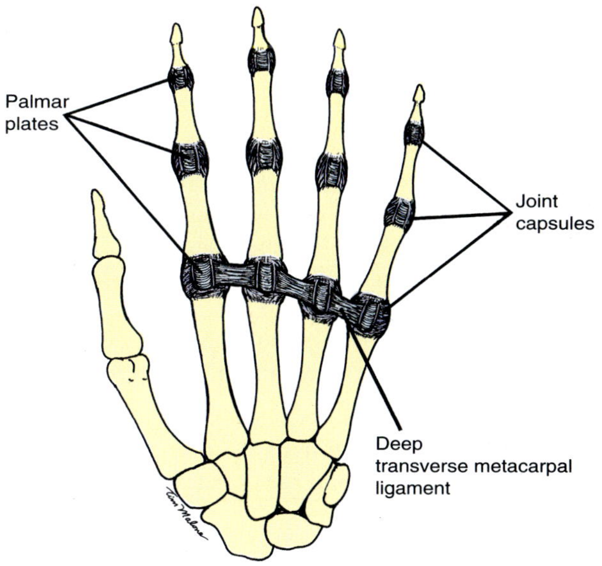

FIGURE 7.2 An anterior (palmar) view of the hand showing joint capsules and palmar plates of the metacarpophalangeal, proximal interphalangeal, and distal interphalangeal joints and the deep transverse metacarpal ligament.

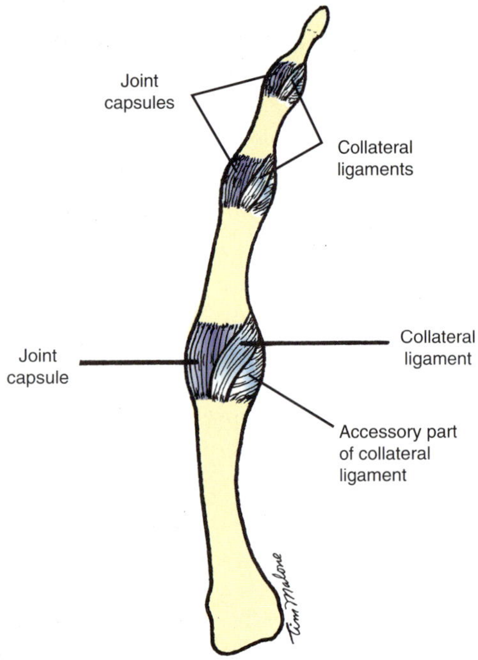

FIGURE 7.3 A lateral view of a finger showing joint capsules and collateral ligaments of the metacarpophalangeal, proximal interphalangeal, and distal interphalangeal joints. The collateral ligaments have two parts: the major cord-like part that is more lateral and a fan-shaped accessory part that is more palmar.

tightening of the cord part of the collateral ligaments, and because of contact between the flatter, almost bicondylar shape of the metacarpal head and the proximal phalange.[1,3] This contact between the metacarpal head and proximal phalanges occurs by about 70 degrees of MCP flexion.[3] A small amount of passive axial rotation is reported at the MCP joints,[2–5] but this motion is not usually measured in the clinical setting.

Arthrokinematics

The concave base of the phalanx slides and rolls on the convex head of the metacarpal in the same direction as movement of the shaft of the phalanx.[3,6] During flexion, the base of the phalanx slides and rolls anteriorly toward the palm, whereas during extension the base of the phalanx slides and rolls dorsally. In abduction, the base of the phalanx slides and rolls in the same direction as the movement of the finger.

Capsular Pattern

Cyriax and Cyriax[7] report that the capsular pattern is an equal restriction of flexion and extension. Kaltenborn[6] notes that all motions are restricted with more limitation in flexion.

Fingers: Proximal Interphalangeal and Distal Interphalangeal Joints

The structure of both the proximal interphalangeal (PIP) and the distal interphalangeal (DIP) joints is very similar (see Fig. 7.1). Each phalanx has a concave base and a convex head. The joint surfaces include the head of the more proximal phalanx and the base of the adjacent, more distal phalanx. Each joint is supported by a joint capsule, a palmar plate, and two collateral ligaments (see Figs. 7.2 and 7.3).[1–3]

Osteokinematics

The PIP and DIP joints of the fingers are classified as synovial hinge joints with 1 degree of freedom: flexion–extension in the sagittal plane.

Arthrokinematics

Motion of the joint surfaces includes a sliding and rolling of the concave base of the more distal phalanx on the convex head of the proximal phalanx. Sliding and rolling of the base of the moving phalanx occurs in the same direction as the movement of the shaft.[3,6] For example, in PIP flexion the base of the middle phalanx slides and rolls toward the palm. In PIP extension, the base of the middle phalanx slides and rolls toward the dorsum of the hand.

Capsular Pattern

The capsular pattern is an equal restriction of both flexion and extension, according to Cyriax and Cyriax.[7] Kaltenborn[6] notes that all motions are restricted with more limitation in flexion.

Thumb: Carpometacarpal Joint

The carpometacarpal (CMC) joint of the thumb is the articulation between the trapezium and the base of the first metacarpal (Fig. 7.4). It is also referred to as the trapeziometacarpal joint. The saddle-shaped trapezium is concave in the sagittal

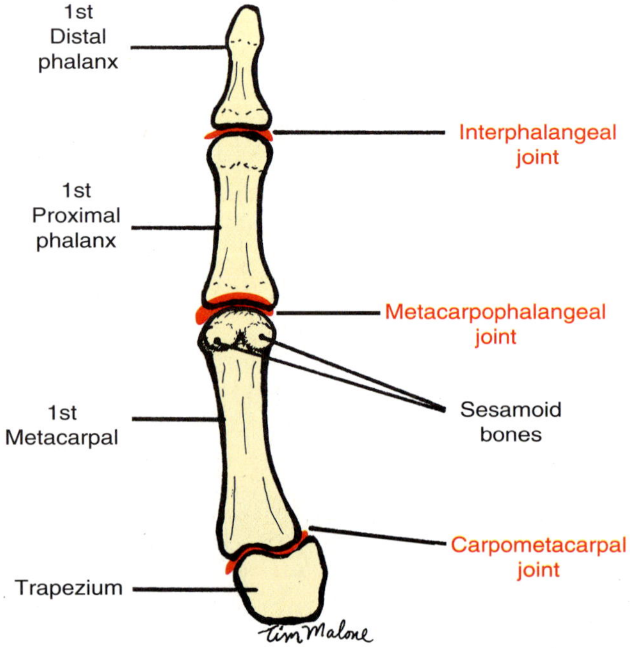

FIGURE 7.4 An anterior (palmar) view of the thumb showing carpometacarpal, metacarpophalangeal, and interphalangeal joints.

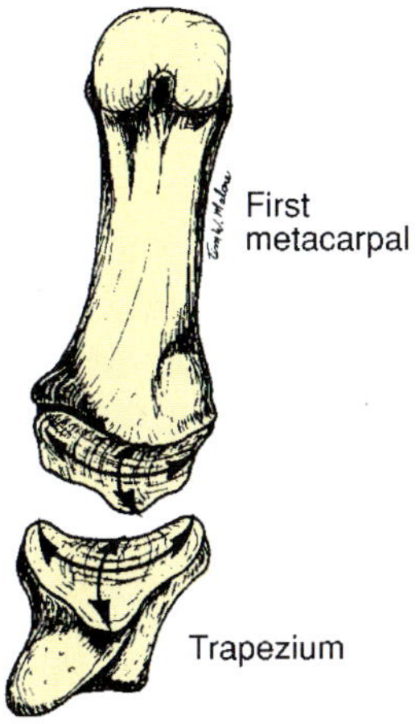

FIGURE 7.5 The saddle-shaped joint surface of the trapezium at the first carpometacarpal (CMC) joint is convex in the frontal plane (flexion–extension) and concave in the sagittal plane (abduction–adduction). The base of the metacarpal of the thumb has a shape that is reciprocal to that of the trapezium. Reproduced with permission from Levangie, PL, and Norkin, CC: Joint Structure and Function: A Comprehensive Analysis, ed 4. FA Davis, Philadelphia, 2005.

plane and convex in the frontal plane (Fig. 7.5).[1,3] The base of the first metacarpal has a reciprocal shape that conforms to that of the trapezium, so that the base of the metacarpal is convex in the sagittal plane and concave in the frontal plane. The joint capsule is thick but lax and is reinforced by ligaments on the radial, ulnar, palmar, and dorsal surfaces (Fig. 7.6).[1–3]

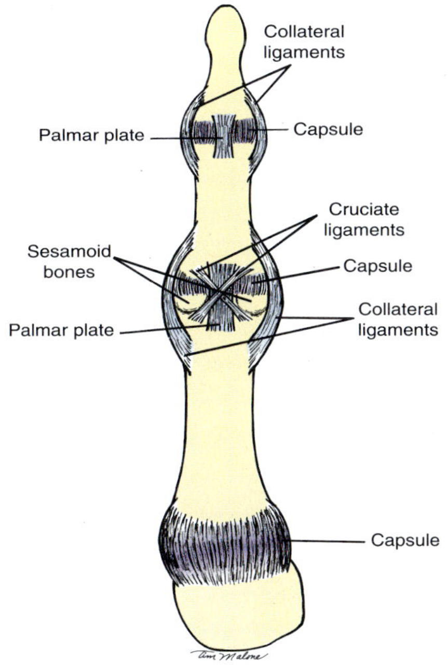

FIGURE 7.6 An anterior (palmar) view of the thumb showing joint capsules, collateral ligaments, palmar plates, and cruciate (intersesamoid) ligaments.

Osteokinematics

The first CMC joint is a saddle joint with 2 degrees of freedom: flexion–extension in the frontal plane parallel to the palm, and abduction–adduction in the sagittal plane perpendicular to the palm.[1–3] These planes of movement for the CMC joint of the thumb are at right angles to the planes of movement of the fingers because the trapezium is anterior to the other carpals, effectively positioning the palmar surface of the thumb medially.[1,8] The laxity of the joint capsule also permits some axial rotation. This rotation allows the thumb to move into position for pulp-to-pulp contact with the fingers during opposition. The sequence of motions that combines with rotation and results in opposition is as follows: abduction, flexion, medial axial rotation (pronation), and adduction.[1,3] Reposition returns the thumb to the starting position.

Arthrokinematics

The concave joint surface of the first metacarpal slides and rolls on the convex surface of the trapezium in the same direction as the metacarpal shaft to produce flexion–extension.[3,6] During flexion, the base of the metacarpal slides and rolls in an ulnar direction. During extension, the base slides and rolls in a radial direction.

To produce abduction–adduction, the convex joint surface of the first metacarpal slides on the concave portion of the trapezium in the opposite direction to the shaft of the metacarpal.[3,6] Therefore, the base of the metacarpal slides toward the dorsal surface of the hand and rolls toward the palmar surface of the hand during abduction. The base of the first metacarpal slides toward the palmar surface of the hand and rolls toward the dorsal surface of the hand during adduction.

Capsular Pattern

The capsular pattern is a limitation of abduction according to Cyriax and Cyriax.[7] Kaltenborn[6] reports limitations in abduction and extension.

Thumb: Metacarpophalangeal Joint

The MCP joint of the thumb is the articulation between the convex head of the first metacarpal and the concave base of the first proximal phalanx (see Fig. 7.4). The joint is reinforced by a joint capsule, palmar plate, two sesamoid bones on the palmar surface, two intersesamoid ligaments (cruciate ligaments), and two collateral ligaments (see Fig. 7.6).

Osteokinematics

The MCP joint is a condyloid joint with 2 degrees of freedom.[1,8] The motions permitted are flexion–extension and a minimal amount of abduction–adduction. Motions at this joint are more restricted than at the MCP joints of the fingers.

Arthrokinematics

At the MCP joint the concave base of the proximal phalanx slides and rolls on the convex head of the first metacarpal in the same direction as the shaft of the phalanx.[3,6] The base of the proximal phalanx moves toward the palmar surface of the thumb in flexion and toward the dorsal surface of the thumb in extension.

Capsular Pattern

The capsular pattern for the MCP joint is a restriction of motion in all directions, but flexion is more limited than extension.[6,7]

Thumb: Interphalangeal Joint

The interphalangeal (IP) joint of the thumb is similar in structure to the IP joints of the fingers. The head of the proximal phalanx is convex, and the base of the distal phalanx is concave (see Fig. 7.4). The joint is supported by a joint capsule, a palmar plate, and two lateral collateral ligaments (see Fig. 7.6).

Osteokinematics

The IP joint is a synovial hinge joint with 1 degree of freedom: flexion–extension.

Arthrokinematics

At the IP joint of the thumb the concave base of the distal phalanx slides and rolls on the convex head of the proximal phalanx, in the same direction as the shaft of the phalanx.[3,6] The base of the distal phalanx moves toward the palmar surface of the thumb in flexion and toward the dorsal surface of the thumb in extension.

Capsular Pattern

The capsular pattern is an equal restriction in both flexion and extension according to Cyriax and Cyriax.[7] Kaltenborn[6] notes that all motions are restricted with more limitation in flexion.

RANGE OF MOTION TESTING PROCEDURES: Fingers

Included in this section are common clinical techniques for measuring joint motions of the fingers and thumb. These techniques, which often place the goniometer on the dorsal surface of the digits, are appropriate for evaluating motions in the majority of people. Groth and Ehretsman found that dorsal placement of the goniometer was preferred by 73% of 231 surveyed therapists in the United States.[9] Similarly, Pratt and Burr, in a survey of 297 occupational therapy and physiotherapy members of the British Association of Hand Therapists in 1999–2000, found that 95% used a dorsal placement when measuring ROM at the MCP, PIP, and DIP joints of the finger.[10] However, swelling and bony deformities sometimes require that the examiner either measure these joints from the lateral aspect or create alternative evaluation techniques. Photocopies, photographs, and tracings of the hand at the beginning and end of the range of motion (ROM) may be helpful.

A summary guide of the detailed ROM measurement procedures included in this chapter is found in Appendix B. This summary information in the appendix may be helpful as a quick reference; the details of the measurement techniques with instructional photographs are presented here.

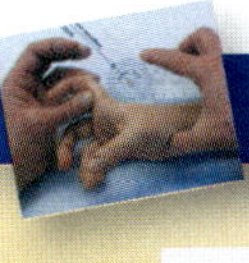

Landmarks for Testing Procedures

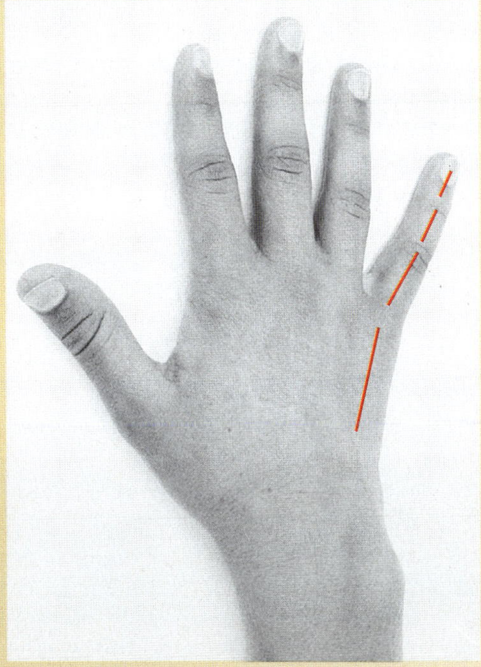

FIGURE 7.7 Posterior view of the right hand showing surface anatomy landmarks for goniometer alignment during measurement of finger range of motion.

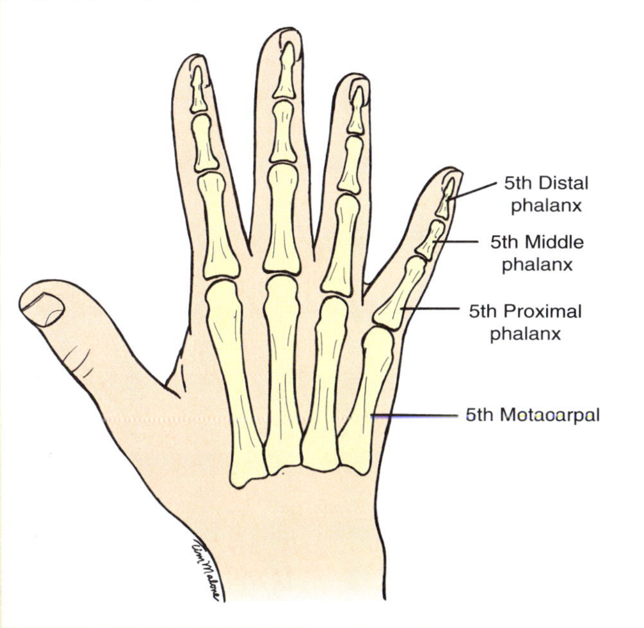

FIGURE 7.8 Posterior view of the right hand showing bony anatomical landmarks for goniometer alignment during the measurement of finger range of motion. The index, middle, ring, and little fingers each have a metacarpal and a proximal, middle, and distal phalanx.

FINGERS: METACARPOPHALANGEAL (MCP) FLEXION

Motion occurs in the sagittal plane around a medial–lateral axis. Normal ROM values for adults vary from 90 to 100 degrees. Metacarpophalangeal flexion appears to increase slightly in an ulnar direction from the index finger to the little finger. This pattern of increasing flexion ROM from the radial to the ulnar side of the hand at the MCP joints allows for a smaller diameter grip on the ulnar side of the hand, and facilitates contact between the thumb and more ulnarly placed fingers during opposition.[1,11] See Research Findings and Tables 7.1 and 7.2 for normal ROM values by age and gender.

Testing Position

Place the individual sitting, with the forearm and hand resting on a supporting surface. Place the forearm midway between pronation and supination, the wrist in 0 degrees of flexion, extension, and radial and ulnar deviation and the MCP joint in a neutral position relative to abduction and adduction. Avoid extreme flexion of the PIP and DIP joints of the finger being examined.

Stabilization

Stabilize the metacarpal to prevent wrist motion. Do not hold the MCP joints of the other fingers in extension because tension in the transverse metacarpal ligament will restrict the motion.

Testing Motion

Flex the MCP joint by pushing on the dorsal surface of the proximal phalanx, moving the finger toward the palm (Fig. 7.9). Maintain the MCP joint in a neutral position relative to abduction and adduction. The end of flexion ROM occurs when resistance to further motion is felt and attempts to overcome the resistance cause the wrist to flex.

Normal End-Feel

The end-feel may be hard because of contact between the palmar aspect of the proximal phalanx and the metacarpal, or it may be firm because of tension in the dorsal joint capsule and the collateral ligaments.

Goniometer Alignment

See Figures 7.10 and 7.11.

1. Center **fulcrum** of the goniometer over the dorsal aspect of the MCP joint.
2. Align **proximal arm** over the dorsal midline of the metacarpal.
3. Align **distal arm** over the dorsal midline of the proximal phalanx.

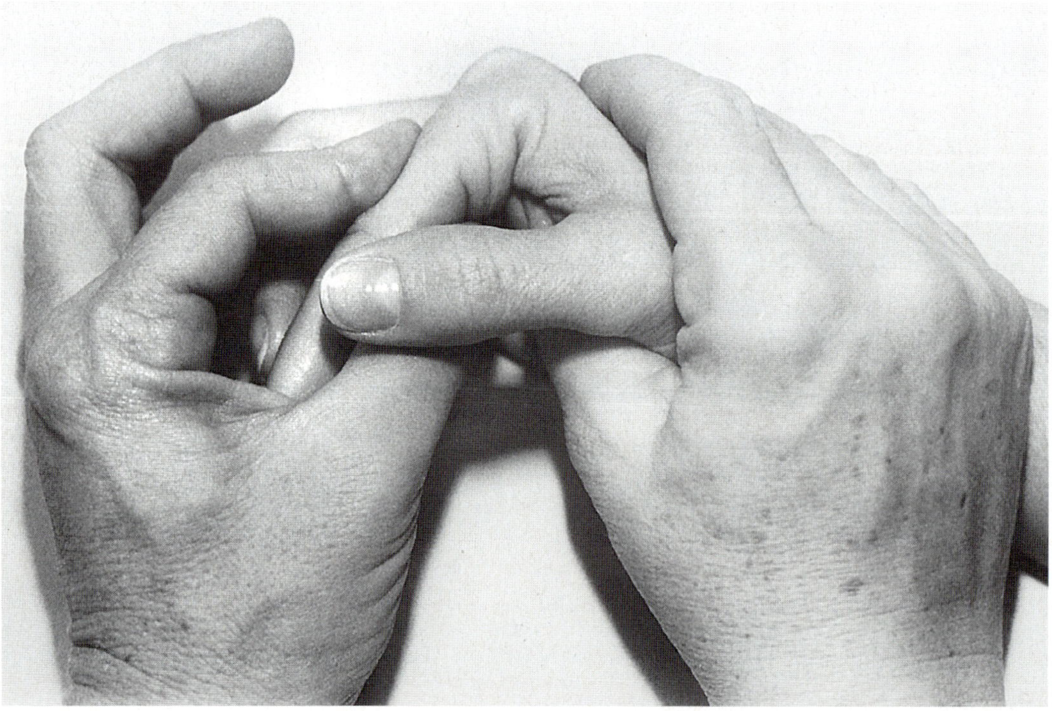

FIGURE 7.9 During flexion of the metacarpophalangeal (MCP) joint, the examiner uses one hand to stabilize the individual's metacarpal and to maintain the wrist in a neutral position. The index finger and the thumb of the examiner's other hand grasp the individual's proximal phalanx to move it into flexion.

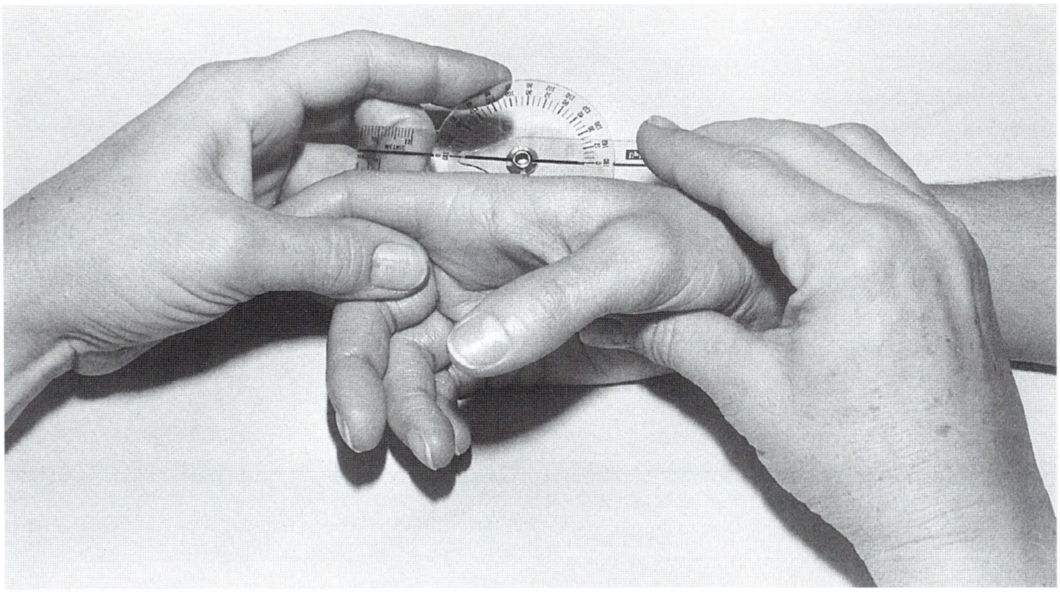

FIGURE 7.10 The alignment of the goniometer at the beginning of metacarpophalangeal (MCP) flexion range of motion. In this photograph, the examiner is using a 6-inch plastic goniometer in which the arms have been trimmed to approximately 2 inches to make it easier to align over the small joints of the hand. Most examiners use goniometers with arms that are 6 inches or shorter when measuring ROM in the hand.

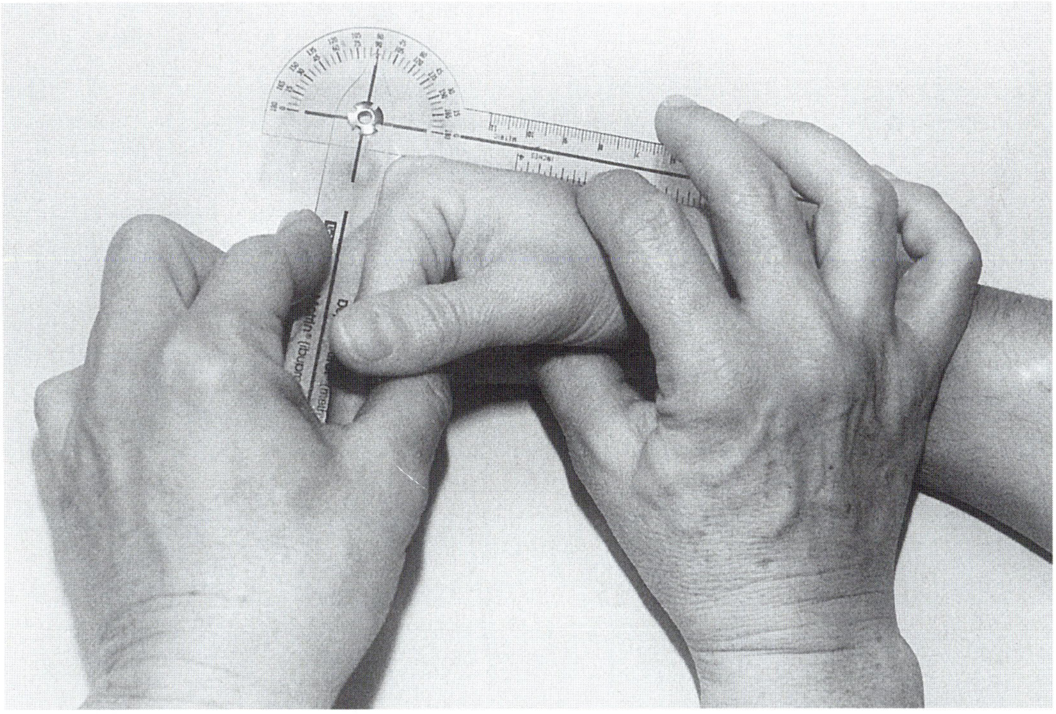

FIGURE 7.11 At the end of metacarpophalangeal (MCP) flexion range of motion, the examiner uses one hand to hold the proximal goniometer arm in alignment and to stabilize the individual's metacarpal. The examiner's other hand maintains the proximal phalanx in MCP flexion and aligns the distal goniometer arm. Note that the goniometer arms make direct contact with the dorsal surfaces of the metacarpal and proximal phalanx, causing the fulcrum of the goniometer to lie somewhat distal and dorsal to the MCP joint.

FINGERS: METACARPOPHALANGEAL EXTENSION

Motion occurs in the sagittal plane around a medial–lateral axis. Normal passive ROM values for adults range from about 20 to 45 degrees. Passive MCP extension ROM is greater than active extension. The little finger is reported to have the greatest amount of MCP extension,[12,13] whereas others report that extension ROM at the MCP joints is equal across all fingers.[11] See Research Findings and Tables 7.1 and 7.2 for normal ROM values by age, gender, and active or passive motion.

Testing Position

Position the individual sitting, with the forearm and hand resting on a supporting surface. Place the forearm midway between pronation and supination; the wrist in 0 degrees of flexion, extension, and radial and ulnar deviation; and the MCP joint in a neutral position relative to abduction and adduction. Avoid extension or extreme flexion of the PIP and DIP joints of the finger being tested. (If the PIP and DIP joints are positioned in extension, tension in the flexor digitorum superficialis and profundus muscles may restrict the motion. If the PIP and DIP joints are positioned in full flexion, tension in the lumbrical, dorsal interossei, and palmar interossei muscles will restrict the motion.)

Stabilization

Stabilize the metacarpal to prevent wrist motion. Do not hold the MCP joints of the other fingers in full flexion because tension in the transverse metacarpal ligament will restrict the motion.

Testing Motion

Extend the MCP joint by pushing on the palmar surface of the proximal phalanx, moving the finger away from the palm (Fig. 7.12). Maintain the MCP joint in a neutral position relative to abduction and adduction. The end of extension ROM occurs when resistance to further motion is felt and attempts to overcome resistance cause the wrist to extend.

Normal End-Feel

The end-feel is firm because of tension in the palmar joint capsule and in the palmar plate.

Goniometer Alignment: Dorsal Aspect

See Figures 7.13 and 7.14 for alignment of the goniometer over the dorsal aspect of the fingers.

1. Center **fulcrum** of the goniometer over the dorsal aspect of the MCP joint.
2. Align **proximal arm** over the dorsal midline of the metacarpal.
3. Align **distal arm** over the dorsal midline of the proximal phalanx.

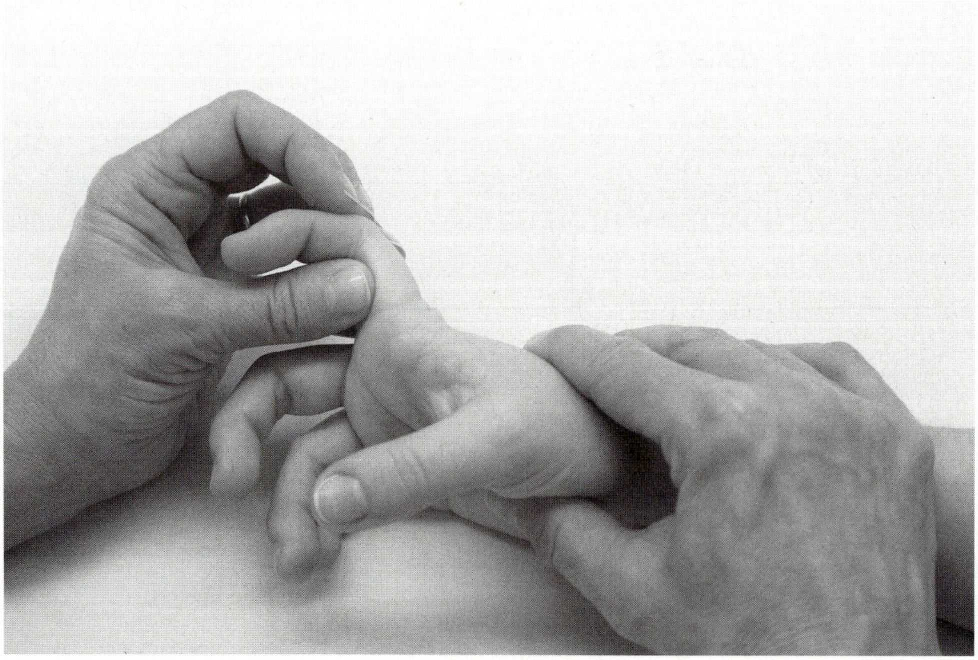

FIGURE 7.12 During metacarpophalangeal (MCP) extension, the examiner uses her index finger and thumb to grasp the individual's proximal phalanx and to move the phalanx dorsally. The examiner's other hand maintains the individual's wrist in the neutral position, stabilizing the metacarpal.

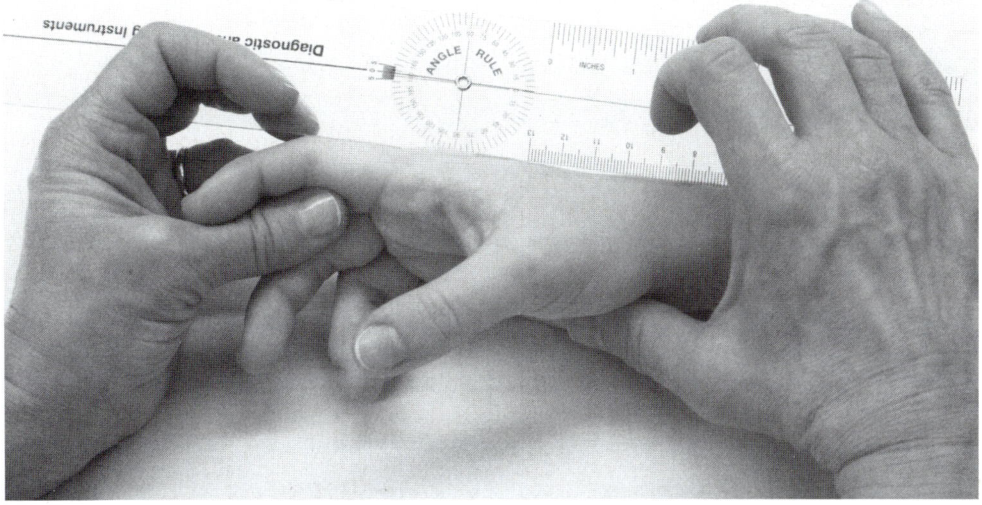

FIGURE 7.13 A full-circle, 6-inch plastic goniometer is being used to measure the beginning range of motion for metacarpophalangeal (MCP) extension. The proximal arm of the goniometer is slightly longer than necessary for optimal alignment. If a goniometer of the right size is not available, the examiner can cut the arms of a plastic model to a suitable length.

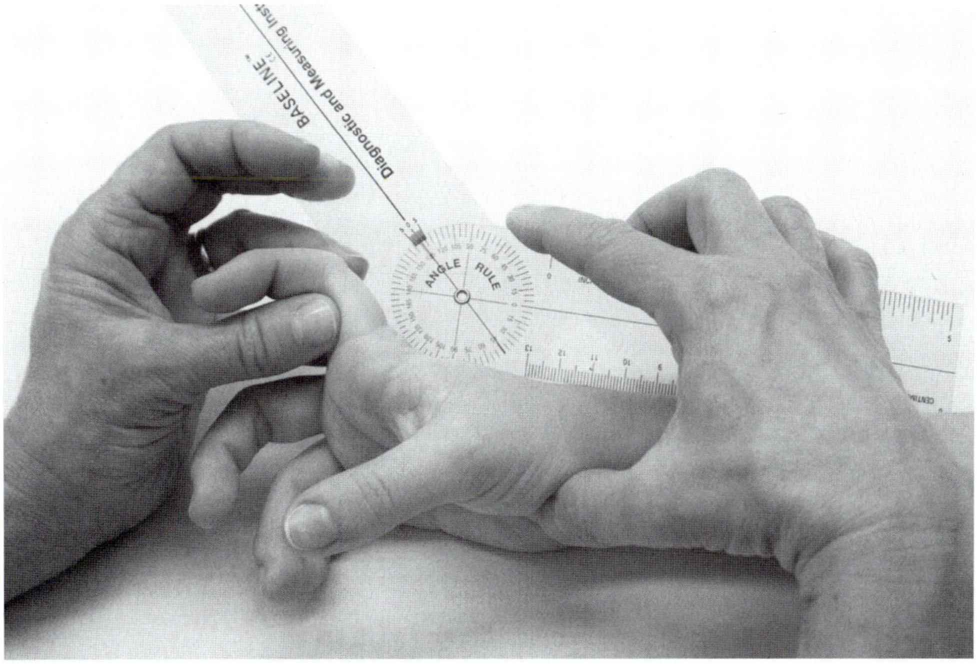

FIGURE 7.14 The alignment of the goniometer at the end of metacarpophalangeal (MCP) extension. The body of the goniometer is aligned over the dorsal aspect of the MCP joint, whereas the goniometer arms are aligned over the dorsal aspect of the metacarpal and proximal phalanx.

Alternative Goniometer Alignment: Palmar Aspect

See Figure 7.15 for alignment of the goniometer over the palmar aspect of the finger. This alignment should not be used if swelling or hypertrophy is present in the palm of the hand.

1. Center **fulcrum** of the goniometer over the palmar aspect of the MCP joint.
2. Align **proximal arm** over the palmar midline of the metacarpal.
3. Align **distal arm** over the palmar midline of the proximal phalanx.

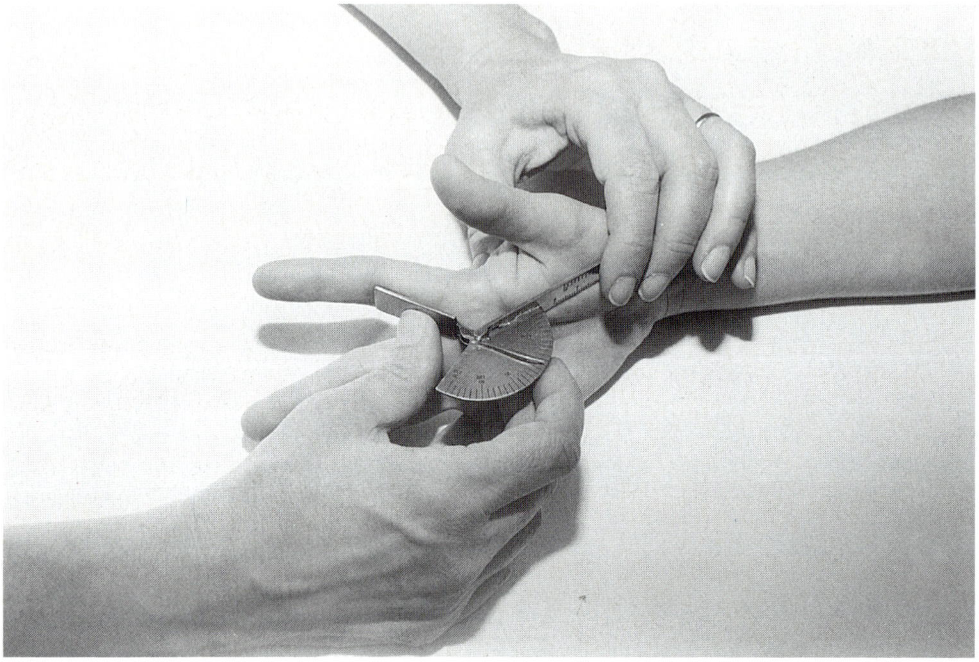

FIGURE 7.15 An alternative alignment of a finger goniometer over the palmar aspect of the proximal phalanx, the metacarpophalangeal joint, and the metacarpal. The shorter goniometer arm must be used over the palmar aspect of the proximal phalanx so that the proximal interphalangeal and distal interphalangeal joints are allowed to relax in flexion.

FINGERS: METACARPOPHALANGEAL ABDUCTION

Motion occurs in the frontal plane around an anterior–posterior axis. No research studies to establish normal abduction ROM values measured with a universal goniometer at the MCP joint have been noted. However, one source states that maximal range of abduction–adduction is 25 degrees.[2] Some values have been reported for the maximal angles between adjacent fingers using tracings[13] and between fingers and the midline of the hand using a gravity-based goniometer.[14] The index and little fingers are generally noted to have more MCP abduction motion than the middle and ring fingers.[1,2]

Testing Position

Position the individual sitting, with the forearm and hand resting on a supporting surface. Place the wrist in 0 degrees of flexion, extension, and radial and ulnar deviation; the forearm in full pronation so that the palm of the hand faces the ground; and the MCP joint in 0 degrees of flexion and extension.

Stabilization

Stabilize the metacarpal to prevent wrist motions.

Testing Motion

Abduct the MCP joint by pushing on the medial surface of the proximal phalanx, moving the finger away from the midline of the hand (Fig. 7.16). Maintain the MCP joint in a neutral position relative to flexion and extension. The end of abduction ROM occurs when resistance to further motion is felt and attempts to overcome the resistance cause the wrist to move into radial or ulnar deviation.

Normal End-Feel

The end-feel is firm because of tension in the collateral ligaments of the MCP joints, the fascia of the web space between the fingers, and the palmar interossei muscles.

Goniometer Alignment

See Figures 7.17 and 7.18.

1. Center **fulcrum** of the goniometer over the dorsal aspect of the MCP joint.
2. Align **proximal arm** over the dorsal midline of the metacarpal.
3. Align **distal arm** over the dorsal midline of the proximal phalanx.

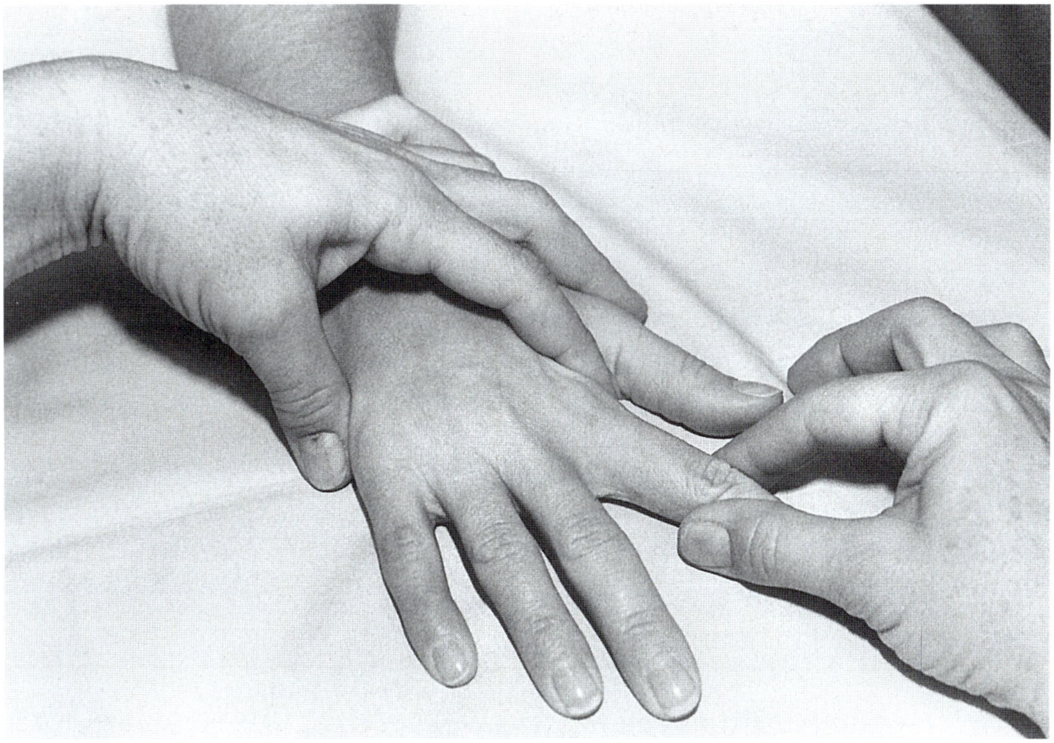

FIGURE 7.16 During metacarpophalangeal (MCP) abduction, the examiner uses the index finger of one hand to press against the individual's metacarpal and prevent radial deviation at the wrist. With the other index finger and thumb holding the distal end of the proximal phalanx, the examiner moves the individual's second MCP joint into abduction.

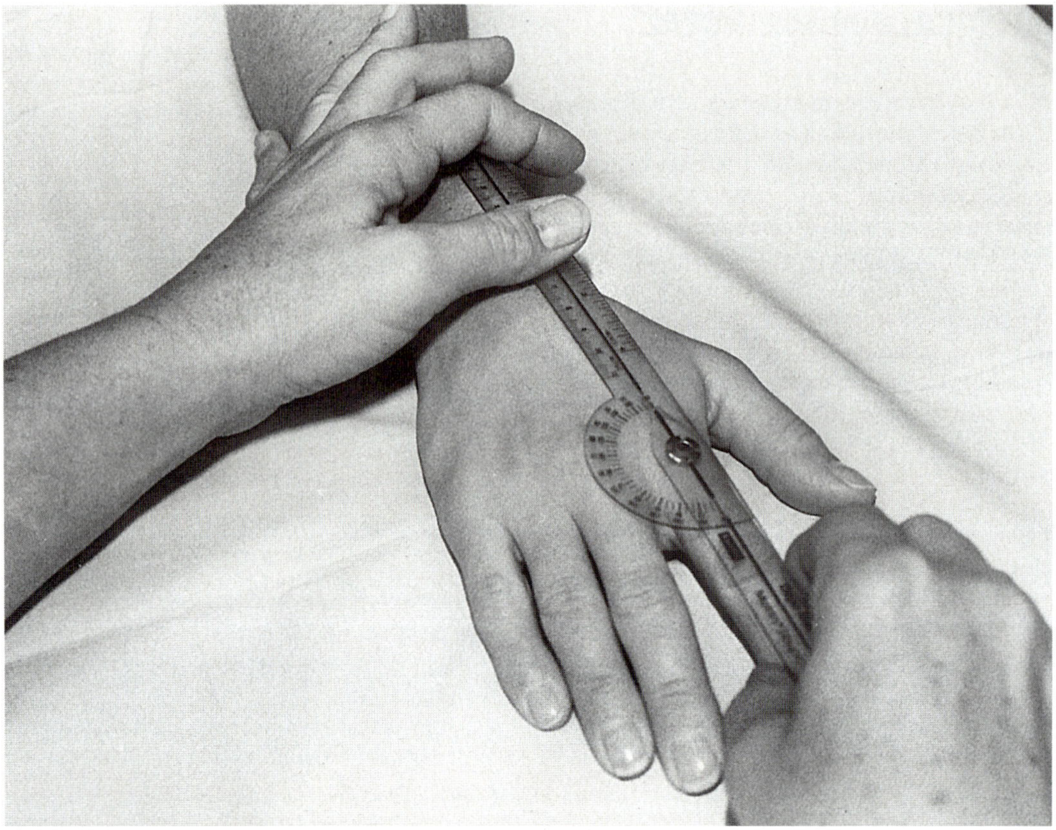

FIGURE 7.17 The alignment of the goniometer at the beginning of metacarpophalangeal abduction range of motion.

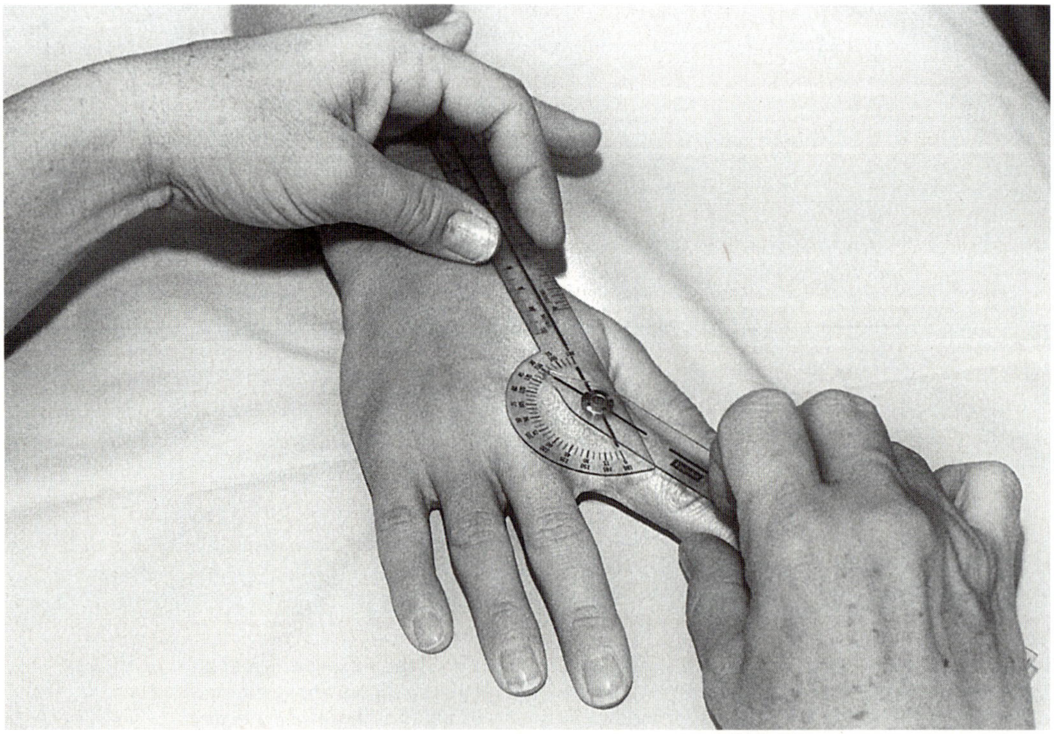

FIGURE 7.18 At the end of metacarpophalangeal (MCP) abduction, the examiner aligns the arms of the goniometer with the dorsal midline of the metacarpal and proximal phalanx rather than with the contour of the hand and finger.

FINGERS: METACARPOPHALANGEAL ADDUCTION

Motion occurs in the frontal plane around an anterior–posterior axis. Metacarpophalangeal adduction is not usually measured and recorded separately from MCP abduction, because it is the return from full abduction to the 0 starting position. There is very little adduction ROM beyond the 0 starting position. At the end of adduction ROM the medial–lateral aspects of the fingers are in contact with the adjoining fingers. No sources were found for normal MCP adduction ROM values. The testing position, stabilization, and goniometer alignment are similar to measuring MCP abduction.

FINGERS: PROXIMAL INTERPHALANGEAL FLEXION

Motion occurs in the sagittal plane around a medial–lateral axis. Normal ROM values for adults range from 100 to 110 degrees. Proximal interphalangeal flexion ROM is similar for all the fingers.[11] See Research Findings and Tables 7.1 and 7.2 for normal ROM values.

Testing Position

Place the individual sitting, with the forearm and hand resting on a supporting surface. Position the forearm in 0 degrees of supination and pronation; the wrist in 0 degrees of flexion, extension, and radial and ulnar deviation; and the MCP joint in 0 degrees of flexion, extension, abduction, and adduction. (If the wrist and MCP joints are positioned in full flexion, tension in the extensor digitorum communis, extensor indicis, or extensor digiti minimi muscles will restrict the motion. If the MCP joint is positioned in full extension, tension in the lumbrical, dorsal interossei, and palmar interossei muscles will restrict the motion.)

Stabilization

Stabilize the proximal phalanx to prevent motion of the MCP joint.

Testing Motion

Flex the PIP joint by pushing on the dorsal surface of the middle phalanx, moving the finger toward the palm (Fig. 7.19). The end of flexion ROM occurs when resistance to further motion is felt and attempts to overcome the resistance cause the MCP joint to flex.

Normal End-Feel

Usually, the end-feel is hard because of contact between the palmar aspect of the middle phalanx and the proximal phalanx. In some individuals, the end-feel may be soft because of compression of soft tissue between the palmar aspect of the middle and proximal phalanges. In other individuals, the end-feel may be firm because of tension in the dorsal joint capsule and the collateral ligaments.

Goniometer Alignment

See Figures 7.20 and 7.21.

1. Center **fulcrum** of the goniometer over the dorsal aspect of the PIP joint.
2. Align **proximal arm** over the dorsal midline of the proximal phalanx.
3. Align **distal arm** over the dorsal midline of the middle phalanx.

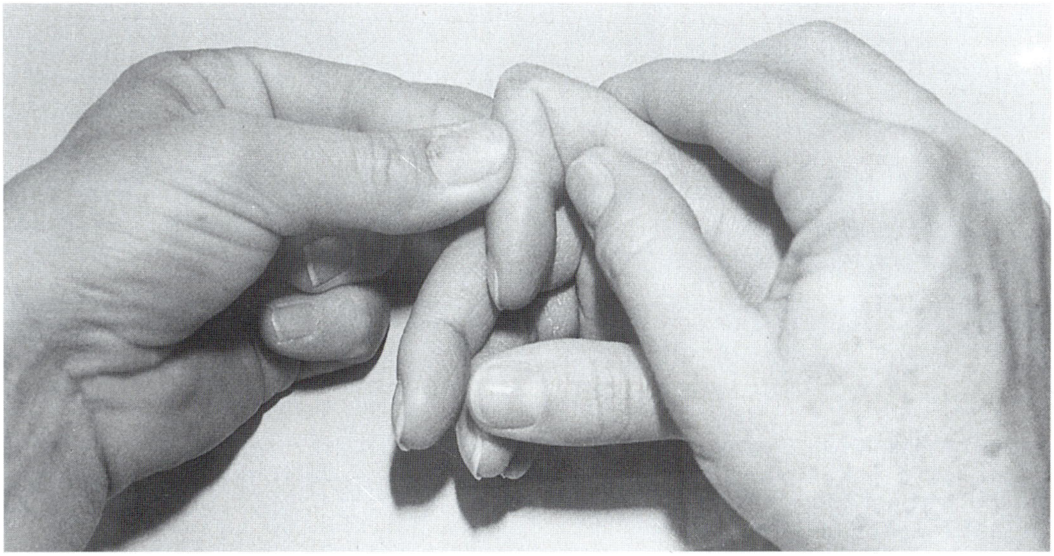

FIGURE 7.19 During proximal interphalangeal (PIP) flexion, the examiner stabilizes the individual's proximal phalanx with her thumb and index finger. The examiner uses her other thumb and index finger to move the individual's PIP joint into full flexion.

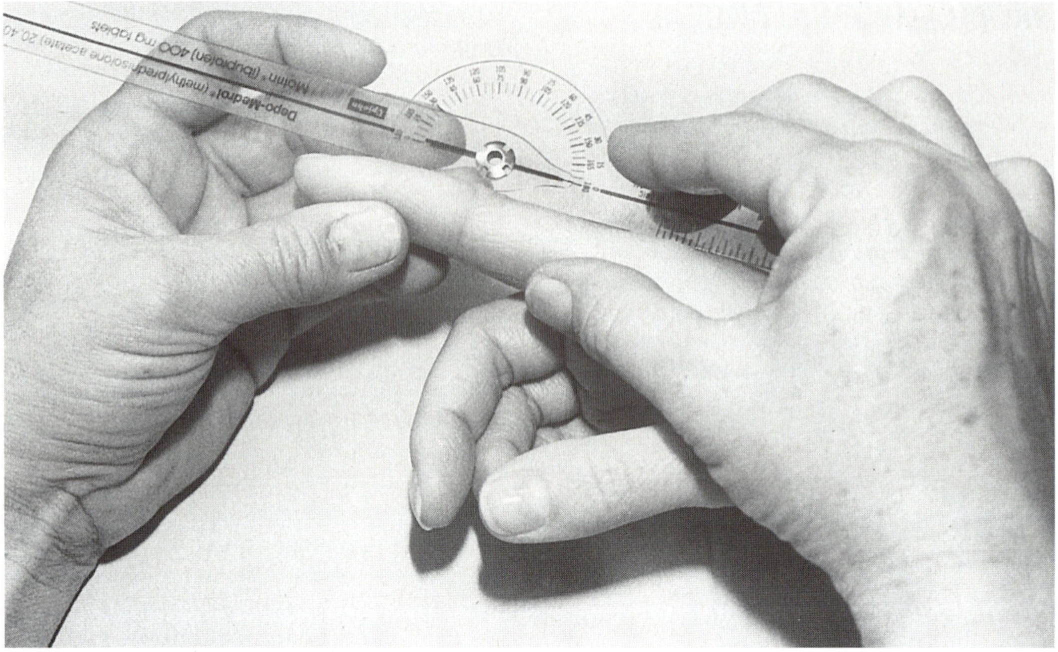

FIGURE 7.20 The alignment of the goniometer at the beginning of proximal interphalangeal (PIP) flexion range of motion.

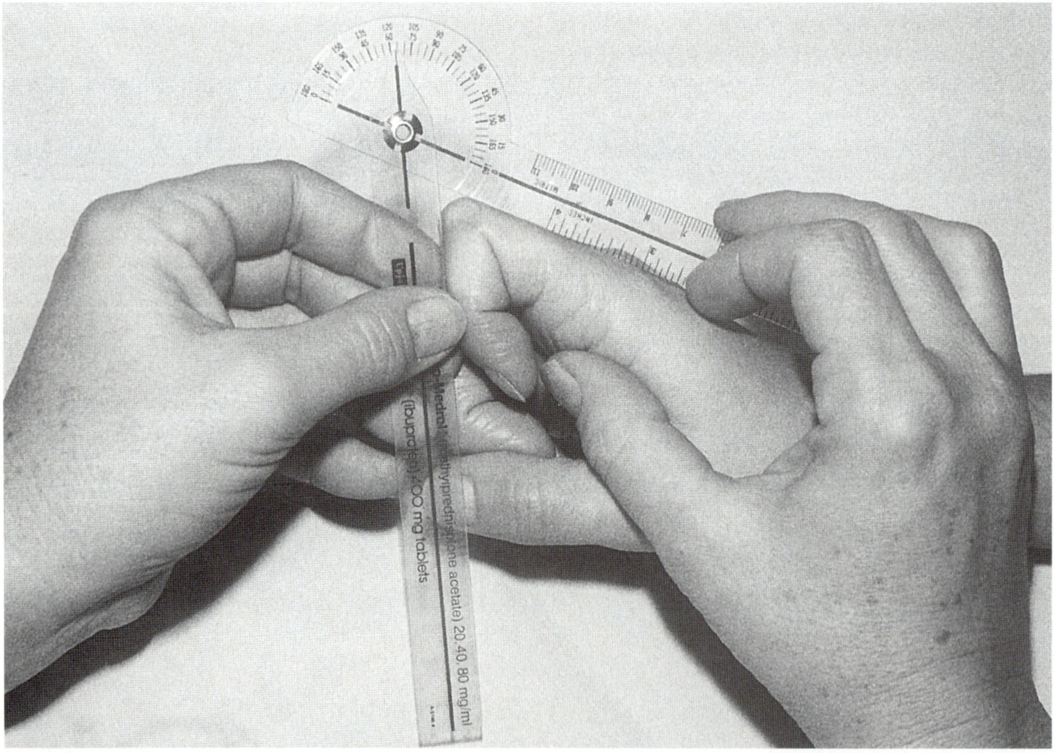

FIGURE 7.21 At the end of proximal interphalangeal (PIP) flexion, the examiner continues to stabilize and align the proximal goniometer arm over the dorsal midline of the proximal phalange with one hand. The examiner's other hand maintains the PIP joint in flexion and aligns the distal goniometer arm with the dorsal midline of the middle phalanx.

FINGERS: PROXIMAL INTERPHALANGEAL EXTENSION

Motion occurs in the sagittal plane around a medial–lateral axis. Proximal interphalangeal extension is usually recorded as the starting position for PIP flexion ROM (see Fig. 7.20). Normal ROM values for adults are generally considered to be about 0 degrees,[15–17] although one study has reported a mean of 7 for active and 16 degrees for passive PIP extension.[11] Proximal interphalangeal extension is generally equal for all fingers.[11] See Research Findings and Tables 7.1 and 7.2 for normal ROM values by age, gender, and active or passive motion.

Testing Position

Place the individual sitting, with the forearm and hand resting on a supporting surface. Position the forearm in 0 degrees of supination and pronation; the wrist in 0 degrees of flexion, extension, and radial and ulnar deviation; and the MCP joint in 0 degrees of flexion, extension, abduction, and adduction. (If the MCP joint and wrist are extended, tension in the flexor digitorum superficialis and profundus muscles will restrict the motion.)

Stabilization

Stabilize the proximal phalanx to prevent motion of the MCP joint.

Testing Motion

Extend the PIP joint by pushing on the palmar surface of the middle phalanx, moving the finger away from the palm. The end of extension ROM occurs when resistance to further motion is felt and attempts to overcome the resistance cause the MCP joint to extend.

Normal End-Feel

The end-feel is firm because of tension in the palmar joint capsule and palmar plate (palmar ligament).

Goniometer Alignment

Refer to Figure 7.20.

1. Center **fulcrum** of the goniometer over the dorsal aspect of the PIP joint.
2. Align **proximal arm** over the dorsal midline of the proximal phalanx.
3. Align **distal arm** over the dorsal midline of the middle phalanx.

FINGERS: DISTAL INTERPHALANGEAL FLEXION

Motion occurs in the sagittal plane around a medial–lateral axis. Normal ROM values for adults vary from 70 to 90 degrees. Distal interphalangeal flexion ROM is generally equal for all fingers.[11] See Research Findings and Tables 7.1 and 7.2 for normal ROM values by age, gender, and active or passive motion.

Testing Position

Position the individual sitting, with the forearm and hand resting on a supporting surface. Place the forearm in 0 degrees of supination and pronation; the wrist in 0 degrees of flexion, extension, and radial and ulnar deviation; and the MCP joint in 0 degrees of flexion, extension, abduction, and adduction. Place the PIP joint in approximately 70 to 90 degrees of flexion. (If the wrist and the MCP and PIP joints are fully flexed, tension in the extensor digitorum communis, extensor indicis, or extensor digiti minimi muscles may restrict DIP flexion. If the PIP joint is extended, tension in the oblique retinacular ligament may restrict DIP flexion.)

Stabilization

Stabilize the middle and proximal phalanx to prevent further flexion of the PIP joint.

Testing Motion

Flex the DIP joint by pushing on the dorsal surface of the distal phalanx, moving the finger toward the palm (Fig. 7.22). The end of flexion ROM occurs when resistance to further motion is felt and attempts to overcome the resistance cause the PIP joint to flex.

Normal End-Feel

The end-feel is firm because of tension in the dorsal joint capsule, collateral ligaments, and oblique retinacular ligament.

Goniometer Alignment

See Figures 7.23 to 7.25.

1. Center **fulcrum** of the goniometer over the dorsal aspect of the DIP joint.
2. Align **proximal arm** over the dorsal midline of the middle phalanx.
3. Align **distal arm** over the dorsal midline of the distal phalanx.

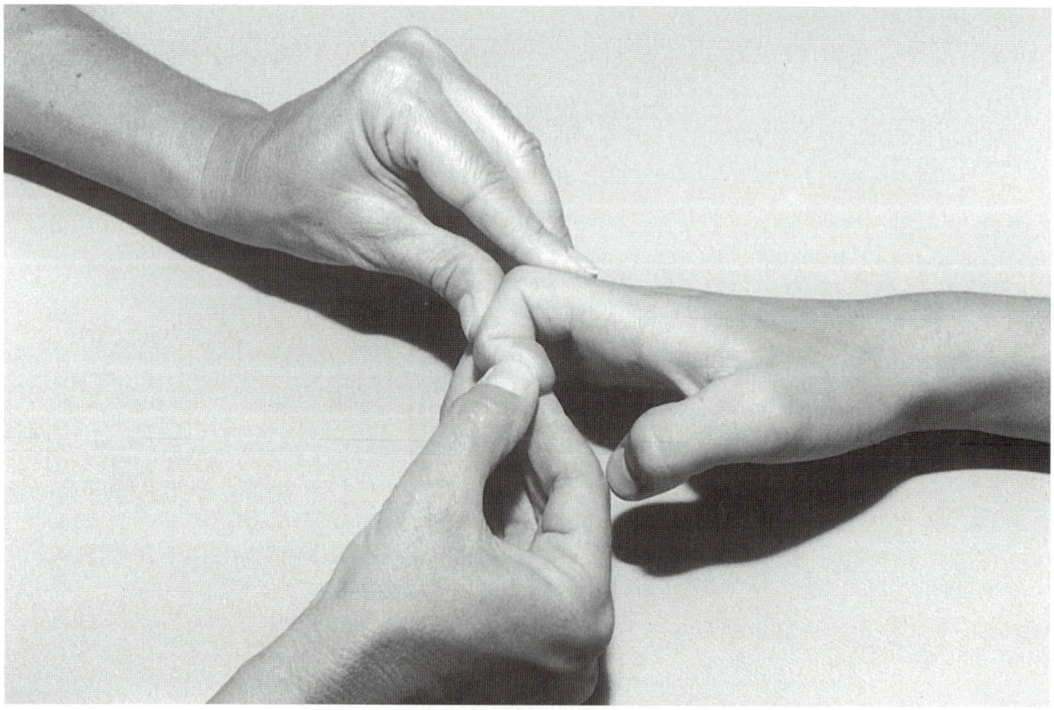

FIGURE 7.22 During distal interphalangeal (DIP) flexion, the examiner uses one hand to stabilize the middle phalanx and keep the proximal interphalangeal joint in 70 to 90 degrees of flexion. The examiner's other hand pushes on the distal phalanx to flex the DIP joint.

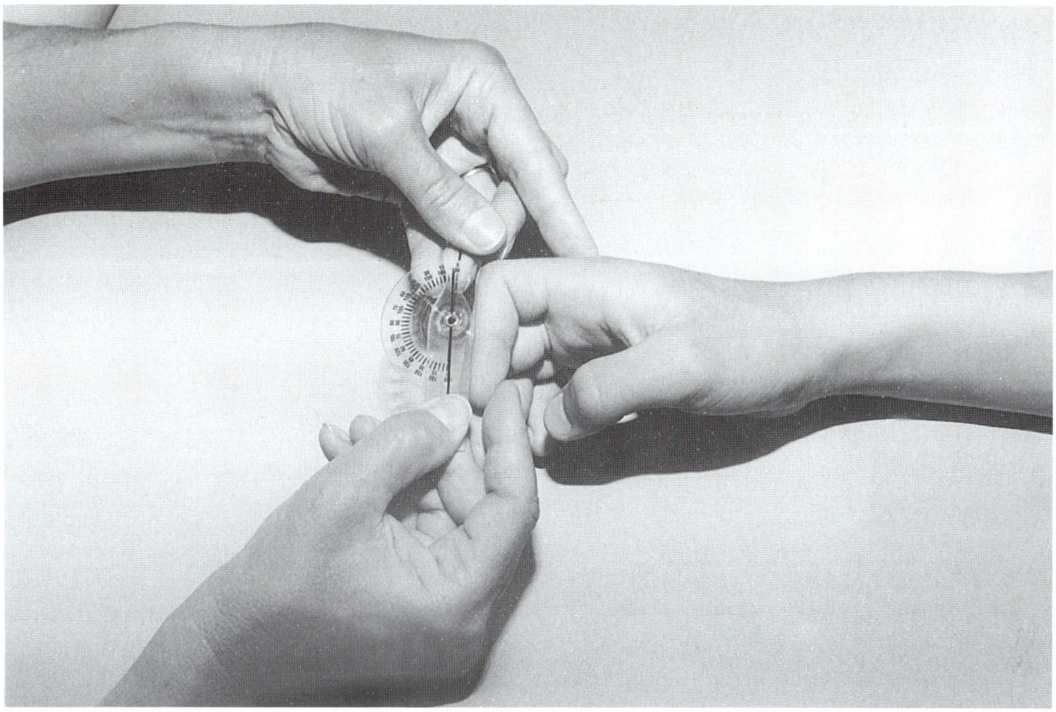

FIGURE 7.23 Measurement of the beginning of distal interphalangeal (DIP) flexion range of motion is being conducted by means of a half-circle plastic goniometer with 6-inch arms that have been trimmed to accommodate the small size of the DIP joint.

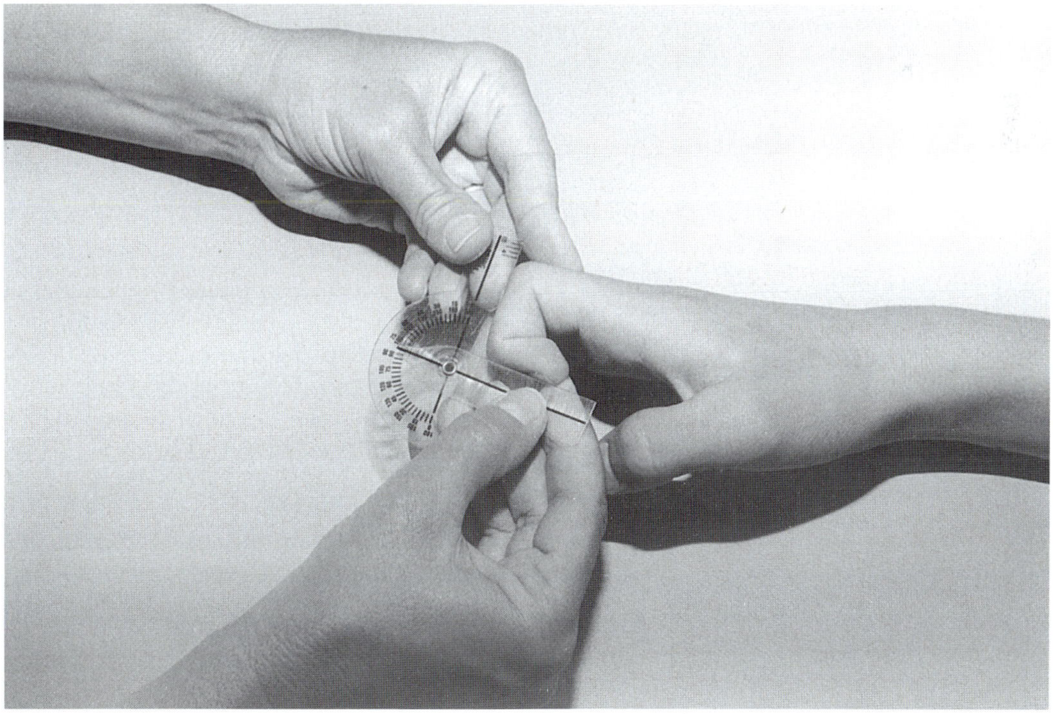

FIGURE 7.24 The alignment of the goniometer at the end of distal interphalangeal (DIP) flexion range of motion. Note that the fulcrum of the goniometer lies distal and dorsal to the proximal interphalangeal joint axis so that the arms of the goniometer stay in direct contact with the dorsal surfaces of the middle and distal phalanges.

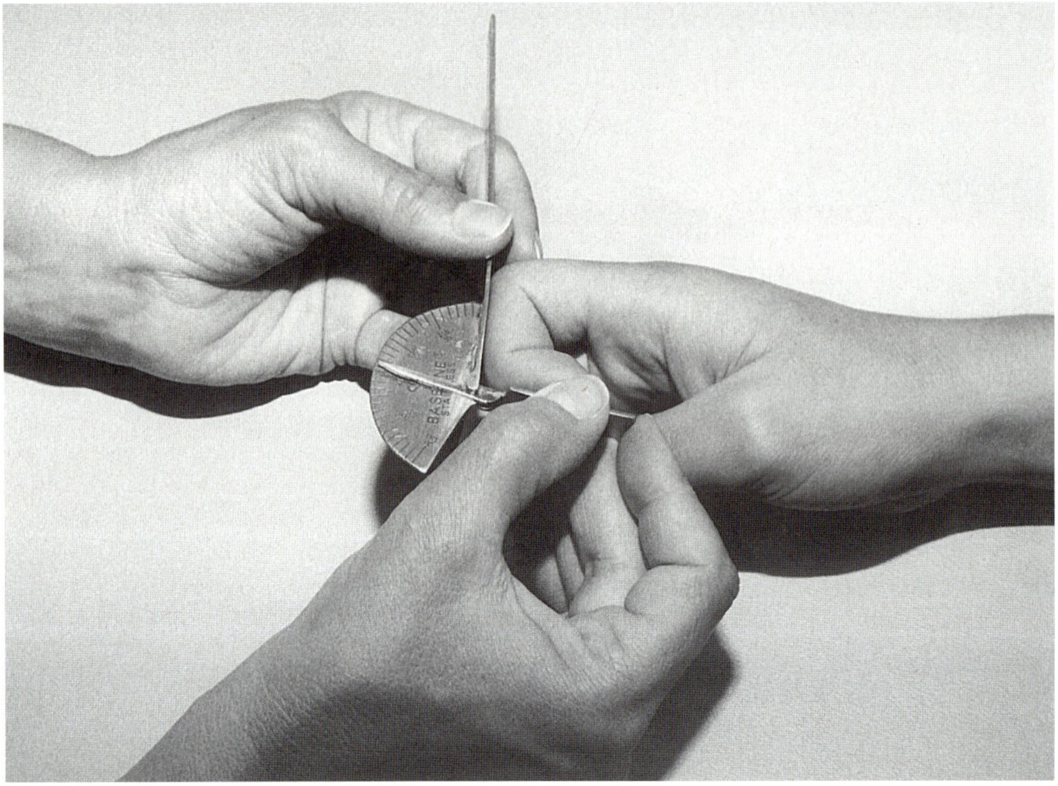

FIGURE 7.25 Distal interphalangeal flexion range of motion also can be measured by using a specialized goniometer that is placed on the dorsal surface of the middle and distal phalanges. This type of goniometer is appropriate for measuring the small joints of the fingers, thumb, and toes.

FINGERS: DISTAL INTERPHALANGEAL EXTENSION

Motion occurs in the sagittal plane around a medial–lateral axis. Distal interphalangeal extension is usually recorded as the starting position for DIP flexion ROM. Normal ROM values for adults are generally considered to be about 0 degrees,[15–17] although one study has reported a mean of 8 for active and 20 degrees for passive DIP extension.[11] Distal interphalangeal extension is generally equal for all fingers.[11] See Research Findings and Tables 7.1 and 7.2 for normal ROM values by age, gender, and active or passive motion.

Testing Position

Position the individual sitting, with the forearm and hand resting on a supporting surface. Place the forearm in 0 degrees of supination and pronation; the wrist in 0 degrees of flexion, extension, and radial and ulnar deviation; and the MCP joint in 0 degrees of flexion, extension, abduction, and adduction. Position the PIP joint in approximately 70 to 90 degrees of flexion. (If the PIP joint, MCP joint, and wrist are fully extended, tension in the flexor digitorum profundus muscle may restrict DIP extension.)

Stabilization

Stabilize the middle and proximal phalanx to prevent extension of the PIP joint.

Testing Motion

Extend the DIP joint by pushing on the palmar surface of the distal phalanx, moving the finger away from the palm. The end of extension ROM occurs when resistance to further motion is felt and attempts to overcome the resistance cause the PIP joint to extend.

Normal End-Feel

The end-feel is firm because of tension in the palmar joint capsule and the palmar plate (palmar ligament).

Goniometer Alignment

Refer to Figure 7.23.

1. Center **fulcrum** of the goniometer over the dorsal aspect of the DIP joint.
2. Align **proximal arm** over the dorsal midline of the middle phalanx.
3. Align **distal arm** over the dorsal midline of the distal phalanx.

FINGERS: COMPOSITE FLEXION OF THE MCP, PIP, AND DIP JOINTS

Composite finger flexion (CFF) is a simple method of quickly assessing multiple joints in a finger to indicate the functional ability to make a fist. However, a disadvantage of CFF is the inability to localize an impairment or response to treatment in a specific joint. Normally, when the MCP, PIP, and DIP joints are maximally flexed, the distance between the fingertip and the distal palmar crease of the hand is zero. In terms of reliability, Ellis and Bruton[18] report that repeated CFF measurements fell within 5 to 6 millimeters 95% of the time when taken by the same tester, and fell within 7 to 9 millimeters 95% of the time when taken by different testers. See Research Findings for more information on reliability.

Testing Position

Place the individual sitting, with the forearm and hand resting on a supporting surface. Position the forearm in neutral supination and pronation and the wrist in 0 degrees of flexion, extension, and radial and ulnar deviation. Alternatively, the forearm could be positioned in full supination.

Stabilization

Stabilize the metacarpals to prevent motion of the wrist.

Testing Motion

Flex the MCP, PIP, and DIP joints by pushing on the dorsal surface of the finger, moving the finger toward the palm. The end of flexion ROM occurs when resistance to further motion is felt and attempts to overcome the resistance cause the wrist to flex.

Normal End-Feel

Usually, the end-feel is soft because of contact between the palmar aspect of the proximal, middle, and distal phalanx and palm of the hand. In other individuals, the end-feel may be firm because of tension in the dorsal joint capsules and the collateral ligaments.

Measurement Method

See Figures 7.26 and 7.27. Measure the perpendicular distance between the distal palmar crease and the tip of the finger.[16,19] Alternatively, the distance between the distal palmar crease and the distal corner of the nailbed on the radial border of the finger can be measured.[18]

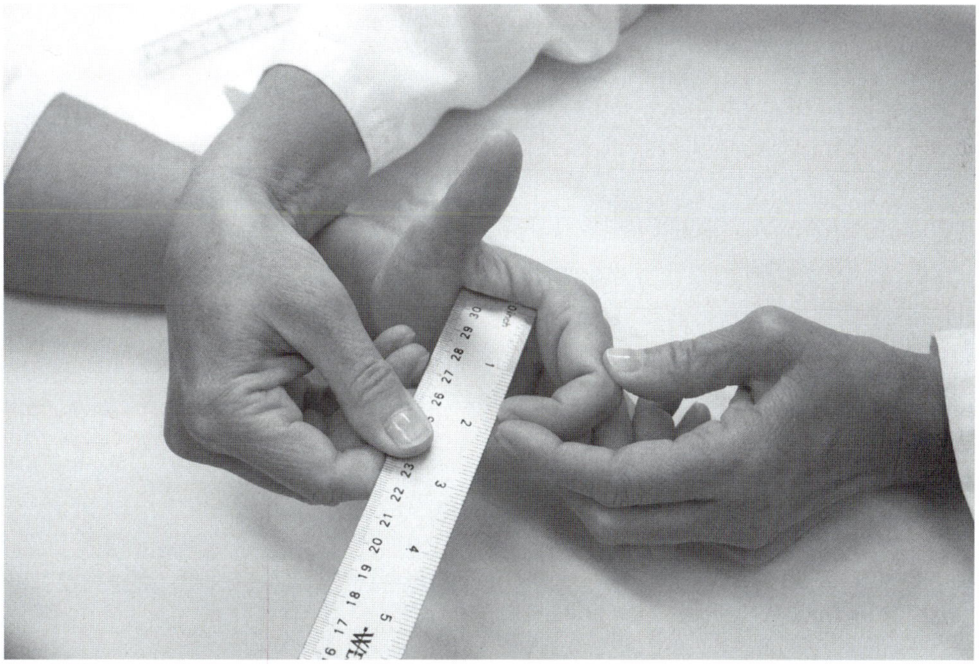

FIGURE 7.26 Composite finger flexion (CFF) is determined by measuring the distance between the distal palmar crease and the tip of the finger at the end of flexion of the MCP, PIP, and DIP joints. Normally, the tip of the finger is able to touch the palm at the distal palmar crease. This individual has limited range of motion.

RANGE OF MOTION TESTING PROCEDURES: Thumb

Landmarks for Testing Procedures

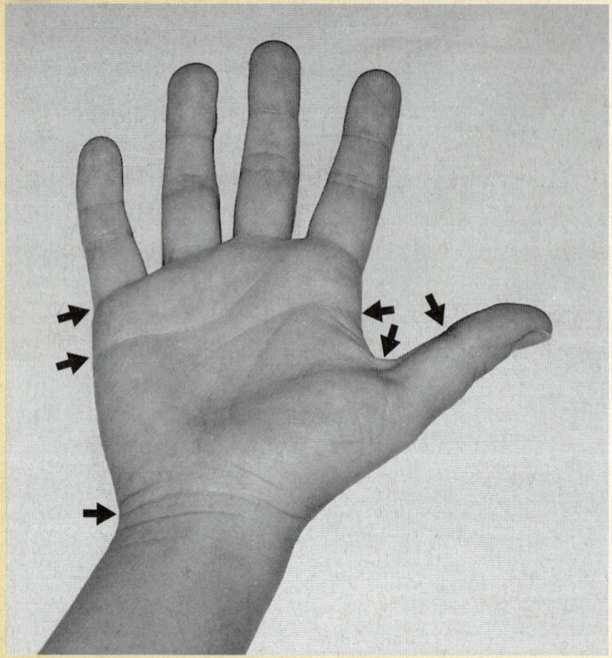

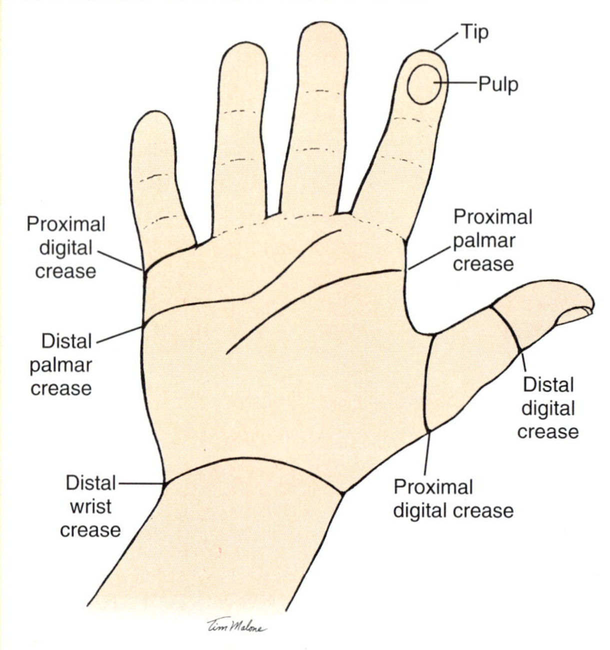

FIGURE 7.27 (A, B) Anterior (palmar) view of the right hand showing the digital and palmar creases used for measuring composite finger flexion and CMC opposition of the thumb.

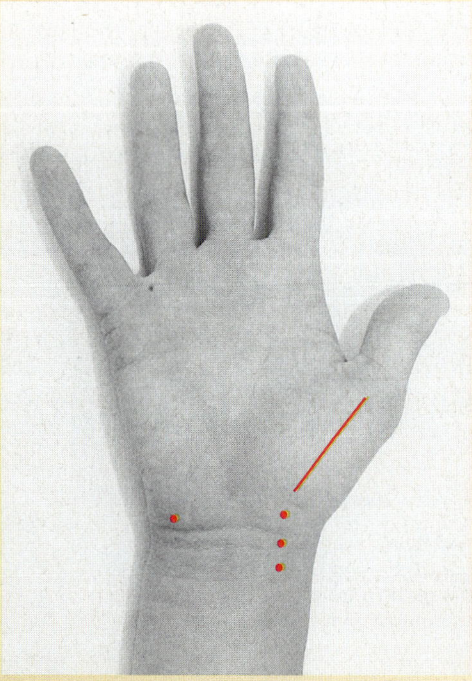

FIGURE 7.28 Anterior (palmar) view of the right hand showing surface anatomy landmarks for goniometer alignment during the measurement of thumb range of motion.

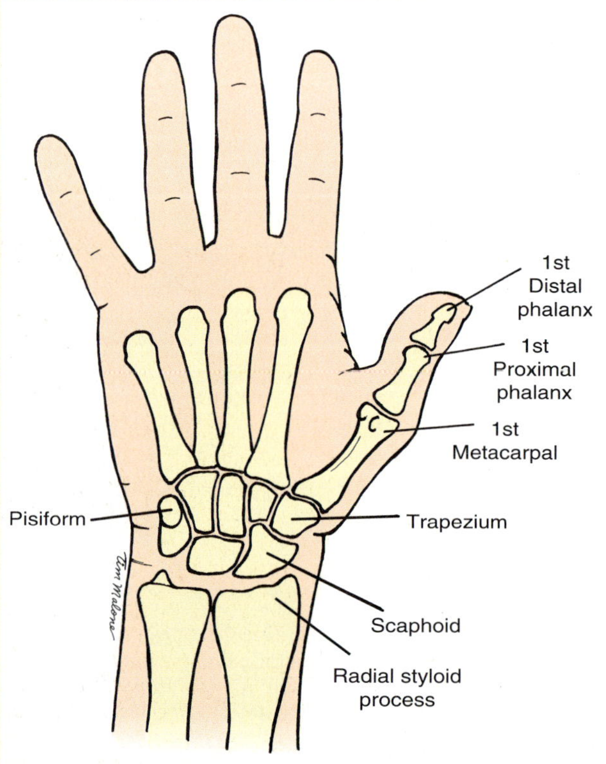

FIGURE 7.29 Anterior (palmar) view of the right hand showing bony anatomical landmarks for goniometer alignment during the measurement of thumb range of motion.

Landmarks for Testing Procedures (continued)

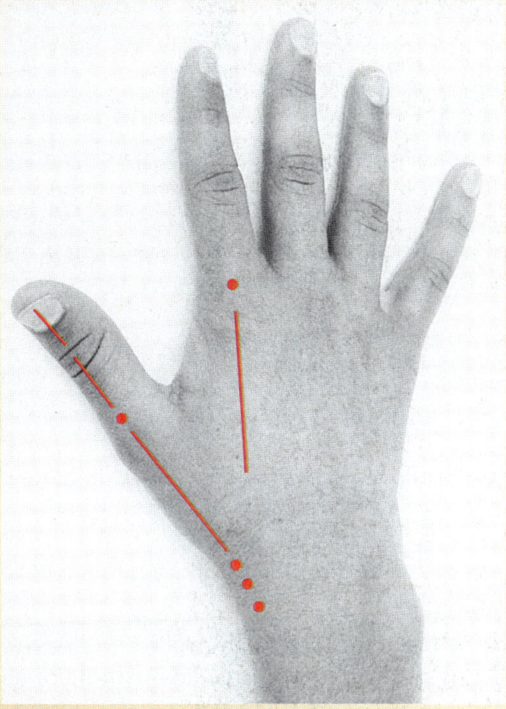

FIGURE 7.30 Posterior view of the right hand showing surface anatomy landmarks for goniometer alignment during the measurement of thumb range of motion.

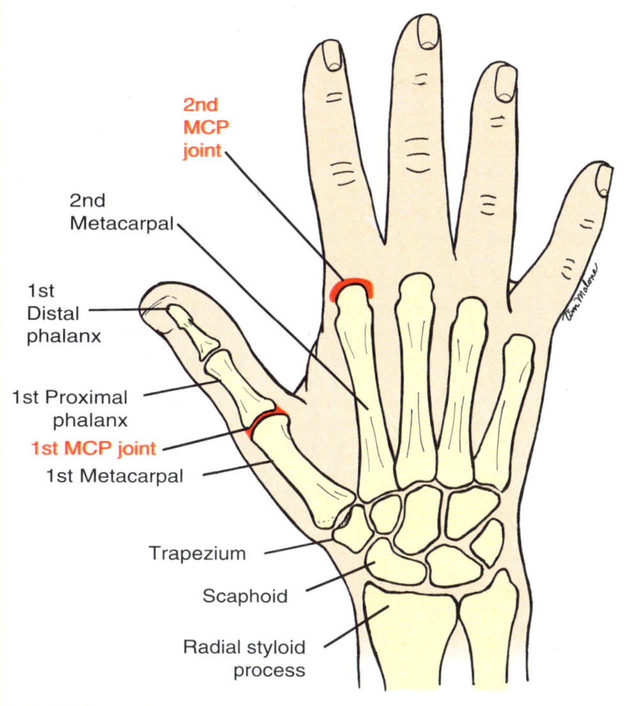

FIGURE 7.31 Posterior view of the right hand showing bony anatomical landmarks for goniometer alignment during the measurement of thumb range of motion.

THUMB: CARPOMETACARPAL FLEXION

Motion occurs in the plane of the hand. When the individual is in the anatomical position, the motion occurs in the frontal plane around an anterior–posterior axis. This motion is sometimes called **radial adduction.** Normal ROM values in adults vary from about 15 to 25 degrees. See Research Findings and Table 7.3. In addition to sources reported in Table 7.3, White, Nolan, and Resteghini[20] report a mean of 25.9 degrees (standard deviation [SD] = 7.4) in a study of 80 adults between the ages of 16 to 62 years using a method similar to this book. Barakat, Field, and Taylor[21] report a mean of 10.2 degrees (SD = 4) in a study of 62 healthy females ranging in age from 18 to 37 years using methods proposed by the International Federation of Societies for Surgery of the Hand (IFSSH).[22]

Testing Position

Position the individual sitting, with the forearm and hand resting on a supporting surface. Place the forearm in full supination; the wrist in 0 degrees of flexion, extension, and radial and ulnar deviation; and the CMC joint of the thumb in 0 degrees of abduction. The MCP and IP joints of the thumb are relaxed in a position of slight flexion. (If the MCP and IP joints of the thumb are positioned in full flexion, tension in the extensor pollicis longus and brevis muscles may restrict the motion.)

Stabilization

Stabilize the carpals, radius, and ulna to prevent wrist motions. Movement of the wrist must be avoided as it will affect the accuracy of the ROM measurement.

Testing Motion

Flex the CMC joint of the thumb by pushing on the dorsal surface of the metacarpal, moving the thumb toward the ulnar aspect of the hand (Fig. 7.32). Maintain the CMC joint in 0 degrees of abduction. The end of flexion ROM occurs when resistance to further motion is felt and attempts to overcome the resistance cause the wrist to deviate ulnarly.

Normal End-Feel

The end-feel may be soft because of contact between muscle bulk of the thenar eminence and the palm of the hand, or it may be firm because of tension in the dorsal joint capsule and the extensor pollicis brevis and abductor pollicis brevis muscles.

Goniometer Alignment

See Figures 7.33 and 7.34.

1. Center **fulcrum** of the goniometer over the palmar aspect of the first CMC joint.
2. Align **proximal arm** with the ventral midline of the radius using the ventral surface of the radial head and radial styloid process for reference.
3. Align **distal arm** with the ventral midline of the first metacarpal.

In the beginning position for flexion and extension, the goniometer will indicate an angle of approximately 30 to 50 degrees rather than 0 degrees, depending on the shape of the hand and wrist position. The difference between the beginning-position degrees and the end-position degrees is the ROM. For example, a measurement that begins at 35 degrees and ends at 15 degrees should be recorded as a ROM of 0 to 20 degrees.

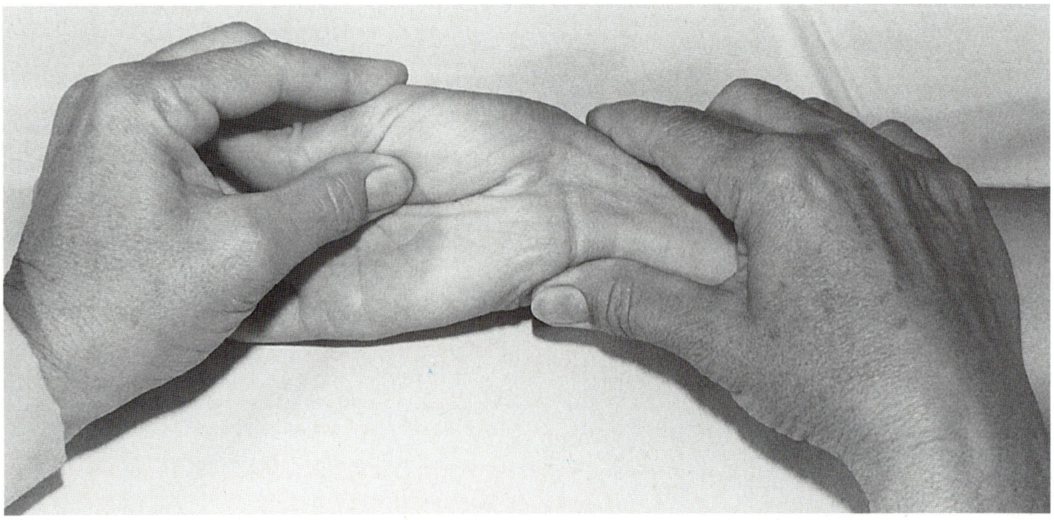

FIGURE 7.32 During carpometacarpal (CMC) flexion, the examiner uses the index finger and thumb of one hand to stabilize the carpals, radius, and ulna to prevent ulnar deviation of the wrist. The examiner's other index finger and thumb flex the CMC joint by moving the first metacarpal medially.

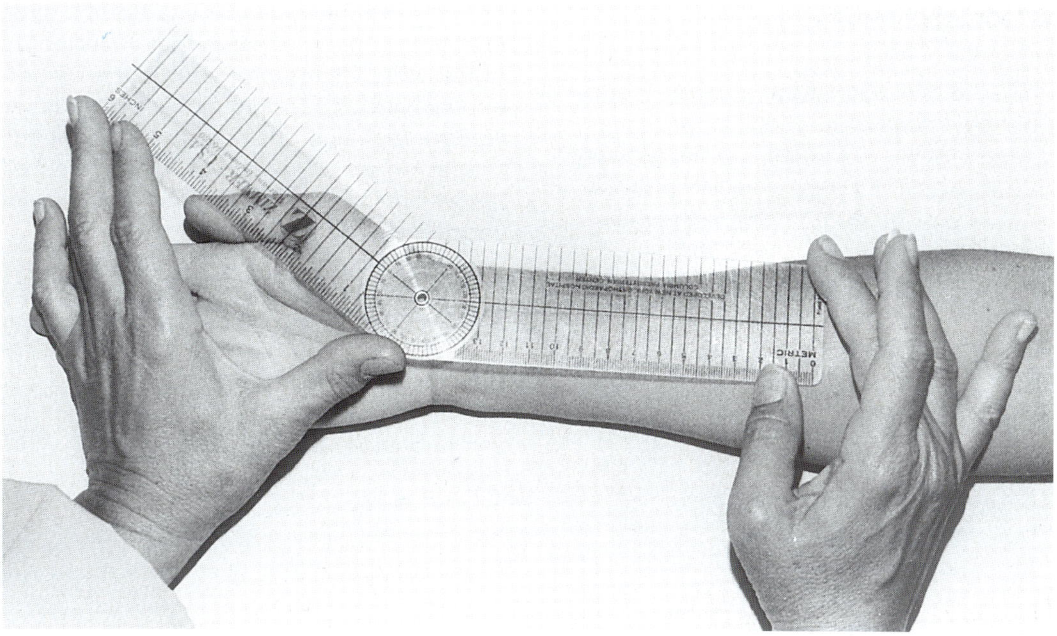

FIGURE 7.33 The alignment of the goniometer at the beginning of carpometacarpal (CMC) flexion range of motion of the thumb. Note that the goniometer does not read 0 degrees.

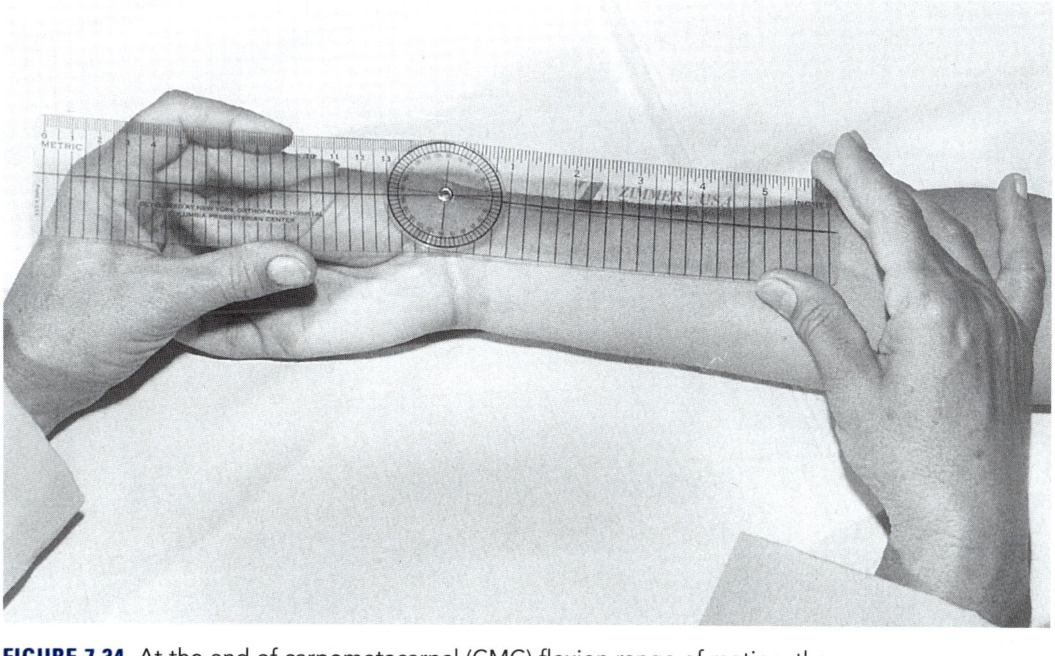

FIGURE 7.34 At the end of carpometacarpal (CMC) flexion range of motion, the examiner uses the hand that was stabilizing the wrist to align the proximal arm of the goniometer with the radius. The examiner's other hand maintains CMC flexion and aligns the distal arm of the goniometer with the first metacarpal. During the measurement, the examiner must be careful not to move the individual's wrist further into ulnar deviation or the goniometer reading will be incorrect (too high).

Alternative Goniometer Alignment

See Figures 7.35 and 7.36.

1. Center **fulcrum** of the goniometer over the palmar aspect of the first CMC joint.
2. Align **proximal arm** with an imaginary line between the palmar surfaces of the trapezium and pisiform. This line is often parallel to the distal wrist crease (refer to Fig. 7.27).
3. Align **distal arm** with the ventral midline of the first metacarpal.

This alternative alignment method avoids errors in ROM measurement due to inadvertent movement of the wrist. The goniometer in the beginning position will indicate an angle of approximately 40 to 70 degrees rather than 0 degrees, depending on the shape and size of the hand. The difference between the beginning-position degrees and the end-position degrees is the ROM.

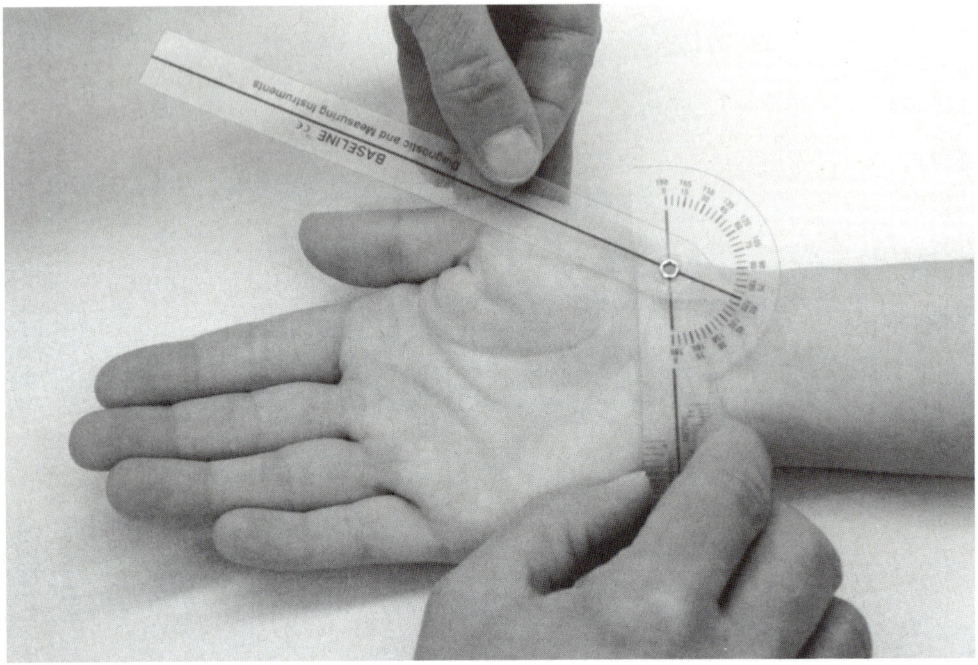

FIGURE 7.35 An alternative method of measuring the beginning of carpometacarpal (CMC) flexion aligns the proximal arm of the goniometer with the palmar surface of the trapezium and pisiform. Note that the goniometer does not read 0 degrees.

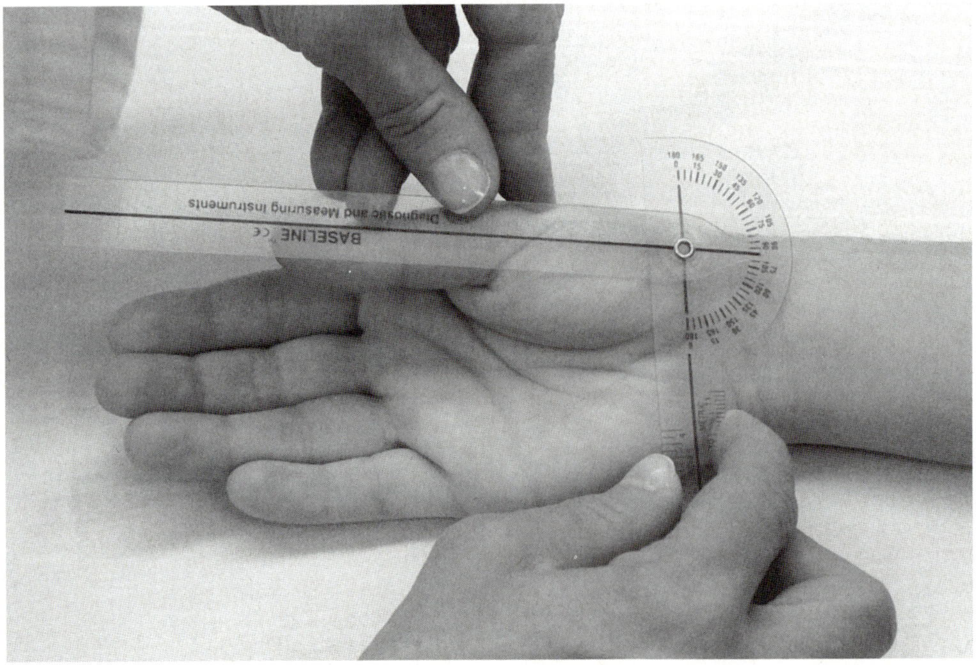

FIGURE 7.36 An alternative method of aligning the goniometer to measure the end of carpometacarpal (CMC) flexion range of motion. The difference between the degrees on the goniometer at the beginning and the end positions is the range of motion.

THUMB: CARPOMETACARPAL EXTENSION

Motion occurs in the plane of the hand. When the individual is in the anatomical position, the motion occurs in the frontal plane around an anterior–posterior axis. This motion is sometimes called **radial abduction.** Reported ROM values for adults usually vary from 15 to 35 degrees depending on the measurement methods. See Research Findings and Table 7.3. In addition to sources reported in Table 7.3, White, Nolan and Resteghini[20] report a mean ROM of 14.9 degrees (SD = 4.7) in a study of 80 adults between the ages of 16 and 62 years using a method similar to this book.

Some authorities such as the IFSSH[22] have reported only the end position of the angle between the thumb and index metacarpal as CMC extension ROM, rather than the change in joint angle at the beginning and end of the motion. This method would result in larger "ROM" values. The IFSSH reports an average about 40 degrees of CMC extension using this method. Barakat and coworkers[21] report a mean of 62.9 degrees (SD = 4.3) of radial abduction (extension) in a study of 62 healthy females between the ages of 18 and 37 years using the methods proposed by the IFSSH.

Testing Position

Position the individual sitting, with the forearm and hand resting on a supporting surface. Place the forearm in full supination; the wrist in 0 degrees of flexion, extension, and radial and ulnar deviation; and the CMC joint of the thumb in 0 degrees of abduction. The MCP and IP joints of the thumb are relaxed in a position of slight flexion. (If the MCP and IP joints of the thumb are positioned in full extension, tension in the flexor pollicis longus muscle may restrict the motion.)

Stabilization

Stabilize the carpals, radius, and ulna to prevent wrist motions. Movement of the wrist must be avoided as it will affect the accuracy of the ROM measurement.

Testing Motion

Extend the CMC joint of the thumb by pushing on the palmar surface of the metacarpal, moving the thumb toward the radial aspect of the hand (Fig. 7.37). Maintain the CMC joint in 0 degrees of abduction. The end of extension ROM occurs when resistance to further motion is felt and attempts to overcome the resistance cause the wrist to deviate radially.

Normal End-Feel

The end-feel is firm because of tension in the anterior joint capsule and the flexor pollicis brevis, adductor pollicis, opponens pollicis, and first dorsal interossei muscles.

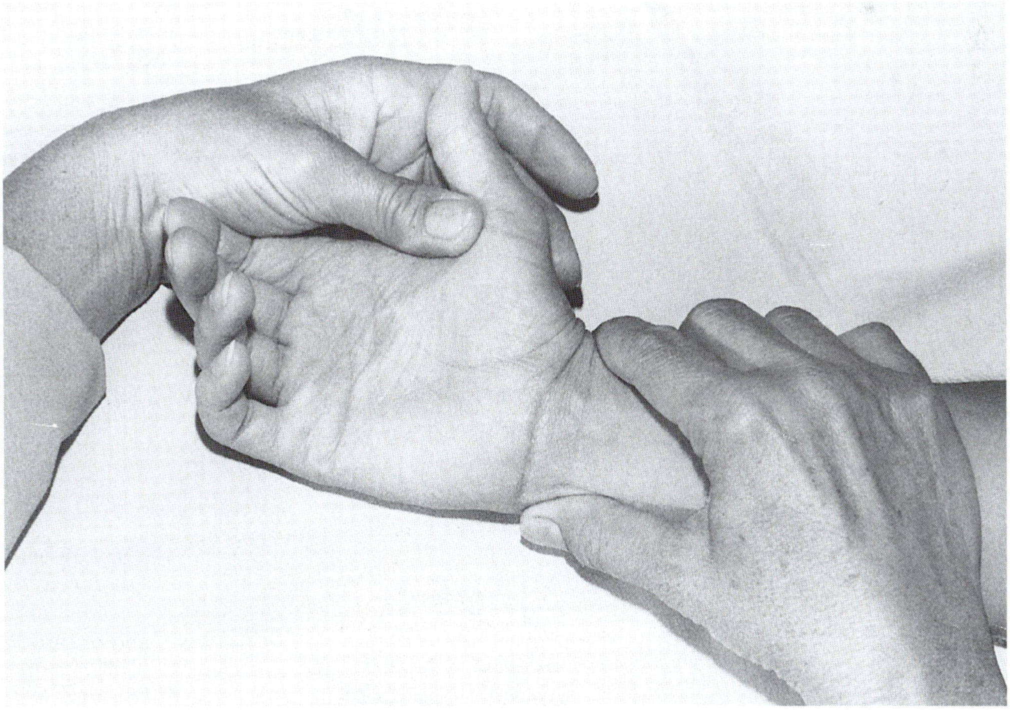

FIGURE 7.37 During carpometacarpal (CMC) extension of the thumb, the examiner uses one hand to stabilize the carpals, radius, and ulna, thereby preventing radial deviation of the individual's wrist. The examiner's other hand is used to pull the first metacarpal laterally into extension.

Goniometer Alignment

See Figures 7.38 and 7.39.

1. Center **fulcrum** of the goniometer over the palmar aspect of the first CMC joint.
2. Align **proximal arm** with the ventral midline of the radius, using the ventral surface of the radial head and the radial styloid process for reference.
3. Align **distal arm** with the ventral midline of the first metacarpal.

In the beginning positions for flexion and extension, the goniometer will indicate an angle of approximately 30 to 50 degrees rather than 0 degrees, depending on the shape of the hand and wrist position. The difference between the beginning-position degrees and the end-position degrees is the ROM. For example, a measurement that begins at 35 degrees and ends at 55 degrees should be recorded as 0–20 degrees.

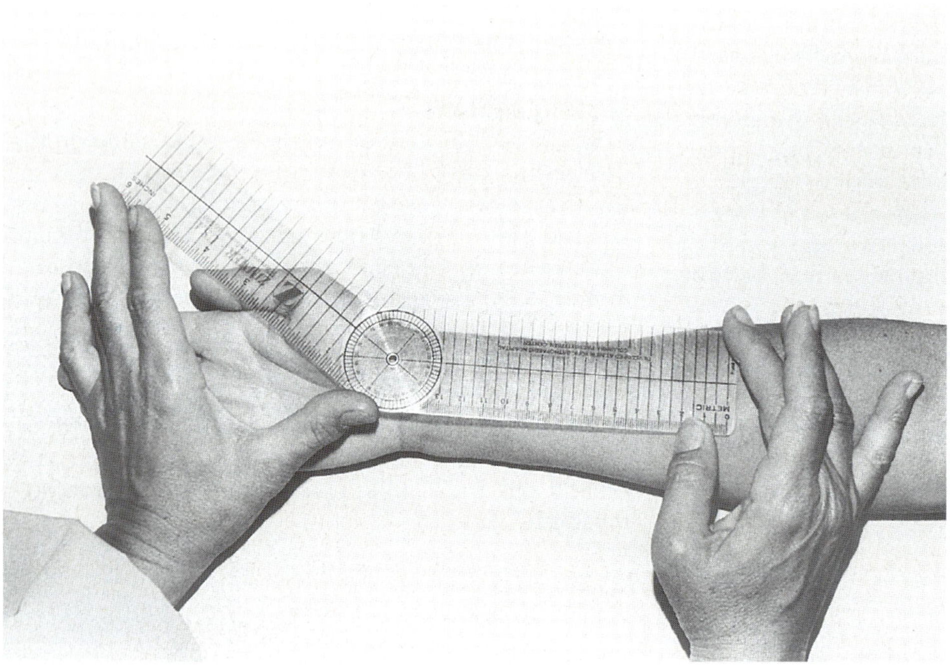

FIGURE 7.38 The goniometer alignment for measuring the beginning of carpometacarpal (CMC) extension range of motion is the same as for measuring the beginning of CMC flexion.

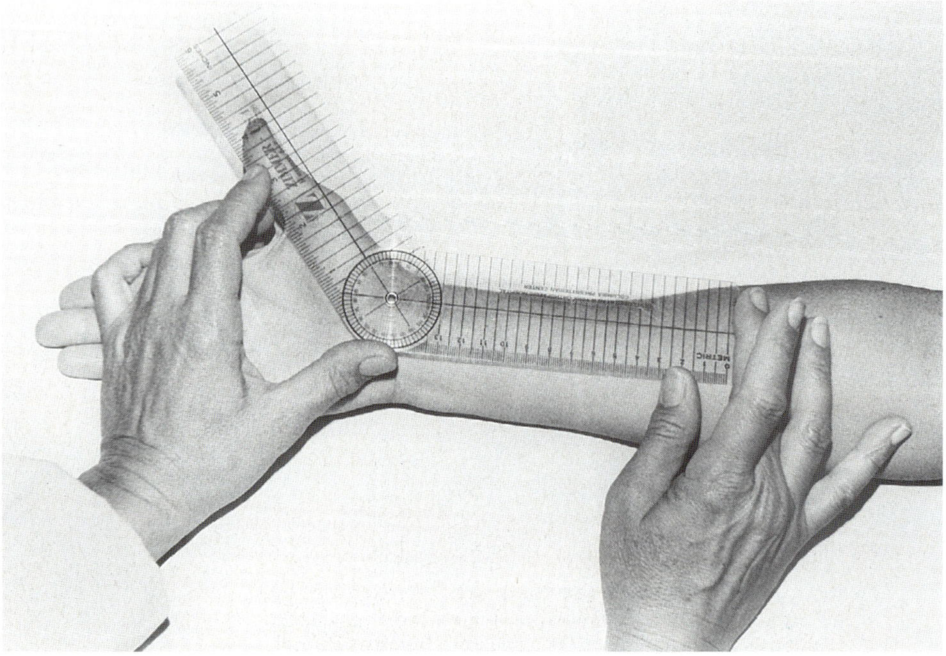

FIGURE 7.39 The alignment of the goniometer at the end of carpometacarpal (CMC) extension range of motion of the thumb. The examiner must be careful to move only the CMC joint into extension and not to change the position of the wrist during the measurement.

Alternative Goniometer Alignment

See Figures 7.40 and 7.41.

1. Center **fulcrum** of the goniometer over the palmar aspect of the first CMC joint.
2. Align **proximal arm** with an imaginary line between the palmar surface of the trapezium and pisiform. This line is often parallel to the distal wrist crease (refer to Fig. 7.27).
3. Align **distal arm** with the ventral midline of the first metacarpal.

This alternative alignment method avoids errors in ROM measurement due to inadvertent movement of the wrist. The goniometer in the beginning position will indicate an angle of 40 to 70 degrees rather than 0 degrees, depending on the shape and size of the hand. The difference between the beginning-position degrees and the end-position degrees is the ROM. For example, a measurement that begins at 50 degrees and ends at 30 degrees should be recorded as a ROM of 0 to 20 degrees.

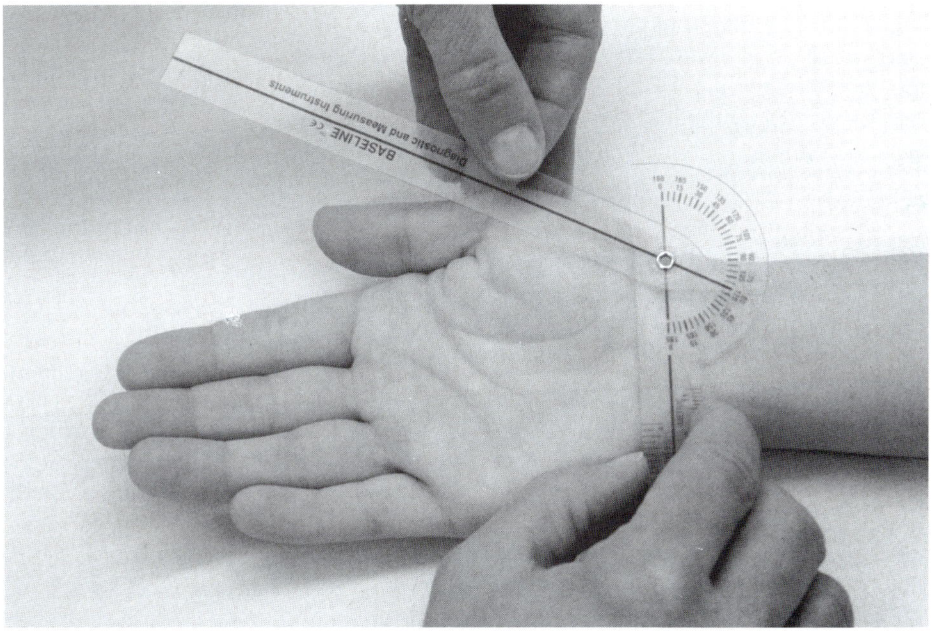

FIGURE 7.40 The alternative method of measuring the beginning of CMC extension is the same as the alternative method for measuring the beginning of CMC flexion.

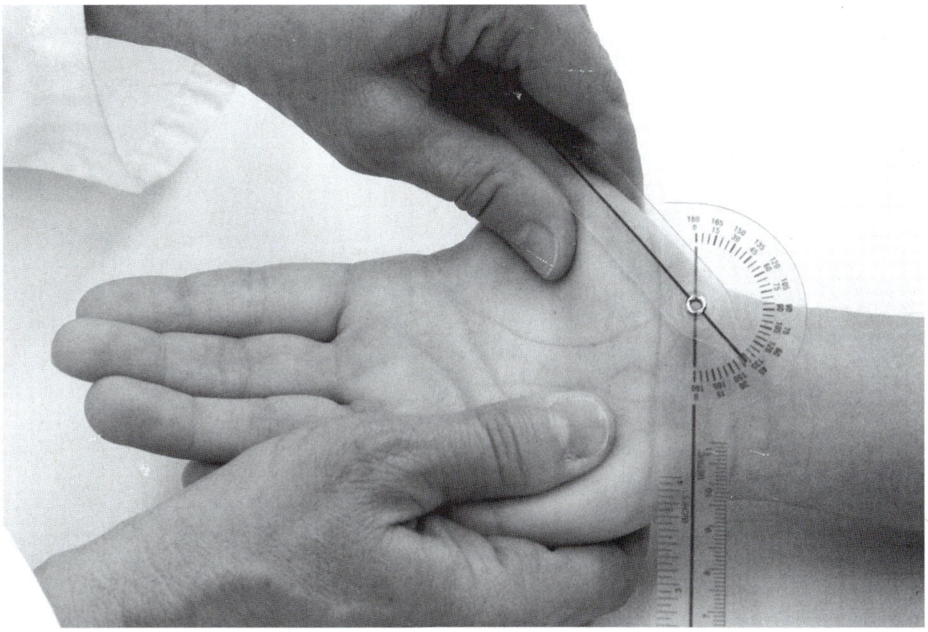

FIGURE 7.41 The alternative method of aligning the goniometer to measure the end of CMC extension ROM.

THUMB: CARPOMETACARPAL ABDUCTION

Motion occurs at a right angle to the palm of the hand. When the individual is in the anatomical position, the motion occurs in the sagittal plane around a medial–lateral axis. This motion is sometimes called **palmar abduction** or **anteposition.** Normal ROM values for adults using the measurement methods presented in this book range from about 40 to 50 degrees.[20,23] The American Academy of Orthopaedic Surgeons reports abduction ROM to be 70 degrees using a different measurement method.[17] See Research Findings and Table 7.3. In addition to sources listed in Table 7.3, Barakat and coworkers[21] report a mean of 61.2 degrees (SD = 4.4) in a study of 62 healthy females using methods proposed by the IFSSH.[22]

Testing Position

Position the individual sitting, with the forearm and hand resting on a supporting surface. Place the forearm midway between supination and pronation; the wrist in 0 degrees of flexion, extension, and radial and ulnar deviation; and the CMC, MCP, and IP joints of the thumb in 0 degrees of flexion and extension.

Stabilization

Stabilize the carpals and the second metacarpal to prevent wrist motions.

Testing Motion

Abduct the CMC joint by moving the metacarpal away from the palm of the hand (Fig. 7.42). The end of abduction ROM occurs when resistance to further motion is felt and attempts to overcome the resistance cause the wrist to flex.

Normal End-Feel

The end-feel is firm because of tension in the fascia and the skin of the web space between the thumb and the index finger. Tension in the adductor pollicis and first dorsal interossei muscles also contributes to the firm end-feel.

Goniometer Alignment

See Figures 7.43 and 7.44.

1. Center **fulcrum** of the goniometer over the lateral aspect of the scaphoid or radial styloid process, so that the proximal and distal arms of the goniometer can be properly positioned over the long axes of the first and second metacarpals.
2. Align **proximal arm** with the lateral midline of the second (index) metacarpal, using the center of the second MCP joint for reference.
3. Align **distal arm** with the dorsal midline of the first (thumb) metacarpal, using the center of the first MCP joint for reference.

Note that the proximal surface of the first metacarpal contacts the trapezium, while the proximal surface of the second metacarpal contacts the trapezoid. Contact of the metacarpals with two different carpals and the palmar position of the trapezium relative to the trapezoid create difficulties in identifying a fulcrum and alignment for the arms of the goniometer in this motion. We suggest using the scaphoid or radial styloid process as the axis, based on which landmark allows the arms of the goniometer to be aligned with the long axes of the first and second metacarpals.

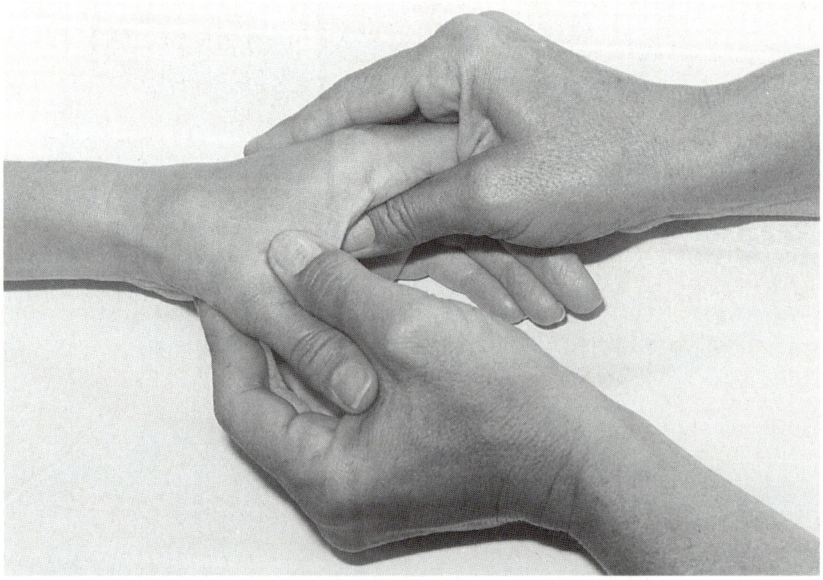

FIGURE 7.42 During carpometacarpal (CMC) abduction, the examiner uses one hand to stabilize the individual's second metacarpal. Her other hand grasps the first metacarpal just proximal to the metacarpophalangeal joint to move it away from the palm and into abduction.

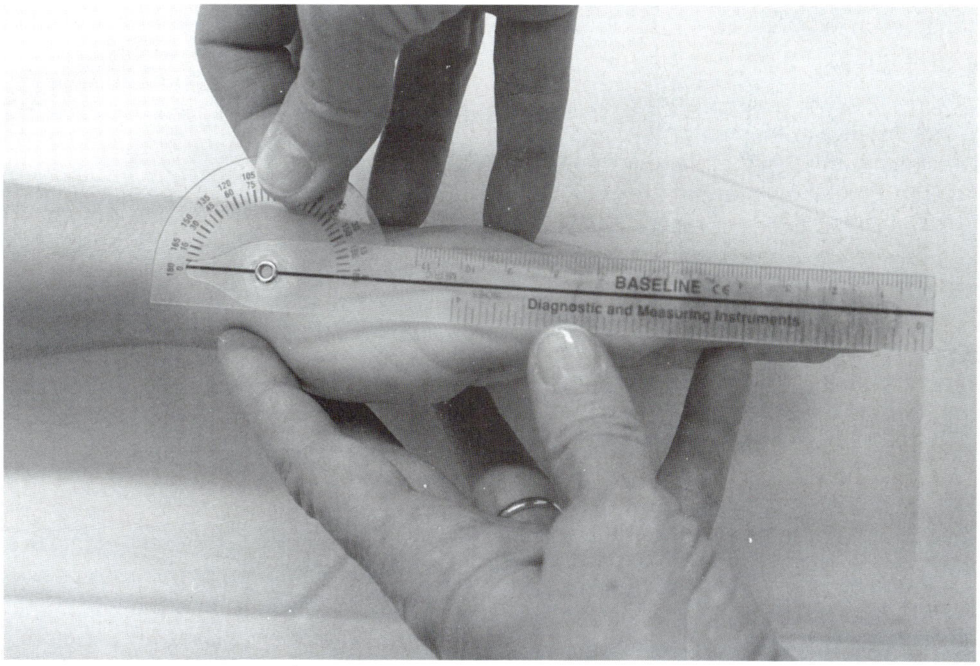

FIGURE 7.43 At the beginning of carpometacarpal (CMC) abduction range of motion, the distal end of the individual's first metacarpal of the thumb is in line with the second metacarpal of the index finger.

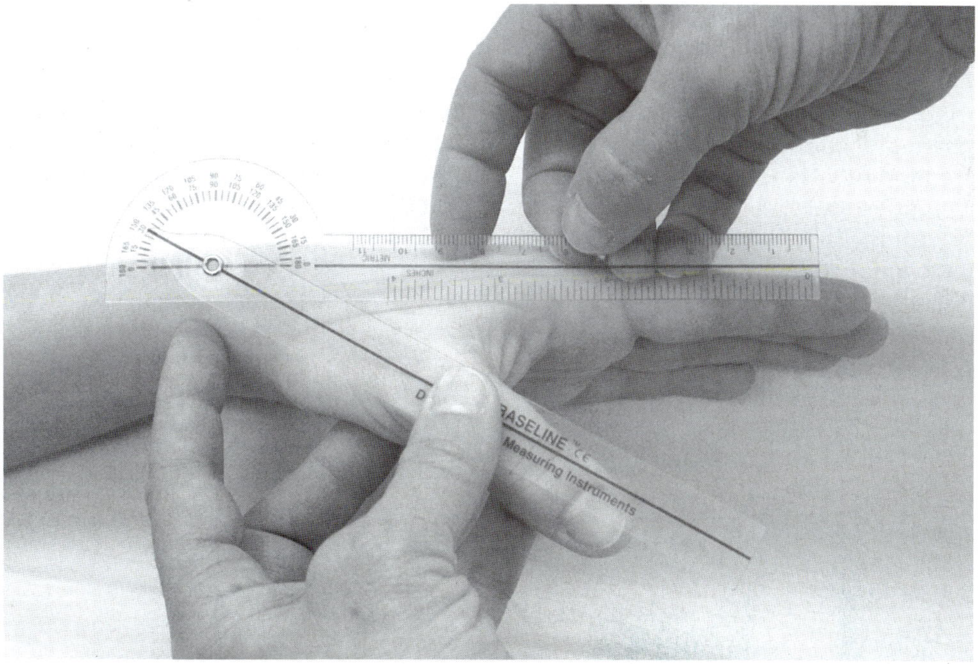

FIGURE 7.44 The alignment of the goniometer at the end of carpometacarpal (CMC) abduction range of motion. The arms of the goniometer are correctly aligned with the first and second metacarpals, not the proximal phalanges.

THUMB: CARPOMETACARPAL ADDUCTION

Motion occurs at a right angle to the palm of the hand. When the individual is in the anatomical position, the motion occurs in the sagittal plane around a medial–lateral axis. Adduction of the CMC joint of the thumb is not often measured and recorded separately because it is the return to the 0 starting position from full abduction.

However, the IFSSH,[22] calling this motion **retroposition,** reports an average of about 15 degrees as measured between the thumb metacarpal and index metacarpal as the thumb passes dorsal to the palm. Barakat and coworkers[21] report a mean of 31 degrees (SD = 4) in a study of 62 healthy females ranging in age from 18 to 37 years using methods proposed by the IFSSH.

THUMB: CARPOMETACARPAL OPPOSITION

This motion is a combination of abduction, flexion, medial axial rotation (pronation), and adduction at the CMC joints of the thumb. Contact between the tip of the thumb and the base of the little finger (proximal digital crease) is usually possible at the end of opposition ROM, providing that some flexion at the MCP and IP joints of the thumb is allowed. If no flexion of the MCP and IP joints of the thumb is allowed, there will be a distance of several centimeters between the thumb and base of the little finger at the end of opposition. Many methods of measuring CMC opposition have been suggested.[15–17,19,22,24–26] It is important for the examiner to record the landmarks that are being used and the amount of motion allowed at the MCP and IP joints of the thumb so that there is consistency between repeated measurements on an individual.

Some researchers have tried to quantify the amount of medial axial rotation (pronation) of the thumb that occurs during opposition. However, results varied widely depending on whether measurements were taken in vivo or in vitro (cadavers), whether isolated metacarpal or total thumb motion was included, and the measurement methods used. Mean axial ROM values vary from about 15 to 55 degrees measured at the metacarpal for motion isolated to the CMC joint, to about 70 to 90 degrees measured at the tip (nail) of the thumb, which includes MCP and IP joint motions.[27–30] No recommendations for the clinical measurement of axial rotation of the thumb are proposed at this time. The procedures that follow are for measuring thumb opposition.

Testing Position

Position the individual sitting, with the forearm and hand resting on a supporting surface. Place the forearm in full supination and the wrist in 0 degrees of flexion, extension, and radial and ulnar deviation.

Stabilization

Stabilize the fifth metacarpal to prevent motion at the fifth CMC joint and wrist.

Testing Motion

Grasp the first metacarpal and move it away from the palm of the hand (abduction) and then in an ulnar direction toward the base of the little finger (flexion and adduction), allowing the first metacarpal to medially rotate (Fig. 7.45). The end of opposition ROM occurs when contact is made between the tip of the thumb and the base of the little finger, if some flexion of the MCP and IP joints of the thumb is allowed (Fig. 7.46). If no flexion is allowed at the MCP and IP joints, the end of opposition will occur when resistance to further motion is felt and attempts to overcome the resistance cause the wrist to deviate or the forearm to pronate.

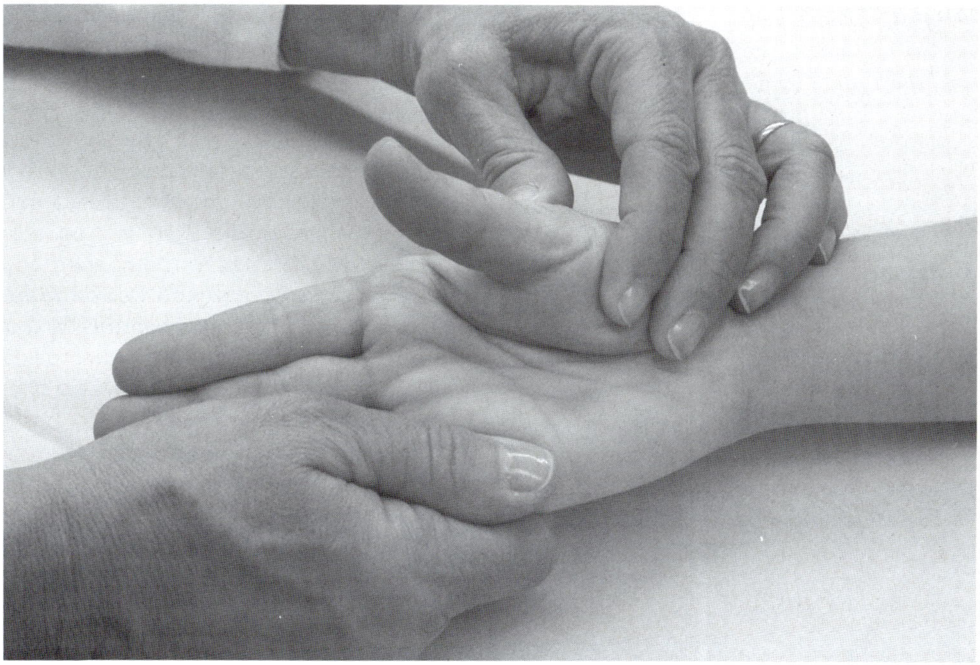

FIGURE 7.45 Midway through the range of motion of carpometacarpal (CMC) opposition, the metacarpal of the thumb is in abduction, flexion, and medial rotation. The fifth metacarpal is stabilized by the examiner.

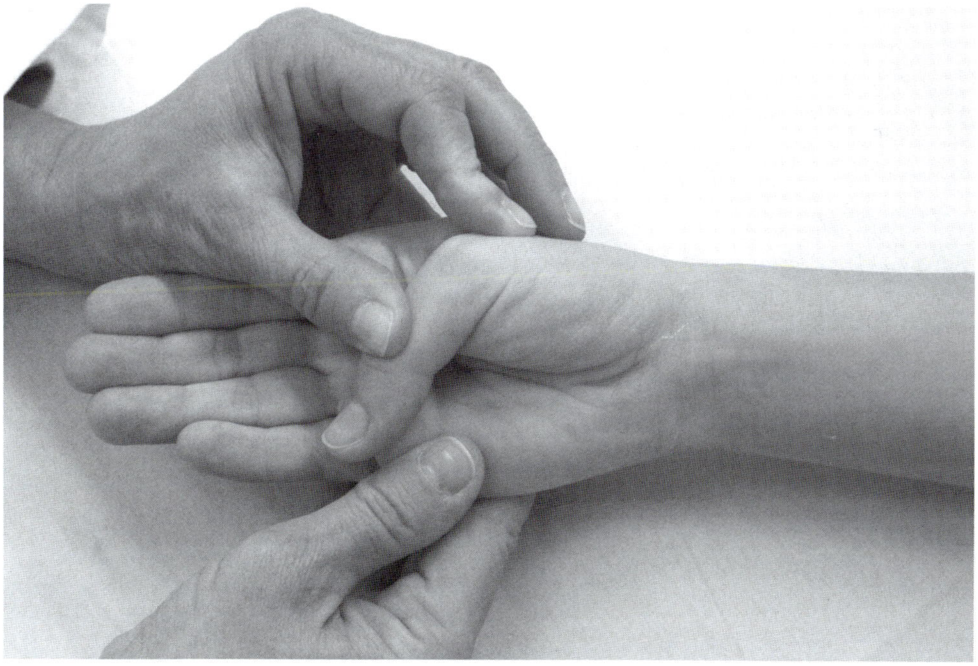

FIGURE 7.46 At the end of the range of opposition the tip of the individual's thumb is normally in contact with the base of the little finger. The thumb has moved through carpometacarpal (CMC) abduction, flexion, medial rotation, and adduction, while the metacarpophalangeal (MCP) joint is allowed to flex.

Normal End-Feel

The end-feel may be soft because of contact between the muscle bulk of the thenar eminence and the palm or between the tip of the thumb with the base of the little finger. In some individuals it may be firm because of tension in the CMC joint capsule, fascia, and skin of the web space between the thumb and the index finger and tension in the adductor pollicis, first dorsal interossei, extensor pollicis brevis, and extensor pollicis longus muscles.

Measurement Method: Linear Distance

The goniometer is not commonly used to measure the angular range of opposition. Instead, a linear ruler is often used to measure the shortest distance between the **tip of the thumb** and the center of the **proximal digital crease of the little finger** at the end of opposition (Fig. 7.47).[15,16]

Alternately, the shortest distance between the center of the **proximal digital crease of the thumb** and the **distal palmar crease directly over the fifth MCP joint** can be measured (Fig. 7.48). In this manner, motion at the MCP and IP joints of the thumb will not affect the measurement of opposition. In both methods, the smaller the distance is between the landmarks, the greater the ROM will be in opposition.

The AMA *Guides to the Evaluation of Permanent Impairment*[17] recommends measuring the largest achievable distance between the **flexion crease of the thumb IP joint** and the **distal palmar crease directly over the third MCP joint.** However, this measurement method seems more consistent with the measurement of CMC abduction than the usual definition of opposition. A distance of less than 8 centimeters is considered impaired.[17]

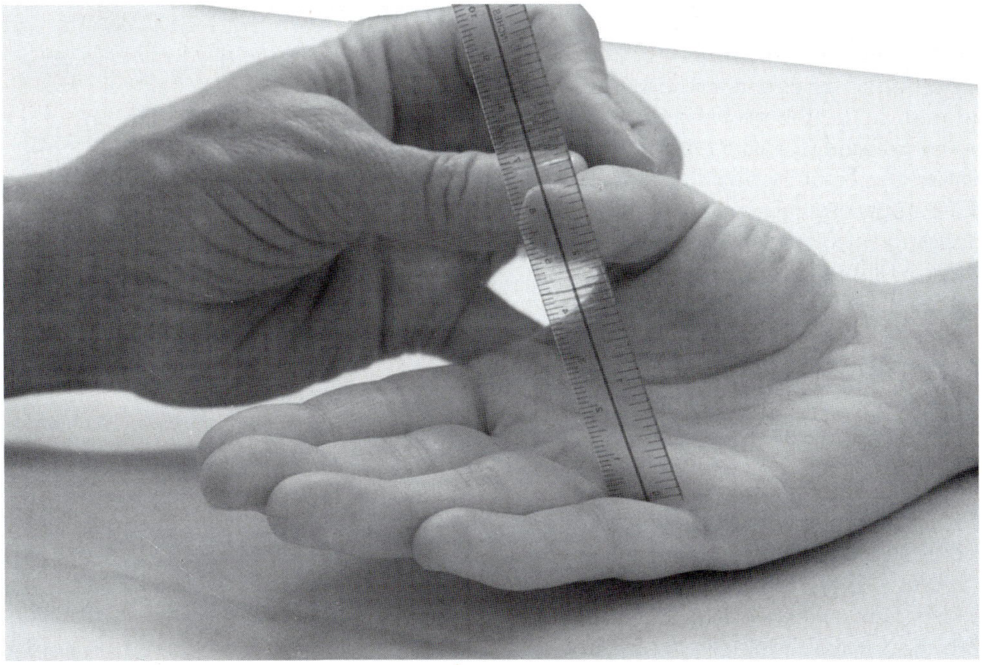

FIGURE 7.47 The range of motion (ROM) in opposition can be determined by measuring the shortest distance between the tip of the thumb and the proximal digital crease of the little finger. The examiner is using the arm of a goniometer to measure, but any ruler would suffice. This individual's hand does not have full ROM in opposition.

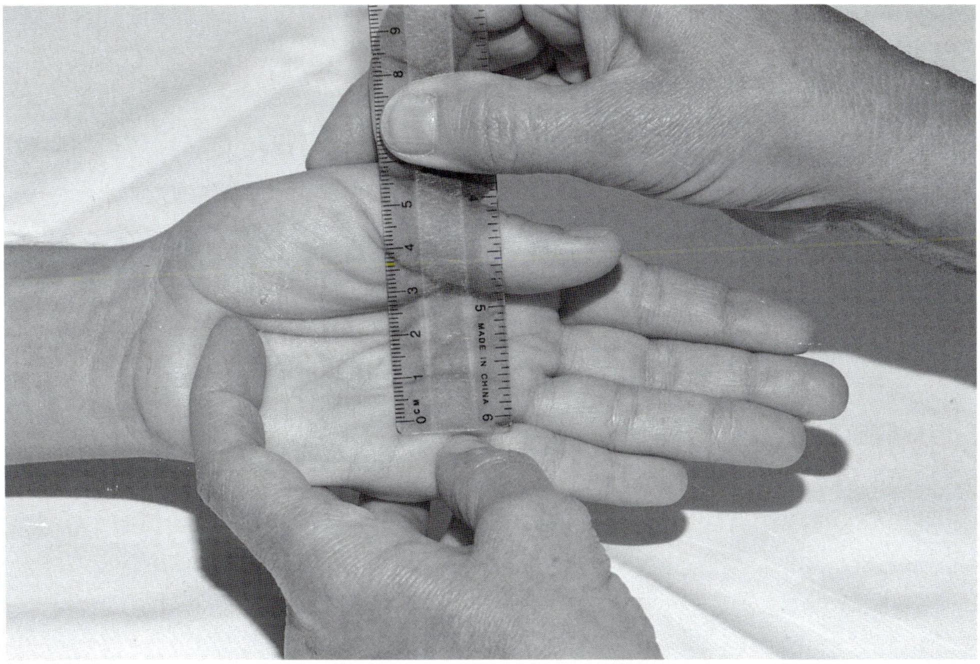

FIGURE 7.48 Another method of measuring thumb opposition is to record the distance between the proximal digital crease of the thumb and the distal palmar crease over the fifth metacarpophalangeal (MCP) joint. This method avoids the inclusion of MCP and IP flexion of the thumb.

Measurement Method: Total Opposition Test

Another clinical method of assessing and describing the composite motion of the thumb during opposition is suggested by Kapandji[26] and the IFSSH.[22] This measurement, called the Total Opposition Test (TOT), is divided into a 10-stage ordinal scale, with each number corresponding to a contact point on the hand that the pulp of the thumb is able to reach (Fig. 7.49). In addition to the first CMC joint, other joints of the thumb and fingers are allowed to flex and move as needed.

The **zero starting position** is with the pulp of the thumb in contact with the lateral side of the proximal phalange of the index finger (Fig. 7.50). In **Stages 1 and 2**, the pulp of the thumb contacts the lateral side of the middle and distal phalanges of the index finger, respectively. **Stages 3 to 6** require contact between the pulp of the thumb with the tips of the index, middle, ring, and little fingers, respectively (Fig. 7.51). The pulp of the thumb then makes contact with the palmar aspect of the DIP crease of the little finger **(Stage 7)**, the PIP crease **(Stage 8)**, the proximal digit crease of the little finger **(Stage 9)**, and the distal palmar crease (Stage 10) near the little finger to complete opposition. Refer to Figure 7.27 for the location of the digital and palmar creases. It is important that the stages are completed in sequence so that true opposition occurs and not just flexion of the thumb to attain Stages 9 and 10.

A mean grade of 9 (SD = 0.5) for the TOT of the right thumb has been reported in a sample of 62 healthy females and 38 healthy males aged 18 to 37 years.[21] The intertester reliability of using this method in patients recovering from burns was excellent with an intraclass correlation coefficient (ICC) value of 0.99 and a minimal detectible difference of 0.3 on the TOT scale.[31]

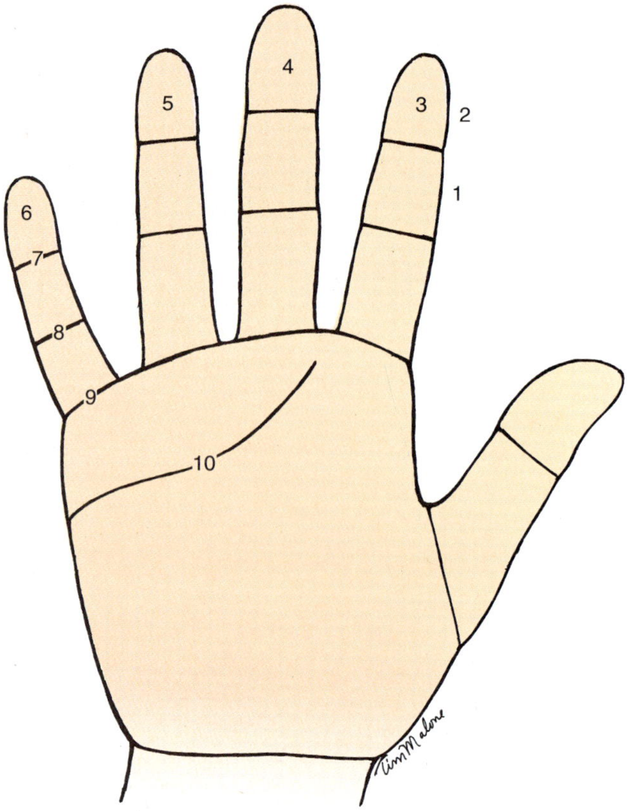

FIGURE 7.49 Illustration of the Total Opposition Test (TOT) showing the 10 stages of numbering thumb opposition.[22,26] The individual moves through the 10 stages in sequence. The score is the highest stage that can be reached using good technique.

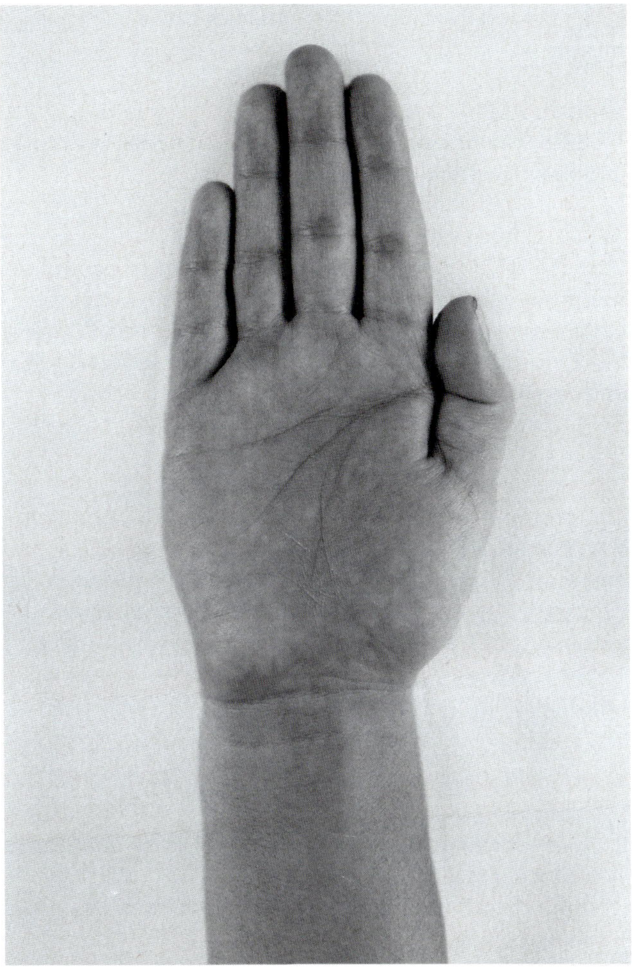

FIGURE 7.50 The starting position for the Total Opposition Test. The thumb is held in contact with the side of the index finger.

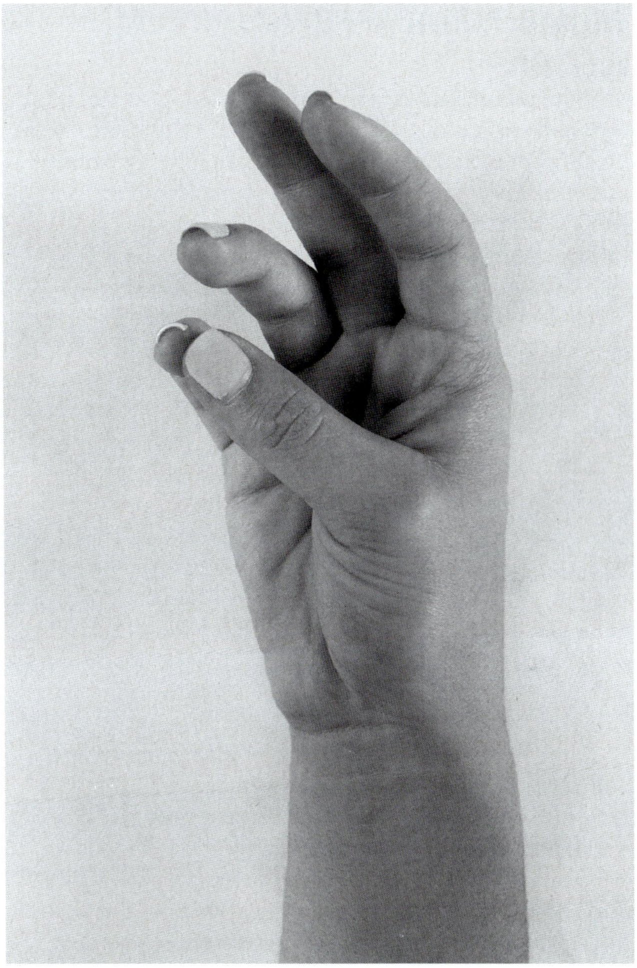

FIGURE 7.51 The individual has moved sequentially through the stages of opposition and is now at Stage 6. The tip of the thumb is in contact with the tip of the little finger.

THUMB: METACARPOPHALANGEAL FLEXION

Motion occurs in the frontal plane around an anterior–posterior axis when the individual is in the anatomical position. Normal ROM values for adults vary from about 50 to 60 degrees. See Research Findings and Table 7.3. In addition to the sources included in Table 7.3, DeSmet and associates[32] report 54.0 degrees (SD = 13.7) of MCP flexion in 101 males and females 16 to 83 years of age. Barakat and coworkers[21] report a mean of 60 degrees (SD = 5.5) in a study of 62 healthy females ranging in age from 18 to 37 years. A bimodal pattern of MCP flexion ROM was report by Hume and associates[33] in 35 males ranging in age from 26 to 28 years, with 85% of the males having a mean of 56 degrees and 15% having a mean of 27 degrees. Other researchers[34,35] have also noted two types of anatomical shape of the metacarpal head of the thumb: round versus flat. The rounded metacarpal head was found to have greater ROM than the flatter metacarpal head.

Testing Position

Position the individual sitting, with the forearm and hand resting on a supporting surface. Place the forearm in full supination; the wrist in 0 degrees of flexion, extension, and radial and ulnar deviation; the CMC joint of the thumb in 0 degrees of flexion, extension, abduction, adduction, and opposition; and the IP joint of the thumb in 0 degrees of flexion and extension. (If the wrist and IP joint of the thumb are positioned in full flexion, tension in the extensor pollicis longus muscle will restrict the motion.)

Stabilization

Stabilize the first metacarpal to prevent wrist motion and flexion of the CMC joint of the thumb.

Testing Motion

Flex the MCP joint by pushing on the dorsal aspect of the proximal phalanx, moving the thumb toward the ulnar aspect of the hand (Fig. 7.52). The end of flexion ROM occurs when resistance to further motion is felt and attempts to overcome the resistance cause the CMC joint to flex.

Normal End-Feel

The end-feel may be hard because of contact between the palmar aspect of the proximal phalanx and the first metacarpal, or it may be firm because of tension in the dorsal joint capsule, the collateral ligaments, and the extensor pollicis brevis muscle.

Goniometer Alignment

See Figures 7.53 and 7.54.

1. Center **fulcrum** of the goniometer over the dorsal aspect of the MCP joint.
2. Align **proximal arm** over the dorsal midline of the metacarpal.
3. Align **distal arm** with the dorsal midline of the proximal phalanx.

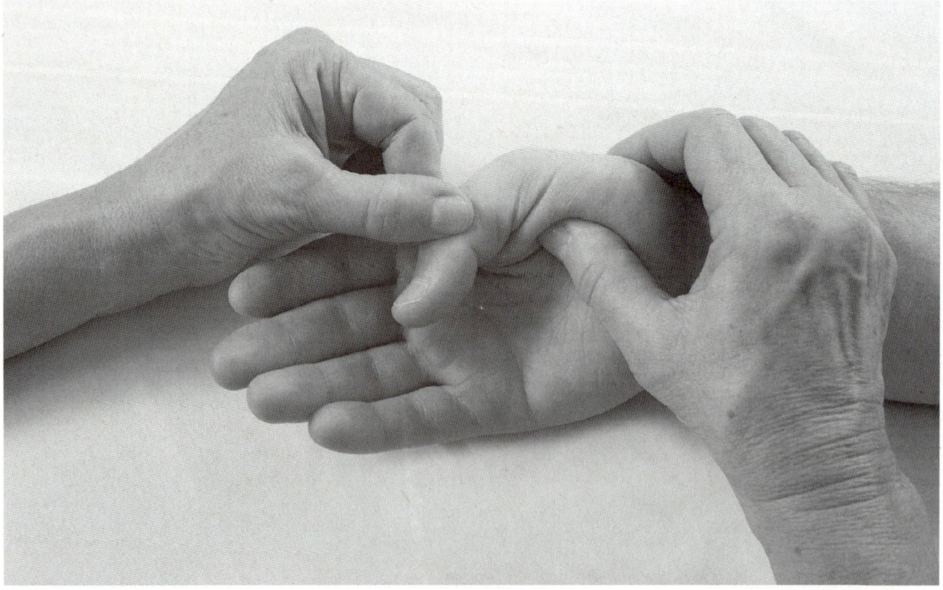

FIGURE 7.52 During metacarpophalangeal (MCP) flexion of the thumb, the examiner uses the index finger and thumb of one hand to stabilize the individual's first metacarpal and maintain the wrist in a neutral position. The examiner's other index finger and thumb grasp the distal end of the proximal phalanx to move it into flexion.

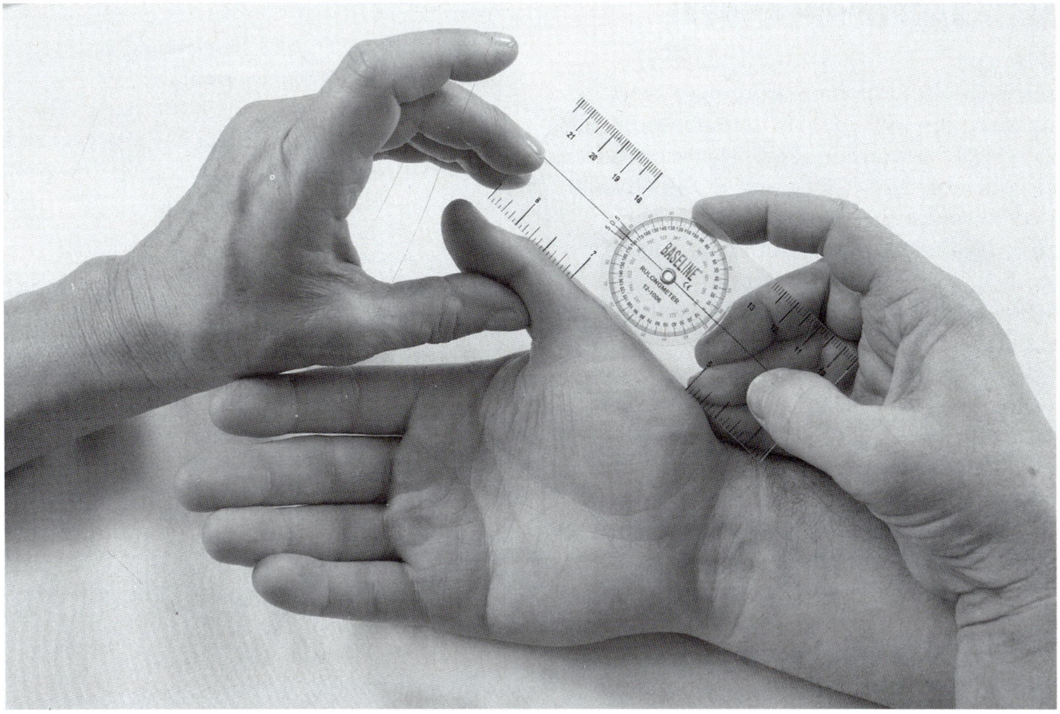

FIGURE 7.53 The alignment of the goniometer on the dorsal surfaces of the first metacarpal and proximal phalanx at the beginning of metacarpophalangeal (MCP) flexion range of motion of the thumb. If a bony deformity or swelling is present, the goniometer may be aligned with the lateral surface of these bones.

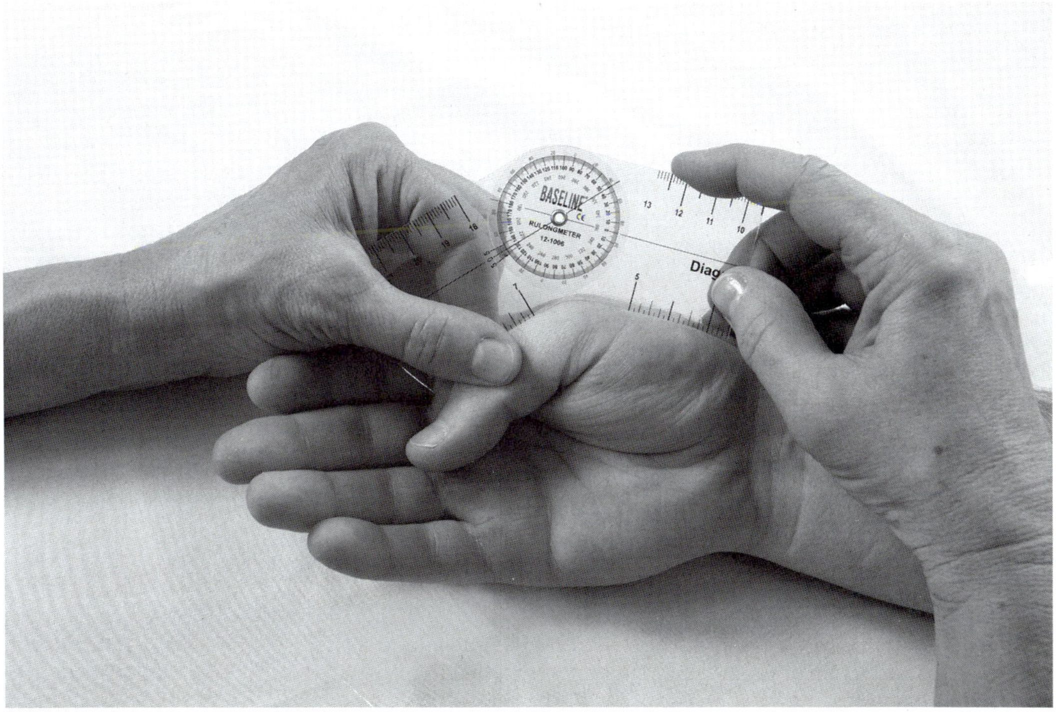

FIGURE 7.54 At the end of metacarpophalangeal (MCP) flexion, the examiner uses one hand to align the proximal arm of the goniometer. The examiner uses her other hand to maintain the proximal phalanx in flexion and align the distal arm of the goniometer.

THUMB: METACARPOPHALANGEAL EXTENSION

Motion occurs in the frontal plane around an anterior–posterior axis when the individual is in the anatomical position. Thumb MCP extension is usually recorded as the starting position for MCP flexion ROM. Normal MCP extension ROM for the thumb is usually considered to be 0 degrees,[15,16,24,25,33] but some sources have reported 8 to 40 degrees depending on the measurement method.[12,17,21,34] Passive MCP extension ROM appears to be greater than active motions.[12] See Research Findings and Table 7.3.

Testing Position

Position the individual sitting, with the forearm and hand resting on a supporting surface. Place the forearm in full supination; the wrist in 0 degrees of flexion, extension, and radial and ulnar deviation; the CMC joint of the thumb in 0 degrees of flexion, extension, abduction, and opposition; and the IP joint of the thumb in 0 degrees of flexion and extension. (If the wrist and the IP joint of the thumb are positioned in full extension, tension in the flexor pollicis longus muscle may restrict the motion.)

Stabilization

Stabilize the first metacarpal to prevent motion at the wrist and at the CMC joint of the thumb.

Testing Motion

Extend the MCP joint by pushing on the palmar surface of the proximal phalanx, moving the thumb toward the radial aspect of the hand. The end of extension ROM occurs when resistance to further motion is felt and attempts to overcome the resistance cause the CMC joint to extend.

Normal End-Feel

The end-feel is firm because of tension in the palmar joint capsule, palmar plate (palmar ligament), intersesamoid (cruciate) ligaments, and flexor pollicis brevis muscle.

Goniometer Alignment

Refer to Figure 7.53.

1. Center **fulcrum** of the goniometer over the dorsal aspect of the MCP joint.
2. Align **proximal arm** over the dorsal midline of the metacarpal.
3. Align **distal arm** with the dorsal midline of the proximal phalanx.

THUMB: INTERPHALANGEAL FLEXION

Motion occurs in the frontal plane around an anterior–posterior axis when the individual is in the anatomical position. Normal ROM values for adults are reported to be about 80 degrees. See Research Findings and Table 7.3. In addition to the sources included in Table 7.3, DeSmet and associates[32] found 79.8 degrees (SD = 10.2) of IP flexion in 101 males and females 16 to 83 years of age. Barakat and coworkers[21] report a mean of 88 degrees (SD = 2.3) in a study of 62 healthy females ranging in age from 18 to 37 years.

Testing Position

Position the individual sitting, with the forearm and hand resting on a supporting surface. Place the forearm in full supination; the wrist in 0 degrees of flexion, extension, and radial and ulnar deviation; the CMC joint in 0 degrees of flexion, extension, abduction, and opposition; and the MCP joint of the thumb in 0 degrees of flexion and extension. (If the wrist and MCP joint of the thumb are flexed, tension in the extensor pollicis longus muscle may restrict the motion. If the MCP joint of the thumb is fully extended, tension in the abductor pollicis brevis and the oblique fibers of the adductor pollicis may restrict the motion through their insertion into the extensor mechanism.)

Stabilization

Stabilize the proximal phalanx to prevent flexion or extension of the MCP joint.

Testing Motion

Flex the IP joint by pushing on the dorsal surface of the distal phalanx, moving the tip of the thumb toward the ulnar aspect of the hand (Fig. 7.55). The end of flexion ROM occurs when resistance to further motion is felt and attempts to overcome the resistance cause the MCP joint to flex.

Normal End-Feel

Usually, the end-feel is firm because of tension in the collateral ligaments and the dorsal joint capsule. In some individuals, the end-feel may be hard because of contact between the palmar aspect of the distal phalanx, the palmar plate, and the proximal phalanx.

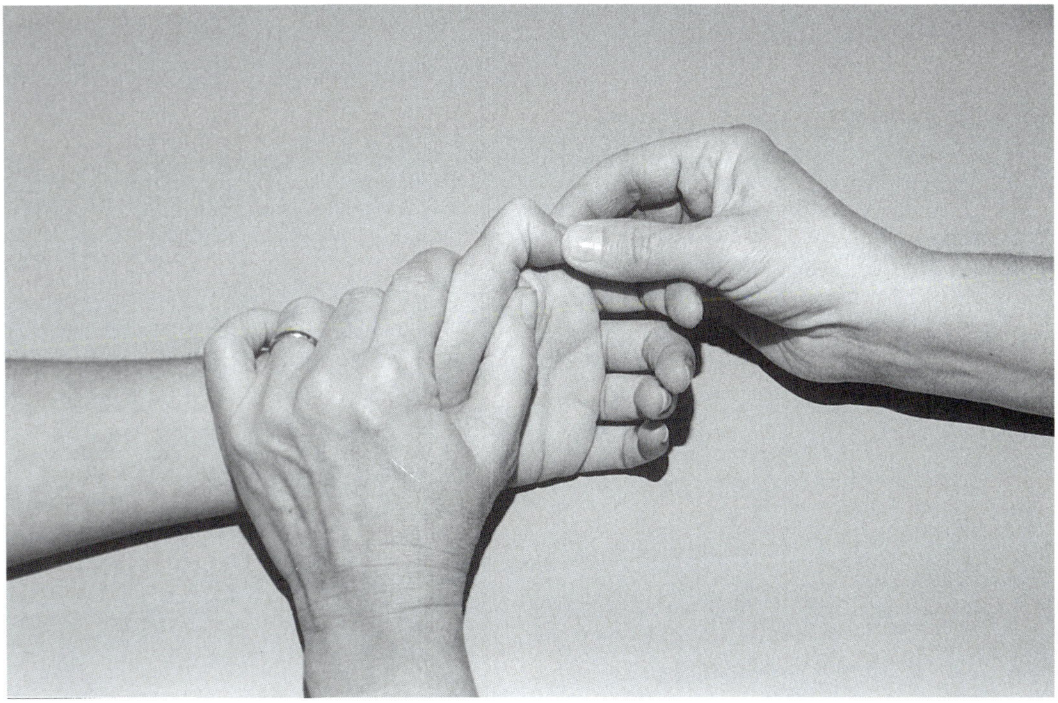

FIGURE 7.55 During interphalangeal (IP) flexion of the thumb, the examiner uses one hand to stabilize the proximal phalanx and keep the metacarpophalangeal joint in 0 degrees of flexion and the carpometacarpal joint in 0 degrees of flexion, abduction, and opposition. The examiner uses her other index finger and thumb to flex the distal phalanx.

Goniometer Alignment

See Figures 7.56 and 7.57.

1. Center **fulcrum** of the goniometer over the dorsal surface of the IP joint.
2. Align **proximal arm** with the dorsal midline of the proximal phalanx.
3. Align **distal arm** with the dorsal midline of the distal phalanx.

In some individuals the angle of the nailbed may make it difficult to place the distal arm on the goniometer on the dorsal surface of the distal phalanx. In this case the axis of the goniometer should be centered over the lateral surface of the IP joint and the arms of the goniometer should be aligned with the lateral longitudinal axes of the proximal and distal phalanx.

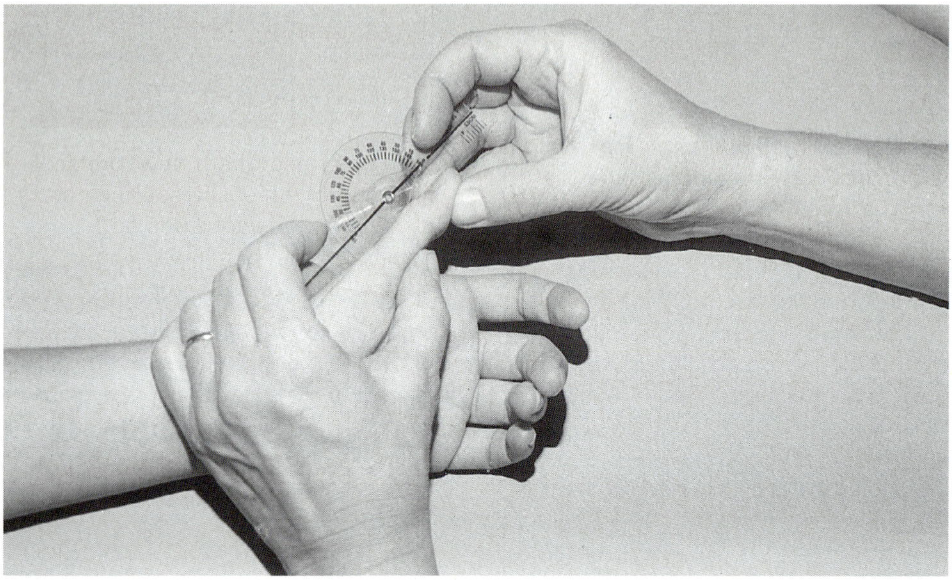

FIGURE 7.56 The alignment of the goniometer at the beginning of interphalangeal (IP) flexion range of motion. The arms of the goniometer are placed on the dorsal surfaces of the proximal and distal phalanges. However, the arms of the goniometer could instead be placed on the lateral surfaces of the proximal and distal phalanges if the nail protruded or if there was a bony prominence or swelling.

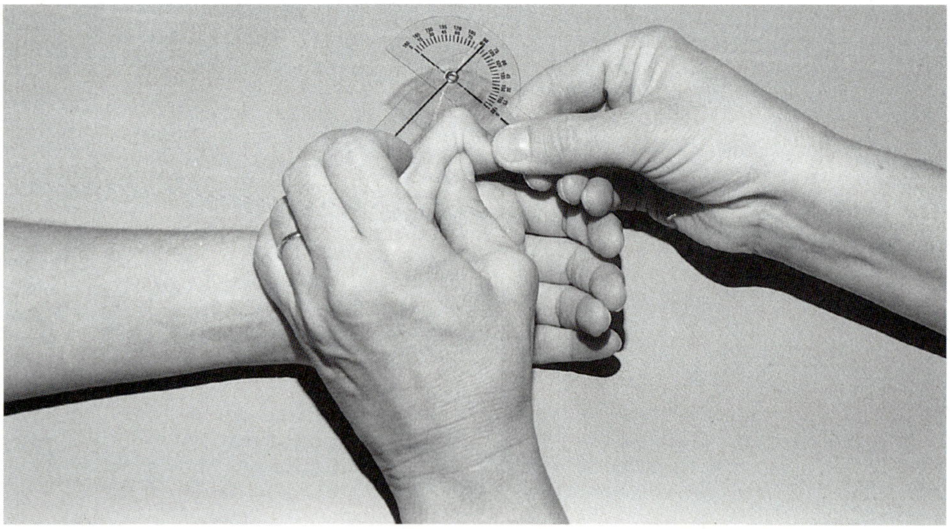

FIGURE 7.57 The alignment of the goniometer at the end of interphalangeal (IP) flexion range of motion. The examiner holds the arms of the goniometer so that they maintain close contact with the dorsal surfaces of the proximal and distal phalanges.

THUMB: INTERPHALANGEAL EXTENSION

Motion occurs in the frontal plane around an anterior–posterior axis when the individual is in the anatomical position. Normal active extension ROM at the IP joint of the thumb varies from about 20 to 30 degrees. Passive extension ROM has been found to be greater than active ROM.[12] See Research Findings and Table 7.3. In addition to the sources cited in Table 7.3, Barakat and coworkers[21] report a mean of 12 degrees (SD = 9.2) in a study of 62 healthy females ranging in age from 18 to 37 years.

Testing Position

Position the individual sitting, with the forearm and hand resting on a supporting surface forearm. Place the forearm in full supination; the wrist in 0 degrees of flexion, extension, and radial and ulnar deviation; the CMC joint of the thumb in 0 degrees of flexion, extension, abduction, and opposition; and the MCP joint of the thumb in 0 degrees of flexion and extension. (If the wrist and MCP joint of the thumb are extended, tension in the flexor pollicis longus muscle may restrict the motion.)

Stabilization

Stabilize the proximal phalanx to prevent extension or flexion of the MCP joint.

Testing Motion

Extend the IP joint by pushing on the palmar surface of the distal phalanx, moving the thumb toward the radial aspect of the hand. The end of extension ROM occurs when resistance to further motion is felt and attempts to overcome the resistance cause the MCP joint to extend.

Normal End-Feel

The end-feel is firm because of tension in the palmar joint capsule and the palmar plate (palmar ligament).

Goniometer Alignment

Refer to Fig 7.56.

1. Center **fulcrum** of the goniometer over the dorsal surface of the IP joint.
2. Align **proximal arm** with the dorsal midline of the proximal phalanx.
3. Align **distal arm** with the dorsal midline of the distal phalanx.

In some individuals the angle of the nailbed may make it difficult to place the distal arm on the goniometer on the dorsal surface of the distal phalanx. In that case the axis of the goniometer should be centered over the lateral surface of the IP joint and the arms should be aligned with the lateral longitudinal axes of the proximal and distal phalanx.

MUSCLE LENGTH TESTING PROCEDURES: Fingers

Landmarks for Testing Procedures

See Figures 7.7 and 7.8 for landmarks for testing procedures of the fingers.

METACARPOPHALANGEAL FLEXORS

A number of muscles perform MCP flexion of the fingers. These muscles include the lumbricals, palmar and dorsal interossei, and the flexor digitorum profundus and superficialis. The lumbrical, palmar interossei, and dorsal interossei muscles cross the MCP, PIP, and DIP joints. The first and second **lumbricals** originate proximally from the radial sides of the tendons of the flexor digitorum profundus of the index and middle fingers, respectively (Fig. 7.58). The third lumbrical originates on the ulnar side of the tendon of the flexor digitorum profundus of the middle finger and the radial side of the tendon of the ring finger. The fourth lumbrical originates on the ulnar side of the tendon of the flexor digitorum profundus of the ring finger and the radial side of the tendon of the little finger. Each lumbrical passes to the radial side of the corresponding finger and inserts distally into the extensor mechanism of the extensor digitorum profundus.

The first **palmar interossei muscle** originates proximally from the ulnar side of the metacarpal of the index finger and inserts distally into the ulnar side of the proximal phalanx and the extensor mechanism of the extensor digitorum profundus of the same finger (Fig. 7.59). The second and third palmar interossei muscles originate proximally from the radial sides of the metacarpal of the ring and little fingers, respectively, and insert distally into the ulnar side of the proximal phalanx and the extensor mechanism of the extensor digitorum profundus of the same fingers.

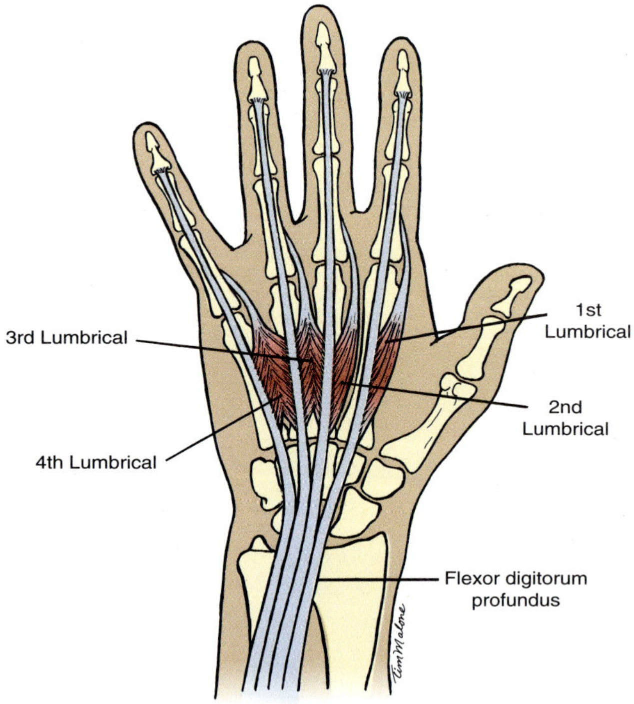

FIGURE 7.58 An anterior (palmar) view of the right hand showing the proximal attachments of the lumbricals. The lumbricals insert distally into the extensor digitorum on the posterior surface of the hand, which can not be seen from this view.

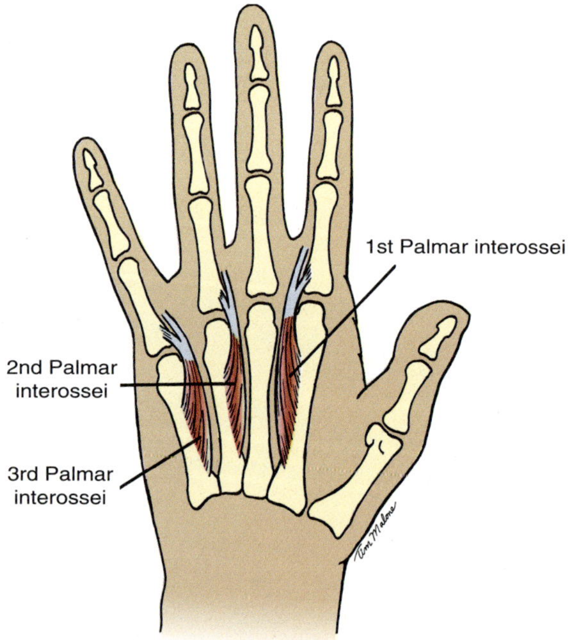

FIGURE 7.59 An anterior (palmar) view of the right hand showing the proximal and distal attachments of the palmar interossei. The palmar interossei also attach distally to the extensor digitorum on the posterior surface of the hand.

The four **dorsal interossei** are bipenniform muscles that originate proximally from two adjacent metacarpals (Fig. 7.60): the first dorsal interossei from the metacarpals of the thumb and index finger, the second from the metacarpals of the index and middle fingers, the third from the metacarpals of the middle and ring fingers, and the fourth from the metacarpals of the ring and little fingers. The dorsal interossei insert distally into the bases of the proximal phalanges and the extensor mechanism of the extensor digitorum profundus of the same fingers.

When these three muscles contract, they flex the MCP joints and extend the PIP and DIP joints. These muscles are passively lengthened by placing the MCP joints in extension and the PIP and DIP joints in full flexion.

The flexor digitorum profundus and flexor digitorum superficialis also flex the MCP joints of the fingers. However, these muscles cross the palmar surfaces of the wrist, MCP, PIP, and DIP joints. If the flexor digitorum profundus and flexor digitorum superficialis muscles are short, they will limit MCP extension with the wrist, PIP, and DIP joints held in extension. Testing the length of the flexor digitorum profundus and flexor digitorum superficialis is presented in Chapter 6. Refer to Muscle Length Testing Procedures: Wrist Flexors.

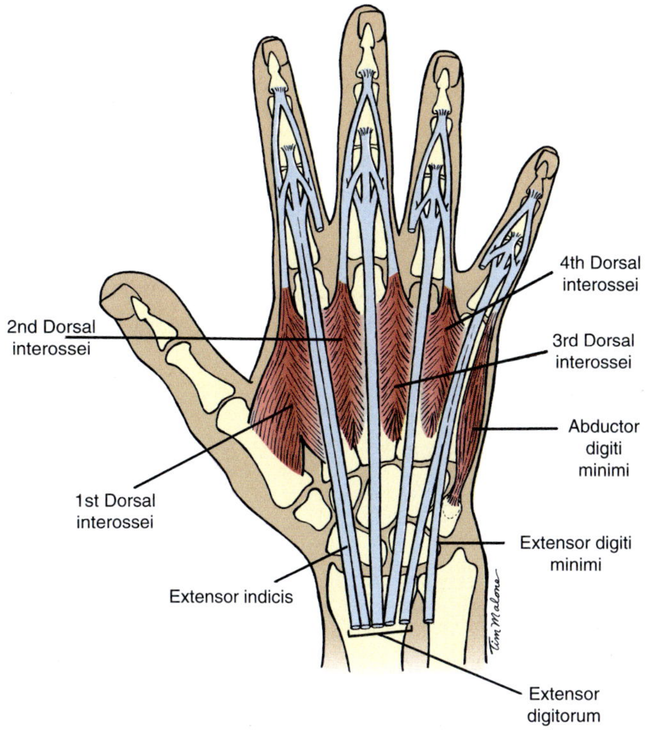

FIGURE 7.60 A posterior view of the right hand showing the proximal attachments of the dorsal interossei on the metacarpals and the distal attachments into the extensor mechanism of the extensor digitorum, extensor indicis, and extensor digiti minimi muscles.

LUMBRICALS, PALMAR INTEROSSEI, AND DORSAL INTEROSSEI MUSCLE LENGTH TEST

Testing Position

Position the individual sitting, with the forearm and hand resting on a supporting surface. Place the forearm midway between pronation and supination and the wrist in 0 degrees of flexion, extension, and radial and ulnar deviation. Flex the MCP, PIP, and DIP joints (Fig. 7.61). The MCP joints should be in a neutral position relative to abduction and adduction.

Stabilization

Stabilize the metacarpals and the carpal bones to prevent wrist motion.

Testing Motion

Hold the PIP and DIP joints in full flexion while extending the MCP joint (Figs. 7.62 and 7.63). All of the fingers may be screened together, but if abnormalities are found, testing should be conducted on individual fingers. The end of flexion ROM occurs when resistance to further motion is felt and attempts to overcome the resistance cause the PIP, DIP, or wrist joints to extend.

Normal End-Feel

The end-feel is firm because of tension in the lumbrical, palmar interossei, and dorsal interossei muscles.

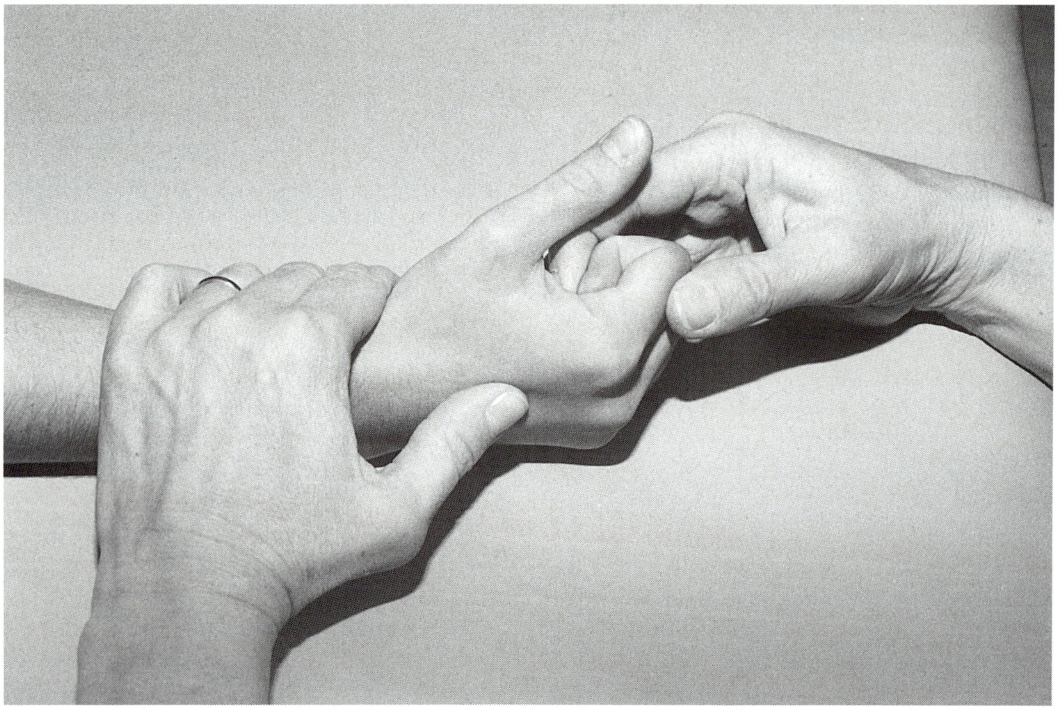

FIGURE 7.61 The starting position for testing the length of the lumbricals and the palmar and dorsal interossei. The examiner uses one hand to stabilize the individual's wrist and the other hand to position the metacarpophalangeal, proximal interphalangeal, and distal interphalangeal joints in full flexion.

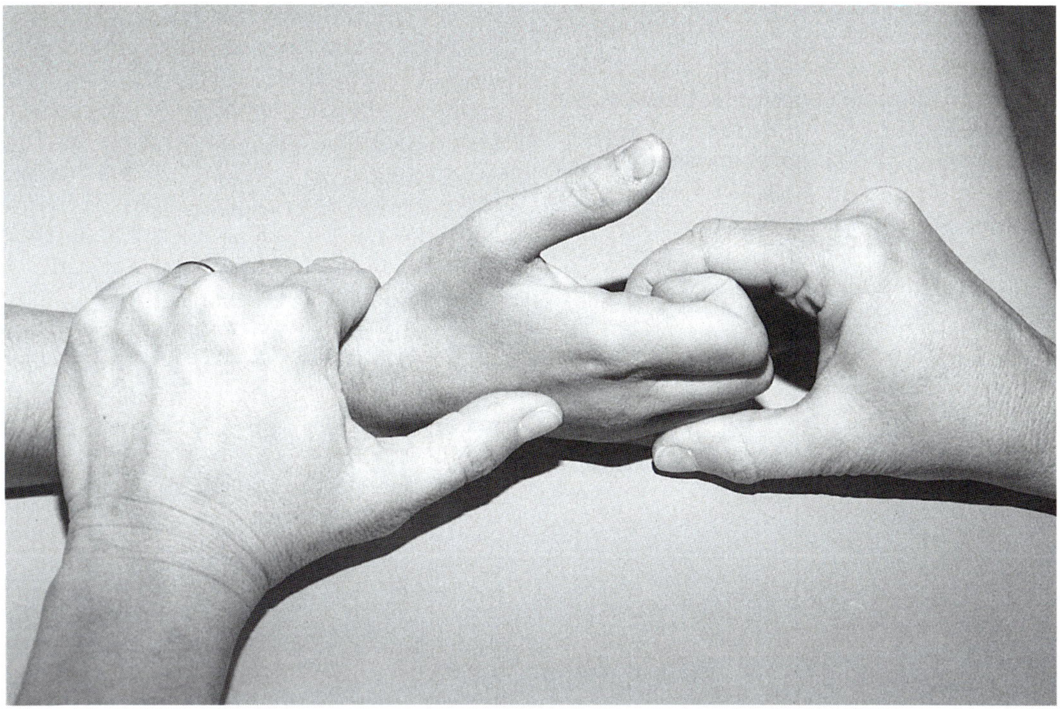

FIGURE 7.62 The end of the motion for testing the length of the lumbricals and the palmar and dorsal interossei. The examiner holds the individual's proximal interphalangeal and distal interphalangeal joints in full flexion while moving the metacarpophalangeal joint into extension.

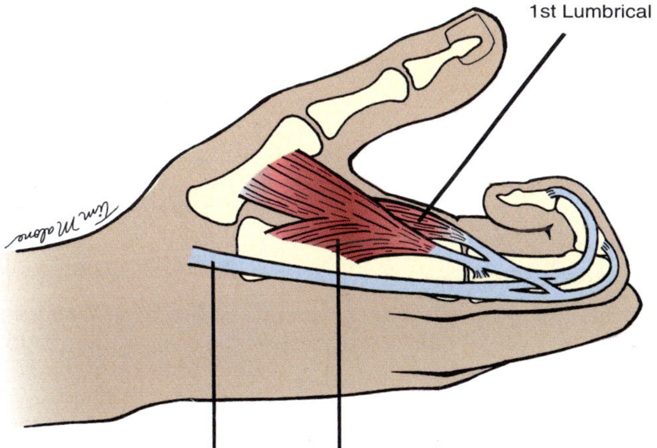

FIGURE 7.63 A lateral view of the right hand showing the first lumbrical and the first dorsal interossei muscles being stretched over the metacarpophalangeal, proximal interphalangeal, and distal interphalangeal joints.

Goniometer Alignment

See Figure 7.64.

1. Center **fulcrum** of the goniometer over the dorsal aspect of the MCP joint.
2. Align **proximal arm** over the dorsal midline of the metacarpal.
3. Align **distal arm** over the dorsal midline of the proximal phalanx.

Interpretation

If the lumbricals and the palmar and dorsal interossei are short in length, they will limit MCP extension when the PIP and DIP joints are positioned in full flexion. If the flexor digitorum profundus and superficialis are short in length, they will limit MCP extension when the wrist, PIP, and DIP joints are positioned in full extension. If MCP flexion is limited regardless of the position of the PIP and DIP joints, the limitation is due to abnormalities of the joint surfaces of the MCP joint or shortening of the palmar joint capsule and the palmar plate. We are not aware of any normative values for this muscle length test.

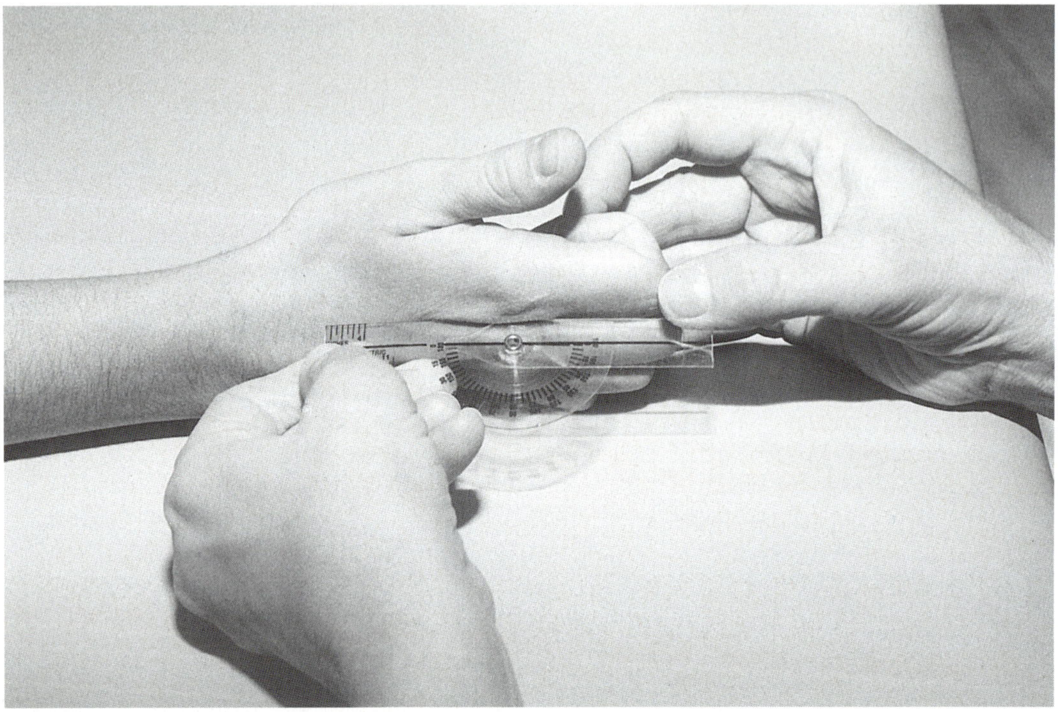

FIGURE 7.64 The alignment of the goniometer at the end of testing the length of the lumbricals and the palmar and dorsal interossei muscles. The arms of the goniometer are placed on the dorsal midline of the metacarpal and proximal phalanx of the finger being tested.

Research Findings

Effects of Age, Gender, and Other Factors

Table 7.1 provides a summary of ROM values for the MCP, PIP, and DIP joints of the fingers. Although the values reported by the sources in Table 7.1 vary, certain trends are evident. The PIP joints, followed by the MCP and DIP joints, have the greatest amount of flexion. The MCP joints have the greatest amount of extension, whereas the PIP joints have the least amount of extension. Total active motion (TAM) is the sum of flexion and extension ROM of the MCP, PIP, and DIP joints of a digit. Normal TAM values range from 290 to 310 degrees for the fingers.

Some differences in ROM values are noted between individual fingers (Table 7.2). Flexion ROM at the MCP joints seems to increase linearly in an ulnar direction from the index finger to the little finger.[11–13] Mallon, Brown, and Nunley[11] report that extension at the MCP joints is approximately equal for all fingers. However, Skvarilova and Plevkova[12] and Smahel and Klimova[13] note that the little finger has the greatest amount of MCP extension. The motions of PIP flexion and extension and DIP flexion are generally equal for all fingers.[11] Some passive extension beyond neutral is possible at the DIP joints, with a minor increase in a radial direction from the little finger toward the index finger.[11]

Only the MCP joints of the fingers have a considerable amount of abduction–adduction. The amount of abduction–adduction varies with the position of the MCP joint. Abduction–adduction ROM is greatest in extension and least in full flexion. In extension the collateral ligaments of the MCP joints are slack and allow full abduction. However, the collateral ligaments tighten and restrict abduction in the fully flexed position.[1,3,4] Some authors note that the index and little fingers have a greater ROM in abduction–adduction than the middle and ring fingers.[1] Others report that the little finger has the greatest MCP abduction.[14]

Table 7.3 presents ROM values for the joints of the thumb. The greatest amount of flexion and extension is reported at the IP joint. Studies by Joseph[35] and Yoshida and coworkers[34] have identified two general anatomical shapes of the metacarpal head of the thumb that may account for some of the variations seen in ROM values at the MCP joint. Metacarpophalangeal joints with a round metacarpal head had greater motion than MCP joints with a flat metacarpal head. Sauseng, Kastenbauer, and Irsigler[37] and Shaw and Morris[38] also present some normative data on MCP and IP flexion of the thumb. Minimal data are available for normal values of motions at the CMC joint.

Age

Goniometric studies focusing on the effects of age on ROM typically exclude the joints of the fingers and thumb. Among the limited number of studies that examined aging effects in the hand, some report less finger and thumb ROM with increasing age, whereas others report no consistent aging effect on thumb ROM.

DeSmet and colleagues[32] found a significant correlation between decreasing MCP and IP flexion of the thumb and increasing age. The 58 females and 43 males who were

TABLE 7.1 Normal Active Finger ROM: Values for Adults in Degrees From Selected Sources

		AAOS[15,16]	AMA[17]	IFSSH[22]	Hume[33] 26–28 yr n = 35 Males	Mallon*[11] 18–35 yr n = 60 Males, 60 Females	Skvarilova†[12] 20–25 yr n = 100 Males, 100 Females		Smahel†[13,36] 18–28 yr n = 52 Males, 49 Females	
Joint	**Motion**				**Mean**	**Mean**	**Mean**	**(SD)**	**Mean**	**(SD)**
MCP	Flexion	90	90	90	100	95	91.0	(6.2)	91.9	(8.0)
	Extension	45	20	30	0	20	25.8	(6.7)	24.8	(7.2)
PIP	Flexion	100	100	105	105	105	107.9	(5.6)	110.7	(5.3)
	Extension	0	0	0	0	7	—	—	—	—
DIP	Flexion	90	70	70	85	68	84.5	(7.9)	81.3	(7.0)
	Extension	0	0	0	0	8	—	—	—	—
Total active motion		—	—		290	303	309.2	(6.6)	308.7	(6.8)

AAOS = American Association of Orthopaedic Surgeons; AMA = American Medical Association; IFSSH = International Federation of Societies for Surgery of the Hand; DIP = Distal interphalangeal; MCP = Metacarpophalangeal; PIP = Proximal interphalangeal; SD = Standard deviation.

*Values were averaged from both genders and all fingers.

† Values were averaged from both genders, both hands, and all fingers and were converted from a 360-degree to a 180-degree recording system.

TABLE 7.2 Normal Individual Finger ROM: Mean Values for Adults in Degrees From Selected Sources

		Mallon[11]		Skvarilova*[12]		Smahel*[13,36]	
		Passive ROM 18–35 yr		Passive ROM 20–25 yr		Active ROM 18–28 yr	
		Male	*Female*	*Male*	*Female*	*Male*	*Female*
Joint	Motion	*n* = 60	*n* = 60	*n* = 100	*n* = 100	*n* = 52	*n* = 49
Index Finger							
MCP	Flexion	94	95	97	97	87	87
	Extension	29	56	55	56	22	26
PIP	Flexion	106	107	115	117	111	113
	Extension	11	19	—	—	—	—
DIP	Flexion	75	75	87	95	78	80
	Extension	22	24	—	—	—	—
Middle Finger							
MCP	Flexion	98	100	102	104	95	94
	Extension	34	54	48	48	20	24
PIP	Flexion	110	112	115	118	111	114
	Extension	10	20	—	—	—	—
DIP	Flexion	80	79	87	98	84	83
	Extension	19	23	—	—	—	—
Ring Finger							
MCP	Flexion	102	103	104	102	94	93
	Extension	29	60	48	49	21	25
PIP	Flexion	110	108	115	119	112	115
	Extension	14	20	—	—	—	—
DIP	Flexion	74	76	83	92	80	78
	Extension	17	18	—	—	—	—
Little Finger							
MCP	Flexion	107	107	107	104	93	93
	Extension	48	62	63	65	27	32
PIP	Flexion	111	110	111	113	104	106
	Extension	13	21	—	—	—	—
DIP	Flexion	72	72	89	102	83	84
	Extension	15	21	—	—	—	—

DIP = Distal interphalangeal; MCP = Metacarpophalangeal; PIP = Proximal interphalangeal; ROM = range of motion.
*Values were converted from a 360-degree to a 180-degree recording system.

included in the study ranged in age from 16 to 83 years. Smahel and Klimova,[13,36] in studies of 101 university students, 60 senior citizens, and 52 pianists, found that the senior citizens had significantly less MCP, PIP, and DIP ranges of motion in the fingers than the university students, except for total abduction (ability to spread fingers) of the MCP joints in females. The mean age differences were 6.3 degrees for active MCP flexion, 6.1 degrees for active MCP extension, 20.4 degrees for passive MCP extension, 9.1 degrees for active PIP flexion, and 9.5 degrees for active DIP flexion. The age differences in ROM were generally greater in males than in females.

Measures of hypermobility that include motions of the thumb and little finger have shown a decrease with age. Beighton, Solomon, and Soskolne[40] used passive apposition of the thumb (with wrist flexion) to the anterior aspect of the forearm and passive hyperextension of the MCP joint of the fifth finger beyond 90 degrees as indicators of hypermobility in a study of 456 men and 625 women in an African village. They

TABLE 7.3 Normal Thumb ROM: Mean Values for Adults in Degrees From Selected Sources

		AAOS[15,16]	AMA[17]	IFSSH[22]	White[23]	Jenkins[39]	Yoshida[34]	Skvarilova*[12]	
					21–92 yr *n* = 48 Males, 48 Females	16–72 yr *n* = 50 Males, 69 Females	18–63 yr *n* = 51 Males, 49 Females	20–25 yr *n* = 100 Males, 100 Females	
Joint	***Motion***				***Passive Mean (SD)***	***Active Mean (SD)***	***Active Mean***	***Active Mean (SD)***	***Passive Mean (SD)***
CMC	Flexion	15		15**	21.7 (6.8)				
	Extension	20	35†	40‡	19.5 (5.7)				
	Abduction	70		40	51.1 (5.5)				
MCP	Flexion	50	60			59 (11)	77	57.0 (10.7)	67.0 (9.0)
	Extension	0	40				35	13.7 (10.5)	22.6 (10.9)
IP	Flexion	80	80	80		67 (11)	81	79.1 (8.7)	85.8 (8.3)
	Extension	20	30	≤ 40			33	23.2 (13.3)	34.7 (13.3)

AAOS = American Association of Orthopaedic Surgeons; AMA = American Medical Association; IFSSH = International Federation of Societies for Surgery of the Hand; DIP = Distal interphalangeal; MCP = Metacarpophalangeal; PIP = Proximal interphalangeal; SD = Standard deviation.

* Values were recalculated to include both thumbs for both genders and were converted from a 360-degree to a 180-degree recording system.

** The IFSSH defines this motion as "movement toward the center of the palm"; calling this motion radial adduction, or the opposite of radial abduction.

† The AMA reports that in this plane of motion the minimal angle of separation between the first and second metacarpal is 15 degrees, whereas the maximal angle of separation between the first and second metacarpals is 50 degrees. The ROM value of 35 degrees is the difference between these two measurements.

‡ The IFSSH reports the maximal angle between the thumb and index metacarpals at the end of the motion rather than the ROM.

found that joint laxity decreased with age. Lamari, Chueire, and Cordeiro,[41] in a study that included similar measures of hypermobility in the thumb/wrist and little finger of 1,120 healthy Brazilian children between the ages of 4 and 7 years, found that lower hypermobility scores were associated with increasing age, even within this limited age range. Overall, 76% of the children were able to apposition the thumb to the forearm and 53% were able to hyperextend the MCP joint of the little finger beyond 90 degrees. Significant age differences were present in both genders for thumb apposition but only in boys for little finger hyperextension.

A study by Allander and associates[42] found that active flexion and passive extension of the MCP joint of the thumb demonstrated no consistent pattern of age-related effects in a study of 517 women and 208 men (between 33 and 70 years of age). These authors stated that the typical reduction in mobility with age resulting from degenerative arthritis found in other joints may be exceeded by an accumulation of ligamentous ruptures that reduce the stability of the first MCP joint.

Similarly, a study by White and associates[23] found no correlation between age and CMC flexion and extension of the thumb in 48 men and 48 women ranging in age from 21 to 96. A negative correlation (–0.22, probability [*p*] = 0.03) between increasing age and abduction ROM at the CMC of the thumb was noted, with a statistically significant but small difference of 4.5 degrees between the group of 35- to 49-year-olds and those older than 65 years.

Gender

Studies that examined the effect of gender on the ROM of the fingers also reported varying results (see Table 7.2). Mallon, Brown, and Nunley[11] found no significant effect of gender on the amount of flexion in any joints of the fingers. However, in this study women generally had more extension at all joints of the fingers than men. Skvarilova and Plevkova[12] found that PIP flexion, DIP flexion, and MCP extension of the fingers were greater in women than in men, whereas MCP flexion of the fingers was greater in men. Smahel and Klimova[13] reported that MCP extension was significantly greater in women versus men in both groups of young and older adults, whereas no gender differences were noted in MCP flexion. In a study of PIP and DIP joint ROM of the fingers, Smahel and Klimova[36] found that women had greater PIP flexion than did men, but they did not differ in DIP flexion.

In regards to the thumb, many studies found no significant ROM differences between males and females. Joseph[35] used radiographs to examine MCP and IP flexion ROM of the thumb in 90 males and 54 females; no significant differences were found between the two groups. He did find two general shapes of MCP joints, round and flat, with the round MCP joints having greater range of flexion. Shaw and Morris[38] noted no gender differences in MCP and IP thumb flexion ROM between 199 males and 149 females aged 16 to 86 years. Likewise, DeSmet and colleagues[32] and Jenkins and associates[39] found no differences in MCP and IP flexion of the thumb because of gender. White and associates[23] found no differences in CMC flexion, extension, and abduction of the thumb because of gender in 48 men and 48 women ranging in age from 21 to 96. White, Nolan, and Resteghini[20] in a study of 160 hands (35 males, 45 females with a mean of 31.5 years) also found no differences because of gender for CMC extension and abduction, although males were found to have an average of 4.6 degrees more CMC flexion than females.

Several studies have reported more motion at the MCP joint or general laxity of the thumb in females compared with males. Allander and associates[42] found that, in some age-groups, females showed more mobility in the MCP joint of the thumb than their male counterparts. Skvarilova and Plevkova[12] noted that MCP flexion and extension of the thumb were greater in females, whereas gender differences were small and unimportant at the IP joint. Yoshida and associates,[34] in a study of 51 healthy men, 49 healthy women, and 70 cadavers, identified two general shapes of the metacarpal head: round and flat. The female gender was associated with greater MCP joint ROM and a higher prevalence of a round metacarpal head, whereas no gender differences were noted in ROM at the IP joint. Beighton, Solomon, and Soskolne,[40] in a study of 456 men and 625 women of an African village; Fairbank, Pynsett, and Phillips,[43] in a study of 227 male and 219 female adolescents; and Lamari and coworkers,[41] in a study of 1,120 young Brazilian children, measured passive apposition of the thumb toward the anterior surface of the forearm and hyperextension of the MCP joints of the fifth or middle fingers. All three studies reported an increase in laxity in females compared with males.

Right Versus Left Sides

The studies that have compared ROM in the right and left joints of the fingers have generally found no significant difference between sides or only a small increase in motion on the left side. Mallon, Brown, and Nunley,[11] in a study in which half of the 120 individuals were right-handed and the other half left-handed, noted no difference between sides in finger motions at the MCP, PIP, and DIP joints. Skvarilova and Plevkova[12] reported only small right–left differences in the majority of the joints of the fingers and thumb in 200 individuals. Only MCP extension of the fingers and thumb and IP flexion of the thumb seemed to have greater ROM values on the left. Smahel and Klimova,[13,36] in studies of 101 university students, 60 senior citizens, and 52 pianists, found that in all three groups MCP joint ROM of the fingers was greater in the left hand. However, in most instances, ROM differences between the left and right hands were not significant for PIP and DIP joints of the fingers.

Similar to findings in studies of the fingers, most studies have reported no difference in ROM between the right and left thumbs. Joseph[35] and Shaw and Morris,[38] in studies of 144 and 248 individuals, respectively, found no significant difference between sides in MCP and IP flexion ROM of the thumb. DeSmet and colleagues[32] examined 101 healthy individuals and also reported no difference between sides for the MCP and IP joints of the thumb. No difference between sides in IP flexion of the thumb was found by Jenkins and associates[39] in a study of 119 subjects. A statistically significant greater amount of MCP flexion was reported for the right thumb than for the left; however, this difference was only 2 degrees. Allander and associates[42] also found no differences attributed to side in MCP motions of the thumb in 720 subjects. White, Nolan, and Resteghini,[20] in a study of 80 healthy adults, found no differences in CMC motions of the thumb between right and left sides or between the dominant and nondominant hands except for a statistically significant greater amount of CMC extension in the dominant hand; however, this difference was less than 1.0 degree.

Testing Position

Mallon, Brown, and Nunley,[11] in addition to establishing normative ROM values for the fingers, also studied passive joint ROM while positioning the next most proximal joint in maximal flexion and extension. The DIP joint had significantly more flexion (18 degrees) when the PIP joint was flexed than when the PIP joint was extended. This finding has been cited as an indication of abnormal tightness of the oblique retinacular ligament.[44] However, the results of Mallon, Brown, and Nunley's study suggest that this finding is normal. The MCP joint had about 6 degrees more flexion when the wrist was extended than when the wrist was flexed, although this difference was not statistically significant. When the wrist was extended, the extensor digitorum, extensor indicis, and extensor digiti minimi were more slack to allow greater flexion of the MCP joint. There was no effect on PIP motion with changes in MCP joint position.

Knutson and associates[45] examined eight subjects to study the effect of seven wrist positions on the torque required to passively move the MCP joint of the index finger. The findings indicated that in many wrist positions, extrinsic tissues (those that cross more than one joint) such as the extensor digitorum, extensor indicis, flexor digitorum superficialis, and flexor digitorum profundus muscles offered greater restraint to MCP flexion and extension than intrinsic tissues (those that cross only one joint). Intrinsic tissues offered greater resistance to passive moment at the MCP joint when the wrist was flexed or extended enough to slacken the extrinsic tissues. Therefore, to evaluate the length or stretch intrinsic tissues at the MCP joint the wrist should be positioned to relax the extrinsic long finger extensor and flexor muscles.

Functional Range of Motion

Joint motion, muscular strength and control, sensation, adequate finger length, and sufficient palm width and depth are necessary for a hand that is capable of performing functional, occupational, and recreational activities. Numerous classification systems and terms for describing functional hand patterns have been proposed. Some common patterns include (1) finger–thumb prehension such as tip (Fig. 7.65), pulp, lateral, and three-point pinch (Fig. 7.66); (2) full-hand prehension, also called a power grip or cylindrical grip (Fig. 7.67); (3) nonprehension, which requires parts of the hand to be used

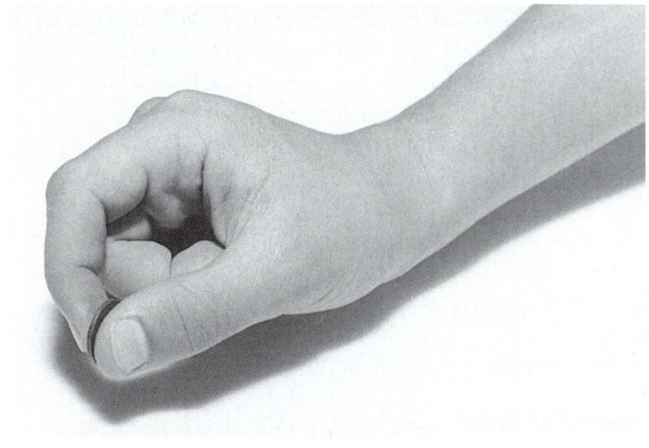

FIGURE 7.65 Picking up a coin is an example of finger–thumb prehension that requires use of the tips or pulps of the digits. In this photograph the pulp of the thumb and the tip of the index finger are being used.

as an extension of the upper extremity; and (4) bilateral prehension, which requires use of the palmar surfaces of both hands.[46] Texts by Casanova and Grunert,[47] Totten and Flinn-Wagner,[48] Mackin and associates,[49] and the American Society of Hand Therapists[19] have reviewed many functional patterns and tests for the hand.

In general, most activities and functional hand patterns utilize positions of flexion at the MCP and IP joints of the digits, with the ring and little fingers in more flexion than the index and middle fingers. However, movement toward extension at the MCP and IP joints is usually needed to initiate prehension and then to release an object. Tables 7.4 and 7.5 summarize the findings of several studies that examined the active ROM of the fingers and thumb during activities of daily living that require various types of finger–thumb prehension or full-hand prehension. These ROM values may be helpful in setting treatment goals for patient with hand impairments and functional limitations.

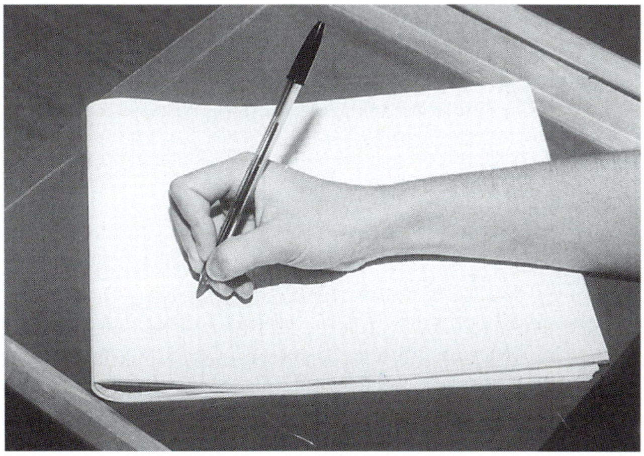

FIGURE 7.66 Writing usually requires finger–thumb prehension in the form of a three-point pinch.

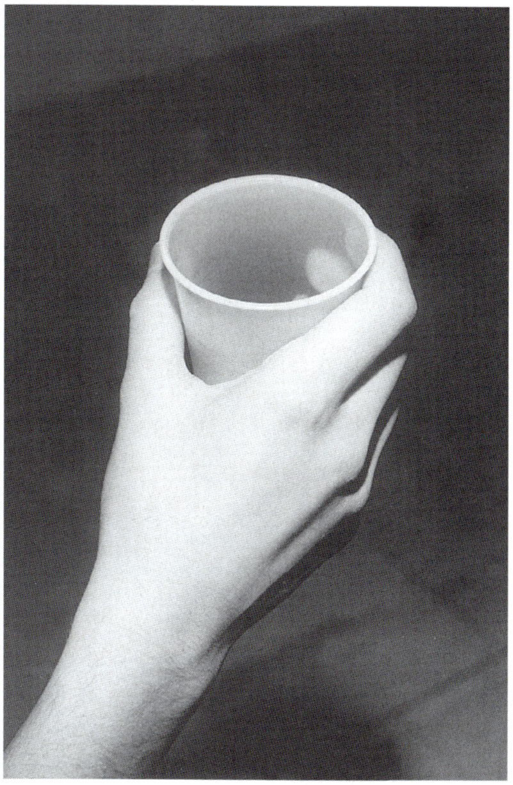

FIGURE 7.67 Holding a cylinder such as a cup requires full-hand prehension (power grip). The amount of metacarpophalangeal and proximal interphalangeal flexion varies, depending on the diameter of the cylinder.

Hume and coworkers[33] used an electrogoniometer to study 35 right-handed young men during the performance of 11 activities of daily living and 4 pinch/grips. The functional position of the fingers and thumb at the completion of each activity was determined and the range of these positions is found in Table 7.4. No significant differences were found between the functional positions of the individual fingers; therefore, the authors presented the findings as a group. Of the activities that were included, holding a soda can (large diameter) required the least amount of finger and thumb flexion, whereas holding a toothbrush (small diameter) required the most. All other activities clustered around a mean of 61 degrees of flexion for the MCP joints, 60 degrees of flexion for the PIP joints, and 39 degrees of flexion for the DIP joints.

Lee and Rim[50] examined the amount of motion required at the joints of the fingers to grip five cylinders of different sizes. Data were collected from four subjects by means of markers and multicamera photogrammetry. Similar to the study by Hume and coworkers,[33] Lee and Rim found that as cylinder diameter decreased, the amount of flexion of the MCP and PIP joints increased. However, DIP joint flexion remained constant at about 40 degrees with all cylinder sizes.

The ROM of the MCP joints of the fingers needed to perform 19 activities of daily living was the focus of a study by

TABLE 7.4 Mean Joint Angles of Fingers and Thumb During Activities of Daily Living in Degrees

Activity	Study			Digit	Joint	Flexion		Extension	
	First Author	*N*	*Measurement Method*			*Min*	*Max*	*Min*	*Max*
11 Activities	Hume*[33]	35	Uniaxial electrogoniometer	Thumb	MCP	10	32		
					IP	2	43		
				Fingers	MCP	33	73		
					PIP	36	86		
					DIP	20	61		
19 Activities	Hayashi**[51]	20	Uniaxial electrogoniometer	2nd	MCP		76		8
				3rd	MCP		91		8
				4th	MCP		96		12
				5th	MCP		96		15
Writing	Hayashi†[51]	20	Uniaxial electrogoniometer	2nd	MCP	30	68		
				3rd	MCP	31	82		
				4th	MCP	36	84		
				5th	MCP	40	90		
Prepare meal	Hayashi†[51]	20	Uniaxial electrogoniometer	2nd	MCP	10	67		
				3rd	MCP	15	81		
				4th	MCP	9	89		
				5th	MCP	12	95		
Wash back	Hayashi†[51]	20	Uniaxial electrogoniometer	2nd	MCP	8	62		
				3rd	MCP	8	80		
				4th	MCP	2	83		
				5th	MCP	4	87		
Make bed	Hayashi†[51]	20	Uniaxial electrogoniometer	2nd	MCP		70		6
				3rd	MCP		82		5
				4th	MCP		84		8
				5th	MCP		85		11
Type on keyboard	Baker‡[52]	20	3D Video system	Thumb	MCP		2		
				2nd	MCP		36		
				3rd	MCP		30		
				4th	MCP		24		
				5th	MCP		17		
				Thumb	IP		18		
				2nd	PIP		36		
				3rd	PIP		44		
				4th	PIP		44		
				5th	PIP		32		

DIP = Distal interphalangeal; IP = Interphalangeal; MCP = Metacarpophalangeal; PIP = Proximal interphalangeal.

* Values indicate joint position at completion of tasks. Minimal and maximum indicate the range of mean values for 11 tasks, which included holding a telephone, can, fork, scissors, toothbrush, and hammer; using a zipper and comb; turning a key; printing with a pen; and unscrewing a jar.

** Values indicate the range of the mean maximum joint angles during all 19 tasks as reported in the text of article. Tasks included the following: open a jar, write, turn key, prepare meal, push open door, place object on overhead shelf, wash walls, do yard work, make bed, carry shopping bag, carry heavy object, change overhead light bulb, blow-dry hair, wash back, put on pullover sweater, use knife, play cards, use a hammer, play Frisbee.

† Values indicate mean minimum and maximum joint angles during the task.

‡ Values indicate mean joint angles during keyboarding for the right hand.

Hayashi and Shimizu.[51] Twenty healthy young adults (10 men and 10 women) were measured with uniaxial electrogoniometers as they moved through the activities. Most activities were performed with the MCP joints in varying amounts of flexion, although a few tasks such as making a bed and heavy household chores (washing walls) required 5 to 15 degrees of MCP extension (see Table 7.4). Mean maximum MCP flexion to perform all activities was 62 degrees for the index finger, 77 degrees for the middle finger, 82 degrees for the ring finger, and 87 degrees for the little finger. These differences in maximum MCP flexion between the fingers were statistically significant, and showed a trend toward increasing flexion from the index to the little finger. No similar trend was noted for maximum MCP extension values.

TABLE 7.5 Mean Angle of Flexion for Fingers and Thumb at Completion of Prehension Activities in Degrees

Activity	Study			Finger			Thumb	
	Name	N	Measurement	MCP Joint	PIP Joint	DIP Joint	MCP Joint	IP Joint
Tip pinch	Hume[33]	35	Uniaxial electrogoniometer	58	76	33	22	25
	Nakomura*[53]	15	2D camera motion system	35	40	60		
Palmar (pad) pinch	Nakomura*	15	2D camera motion system	35	40	50		
Lateral (key) pinch	Hume	35	Uniaxial electrogoniometer	62	76	46	20	16
Precision (3 point) grasp	Hume	35	Uniaxial electrogoniometer	33	39	26	10	28
Power grip	Hume	35	Uniaxial electrogoniometer	72	78	50	23	36

DIP = Distal interphalangeal; IP = Interphalangeal; MCP = Metacarpophalangeal; PIP = Proximal interphalangeal.
* Values extrapolated from graphs for index finger.

Baker and associates[52] studied finger, thumb, and wrist movements of 20 healthy expert typists using a standard (flat) computer keyboard. Range of motion and angular velocity were recorded with a Vicon motion-measurement system. Mean MCP flexion of the fingers ranged from 15 to 37 degrees, with a trend toward progressively smaller MCP flexion from the index to the little finger (Table 7.4). This trend may be related to the pronated wrist position and the practice of some typists to hyperextend the MCP joints of the little and ring fingers while holding the fingers above the keyboard to avoid unintended key strikes. Mean PIP flexion of the fingers ranged from 14 to 48 degrees; PIP flexion of the middle and ring fingers was greater than flexion of the index and little fingers. The thumb had significantly less MCP and IP flexion than the fingers.

A study by Nakamura and coworkers[53] examined the proportion and pattern of movements between the MCP, PIP, and DIP joints of the index finger during tip pinch and palmar (pulp) pinch with the thumb, during the grasping of two discs of different sizes, and during pure finger extension (hand opening). Fifteen healthy subjects (4 males and 11 females) ranging in age from 21 to 46 years were measured with a two-dimensional camera motion system. Range-of-motion values during the two pinch tasks were presented in graphs and the mean maximal flexion angles at the completion of the pinch tasks are summarized in Table 7.5. In this study, the DIP joint had the most flexion, followed by the PIP and MCP joints.

Reliability and Validity

Reliability of Goniometric Measurements

Many studies have been conducted to assess the reliability of goniometric measurements in the hand. Most studies found that measurements of all joints of the fingers and MCP and IP joints of the thumb that were taken with universal goniometers and specialized finger goniometers were highly reliable. Several studies[54–57] found that measurement of DIP flexion can be slightly less reliable than that of more proximal joints, most likely due to difficulty placing the arms of a goniometer over the small phalanges. Measurements of the CMC joint of the thumb seem to be the least reliable. Measurements taken over the dorsal surface of the digits appear to be similar to those taken laterally.

Consistent with other regions of the body, measurements of finger and thumb ROM taken by one examiner are more reliable than measurements taken by several examiners. Research studies generally support the opinions of Bear-Lehman and Abreu[58] and Adams, Greene, and Topoozian[19] that the margin of error is generally accepted to be about 5 degrees for goniometric measurement of joints in the hand, provided that measurements are taken by the same examiner and that standardized techniques are employed. Visual estimates are much less reliable than goniometric measurements and are not recommended. The findings of many of the following studies are presented in more detail in Tables 7.6 and 7.7 for the fingers and Tables 7.8 and 7.9 for the thumb; studies of healthy populations are presented first, followed by studies of patient populations.

Fingers

Healthy Populations The reliability of goniometric measurements of finger ROM in healthy people has been the focus of several studies. Lewis, Fors, and Tharion[56] examined the reliability of measuring active and passive ROM at the MCP, PIP, and DIP joints of the middle finger in 20 healthy adults, three times by each of seven therapists. Measurements were taken with a Rolyan hyperextension finger goniometer over the dorsal surface of the finger. Active ROM measurements were taken with the subjects making a closed fist followed by active full extension, whereas passive ROM measurements were taken at individual joints with extrinsic tissues relaxed. The reliability of active measurements was better

TABLE 7.6 Intratester Reliability of Finger ROM Measurements for Healthy and Patient Populations

Study	N	Sample	Methods	Joint/Motion	r	ICC	Absolute Measures (degrees)
Healthy Populations							
Burr et al[55]	1	Healthy adult	40 testers (hand therapists), 3 devices applied dorsally 3 times: EMS plastic goniometer with shortened arms, Rolyan plastic goniometer, Dexter computerized system	Static positions of second and third digits EMS goniometer: PIP DIP Rolyan goniometer PIP DIP Dexter system PIP DIP			Median difference between max and min measurements: 2, 2 2, 3 2, 6 2, 4 2, 2 2, 5
Ellis et al[54]	1	Healthy adult	40 testers (PT, OT), using 2 devices: Rolyan dorsal finger goniometer, wire tracing	2 static positions, third digit Goniometer: MCP PIP DIP Wire tracing: MCP PIP DIP			95% CI of difference between measurements:* 3.8, 4.3 4.7, 4.3 6.4, 6.1 8.9, 8.0 10.9, 8.1 9.8, 10.5
Ellis and Bruton[18]	1	Healthy adult	51 testers (PT, OT), using Rolyan dorsal finger goniometer for PIP angle, and ruler for composite finger flexion (CFF)	3 static positions, PIP joint angles Goniometer: second digit third digit fourth digit Ruler CFF: second digit third digit fourth digit			95% CI of difference between 2 measurements:* 5 degrees 4 degrees 4 degrees 5 mm 5 mm 6 mm
Hamilton and Lachenbruch[61]	1	Healthy adults	7 testers (PT), 3 types of goniometers: dorsal finger, lateral universal and pendulum	Static position of MCP, PIP, and DIP joints of 4 fingers			Variance: Dorsal = 2.2 Lateral = 2.8 Pendulum = 2.2
Lewis et al[56]	20	Healthy adults	AROM and PROM, 7 testers (OT, PT), Rolyan dorsal plastic goniometer	Third digit, AROM MCP joint PIP joint DIP joint PROM MCP joint PIP joint DIP joint		 .64–.93, $\bar{x}$ = .80 .68–.94, $\bar{x}$ = .83 .78–.99, $\bar{x}$ = .92 .57–.84, $\bar{x}$ = .74 .43–.93, $\bar{x}$ = .76 .72–.99, $\bar{x}$ = .89	Method error: 1.2–3.5, $\bar{x}$ = 2.2 1.3–4.3, $\bar{x}$ = 2.2 0.7–7.1, $\bar{x}$ = 2.9 1.7–3.9, $\bar{x}$ = 2.1 1.4–5.2, $\bar{x}$ = 2.7 0.9–5.5, $\bar{x}$ = 3.3

TABLE 7.6 Intratester Reliability of Finger ROM Measurements for Healthy and Patient Populations (continued)

Study	N	Sample	Methods	Joint/Motion	r	ICC	Absolute Measures (degrees)
Healthy Populations							
Macionis[57]	24	Healthy adults	24 testers (medical students), Jamar dorsal plastic goniometer (and paper strip method not reported here)	2 static splinted positions, fourth digit Extended position: MCP joint PIP joint DIP joint Flexed position: MCP joint PIP joint DIP joint		 .89, .89 .86, .90 .87, .91 .91, .93 .87, .89 .85, .86	SEM: 2.9, 3.1 3.3, 4.2 3.3, 3.6 2.4, 2.8 3.2, 3.6 3.4, 3.8
Stam et al[60]	20	Healthy subjects	Testers not defined, joint angles measured holding cylinders 3.2 and 7.5 centimeters in diameter, with goniometer and Compangle	2 static positions Goniometer MCP PIP DIP Compangle MCP PIP DIP		 .74, .83 .80, .80 .58, .63 .76, .83 .89, .90 .73, .71	SEM: 4.3, 4.8 4.8, 3.7 5.9, 4.2 3.9, 4.3 3.0, 2,5 4,3, 3.3
Weiss et al[62]	8	Healthy adults	AROM, 1 tester (PT), 2 methods: metal dorsal goniometer, Exos Handmaster	6 static positions of MCP, PIP and DIP joints of second digit Goniometer: Exos:	 .98 .93	 .98 .99	Mean differences: 0.8 0.5
Patient Populations							
Brown et al[64]	30	Patients with orthopedic injuries	3 testers (OT, PT), Jamar dorsal finger goniometer, and Dexter Hand Evaluation System	MCP, PIP, and DIP joints for Total Active Motion (TAM) Goniometer: Dexter:		 .97–.98 .98–.99	
Flower and LaStayo[65]	7	Patients with fused PIP joints	1 tester (PT), metal dorsal finger goniometer	PIP extension of fingers		.98	
Glasgow et al[67]	10	Patients with traumatic hand injury	2 testers (therapists), Smith and Nephew metal finger goniometer	PROM with 500 g torque applied, flexion, various joints		.99, .99	

r = Pearson product-moment correlation coefficient; ICC = Intraclass correlation coefficient; DIP = Distal interphalangeal; IP = Interphalangeal; MCP = Metacarpophalangeal; PIP = Proximal interphalangeal; AROM = active range of motion; PROM = passive range of motion; PT = Physical therapist or physiotherapist; OT = Occupational therapist; SD = Standard deviation (of the repeated measurements); SEM = Standard error of the repeated measurements; MDC = Minimal detectable change; SDD = Smallest detectable difference; 95% CI = 95 percent confidence interval.

* Also called the repeatability coefficient or MDC; the two numbers are for the first and second static positions.

TABLE 7.7 Intertester Reliability of Finger ROM Measurements for Healthy and Patient Populations

Study	n	Sample	Methods	Joint/Motion	r	ICC	Absolute Measures (degrees)
Healthy Populations							
Bruton, et al[77]	1	Healthy adult	40 testers (PT, OT), using 2 methods: Rolyan dorsal finger goniometer, visual estimate	2 static splinted positions of MCP joints of third digit Goniometer: Visual: Goniometer: Visual:			SD: 1.1, 1.7 15.7, 18.0 95% CI of difference between 2 measurements*: 4.4, 5.9 44.5, 51.0
Burr et al[55]	1	Healthy adult	40 testers (hand therapists), 3 devices applied dorsally 3 times: EMS plastic goniometer with shortened arms, Rolyan plastic goniometer, Dexter computerized system	Static splint of second and third digits EMS goniometer: PIP DIP Rolyan Goniometer: PIP DIP Dexter system: PIP DIP			SD of means: 2–3, $\bar{x}$ = 2.5 3–5, $\bar{x}$ = 4.3 2–6, $\bar{x}$ = 4.0 3–4, $\bar{x}$ = 3.3 2–4, $\bar{x}$ = 3.0 3–6, $\bar{x}$ = 4.3
Ellis et al[54]	1	Healthy adult	40 testers (PT, OT), using 2 devices: Rolyan dorsal finger goniometer, wire tracing	2 static splinted positions of third digit Goniometer: MCP PIP DIP Wire tracing: MCP PIP DIP			95% CI of difference between measurements:* 4.4, 5.9 7.2, 6.0 9.8, 9.9 10.3, 10.4 12.3, 9.5 11.9, 13.2
Ellis and Bruton[18]	1	Healthy adult	51 testers (PT, OT), using 2 devices: Rolyan dorsal finger goniometer for PIP angle, and ruler for composite finger flexion (CFF)	3 static splinted positions Goniometer: second digit third digit fourth digit Ruler CFF: second digit third digit fourth digit			95% CI of difference between measurements:* 7 degrees 7 degrees 9 degrees 7 mm 8 mm 9 mm

TABLE 7.7 Intertester Reliability of Finger ROM Measurements for Healthy and Patient Populations (continued)

Study	*n*	Sample	Methods	Joint/Motion	*r*	ICC	Absolute Measures (degrees)
Healthy Populations							
Lewis et al[56]	20	Healthy adults	AROM and PROM, 7 testers (OT, PT), Rolyan dorsal plastic goniometer	Third digit AROM MCP joint PIP joint DIP joint PROM MCP joint PIP joint DIP joint		 .61–.70, x = .67 .55–.73, x = .67 .80–.88, x = .85 .37–.54, x = .48 .48–.62, x = .56 .24–.29, x = .35	
Marcionis[57]	24	Healthy adults	24 testers (medical students), Jamar dorsal plastic goniometer (and paper strip method)	2 static splinted positions of fourth digit Extended position: MCP joint PIP joint DIP joint Flexed position: MCP joint PIP joint DIP joint		 .86, .87 .80, .84 .86, .88 .86, .88 .80, .86 .75, .83	 SEM: 3.2, 3.5 4.0, 4.9 3.8, 3.8 3.1, 3.0 3.9, 4.1 4.2, 4.4
Patient Populations							
Brown et al[64]	30	Patients with orthopedic injuries	3 testers (OT, PT), Jamar dorsal finger goniometer, and Dexter Hand Evaluation System	MCP, PIP, and DIP joints for Total Active Motion (TAM), Goniometer: Dexter:		 .97–.98 .98–.99	
Edgar et al[31]	21	Burn survivors	AROM, 4 testers (PT), measured composite finger flexion (CFF) and hand span with ruler	CFF Hand span		.94 .98	MDD = 7 mm MDD = 10 mm
Engstrand et al[66]	13	Patients with Dupuytren's disease	AROM, 8 testers (OT), plastic 360-degree shortened goniometer applied dorsally	Second to fifth digits MCP extension PIP extension DIP extension MCP flexion PIP flexion DIP flexion TAE TAF		 .95 .97 .96 .83 .92 .91 .95 .90	 SEM = 2, Diff = 3 SEM = 2, Diff = 7 SEM = 2, Diff = 3 SEM = 1. Diff = 4 SEM = 1, Diff = 4 SEM = 1, Diff = 11 SEM = 3, Diff = 8 SEM = 2, Diff = 18

(table continues on page 244)

TABLE 7.7 Intertester Reliability of Finger ROM Measurements for Healthy and Patient Populations (continued)

Study	*n*	Sample	Methods	Joint/Motion	*r*	ICC	Absolute Measures (degrees)
Patient Populations							
Glasgow et al[67]	10	Patients with traumatic hand injury	PROM with 500 g torque applied, 2 testers (therapists), Smith and Nephew metal finger goniometer	Flexion of MCP or IP joints		.99	
Groth et al[63]	1	Patient with multiple second and third digit fractures	AROM, 6 testers (OT, PT), using dorsal DeVore and lateral 6-inch plastic goniometer	Flexion and extension of PIP and DIP joints of second and third digits Dorsal: Lateral:		 .99 .86	SD: 4.5 5.0

r = Pearson correlation coefficient; ICC = Intraclass correlation coefficient; DIP = Distal interphalangeal; IP = Interphalangeal; MCP = Metacarpophalangeal; PIP = Proximal interphalangeal; PT = Physical therapist or physiotherapist; AROM = Active range of motion; PROM = Passive range of motion; OT = Occupational therapist; SD = Standard deviation (of the repeated measurements); SEM = Standard error of the repeated measurements, but Engstrand refers to this as standard error of the mean; MDC = Minimal detectable change; SDD = Smallest detectable difference; 95% CI = 95 percent confidence interval; TAE = Total active extension; TAF = Total active flexion; Diff = Difference between the highest and lowest measurement $\bar{x}$ = mean.

* Also called the repeatability coefficient; the two numbers listed are for the first and second static positions.

than passive measurements. Intratester reliability as indicated by ICC values ranged from 0.43 to 0.99, with mean measurement errors ranging from 2.2 to 3.3 degrees; differences in ROM greater than 4 degrees were present less than 5% of the time. Intertester ICC values ranged from 0.24 to 0.95, with differences between testers greater than 5 degrees 80% of the time. The results support the findings of other studies that intratester reliability is better than intertester reliability, and that one can have confidence that a repeated measurement by the same therapist will be within 5 to 6 degrees of earlier measurements 95% of the time.

Goldsmith and Juzl[59] studied the intratester reliability of measuring active ROM of the MCP, PIP, and DIP joints of the fingers in 12 healthy subjects and the intertester reliability in 12 patients with hand conditions. A universal goniometer adapted for measuring the hand (one short arm) was applied over the dorsal surface. The two therapists each took three measurements of flexion and extension at each joint in one session to assess intratester reliability, and one measurement of flexion and extension at each involved joint in one session to assess intertester reliability. Both intratester and intertester reliability were high, with correlation coefficients greater than 0.99. When agreement was defined as within 3 degrees, the percentage of agreement was 93.9% to 94.6% for intratester reliability and 67.7% for intertester reliability. When agreement was defined as within 5 degrees, the percentage of agreement was 99.7% to 100% for intratester reliability and 87.1% for intertester reliability.

More studies have examined the reliability of goniometric measurement of finger joints held in static positions. Cylinders, hand splints, wax hand models, and wire-fixated cadavers have been used to maintain consistent joint angles and simulate limited ROM found in injured hands. For example, the intratester reliability of measuring the angle of finger joints while grasping two cylinders, with diameters of 3.2 and 7.5 centimeters, was studied by Stam and coworkers[60] in 20 healthy subjects. Measurements were taken twice, 1 week apart, with both a conventional goniometer and a new device (Compangle). The Compangle had two legs similar to a compass with feet placed on the bones that are proximal and distal to the joint. The new device was shown to have better intratester reliability than the goniometer. Depending on the joint being measured, ICC values for the goniometer and Compangle ranged from 0.58 to 0.83 and from 0.71 to 0.90, respectively. Standard error of the measurement (SEM) ranged from 3.7 to 5.9 degrees for the goniometer and from 2.5 to 4.3 degrees for the Compangle.

Hamilton and Lachenbruch[61] had seven testers take measurements of MCP, PIP, and DIP flexion in one healthy subject whose fingers were held in a fixed position. A single daily measurement was taken by each tester on four different days with each of the three types of goniometers. These authors found intratester reliability to be higher than intertester reliability. Mean intratester variances for the repeated measurements for all devices were about 2 to 3 degrees. No degree values for intertester variances were provided. No significant differences existed between measurements taken with a dorsal (over-the-joint) finger goniometer, a universal goniometer on the lateral surface, or a pendulum goniometer.

Weiss and associates[62] compared measurements of index finger MCP, PIP, and DIP joints in six static positions taken by a dorsal metal finger goniometer with those taken by the Exos Handmaster (a Hall-effect instrumented exoskeleton). Eight healthy subjects were measured with each device during one session by one examiner (occupational therapist) and again within 2 weeks of the initial session. Intratester reliability was high for both devices, with ICCs ranging from 0.98 to 0.99. Mean differences between sessions for each instrument were less than 1 degree. Measurements taken by the finger goniometer and those taken by the Exos Handmaster were significantly different from each other (mean difference = 7 degrees) but were highly correlated (Pearson product-moment correlation coefficient $r = 0.89–0.94$).

Ellis, Bruton, and Goddard[54] placed one healthy adult in two splints while 40 therapists measured the MCP, PIP, and DIP joints of the middle finger by means of a dorsal finger goniometer and a wire tracing. Each therapist measured each joint three times with each device. The goniometer consistently produced smaller ranges and smaller standard deviations than the wire tracing, indicating better reliability for the goniometer. The 95% confidence limit for the difference between two measurements ranged from 3.8 to 6.4 degrees (intratester) and 4.4 to 9.9 degrees (intertester) for the goniometer. Using the wire tracing method, the 95% confidence limit for the difference between two measurements ranged from 8.0 to 10.5 degrees (intratester) and 9.5 to 13.2 degrees (intertester). Both methods had more variability when distal joints were measured, possibly because of the shorter phalanges used to align the goniometer or wire. Intratester reliability was always higher than intertester reliability.

Burr and associates[55] compared the intratester and intertester reliability of three types of goniometers applied dorsally to the index and middle fingers: (1) the 180-degree plastic Electro-Medical Supplies (EMS) goniometer with arms shortened to 9 and 5 centimeters, (2) the plastic Rolyan hyperextension goniometer, and (3) the Dexter Computerized Assessment goniometer. Forty hand therapists measured the PIP and DIP joints of one healthy subject whose hand was immobilized in a splint; they did so three times with each of the three devices. Reliability was best for the EMS goniometer (which more therapists used), followed by the Dexter computerized goniometer and Rolyan hyperextension goniometer. There were significant differences between the devices in three out of the four joint measurements, with the Rolyan goniometer resulting in about 2 to 4 degrees lower median values than the other two goniometers. Similar to other studies, intratester was better than intertester reliability. The authors noted that testers were less consistent (less reliable) when measuring more flexed joints regardless of whether the joints were the PIP or DIP joints.

Macionis[57] examined the intratester and intertester reliability of measuring angles of the MCP, PIP, and DIP joints of the fourth digit held in two static finger positions of flexion and extension in 24 healthy medical students. The students participated in groups of 12 as both subjects and testers. Measurements were made twice by each tester with a dorsally placed plastic finger goniometer (Jamar EZ Read), and twice with an unusual system of dorsally applied paper strips with angles read by a computerized imaging system. Reliability was similar for both methods, with ICCs ranging from 0.73 to 0.93 for the goniometer and from 0.69 to 0.90 for the paper strip system. Standard error of measurement (SEM) values for both systems ranged from 2.4 to 4.9 degrees, resulting in minimal detectible change (also called minimal detectible difference or repeatability coefficient) of greater than 5 degrees for repeated measurements by both the same tester and different testers. Similar to other studies, Macionis reported intratester reliability to be better than intertester reliability, and measurements of the DIP joint slightly less consistent than the more proximal joints.

The distance between the fingertip pulp and distal palmar crease has been suggested as a simple and quick method of estimating total finger flexion ROM at the MCP, PIP, and DIP joints.[16,19] Ellis and Bruton[18] examined the intratester and intertester reliability of composite finger flexion (CFF) and compared it with dorsal goniometric measures of PIP flexion of the index, middle, and ring fingers. One hand was splinted in three positions and measured with a ruler and goniometer three times by 51 therapists at 18 hospital sites. Intratester goniometric measurements fell within 4 to 5 degrees of each other 95% of the time, whereas intertester goniometric measurements fell within 7 to 9 degrees of each other 95% of the time. Composite finger flexion measures fell within 5 to 6 millimeters of each other 95% of the time for intratester measurements and within 7 to 9 millimeters of each other for intertester measurements. After scaling the two methods to allow comparison, the goniometer provided better reliability than CFF for measurements taken by the same tester, but both methods were equally reliable for measurements taken by different testers. The authors suggested that CFF may be a useful alternative when multiple joint measures are needed or when goniometry is impractical.

Patient Populations The intratester and intertester reliability of measuring finger ROM with goniometers has been found to be very high in studies of patients with traumatic hand injuries, orthopedic conditions, fused joints, and Dupuytren disease. Intraclass correlation coefficient (ICC) values generally ranged from 0.98 to 0.99 for repeated measurements by the same tester, and ranged from 0.83 to 0.99 for repeated measurements made by different testers.

Groth and coworkers[63] had 39 therapists measure the PIP and DIP joints of the index and middle fingers of one patient with a crushing injury, both dorsally and laterally, using either a 6-inch plastic universal goniometer or a DeVore metal finger goniometer. No significant difference in measurements was found between the two instruments. No differences were found between the dorsal and lateral measurement methods for seven of the eight joint motions, with mean differences ranging from 2 to 0 degrees. In a subset of six therapists, intertester reliability was high for both methods, with ICCs ranging from 0.86 for lateral methods to 0.99 for dorsal methods.

Brown and colleagues[64] evaluated the ROM of the MCP, PIP, and DIP joints of two fingers in 30 patients with upper-extremity orthopedic injuries to calculate total active motion (TAM) by means of the dorsal finger goniometer and the computerized Dexter Hand Evaluation and Therapy System. Three therapists measured each finger three times with each device during one session. Means of the three measurements were used for intertester analyses. Intratester and intertester reliability were high for both methods, with ICCs ranging from 0.97 to 0.99. The mean difference between methods ranged from 0.1 degrees to 2.4 degrees.

A preliminary reliability study was conducted by Flower and LaStayo[65] on seven patients with fused PIP joints using a dorsally applied metal finger goniometer. Measurements were taken twice of PIP extension over a 2- to 8-week period by one therapist. Intratester reliability was excellent with ICC values of 0.98 degrees.

The intertester reliability of measuring finger motions in patients with Dupuytren disease was likewise found to be high in a study by Engstrand, Krevers, and Kvist.[66] Eight occupational therapists measured the MCP, PIP, and DIP joints of the affected fingers of 12 patients, using a dorsally applied 360-degree plastic goniometer shortened to accommodate the fingers. Intertester reliability was good to excellent as indicated by ICC values ranging from 0.83 to 0.97 and SEM values of less than 3 degrees. The mean difference between the highest and lowest measurement for each joint and motion ranged from 3 to 11 degrees, with an overall mean of 5.3 degrees.

The reliability of goniometric passive ROM measurements using a prescribed amount of torque (500 grams) to move a joint has been reported by Glasgow, Wilton, and Tooth[67] in a study of 10 patients with various traumatic finger and thumb injuries. Two therapists took 10 repeated measurements of one joint per patient using a Smith and Nephew metal specialized finger goniometer (placed dorsally). Intratester and intertester reliability was excellent, with all ICC values greater than 0.99.

Edgar and colleagues[31] studied the reliability of linear measures of motion in the form of composite finger flexion (CFF) and hand span in up to 21 burn survivors. Composite finger flexion was determined by measuring the distance between the tip of the finger and the distal palmar crease of the affected finger while the subjects made a fist. Hand span was measured from the tips of the little finger and thumb during maximal combined abduction. Other body joints and motions were included but those results are not reported here. Within a 60-minute period active ROM was assessed by two of four possible physical therapists twice. Intratester reliability for CCF was excellent, with an ICC value of 0.99. Intertester reliability for CFF and hand span was also excellent, with ICC values of 0.94 and 0.98 and minimal detectible differences of 0.7 and 1.0 centimeters, respectively.

Thumb

Healthy Populations Barakat and coworkers[21] took repeated ROM measurements at the CMC, MCP, and IP joints of the right thumb in a subsample of 10 women who were participating in a normative ROM study of 64 women. Intratester reliability was measured twice by one tester, and intertester reliability was measured by two testers using goniometric methods of measuring end ROM positions described by the International Federation of Societies for Surgery of the Hand.[22] Intratester and intertester reliability for CMC flexion (called radial adduction in the article) was very poor, with correlation values of 0.04 and 0.02, respectively, which was attributed to difficulties keeping the stationary arm of the goniometer aligned with the palmar aspect of the index finger during the thumb motion. When CMC flexion was excluded, the mean intratester correlation improved substantially to 0.93 and intertester correlation to 0.82 for all other motions and joints of the thumb. Refer to Tables 7.8 and 7.9.

The reliability of four methods of measuring active ROM for thumb CMC (palmar) abduction was studied by Itoh and associates[68] in 30 healthy adults (15 men, 15 women). Two testers, an orthopedic surgeon and a hand surgeon, measured each subject twice on one day and then again 3 weeks later. The methods used were (1) a ruler to measure between the tip of the thumb nail and radial edge of flexion crease of index finger PIP joint, (2) a ruler to measure between the ulnar edge of flexion crease of thumb IP joint and the radial edge of proximal palmar crease, (3) a goniometer to measure the angle between the metacarpals of the thumb and index finger, (see below) and (4) a goniometer to measure the angle between the proximal phalanges of the thumb and index finger. Methods 1 and 2, which used a ruler for measurement, had fair to good intratester reliability, with ICC values between 0.74 and 0.89 and intertester reliability with ICC values of 0.81 and 0.79. The reliability of Methods 3 and 4, which used goniometers to measure the angles, was much less. Correlations for measuring the angle between the metacarpals of the thumb and index finger (Method 3) were 0.71 and 0.37 for intratester, and 0.42 for intertester. Correlations for measuring the angle between the proximal phalanges of the thumb and index finger (Method 4) were 0.30 and 0.28 for intratester, and 0.28 for intertester. The authors recommended using distance measurements over joint angle measurements as the distance measurement were more reproducible. Difficulty locating the fulcrum for angular measurements seemed to contribute to less accurate and repeatable measurement of thumb CMC abduction.

De Kraker and associates[69] also examined the reliability of measuring active and passive thumb CMC (palmar) abduction ROM in a study of six methods: (1) conventional goniometery measuring the angle between the metacarpals of the thumb and index finger, (2) Pollexograph angle aligned with tip of thumb, (3) Pollexograph angle aligned with thumb metacarpal, (4) American Medical Association (AMA) distance method for opposition between distal palmar crease over third digit MCP joint to flexor crease of thumb IP joint, (5) American Society of Hand Therapists (ASHT) distance method between distal palmar crease over third digit MCP joint to tip of the thumb, and (6) intermetacarpal distance (IMD) between first and second metacarpal heads with dorsal calliper. Measurements were taken by two testers (hand therapist and trainee in plastic surgery) in 25 healthy adults. Distance measurements with a dorsally applied calliper provided the highest intratester and intertester reliability. Angular measurements using the Pollexograph aligned with the metacarpal or tip of the thumb were more reliable than measurements made with a conventional goniometer. There were no consistent differences in the reliability of measuring active versus passive ROM.

The abduction angle of the CMC joint of the thumb and the flexion angles of the PIP joint of the index finger and the MCP joint of the little finger were measured by 30 testers (10 physiotherapy students, 10 physiotherapists, and 10 hand therapists) in a study by Carvalho, Mazzer, and Barbier.[70] Measurements were made with a 180-degree plastic goniometer on the dorsal surface of a wax hand model, and from a digital photograph of the model using two photogrammetric software programs (CorelDRAW and ALCimagem). Measurements were repeated three times for each method by each tester. Intratester reliability was excellent (ICC greater than 0.97) for each group of testers and method in all joint angles combined. Intertester reliability was excellent (ICC greater than 0.99) for each group of testers in all situations combined, as was the reliability of all methods in all situations combined. Interestingly, intra- and intertester reliability as noted by the ICC was generally the highest for measuring the CMC abduction angle of the thumb and least for measuring flexion angle of the PIP joint of the index finger, although the standard deviations of the mean measurements were the smallest for the PIP joint (2.6–2.9 degrees, depending on the method) and greatest for the CMC joint (6.0–7.2 degrees). Goniometric and photometric measurements could not be interchanged as they varied for some of the angles.

Patient Population Sauseng and coworkers,[37] in a study of 50 patients with type 1 diabetes mellitus and 44 healthy controls, measured active ROM of the thumb MCP joint, thumb IP joint, fifth digit MCP joint, wrist, ankle, and first metatarsal phalangeal joint using a pocket goniometer. Each motion was measured three times by one tester. The coefficients of variation for the measurements were between 1.3% and 8.2%. The ROM of all tested joints was significantly lower in the diabetic versus the control group except for the first IP and MCP joints.

The reliability of measuring thumb CMC opposition was examined as part of a study by Edgar and colleagues[31] of 21 burn survivors. Opposition was measured using a 0- to 10-point scale by Kapandji[26] in which the thumb sequentially touches the index, middle, ring, and little fingers. Two physical therapists assessed the motion twice within a 60-minute period. Intertester reliability was excellent, with an ICC value of 0.99 and a minimal detectible difference of 0.3 on the scale.

Validity of Goniometric Measurements

Goniometric measurements of the fingers have been compared to radiographs, digital photographs, video motion analysis, and disability measures in patient populations. In a study by Groth and coworkers,[63] active ROM of the PIP and DIP joints of the index and middle fingers of one patient who had sustained a crush injury with multiple fractures was measured by 39 therapists over a 3-day period. Measurements were made dorsally and laterally using either a DeVore metal finger goniometer or a 6-inch plastic universal goniometer. Prior to the goniometer measurements, radiographs were taken. In terms of concurrent validity, there were significant differences in measurements obtained from radiographs versus those from goniometers except for laterally measured index finger PIP extension and flexion. Differences between radiographic and mean goniometric measurements ranged from 1 to 2 degrees for laterally and dorsally measured index finger PIP motions, to 14 degrees for laterally and dorsally measured middle finger PIP motions. The authors noted that concurrent validity was inconclusive because some of these differences may have been due to variations in the patient instructions for performing active motion, patient positioning, and patient fatigue with multiple active measurements.

Kato and coworkers[71] compared the accuracy of three therapists measuring PIP joint angles using three types of universal goniometers to lateral x-ray films in 16 fingers fixated with Kirschner wires from four cadavers. Each examiner used a 6-inch plastic goniometer with 6-inch arms, a plastic goniometer with a 3.5-inch and a 1-inch arm, and a metal goniometer with 1.5-inch arms to take measurements on the lateral and dorsal surfaces of the fingers. Intertester reliability was good with Pearson product-moment correlation coefficients (r) ranging from 0.80 to 0.82. The mean angle discrepancies between the goniometers and x-rays ranged from 1.2 to 3.3 degrees (SD = 3.5–6.0 degrees) for the lateral method and from 0.5 to 2.9 degrees (SD = 3.5–6.4 degrees) for the dorsal method. There was no difference in angle discrepancies between types of goniometers using the lateral method. However, with two testers using the dorsal method the angle discrepancy was greater with the plastic goniometer with 6-inch arms, perhaps because the arms were longer than the other two goniometers. The authors recommend using any of the three types of goniometers with the lateral measurement method and goniometers with short arms with the dorsal method.

In a study by Georgeu, Mayfield, and Logan,[72] one therapist measured full active flexion and extension of the MCP, PIP, and DIP joints of the little or ring finger in 20 patients. A digital camera, aligned with the MCP joint with the hand placed in a stabilizing device, was integrated with a computer to also determine ROM. There was a high correlation

TABLE 7.8 Intratester Reliability of Thumb ROM Measurements for Healthy Populations

Study	*N*	Sample	Methods	Motion	*r*	ICC	Absolute Measures (degrees)
Barakat et al[21]	10	Healthy women	1 tester (not defined), goniometer	CMC flexion*		.04	
				CMC, MCP, IP motions excluding CMC flexion		.93	
Carvalho et al[70]	1	Wax hand model	30 testers (PT students, PT, hand therapists), 180° plastic goniometer, 3 measurements per tester per joint	CMC abduction, axis on radial styloid, arms on lateral midline of first and second metacarpals		.72, 57, .87, x = .72	
de Kraker et al[69]	25	Healthy adults	2 testers (hand therapist, trainee in plastic surgery), 3 angular methods: goniometer first and second metacarpal, Pollexograph-thumb tip, Pollexograph-thumb metacarpal.	AROM, PROM, CMC abduction			
				Goniometry:		.55, .76	SEM = 4.3, 3.5 SDD = 11.8, 9.7
				Pollexograph-tip:		.71, .82	SEM = 2.5, 2.0 SDD = 7.0, 5.5
				Pollexograph-metacarpal:		.82, .81	SEM = 2.2, 2.7 SDD = 6.4, 7.5
			3 distance methods: AMA thumb IP crease to third distal palmar crease, ASHT thumb tip to third distal palmar crease, intermetacarpal distance (IMD) dorsal first MC head to second MC head.	AMA:		.72, .65	SEM = 4.1, 3.9 mm SDD = 11.4, 10.9 mm
				ASHT:		.78, .72	SEM = 4.4, 4.5 mm SDD = 12.3, 12.6 mm
				IMD:		.95, .92	SEM = 1.2, 1.4 mm SDD = 3.3, 4.1 mm
Itoh et al[68]	30	Healthy adults	2 testers (1 orthopedic surgeon, 1 hand surgeon), 2 measurement methods using ruler, 2 measurement methods using goniometer	AROM CMC abduction (palmar):			
				Distance tip of thumb to PIP crease of second digit;		.76, .88	
				Distance thumb IP crease to PIP crease of second digit;		.74, .89	
				Goniometer aligned with first and second metacarpals;		.71, .37	
				Goniometer aligned with first and second proximal phalanges		.30, .28	

r = Pearson correlation coefficient; ICC = Intraclass correlation coefficient; DIP = Distal interphalangeal; IP = Interphalangeal; MCP = Metacarpophalangeal; PIP = Proximal interphalangeal; AROM = Active range of motion; PROM = Passive range of motion; PT = Physical therapist or physiotherapist; OT = Occupational therapist; AMA = American Medical Association; ASHT = American Society of Hand Therapists; SEM = Standard error of the repeated measurements; SDD = Smallest detectable difference.

* Barakat et al called this "radial adduction," which appears to be equivalent to flexion in the terminology that has been used in this book.

TABLE 7.9 Intertester Reliability of Thumb ROM Measurements for Healthy and Patient Populations

Study	*N*	Sample	Methods	Motion	*r*	ICC	Absolute Measures (degrees)
Barakat et al[21]	10	Healthy women	1 tester (not defined), goniometer	CMC flexion* CMC, MCP, IP motions excluding CMC flexion	.02 .82		
Carvalho et al[70]	1	Wax hand model	30 testers (hand PT, general PT, PT students), 180° plastic goniometer, 3 measurements per tester per joint	Thumb CMC abduction, axis on radial styloid, arms on lateral midline of first and second metacarpals		.90	SD: 4.6–9.5, x = 6.7
de Kraker et al[69]	25	Healthy adults	2 testers (hand therapist, trainee in plastic surgery), 3 angular methods: goniometer first and second metacarpal, Pollexograph-thumb tip, Pollexograph-thumb metacarpal. 3 distance methods: AMA thumb IP crease to third distal palmar crease, ASHT thumb tip to third distal palmar crease, intermetacarpal distance (IMD) dorsal first MC head to second MC head.	AROM, PROM, CMC abduction			
				Goniometry:		.31, .37	SEM = 5.2, 5.9 SDD = 14.4, 16.5
				Pollexograph-tip:		.66, .59	SEM = 2.6, 3.3 SDD = 7.1, 9.0
				Pollexograph-metacarpal:		.57, .61	SEM = 3.7, 3.5 SDD = 10.3, 9.7
				AMA:		.24, .52	SEM = 6.6, 5.0 mm SDD = 18.4, 13.9 mm
				ASHT:		.55, .52	SEM = 5.6, 6.2 mm SDD = 15.6, 17.2 mm
				IMD:		.82, .79	SEM = 2.2, 2.4 mm SDD = 6.1, 6.5 mm
Itoh et al[68]	30	Healthy adults	2 testers (1 orthopedic surgeon, 1 hand surgeon), 2 measurement methods using ruler, 2 measurement methods using goniometer	AROM CMC abduction:			
				Distance tip of thumb to PIP crease of second digit;	.81		
				Distance IP crease of thumb to PIP crease of second digit;	.79		
				Goniometer aligned with first and second metacarpals;	.42		
				Goniometer aligned with first and second proximal phalanges	.28		
Edgar et al[31]	21	Burn survivors	AROM, 4 testers (PT), measured thumb opposition with 0- to 10-point scale twice	Kapandji total opposition scale (TOT)		.99	MDD = 0.3 of TOT scale points

r = Pearson product-moment correlation coefficient; ICC = Intraclass correlation coefficient; PT = Physical therapist or physiotherapist; OT = Occupational therapist; AMA = American Medical Association; ASHT = American Society of Hand Therapists; CMC = Carpometacarpal; MCP = Metacarpophalangeal; IP = Interphalangeal; PIP = Proximal interphalangeal; AROM = Active range of motion; PROM = Passive range of motion; TOT = Total Opposition Test; MDD = Minimal detectible difference; SD = Standard deviation of the repeated measurements; SEM = Standard error of the repeated measurements; SDD = Smallest detectable difference.

* Barakat et al called this "radial adduction," which appears to be equivalent to flexion in the terminology that has been used in this book.

between the two methods ($r^2 = 0.98$). The photograph-computer method averaged 1 degree greater than the goniometer method but was not significantly different.

A marker-based motion-capture system (Vicon) was compared with a manual goniometer for the measurement of three static flexion postures (30, 60, and 90 degrees) of the finger MCP and PIP joints in five healthy college students. Cook and associates[73] found that the motion system and goniometric measurements varied an average of –1.8 degrees at the MCP joint and +3.5 degrees at the PIP joint in the second to fifth digits. Generally, greater flexion postures resulted in greater differences between methods, which the authors attributed to difficulties in placing and reading the goniometer and movement of the markers in the capture system as the skin shifted. The use of goniometers in the clinical setting and the motion-capture system in the research setting for the investigation of finger-intensive activities was supported.

Goodson and associates[74] measured ROM of the wrist, MCP, and IP joints of the fingers with goniometers applied to the dorsal surface, pinch/grip strength, and pain and disability scoring (Cochin scale) in 10 patients with rheumatoid arthritis, 10 patients with osteoarthritis, and 10 healthy control subjects. Range of motion and pinch/grip measurements were able to clearly discriminate between patient groups, which pain and disability scales were unable to do. Patients with rheumatoid arthritis had the greatest reduction in ROM of the MCP, followed by wrist and PIP joints. Patients with osteoarthritis had the greatest reduction in ROM at the DIP followed by the PIP joints. In the rheumatoid arthritis group, ROM of the MCP joints correlated with disability scores ($r^2 = 0.31$) and time since initial diagnosis ($r^2 = 0.32$). Wrist ROM was also related to time since diagnosis ($r^2 = 0.37$). The authors concluded that ROM and pinch/grip strength may more accurately reflect functional impairment associated with arthritis than pain and disability measures.

Field[75] studied 100 patients with Colles fractures of the wrist for the development of algodystrophy (complex regional pain syndrome). Range of motion of the PIP, DIP, and MCP joints of the fingers was measured at 1, 5, and 9 weeks on the dorsal surfaces with a finger goniometer and summed to generate a total ROM value for the hand. Pain response to pressure was assessed with a dolorimeter. Swelling was assessed using a water displacement method. Differences between the affected and unaffected hands were used in statistical tests. At 9 weeks' postfracture, 24 patients were diagnosed with algodystrophy. Goniometry ROM measurements at 1 week showed a sensitivity of 96% and a specificity of 59% in predicting the development of algodystrophy. The cutoff for a positive test appeared to be about 70 degrees of ROM loss in the affected hand. The combination of dolorimetry and goniometry resulted in a sensitivity of 96% and improved specificity to 73%.

MacDermid and coworkers[76] studied the validity of using fingertip pulp-to-palm distance versus total finger flexion (also called composite finger flexion) to predict disability as measured by an upper-extremity disability score (Disabilities of the Arm, Shoulder, and Hand, or DASH). Active MCP, PIP, and DIP flexion of the most severely affected finger was measured in 50 patients by one examiner who used a dorsally placed electrogoniometer NK Hand Assessment System. A micrometer tool was used to measure pulp-to-palm distance in the same patients. The correlation between pulp-to-palm distance and total active flexion was –0.46 to –0.51, indicating that the measures were related but were not interchangeable. The relationship between DASH scores and total active flexion was stronger ($r = 0.45$) than the relationship between DASH scores and pulp-to-palm distances ($r = 0.21–0.30$). The authors suggested that total active motion is a more functional measure than pulp-to-palm distance, and that pulp-to-palm distance "should only be used to monitor individual patient progress and not to compare outcomes between patients or groups of patients."[76]

Reliability and Validity of Visual Estimates

Visual estimates of joint angle positions of the fingers have been found to have much poorer reliability and validity than goniometric measurements. The intertester reliability of visual estimates and goniometric measurements of the MCP joint of the third digit was studied by Bruton, Ellis, and Goddard.[77] One healthy subject had the MCP joint held in two positions by removable static splints while 40 therapists estimated the joint angle and then took one dorsal goniometric measurement. The visual estimates produced much larger ranges and standard deviations of the static positions than goniometry. The mean standard deviations of the visual estimates were 15.7 and 18.0 degrees for the two positions, whereas mean standard deviations for the goniometry were 1.1 and 1.7 degrees. The 95% limit on the differences between two measurements by difference observers was 45 to 51 degrees for the visual estimates, versus 5 to 6 degrees for the goniometer. No differences in tester characteristics such as occupation, years of clinical and specialist experience, and use of the measurement tools had an effect on reliability.

Rose and associates[78] explored the validity of visual estimates by conducting a study in which 71 plastic surgeons and therapists of varying seniority and experience visually estimated the static angles of the MCP and IP joints of the fingers and thumb of a resin cast of an adult male hand. The gold standard for comparison was a computer-based goniometer of the hand assessment and treatment system (HAT) that has been shown to vary less than 1 degree on repetitive measurements. The visual estimates were inaccurate by a mean of about 25% and median of 22%. The most accurate visual estimates were of the thumb IP joint and fifth digit DIP joint with median errors of 18%. Consultant surgeons were the most accurate and physiotherapists the least. Hand surgery experience and a stated interest in hand surgery correlated with more accurate estimations. The authors concluded that although visual accuracy improves with experience, it is an inaccurate technique, and therefore goniometers should be used for measuring joint angles in the hand.

REFERENCES

1. Austin, NM: The Wrist and Hand Complex. In Levangie, PL, and Norkin, CC: Joint Structure and Function: A Comprehensive Analysis, ed 5. FA Davis, Philadelphia, 2011.
2. Standring, S (ed): Gray's Anatomy, ed 39. Elsevier, New York, 2005.
3. Neumann, DA: Kinesiology of the Musculoskeletal System, ed 2. Mosby, St. Louis, 2010.
4. Tubiana, R, Thomine, JM, and Mackin, E (eds): Examination of the Hand and Upper Limb, ed 2. Martin Dunitz, London, 1998.
5. Krishnan, J, and Chipchase, L: Passive axial rotation of the metacarpophalangeal joint. J Hand Surg 22B:270, 1997.
6. Kaltenborn, FM: Manual Mobilization of the Joints: The Extremities, ed 7. Olaf Norlis Bokhandel, Oslo, Norway, 2011.
7. Cyriax, JH, and Cyriax, PJ: Illustrated Manual of Orthopaedic Medicine. Butterworths, London, 1983.
8. Ranney, D: The hand as a concept: Digital differences and their importance. Clin Anat 8:281, 1995.
9. Groth, GN, and Ehretsman, RL: Goniometry of the proximal and distal interphalangeal joints, part I: A survey of instrumentation and placement preferences. J Hand Ther 14:18, 2001.
10. Pratt, AL, and Burr, N: A review of goniometry use within current hand therapy practice. Br J Hand Ther 6:45, 2001.
11. Mallon, WJ, Brown, HR, and Nunley, JA: Digital ranges of motion: Normal values in young adults. J Hand Surg Am 16:882, 1991.
12. Skvarilova, B, and Plevkova, A: Ranges of joint motion of the adult hand. Acta Chir Plast 38:67, 1996.
13. Smahel, Z, and Klimova, A: The influence of age and exercise on the mobility of hand joints: 1: Metacarpophalangeal joints of the three-phalangeal fingers. Acta Chir Plast 46:81, 2004.
14. Gurbuz, H, Mesut, R, and Turan, FN: Measurement of active abduction of metacarpophalangeal joints via electronic digital inclinometric technique. Ital J Anat Embryol 111:9, 2006.
15. American Academy of Orthopaedic Surgeons: Joint Motion: Methods of Measuring and Recording. AAOS, Chicago, 1965.
16. Greene, WB, and Heckman, JD (eds): The Clinical Measurement of Joint Motion. American Academy of Orthopaedic Surgeons, Rosemont, Ill., 1994.
17. Cocchiarella, L, and Andersson, GBJ (eds): American Medical Association: Guides to the Evaluation of Permanent Impairment, ed 5. AMA, Chicago, 2001.
18. Ellis, B, and Bruton, A: A study to compare the reliability of composite finger flexion with goniometry for measurement of range of motion in the hand. Clin Rehabil 16:562, 2002.
19. Adams, LS, Greene, LW, and Topoozian, E: Range of Motion. In American Society of Hand Therapists: Clinical Assessment Recommendations, ed 2. ASHT, Chicago, 1999.
20. White, J, Nolan, DP, and Resteghini, JM: Normative range of motion values for the carpometacarpal (CMC) joint of the thumb with reference to hand dominance, side, and gender. Phys Ther 2012. Retrieved from http://apps.apta.org/custom/abstracts/pt2012/1175-RR.html.
21. Barakat, MJ, Field, J, and Taylor, J: The range of movement of the thumb. Hand 8:179, 2013.
22. International Federation of Societies for Surgery of the Hand (IFSSH): Terminology of Hand Surgery, ed 4. Chapter 5: Atlas of Surface Anatomy and Joint Motion. IFSSH, 2001. Retrieved from http://www.ifssh.info/TerminalolgyofHandSurgery.html.
23. White, J, et al: The influence of age and gender on normative range of motion values of the carpometacarpal joint of the thumb. J Hand Ther 27(2):e1, 2014. Retrieved from http://dx.doi.org/10.1016/j.jht.2014.01.002.
24. Clarkson, HM: Joint Motion and Function Assessment. Lippincott Williams & Wilkins. Philadelphia, 2005.
25. Reese, NB, and Bandy, WD: Joint Range of Motion and Muscle Length Testing. WB Saunders, Philadelphia, 2002.
26. Kapandji, A: Clinical test of apposition and counter-apposition of the thumb. Ann Chir Main 5:67, 1986.
27. Cooney, WP, et al: The kinesiology of the thumb trapeziometacarpal joint. J Bone Joint Surg Am 6:1371, 1981.
28. Zancoll, EC, Ziadenberg, C, and Zancolli, E, Jr: Biomechanics of the trapeziometacarpal joint. Clin Orthop Relat Res 220:14, 1987.
29. Coert, JH, et al: Quantifying thumb rotation during circumduction utilizing a video technique. J Orthop Res 21:1151, 2003.
30. Cheema, TA, et al: Measurement of rotation of the first metacarpal during opposition using computed tomography. J Hand Surg 31A:76, 2006.
31. Edgar, D, et al: Goniometry and linear assessments to monitor movement outcomes: Are they reliable tools in burn care? Burns 35:58, 2009.
32. DeSmet, L, et al: Metacarpophalangeal and interphalangeal flexion of the thumb: Influence of sex and age, relation to ligamentous injury. Acta Orthop Belg 59:357, 1993.
33. Hume, M, et al: Functional range of motion of the joints of the hand. J Hand Surg Am 15:240, 1990.
34. Yoshida, R, et al: Motion and morphology of the thumb metacarpophalangeal joint. J Hand Surg Am 28:753, 2003.
35. Joseph, J: Further studies of the metacarpophalangeal and interphalangeal joints of the thumb. J Anat 85:221, 1951.
36. Smahel, Z, and Klimova, A: The influence of age and exercise on the mobility of hand joints: 2: Interphalangeal joints of the three-phalangeal fingers. Acta Chir Plast 46:122, 2004.
37. Sauseng, S, Kastenbauer, T, and Irsigler, K: Limited joint mobility in selected hand and foot joints in patients with type 1 diabetes mellitus: A methodology comparison. Diab Nutr Metab 15:1, 2002.
38. Shaw, SJ, and Morris, MA: The range of motion of the metacarpophalangeal joint of the thumb and its relationship to injury. J Hand Surg Br 17:164, 1992.
39. Jenkins, M, et al: Thumb joint motion: What is normal? J Hand Surg Br 23:796, 1998.
40. Beighton, P, Solomon, L, and Soskolne, CL: Articular mobility in an African population. Ann Rheum Dis 32:413, 1973.
41. Lamari, NM, Chueire, AG, and Cordeiro, JA: Analysis of joint mobility patterns among preschool children. Sao Paulo Med 123:119, 2005.
42. Allander, E, et al: Normal range of joint movements in shoulder, hip, wrist and thumb with special reference to side: A comparison between two populations. Int J Epidemiol 3:253, 1974.
43. Fairbank, JCT, Pynsett, PB, and Phillips, H: Quantitative measurements of joint mobility in adolescents. Ann Rheum Dis 43:288, 1984.
44. Nicholson, B: Clinical Evaluation. In Stanley, BG, and Tribuzi, SM: Concepts in Hand Rehabilitation. FA Davis, Philadelphia, 1992.
45. Knutson, JS, et al: Intrinsic and extrinsic contributions to the passive moment at the metacarpophalangeal joint. J Biomech 33:1675, 2000.
46. Melvin, J: Rheumatic Disease in Adult and Child: Occupational Therapy and Rehabilitation, ed 3. FA Davis, Philadelphia, 1989.
47. Casanova, JS, and Grunert, BK: Adult prehension: Patterns and nomenclature for pinches. J Hand Ther 2:231, 1989.
48. Totten, PA, and Flinn-Wagner, S: Functional evaluation of the hand. In Stanley, BG, and Tribuzi, SM (eds): Concepts in Hand Rehabilitation. FA Davis, Philadelphia, 1992.
49. Mackin, E, et al: Hunter, Mackin & Callahan's Rehabilitation of the Hand and Upper Extremity, ed 5. Elsevier, St Louis, 2002.
50. Lee, JW, and Rim, K: Measurement of finger joint angles and maximum finger forces during cylinder grip activity. J Biomed Eng 13:152, 1991.
51. Hayashi, H, and Shimizu, H: Essential motion of metacarpophalangeal joint during activities of daily living. J Hand Ther 26:69, 2013.
52. Baker, NA, et al: Kinematics of the finger and hands during computer keyboard use. Clin Biomech 22:34, 2007.
53. Nakamura, M, et al: Analysis of voluntary finger movements during hand tasks by a motion analyzer. J Electromyogr Kinesiol 8:295, 1998.
54. Ellis, B, Bruton, A, and Goddard, JR: Joint angle measurement: A comparative study of the reliability of goniometry and wire tracing for the hand. Clin Rehabil 11:314, 1997.
55. Burr, N, Pratt, AL, and Stott, D: Inter-rater and intra-rater reliability when measuring interphalangeal joints. Physiotherapy 89:641, 2003.
56. Lewis, E, Fors, L, and Tharion, WJ: Interrater and intrarater reliability of finger goniometric measurements. Am J Occup Ther 64:555, 2010.
57. Macionis, V: Reliability of the standard goniometry and diagrammatic recording of finger joint angles: A comparative study with healthy subjects and non-professional raters. BMC Musculoskelet Dis 14:17, 2013.
58. Bear-Lehman, J, and Abreu, BC: Evaluating the hand: Issues in reliability and validity. Phys Ther 69:1025, 1989.
59. Goldsmith, N, and Juzl, E: Inter-rater reliability of two trained raters using a goniometer for the measurement of finger joints. Br J Hand Ther 3:12, 1998.
60. Stam, HJ, et al: The Compangle: A new goniometer for joint angle measurement of the hand. A technical note. Eur Medicophys 42:37, 2006.
61. Hamilton, GF, and Lachenbruch, PA: Reliability of goniometers in assessing finger joint angle. Phys Ther 49:465, 1969.
62. Weiss, PL, et al: Using the Exos Handmaster to measure digital range of motion: Reliability and validity. Med Eng Phys 16:323, 1994.
63. Groth, G, et al: Goniometry of the proximal and distal interphalangeal joints. Part II: Placement preferences, interrater reliability, and concurrent validity. J Hand Ther 14:23, 2001.

64. Brown, A, et al: Validity and reliability of the Dexter Hand Evaluation and Therapy System in hand-injured patients. J Hand Ther 13:37, 2000.
65. Flower, KR, and LaStayo, PC: Effect of total end range time on improving passive range of motion. J Hand Ther 7:150, 1994. (Reprinted in J Hand Ther 25:48, 2012.)
66. Engstrand, C, Krevers, B, and Kvist, J: Interrater reliability in finger joint goniometer measurement in Dupuytren's disease. Am J Occup Ther 66:98, 2012.
67. Glasgow, C, Wilton, J, and Tooth, L: Optimal daily total end range time for contracture: Resolution in hand splinting. J Hand Ther 16:207, 2003.
68. Itoh, S, et al: Reproducibility of measurements of thumb abduction. Hand Surg 15:7, 2010.
69. De Kraker, M, et al: Palmar abduction: Reliability of 6 measurements methods in healthy adults. J Hand Surg Am 34:523, 2009.
70. Carvalho, RMF, Mazzer, N, and Barbier, CH: Analysis of the reliability and reproducibility of goniometry compared to hand photogrammetry. Acta Orthop Bras (online) 30:139, 2012.
71. Kato, M, et al: The accuracy of goniometric measurements of proximal interphalangeal joints in fresh cadavers: Comparison between methods of measurement, types of goniometers, and fingers. J Hand Ther 20:12, 2007.
72. Georgeu, GA, Mayfield, S, and Logan, AM: Lateral digital photography with computer-aided goniometry versus standard goniometry for recording finger joint angles. J Hand Surg Br 27:184, 2002.
73. Cook, JR, et al: Measurement of wrist and finger postures: A comparison of goniometric and motion capture techniques. J Appl Biomech 23:70, 2007.
74. Goodson, A, et al: Direct, quantitative clinical assessment of hand function: Usefulness and reproducibility. Man Ther 12:144, 2007.
75. Field, J: Measurement of finger stiffness in algodystrophy. Hand Clin 19:511, 2003.
76. MacDermid, JC, et al: Validity of pulp-to-palm distance as a measure of finger flexion. J Hand Surg Br 26:432, 2001.
77. Bruton, A, Ellis, B, and Goddard, J: Comparison of visual estimation and goniometry for assessment of metacarpophalangeal joint angle. Physiotherapy 85:201, 1999.
78. Rose, V, et al: Visual estimation of finger angles: Do we need goniometers? J Hand Surg Br 27:382, 2002.

PART III

LOWER-EXTREMITY TESTING

OBJECTIVES

On completion of Part III, you will be able to:

1. **Identify:**

   appropriate planes and axes for each lower-extremity joint motion
   normal ranges of motion for each lower-extremity joint
   structures that limit the end of the range of motion (ROM)
   expected normal end-feels

2. **Describe:**

   testing positions used for each lower-extremity joint motion and muscle length test
   goniometer alignment for each motion and muscle length test
   capsular pattern of restricted motion
   range of motion necessary for selected functional activities at each major lower-extremity joint

3. **Explain:**

   how age, gender, and other variables may affect the ROM
   how sources of error in measurement may affect testing results

4. **Perform a goniometric measurement of joint ROM and muscle length testing for the hip, knee, ankle, and foot that includes:**

   a clear explanation of the testing procedure
   proper positioning of the individual in testing position
   adequate stabilization
   use of appropriate testing motion
   correct determination of the end of the motion
   correct identification of the end-feel
   palpation of the appropriate bony landmarks
   accurate alignment of the goniometer and correct reading and recording of goniometric measurements

5. **Plan goniometric measurements of the hip, knee, ankle, and foot that are organized by body position.**

6. **Assess the intratester and intertester reliability of the reader's goniometric measurements of the lower-extremity joints using the statistical methods described in Chapter 3.**

CHAPTER 8

The Hip

Erin Hartigan, PT, DPT, PhD, OCS, ATC
D. Joyce White, PT, DSc

Structure and Function

Iliofemoral Joint

The hip joint, more specifically called the iliofemoral joint, links the lower extremity with the trunk. The proximal joint surface is the acetabulum, which is formed superiorly by the ilium, posteroinferiorly by the ischium, and anteroinferiorly by the pubis (Fig. 8.1). The concave acetabulum faces laterally, inferiorly, and anteriorly and is deepened by a fibrocartilaginous acetabular labrum.[1] The distal joint surface is the convex head of the femur. The joint is enclosed by a strong, thick capsule, which is reinforced anteriorly by the iliofemoral and pubofemoral ligaments (Fig. 8.2) and posteriorly by the ischiofemoral ligament (Fig. 8.3).

Osteokinematics

The hip is a synovial ball-and-socket joint with 3 degrees of freedom. Motions permitted at the joint are flexion–extension in the sagittal plane around a medial–lateral axis, abduction–adduction in the frontal plane around an anterior–posterior axis, and medial and lateral rotation in the transverse plane around a vertical or longitudinal axis.[1] The axis of motion goes through the center of the femoral head.

Arthrokinematics

In an open kinematic (non-weight-bearing) chain, the convex femoral head rolls in the same direction and slides in the opposite direction to movement of the shaft of the femur. In flexion, the femoral head rolls anteriorly and slides posteriorly and inferiorly on the acetabulum, whereas in extension, the femoral head rolls posteriorly and slides anteriorly and

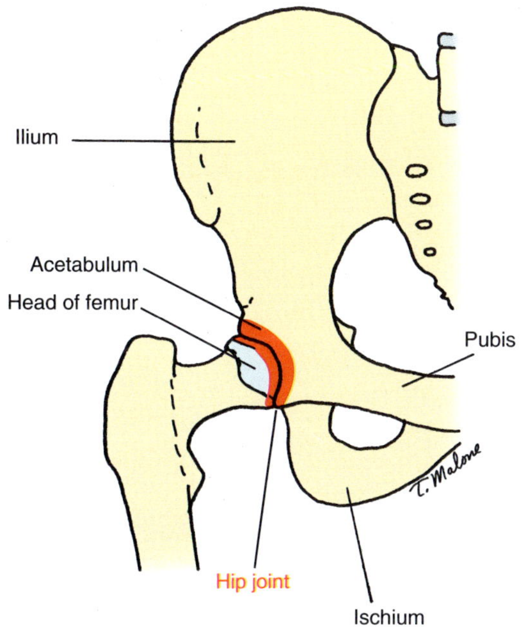

FIGURE 8.1 An anterior view of the right hip joint.

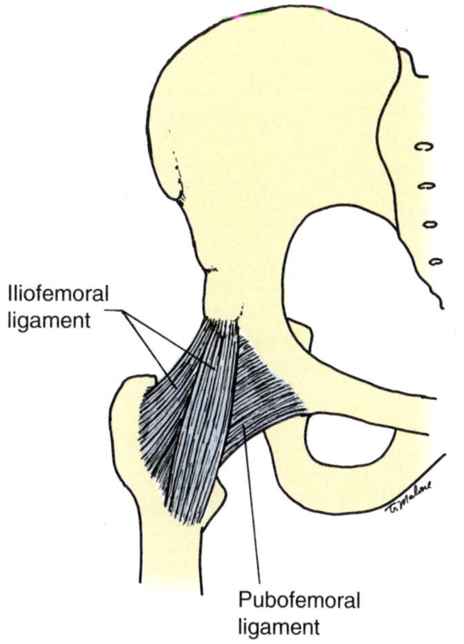

FIGURE 8.2 An anterior view of the right hip joint showing the iliofemoral and pubofemoral ligaments.

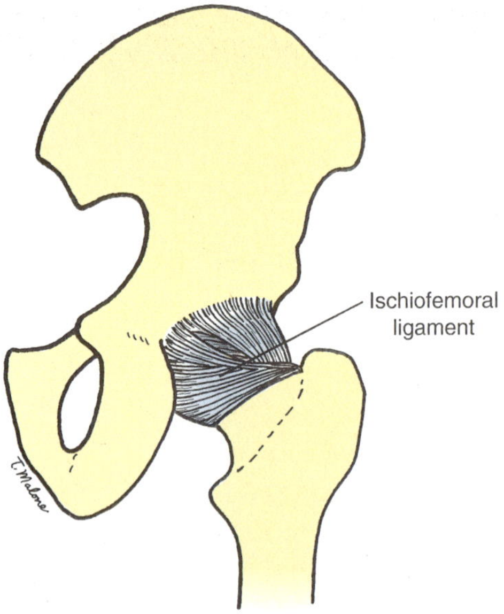

FIGURE 8.3 A posterior view of the right hip joint showing the ischiofemoral ligament.

superiorly. In medial rotation, the femoral head rolls anteriorly and slides posteriorly on the acetabulum. During lateral rotation, the femoral head rolls posteriorly and slides anteriorly. In abduction, the femoral head rolls superiorly and slides inferiorly, whereas in adduction, the femoral head rolls inferiorly and slides superiorly. Refer to Chapter 1 for the explanations of slide, spin, and roll (e.g., Figs. 1.2, 1.3, and 1.4, respectively).

Capsular Pattern

The capsular pattern is characterized by a marked restriction of medial rotation accompanied by limitations in flexion and abduction. A slight limitation may be present in extension, but little or no limitation is present in lateral rotation and adduction.[2]

RANGE OF MOTION TESTING PROCEDURES: Hip

Landmarks for Testing Procedures

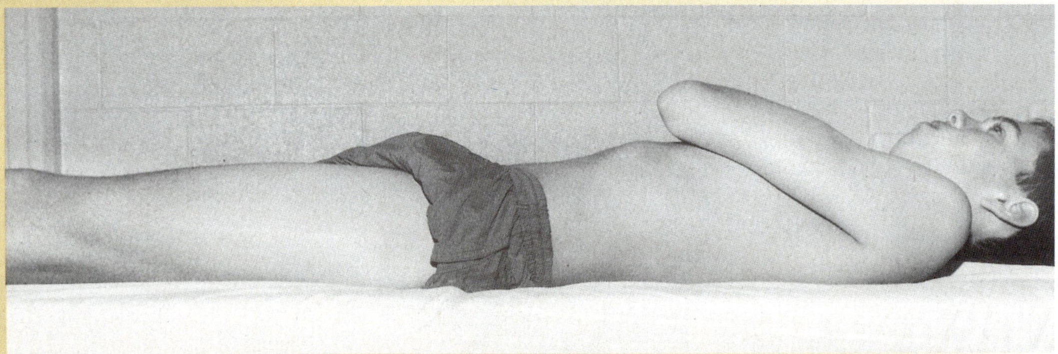

FIGURE 8.4 A lateral view of the hip showing surface anatomy landmarks for aligning the goniometer for measuring hip flexion and extension.

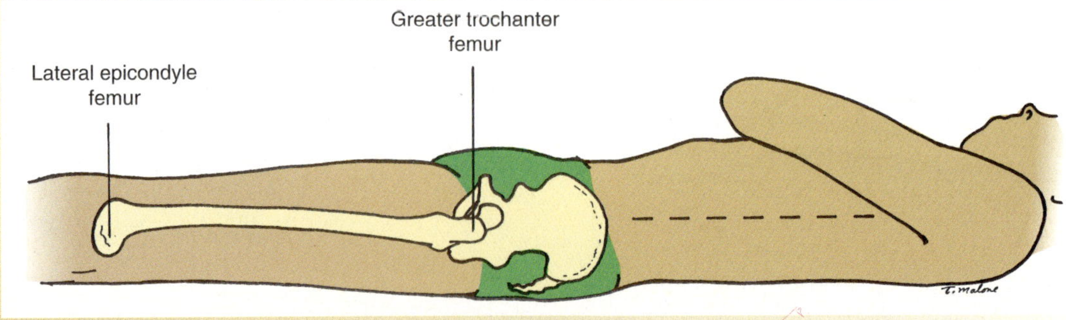

FIGURE 8.5 A lateral view of the hip showing bony anatomical landmarks for aligning the goniometer.

Landmarks for Testing Procedures (continued)

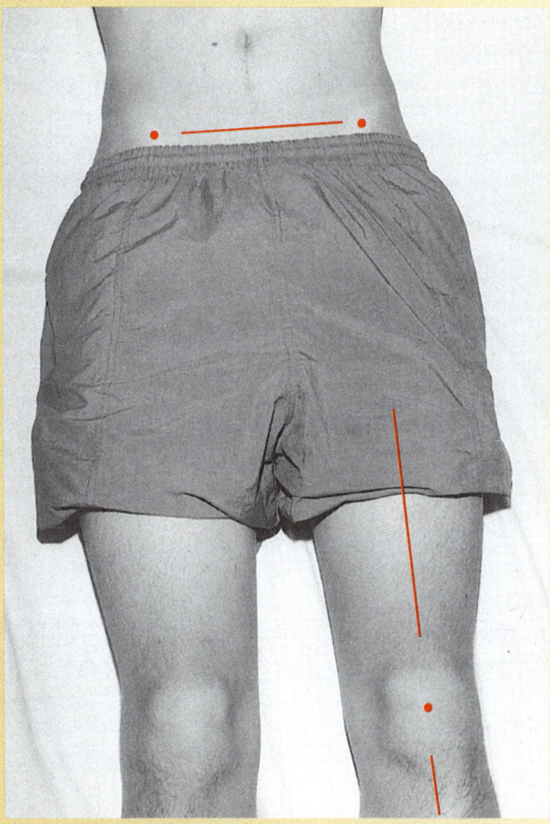

FIGURE 8.6 An anterior view of the hip showing surface anatomy landmarks for aligning the goniometer.

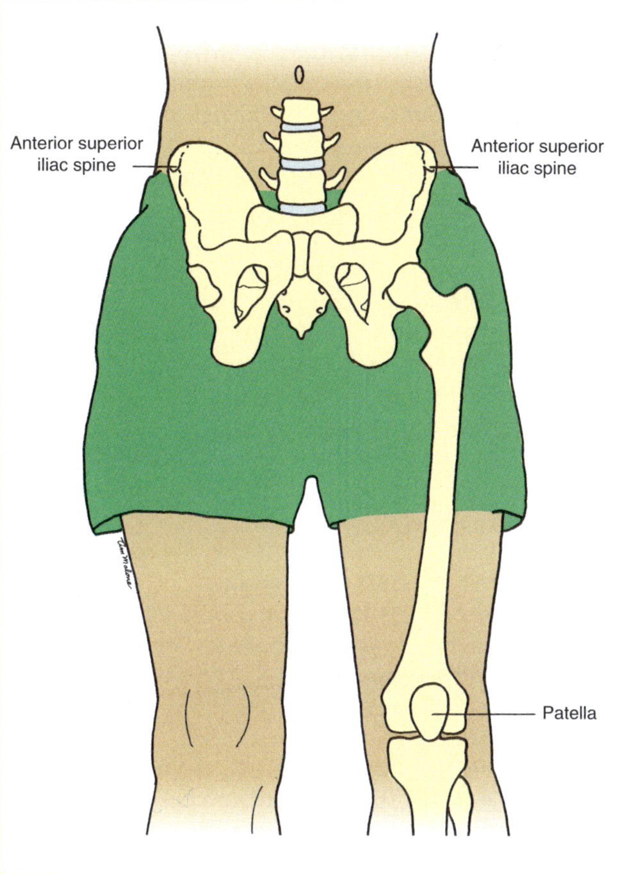

FIGURE 8.7 An anterior view of the pelvis showing the anatomical landmarks for aligning the goniometer for measuring abduction and adduction.

HIP FLEXION

Motion occurs in the sagittal plane around a medial–lateral axis. Hip flexion range of motion (ROM) values for adults generally vary from 120 to 140 degrees.[3–7] Hip flexion ROM tends to decrease from toddler to senior age although differences are generally small, ranging from about 4 degrees (males) to 10 degrees (females).[6] Refer to Research Findings and Tables 8.2 to 8.5 for normal ROM values by age and gender.

Testing Position

Place the individual in the supine position, with the pelvis in neutral, knees extended, and both hips in 0 degrees of abduction, adduction, and rotation. Clinically, while resting in supine the pelvis is often tilted and the thigh may be externally rotated. Verify that the pelvis is in neutral alignment by palpating the anterior superior iliac spine (ASIS) and posterior superior iliac spine (PSIS) and positioning the ASIS vertically in line with the PSIS if needed. Confirm that the hip is in 0 degrees of rotation by palpating the medial and lateral femoral epicondyles and observing the patella. The patella should be facing anteriorly, but confirmation of neutral hip rotation is more accurately assessed by the epicondyles, as the patella can be misaligned.

Stabilization

Stabilize the ipsilateral pelvis with one hand to prevent posterior tilting or rotation. Keep the contralateral lower extremity flat on the table in the neutral position to provide additional stabilization.

Testing Motion

Flex the hip by lifting the thigh off the table. Allow the knee to flex passively during the motion to reduce tension in the hamstring muscles. Maintain the extremity in neutral rotation and abduction and adduction throughout the motion (Fig. 8.8). The end of the ROM occurs when resistance to further motion is felt and attempts at overcoming the resistance cause posterior tilting of the pelvis. Therefore, position your thumb and fingers accordingly to note this posterior tilting motion of the pelvis as the PSIS moves inferiorly and the ASIS moves superiorly.

Normal End-Feel

The end-feel is usually soft because of contact between the muscle bulk of the anterior thigh and the lower abdomen. However, the end-feel may be firm because of tension in the posterior joint capsule and/or the gluteus maximus muscle.

Goniometer Alignment

See Figures 8.9 and 8.10.

1. Center **fulcrum** of the goniometer over the lateral aspect of the hip joint, using the greater trochanter of the femur for reference.
2. Align **proximal arm** with the lateral midline of the pelvis.
3. Align **distal arm** with the lateral midline of the femur, using the lateral epicondyle as a reference.

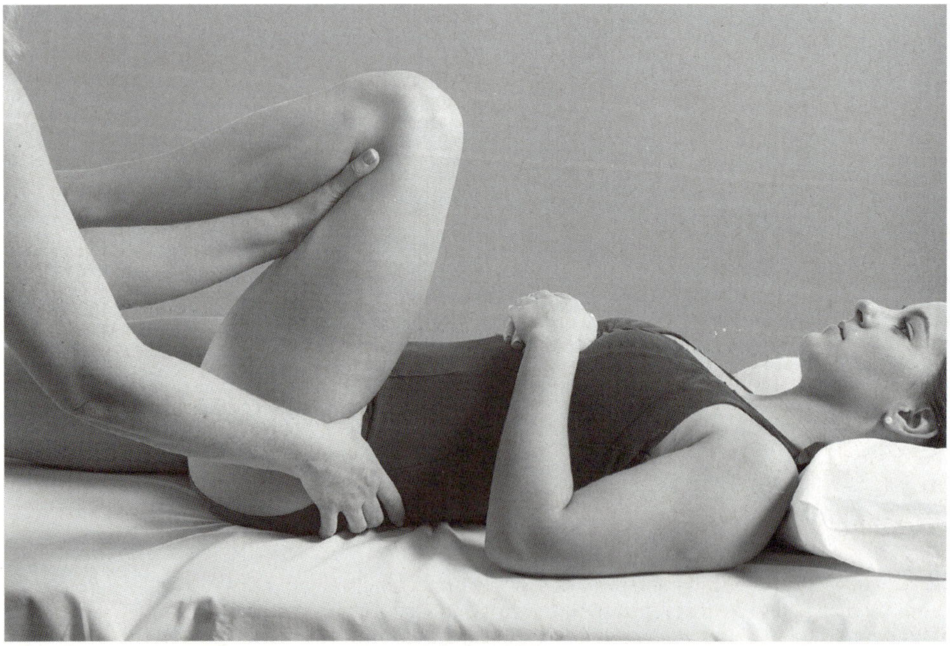

FIGURE 8.8 Assessment of end-feel and estimation of the end of left hip flexion passive ROM. The placement of the examiner's hand on the pelvis allows the examiner to stabilize the pelvis and to detect any pelvic motion.

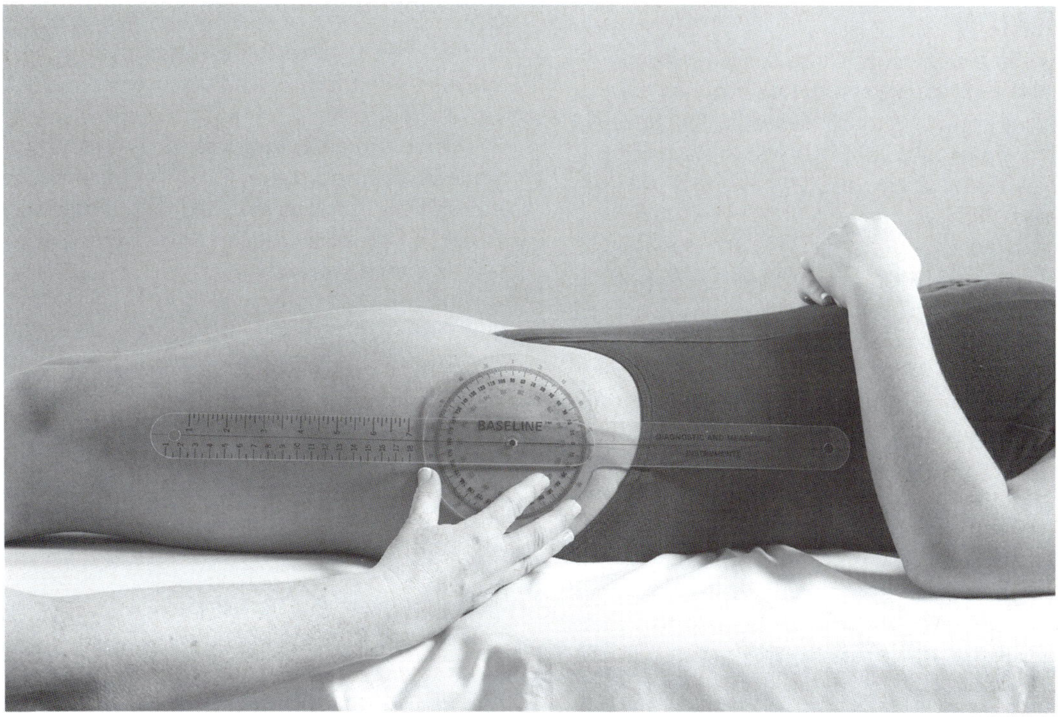

FIGURE 8.9 Goniometer alignment in the supine starting position for measuring hip flexion ROM.

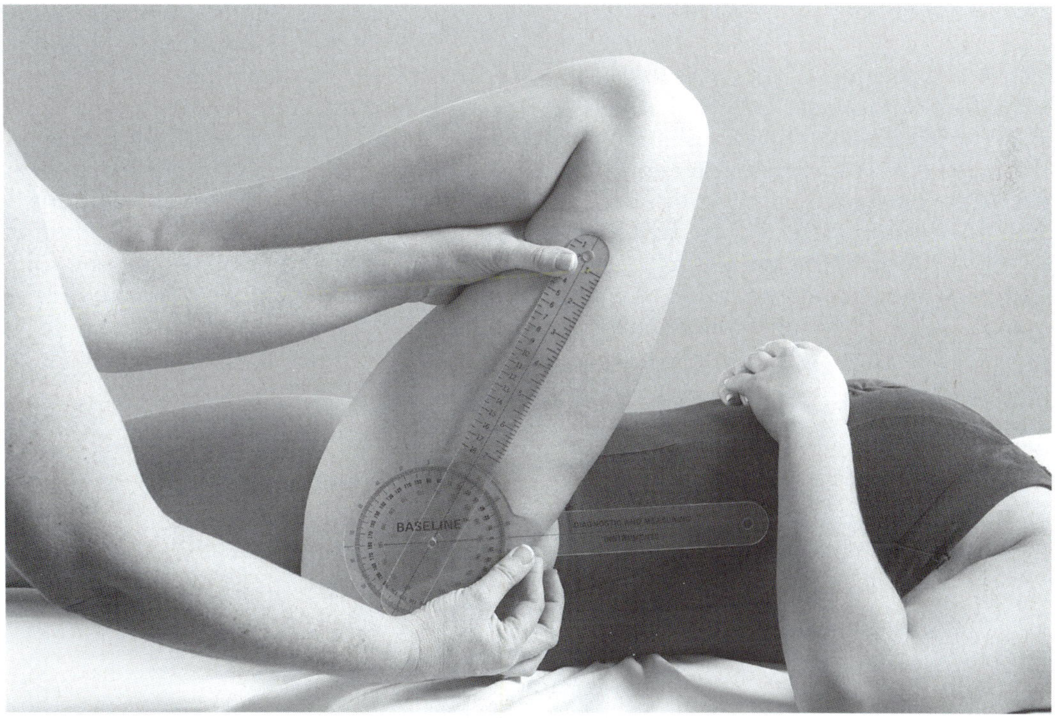

FIGURE 8.10 The goniometric measurement at the end of hip flexion ROM. The examiner uses one hand to align the distal goniometer arm and to maintain the hip in flexion. The examiner's other hand shifts from stabilizing the pelvis to hold the proximal goniometer arm aligned with the lateral midline of the pelvis.

HIP EXTENSION

Motion occurs in a sagittal plane around a medial–lateral axis. Normal hip extension ROM values for adults vary from about 18 to 30 degrees.[3,4–6,8] Refer to Research Findings and Tables 8.2 to 8.5 for normal ROM values by age and gender.

Testing Position

Place the individual in the prone position, with both knees extended and the hip to be tested in 0 degrees of abduction, adduction, and rotation. Clinically, while resting in the prone position the pelvis is often tilted and the thigh may be abducted and rotated. Verify that the pelvis is in neutral alignment by palpating the anterior superior iliac spine (ASIS) and posterior superior iliac spine (PSIS), and positioning the ASIS vertically in line with the PSIS. Confirm that the hip is in 0 degrees of rotation by palpating the medial and lateral femoral epicondyles. If necessary, a small pillow may be placed under the abdomen for comfort, but be sure to avoid placing the individual in hip flexion and/or lumbar flexion. No pillow should be placed under the head.

Stabilization

Hold the ipsilateral pelvis with one hand to prevent an anterior tilt and to feel for the end ROM. Keep the contralateral extremity flat on the table to provide additional pelvic stabilization.

Testing Motion

Extend the hip by raising the lower extremity from the table (Fig. 8.11). Maintain the knee in extension throughout the movement to ensure that tension in the two-joint rectus femoris muscle does not limit the hip extension ROM. The end of the ROM occurs when resistance to further motion of the femur is felt and attempts at overcoming the resistance cause anterior tilting of the pelvis and/or extension of the lumbar spine. Therefore, position your thumb and fingers accordingly to note this anterior tilting motion of the pelvis as the PSIS moves superiorly and the ASIS moves inferiorly.

Once the examiner has determined the end-feel and estimated the ROM, an assistant could help support the thigh at the end of the motion, making it easier for the examiner to align the goniometer and take the measurement.

Normal End-Feel

The end-feel is firm because of tension in the anterior joint capsule and the iliofemoral ligament and, to a lesser extent, the ischiofemoral and pubofemoral ligaments. Tension in various muscles that flex the hip, such as the iliopsoas, sartorius, tensor fasciae latae, gracilis, and adductor longus, may contribute to the firm end-feel.

Goniometer Alignment

See Figures 8.12 and 8.13.

1. Center **fulcrum** of the goniometer over the lateral aspect of the hip joint, using the greater trochanter of the femur for reference.
2. Align **proximal arm** with the lateral midline of the pelvis.
3. Align **distal arm** with the lateral midline of the femur, using the lateral epicondyle as a reference.

Alternative Testing Position: Side-Lying

If the individual is unable to assume a comfortable prone position, the testing position may be altered to side-lying with the leg being tested in the upper position. In the side-lying position, the bottom limb should be in slight hip and knee flexion for comfort and stability. The stabilization, testing motion, end-feel, and goniometer alignment are the same as for the prone testing position procedure.

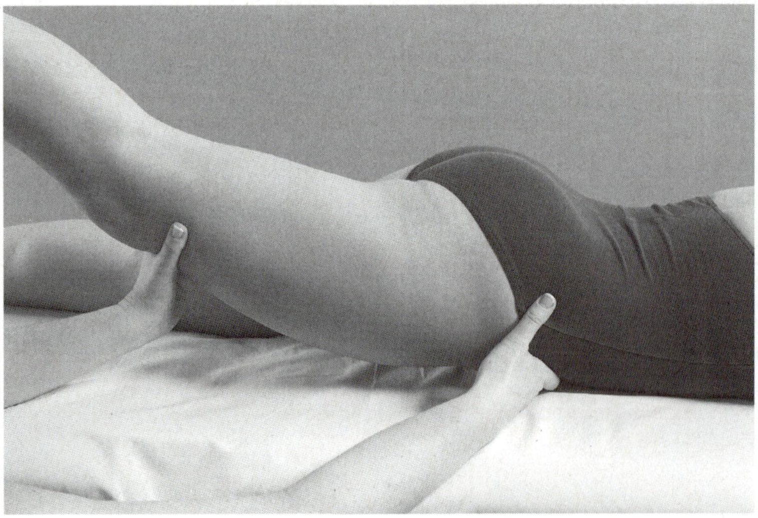

FIGURE 8.11 Assessment of end-feel and estimation of hip extension passive ROM. The examiner uses one hand to support the distal femur, while the other hand grasps the pelvis at the level of the anterior superior iliac spine to stabilize and detect pelvic tilting.

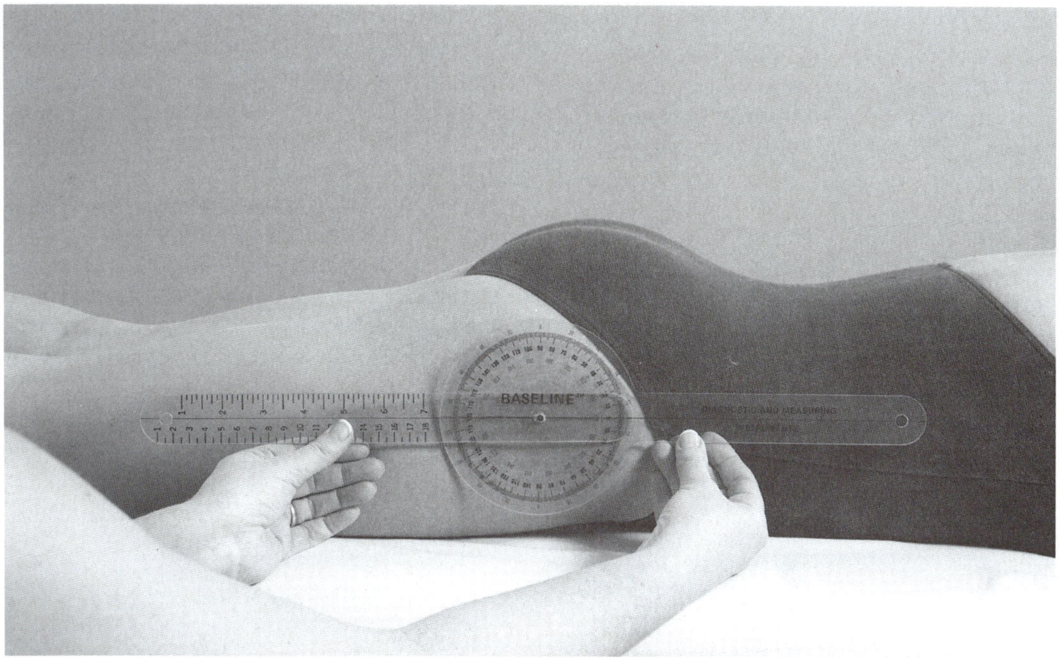

FIGURE 8.12 Goniometer alignment in the prone starting position for measuring hip extension ROM.

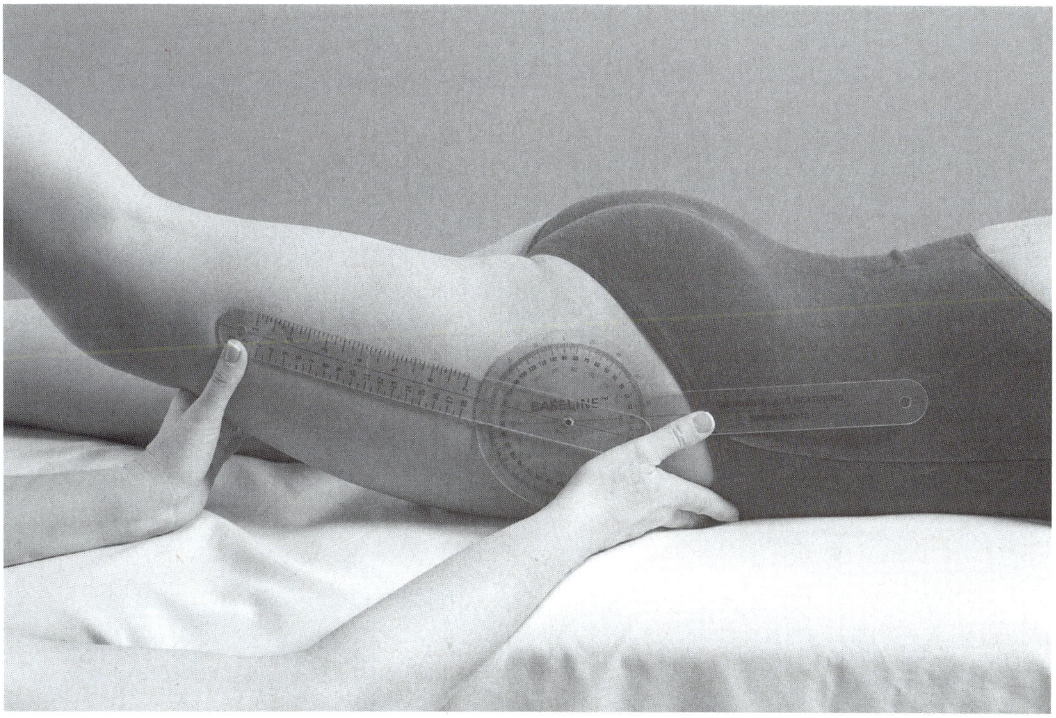

FIGURE 8.13 The goniometric measurement at the end of hip extension passive ROM. The examiner uses one hand to hold the proximal goniometer arm in alignment. The examiner's other hand supports the femur and keeps the distal goniometer arm in alignment.

HIP ABDUCTION

Motion occurs in the frontal plane around an anterior–posterior axis. Normal abduction ROM values for adults vary from about 40 to 55 degrees.[4,5,8] Refer to Research Findings and Tables 8.2 to 8.5 for normal ROM values by age and gender.

Testing Position

Place the individual in the supine position, with knees extended and hips in 0 degrees of flexion, extension, and rotation. Confirm that the hip is in neutral rotation by palpating the medial and lateral femoral epicondyles to ensure that they are level and the patella faces anteriorly. Position the individual at the edge of the plinth opposite to the limb being tested to allow the table to support the limb at the end of the ROM.

Stabilization

Keep a hand on the iliac crest of the pelvis to prevent lateral tilting in the superior direction (elevation) and rotation. Watch for lateral flexion of the trunk.

Testing Motion

Abduct the hip by moving the lower extremity laterally (Fig. 8.14). Do not allow lateral rotation or flexion of the hip as you move the hip into abduction. The end of the ROM occurs when resistance to further motion of the femur is felt and attempts to overcome the resistance cause lateral pelvic tilting, pelvic rotation, and/or lateral flexion of the trunk.

Normal End-Feel

The end-feel is firm because of tension in the inferior (medial) joint capsule, pubofemoral ligament, ischiofemoral ligament, and inferior band of the iliofemoral ligament. Passive tension in the adductor magnus, adductor longus, adductor brevis, pectineus, and gracilis muscles may contribute to the firm end-feel.

Goniometer Alignment

See Figures 8.15 and 8.16.

1. Center **fulcrum** of the goniometer over the anterior superior iliac spine (ASIS) of the extremity being measured.
2. Align **proximal arm** with an imaginary horizontal line extending from one ASIS to the other.
3. Align **distal arm** with the anterior midline of the femur, using the midline of the patella for reference. Palpate the midpoint between the femoral epicondyles to confirm that the midline of the patella is not displaced medially or laterally.

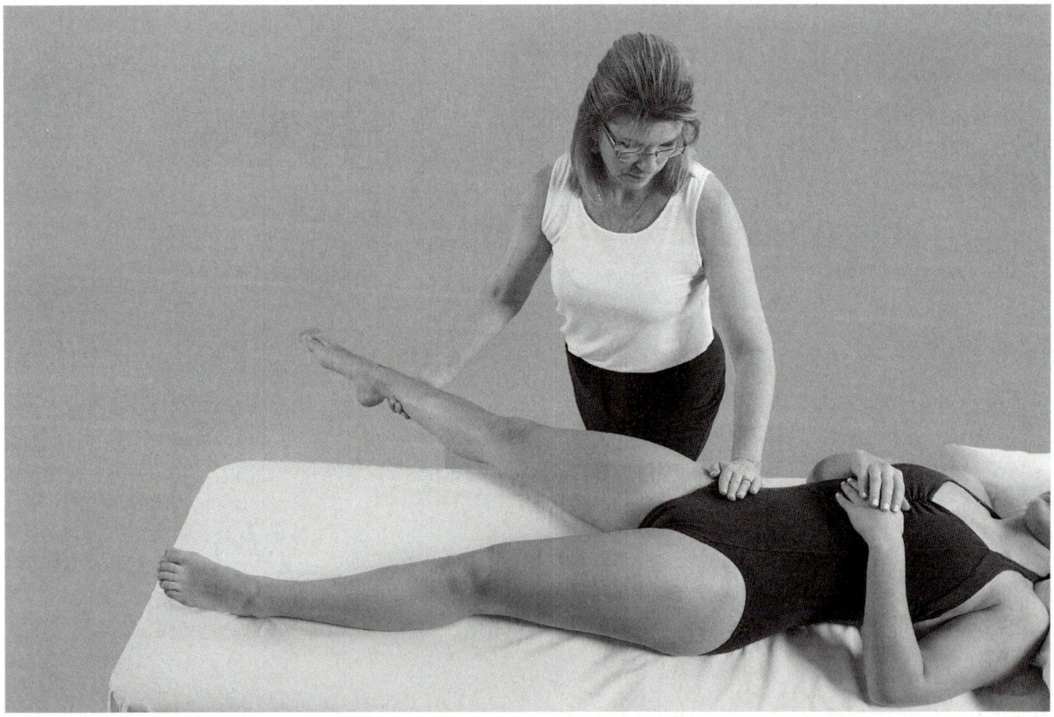

FIGURE 8.14 Assessment of end-feel and estimation of the end of right hip abduction passive ROM. The individual is positioned close to the left side of the plinth to maximize space for the right limb to move into hip abduction. The examiner uses one hand to move the leg into abduction. The examiner's grip on the lower leg is designed to prevent medial or lateral rotation of the hip. The examiner's other hand not only stabilizes the pelvis but is used to detect pelvic motion.

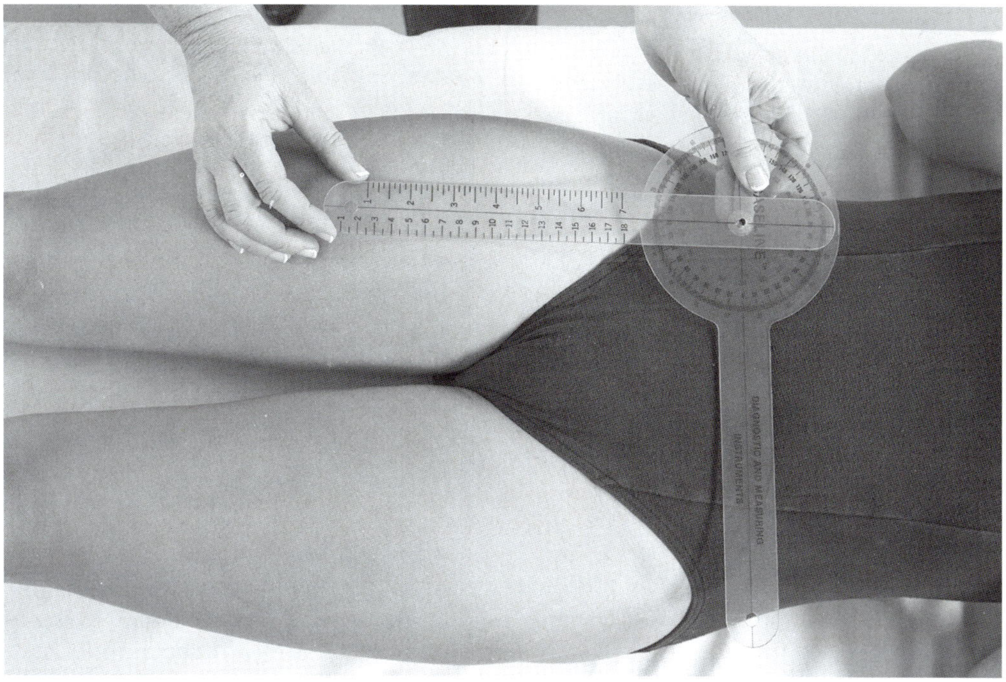

FIGURE 8.15 In the starting position for measuring hip abduction ROM, the goniometer is at a 90-degree angle. This position is considered to be the 0-degree starting position. Ideally, the goniometer will have two scales and the start position can be read as 0 degrees or 90 degrees. If there is only one scale, the examiner must do math to transpose the reading from 90 degrees to 0 degrees. For example, an actual reading of 90 to 120 degrees on the goniometer will be recorded as 0–30 degrees.

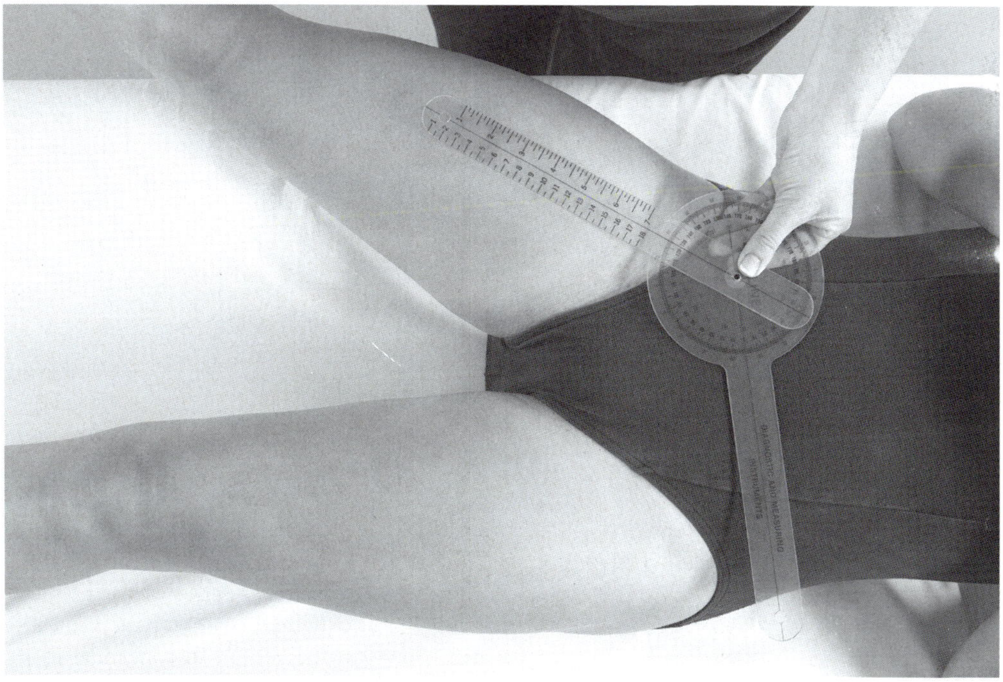

FIGURE 8.16 The goniometric measurement indicating the end of right abduction passive ROM. The examiner has determined the end-feel and has moved the right hand from stabilizing the pelvis to hold the goniometer in correct alignment. The examiner may also place the individual's index fingers over the right and left ASIS to help assure accurate goniometric alignment.

HIP ADDUCTION

Motion occurs in a frontal plane around an anterior–posterior axis. Normal adduction ROM for adults is generally 20 to 25 degrees.[8,9] Refer to Research Findings and Tables 8.2 to 8.5 for normal ROM values by age and gender.

Testing Position

Place the individual in the supine position, with both knees extended and the hip being tested in 0 degrees of flexion, extension, and rotation. Confirm that the hip is in neutral rotation by palpating the medial and lateral femoral epicondyles to ensure that they are level and the patella faces anteriorly. Abduct the contralateral extremity to provide sufficient space to complete the full ROM in adduction.

Stabilization

Stabilize the ipsilateral pelvis to prevent lateral tilting in the caudal direction and rotation. Watch for lateral flexion of the trunk.

Testing Motion

Adduct the hip by moving the lower extremity medially toward the contralateral lower extremity (Fig. 8.17). The examiner's hand is used to move the extremity into adduction and to maintain the hip in neutral flexion and rotation. The end of the ROM occurs when resistance to further adduction is felt and attempts to overcome the resistance cause lateral pelvic tilting, pelvic rotation, and/or lateral trunk flexion.

Normal End-Feel

The end-feel is firm because of tension in the superior (lateral) joint capsule and the superior band of the iliofemoral ligament. Tension in the gluteus medius and minimus and the tensor fasciae latae muscles may also contribute to the firm end-feel.

Goniometer Alignment

See Figures 8.18 and 8.19.

1. Center **fulcrum** of the goniometer over the ASIS of the extremity being measured.
2. Align **proximal arm** with an imaginary horizontal line extending from one ASIS to the other.
3. Align **distal arm** with the anterior midline of the femur, using the midline of the patella for reference. Palpate the midpoint between the femoral epicondyles to confirm that the midline of the patella is not displaced medially or laterally.

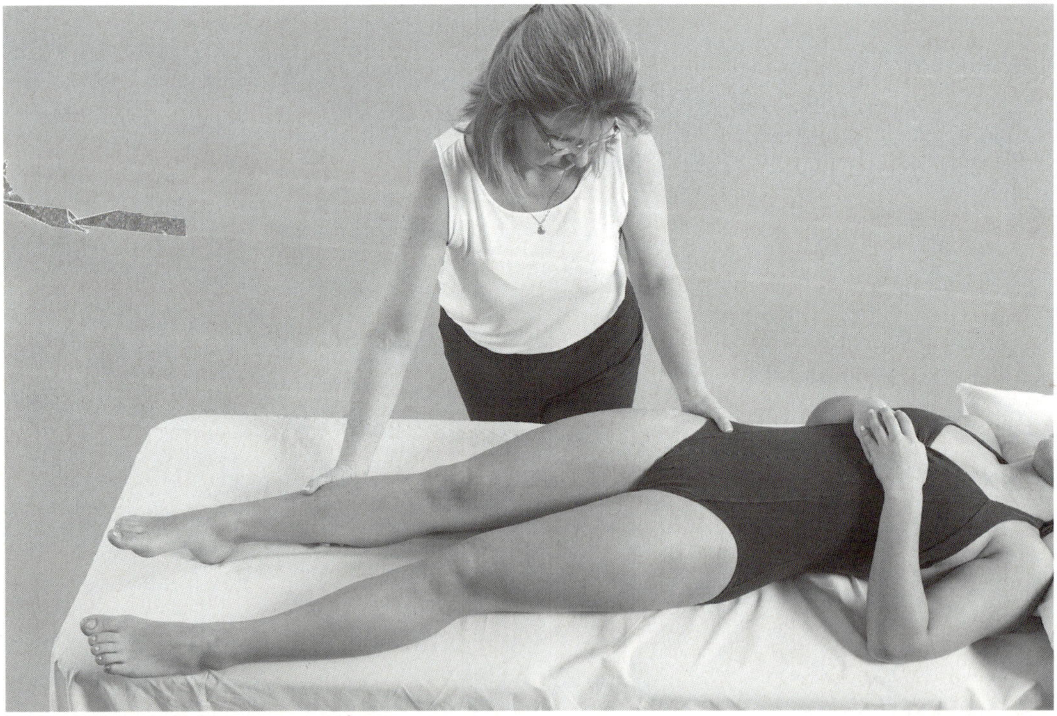

FIGURE 8.17 Assessment of end-feel and estimation of the end of the right hip adduction passive ROM. The examiner positioned the left limb in hip abduction to allow space for right hip adduction to occur. The examiner moves the hip in adduction with one hand and stabilizes the pelvis with the other hand.

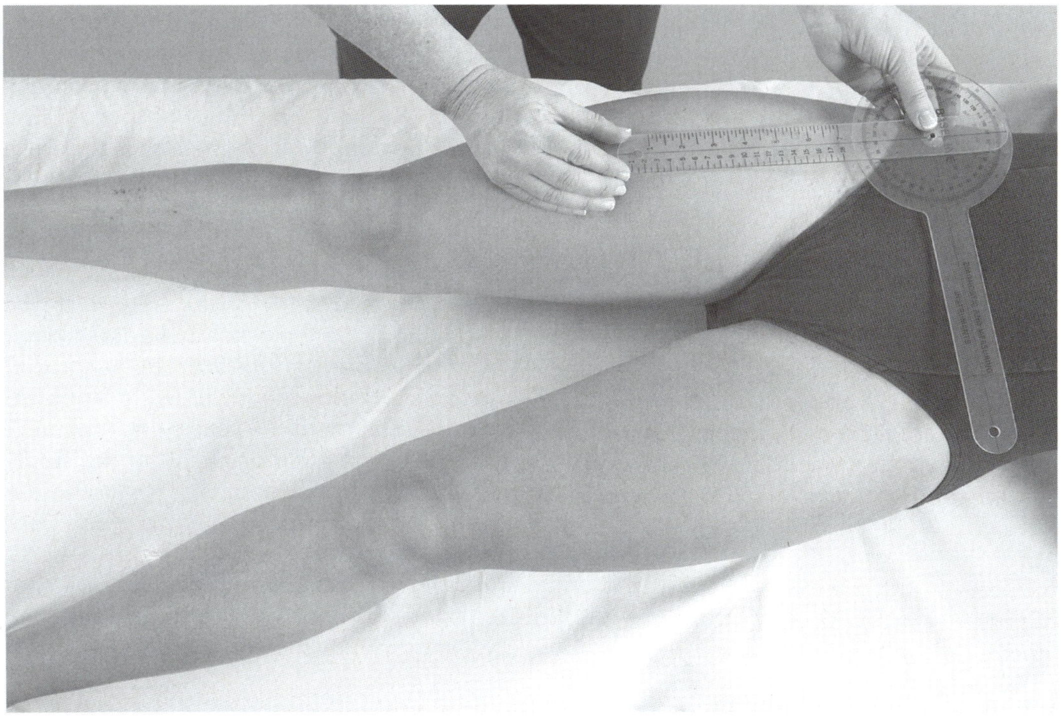

FIGURE 8.18 In the starting position for measuring hip adduction ROM, the goniometer is at a 90-degree angle. This position is considered to be the 0-degree starting position. Ideally, the goniometer will have two scales and the start position can be read as 0 degrees or 90 degrees. If there is only one scale, the examiner must do math to transpose the reading from 90 degrees to 0 degrees. For example, an actual reading of 90 to 60 degrees will be recorded as 0–30 degrees.

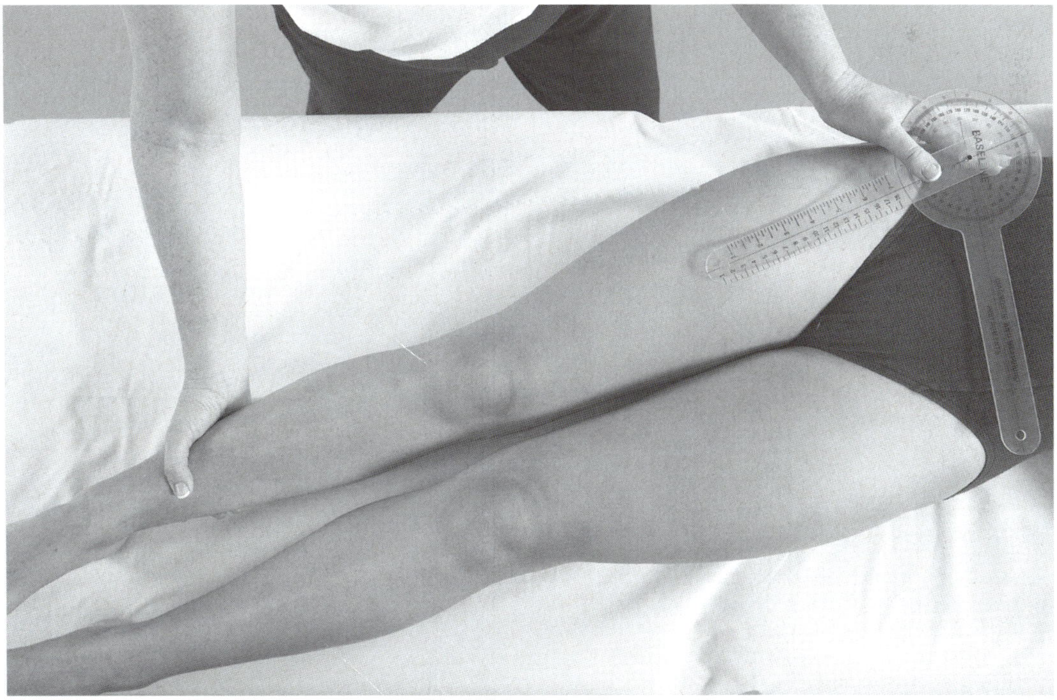

FIGURE 8.19 The goniometric measurement indicating the end of the right hip adduction passive ROM. The examiner uses one hand to hold the fulcrum of the goniometer over the individual's anterior superior iliac spine. The examiner prevents hip rotation by maintaining a firm grasp at the individual's lower leg with the other hand.

HIP MEDIAL (INTERNAL) ROTATION

Motion occurs in a transverse plane around a vertical axis when the individual is in anatomical position. Normal medial rotation ROM values for adults vary from about 30 to 45 degrees, with greater ranges noted in the prone position.[3–5,8] Refer to Research Findings and Tables 8.2 to 8.5 for normal ROM values by age and gender.

Testing Position

Seat the individual on a firm surface, with the knees flexed to 90 degrees over the edge of the surface. Place the hip in 0 degrees of abduction and adduction and in 90 degrees of flexion. If the femur is not in 90 degrees of flexion, then place a towel roll under the distal end of the femur to maintain the femur in a horizontal plane.

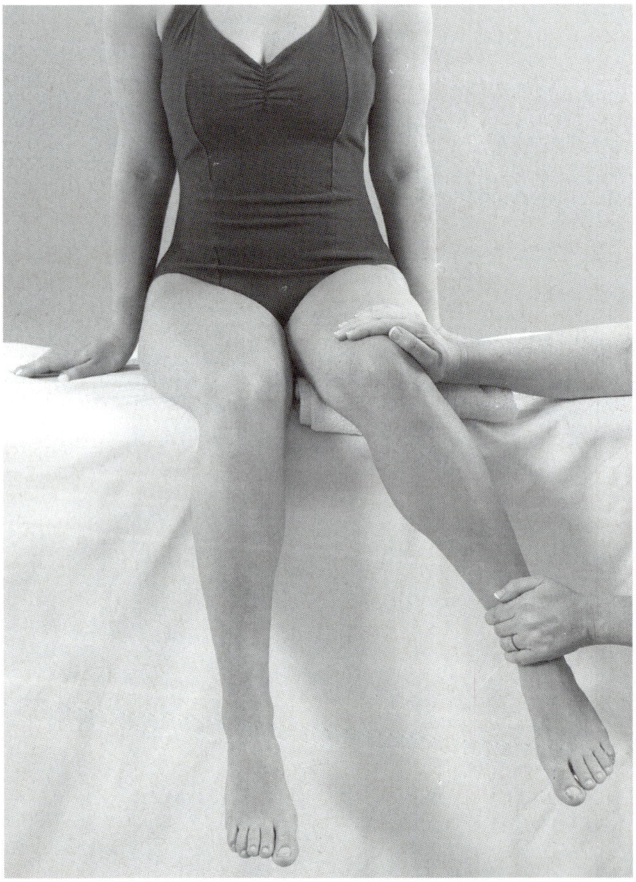

FIGURE 8.20 Assessment of end-feel and estimation of the left hip medial rotation passive ROM. A towel roll is placed under the distal femur to maintain the femur in a horizontal position. The individual uses his or her arms to maintain proper upright sitting posture. One of the examiner's hands is placed on the distal femur to prevent hip flexion, adduction, and abduction. The other hand moves the lower leg laterally while the examiner watches for pelvis motion. To confirm the end ROM, the examiner moves a hand to stabilize the ipsilateral pelvis to determine the end-feel.

Stabilization

Stabilize the distal end of the femur to prevent abduction, adduction, or further flexion of the hip. Instruct the individual to use proper sitting posture as weight-bearing through the ischial tuberosities assists with stabilization and helps to avoid rotations and lateral tilting of the pelvis.

Testing Motion

Place one hand at the distal femur to provide stabilization, and use the other hand at the distal tibia to move the lower leg laterally. The hand performing the motion also holds the lower leg in a neutral position to prevent rotation of the tibia on the femur (Fig. 8.20). The end of the ROM occurs when resistance is felt and attempts at further motion cause lateral tilting (elevation or hiking) or rotations of the pelvis or lateral flexion of the trunk. If the individual reports discomfort in the knee joint during testing, then do not put forces across the knee joint but rather passively medially rotate the hip by moving the distal end of the femur.

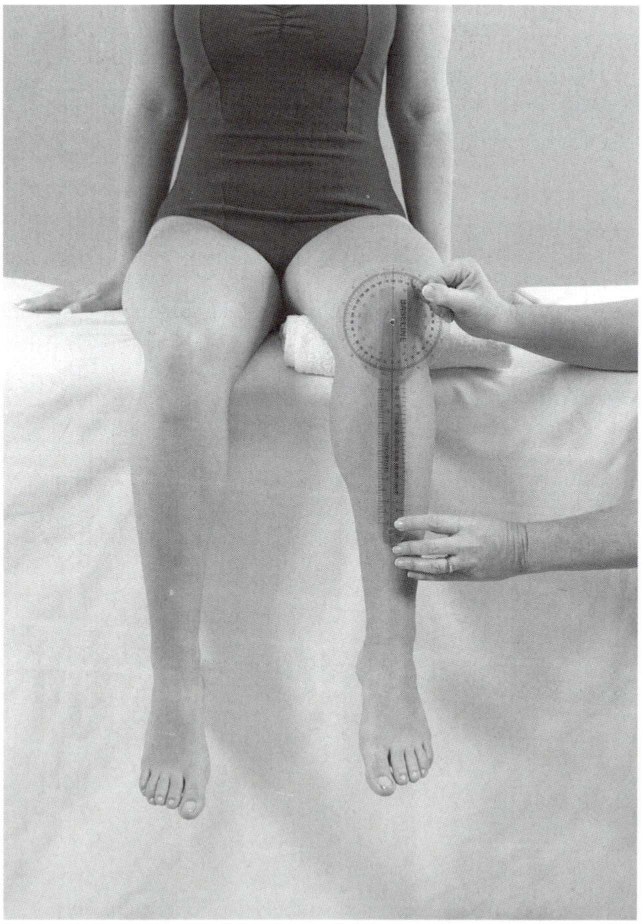

FIGURE 8.21 In the starting position for measuring hip medial rotation, the fulcrum of the goniometer is placed over the midpoint of the patella. Both arms of the instrument are together.

Normal End-Feel

The end-feel is firm because of tension in the posterior joint capsule and the ischiofemoral ligament. Tension in the following muscles may also contribute to the firm end-feel: piriformis, obturator internus, obturator externus, gemellus superior, gemellus inferior, quadratus femoris, gluteus medius (posterior fibers), and gluteus maximus.

Goniometer Alignment

See Figures 8.21 and 8.22.

1. Center **fulcrum** of the goniometer over the anterior aspect of the patella.
2. Align **proximal arm** so that it is perpendicular to the floor or parallel to the supporting surface. Goniometers with a level attached to the proximal arm are helpful for novices.
3. Align **distal arm** with the anterior midline of the lower leg, using the crest of the tibia and a point midway between the two malleoli for reference.

Alternative Testing Position: Prone

Position the individual prone with both legs extended. Place a strap across the pelvis for stabilization. Flex the knee to 90 degrees in the leg to be tested. (The other leg should remain flat on the table with the knee extended.) Goniometer alignment is the same as in the sitting position (Fig. 8.23).

➧ **NOTE:** This position should only be used if the rectus femoris is of normal length; if it isn't, then the sitting position should be used.

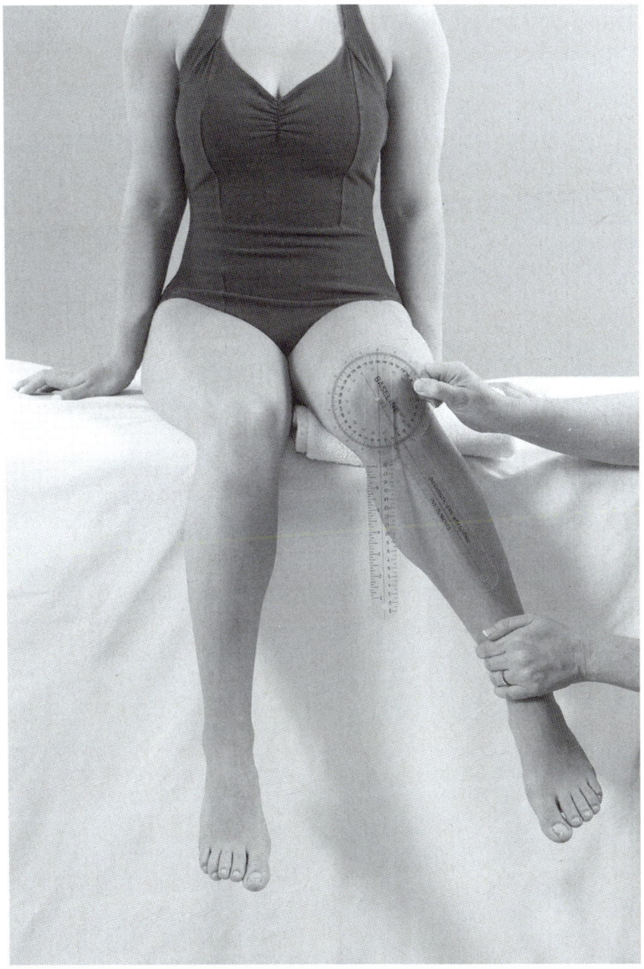

FIGURE 8.22 The goniometric measurement indicating the end of left hip medial rotation passive ROM. The proximal arm of the goniometer is perpendicular to the floor while the distal arm maintains alignment with the anterior midline of the lower leg.

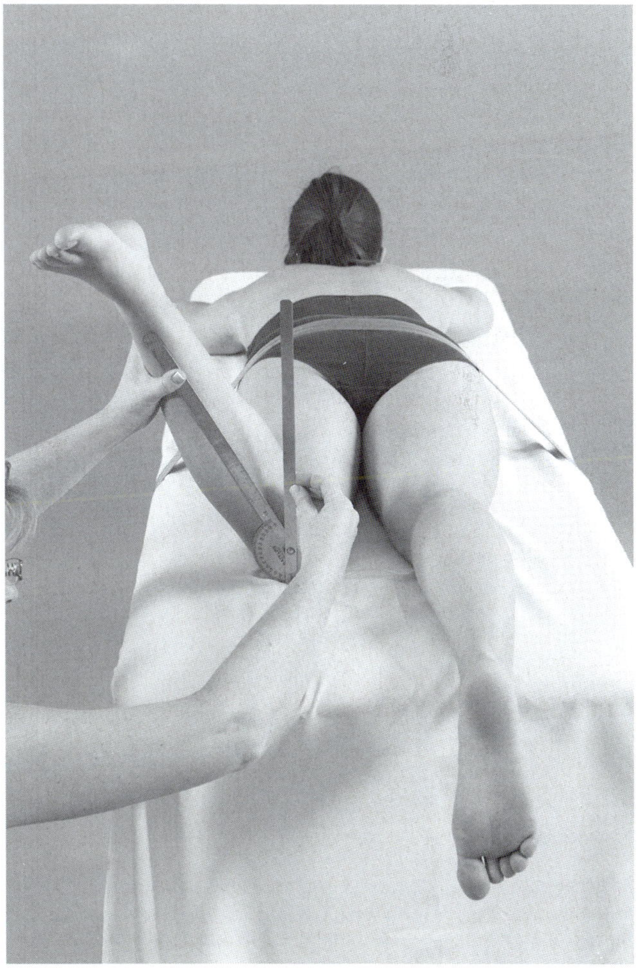

FIGURE 8.23 Left hip medial rotation passive ROM in the alternate prone testing position with the goniometer aligned at the end of the motion. Note that a strap is placed across the pelvis for stabilization.

HIP LATERAL (EXTERNAL) ROTATION

Motion occurs in a transverse plane around a longitudinal axis when the individual is in anatomical position. Normal lateral rotation ROM values for adults vary from about 32 to 50.[3–5,8] Refer to Research Findings and Tables 8.2 to 8.5 for normal ROM values by age and gender.

Testing Position

Seat the individual on a firm surface with knees flexed to 90 degrees over the edge of the surface. Place the hip in 0 degrees of abduction and adduction and in 90 degrees of flexion. If the femur is not in 90 degrees of flexion, then place a towel roll under the distal end of the femur to maintain the femur in a horizontal plane. Flex the contralateral knee beyond 90 degrees to allow the hip being measured to complete its full range of lateral rotation.

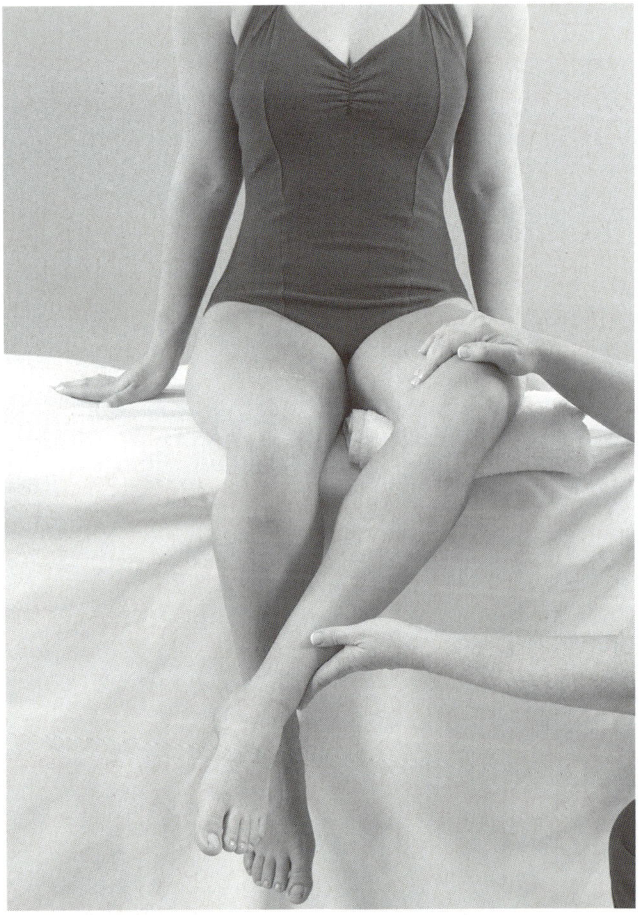

FIGURE 8.24 Assessment of end-feel and estimation of the left hip lateral rotation passive ROM. A towel roll is placed under the distal femur to maintain the femur in a horizontal position. The individual uses arm support to maintain proper upright sitting posture. The examiner places one hand on the distal femur to prevent hip flexion and hip abduction. The individual flexes the right knee to allow the left lower extremity to complete the lateral rotation ROM. The examiner's other hand moves the lower leg medially while the examiner watches for pelvis motion. To confirm the end ROM, the examiner moves a hand to stabilize the ipsilateral pelvis to determine the end-feel.

Stabilization

Stabilize the distal end of the femur to prevent abduction or further flexion of the hip. Instruct the individual to use proper sitting posture as weight-bearing through the ischial tuberosities assists with stabilization and helps to avoid rotations and lateral tilting of the pelvis.

Testing Motion

Place one hand at the distal femur to provide stabilization, and place the other hand on the distal leg to move the lower leg medially (Fig. 8.24). The hand on the lower leg also prevents rotation of the tibia on the femur. The end of the motion occurs when resistance is felt and attempts at overcoming the resistance cause lateral tilting (depression or dropping) or rotations of the pelvis, or trunk lateral flexion. If the individual reports discomfort in the knee joint during testing, then do not apply forces cross the knee joint, but rather passively laterally rotate the hip by moving the distal end of the femur.

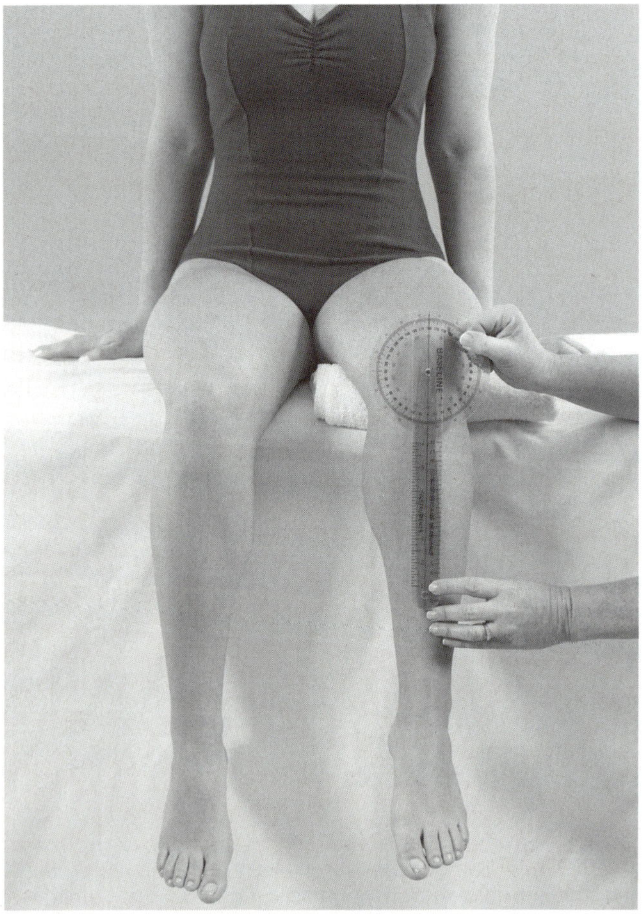

FIGURE 8.25 In the starting position for measuring hip lateral rotation, the fulcrum of the goniometer is placed over the midpoint of the patella. Both arms of the instrument are together.

Normal End-Feel

The end-feel is firm because of tension in the anterior joint capsule, iliofemoral ligament, and pubofemoral ligament. Tension in the anterior portion of the gluteus medius, gluteus minimus, adductor magnus, adductor longus, pectineus, and piriformis muscles also may contribute to the firm end-feel.

Goniometer Alignment

See Figures 8.25 and 8.26.

1. Center **fulcrum** of the goniometer over the anterior aspect of the patella.
2. Align **proximal arm** so that it is perpendicular to the floor or parallel to the supporting surface. Goniometers with a level attached to the proximal arm are helpful for novices.
3. Align **distal arm** with the anterior midline of the lower leg, using the crest of the tibia and a point midway between the two malleoli for reference.

See Appendix B for a summary of hip range of motion measurement procedures using a goniometer.

Alternative Testing Position: Prone

Position the individual prone with both legs extended. Place a strap across the pelvis for stabilization. Flex the knee to 90 degrees in the leg to be tested. The other leg should remain flat on the table with the knee extended. Goniometer alignment is the same as in the sitting position (Fig. 8.27).

➧ **NOTE:** This position should be used only if the rectus femoris is of normal length. If the rectus is short then the seated position should be used.

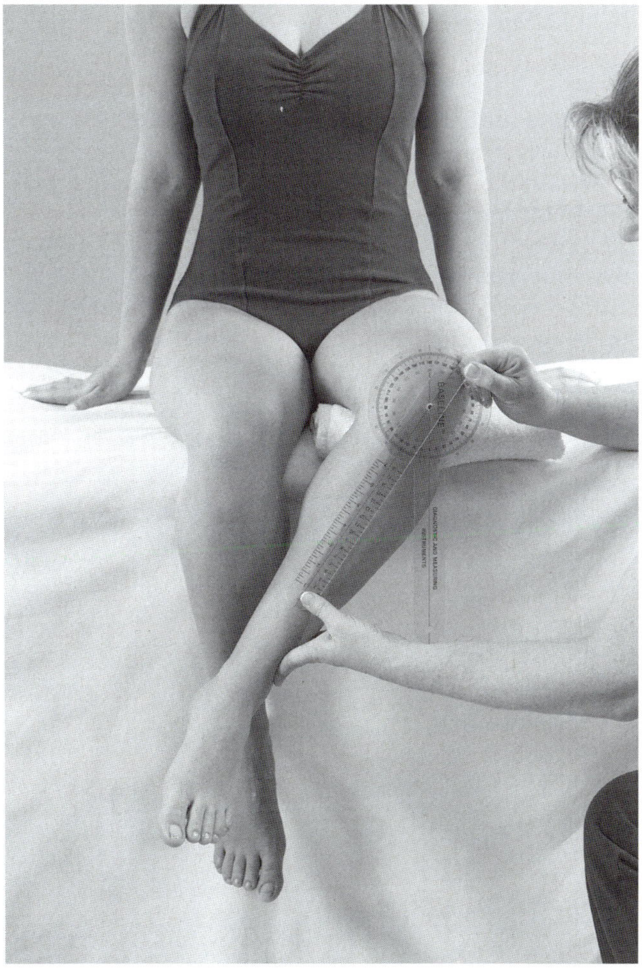

FIGURE 8.26 The goniometric measurement indicating the end of left hip lateral rotation passive ROM. The proximal arm of the goniometer is perpendicular to the floor while the distal arm maintains alignment with the anterior midline of the lower leg.

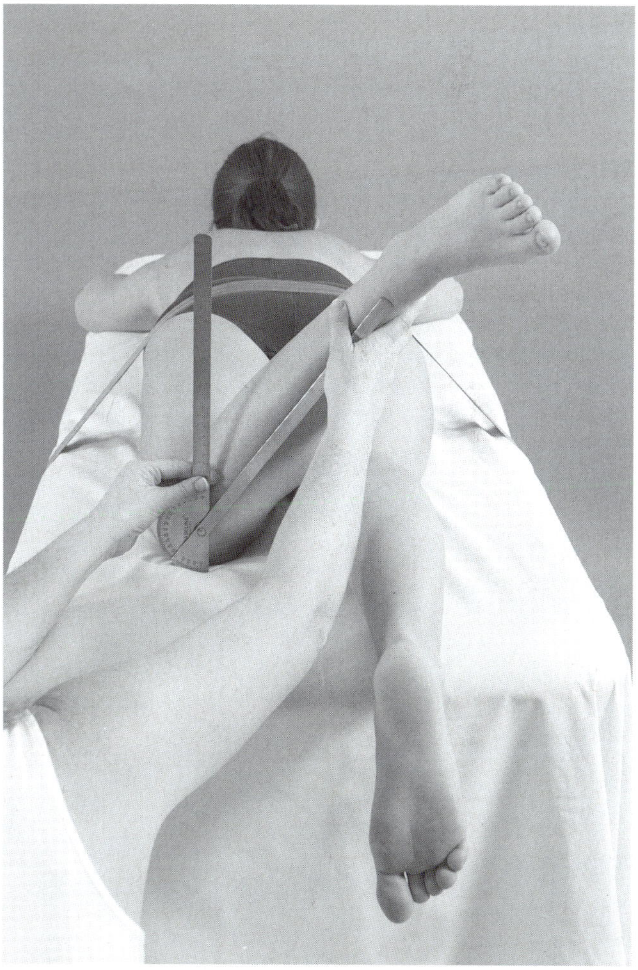

FIGURE 8.27 Right hip lateral rotation passive ROM in the alternate prone testing position with the goniometer aligned at the end of the motion. Note that a strap is placed across the pelvis for stabilization.

MUSCLE LENGTH TESTING PROCEDURES: Hip

Landmarks for Testing Procedures

See Figures 8.4 through 8.7.

Knowledge of gross anatomy and physiology is essential to determine through clinical reasoning which structures may be responsible for impaired ROM. Because many muscles that act at the hip cross more than the hip joint, muscle length testing is warranted when ROM is impaired. Muscle length testing can help to differentiate whether two joint muscles are short and thus contribute to joint ROM limitations. The first step is to isolate one joint at a time to ensure that motion is not impaired by structures that cross only one joint. The examiner then tests muscles that cross more than one joint by passively bringing the muscle's origin and insertion away from each other, which tests the length of the muscle over all joints.

HIP FLEXORS

The iliacus and psoas major muscles flex the hip in the sagittal plane of motion. The rectus femoris flexes the hip in the sagittal plane but also extends the knee. Other muscles, because of their attachments, create hip flexion in combination with other motions. The sartorius flexes, abducts, and laterally rotates the hip while flexing the knee. The tensor fascia lata abducts, flexes, and medially rotates the hip and extends the knee. Several muscles that primarily adduct the hip, such as the pectineus, adductor longus, and adductor brevis, also lie anterior to the axis of the hip joint and can contribute to hip flexion. Short muscles that flex the hip limit hip extension ROM. Hip extension can also be limited by abnormalities of the joint surfaces, shortness of the anterior joint capsule, and short iliofemoral and ischiofemoral ligaments.

The anatomy of the major muscles that flex the hip is illustrated in Figure 8.28. The **iliacus** originates proximally from the upper two-thirds of the iliac fossa, the inner lip of the iliac crest, the lateral aspect (ala) of the sacrum, and the sacroiliac and iliolumbar ligaments (see Fig. 8.28A). It inserts distally on the lesser trochanter of the femur. The **psoas major** originates proximally from the sides of the vertebral bodies and intervertebral discs of T12–L5 and the transverse processes of L1–L5 (see Fig. 8.28A). It inserts distally on the lesser trochanter of the femur These two muscles are commonly referred to as the **iliopsoas.** If the iliopsoas is short, it limits hip extension without pulling the hip in another direction of motion; the thigh remains in the sagittal plane. Knee position does not affect the length of the iliopsoas muscle.

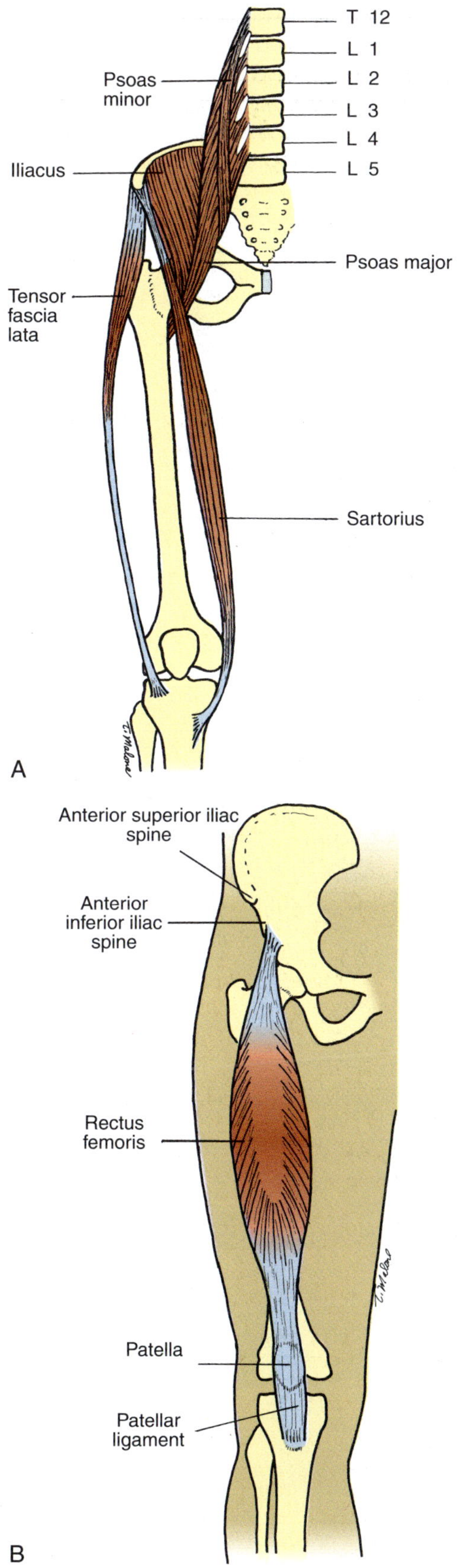

FIGURE 8.28 An anterior view of the hip flexor muscles.

The **rectus femoris** arises proximally from two tendons: the anterior tendon from the anterior inferior iliac spine and the posterior tendon from a groove superior to the brim of the acetabulum (see Fig. 8.28B). It inserts distally into the base of the patella and into the tibial tuberosity via the patellar ligament. A short rectus femoris limits hip extension and knee flexion. If the rectus femoris is short and hip extension is attempted, the knee passively moves into extension to accommodate the shortened muscle. Sometimes, when the rectus femoris is shortened and hip extension is attempted, the knee remains flexed but hip extension is limited.

The **sartorius** arises proximally from the ASIS and the upper aspect of the iliac notch (see Fig. 8.28A). It inserts distally into the proximal aspect of the medial tibia. If the sartorius is short, it limits hip extension, hip adduction, and knee extension. If the sartorius is short and hip extension is attempted, the hip passively moves into hip abduction and knee flexion to accommodate the short muscle.

The **tensor fascia lata** arises proximally from the anterior aspect of the outer lip of the iliac crest and the lateral surface of the ASIS and iliac notch (see Fig. 8.28A). It inserts distally into the iliotibial band of the fascia lata about one-third of the distance down the thigh. The iliotibial band inserts into the lateral anterior surface of the proximal tibia. When the tensor fascia lata is short, it can limit hip adduction, extension and lateral rotation, and knee flexion. If hip extension is attempted, the hip passively moves into abduction and medial rotation to accommodate the short muscle.

The **pectineus** originates from the pectineal line of the pubis and inserts in a line from the lesser trochanter to the linea aspera of the femur. The **adductor longus** arises proximally from the anterior aspect of the pubis and inserts distally into the linea aspera of the femur. The **adductor brevis** originates from the inferior ramus of the pubis. It inserts into a line that extends from the lesser trochanter to the linea aspera, the proximal part of the linea aspera just posterior to the pectineus, and proximal part of the adductor longus. Shortness of these muscles limits hip abduction and extension. If these muscles are short and hip extension is attempted, the hip passively moves into adduction to accommodate the shortened muscles.

THOMAS TEST

The Thomas test evaluates the length of the one- and two-joint muscles that flex the hip. The Thomas test can be completed in two sequences to identify one-joint from two-joint muscle shortness.

Testing Position

Place the individual in the sitting position at the end of the examining table, with the lower thighs, knees, and legs off the table. Assist the individual into the supine position by supporting the back and flexing the hips and knees (Fig. 8.29). This sequence is used to avoid placing strain on the individual's lower back. Once supine, flex the hips by bringing the knees toward the chest just enough to flatten the low back and pelvis against the table (Fig. 8.30). In this position, the pelvis is in about 10 degrees of posterior pelvic tilt.

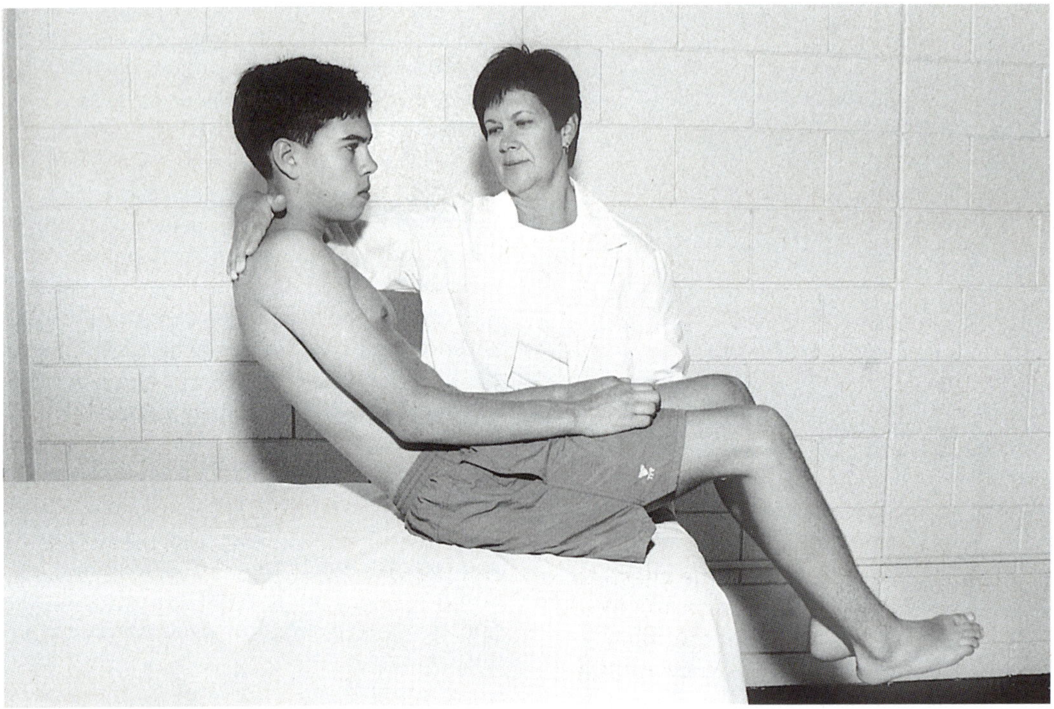

FIGURE 8.29 The examiner assists the individual into the starting position for testing the length of the hip flexors.

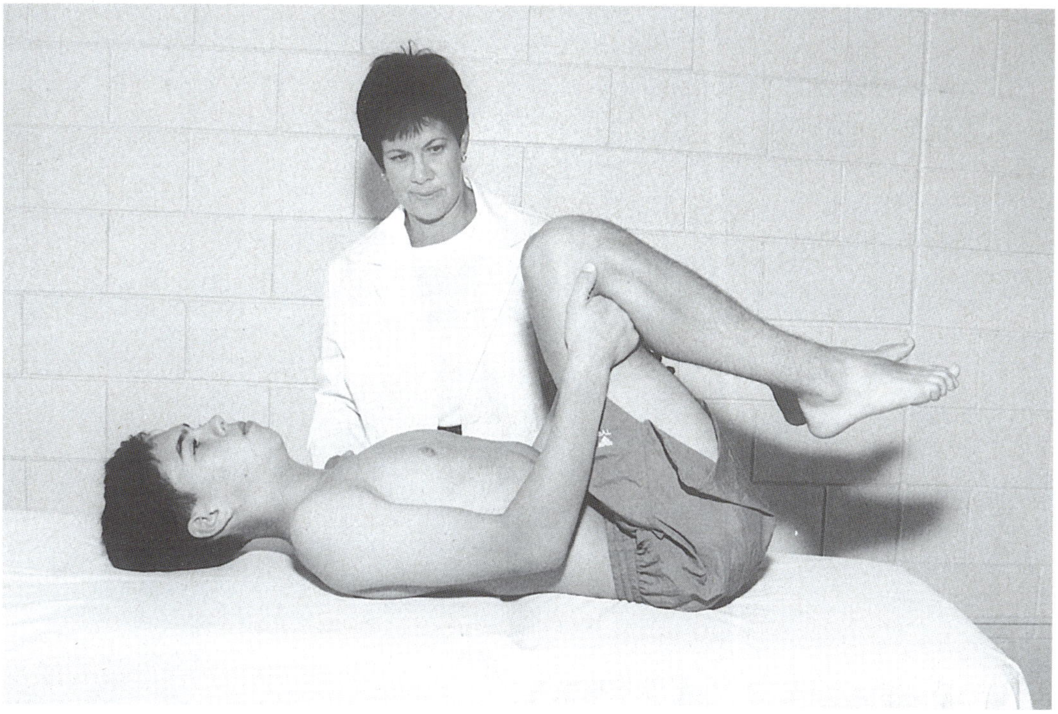

FIGURE 8.30 The starting position for testing the length of the hip flexors. Both knees and hips are flexed so that the low back and pelvis are flat on the examining table.

Stabilization

Either the examiner or the individual holds the hip not being tested in flexion (knee toward the chest) to maintain the low back and pelvis flat against the examining table. If the individual cannot reach the thigh, then a towel or sheet placed behind the knee can be used to hold the thigh in flexion.

Testing Motion

Passively extend the hip being tested by slowly lowering the thigh toward the examining table. Be sure the lower extremity remains in the sagittal plane by keeping the hip from rotating, abducting, or adducting. The examiner confirms that the thigh and lower leg are relaxed and not being actively held in flexion. Often individuals require extra cues to relax the muscles in the limb being tested. See Figures 8.31 and 8.32.

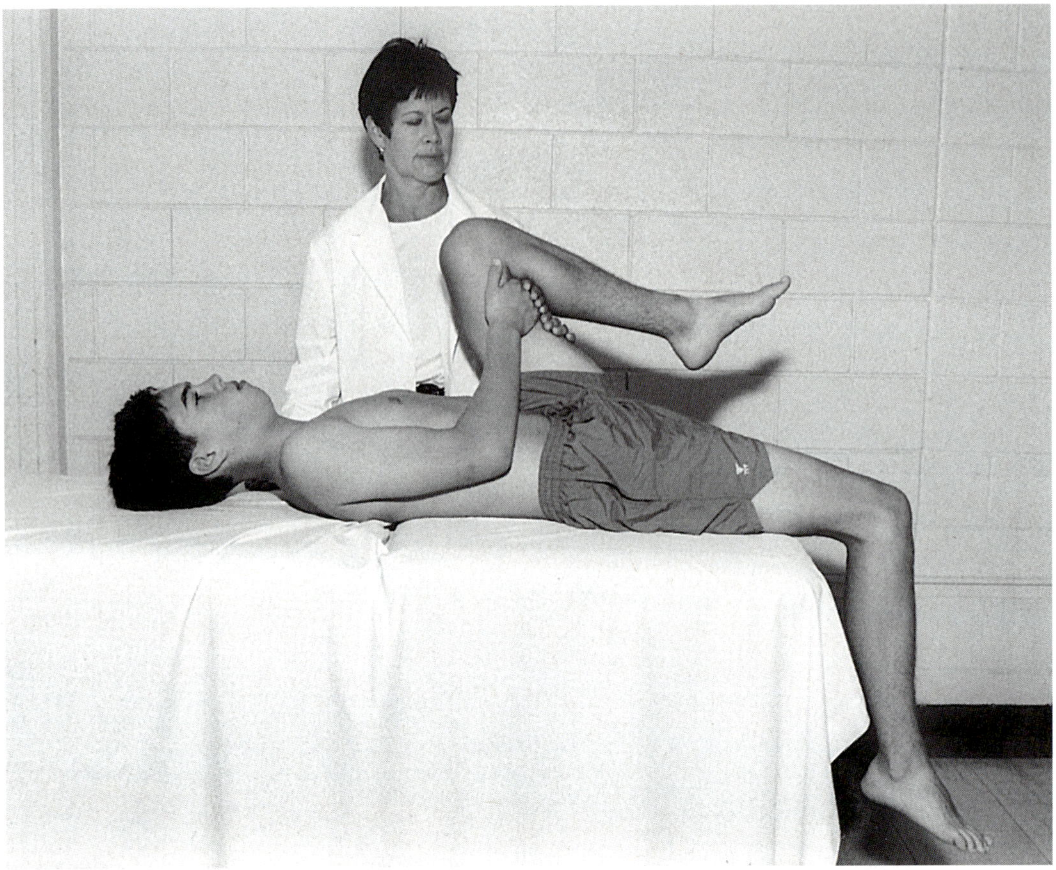

FIGURE 8.31 The end of the motion for testing the length of the right hip flexors. The individual has normal length of the right hip flexors: The hip is able to extend to 10 degrees (thigh is flat on table), the knee remains in 80 degrees of flexion, and the lower extremity remains in the sagittal plane. Ordinarily the examiner would stand on the side of the hip being tested, but she has moved to the other side so that a photograph could be taken.

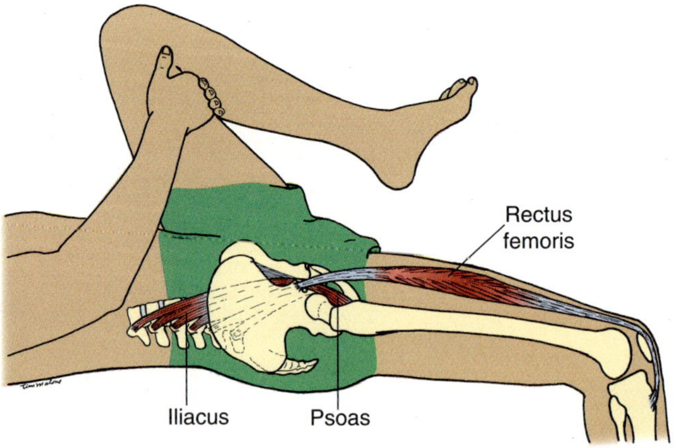

FIGURE 8.32 A lateral view of the hip showing the hip flexors at the end of the Thomas test.

Normal End-Feel

When the knee remains flexed at the end of hip extension ROM, the end-feel is firm usually owing to tension in the rectus femoris. When the knee is passively held in extension at the end of hip extension ROM, the end-feel is firm owing to tension in the iliopsoas muscle and possibly the anterior joint capsule, iliofemoral ligament, pubofemoral ligament, and ischiofemoral ligament. If one or more of the following muscles are abnormally short in length, they may also contribute to a firm end-feel: sartorius, tensor fascia lata, pectineus, adductor longus, and adductor brevis.

Goniometer Alignment

See Figure 8.33.

1. Center **fulcrum** of the goniometer over the lateral aspect of the hip joint, using the greater trochanter of the femur for reference.
2. Align **proximal arm** with the lateral midline of the pelvis.
3. Align **distal arm** with the lateral midline of the femur, using the lateral epicondyle for reference.

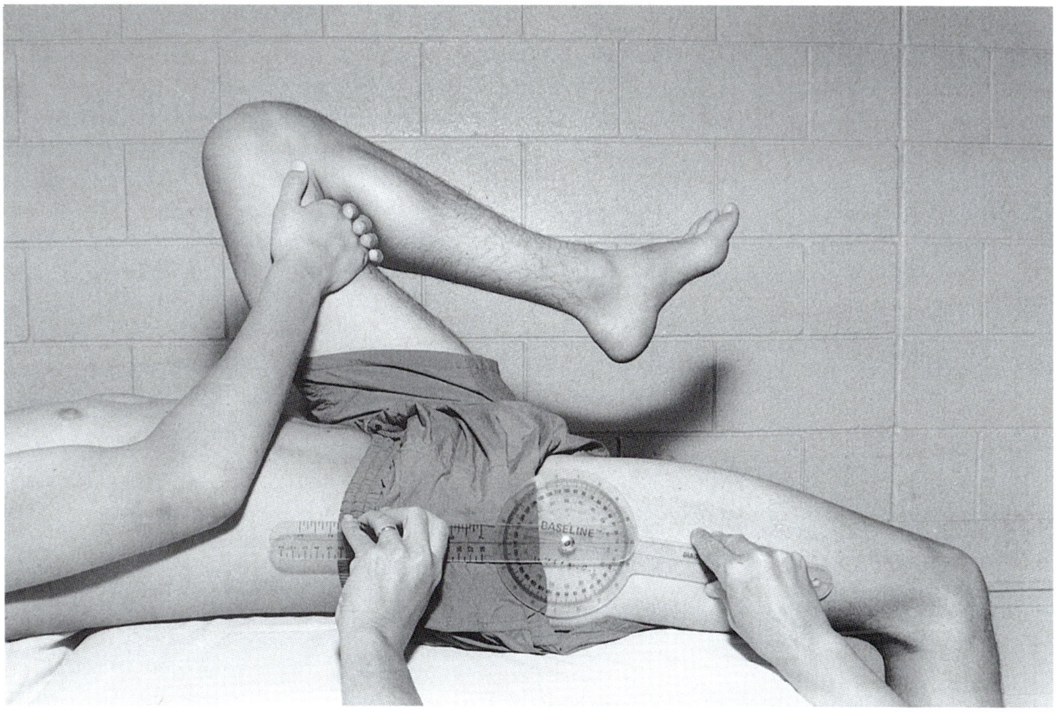

FIGURE 8.33 Goniometer alignment for measuring the length of the hip flexors.

Interpretation

If the thigh lies flat on the examining table and the knee remains in at least 80 degrees of flexion, the iliopsoas and rectus femoris muscles are of normal length[10] (Figs. 8.31, 8.32, and 8.33). At the end of the test, the hip is in approximately 10 degrees of extension because the pelvis is being held in 10 degrees of posterior tilt. At this point, the test would be considered negative and no further testing is needed. Research conducted on 20 healthy Finnish students (12 women, 8 men), aged 18 to 45 years, provided normative values for passive ROM of hip and knee joints at the end range of the Thomas test position: 6 to 7 degrees for hip extension and 118 to 120 degrees for knee flexion.[11]

If the thigh does not lie flat on the table with the knee in at least 80 degrees of flexion then further testing is needed to determine the cause (Fig. 8.34). Information as to which muscles are short can be gained by varying the position of the knee and carefully observing passive motions of the hip and knee while hip extension is attempted. Repeat the starting position by flexing the hips and bringing the knee toward the chest. Extend the hip by lowering the thigh toward the examining table, but this time support the knee in extension (Fig. 8.35). When the knee is held in extension, the rectus femoris is slack over the knee joint. If the hip extends with the knee held in extension so that the thigh is able to lie on the examining table, then the iliopsoas, anterior joint capsule, iliofemoral ligament, and ischiofemoral ligament are not limiting the hip extension, and the rectus femoris can be ascertained as being short. If the hip cannot extend with the knee held in extension and the thigh does not lie on the examining table, one-joint hip flexors such as the iliopsoas and/or joint structures such as the anterior joint capsule, iliofemoral ligament, and ischiofemoral ligament may be short.

Several situations may affect the results of the Thomas test and lead to false-positive and false-negative findings. Pulling the stabilizing knee too far toward the individual's chest will cause a reversal of the lumbar lordosis (e.g., flexion of the lumbar spine) and the pelvis to go into an exaggerated posterior tilt. This low-back and pelvic position creates the appearance of tightness in the hip flexors of the limb being tested when, in fact, no tightness is present. An example of a false-negative finding (e.g., concluding that the rectus femoris is of normal length when in fact the muscle is tight) would occur if stabilization was not maintained and the pelvis rolled into an anterior tilt resulting in the appearance of normal hip extension.

The end position of the Thomas test can also be used to determine whether other structures may be tight and need to be tested. When the hip is extending toward the examining table, observe carefully to see whether the lower extremity stays in the sagittal plane. If the examiner is unable to maintain a neutral hip and the hip moves into the frontal or transverse planes, then other structures such as the sartorius, tensor fascia lata, pectineus, and adductor longus and brevis should be investigated for potential shortening (Table 8.1).

TABLE 8.1 Position of Hip at End of Thomas Test in Relation to Possible Short Structures

Hip Rests in:	Possible Short Structures	Follow-Up Tests
~10° extension with thigh on table, knee flexed at least 80°	Normal length of iliopsoas and rectus femoris	
Flexion with thigh off table, knee fully extended	2-joint muscle: iliopsoas Inert joint structures: anterior joint capsule, iliofemoral, ischiofemoral, and pubofemoral ligaments	Joint play assessment of hip
~10° extension with thigh on table, knee flexed less than 80°	2-joint muscle: rectus femoris	Ely test
Medial rotation and/or abduction	2-joint muscle: tensor fascia lata 1-joint muscles: gluteus medius, minimus, and maximus Inert structures: superior (lateral) joint capsule and the superior band of the iliofemoral ligament	Ober or Modified Ober test Hip lateral rotation PROM Hip adduction PROM Joint play assessment of hip
Lateral rotation and abduction	2-joint muscle: sartorius muscle 1-joint muscles: piriformis, obturators (internus and externus), gemelli (superior and inferior), quadratus femoris, gluteus medius, minimus, and gluteus maximus Inert structures: posterior joint capsule and the ischiofemoral ligament	Hip medial rotation PROM Hip adduction PROM Joint play assessment of hip
Adduction	2-joint muscle: gracilis 1-joint muscles: adductor magnus, adductor longus, adductor brevis, and pectineus Inert structures: inferior (medial) joint capsule, pubofemoral ligament, ischiofemoral ligament, and inferior band of the iliofemoral ligament	Hip abduction PROM Joint play assessment of hip

PROM = Passive range of motion; ° = degrees; ~ = approximately.

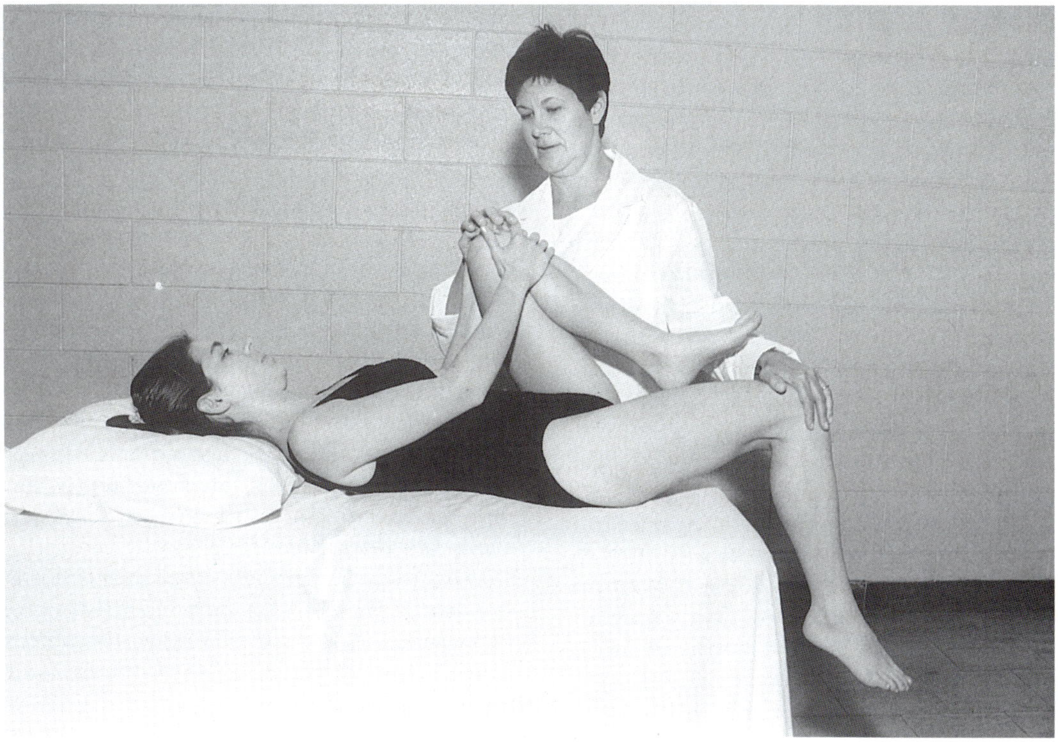

FIGURE 8.34 This individual has restricted hip extension. Her thigh is unable to lie on the table with the knee flexed to 80 degrees. Further testing is needed to determine which structures are short.

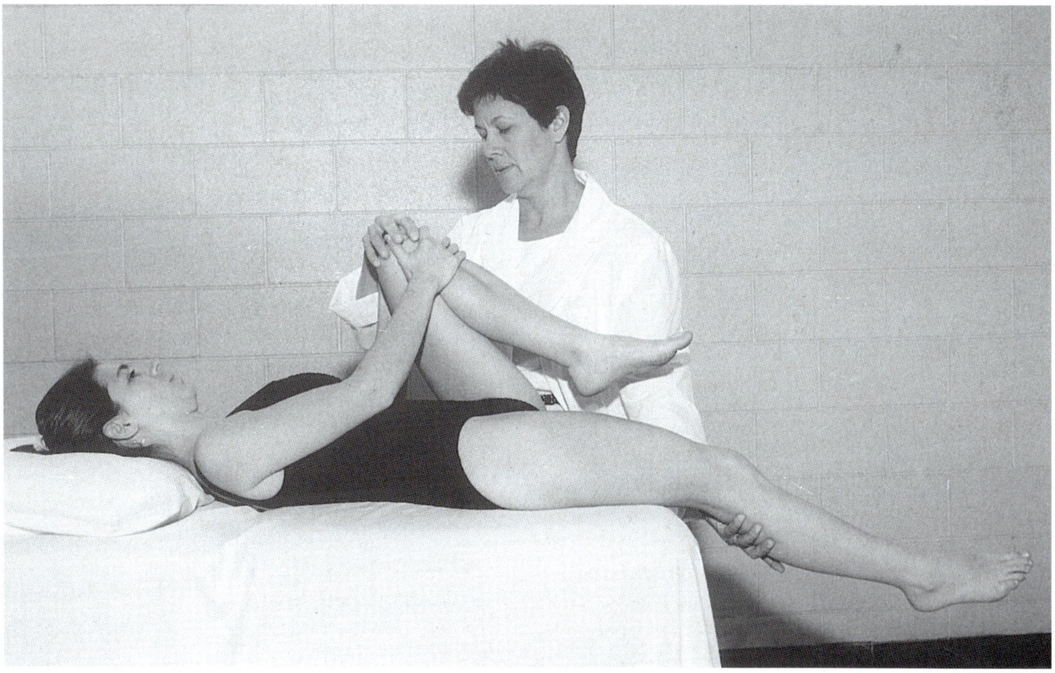

FIGURE 8.35 Because the individual had restricted hip extension at the end of the testing motion (see Fig. 8.34), the testing motion needs to be modified and repeated. This time, the knee is held in extension when the extremity is lowered toward the table. At the end of the test, the hip extends to 10 degrees, and the thigh lies flat on the table. Therefore, one may conclude that the rectus femoris is short and that the iliopsoas, anterior joint capsule, and iliofemoral and ischiofemoral ligaments are of normal length.

HIP EXTENSORS

Four muscles act as hip extensors: the gluteus maximus and three hamstring muscles. The **gluteus maximus** muscle originates at the posterior ilium, sacrum, coccyx, and aponeurosis of the erector spinae and inserts into the distal portion of the iliotibial tract of the tensor fascia lata and the gluteal tuberosity on the distal femur. Contraction of this one-joint muscle acts to extend the hip and can also laterally rotate and abduct the thigh. The hamstring muscles, composed of the semitendinosus, semimembranosus, and biceps femoris, cross two joints—the hip and the knee. When they contract, they extend the hip and flex the knee. The **semitendinosus** originates proximally from the ischial tuberosity and inserts distally on the proximal aspect of the medial surface of the tibia (see Fig. 8.36A). The **semimembranosus** originates from the ischial tuberosity and inserts on the posterior medial aspect of the medial condyle of the tibia (see Fig. 8.36B). The long head of the **biceps femoris** originates from the ischial tuberosity and the sacrotuberous ligament, whereas the short head of the biceps femoris originates proximally from the lateral lip of the linea aspera, the lateral supracondylar line, and the lateral intermuscular septum (see Fig. 8.36A). The biceps femoris inserts on the head of the fibula with a small portion extending to the lateral condyle of the tibia and the lateral collateral ligament.

Because the hamstring muscles cross the hip and knee joints, they can limit both hip flexion and knee extension. Hip flexion is limited when the hamstrings are short and the knee is held in full extension. However, if hip flexion is limited when the knee is flexed, abnormalities of the joint surfaces, shortness of the posterior joint capsule, or a short gluteus maximus may be present.

Hamstring length can be measured using either the straight leg raising (SLR) method, wherein the angle between the pelvis and the thigh is measured, or by the distal hamstring length method, wherein the angle between the thigh and the lower leg is measured. The SLR test is presented in the following section, and the distal hamstring length test, also called the popliteal angle (or PA) test, is covered in Chapter 9.

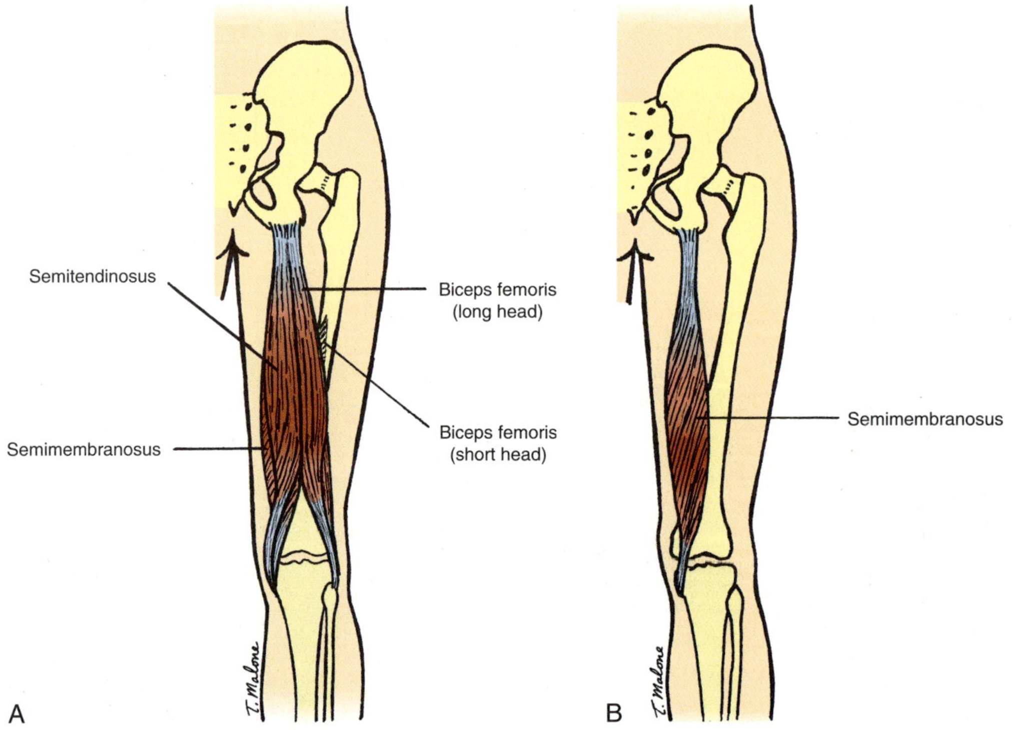

FIGURE 8.36 (A, B) A posterior view of the hip showing the hamstring muscles.

STRAIGHT LEG RAISING (SLR) TEST

The straight leg raise (SLR) evaluates the length of the hamstring muscles.

Testing Position

Place the individual supine with both knees extended and hips in 0 degrees of flexion, extension, abduction, adduction, and rotation (Fig. 8.37). If possible, remove clothing to expose the ilium and low back so the pelvis and lumbar spine can be observed during the test.

Stabilization

Hold the knee of the lower extremity being tested in full extension. Keep the other lower extremity flat on the examining table to stabilize the pelvis and prevent the pelvis from tilting posteriorly and the lumbar spine from flexing. Usually, the weight of the lower extremity provides adequate stabilization, but a strap securing the thigh to the examining table can be added if necessary.

Testing Motion

Passively flex the hip by lifting the lower extremity off the table (Figs. 8.38 and 8.39). The examiner keeps the knee in full extension by applying firm pressure to the anterior thigh while flexing the hip. As the hip flexes, the pelvis and low back should flatten against the examining table. The end of the testing motion occurs when resistance is felt from tension in the posterior thigh and further flexion of the hip causes knee flexion, posterior pelvic tilt, or lumbar flexion.

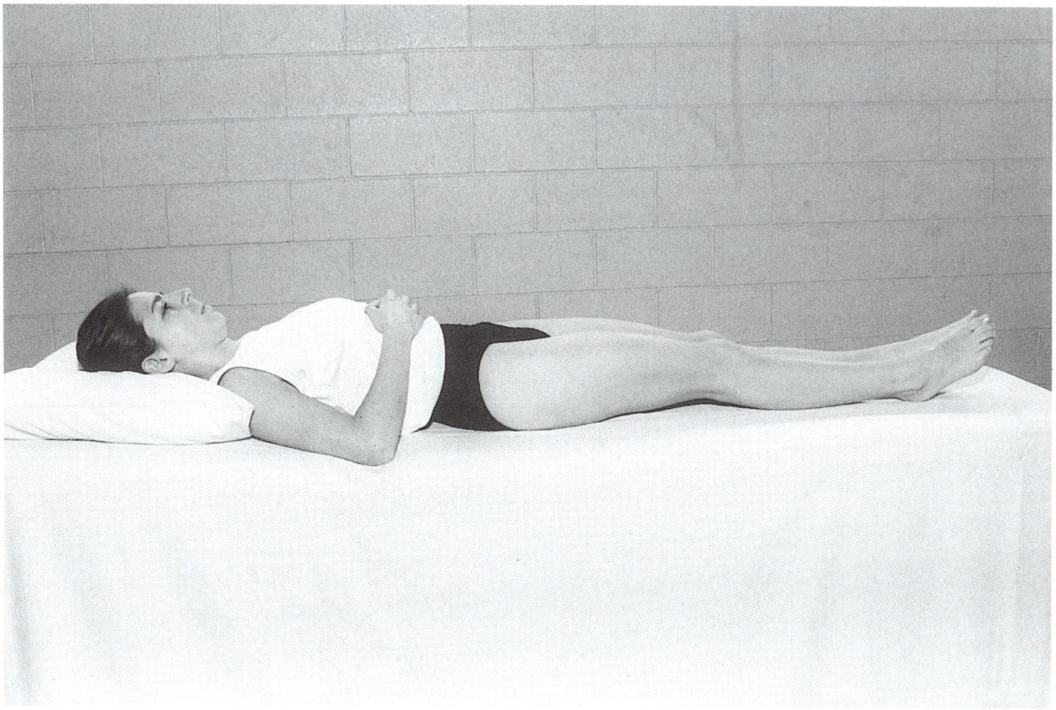

FIGURE 8.37 The starting position for testing the length of the hamstring muscles with the straight leg raising (SLR) test.

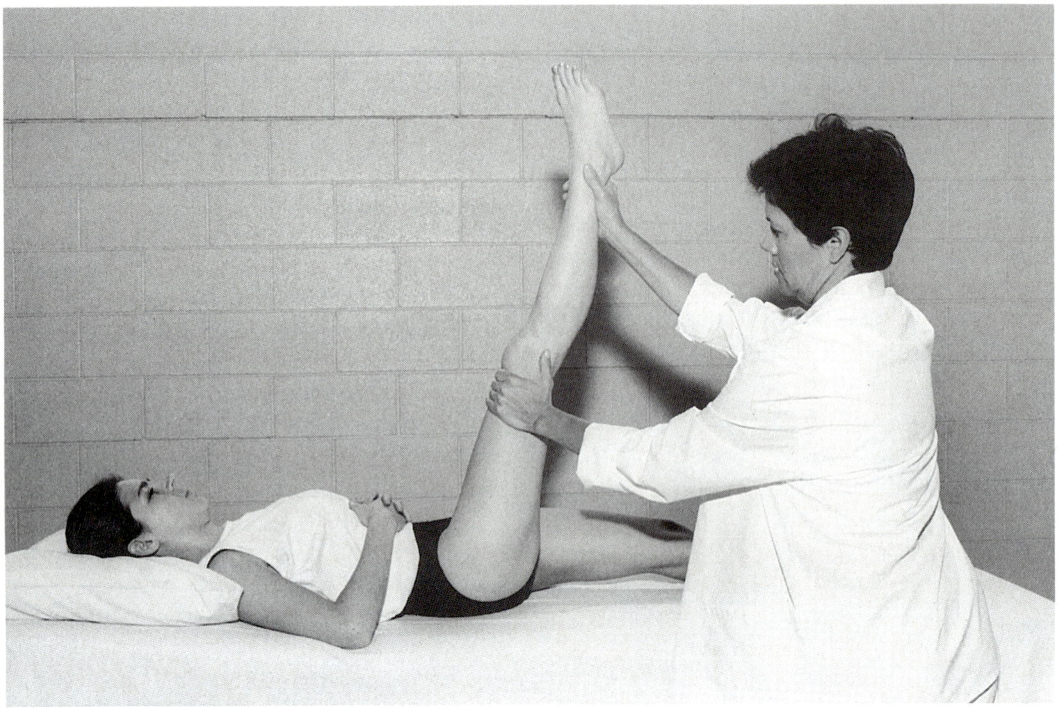

FIGURE 8.38 The end of the testing motion for the straight leg raising test, which evaluates the length of the hamstring muscles. The individual has normal length of the hamstrings: the hip can be passively flexed to 70 to 80 degrees with the knee held in full extension.

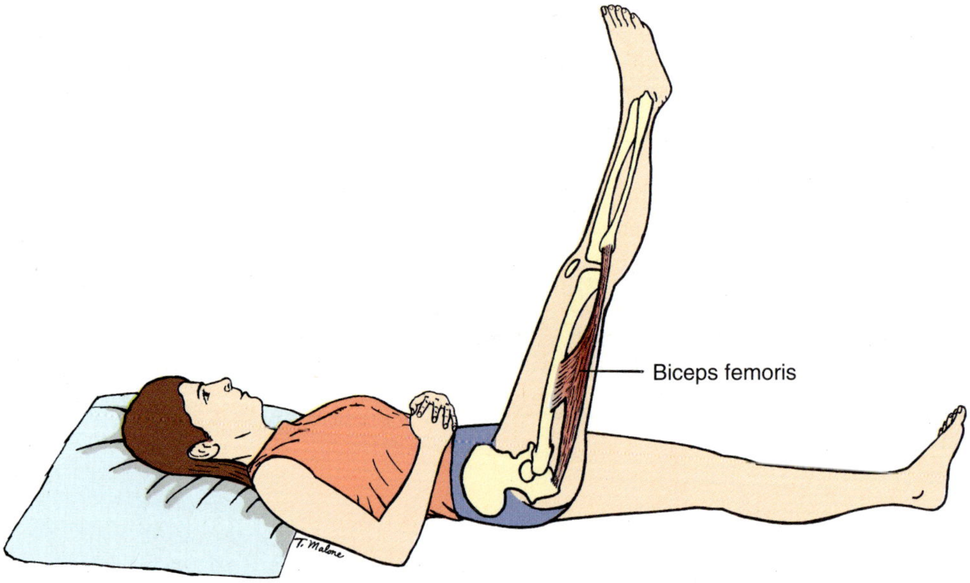

FIGURE 8.39 A lateral view of the hip showing the biceps femoris at the end of the testing motion for the straight leg raising test.

Normal End-Feel

The end-feel is firm owing to tension in the semimembranosus, semitendinosus, and biceps femoris muscles.

Goniometer Alignment

See Figure 8.40.

1. Center **fulcrum** of the goniometer over the lateral aspect of the hip joint, using the greater trochanter of the femur for reference.
2. Align **proximal arm** with the lateral midline of the pelvis.
3. Align **distal arm** with the lateral midline of the femur, using the lateral epicondyle for reference.

Interpretation

If hip flexion measurements are between 68 and 80 degrees, then the SLR test is considered negative or normal.[10,12] In a study of 214 adults (106 men and 106 women) aged 20 to 79 years, Youdas and associates[12] measured hip flexion ROM using the SLR test and found that females had a mean hip flexion range of 76.3 (standard deviation [SD] = 9.5) degrees and males had a mean range of 68.5 (SD = 6.8) degrees. These findings are in agreement with other sources that suggest that hip flexion between 70 and 80 degrees with the knee extended indicates normal length of the hamstring muscles.[10]

To ensure that the correct interpretation of restricted hip motion is a true positive result owing to tightness of the two joint muscles, flex the knee and confirm that the hip can move into greater hip flexion ROM. Flexing the knee puts the hamstrings on slack. If the amount of hip flexion does not increase when the knee is flexed, then the one-joint muscle that extends the hip (gluteus maximus) or inert hip joint structures could be restricting the motion. If the examiner allows posterior tilting of the pelvis while performing the SLR, then the hamstrings may be incorrectly interpreted as having normal flexibility (i.e., false negative) when in fact they may be short in length.

Shortness of muscles in the hip and lumbar region can also influence the results of the SLR test. If the individual has short hip flexors on the side that is not being tested, the pelvis may be in an anterior tilt when that lower extremity is lying on the examining table. If an anterior pelvic tilt is present, then the distance that the leg being tested can lift off the examining table is decreased. Thus, an anteriorly titled pelvis can give the appearance of less hamstring length than is actually present. To remedy this potential false-positive SLR test result, position the pelvis in neutral: have the individual flex the hip not being tested by resting the foot on the table or by supporting the posterior thigh with a pillow (Fig. 8.41). This position slackens the short hip flexors on the hip not being tested and allows the low back and pelvis to flatten against the examining table. Be careful to avoid an excessive amount of posterior pelvic tilt and lumbar flexion.

If the patient has short lumbar extensors, the low back has an excessive lordotic curve and the pelvis is in an anterior tilt. As mentioned, the distance that the leg can lift off the examining table is decreased if the pelvis is in an anterior tilt, giving the appearance of less hamstring length than is actually present. In this case, the examiner needs to carefully align the proximal arm of the goniometer with the lateral midline of the pelvis when measuring hip flexion ROM and not be misled by the height of the lower extremity from the examining table.

There is some evidence that gender and age influence the length of the hamstring muscles. Youdas and colleagues[12] found gender differences in two methods of measuring hamstring length (straight leg raising and popliteal angle) in 214 adults aged 20 to 79 years. Women had approximately 8 degrees more hip motion than men in the SLR test, and 11 degrees more knee motion than men in the popliteal angle test.[12] In a study of older adults by James and Parker,[13] men and women had similar mean values in hip flexion ROM with the knee extended in the group aged 70 to 74 years, but in the group aged 70 to older than 85 years, men had about a 25% decrease in ROM, whereas women had a decrease of only about 11%.

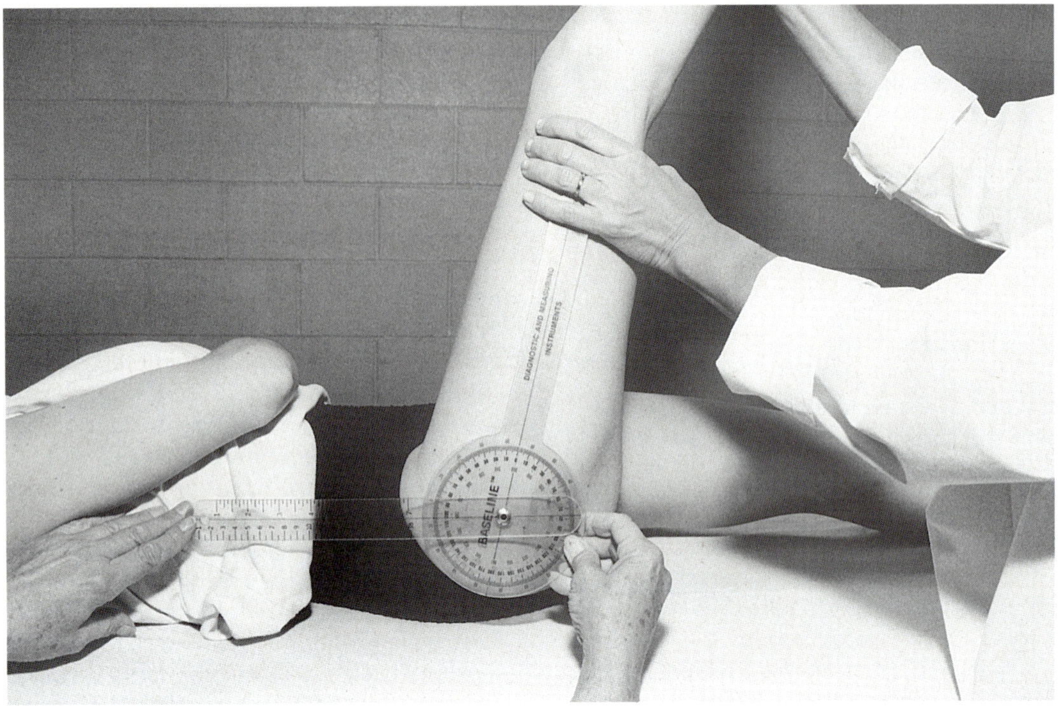

FIGURE 8.40 Goniometer alignment for measuring the length of the hamstring muscles. It appears that the knee has been allowed to flex slightly, so that the test needs to be repeated with the knee carefully held in extension before an accurate measurement can be made. Another examiner will need to take the measurement while the first examiner supports the leg being tested.

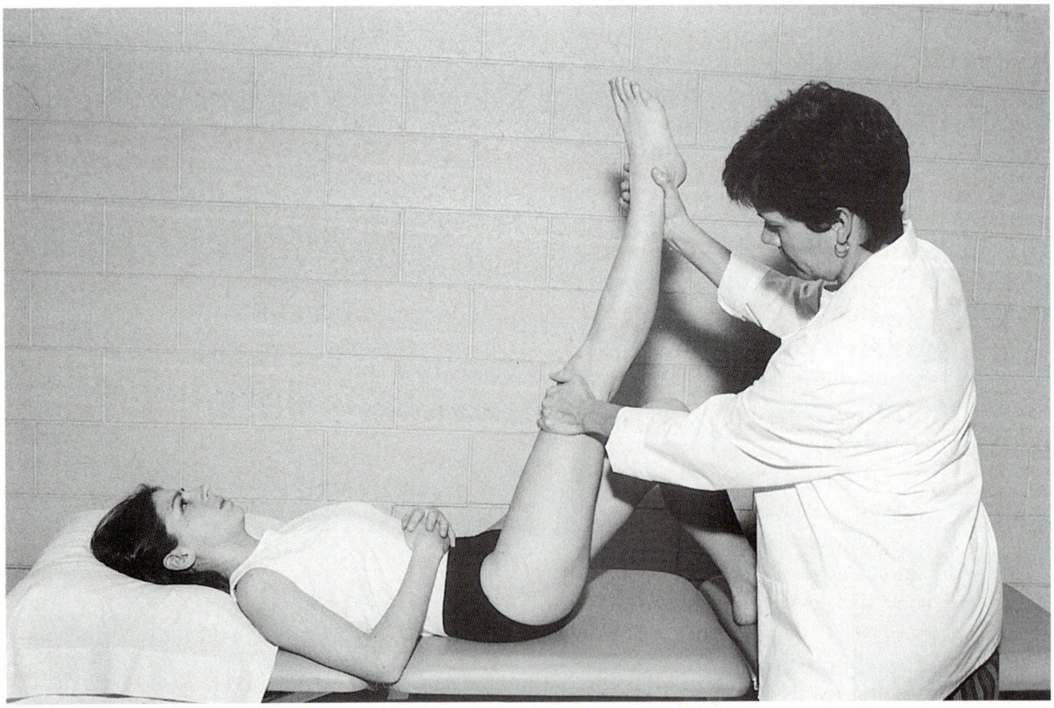

FIGURE 8.41 If an individual has shortness of the contralateral hip flexors, flex the contralateral hip to prevent an anterior pelvic tilt.

HIP ABDUCTORS

The tensor fascia lata, gluteus medius, and gluteus minimus abduct the hip with assistance from the gluteus maximus. The **tensor fascia lata** crosses both the hip and knee joints. When the tensor fascia lata contracts, the hip abducts, flexes, and medially rotates and the knee extends. The tensor fascia lata arises proximally from the anterior aspect of the outer lip of the iliac crest and the lateral surface of the ASIS and the iliac notch (Fig. 8.42). This muscle attaches distally into the iliotibial band (ITB) about one-third of the way down the thigh. The iliotibial band inserts into the lateral tuberosity of the tibia, the head of the fibula, the lateral condyle of the femur, and the lateral patellar retinaculum. If the tensor fascia lata is short, it limits hip adduction and to a lesser extent hip extension, hip lateral rotation, and knee flexion. The length of the tensor fascia lata and iliotibial band is evaluated with the Ober and Modified Ober tests. Shortening of this structure has been cited as a contributing cause of low-back pain,[14] ITB friction syndrome,[15] and patellofemoral pain owing to abnormal lateral tracking and tilting of the patella.[16]

The gluteus medius and minimus cross only the hip joint. The **gluteus medius** originates from the ilium below the iliac crest and the **gluteus minimus** attaches inferior to gluteus medius on the ilium: Both the gluteus medius and minimus lie under the gluteus maximus and insert at the greater trochanter of the femur. If these one-joint muscles are short, they may limit hip adduction. They are evaluated by measuring hip adduction ROM.

OBER TEST

The Ober test examines the length of the tensor fascia lata and the iliotibial band that act to abduct the hip.

Testing Position

Place the individual in the side-lying position, with the hip being tested uppermost. Position the posterior aspect of the individual near the edge of the examining table, so that the examiner can stand directly behind the individual. The bottom hip and knee are in a flexed position to stabilize the trunk, flatten the lumbar curve, and keep the pelvis in a slight posterior tilt. Initially extend the uppermost knee and place the hip in 0 degrees of flexion, extension, adduction, abduction, and rotation. At least 0 degrees of hip extension are needed to perform length testing of the tensor fascia lata and iliotibial band. If the iliopsoas is tight, it prevents the proper positioning of the tensor fascia lata over the greater trochanter. If the rectus femoris is short, the knee may be extended during the test,[10] but extreme care must be taken to avoid rotation of the hip as the leg is lowered into adduction. This change in test position is called a Modified Ober test.

Stabilization

Place one hand on the iliac crest to stabilize the pelvis. Firm pressure is required to prevent the pelvis from laterally tilting during the testing motion. Having the individual flex the bottom hip and knee can also help to stabilize the trunk and pelvis.

Testing Motion

Support the leg being tested by holding the medial aspect of the knee and the lower leg. Flex the hip and the knee to 90 degrees (Fig. 8.43). Keep the knee flexed and move the hip into abduction and then into extension to position the tensor fascia lata over the greater trochanter of the femur (Fig. 8.44). Test the length of the tensor fascia lata and iliotibial band by lowering the leg into hip adduction and bringing it down toward the examining table (Figs. 8.45 and 8.46). Do not allow the pelvis to tilt laterally (an inferior pelvic drop places the hip in abduction), the hip to flex, or the hip to medially rotate because these motions slacken the muscle. Keep the knee flexed and the hip in neutral rotation.

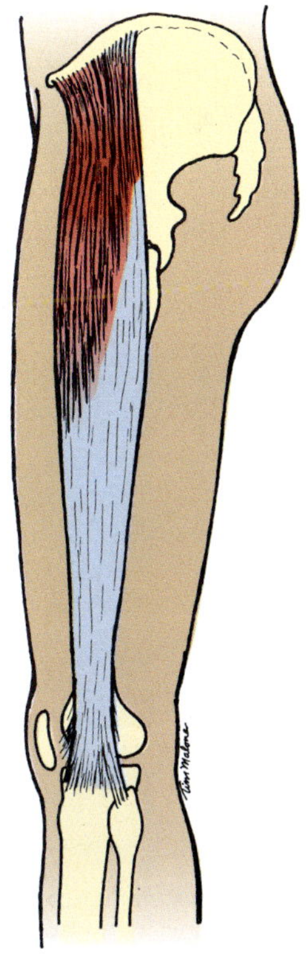

FIGURE 8.42 A lateral view of the left hip showing the tensor fascia lata muscle (in red) and the iliotibial band.

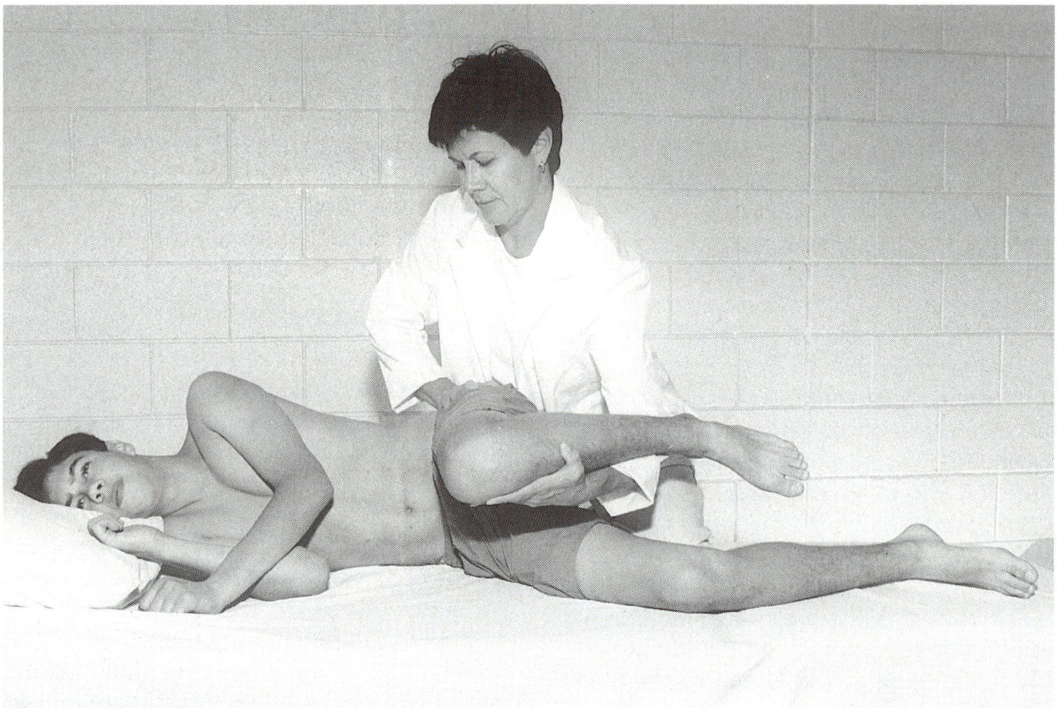

FIGURE 8.43 The first step in the testing motion for the length of the tensor fascia lata and iliotibial band is to flex the hip and knee.

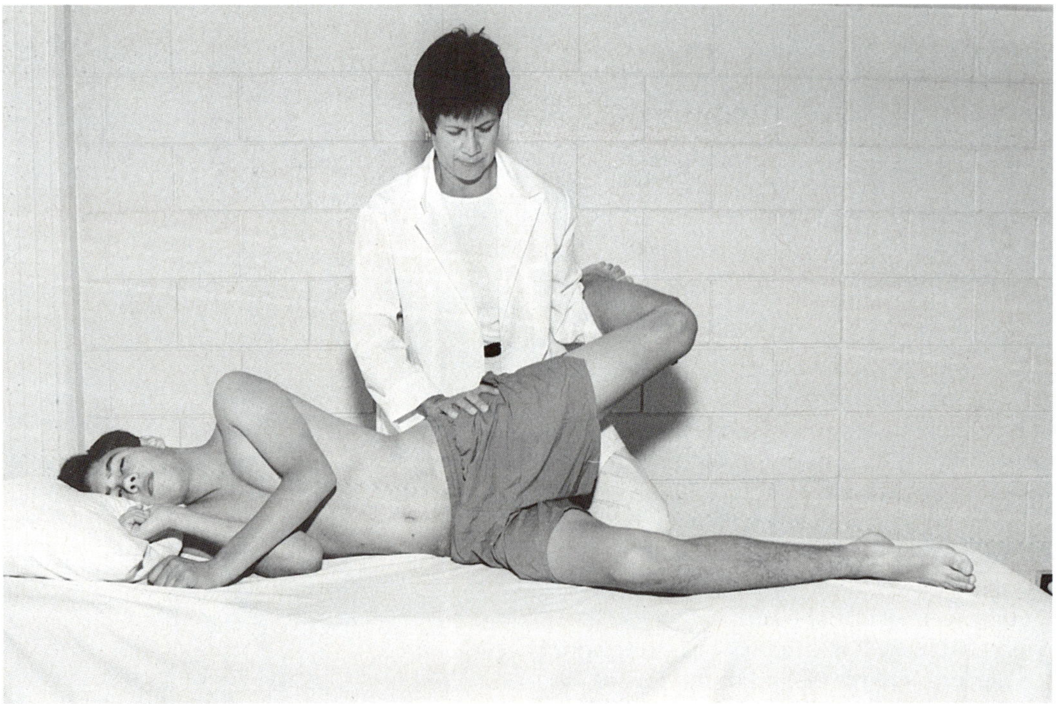

FIGURE 8.44 The next step in the testing motion for the length of the tensor fascia lata and iliotibial band is to abduct and extend the hip.

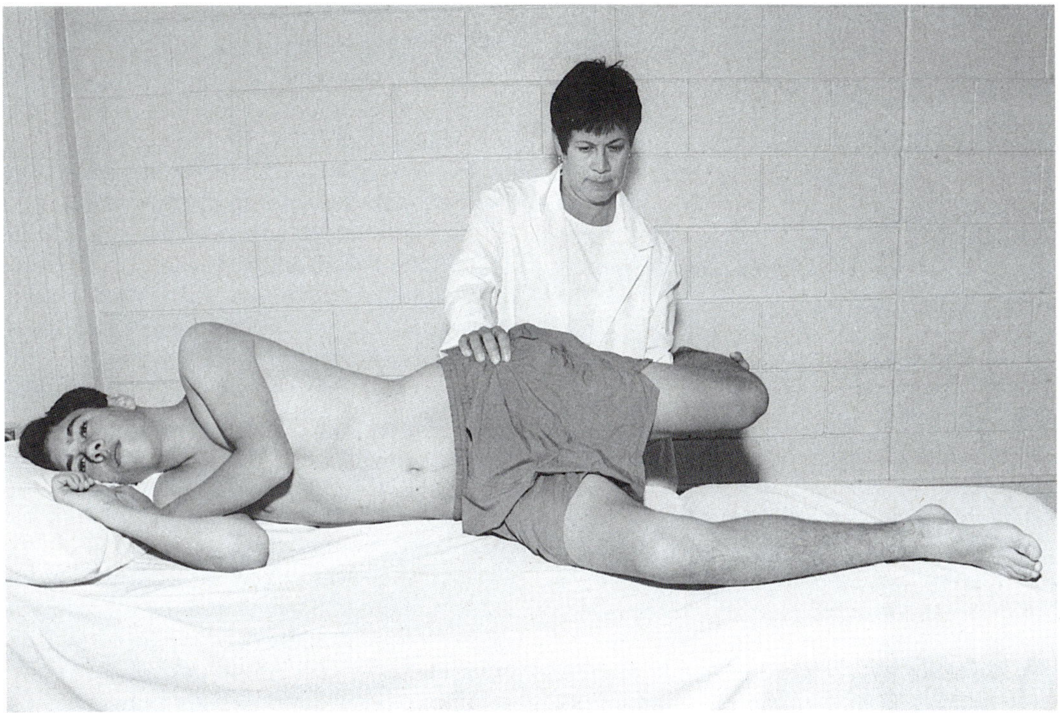

FIGURE 8.45 The end of the testing motion for the Ober test, which evaluates the length of the tensor fascia lata and iliotibial band. The examiner is firmly holding the iliac crest to prevent a lateral tilt of the pelvis while the hip is lowered into adduction. No flexion or medial rotation of the hip is allowed. This individual has a normal length of the tensor fascia lata and iliotibial band; the thigh drops to slightly below horizontal.

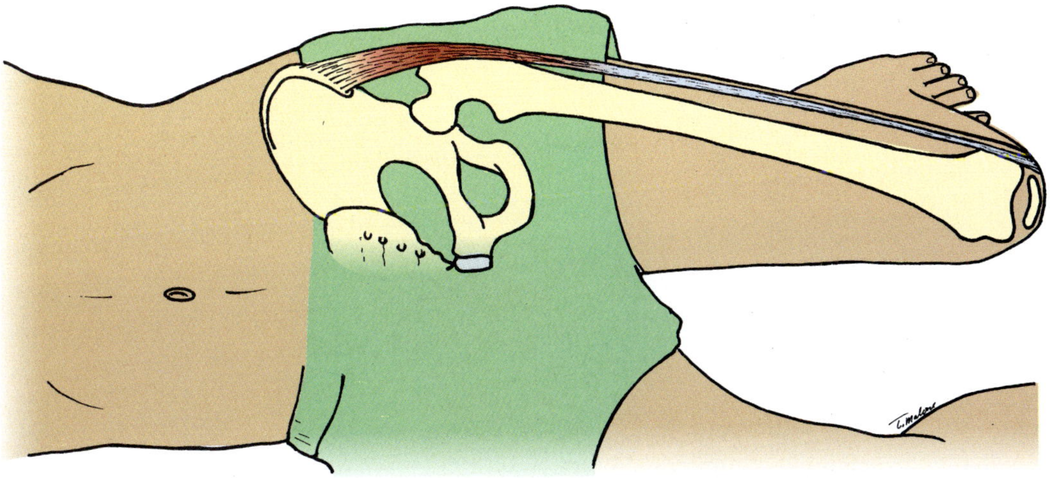

FIGURE 8.46 An anterior view of the hip showing the tensor fascia lata and iliotibial band at the end of the Ober test.

Normal End-Feel

The end-feel is firm owing to tension in the tensor fascia lata and iliotibial band.

Goniometer Alignment

See Figure 8.47.

1. Center **fulcrum** of the goniometer over the ASIS of the extremity being measured.
2. Align **proximal arm** with an imaginary line extending from one ASIS to the other.
3. Align **distal arm** with the anterior midline of the femur, using the midline of the patella for reference.

Interpretation

If the thigh drops slightly below horizontal (10 degrees of hip adduction), the test is negative and the tensor fascia lata and iliotibial band are of normal length.[10] If the thigh remains above horizontal in hip abduction, the tensor fasciae lata, iliotibial band, and/or the gluteus medius, minimus, hip joint structures may be short. Some authors have stated that the tensor fasciae latae is of normal length when the hip adducts to the examining table.[17,18] However, according to Kendall and colleagues,[10] stabilization of the pelvis to prevent a lateral tilt and avoidance of hip flexion and medial rotation will limit hip adduction to 10 degrees during the testing motion, which causes the thigh to drop only slightly below the horizontal position. More conservative hip adduction values have been reported as normal by Cade and associates,[19] who found that only 7 of 50 young female subjects had a negative Ober test when the horizontal leg position or 0 degrees of adduction was used as the test parameter.

Gajdosik, Sandler, and Marr[20] used a universal goniometer centered over the ipsilateral ASIS and aligned with the anterior midline of the femur to determine the effects of knee position and gender on Ober test values for 49 adults aged 20 to 43 years. The 26 women in the study had a mean of 6 degrees of abduction (SD = 5 degrees), and the 23 men had a mean of 4 degrees of abduction (SD = 5) with the difference between genders being statistically significant.[20]

According to Wang and colleagues,[21] a normal value for 36 healthy subjects with a mean age of 24.3 years was found to be 17.8 degrees of adduction measured at the lateral femoral epicondyle at the knee with an inclinometer. Reese and Bandy[22] also used an inclinometer over the distal femur to measure the hip adduction position in 61 healthy subjects with a mean age of 24 years and a mean value of 18.9 degrees of adduction (SD = 7.6 degrees) was reported. Hip adduction angles were similar between the inclinometer studies, yet goniometric values were much less than those reported using an inclinometer. These differences may be related to the fact that the goniometers were aligned with the anterior midline of the femur, whereas the inclinometers were placed on the lateral distal thigh, therefore reflecting the contour of the thigh.

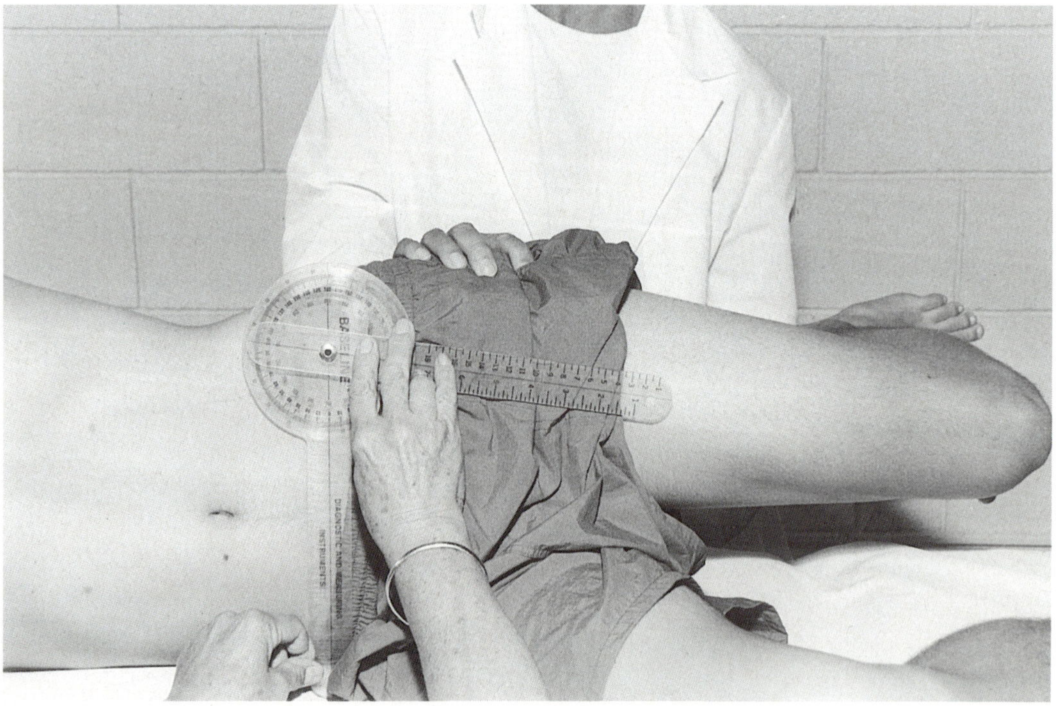

FIGURE 8.47 Goniometer alignment for measuring the length of the tensor fascia lata and iliotibial band. The examiner stabilizes the pelvis and positions the leg being tested while another examiner takes the measurement. If another examiner is not available, a visual estimate will have to be made.

MODIFIED OBER TEST

The Modified Ober test evaluates the length of the hip abductors. This test was first proposed by the Kendalls in 1952 to reduce strain in the medial aspect of the knee joint, to reduce tension on the patella, and to reduce the influence of a tight two-joint rectus femoris muscle.[10]

Testing Position

The starting position is the same as for the Ober test except that the knee is held in extension throughout the test.

Stabilization

Stabilization is the same as in the Ober test.

Testing Motion

The testing motion is the same as for the Ober test, but medial rotation may be more of a concern and must be prevented. The end of the test occurs when the pelvis begins to tilt laterally or the leg stops moving into hip adduction (Fig. 8.48).

Normal End-Feel

The end-feel is firm and the same as in the Ober test.

Goniometer Alignment

Goniometer alignment is the same as in the Ober test (see Fig. 8.47).

Interpretation

A positive and negative test result for the Modified Ober test is determined in the same manner as for the Ober test.[10] However, Gajdosik, Sandler, and Marr[20] suggest that the two tests yield different values and should not be used interchangeably. Gajdosik and colleagues[20] measured 49 healthy adults (26 women, 23 men) using a goniometer and found that hip adduction movement was significantly more restricted for both genders with the knee flexed during the Ober test (mean hip abduction angle: 4 degrees for men and 6 degrees for women) than with the knee extended during the Modified Ober test (mean hip adduction angle: 9 degrees for men and 4 degrees for women). Reese and Bandy[22] determined the mean hip adduction position in 61 individuals (17 males, 44 females) with an inclinometer over the lateral femoral epicondyle. These researchers[22] also found a greater amount of hip adduction during the Modified Ober test (23.4 degrees [SD = 7.0 degrees]) than during the traditional Ober test (18.6 degrees [SD = 6.9 degrees]). Additionally, the inclinometer method does not appear to produce similar values compared with the goniometry method when performing the traditional Ober test or the Modified Ober test.

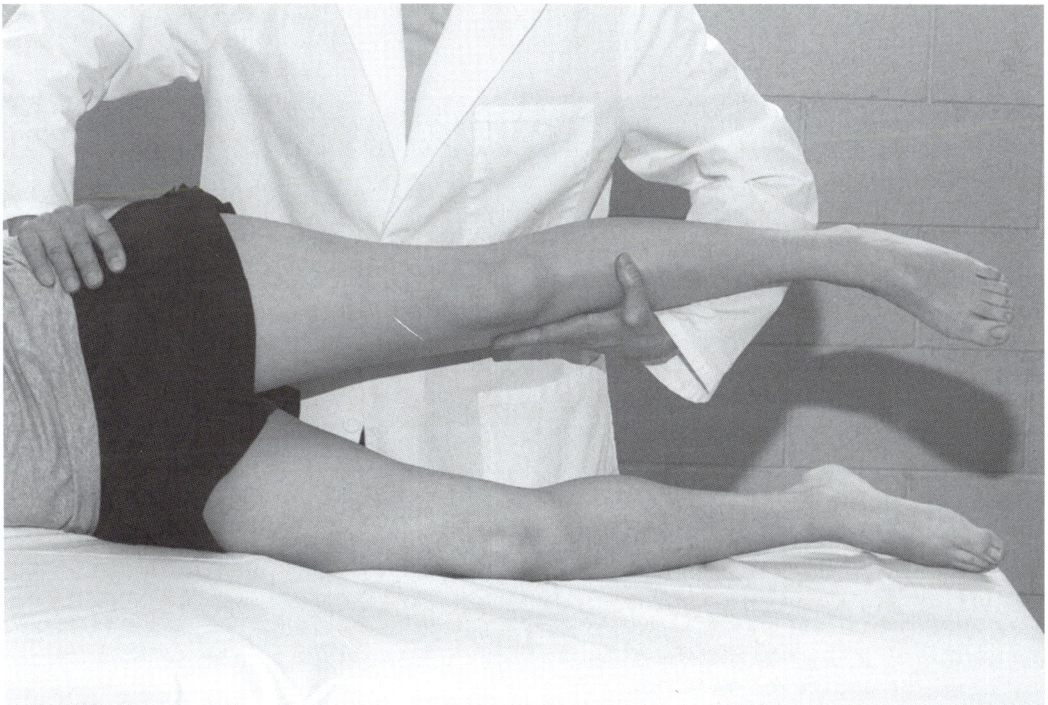

FIGURE 8.48 The extended position of the knee is shown at the end of the Modified Ober test.

Research Findings

Effects of Age, Gender, and Other Factors

Currently the physical therapy profession emphasizes evidence-based practice and endorses the International Classification of Functioning, Disability and Health (ICF), which stresses health and function rather than disability and cause. The following research findings provide evidence of normal hip ROM values for infants through old age (see Tables 8.2 and 8.3), modifiable and nonmodifiable factors that impact hip mobility, ranges needed for functional tasks, and the reliability of various measurement techniques. When appropriate, the age, gender, measurement instrument used, and number of subjects measured to obtain ROM values are noted; however, the American Academy of Orthopaedic Surgeons (AAOS)[3] and the American Medical Association (AMA)[4] sources did not report this information.

Age

Research indicates that age affects hip ROM[6,7,23–30] and that the effects are motion specific. Passive ROM values for neonates are comparatively larger than the passive ROM values of older children and adults in most hip motions except for extension, which is limited.[23–27,30] The marked limitation in hip extension passive ROM in newborns and infants results in an inability to extend the hip from full flexion to the neutral position of 0; thus, the limited hip extension values occur as reported in Table 8.3.[25,27,30]

The term "physiological limitation of motion" has been used to describe the normal hip extension limitation of motion in infants.[24,31] Movement into extension evolves without the need for intervention and should not be considered pathological in newborns and infants.[31] The inability to passively extend the hip has been attributed to the flexed position of the hip in the womb and to the increased flexor tone that is present in neonates and infants. In a longitudinal study, Broughton, Wright, and Menelaus[26] found that hip extension limitations in infants were 34.1 degrees at birth, decreased to 18.9 degrees at 3 months, and then to 7.5 degrees by 6 months of age. Cross-sectional studies also suggest that limitations in hip extension motion continue to resolve as the infant gets older. For example, 100% of the 9- and 12-month-old infants tested (n = 50) had some degree of hip extension limitation; 89% of infants had limitations at 18 months of age; and 72% had limitations at 24 months.[28] By 2 years of age, the hip typically moves into hip extension[28] and hip ROM values begin to approach adult values by early adolescence.[6,29,32] In fact, hip extension ROM in children who were less than 10 years old averages about 27 degrees in side-lying[6] and 20 degrees in prone position[29,32] (see Tables 8.2 and 8.3).

Boone and Azen[9] reported a trend of increasing passive hip extension ROM from birth until approximately age 30 to 39 years before the typical reduction with aging becomes apparent. Active hip range of motion also appears to decrease as people approach old age. Walker and colleagues[33] compared active hip extension ROM between those aged 60 to 69 years and 75 to 84 years (30 women and 30 men). Though no differences were found between age-groups, both groups were unable to attain a neutral starting position for hip flexion. The

TABLE 8.2 Normal Hip ROM Values for Young to Older Adults in Degrees From Selected Sources

	AAOS[3]	AMA[4]	Boone and Azen[9] *	Kumar et al[7]	Roach and Miles[5]		
			19–54 yr n = 56 Males	25–75 yr n = 104 Males and Females	25–39 yr n = 433 Males and Females	40–59 yr n = 727 Males and Females	60–74 yr n = 523 Males and Females
Motion			*Mean (SD)*	*Mean (SD)*	*Mean (SD)*	*Mean (SD)*	*Mean (SD)*
Flexion	120	100	121.3 (6.4)	137.0 (6.9)	122 (12)	120 (14)	118 (13)
Extension	20	30	12.1 (5.4)	—	22 (8)	18 (7)	17 (8)
Abduction		40	40.5 (6.0)	42.0 (5.1)	44 (11)	42 (11)	39 (12)
Adduction		20	25.6 (3.6)	—	—	—	—
Medial rotation	45	40†	44.4 (4.3)	27.2 (6.9)	33 (7)	31 (8)	30 (7)
Lateral rotation	45	50†	44.2 (4.8)	30.5 (5.2)	34 (8)	32 (8)	29 (9)

AAOS = American Academy of Orthopaedic Surgeons; AMA = American Medical Association.

SD = standard deviation.

* Active range of motion presented.

† Tested with individuals in the supine position.

TABLE 8.3 Normal Hip ROM Values for Newborns and Children in Degrees From Selected Sources

	Drews et al[27]	Schwarze and Denton[25]	Watanabe et al[30]	Sankar et al[29]			
	12 hr–6 days *n* = 54	1–3 days *n* = 1,000	4 weeks *n* = 62	2–5 yr *n* = 41 Males	2–5 yr *n* = 22 Females	6–10 yr *n* = 67 Males	6–10 yr *n* = 39 Females
Motion	***Mean (SD)***	***Mean***	***Mean***	***Mean (SD)***	***Mean (SD)***	***Mean (SD)***	***Mean (SD)***
Flexion	—	—	138	118 (12)	121 (10)	118 (9)	122 (13)
Extension	Lacking 28.3 (6.0)*	Lacking 20	Lacking 12	21 (5)	21 (5)	19 (4)	21 (5)
Abduction	55.5 (9.5)†	78†	51	51 (11)	53 (15)	43 (12)	51 (12)
Adduction	6.4 (3.9)†	15†	—	17 (5)	18 (5)	15 (5)	18 (6)
Medial rotation	79.8 (9.3)†	58	24	Hip flexed: 45 (13) Hip extended: 47 (9)	Hip flexed: 47 (11) Hip extended: 51 (9)	Hip flexed: 40 (10) Hip extended: 44 (11)	Hip flexed: 41 (11) Hip extended: 48 (5)
Lateral rotation	113.7 (10.4)†	80	66	Hip flexed: 51 (11) Hip extended: 47 (10)	Hip flexed: 49 (12) Hip extended: 50 (12)	Hip flexed 51 (11) Hip extended: 42 (10)	Hip flexed: 49 (12) Hip extended: 47 (11)

SD = Standard deviation.

* Tested with individuals in the side-lying position.

† Tested with individuals in the supine position.

mean starting position for both older adult groups for measurements of hip flexion ROM was 11 degrees instead of 0 degrees.[33] Others have also reported that hip extension was the only active hip ROM in which the difference between the youngest (25–39 years) and the oldest groups (60–74 years) constituted a decrease of more than 20% of the available arc of motion.[5]

Hip medial and lateral rotation ROM also appears to decrease as one ages. Neonates have larger medial rotation and much larger hip lateral ROM values compared with the same motions of older children and adults (see Tables 8.2, 8.3, and 8.4). A study of 720 individuals between 33 and 70 years of age found that older groups had significantly less passive hip rotation ROM than younger groups.[34] Furthermore, decreases have been reported in both active and passive hip medial and lateral ROM in individuals between 70 and 92 years of age.[13]

The relationship between hip lateral and medial rotation in infants also appears to differ from that found in a majority of older children and adults. Hip lateral rotation values for neonates are considerably greater than medial rotation[23] with differences holding through childhood. After that, differences resolve as a study of 1,140 children aged 8 to 9 years demonstrates, with 90% of the children having less than 10 degrees' difference between passive lateral and medial hip rotation.[35]

Neonates also have much larger hip abduction ROM values compared with the same motions of adults and older children.[4,5,7,9,25,27,29,30] Similar to hip rotation ROM findings, evidence also supports reduced hip abduction and adduction with aging. For example, individuals who were 60 to 84 years old[33] presented with hip rotation, abduction, and adduction values being 14 to 25 degrees less than the average hip ROM values published by the American Academy of Orthopaedic Surgeons.[3] Walker and colleagues[33] found that hip abduction decreased the most with age and was 33.4% less in the oldest group of men and women (aged 85 to 92 years) compared with the youngest group (aged 70 to 74 years). In contrast, hip flexion with the knee either extended or flexed was least affected by age, with a significant reduction occurring only in those older than 85 years of age.[33]

Though most passive hip ROM appears to decrease slightly over time, Roach and Miles[5] found very little difference in active hip ROM in those between 25 and 74 years of age. Furthermore, differences in active ROM in individuals between 25 and 74 years of age represented a loss of less than 10% of the arc of motion.[5] Given the apparent clinical insignificance in ROM differences between age-groups, Roach and Miles[5] suggest that any substantial loss of mobility should be viewed as abnormal and not attributable to aging. Nonaka and colleagues[36] found that hip mobility decreased with advancing age but knee mobility remained unchanged. Because most activities of daily living can be performed without maximal lengthening of hip joint muscles, the researchers[36] argue that altered activity drives the loss of ROM and not age. These authors[36] suggest that a decrease in physical activities results in shortening of muscles and/or connective tissue, and in turn leads to reduced hip motion. Though better controlled longitudinal studies are needed to confirm whether changes in activity and life style influence reduced hip mobility over time, evidence from cross-sectional studies provides support for the use of age-appropriate norms.

Gender

The effects of gender on hip ROM appear to be age and motion specific and account for only a relatively small amount of total variance in measurement. Gender effects have not been reported in neonates and infants. For example, no significant gender differences were found in any hip passive ROM measures in 60 neonates (26 females and 34 males)[23] and no gender differences were reported for hip rotation in 86 infants and young children (aged 9 to 24 months).[28] However, results are contradictory regarding gender differences in adolescents and adults.[32,34,37,38]

In general, evidence suggests that gender does influence hip mobility in adolescents and adults, with females having greater mobility compared with males; however, motion, age, and cultural influences may affect gender differences (see Tables 8.4 and 8.5). A population study of Swedish and Icelandic individuals between 33 and 70 years that included 517 female and 203 males reported that females have greater hip joint mobility than males.[34] Results from this population study by Allander and colleagues determined that in five of eight age-groups spanning from 33 to 70 years, females had a greater hip mobility than males.[34] Researchers from Norway also found age and motion-specific differences when assessing passive ROM in 761 healthy females and males aged 4 to 104 years.[32] Females of all age-groups had greater passive hip ROM than males for passive total ROM, total rotation, medial rotation, adduction, and abduction; however, only medial rotation and abduction motions reached statistically significant differences (see Table 8.4).[32] Female children from Norway who were in the 11- and 15-year-old age-groups and female adults also had significantly greater hip flexion than males.[32]

Healthy individuals residing in the United States also appear to present with differences in hip ROM between genders in both children and adults; however, differences were motion and age specific and results from the two studies were not completely complementary.[13,39] One study concluded that women had greater mobility than men in all hip motions except abduction,[13] whereas the other study[39] found significant differences between genders only in certain age-groups and these gender differences were motion specific. Specifically, female children (1 to 9 years of age), young adult females (21 to 29 years of age), and older adult females (61 to 69 years of age) had significantly more hip flexion than their male counterparts.[39]

Several research findings indicate that females have greater hip lateral rotation than males.[33,34,40] Walker and colleagues[33] found that 30 females aged 60 to 84 years had 14 degrees more ROM in hip medial rotation than their male counterparts. Simoneau and coworkers[40] reported that females (mean age of 21.8 years) had higher mean values in both medial and lateral rotation than age-matched male individuals.

The Thomas test has also been investigated to test for gender differences.[41] The mean knee joint angle for all participants was 50 degrees (SD = 12 degrees) with scores occurring

TABLE 8.4 Age and Gender Effects on Hip ROM in Children and Adolescents: Normal Values in Degrees

		Svenningsen[32]			Soucie[6]	
	Females Males	4 yr n = 52 n = 51	8 yr n = 52 n = 52	15 yr n = 57 n = 57	2–8 yr n = 39 n = 55	9–19 yr n = 56 n = 48
Motion		**Mean**	**Mean**	**Mean**	**Mean**	**Mean**
Flexion	Females	151	146	141	141	135
	Males	149	146	138	131	135
Extension	Females	29	27	26	26	21
	Males	28	27	25	28	18
Abduction	Females	55	50	46		
	Males	53	47	42		
Adduction	Females	30	28	28		
	Males	30	28	29		
Medial rotation	Females	60	57	48		
	Males	51	51	41		
Lateral rotation	Females	44	43	42		
	Males	48	42	43		

Group means presented in degrees. The circles indicate significant differences between genders. Soucie and colleagues[6] did not report statistics on gender differences.

TABLE 8.5 Age and Gender Effects on Hip ROM in Adults: Normal Values in Degrees

		Svenningsen[32]	Soucie[6]	
	Females Males	23 yr *n* = 104 *n* = 102	20–44 yr *n* = 143 *n* = 114	45–69 yr *n* = 123 *n* = 96
Motion		***Mean***	***Mean***	***Mean***
Flexion	Females	141	134	131
	Males	137	130	127
Extension	Females	26	18	17
	Males	23	17	14
Abduction	Females	42		
	Males	40		
Adduction	Females	30		
	Males	29		
Medial rotation	Females	52		
	Males	38		
Lateral rotation	Females	41		
	Males	43		

The circles indicate significant differences between genders. Soucie and colleagues[6] did not report statistics on gender differences.

over a large range in men (range 20–95 degrees) and women (range 14–85 degrees). On average, women demonstrated greater rectus femoris muscle length with a larger flexion angle at the knee joint compared with men during modified Thomas testing.[41]

There is evidence that suggests that hip mobility in females is not always greater than it is in males. Boone et al[39] and Svenningson et al[32] reported that females demonstrate less mobility than males for certain motions during specific ages. Boone et al[39] reported that young and older adult females demonstrate less hip extension than males. Females also had less hip adduction and lateral rotation than males but these differences were observed only in children and young adults. Svenningsen and colleagues[32] also found that males had higher lateral rotation than females in the 4-year-old children and adult (mean of 23 years old) groups (see Tables 8.4 and 8.5).

Still other researchers report no differences in hip mobility between genders. Hip ROM appears to be similar between genders in healthy older adults aged 65 to 85 years from China,[42] as well as healthy and diabetic individuals aged 21 to 71 years from Nigeria.[43] The Chinese researchers used a photographic method to measure hip motion. Additionally, gender comparisons of total hip rotation in other studies indicate no differences between male and female adolescents[37] and adults.[34] Males and females also had no significant differences for either the Ober or Modified Ober tests.[44]

Though research findings may differ, it appears that evidence supports the use of age and gender appropriate norms. However, caution should be used when interpreting mean differences that are statistically significantly different between genders and across different age ranges, as there is limited data on clinically meaningful differences in hip ROM values.

Body Mass Index

Increases in body mass index (BMI) seem to decrease ROM at the hip.[45–48] The association between BMI and hip ROM may be affected by pubertal degree of maturation because BMI values depend on the pubertal status, especially in females.[45] Because the degree of pubertal maturation has a greater influence on BMI than age in both genders, and even more so in females,[45] pubertal status should be considered along with age when assessing ROM.

A threshold or specific magnitude of BMI may drive the relationship between increased BMI and loss of hip mobility. Bennell and associates[49] found no relationship between BMI and active ROM in hip rotation in a study comparing 77 novice ballet dancers and 49 age-matched controls between the ages of 8 and 11 years; however, the mean BMI values were 16.3 and 18.3 for dancers and controls, respectively. Conversely, in an older and heavier population, Kettunen and colleagues[46] found that former elite athletes (long-distance runners, soccer players, weight lifters, and shooters) with a high BMI (≥ 28.1) had smaller passive hip rotation ROM compared with former elite athletes with a low BMI (< 24).

Researchers have investigated the relationship between BMI and hip flexion ROM. Escalante and coworkers[47] determined that there was a loss of at least 1 degree of passive ROM in hip flexion for each unit increase in BMI in a group of

687 community-dwelling elders who were 65 to 78 years of age. Individuals who were severely obese had an average of 18 degrees less hip flexion than nonobese individuals as measured in the supine position with an inclinometer. Body mass index explained a higher proportion of the variance in hip flexion ROM than did age, gender, ethnicity, pain, self-reported arthritis, and diabetes mellitus.[47] Lichtenstein and associates[48] studied interrelationships among the variables reported by Escalante and coworkers[47] and concluded that BMI could be considered a primary direct determinant of hip flexion passive ROM. The known association between hip flexion ROM and walking velocity suggests that reducing BMI may lead to increased walking velocity.[47] Because walking velocity is associated with quality of life[50] and walking velocity has the ability to predict future health status,[51,52] interventions to decrease BMI and in turn improve hip flexion ROM seem warranted.

Methodological Differences Known to Influence Hip Range of Motion

Measurement Device

Evidence suggests that similar methodology and the same devices should be used to measure hip ROM.[53,54] For example, measurements of active ROM of hip adduction, abduction, and extension taken with the Ortho Ranger and goniometer were poorly correlated (Pearson product- moment correlation coefficient [*r*] range: 0.07 to 0.57); therefore, these two instruments should not be used interchangeably.[53] Likewise, comparisons of measurements taken with the goniometer and inclinometer indicate that in some positions, the active hip ROM values were statistically different between the two devices.[54] In another study,[55] passive hip extension and medial and lateral rotation ROM measured with a goniometer and inclinometer differed between 3 and 5 degrees. Conversely, Clapis, Davis, and Davis[56] compared goniometer and inclinometer measurements using the modified Thomas test to assess sagittal plane hip angles in 42 healthy individuals. The hip flexion measurements were not significantly different between those taken with the goniometer and inclinometer, and measurements taken with each device were strongly correlated with each other ($r = 0.89$ and 0.92 for testers 1 and 2, respectively). Thus, these authors concluded that the goniometer and inclinometer can be used interchangeably to measure hip flexion during the Thomas test.[56]

Active and Passive Motion

The use of active or passive motion during joint measurement may affect ROM values. Norms for active and passive ROM values may not be comparable and thus not used interchangeably. Active hip mobility requires the individual's ability to follow commands, stabilize the trunk, and move the limb through the available range of motion of the joint. During passive hip mobility, the individual relaxes and does not assist with the movement of the limb; thus, impaired motor control and/or strength would not influence the motion.[57] There is a paucity of evidence that compares active and passive hip ROM in the same individual.[54] However, ranges may be different, especially in older adults. For example, active ROM for hip extension was lacking 11 degrees for the 60 individuals between 60 and 84 years,[33] whereas passive hip extension ROM was 17 degrees for the 523 individuals aged 60 to 74 years.[5] Though hip extension ROM was vastly different between these two studies,[5,33] the active ROM and passive ROM were not measured in the same group; therefore, the reason for the differences cannot be determined.

Testing Position

Variations in testing position do not seem to affect hip ROM measures in neonates but may affect ROM values in adults. Passive ROM measurements of hip medial and lateral rotation taken from 100 neonates were no different in the prone position compared with measurements taken in the supine position.[25] However, in adults, evidence suggests that hip ROM values are dependent on position (see Table 8.6).[40,54] Active lateral hip rotation measured in the sitting position in 60 healthy college students was statistically less than in the prone position; however, different positions had little effect on medial rotation.[40] Active and passive hip ROM values were also measured in a smaller sample size with a greater age range (two males and seven females aged 21 to 43 years).[54] Findings indicated that lateral as well as medial rotation ROM were significantly less when measured in the sitting and supine positions compared with the prone position for both active and passive ROM.[54] A longitudinal study of 326 healthy individuals from India aged 1 to 75 years also confirms that passive hip medial and lateral rotation is greater in prone than in seated or supine position.[58] Bierma-Zeinstra and colleagues[54] also reported greater hip adduction when measured in side-lying than in supine position; however, passive hip abduction did not differ between positions.

Hip and knee position also appears to influence hip extension and abduction ROM measures in adults. Van Dillen and coworkers[59] compared the effects of knee and hip position on passive hip extension ROM in 10 patients with low-back pain and 35 healthy individuals. Both groups had less hip extension when the hip was in neutral abduction than when the hip was fully abducted. Both groups also displayed less hip extension ROM when the knee was flexed to 80 degrees than when the knee was fully extended.[59] This finding lends support for Kendall and colleagues,[10] who maintain that changing the knee joint angle during the Thomas test affects the passive hip extension ROM. Gajdosik, Sandler, and Marr[20] found that changing the position from knee flexion in the Ober test to knee extension in the Modified Ober test increased the angle of hip adduction in 49 subjects. Because the testing position may affect hip ROM, the position of the individual (e.g., supine, sitting, prone) should be standardized and reported.

Dance and Sports

A sampling of articles related to the effects of ballet and other forms of dance and ice hockey illustrate that ROM requirements depend on activity, and changes in ROM may be specific to the particular activity. Because dancers require positions in which their hips are externally rotated and their

TABLE 8.6 Effects of Position on Hip Rotation ROM: Normal Values in Degrees

Author	Motion	Position		
		Seated	*Prone*	*Supine*
Simoneau et al[40]	Lateral rotation*	36 (7)	45 (10)	—
	Medial rotation*	33 (7)	36 (9)	—
Bierma-Zeinstra et al[54]	Lateral rotation*	33.9	47.0	33.1
	Medial rotation*	33.6	46.3	36.0
	Lateral rotation†	37.6	51.9	34.2
	Medial rotation†	38.8	53.2	39.9
Kumar et al[7]	Lateral rotation†	30.5 (5.2)	38.0 (10.3)	25.9 (7.1)
	Medial rotation†	27.2 (6.9)	32.2 (11.2)	20.5 (5.8)

Group means (standard deviation) presented in degrees.
* Active ROM measured with a universal goniometer.
† Passive ROM measured with a universal goniometer.

feet are "turned out," studies have investigated the motion of this turned out position.[49,60] Bennell and colleagues[49] studied 77 individuals aged 8 to 11 years who were trained in ballet and found no significant difference in the degree of turnout compared with the 49 age-matched controls. Even though the degree of turnout angle was no different between groups, passive hip lateral and medial rotation was significantly less in the dancers than in the controls.[49] Interestingly, hip lateral rotation accounted for 60% of the degree of turnout angles in the ballet dancers compared with 80% in the control group. The relatively large percentage of nonhip lateral rotation (e.g., external rotation achieved from below the hip during turnout) increases torsional forces on the medial aspect of the knee, ankle, and foot in the young dancers and may put this group at risk of injury.[49] Gilbert, Gross, and Klug[60] also reported turnout angles that were significantly greater (between 13 and 17 degrees) than the sum of bilateral hip lateral rotation ROM in a small study of 20 female ballet dancers aged 11 to 14 years. These findings indicated that subjects used motion at anatomical locations other than the hip to achieve turnout angles.

Steinberg and colleagues[61] compared passive hip ROM in 1320 females who participated in dancing classes (ballet, modern dance, and jazz) and 223 nondancers of similar age (8 to 16 years). Passive hip medial and lateral rotation significantly decreased in both groups with increasing age, whereas active hip extension ROM increased only in the dancer group. Similar to Gilbert and colleagues' findings,[60] passive hip lateral rotation did not increase with age or years of experience with dance classes.[61] Given the evidence, assessing hip rotation in dancers seems warranted. Perhaps implementing interventions focused on increasing or maintaining hip rotation should be considered for dancers.

Participation in ice hockey also appears to impact hip mobility. Tyler and colleagues[62] found that a group of 25 professional male ice hockey players had about 10 degrees less hip extension ROM than a group of 25 matched controls. These authors postulated that the loss of hip extension in the hockey players was probably due to tight anterior hip capsule structures and short iliopsoas muscles. The flexed hip and knee posture assumed by the players during skating probably contributed to the muscle shortness and loss of hip extension ROM noted during the Thomas test.[62] Though there is no conclusive link between decreased hip extension ROM and the high rate of hip flexor, abdominal, and groin strains in hockey,[63,64] attention to hip ROM in hockey players, as in dancers, appears warranted.

Health Conditions

Reduced hip ROM is also associated with health conditions and running and leg injuries. Interestingly, in a study of 100 healthy adults aged 20 to 41 years, only 27% had greater lateral rotation than medial rotation, whereas 48% of 50 patients with back problems had greater hip lateral rotation than medial rotation.[65] Whether the relative decrease in the amount of medial hip rotation relative to lateral rotation is a process of aging, a result of low-back pain, or predisposes an individual to back pain is uncertain.

Evidence is mounting that hip pathology influences hip rotation and may be predictive of hip diagnoses, as well as success or failure after certain treatments. For example, limited hip ROM (medial rotation < 15 degrees, hip flexion < 115 degrees) and hip pain are standard criteria used to diagnose hip osteoarthritis (OA).[66,67] More recent evidence includes limited hip medial rotation (≤ 25 degrees) as a variable related to diagnose hip OA.[68] Evidence also indicates that less hip abduction and lateral and medial hip rotation is associated with greater radiographic severity of hip OA and greater self-reported dysfunction.[69] Reduced hip mobility also relates to functional limitations, with low ROM associated with higher levels of disability.[70] Therefore, baseline measures and changes in hip ROM should be monitored to determine the efficacy of treatment in individuals with hip OA.

Hip mobility should also be monitored in elders because ROM values relate to functional outcomes and risk of falls. As mentioned in the section on aging, hip extension ROM decreases as one enters old age.[36] Hip extension ROM averaged only 4 degrees for 111 nursing home residents.[71] Reduced hip extension is of concern, as hip extension ROM was the only joint parameter that was significantly reduced in elderly fallers compared with elderly non-fallers and young adults.[72] Additionally, reduced lower-extremity passive ROM values predicted function in elderly living in assisted living residences and in skilled nursing facilities (22 men; 58 women; mean age of 81 years).[73] Therefore, assessing hip ROM and extension in particular in elders is warranted. Evidence suggests that increasing hip extension ROM may improve the health status and reduce the risk of falls in individuals with hip OA and residents of nursing homes and assisted living and skilled nursing facilitates.

Men and women with diabetes appear to have less hip flexion (92 degrees) than age-matched controls aged 21 to 72 years (111.0 degrees).[43] An average of 92 degrees is less than the motion required to squat down, don socks, and stoop.[74] If hip ROM is assessed and deficits are addressed, then increased mobility may, in turn, improve functional outcomes for individuals with diabetes.

A systematic review and meta-analysis concluded that the risk of developing metatarsal stress syndrome (MTSS) varies by gender, and increased passive lateral hip rotation ROM is significantly associated with increased risk of MTSS in male runners but not in females.[75] Additionally, a prospective study that followed 230 high school runners aged 15 years for 3 years found a statistically significant relationship between increased passive medial hip rotation angle in sitting and MTSS in females but not in males.[76] A retrospective study that included males and females found significantly greater passive hip medial rotation measured in prone position on the injured side than on the uninjured side (6.5-degree difference) of unilaterally injured runners.[77] Thus, hip ROM should be evaluated in runners and clinical decisions should factor in potential gender differences.

Hip ROM values are also used in clinical prediction rules to predict how interventions will alter functional outcomes in individuals with low-back pain. For example, a straight leg raise greater than 91 degrees is one of the variables that predicts successful outcomes if the treatment plan includes lumbar stabilization exercises.[78] One of the variables to predict a favorable outcome after a lumbar spine manipulation in individuals with acute low-back pain is greater than 35 degrees of medial rotation in either hip.[79] Alternatively, individuals who have a decreased average total hip rotation ROM or decreased hip medial rotation ROM discrepancy between sides are unlikely to respond favorably to a lumbar spine manipulation.[80]

Likewise, hip mobility is a known predictor of outcomes in individuals with knee pathologies. Side-to-side hip medial rotation difference of greater than 14 degrees is a predictor that individuals with patellofemoral pain syndrome are more likely to respond to lumbar spine manipulation.[81] Passive hip medial rotation less than 17 degrees is a predictor that individuals with knee OA are more likely to respond to hip mobilization.[82] Thus, hip medial rotation may be an important objective measure when individuals present with specific knee pathologies as well as hip pathologies.

Functional Range of Motion

Adequate ROM at the hip is important for meeting mobility demands such as walking, ascending and descending stairs, and performing many activities of daily living that require sitting and bending. During gait, most hip motion occurs in the sagittal plane, with less motion in the frontal plane and subtle motion happening in the transverse plane.[83] An arc of motion from about 20 degrees of hip extension to 25 degrees of hip flexion occurs in the sagittal plane during gait.[84] Small arcs of motion occur in the frontal plane, with hip abduction peaking at

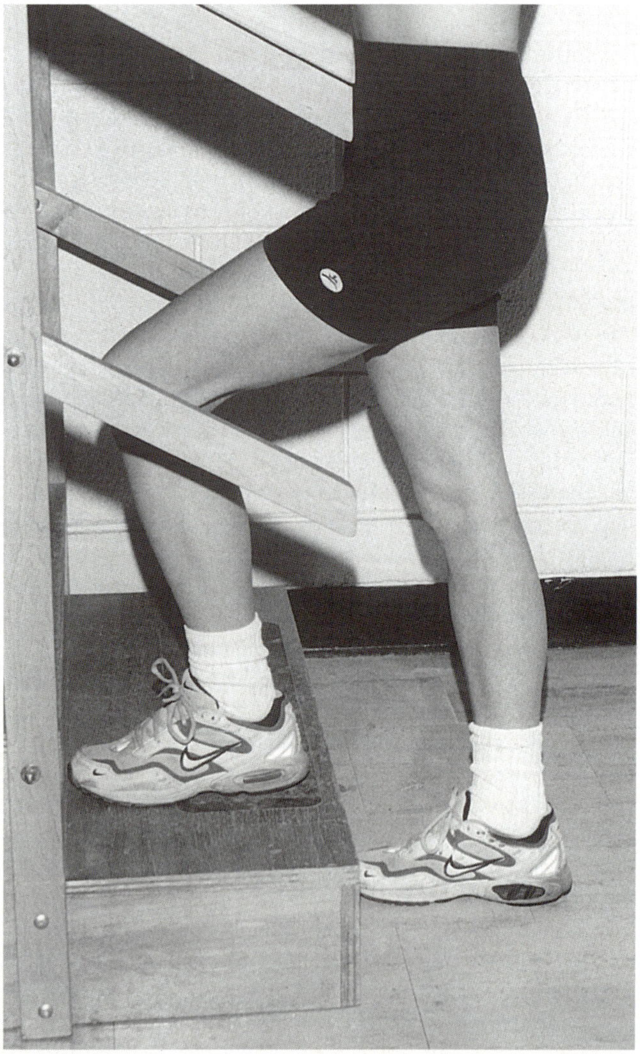

FIGURE 8.49 Ascending stairs requires between 47 and 66 degrees of hip flexion, depending on stair dimensions.[89]

approximately 5 degrees and hip adduction peaking at approximately 10 degrees in both men and women.[85] Even smaller arcs of motion occur in the transverse plane, with total hip rotation (e.g., hip medial and lateral rotation) averaging 8 degrees.[86]

Though hip extension occurs during gait, Lee and colleagues[87] report that both healthy children and children diagnosed with cerebral palsy (CP) can ambulate with hip flexion contractures. Children with limited hip extension mobility were able to ambulate likely owing to compensatory mobility at the pelvis, lumbar spine, knee, and ankle joints. Lee and colleagues[87] also tested convergent validity to determine which hip mobility test was most highly correlated with maximum hip extension measured during the stance phase of gait. Related hip mobility during gait correlated with prone hip extension measures (e.g., Staheli test) in individuals with CP, whereas the supine hip extension (e.g., Thomas test) was found to be the most valid measure of hip flexion contractures during gait for children without CP who acted as controls.[86]

According to Magee,[74] ideal functional hip ranges are 120 degrees of flexion, 20 degrees of abduction, and 20 degrees of lateral rotation; however, the mobility needs vary depending on the task.[74,88–90] Approximately 65 degrees of hip flexion ROM is needed to ascend and 40 degrees to descend stairs (Fig. 8.49), with 18-centimeter risers (7.1 inches) and a tread length of 28.5 centimeters (11.2 inches) as noted in a study of 16 males and 17 females adults.[90] Other researchers report a range of 47 to 66 degrees of hip flexion to ascend stairs and a range of 26 to 45 degrees to descend stairs of varying heights by tall to short adult females.[89] Slight hip extension is required to ascend and descend stairs with a low riser height (12.7 centimeters, 5 inches) and large tread depth (41.9 centimeters, 16.5 inches).

Other functional and self-care activities require a larger ROM at the hip than walking and stairs. For example, sitting requires at least 90 to 112 degrees of hip flexion with the knees flexed (Fig. 8.50).[74] Additional hip flexion ROM is necessary for putting on socks (120 degrees), squatting (115 degrees), and stooping (125 degrees)[74] (Fig. 8.51).

The daily activities of various cultures may require different sets of functional ROM values. The squatting position used for toileting in non-Western cultures and the various praying and resting positions of different cultures (e.g., Muslim prayer

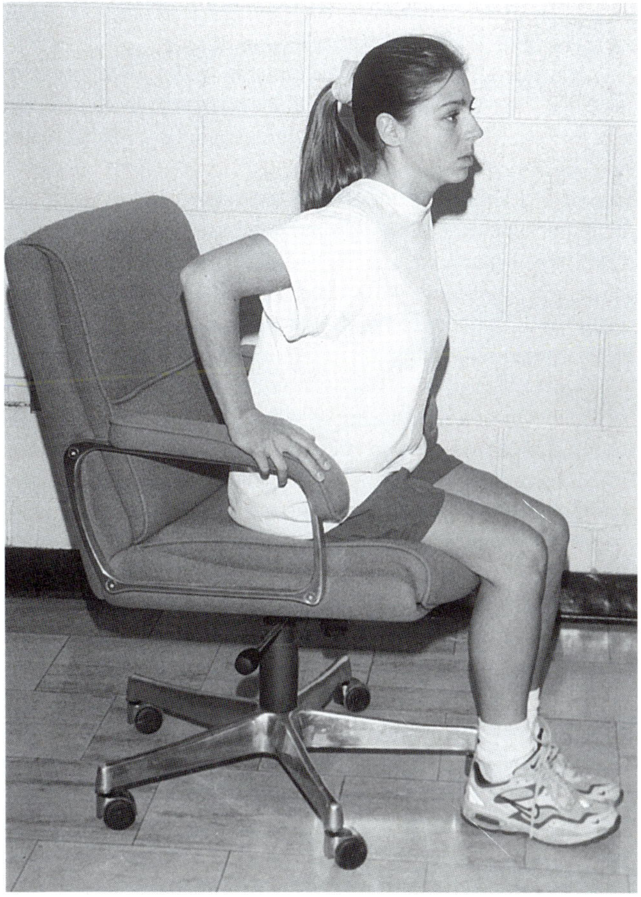

FIGURE 8.50 Sitting in a chair with an average seat height requires 112 degrees of hip flexion.[74]

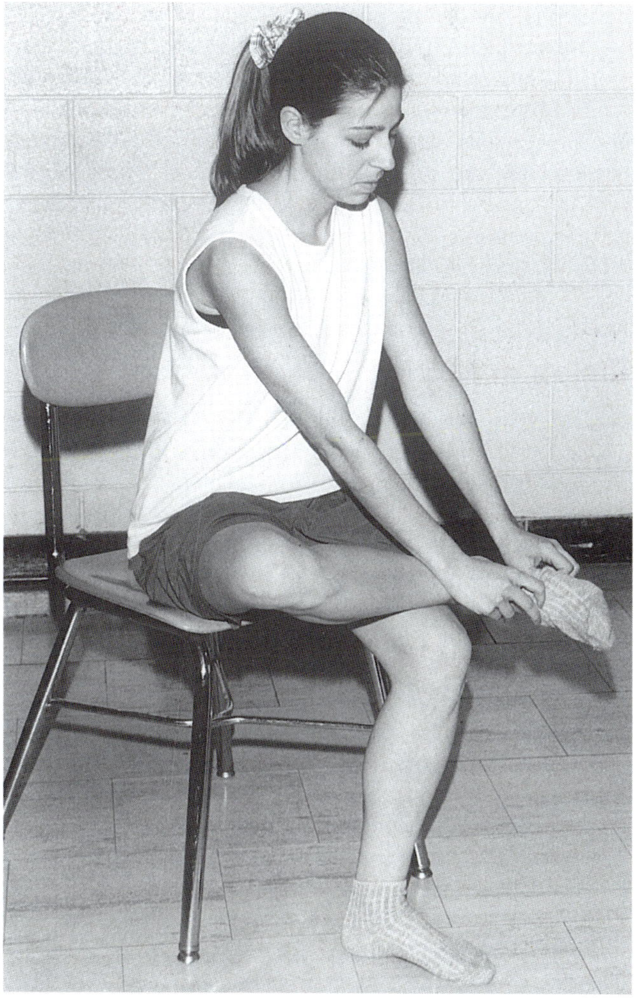

FIGURE 8.51 Putting on socks requires 120 degrees of flexion, 20 degrees of abduction, and 20 degrees of lateral rotation.[74]

movements, cross-legged sitting, kneeling) may involve additional ROM values at the hips. Evidence to guide functional ROM requirements for hip joint implants in non-Western cultures report that squatting requires a range of 130 degrees to full range of hip flexion, 5 to 36 degrees of hip lateral rotation, and 10 to 30 degrees of hip abduction.[91] Sitting cross-legged requires a range of 90 to 100 degrees of hip flexion, 35 to 60 degrees of lateral rotation, and 40 to 45 degrees of hip abduction.[91] Similar hip ROM values were found in a study of 30 healthy individuals from India with a mean of 83 degrees of hip flexion, 34 degrees of hip abduction, and 37 degrees of hip lateral rotation needed to sit cross-legged.[92] These 30 individuals also had a mean of 95 degrees of hip flexion required for squatting with the heels down.[92] In another study, the hip mobility of 44 healthy individuals from India were measured while they sat cross-legged and results were also similar: a mean of 91 degrees of hip flexion, 39 degrees of hip abduction, and 49 degrees of lateral rotation.[93]

Given the wide variation in functional ROM of the hip joint during different tasks, the clinician should consider the needs of each individual. For example, the clinician needs to obtain the cultural, art/sport, employment, and recreational requirements to formulate ROM goals specific for each individual. Consideration should also be given to the health condition of the individual as well as including the assessment of any potential compensatory strategies utilized after certain health conditions, diagnoses, or impairments. These considerations are important because compensations can lead to reductions in hip ROM when certain functional activities or movement patterns are avoided.

Reliability and Validity of Hip Range of Motion Measurements

Studies of the reliability of hip ROM have examined active and passive motion and different types of measuring instruments in different age-groups and populations.[94–99] A sampling of intratester and intertester reliability studies is provided in Table 8.7 and Table 8.8, respectively. Whenever possible, relative reliability, such as the intraclass correlation coefficient (ICC) and Pearson product moment correlation coefficient (r), as well as absolute measures of reliability in units of degrees are included.

Comparisons among hip reliability studies are difficult because of wide variations in measurement methods and study populations; however, some generalizations can be made. Although hip ROM measurements overestimate true hip ROM due to the difficulty in stabilizing pelvic motion,[65,100,101] measurements of hip mobility appear to be acceptable for clinical practice. Measurement devices are more reliable than visual estimations;[95,102,103] therefore, devices are recommended over visual assessment of hip ROM. Ideally, the same tester should measure an individual over time because intratester measurements are usually more reliable than intertester measurements.[54,104,105] Passive ROM measures may be less variable and more reliable than active ROM.[54] Of course, for active ROM to be reproducible the individual being tested needs to have no marked weakness or pain.[54]

Some researchers recommend stringent standardization of the measurement techniques and the use of an assistant/helper to support the limb during hip ROM measurements to improve reliability; however, reliability values vary between studies regardless of whether an assistant was used[101,106] or not.[11] Furthermore, acceptable intertester reliability has been reported prior to standardization when using a goniometer to measure passive hip motion in individuals with hip OA.[107] Neither the goniometer nor inclinometer has a clear advantage in terms of reliability; however, researchers recommend that the same instrument should be used in all subsequent measurements of ROM to track an individual's progress.[54,55] Brief summaries of a number of studies are discussed to provide the reader with a sense of the varying methods and findings of research on the reliability of hip ROM measurements. No discernible ROM differences between limbs is apparent;[55] therefore, if a study reported reliability results for both limbs, only the reliability measuring ROM in the right hip is included in Tables 8.7 through 8.11.

Reliability of Active ROM Hip Measurements

Several research studies[33,40,53,54,104] investigated the reliability of active ROM hip measurements in healthy adults. Boone and associates[104] conducted a study in which four physical therapists used a goniometer to measure active hip abduction ROM in 12 healthy male volunteers aged 26 to 54 years. Acceptable reliability was obtained when three measurements of active hip abduction were taken by the same tester at each of four sessions scheduled on a weekly basis for 4 weeks (intratester $r = 0.75$); however, reliability decreased if the measurements were taken by different testers (intertester $r = 0.55$).[104] Because the absolute error was higher when measurements were obtained by two testers, larger gains in active ROM were needed to determine improvements. For example, if each measurement was taken by a different tester, an increase in motion needed to exceed 6 degrees to suggest improvements in active hip abduction ROM over time, whereas if one tester repeated the measurements, an increase exceeding 4 degrees indicated improvement.[104] Boone and colleagues[104] also reported that one measurement was as reliable as taking the average of repeated measurements in onc session for hip abduction active ROM.[104]

Clapper and Wolf[53] compared the reliability of the Ortho Ranger, an electronic computed pendulum inclinometer, with a goniometer in a study of active hip motion involving 10 healthy males and 10 healthy females. The goniometer showed significantly less variation than the Ortho Ranger, except for measurements of hip lateral rotation (see Table 8.7). The authors[53] concluded that the goniometer was a more reliable instrument than the Ortho Ranger.

Simoneau and colleagues[40] created three teams of two testers each to determine the intertester reliability of active

TABLE 8.7 Intratester Reliability of Hip ROM Measurements Using Goniometers and Inclinometers for Healthy and Patient Populations

Study	N	Sample	Methods	Motion	r	ICC	Absolute Reliability
Healthy Populations							
Aalto et al[11]	20	Healthy adults (18–45 yr)	PROM, 2 testers (PT), goniometer, Sitting	Medial rotation		Tester 1; 2 .95; .95	CV (%) 8.4; 4.2
Clapper and Wolf[53]	20	Healthy adults (23–40 yr)	AROM, 1 tester (PT) Goniometer,				
			Supine	Flexion		.95	
			Prone	Extension		.83	
			Standing	Abduction		.86	
			Standing	Adduction		.80	
			Supine	Medial rotation		.92	
			Supine	Lateral rotation		.80	
Clapper and Wolf[53]	20	Healthy adults (23–40 yr)	AROM, 1 tester (PT), Ortho Ranger,				
			Supine	Flexion		.89	
			Prone	Extension		.72	
			Standing	Abduction		.79	
			Standing	Adduction		.77	
			Supine	Medial rotation		.86	
			Supine	Lateral rotation		.86	
Ellison et al[65]	22	Healthy adults (20–41 yr)	PROM, 3 testers (PT), inclinometer, prone	Medial rotation		.99	
				Lateral rotation		.96	
Prather et al[106]	28	Healthy adults (18–51 yr)	PROM, 28 testers (15 PT, 13 physicians),* goniometer				CV (%)
			Supine	Flexion		.95	3
			Prone	Extension		.83	16
			Supine	Abduction		.85	10
			Supine	Adduction		.88	16
			Supine	Medial rotation		.88	14
			Supine	Lateral rotation		.95	7
			Prone	Medal rotation		.94	10
			Prone	Lateral rotation		.85	8
Steinberg et al[61]	20	Healthy females (8–16 yr)	PROM, 2 testers (physicians), goniometer				
			Supine	Flexion	.96		
			Prone	Extension	.91		
			Prone	Medial rotation	.90		
			Prone	Lateral rotation	.90		
Patient Populations							
Cadenhead et al[111]	6	Adults with cerebral palsy (20–44 yr)	PROM, 1 tester (PT),* goniometer				
			Prone	Extension		.98	
			Supine	Abduction		.97	
			Supine	Lateral rotation		.79	
Ellison et al[65]	15	Adults with low-back pain (23-61 yr)	PROM, 3 testers (PT), inclinometer, prone	Medial rotation		.96	
				Lateral rotation		.96	

(table continues on page 298)

TABLE 8.7 Intratester Reliability of Hip ROM Measurements Using Goniometers and Inclinometers for Healthy and Patient Populations (continued)

Study	N	Sample	Methods	Motion	r	ICC	Absolute Reliability
Patient Populations							
Fosang et al[110]	18	Children with cerebral palsy (2–10 yr)	PROM, 6 testers (PT), goniometer, Supine	Abduction		Range = .58–.83	SEM (°): 3.7–6.9
Mutlu et al[99]	38	Children with cerebral palsy (18–108 mo)	PROM, 3 testers (PT), goniometer,		Tester 1; 2; 3	Tester 1; 2; 3	
			Supine	Abduction	.54; .32; .53	.70; .48; .69	
			Sitting	Lateral rotation	.75; .72; 67	.85; .84; .80	
Nussbaumer et al[101]	30	Healthy adults and adults with femoroacetabular impingement (35 ± 11 yr)	PROM, 1 tester (human movement scientist),* goniometer				CV (%); SEM (°)
			Supine	Flexion		.92	3.12; 3.94
			Supine	Abduction		.92	5.84; 2.36
			Supine	Adduction		.84	6.73; 2.36
			Supine	Medial rotation		.95	7.74; 2.42
			Supine	Lateral rotation		.91	5.23; 2.53
Pua et al[108]	22	Adults with hip osteoarthritis (50–84 yr)	PROM, 1 tester (PT), extendable goniometer or electronic inclinometer				SEM; MDC (°)
			Supine, inclinometer	Flexion		.97	3.5; 8.2
			Supine, inclinometer	Extension		.89	4.7; 11.0
			Supine, goniometer	Abduction		.94	3.2; 7.3
			Seated, inclinometer	Medial rotation		.93	3.4; 7.8
			Seated, inclinometer	Lateral rotation		.96	3.1; 7.1

ICC = Interclass correlation coefficient; CV = Coefficient of variation; MDC = Minimal detectable change; SEM = Standard error of measurement; PROM: Passive range of motion; AROM = Active range of motion; *r* = Pearson product-moment correlation coefficient; PT = Physical therapist(s); ° = degrees.

* Indicates that the tester had an assistant helping to take the measurement.

hip medial and lateral rotation measures in 60 healthy, college-aged individuals. Range of motion was measured with a goniometer and the pelvis was stabilized with a gait belt. Hip internal rotation was performed bilaterally when the individual was in the seated and prone position. The ICC values for each team ranged from 0.76 to 0.98 and the difference between the means of each tester for each measurement was less than 1 degree for all conditions (e.g., medial and lateral hip ROM measured in seated and prone positions). The combined ICCs (aggregate of all individuals) for the six testers were 0.90 or greater[40] (see Table 8.8).

Bierma-Zeinstra and associates[54] measured nine healthy individuals (two males and seven females) between 21 and 43 years to compare the intra- and intertester reliability of active hip ROM measurements taken with an electronic inclinometer and a goniometer. Measurements were taken in different positions: hip medial and lateral rotation in prone, supine, and sitting positions; hip abduction and adduction in side-lying and supine positions. To examine intratester variability within one investigator, one tester took 10 repeated measurements on each subject. Error was reported as standard deviations (SDs) in degrees and ranges were similar between the goniometer and inclinometer (2 to 4 degrees and 3 to 6 degrees, respectively). To examine intertester reliability, 10 different observers measured hip rotation in the sitting position. Intertester variability (SD between investigators) was 4 to 5 degrees for the goniometer and 3 to 4 degrees for the inclinometer. The devices with the least variability during active ROM measures were contradictory: Lower intratester errors were reported for the inclinometer for lateral rotation in prone position but the goniometer had lower errors during medial rotation in prone position.

TABLE 8.8 Intertester Reliability of Hip ROM Measurements Using Goniometers and Inclinometers for Healthy and Patient Populations

Study	N	Sample	Methods	Motion	ICC	Absolute Reliability
Healthy Populations						
Aalto et al[11]	20	Healthy adults (18–45 yr)	PROM, 2 testers (PT), goniometer, sitting	Medial rotation	.91	CV (%) = 11.1
Drews [27]	9	Healthy infants (12 hr–6 days)	PROM, side-lying,			
			Goniometer	Extension	.56	
			Inclinometer	Extension	.74	
Ellison et al[65]	22	Healthy adults (20–41 yr)	PROM, 3 testers (PT), inclinometer, prone	Medial rotation	.99	
				Lateral rotation	.96	
Prather et al[106]	28	Healthy adults (18–51 yr)	PROM, 28 testers (15 PT, 13 physicians)*, goniometer			Mean absolute difference (°); CV (%)
			Supine	Flexion	.87	6.5; 5
			Prone	Extension	.44	5.5; 28
			Supine	Abduction	.34	8.9; 20
			Supine	Adduction	.54	5.1; 38
			Supine	Medial rotation	.75	6.4; 20
			Supine	Lateral rotation	.63	9.1; NA
			Prone	Medial rotation	.79	6.5; 18
			Prone	Lateral rotation	.18	8.2; 18
Simoneau et al[40]	60	Healthy adults (18–27 yr)	AROM, 6 testers, goniometer			
			Prone	Medial rotation	.94	
			Seated	Medial rotation	.91	
			Prone	Lateral rotation	.93	
			Seated	Lateral rotation	.90	
Patient Populations						
Ellison et al[65]	15	Adults with low-back pain (23–61 yr)	PROM, 3 testers (PT), inclinometer, prone	Medial rotation	.96	
				Lateral rotation	.95	
Fosang et al[110]	18	Children with cerebral palsy (2–10 yr)	PROM, goniometer, 6 testers (PT), supine	Abduction	.62	SEM (°) = 5.6
McWhirl and Glanzman	25	Children with cerebral palsy (2–18 yr)	PROM, 2 testers (PT),* goniometer, supine	Abduction	.91	Mean absolute difference (°) 3.6
Mutlu et al[99]	38	Children with cerebral palsy (18–108 mo)	PROM, 3 testers (PT), goniometer		First measure; second measure	
			Supine	Abduction	.77; .61	
			Sitting	Lateral rotation	.91; .92	
Owen et al[114]	101	Children with fractured femur (4–10 yr)	Goniometer, 4 clinical sites, number of testers not provided			Mean difference (°)
				Flexion	.48	–1.5
				Abduction	.28	1.8
				Adduction	.20	–1.9
				Medial rotation	.41	2.3
				Lateral rotation	.06	–3.4

(table continues on page 300)

TABLE 8.8 Intertester Reliability of Hip ROM Measurements Using Goniometers and Inclinometers for Healthy and Patient Populations (continued)

Study	N	Sample	Methods	Motion	ICC	Absolute Reliability
Patient Populations						
Poulsen et al[109]	48	Adults with hip osteoarthritis (65.6 ± 8 yr)	PROM, 2 testers (physician), goniometer			Mean difference; SEM (°)
			Supine	Flexion	.73	7; 8
			Prone (assumed)	Extension	.68	2; 4
			Supine	Abduction	.63	3; 6
			Supine	Adduction	.65	0; 4
			Supine	Medial rotation	.63	−8; 9
			Supine	Lateral rotation	.53	−4; 6
Poulsen et al[109]	61	Adults with hip osteoarthritis (65.6 ± 8 yr)	PROM, 2 testers (chiropractor), goniometer			Mean difference; SEM (°)
			Supine	Flexion	.79	4; 7
			Prone (assumed)	Extension	.33	−6; 5
			Supine	Abduction	.45	7; 8
			Supine	Adduction	.14	3; 6
			Supine	Medial rotation	.44	2; 10
			Supine	Lateral rotation	.48	2; 8

ICC = Interclass correlation coefficient; CV = Coefficient of variation; PROM = Passive range of motion; AROM = Active range of motion; SEM = Standard error of the measurement; ° = degrees.

* Indicates that the tester had an assistant helping to take the measurement.

Walker and colleagues[33] tested the reliability of active hip ROM measurements by having four testers measure four individuals on one day. The testers measured hip flexion, abduction, adduction, and medial and lateral rotation. All Pearson product moment correlation coefficients for intratester reliability were high ($r = 0.81–0.99$). The two testers with the highest intratester reliability were then chosen to obtain all measurements for a larger study that included measuring active hip ROM in 60 healthy adults between 60 and 84 years old. Though specific mean intertester variability between these two testers was not reported for each hip motion, combined error was reported to be 6 degrees (SD = 5 degrees) for all motions measured including upper- and lower-extremity motions.[33]

Reliability of Passive ROM Hip Measurement

Numerous studies have investigated the reliability of measuring passive ROM at the hip.[11,27,54,55,61,65,95,97,101–103,105,106,108–111] Selected studies below summarize the reliability of passive hip ROM, from adults to children, first in healthy populations[11,54,55,61,65,101–103,105,106] and then in patient populations.[95,97,101,103,108,109,111]

Healthy Populations

Van Trijffel and colleagues[102] conducted a systematic review of studies of intertester reliability of passive hip ROM in humans. Studies were excluded if the hip joint was replaced (arthroplasty), had restrictions in passive ROM that were due to pain or instability, or if abnormal tone was present (e.g., neurological condition). Seven studies met the inclusion criteria and consistently reported low reliability for most hip motions regardless if measurements were taken with a goniometer or inclinometer (ICCs or r values < 0.75). Goniometric measurements of hip flexion and goniometric and inclinometer measures of medial rotation appear to be most reliable, whereas visual estimations of all hip motions were not reliable (ICCs < 0.56). Chevillotte and colleagues[103] also reported that intertester ICCs for visual estimations of hip motion ranged from 0.0 to 0.45 for healthy individuals (20 hips), suggesting that visual estimations of hip motion are not reliable.

Aalto and colleagues[11] reported on the intratester and intertester reliability when two physical therapists obtained medial rotation ROM measurements taken on healthy adults. Passive movement, including stretching, was performed until a firm or bony end was reached, compensatory motion occurred, and/or the individual reported discomfort. Although repeated stretching increased passive ROM in hip medial rotation, the measurements after eight bouts of stretching were not more reliable than measurements taken prior to stretching. Because intratester reliability was greater than intertester reliability, the authors recommended that the same physical therapist take repeated measurements (see Tables 8.7 and 8.8).

Bierma-Zeinstra and associates[54] also compared the reliability of passive hip medial and lateral rotation ROM in sitting and prone with the inclinometer and goniometer. The variability within the testers was reported as standard deviations (SD) in degrees and ranges were similar for the goniometer and inclinometer (2 to 4 degrees and 3 to 4 degrees, respectively). Intertester variability (SD between testers) was determined using 10 examiners who measured hip flexion and medial and lateral rotation in sitting position with the inclinometer and goniometer. Variability was 5 degrees for the goniometer and 4 degrees for the inclinometer. Results from this study indicate that systematic differences occur between the goniometer and inclinometer measures in passive hip ROM.

Ekstrand and associates[105] used a flexometer (gravity inclinometer) to measure the passive ROM of hip flexion, extension, and abduction in healthy men in two testing series. Both series included a physical therapist and an orthopedic surgeon working as a team. In the first series, series A, the testing procedures were standardized similar to measurements obtained in clinical practice. In the second series, series B, procedures were more rigidly standardized, including marking anatomical landmarks, securing hard boards over the examining bench, and altering the bench height. The intertester error in series A, expressed as the interassay (CV percentage), was higher than the error in series B (Table 8.8). These results suggest that error decreases and reliability improves when rigid standardization such as better fixation and precise identification and marking of the anatomical landmarks are used.

Roach and colleagues[55] measured passive ROM of hip extension and medial and lateral rotation in 30 healthy subjects using a goniometer and inclinometer. The average intratester ICCs were 0.80 for the goniometer and 0.90 for the inclinometer.

Steinberg and associates[61] calculated intratester reliability coefficients on ROM measurements on 20 healthy females prior to completing a large longitudinal study. Intratester Pearson product moment correlation coefficient values were high for all hip motions tested on 2 consecutive days. The intertester reliability was also compared between the two surgeon examiners, and as expected intratester reliability was greater than intertester reliability: Intratester r values ranged from 0.90 to 0.96 and intertester r values ranged from 0.74 to 0.95 (see Table 8.7).

Prather and colleagues[106] conducted a study on 28 healthy adults to determine intratester and intertester reliability of goniometric measurement of passive hip ROM. Fifteen physicians and 13 physical therapists had acceptable intratester reliability for all hip motions (ICC = 0.83 to 0.95; see Table 8.7); however, intertesting was not as reliable (ICC = 0.18 to 0.87; see Table 8.8). Passive hip motions were measured in both limbs and ICC values were not influenced by the side tested; therefore, the ICCs for the right and left hips were reported with the limbs combined.

Ellison and coworkers[65] used an inclinometer and a goniometer to measure passive hip rotation in prone position with the test hip in neutral and the knee flexed to 90 degrees and the opposite hip in 30 degrees of abduction in healthy individuals. The high intratester and intertester ICCs for the hip rotation indicate that each instrument was reliable, but the testers preferred the inclinometer because it was easier to use. The ICC values for the right limbs of measurements using an inclinometer can be found in Tables 8.7 and 8.8. Intraclass correlation coefficients for the goniometer were not reported.

Patient Populations

Adults

Researchers have examined the reliability of passive hip ROM in adults with various medical conditions. Many studies have focused on patients with osteoarthritis (OA) of the hip. Chevillotte and colleagues[103] reported on the reliability of passive hip ROM for individuals with hip OA pre– and post–total hip arthoplasty when measured by expert testers (orthopedic surgeons) and trainees. Intertester reliability of visual estimates was poor, with ICC values ranging from 0.12 to 0.56 for both groups: individuals with hip OA who were scheduled for a total hip arthroplasty (21 hips) and those who were at least 12 months post–total hip arthroplasty (21 hips). Though variability decreased when the measurements were repeated by the same expert tester, the errors during visual estimation, regardless of intratester or intertester comparisons, were substantial and therefore were not recommended for clinical practice.[103]

Conversely, Holm and associates[95] found no significant differences between goniometric measurements and visual estimates or intratester differences between sessions with the exception of hip abduction ROM. This study included 25 individuals with hip OA (6 males, 19 females; mean age 68.5 years). Goniometric measurements were obtained by two teams of two physical therapists assisting each other and a single experienced physical therapist using a half-circle metal goniometer. One orthopedic surgeon also made visual estimates. Measurements were taken on two occasions with a week between sessions. Concordance, expressed as the standardized agreement index, between visual estimates made by the orthopedic surgeon and goniometric measurements made by two experienced physical therapists was 0.77 to 0.83, which indicates good agreement. Goniometric measurements taken by the two therapists were significantly different from measurements made by the single therapists, except for medial rotation. The authors[95] concluded that to obtain the most accurate results, measurements should be performed by two people assisting each other, with hip flexion motion being most reproducible.

Sutlive and colleagues[68] investigated the intertester reliability of measuring passive hip ROM in 30 patients with unilateral hip pain and possible OA by teams of two physical therapy doctoral students using standardized measurement methods. Universal goniometers were used for most hip ROM measurements, whereas inclinometers were used for hip rotations. The ICC values were acceptable, ranging from 0.54 for adduction to 0.85 for flexion and abduction and 0.88 for medial rotation. Absolute errors were reasonable, with standard error of measurement (SEM) values ranging from 0.7 to 2.0 degrees and minimal detectable change (MDC) values ranging from 1.9 to 5.5 degrees. These results suggest that doctoral physical therapy students demonstrated reproducible hip ROM measurements that were clinically acceptable.[68]

Croft and associates[97] had six clinicians use a fluid-filled inclinometer called a Plurimeter to take passive hip flexion and rotation ROM measurements of both hips in six patients with osteoarthritis involving only one hip joint. The results showed that the degree of agreement among testers was greatest for measurements of hip flexion.[97]

Pua and colleagues[108] reported on the intratester reliability of one physical therapist with 7 years of clinical experience who measured passive hip ROM in individuals with hip OA. Hip abduction ROM was measured using an extendable goniometer with the contralateral hip in 10 degrees of hip abduction. Hip flexion, extension, and rotations were measured using an electric inclinometer. Individuals returned for retesting an average of 19 days after the initial measurements. The intratester ICCs and absolute measurement errors indicate acceptable reliability and the minimum detectable changes were less than 11 degrees for all motions (see Table 8.7).[1]

Cibere and colleagues[106] investigated whether standardization (e.g., consensus about technique, landmarks) would influence the intertester reliability of hip ROM measured with a goniometer. Passive hip ROM of six individuals with hip OA (63 years; range 49–65 years) was measured by physicians (rheumatologists and orthopedic surgeons). The reliability coefficient (*Rc*) was calculated as $Rc = 1 - \text{variance}_{\text{doctor}}$, where $\text{variance}_{\text{doctor}}$ was the proportion of the total variance attributed to the doctors. Prestandardization *Rc*s were greater than 0.87 for hip flexion, abduction, medial rotation in sitting and supine positions, and lateral rotation in supine position. After standardization instructions, *Rc* for hip lateral rotation in sitting position improved from 0.55 to 0.80, whereas hip adduction decreased from 0.72 to 0.56. Therefore, the intertester reliability between these two disciplines was acceptable for most hip measurements, even prior to standardizing the protocols.[106]

Cliborne and associates[112] investigated the intratester reliability of hip flexion in 22 individuals with osteoarthritis of the knee (mean age = 61.2 years) and 17 individuals without symptoms. Results indicated that intratester reliability for hip flexion for two pairs of testers using an inclinometer was excellent, with an ICC of 0.94. Poulsen and colleagues[109] reported on the intertester reliability of two orthopedists and two chiropractors measuring six hip motions in patients with OA. Hip ROMs were measured once by each tester with a goniometer and the value was recorded to the nearest 5 degrees. An assistant helped hold the limb during hip extension measurements. Results for reproducibility were fair to poor between the pair of orthopedists and the pair of chiropractors. Absolute differences between the ROM measurements of both practitioner groups were variable and hip medial rotation had the worst standard error of the measurement (see Table 8.8).

The reliability of measuring hip ROM in patients with orthopedic conditions other than OA has also been studied. Nussbaumer and colleagues[101] tested the intratester reliability of goniometric measurements of passive hip ROM in individuals with femoroacetabular impingement and healthy people. Because ICCs for test-retest measurements were similar between groups, the results were combined and are reported in Table 8.7. Findings suggest that goniometric values can be used with confidence in the clinic.

Cibulka and colleagues[113] measured passive medial and lateral hip rotation in 100 individuals with low-back pain, and determined that goniometric measurements of rotation taken in the prone position were more reliable than those taken in the sitting position.

Six adults with cerebral palsy (CP) were the subjects in a reliability study conducted by Cadenhead and associates.[111] The investigators tested the intratester reliability of hip ROM measurements taken by a physical therapist and found the reliability to be acceptable for clinical use (see Table 8.7).

Infants and Children

Researchers have also investigated the reliability of hip ROM measurement in healthy infants[27] and in children with spastic cerebral palsy[94,99,110] and femoral fractures.[114]

Drews[27] measured hip extension ROM in healthy infants while they were positioned in side-lying and found better intertester reliability when using an inclinometer compared with a goniometer (see Table 8.8).

Fosang and associates[110] tested the intratester and intertester reliability of passive hip abduction ROM in children with cerebral palsy. The six testers were physical therapists with between 4 and 21 years of clinical practice treating children. The therapists worked in pairs to take measurements of each child twice daily over 6 days. The authors cautioned that given the wide error margins for reliability measures, potentially large changes in hip abduction ROM are needed to assure that changes are not the result of measurement error alone (see Tables 8.7 and 8.8).

Mutlu and associates[99] conducted a study in which passive ROM was measured in children with spastic cerebral palsy. Three physical therapists used a goniometer to measure hip ROM once in each session on two different occasions 1 week apart. Given the intratester reliability and intertester reliability (see Tables 8.7 and 8.8, respectively), Mutlu and colleagues[99] concluded that experience played a role in goniometric reliability and measurements were appropriate for use in the clinic.

McWhirk and Glanzman[94] found that the intertester reliability for hip abduction ROM was high when measured in 25 children aged 2 to 18 years with spastic cerebral palsy (ICC = 0.91; 95% CI for mean absolute difference = 3.5 ± 1.5 degrees). Of note is that two therapists with differing levels of pediatric experience (10 years and 1 year) assisted each other during the measurements when achieving these high levels of intertester reliability.

Owen and colleagues[114] reported on active hip ROM in 82 children who incurred a femoral shaft fracture and were treated with an external fixator or a spica cast. Testers measured active hip ROM at 15 and 24 months post-fracture using goniometric protocols established by the AAOS. It was unclear whether comparisons for intertester reliability were made within one time frame or between 15 and 24 months' post-fracture. Even using standardized protocols for active hip ROM, relative intertester reliability was low (see Table 8.8). Based on calculation of 95% limits of agreement the authors concluded that true change occurs only when differences exceed 30 degrees for most hip motions.[114] However, the limits of agreement appeared to be determined using the standard deviations of the means, which is more indicative of biological variation.

Reliability and Validity of Muscle Length Testing

Muscle length testing in the clinical setting is typically graded as positive (short) or negative (within normal limits). Objective values in degrees of joint angle at the end of the tests are less frequently measured. However, the reliability of the objective measures indicates whether the muscle length tests are appropriate for clinical use.

Reliability of the Thomas Test

Evidence from reliability studies suggests that using a goniometer[21,56,115–117] and inclinometer[56] to measure hip flexor shortness during the Thomas test is appropriate for clinical use with healthy individuals. However, others have reported less favorable results in healthy individuals[41,59] and in those with an orthopedic or neurological impairment, suggesting that this test may be less suitable for clinical use in certain individuals.[94,96,98,99,118,119] As in other measurement procedures, intratester reliability is usually better than intertester reliability.

Healthy Population

Aalto and colleagues[11] reported acceptable intratester reliability for the Thomas test using healthy individuals. Two well-trained physical therapists each performed the testing independently. This study's protocol positioned the individual's opposite hip in maximal flexion and the tester used a goniometer to measure passive sagittal plane hip ROM without assistance. Though the intratester ICCs were high for both testers, the absolute differences were variable between testers (see Table 8.9). The intertester ICCs were not as favorable, suggesting that the same tester should repeat the measurements (Table 8.10).

Winters and colleagues[115] reported that within-session ICCs were 0.98 for both intratester and intertester reliability, indicating excellent reliability. An investigator performed a modified Thomas test with assistance on 20 healthy individuals without low-back pain or lumbar quadrant symptoms. Additional details about the demographics of the testers and individuals tested were not disclosed. Harvey[116] reported on the intratester reliability during the modified Thomas test in 117 elite athletes (e.g., tennis, basketball, rowing, and running). The athlete held one limb in maximal hip flexion while the opposite limb was lowered toward the floor. A goniometer was used to measure hip flexion, hip abduction, and knee flexion of the lowered limb. Though specific ICCs for each motion were not provided, the ICC range (0.91–0.94) suggests that the Thomas test is highly reliable for clinical use.[1] Furthermore, the results suggest that these elite athletes have short one-joint and two-joint hip flexors.

Clapis and colleagues[56] reported on the reliability of goniometer and inclinometer measurements during the modified Thomas test and found that the relative intertester reliability was high (> 0.89) and the absolute error was low (SEM < 2.1 degrees) in healthy adults (see Table 8.10).

Godges and colleagues[117] measured passive hip extension ROM with a goniometer during a modified Thomas test. Modifications included the use of bilateral leg braces locking the knees at 90 degrees of flexion. One tester had two assistants (one to assist with the limb placement, one to read standardized instructions) during the measurement. The relative reliability was acceptable for measurements taken prior to and following an intervention: One group was assigned to hip stretching and another was assigned to trunk strengthening (see Table 8.9).

Wang and colleagues[21] performed intratester reliability testing on healthy individuals and also used a knee brace to control for the knee position: knee extended to measure iliopsoas and knee flexed to 90 degrees to measure rectus femoris ROM. The tester had assistance and measurements were repeated within 1 or 2 days. The ICCs were 0.97, indicating excellent intratester reliability (see Table 8.9). Although the two aforementioned studies report acceptable relative reliability, a Thomas test protocol that requires a knee brace is not commonly performed in a clinical setting.

Van Dillen and colleagues[59] measured test-retest reliability on healthy individuals and found that the relative intratester reliability of goniometric values measured during the Thomas test was acceptable for clinical use (Table 8.9). However, the sample size was small and the measurement was obtained using three examiners: One examiner palpated the lumbar spine, assured the spine was flat, and determined when lumbar motion occurred; a second examiner controlled the limb during the passive ROM; and a third examiner read and recorded the goniometric findings. The occupation and experience of the examiners were not provided.

Peeler and Anderson[41] reported on the intratester and intertester reliability of measuring sagittal plane hip ROM values and scoring the Thomas test as pass or fail. Three testers, who were certified athletic trainers with 6 to 22 years of experience, performed test-retest assessments 7 to 10 days apart in healthy individuals. The protocol was modified as the individual was instructed to hold a bent knee to the chest while the opposite knee was to remain at 90 degrees with the thigh resisting flat on the table. The knee angle of the lower leg was

TABLE 8.9 Intratester Reliability of Muscle Length Testing Using the Thomas Test for the Hip Flexors

Study	*N*	Sample	Methods	*r*	ICC	Absolute Reliability
Healthy Populations						
Aalto et al[11]	20	Healthy adults (18–45 yr)	2 testers (PT), goniometer Hip extension angle Knee flexion angle		Tester 1; 2 .96; .95 .87; .81	CV (%): Tester 1; 2 9.3; 29.1 4.3; 3.3
Godges et al[117]	25	Healthy males (19–24 yr)	1 tester, 2 assistants,* goniometer, knee braced at 90° flexion		Pre-; post-intervention: .80; .88	
Kilgour et al[98]	25	Healthy children (6–17 yr)	1 tester, 2 assistants* (PT), goniometer, knee extended		(range for 2 limbs and 2 sessions) .09–.91	Mean absolute difference (°) intrasession: 0.7 intersession: 1.3
Peeler et al[41]	54	Healthy adults (18–45 yr)	3 testers (ATC), goniometer in degrees		Tester 1; 2; 3: .65; .72; .67	
Peeler et al[41]	54	Healthy adults (18–45 yr)	3 testers (ATC), Pass/Fail score		κ statistics for tester 1; 2; 3: .54; .39; .28	
Van Dillen[59]	10	Healthy adults (31 ± 11 yr old)	1 tester, 2 assistants,* goniometer, 2 positions: 80° knee flexion 0° knee flexion		.70 .72	
Wang et al[127]	10	Individuals' details not provided	1 tester, goniometer, 2 positions: Knee braced at 90° flexion Knee braced at 0° flexion		.97 .97	
Patient Populations						
Bartlett et al[119]	14	Children/young adults with myelomeningocele (4–19 yr)	2 testers, goniometer	.93		Mean difference (°) 5.1
Bartlett et al[119]	14	Children/young adults with spastic diplegia (6–20 yr)	2 testers, goniometer	.89		Mean difference (°) 3.2
Glanzman et al[120]	25	Children with cerebral palsy (6–18 yr)	1–2 testers, goniometer, 1 person measuring 2 persons measuring		.98 .98	
Kilgour et al[98]	25	Children with spastic diplegia (6–17 yr)	1 tester, 2 assistants* (PT), goniometer, knee extended		range: 2 limbs and 2 sessions .17–.66	Mean absolute difference (°) intrasession: 1.0 intersession: 1.2
Mutlu et al[99]	38	Children with spastic cerebral palsy (18–108 mo)	3 testers (PT), goniometer	Tester 1; 2; 3; .88, .99, .61	Tester 1; 2; 3; .92, .99, .73	
Pandya et al[96]	150	Children/young adults with Duchenne muscular dystrophy (under 1–20 yr)	5 testers (PT), goniometer, knee extended		.85	
Pua et al[131]	22	Adults with hip osteoarthritis (50–84 yr)	1 tester (PT), goniometer, Knee flexed 80° Knee unconstrained		.86 .89	SEM; MDC (°) 4.5; 10.5 4.7; 11.0

ICC = Interclass correlation coefficient; CV = Coefficient of variation; MDC = Minimal detectable change; SEM = Standard error of measurement; *r* = Pearson product-moment correlation coefficient; ATC = athletic trainer certified; PT = Physical therapist(s). K statistic = Kappa statistic; ° = degrees.

*An assistant provided help during the assessment.

TABLE 8.10 Intertester Reliability of Muscle Length Testing Using the Thomas Test for the Hip Flexors

Study	N	Sample	Methods	r	ICC	Absolute Reliability
Healthy Populations						
Aalto et al[11]	20	Healthy adults (18–45 yr)	2 testers (PT), goniometer, Hip extension Knee flexion		 .87 .62	CV (%) 79.8 9.4
Bartlett et al[119]	15	Healthy children and young adults (3–20 yr)	2 testers, goniometer			Mean difference (°) 1.9
Clapis et al[56]	42	Healthy adults (18–36 yr)	2 testers (PT), Goniometer Inclinometer		 .92 .89	SEM (°) 1.9 2.1
Lee et al[86]	37	Healthy children (5–15 yr)	3 testers, goniometer		.21	Mean absolute difference (°) 1.2
Peeler et al[41]	54	Healthy adults (18–45 yr)	3 testers (ATC) Goniometer in degrees Pass/Fail scores		 .50 κ statistics .33	SEM (°); CV (%); 7; 19
Patient Populations						
Ashton et al[118]	4	Children with spastic cerebral palsy (2 mild, 2 moderate) (10–13 yr)	16 testers (PT), goniometer Specific instruction Nonspecific instruction		Mild CP; moderate CP .55; .70 .53; .70	
Bartlett et al[119]	15	Children/young adults with myelomeningocele (4–19 yr)	2 testers, goniometer	.90		Mean difference between 2 testers (°) 6.4
Bartlett et al[119]	15	Children/young adults with spastic diplegia (6–20 yr)	2 testers, goniometer	.70		Mean difference between 2 testers (°) 9.2
Currier et al[82]	25	Adults with knee osteoarthritis (51–79 yr)	2 testers (PT student) Hip extension, inclinometer Knee flexion, goniometer		 .20 .07	SEM (°); CV (%) 4.5; 24 8.2; 4
Lee et al[86]	36	Children with cerebral palsy (5–19 yr)	3 testers, goniometer		.50	Mean absolute difference (°) 5.8
McWhirk and Glanzman[94]	25	(46 hips) Children with cerebral palsy (2–18 yr)	2 testers (PT), goniometer		.58	Mean absolute difference (°) 4.0
Mutlu et al[99]	38	Children with spastic CP (18–108 mo, mean 53 mo)	3 testers (PTs, goniometer		.95	
Owen et al[114]	101	Children, post-fractured femur (4–10 yr)	4 clinical sites, number of testers not provided, goniometer		.19	Mean difference (°); 95% LOA (°) .02; –28.8 to 28.8
Pandya et al[96]	21	Children/young adults with Duchenne muscular dystrophy (< 1–20 yr)	5 testers (PT), goniometer, knee extended		.74	

ICC = Interclass correlation coefficient; CV = Coefficient of variation; MDC = Minimal detectable change; SEM = Standard error of measurement; *r* = Pearson product moment correlation coefficient; LOA = Limits of agreement; ATC = Athletic trainer certified; PT = Physical therapist(s); ° = degrees.

*An assistant provided help during the assessment.

measured with the axis of rotation of the goniometer aligned over the head of the fibula. A passing score was assigned if the test knee remained in a stationary 90-degree position, whereas a failing score was assigned if the knee extended to less than 90 degrees. Both intratester and intertester reliability results indicated that the goniometric method was more consistent than the pass/fail method (see Tables 8.9 and 8.10). However, the high absolute errors bring into question the clinical use of this modified Thomas test to measure two-joint muscle mobility, even when clinicians have experience and are similarly trained. For example, the minimum detectable difference of 19 degrees suggests that a 19-degree difference in knee flexion ROM is needed to assume that a real difference occurs between the test and retest scores.

Patient Populations

The clinical utility for measuring sagittal plane hip ROM using the Thomas test for individuals with hip osteoarthritis (OA) is inconclusive because reliability results vary. Pua and colleagues[108] reported on the intratester reliability of hip flexion measured with an extendable goniometer in people with hip OA. An experienced physical therapist measured passive hip flexion, first with the knee constrained at approximately 80 degrees of flexion, and then with the knee hanging freely, unconstrained. Good ICCs for intratester reliability were obtained (Table 8.9). A large amount of time elapsed between the test and retest measurements (median of 19 days). Currier and colleagues[82] reported on the reliability of the Thomas test in individuals who had knee OA. Results suggest that the hip extension measured with a gravity inclinometer is not reliable between two physical therapy students; however, the knee ROM values measured with a goniometer appear to be more reproducible between testers (Table 8.10).

Investigators have reported on the reliability of using the Thomas test for children with various medical diagnoses[86,94,96,98,99,114,118–121] and in some studies have included healthy children as controls. The most numerous reliability studies in patient populations have focused on children with spastic cerebral palsy. Kilgour and colleagues[98] reported on the reliability of one pediatric physical therapist who measured children with and without spastic diplegia. The therapist had 30 years of experience and performed the Thomas test while assisted by a holder and recorder. Measurements were repeated within one session and 7 days later to test intratester intrasession and intersession reliability, respectively. Relative and absolute reliability was reported for children with and without spastic diplegia and the absolute difference was calculated using the initial measurements from Session 1 and Session 2 (see Table 8.10). Although the range for the ICCs was large, the absolute errors were low for both groups. Averaging measures did not improve reliability compared with single measures. The therapists also measured a fixed joint on a mannequin. Variation of the fixed joint measurements was very low, yet the variation in both groups was high, indicating that a major source of error in the study may be due to difficulty in determining the correct end-range joint positioning. Additionally, the similar measurement variability seen in children with and without spastic diplegia indicates that measurement error was not influenced by the presence of spasticity. Given the results, the authors concluded that the Thomas test can be used clinically for children with and without spasticity and that there was no need for taking multiple measurements within one session.

Bartlett and colleagues[119] investigated whether two therapists who were experienced users of the goniometer had acceptable intratester reliability. The therapists participated in detailed training sessions to ensure uniform testing procedures during the Thomas test. Children with spastic diplegia and meningomyelocele were measured initially and again after a 45-minute wait. Acceptable relative reliability was found for both groups; however, the absolute differences between the initial and follow-up measurements were larger for the children with meningomyelocele[119] (see Table 8.9). Bartlett and colleagues[119] also assessed the intertester reliability of using the Thomas test on children and young adults in three groups: those with spastic diplegia, meningomyelocele, and healthy controls. Intertester absolute differences (value of tester 2 minus value of tester 1) indicated that less difference was found in the healthy group (see Table 8.10). Because the Thomas test was not as reliable and reproducible in those with medical diagnoses, the authors recommended use of the Thomas test for individuals without spasticity.

Lee and colleagues[86] report variable and less than acceptable ICCs for intertester reliability for children with and without cerebral palsy. However, they[86] concluded that the mean absolute differences support the clinical utility of the Thomas test for children with and without cerebral palsy (see Table 8.10).

Ashton and colleagues[118] investigated whether intertester reliability would differ when physical therapists used specific or nonspecific measurement instructions during the Thomas test when measuring children with spastic diplegia. Results indicated that the type of instructions did not influence reliability (see Table 8.10). Because the relative reliability of the Thomas test was low, the authors summarized that the measurements were not sufficiently reliable for studying children with cerebral palsy.

McWhirk and Glanzman[94] found low intertester reliability when different therapists used the Thomas test to measure hip extension in children with spastic cerebral palsy. Two physical therapists (10 years versus 1 year of experience) assisted each other to help support and stabilize the limbs during the measurements. Though the relative reliability results were low, the absolute error suggests that a less experienced and more experienced therapist can produce measures within 6 degrees during the same session (Table 8.10). The results[94] demonstrated that therapists with differing levels of pediatric experience can achieve moderate to high levels of intertester reliability when using a strict protocol and a second person to assist.

Others have reported more favorable results, thus supporting the Thomas test for children with cerebral palsy. Glanzman and colleagues[120] reported that the relative intratester reliability was acceptable for muscle length testing using the Thomas test for clinical use in children with cerebral palsy (see Table 8.10). These investigators reported that relative reliability was no different when the tester performed the measurement with and without an assistant. Mutlu and associates[99] also reported high intra- and intertester reliability for the Thomas test (see Tables 8.9 and 8.10, respectively). Three physical therapists measured children with cerebral palsy on two different occasions 1 week apart, suggesting that the Thomas test can be used clinically for children with spastic diplegia.[99] However, Stuberg and colleagues[121,122] reported less intratester variability compared with intertester variability and concluded that the same tester should repeat the Thomas test when assessing hip extension in children with moderate to severe hypertonicity.

In a study by Pandya and colleagues,[96] five physical therapists used goniometers to measure passive hip extension using a Thomas test in 105 children and adolescents who had Duchenne muscular dystrophy. The children and adolescents were recruited from four clinics and each therapist took measurements three times within a 1-month period. Intratester reliability was better than the intertester reliability (Tables 8.9 and 8.10); therefore, the investigators concluded that the same examiner should take follow-up measurements to assess the results of therapeutic intervention for those diagnosed with Duchenne muscular dystrophy.

Owen and colleagues[114] studied the intertester reliability of the Thomas test in children with femur fracture who were treated with a hip spica cast or an external fixator. To be eligible for this study, the child needed to be able to actively extend the hip. Four international sites participated in the data collections. The reported limits of agreement suggest that differences between two measurements obtained by different examiners would need to exceed 29 degrees to be 95% confident that the differences represent a true change in hip extension. Given children's average hip extension ROM, this high value of change may be unlikely[114] (see Table 8.10).

Reliability of the Straight Leg Raise (SLR) Test

In general, evidence suggests that measurements of hamstring muscle length via the SLR test have acceptable intratester and intertester reliability and thus are clinically useful.[12,123–125] (Tables 8.11 and 8.12, respectively). Hanten and Chandler[125] obtained measurements on healthy females only and reported on the ICCs of retest measures that occurred immediately within the same session. A fluid-filled goniometer was placed on the lateral thigh, 10 centimeters proximal to the lateral femoral condyle, and straps were used to stabilize the opposite limb in 20 degrees of hip flexion. High intratester ICCs were reported when measuring the passive SLR angle[125] (see Table 8.11).

Gajdosik and colleagues[123] reported on the test-retest reliability in healthy males using a goniometer and found moderate ICC levels with and without straps. In addition to assessing the repeatability of the SLR test, Gajdosik and colleagues[123] tested whether stabilization straps improved the reliability of SLR values in 15 healthy males. The tests were repeated after 30 minutes of rest. The examiner performed the SLR using stabilization straps and using the traditional method of having the individual maintain a flat back (posterior pelvic tilt). The ICCs for both methods were acceptable, the measures were highly correlated with each other (Pearson correlation: $r = 0.70$), and the values were not significantly different; therefore, straps are not necessary[123] (see Table 8.11).

Ylinen, Kautiainen, and Hakkinen[126] tested whether the active SLR, passive manual SLR (e.g., maximum tolerated stretch, not passive ROM), and instrumented SLR were reliable measures. Men with decreased hamstring flexibility who played recreational sports four times per week on average were recruited. Test-retest reproducibility on the same day indicates an acceptable range of relative and absolute reliability (see Table 8.11). The coefficient of reproducibility reported is the expected absolute difference between the same-day test-retest values. The researchers[126] also compared measurement methods to investigate the validity of the methods and test whether the methods were sensitive to changes in the SLR test. Therefore, the males were tested at baseline and 4 weeks after participating in a home-based, right-leg-stretching program with the left leg serving as the control. Findings indicated that the values for the SLR in the stretched limb were significantly different between the three testing methods, with the instrumented SLR showing good sensitivity to changes, whereas the active and passive manual SLR showed a poor ability to detect change. Thus, the authors[126] concluded that although ICCs appear to be acceptable for active, manual, and instrumented SLR methods, the instrumented SLR was able to differentiate changes between the stretched and unstretched limb. A limitation of this study was that the order of testing was active, passive, then instrumented SLR.[126] Furthermore, clinically instrumented SLR devices are not typically available to test systematic changes over time.

Wang and colleagues[127] reported high ICCs for the SLR, with a brace locking the knee in extension, when retesting occurred 1 to 2 days later (see Table 8.11).

Hsieh, Walker, and Gillia[128] investigated whether three methods to measure a passive SLR resulted in different reliability values. High ICCs were reported when using a goniometer, flexometer (gravity-type goniometer), or tape measure to take the measurement within the same session. However, the tape measure values were not as reliable when the retest measurements were performed on a different day with an average of 3 days between tests (intersession reliability)[128] (see Table 8.11).

Aalto and colleagues[11] reported that SLR values in healthy adults remained stable over a 2-day period and a

TABLE 8.11 Intratester Reliability of Muscle Length Testing Using the Straight Leg Raise (SLR) for the Hip Extensors

Study	N	Sample	Methods	ICC	Absolute Reliability
Healthy Populations					
Aalto et al[11]	20	Healthy adults (18–45 yr)	Passive, 2 testers (PT), goniometer	(Tester 1; 2)	CV (%) (Tester 1; 2)
			Intraday	.94; .96	3.6; 2.9
			Interday	.79; 99	6.4; 2.6
Gajdosik et al[123]	15	Healthy males (mean 23 yr)	Passive, 1 tester,* gravity pendulum goniometer,		
			No straps	.88	
			Straps	.83	
Hanten and Chandler[125]	75	Healthy females (18–29 yr)	Passive, fluid- filled inclinometer	.91	
Hsieh et al[128]	10	Healthy adults (26–30 yr)	1 tester (PT),*	Intra; Intersession	SD of intrasession measurement error (°)
			Goniometer	.95; .88	1.9
			Flexometer	.97; .88	1.5
			Tape measure	.99; .74	1.5
Kilgour et al[98]	25	Healthy children (6–17 yr)	1 tester (PT),* goniometer	(range for 2 limbs and 2 sessions)	Mean absolute difference (°)
			Intrasession	.99–.99	2.4
			Intersession	.52–.61	8.1
Lindell et al[129]	20	Healthy adults (22–55 yr)	Active, 2 testers		SEM; mean difference (°)
			PT	.99	2; 0
			Research assistant	.97	3; 0
Ylinen et al[126]	12	Healthy males (mean 34 yr)	Digital protractor, knee braced	.91	Coefficient of reproducibility 7
Youdas et al[12]	43	Healthy adults (20–79 yr old)	Passive, 2 testers (PT), goniometer	.98	
Wang et al[127]	10	Healthy adults (18–37 yr old)	1 tester,* goniometer, knee braced in extension	.90	
Patient Populations					
Kilgour et al[98]	25	Children with cerebral palsy (6–17 yr)	1 tester (PT),* goniometer	(range for 2 limbs and 2 sessions)	Mean absolute difference (°)
			Intrasession	.95–.98	4.2
			Intersession	.62–.63	6.6

ICC = Interclass correlation coefficient; CV = Coefficient of variation; SD = Standard deviation; SEM = Standard error of measurement; PT = Physical therapist(s); ° = degrees.

*An assistant provided help during the assessment.

separate fixing protocol was not required to detect changes over time. These authors[11] concluded that using the goniometer to measure passive SLR was repeatable for one tester, and between testers, within the same session (intraday) and over 2 days (interday) (see Tables 8.11 and 8.12, respectively). There was, however, no mention of how the tester stabilized the pelvis.

Youdas and colleagues[12] reported acceptable intratester reliability when experienced physical therapists used a goniometer to measure the passive SLR angle on both limbs for a large number of individuals tested over a large age span (see Table 8.11).

Lindell, Eriksson, and Strender[129] tested whether trained and untrained individuals could perform the active SLR test reliably. Healthy individuals were tested three times during one session: twice by one tester and once by another. The intratester reliability appeared acceptable (see Table 8.11). Intertester reliability statistics were calculated from measurements on healthy adults and adults with neck and/or back pain. The researchers[129] used strict criteria for reliability and given

TABLE 8.12 Intertester Reliability of Muscle Length Testing Using the Straight Leg Raise (SLR) for the Hip Extensors

Study	N	Sample	Methods	ICC	Absolute Reliability
Healthy Populations					
Aalto et al[11]	20	Healthy adults (18–45 yr)	Passive, 2 testers (PT), goniometer		CV (%)
			Intraday	.94	5.2
			Interday	.94	5.7
Lindell et al[129]	20	Healthy adults (2–55 yr)	Active, 2 testers (PT, research assistant), goniometer	.84	SEM; mean difference (°) 5; 4
Patient Populations					
Lindell et al[129]	30	Adults with neck and/or back pain > 4 weeks (20–63 yr)	Active, 2 testers (PT, research assistant), goniometer	.96	SEM; mean difference (°) 4; 2
Piva et al[124]	30	Adults with patellofemoral pain syndrome (29 ± 8.4 yr)]	Passive, 4 testers (PT), gravity goniometer on lower half of anterior tibia	.92	SEM (°) 4.3

ICC = Interclass correlation coefficient; CV = Coefficient of variation; SEM = Standard error of measurement; PT = Physical therapist(s); ° = degrees.

the relative and absolute differences between testers, the use of an untrained examiner to measure the active SLR was not supported (see Table 8.12).

Piva and colleagues[124] conducted a multicenter study and four physical therapists (one pair working together from each site) obtained two SLR measures on individuals diagnosed with patellofemoral pain syndrome. Measurements were obtained using a gravity goniometer (e.g., inclinometer) and the average SLR trials were recorded. Intertester ICCs were acceptable for each pair of physical therapists[124] (see Table 8.12).

Kilgour and colleagues[98] investigated the reliability of using the SLR to measure hamstring length in children with and without cerebral palsy. Repeated measurements were obtained within one session and 7 days later to assess intrasession and intersession reliability, respectively (see Table 8.11). Because intersession variation in measures was similar for both groups, the researchers concluded that variability was not influenced by the presence of spasticity. Furthermore, averaging the two measures did not improve intersession reliability compared with the use of a single measure, indicating that repeated measures may not be necessary.[98]

Stuberg and colleagues[121] examined the reliability of using a goniometer to measure the SLR in children with moderate to severe hypertonicity (e.g., cerebral palsy; Reye, Sanfilippo, and Dandy-Walker syndromes; and trisomy 18). Results indicate that intratester differences were 7.6 degrees and percentage of agreement between testers at 5 degrees was only 30% for the SLR.[121]

Reliability of the Ober and Modified Ober Tests

The reliability of the Ober and Modified Ober tests appears to be clinically acceptable when measured with a goniometer or inclinometer for healthy adults and those with knee pain.[20,22,44,124,130] The use of a strict testing protocol and another person either to stabilize or to help hold the test limb has been suggested to improve the consistency of the testing.[20]

Gajdosik and colleagues[20] assessed the intratester reliability of measurements of the Ober and Modified Ober tests using three repeated measurements in one session. The healthy individuals being tested were positioned in side-lying position with the bottom hip and knee flexed to 45 degrees to help stabilize the pelvis. One therapist administered the test while an assistant positioned the goniometer to align with a line drawn to mark the midline of the thigh and read the goniometer. The ICCs for men were slightly lower than for women for the Ober test and the Modified Ober test (Table 8.13), perhaps because the heavier limb of men relative to women influencing the ability to stabilize the pelvis.[20]

Reese and Bandy[22] used an inclinometer on the distal thigh to determine the intratester reliability of the repeated measurements of the Ober and Modified Ober tests in healthy adults. Intratester reliability was indicated as acceptable based on relative and absolute reliability, suggesting that both tests are acceptable for clinical use[22] (see Table 8.13).

Herrington and colleagues[44] used a pressure biofeedback device to detect onset of motion of the pelvis. Though there was a small sample size of only five healthy subjects, the relative and absolute reliability measures indicate that the methodology used here is acceptable for clinical use[44] (see Table 8.13).

Piva and colleagues[124] used an inclinometer to measure the frontal plane hip angle in adults with patellofemoral pain

TABLE 8.13 Intratester Reliability of Muscle Length Testing Using the Ober and Modified Ober Tests for the Hip Abductors

Study	N	Sample	Methods	r	ICC	Absolute Reliability
Healthy Populations						
Gajdoski et al[20]	49	Healthy adults (20–43, mean 27 yr)	2 testers,* goniometer		Men; women	
			Ober		.83; .87	
			Modified Ober		.82; .92	
Reese and Bandy[2]	61	Healthy adults (21–30, mean 24 yr)	1 tester (PT),* inclinometer			Mean absolute difference (°) between days
			Ober		.90	.6
			Modified Ober		.91	.4
Herrington et al[44]	5	Healthy adults (18–34 yr)	Fluid goniometer, pressure biofeedback unit at pelvis			SEM (°)
			Ober	.96		1.3
			Modified Ober	.97		1.1
Patient Populations						
Melchione and Sullivan[130]	10	Adolescents/adults with knee pain (16–43 yr)	2 testers (PTs), inclinometer, Modified Ober Knee in 5° of flexion; special leveling device on pelvis		.94	SEM (°) 1.0

r = Pearson product moment correlation coefficient; ICC = Interclass correlation coefficient; SEM = Standard error of measurement; PT = Physical therapist(s); ° = degrees.

TABLE 8.14 Intertester Reliability of Muscle Length Testing Using the Ober and Modified Ober Tests for the Hip Abductors

Study	N	Sample	Methods	ICC	Absolute Reliability
Patient Populations					
Melchione and Sullivan[130]	10	Adolescents/adults with knee pain (16–43 yr)	2 testers (PT), inclinometer, Modified Ober with knee in 5° of flexion; special levelling device on pelvis	.73	SEM (°) 2.0
Piva et al[124]	30	Adults with patellofemoral pain syndrome (mean 29 yr)	4 testers (PT), gravity inclinometer, Ober	.97	SEM (°) 2.1

ICC = Interclass correlation coefficient; SEM = Standard error of measurement; PT = Physical therapist(s).

syndrome. The relative and absolute relativity measures indicate that the Ober test is acceptable for clinical use in this population[1] (see Table 8.14).

Melchione and Sullivan[130] developed a specialized level device to attach to the pelvis to provide feedback while performing a modified version of the Ober test (5 degrees of knee flexion). These researchers recruited individuals with anterior knee pain to test the reliability of this new methodology. The relative and absolute reliability measures indicate that the methodology used here is acceptable for clinical use, even when a different tester obtains the follow-up measurement (Table 8.13 and Table 8.14, respectively).

REFERENCES

1. Martin, RL: The Hip Complex. In Levangie, P, and Norkin, CC: Joint Structure and Function: A Comprehensive Analysis, ed 5. FA Davis, Philadelphia, 2011.
2. Cyriax, JH, and Cyriax, P: Illustrated Manual of Orthopaedic Medicine. Butterworths, London, 1983.
3. Greene, WB, and Heckman, JD (eds): The Clinical Measurement of Joint Motion. American Academy of Orthopaedic Surgeons, Rosemont, IL, 1994.
4. Cocchiarella, L, and Andersson, GBL (eds): Guides to the Evaluation of Permanent Impairment, ed 5. American Medical Association, Chicago, 2000.
5. Roach, KE, and Miles, TP: Normal hip and knee active range of motion: The relationship to age. Phys Ther 71(9):656, 1991.
6. Soucie, JM, et al: Range of motion measurements: Reference values and a database for comparison studies. Haemophilia 17(3):500, 2011.
7. Kumar, S, et al: Normal range of motion of hip and ankle in Indian population. Acta Orthop Traumatol Turc 45(6):421, 2011.
8. Rodinelli, RD (ed): Guides to Evaluation of Permanent Impairment, ed 6. American Medical Association, Chicago, 2007.
9. Boone, DC, and Azen, SP: Normal range of motion of joints in male subjects. J Bone Joint Surg Am 61(5):756, 1979.
10. Kendall, FP: Muscles: Testing and Function With Posture and Pain, ed 5. Lippincott Williams & Wilkins, Baltimore, 2005.
11. Aalto, TJ, et al: Effect of passive stretch on reproducibility of hip range of motion measurements. Arch Phys Med Rehabil 86(3):549, 2005.
12. Youdas, JW, et al: The influence of gender and age on hamstring muscle length in healthy adults. J Orthop Sports Phys Ther 35(4):246, 2005.
13. James, B, and Parker, AW: Active and passive mobility of lower limb joints in elderly men and women. Am J Phys Med Rehabil 68(4):162, 1989.
14. Ober, F: The role of the iliotibial band and fascia lata as a factor in the causation of lower back disabilities and sciatica. J Bone Joint Surg Am 18:105, 1936.
15. Noble, H, Hajeck, MR, and Porter, M: Diagnosis and treatment of iliotibial band tightness in runners. Phys Sports Med 10:67, 1982.
16. McConnell, J: The physical therapist's approach to patellofemoral disorders. Clin Sports Med 21(3):363, 2002.
17. Hoppenfeld, S: Physical Examination of the Spine and Extremities. Appleton-Century-Crofts, New York, 1976.
18. Gose, JC, and Schweizer, P: Iliotibial band tightness. J Orthop Sports Phys Ther 10(10):399, 1989.
19. Cade, D, et al: Indirectly measuring length of the iliotibial band and related hip structures: A correlational analysis of four adduction tests. Abstract Platform Presentation, APTA Combined Sections Meeting. J Orthop Sports Phys Ther 31:A22, 2001.
20. Gajdosik, RL, Sandler, MM, and Marr, HL: Influence of knee positions and gender on the Ober test for length of the iliotibial band. Clin Biomech 18(1):77, 2003.
21. Wang, TG, et al: Assessment of stretching of the iliotibial tract with Ober and modified Ober tests: An ultrasonographic study. Arch Phys Med Rehabil 87(10):1407, 2006.
22. Reese, NB, and Bandy, WD: Use of an inclinometer to measure flexibility of the iliotibial band using the Ober test and the modified Ober test: Differences in magnitude and reliability of measurements. J Orthop Sports Phys Ther 33(6):326, 2003.
23. Forero, N, Okamura, LA, and Larson, MA: Normal ranges of hip motion in neonates. J Pediatr Orthop 9(4):391, 1989.
24. Waugh, KG, et al: Measurement of selected hip, knee, and ankle joint motions in newborns. Phys Ther 63(10):1616, 1983.
25. Schwarze, DJ, and Denton, JR: Normal values of neonatal lower limbs: An evaluation of 1,000 neonates. J Pediatr Orthop 13(6):758, 1993.
26. Broughton, NS, Wright, J, and Menelaus, MB: Range of knee motion in normal neonates. J Pediatr Orthop 13(2):263, 1993.
27. Drews, J, Vraciu, JK, and Pellino, G: Range of motion of the joints of the lower extremities of newborns. Phys Occup Ther Pediatr 4:49, 1984.
28. Phelps, E, Smith, LJ, and Hallum, A: Normal ranges of hip motion of infants between nine and 24 months of age. Dev Med Child Neurol 27(6):785, 1985.
29. Sankar, WN, Laird, CT, and Baldwin, KD: Hip range of motion in children: What is the norm? J Pediatr Orthop 32(4):399, 2012.
30. Watanabe, H, et al: The range of motions of the extremities in healthy Japanese people: The difference according to age. Nippon Seikeigeka Gakkai Zasshi 53:275, 1979.
31. Walker, JM: Musculoskeletal development: A review. Phys Ther 71(12):878, 1991.
32. Svenningsen, S, et al: Hip motion related to age and sex. Acta Orthop Scand 60(1):97, 1989.
33. Walker, JM, et al: Active mobility of the extremities in older subjects. Phys Ther 64(6):919, 1984.
34. Allander, E, et al: Normal range of joint movements in shoulder, hip, wrist and thumb with special reference to side: A comparison between two populations. Int J Epidemiol 3(3):253, 1974.
35. Kozic, S, et al: Femoral anteversion related to side differences in hip rotation. Passive rotation in 1,140 children aged 8–9 years. Acta Orthop Scand 68(6):533, 1997.
36. Nonaka, H, et al: Age-related changes in the interactive mobility of the hip and knee joints: A geometrical analysis. Gait Posture 15(3):236, 2002.
37. Fairbank, JC, Pynsent, PB, and Phillips, H: Quantitative measurements of joint mobility in adolescents. Ann Rheum Dis 43(2):288, 1984.
38. Beighton, P, Solomon, L, and Soskolne, CL: Articular mobility in an African population. Ann Rheum Dis 32(5):413, 1973.
39. Boone, D, Walker, JM, and Perry, J: Age and sex differences in lower extremity joint motion. Paper presented at the National Conference of the American Physical Therapy Association, Washington, DC, 1981.
40. Simoneau, GG, et al: Influence of hip position and gender on active hip internal and external rotation. J Orthop Sports Phys Ther 28(3):158, 1998.
41. Peeler, JD, and Anderson, JE: Reliability limits of the modified Thomas test for assessing rectus femoris muscle flexibility about the knee joint. J Athl Train 43(5):470, 2008.
42. Hu, H, et al: Measurements of voluntary joint range of motion in the Chinese elderly living in Bejiing area by a photographic method. Int J Indust Ergon 36:861, 2006.
43. Sanya, AO, and Obi, CS: Range of motion in selected joints of diabetic and non-diabetic subjects. Afr J Health Sci 6(1):17, 1999.
44. Herrington, L, Rivett, N, and Munro, S: The relationship between patella position and length of the iliotibial band as assessed using Ober's test. Man Ther 11(3):182, 2006.
45. Bini, V, et al: Body mass index in children and adolescents according to age and pubertal stage. Eur J Clin Nutr 54(3):214, 2000.
46. Kettunen, JA, et al: Factors associated with hip joint rotation in former elite athletes. Br J Sports Med 34(1):44, 2000.
47. Escalante, A, et al: Determinants of hip and knee flexion range: Results from the San Antonio Longitudinal Study of Aging. Arthritis Care Res 12(1):8, 1999.
48. Lichtenstein, MJ, et al: Modeling impairment: Using the disablement process as a framework to evaluate determinants of hip and knee flexion. Aging (Milano) 12(3):208, 2000.
49. Bennell, K, et al: Hip and ankle range of motion and hip muscle strength in young female ballet dancers and controls. Br J Sports Med 33(5):340, 1999.
50. Schmid, A, et al: Improvements in speed-based gait classifications are meaningful. Stroke 38(7):2096, 2007.
51. Studenski, S, et al: Physical performance measures in the clinical setting. J Am Geriatr Soc 51(3):314, 2003.
52. Purser, JL, et al: Walking speed predicts health status and hospital costs for frail elderly male veterans. J Rehabil Res Dev 42(4):535, 2005.
53. Clapper, MP, and Wolf, SL: Comparison of the reliability of the Orthoranger and the standard goniometer for assessing active lower extremity range of motion. Phys Ther 68(2):214, 1988.
54. Bierma-Zeinstra, SM, et al. Comparison between two devices for measuring hip joint motions. Clin Rehabil 12(6):497, 1998.
55. Roach S, et al: Concurrent validity of digital inclinometer and universal goniometer in assessing passive hip mobility in healthy subjects. Int J Sports Phys Ther 8(5):680, 2013.
56. Clapis, PA, Davis, SM, and Davis, RO: Reliability of inclinometer and goniometric measurements of hip extension flexibility using the modified Thomas test. Physiother Theory Pract 24(2):135, 2008.
57. Cyriax, J: Textbook of Orthopaedic Medicine: Vol. 1: Diagnosis of Soft Tisse Lesions, ed 8. Bailliere Tindall, London, 1982.
58. Kumar, D, et al: Differences in the association of hip cartilage lesions and cam-type femoroacetabular impingement with movement patterns: A preliminary study. PM R 2014.
59. Van Dillen, LR, et al: Effect of knee and hip position on hip extension range of motion in individuals with and without low back pain. J Orthop Sports Phys Ther 30(6):307, 2000.
60. Gilbert, CB, Gross, MT, and Klug, KB: Relationship between hip external rotation and turnout angle for the five classical ballet positions. J Orthop Sports Phys Ther 27(5):339, 1998.

61. Steinberg, N, et al: Range of joint movement in female dancers and non-dancers aged 8 to 16 years: Anatomical and clinical implications. Am J Sports Med 34(5):814, 2006.
62. Tyler, TF, et al: Groin injuries in sports medicine. Sports Health 2(3):231, 2010.
63. Emery, CA, Meeuwisse, WH, and Powell, JW: Groin and abdominal strain injuries in the National Hockey League. Clin J Sport Med 9(3):151, 1999.
64. Shindle, MK, et al: Hockey injuries: A pediatric sport update. Curr Opin Pediatr 22(1):54, 2010.
65. Ellison, JB, Rose, SJ, and Sahrmann, SA: Patterns of hip rotation range of motion: A comparison between healthy subjects and patients with low back pain. Phys Ther 70(9):537, 1990.
66. Altman, RD: The classification of osteoarthritis. J Rheumatol Suppl 43:42, 1995.
67. Altman, R, et al: The American College of Rheumatology criteria for the classification and reporting of osteoarthritis of the hip. Arthritis Rheum 34(5):505, 1991.
68. Sutlive, TG, et al: Development of a clinical prediction rule for diagnosing hip osteoarthritis in individuals with unilateral hip pain. J Orthop Sports Phys Ther 38(9):542, 2008.
69. Arokoski, MH, et al: Physical function in men with and without hip osteoarthritis. Arch Phys Med Rehabil 85(4):574, 2004.
70. Steultjens, MP, et al: Range of joint motion and disability in patients with osteoarthritis of the knee or hip. Rheumatology (Oxford) 39(9):955, 2000.
71. Mollinger, LA, and Steffen, TM: Knee flexion contractures in institutionalized elderly: Prevalence, severity, stability, and related variables. Phys Ther 73(7):437, 1993.
72. Kerrigan, DC, et al: Reduced hip extension during walking: Healthy elderly and fallers versus young adults. Arch Phys Med Rehabil 82(1):26, 2001.
73. Beissner, KL, Collins, JE, and Holmes, H: Muscle force and range of motion as predictors of function in older adults. Phys Ther 80(6):556, 2000.
74. Magee, DJ. Orthopedic Physical Assessment, ed 4. Saunders, Philadelphia, 2002.
75. Newman, P, et al: Risk factors associated with medial tibial stress syndrome in runners: A systematic review and meta-analysis. Open Access J Sports Med 4:229, 2013.
76. Yagi, S, Muneta, T, and Sekiya, I: Incidence and risk factors for medial tibial stress syndrome and tibial stress fracture in high school runners. Knee Surg Sports Traumatol Arthrosc 21(3):556, 2013.
77. Zifchock, RA, et al: Side-to-side differences in overuse running injury susceptibility: A retrospective study. Hum Mov Sci 27(6):888, 2008.
78. Hicks, GE, et al: Preliminary development of a clinical prediction rule for determining which patients with low back pain will respond to a stabilization exercise program. Arch Phys Med Rehabil 86(9):1753, 2005.
79. Childs, JD, et al: A clinical prediction rule to identify patients with low back pain most likely to benefit from spinal manipulation: A validation study. Ann Intern Med 141(12):920, 2004.
80. Fritz, JM, et al: Factors related to the inability of individuals with low back pain to improve with a spinal manipulation. Phys Ther 84(2):173, 2004.
81. Iverson, CA, et al: Lumbopelvic manipulation for the treatment of patients with patellofemoral pain syndrome: Development of a clinical prediction rule. J Orthop Sports Phys Ther 38(6):297, 2008.
82. Currier, LL, et al: Development of a clinical prediction rule to identify patients with knee pain and clinical evidence of knee osteoarthritis who demonstrate a favorable short-term response to hip mobilization. Phys Ther 87(9):1106, 2007.
83. Perry, CJ, et al: The effects of anterior load carriage on lower limb gait parameters during obstacle clearance. Gait Posture 32(1):57, 2010.
84. Ranchos Los Amigos Medical Center: The Pathokinesiology Service and the Physical Assesment Department: Observational Gait Analysis Handbook. Downey, CA, 1989.
85. Weisl, H: The movements of the sacroiliac joint. Acta Anat (Basel) 23(1):80, 1955.
86. Thorstensson, A, et al: Trunk movements in human locomotion. Acta Physiol Scand 121(1):9, 1984.
87. Lee, KM, et al: Reliability of physical examination in the measurement of hip flexion contracture and correlation with gait parameters in cerebral palsy. J Bone Joint Surg Am 93(2):150, 2011.
88. McFadyen, BJ, and Winter, DA: An integrated biomechanical analysis of normal stair ascent and descent. J Biomech 21(9):733, 1988.
89. Livingston, LA, Stevenson, JM, and Olney, SJ: Stairclimbing kinematics on stairs of differing dimensions. Arch Phys Med Rehabil 72(6):398, 1991.
90. Protopapadaki, A, et al: Hip, knee, ankle kinematics and kinetics during stair ascent and descent in healthy young individuals. Clin Biomech (Bristol, Avon) 22(2):203, 2007.
91. Mulholland, SJ, and Wyss, UP: Activities of daily living in non-Western cultures: Range of motion requirements for hip and knee joint implants. Int J Rehabil Res 24(3):191, 2001.
92. Hemmerich, A, et al: Hip, knee, and ankle kinematics of high range of motion activities of daily living. J Orthop Res 24(4):770, 2006.
93. Kapoor A, et al: Range of movements of lower limb joints in cross-legged sitting posture. J Arthroplasty 23(3):451, 2008.
94. McWhirk, LB, and Glanzman, AM: Within-session interrater reliability of goniometric measures in patients with spastic cerebral palsy. Pediatr Phys Ther 18(4):262, 2006.
95. Holm, I, et al: Reliability of goniometric measurements and visual estimates of hip ROM in patients with osteoarthrosis. Physiother Res Int 5(4):241, 2000.
96. Pandya, S, et al: Reliability of goniometric measurements in patients with Duchenne muscular dystrophy. Phys Ther 65(9):1339, 1985.
97. Croft, PR, et al: Interobserver reliability in measuring flexion, internal rotation, and external rotation of the hip using a plurimeter. Ann Rheum Dis 55(5):320, 1996.
98. Kilgour, G, McNair, P, and Stott, NS: Intrarater reliability of lower limb sagittal range-of-motion measures in children with spastic diplegia. Dev Med Child Neurol 45(6):391, 2003.
99. Mutlu, A, Livanelioglu, A, and Gunel, MK: Reliability of goniometric measurements in children with spastic cerebral palsy. Med Sci Monit 13(7):CR323, 2007.
100. Bohannon, RW, Gajdosik, RL, and LeVeau, BF: Relationship of pelvic and thigh motions during unilateral and bilateral hip flexion. Phys Ther 65(10):1501, 1985.
101. Nussbaumer, S, et al: Validity and test-retest reliability of manual goniometers for measuring passive hip range of motion in femoroacetabular impingement patients. BMC Musculoskelet Disord 11:194, 2010.
102. van Trijffel, E, et al: Inter-rater reliability for measurement of passive physiological movements in lower extremity joints is generally low: A systematic review. J Physiother 56(4):223, 2010.
103. Chevillotte, CJ, et al: Variability in hip range of motion on clinical examination. J Arthroplasty 24(5):693, 2009.
104. Boone, DC, et al: Reliability of goniometric measurements. Phys Ther 58(11):1355, 1978.
105. Ekstrand, J, et al: Lower extremity goniometric measurements: A study to determine their reliability. Arch Phys Med Rehabil 63(4):171, 1982.
106. Prather, H, et al: Reliability and agreement of hip range of motion and provocative physical examination tests in asymptomatic volunteers. PM R 2(10):888, 2010.
107. Cibere, J, et al: Reliability of the hip examination in osteoarthritis: Effect of standardization. Arthritis Rheum 59(3):373, 2008.
108. Pua, YH, et al: Intrarater test-retest reliability of hip range of motion and hip muscle strength measurements in persons with hip osteoarthritis. Arch Phys Med Rehabil 89(6):1146, 2008.
109. Poulsen, E, et al: Reproducibility of range of motion and muscle strength measurements in patients with hip osteoarthritis—an inter-rater study. BMC Musculoskelet Disord 13:242, 2012.
110. Fosang, AL, et al: Measures of muscle and joint performance in the lower limb of children with cerebral palsy. Dev Med Child Neurol 45(10):664, 2003.
111. Cadenhead, SL, McEwen, IR, and Thompson, DM: Effect of passive range of motion exercises on lower-extremity goniometric measurements of adults with cerebral palsy: A single-subject design. Phys Ther 82(7):658, 2002.
112. Cliborne, AV, et al: Clinical hip tests and a functional squat test in patients with knee osteoarthritis: Reliability, prevalence of positive test findings, and short-term response to hip mobilization. J Orthop Sports Phys Ther 34(11):676, 2004.
113. Cibulka, MT, et al: Unilateral hip rotation range of motion asymmetry in patients with sacroiliac joint regional pain. Spine (Phila Pa 1976) 23(9):1009, 1998.
114. Owen, J, Stephens, D, and Wright, JG: Reliability of hip range of motion using goniometry in pediatric femur shaft fractures. Can J Surg 50(4):251, 2007.
115. Winters, MV, et al: Passive versus active stretching of hip flexor muscles in subjects with limited hip extension: A randomized clinical trial. Phys Ther 84(9):800, 2004.

116. Harvey, D: Assessment of the flexibility of elite athletes using the modified Thomas test. Br J Sports Med 32(1):68, 1998.
117. Godges, JJ, MacRae, PG, and Engelke, KA: Effects of exercise on hip range of motion, trunk muscle performance, and gait economy. Phys Ther 73(7):468, 1993.
118. Ashton, BB, Pickles, B, and Roll, JW: Reliability of goniometric measurements of hip motion in spastic cerebral palsy. Dev Med Child Neurol 20(1):87, 1978.
119. Bartlett, MD, et al: Hip flexion contractures: A comparison of measurement methods. Arch Phys Med Rehabil 66(9):620, 1985.
120. Glanzman, AM, Swenson, AE, and Kim, H: Intrarater range of motion reliability in cerebral palsy: A comparison of assessment methods. Pediatr Phys Ther 20(4):369, 2008.
121. Stuberg, WA, Fuchs, RH, and Miedaner, JA: Reliability of goniometric measurements of children with cerebral palsy. Dev Med Child Neurol 30(5):657, 1988.
122. Stuberg, WA, and Metcalf, WK: Reliability of quantitative muscle testing in healthy children and in children with Duchenne muscular dystrophy using a hand-held dynamometer. Phys Ther 68(6):977, 1998.
123. Gajdosik, RL, et al: Comparison of four clinical tests for assessing hamstring muscle length. J Orthop Sports Phys Ther 18(5):614, 1993.
124. Piva, SR, et al: Reliability of measures of impairments associated with patellofemoral pain syndrome. BMC Musculoskelet Disord 7:33, 2006.
125. Hanten, WP, and Chandler, SD: Effects of myofascial release leg pull and sagittal plane isometric contract-relax techniques on passive straight-leg raise angle. J Orthop Sports Phys Ther 20(3):138, 1994.
126. Ylinen, JJ, Kautiainen, HJ, and Hakkinen, AH: Comparison of active, manual, and instrumental straight leg raise in measuring hamstring extensibility. J Strength Cond Res 24(4):972, 2010.
127. Wang, SS, et al: Lower extremity muscular flexibility in long distance runners. J Orthop Sports Phys Ther 17(2):102, 1993.
128. Hsieh, CY, Walker, JM, and Gillis, K: Straight-leg-raising test. Comparison of three instruments. Phys Ther 63(9):1429, 1983.
129. Lindell, O, Eriksson, L, and Strender, LE: The reliability of a 10-test package for patients with prolonged back and neck pain: Could an examiner without formal medical education be used without loss of quality? A methodological study. BMC Musculoskelet Disord 8:31, 2007.
130. Melchione, WE, and Sullivan, MS: Reliability of measurements obtained by use of an instrument designed to indirectly measure iliotibial band length. J Orthop Sports Phys Ther 18(3):511, 1993.
131. Pua, YH, et al: Association of physical performance with muscle strength and hip range of motion in hip osteoarthritis. Arthritis Rheum 61(4):442, 2009.

CHAPTER 9

The Knee

Cynthia C. Norkin, PT, EdD

Structure and Function

Tibiofemoral and Patellofemoral Joints

The knee is composed of two distinct articulations enclosed within a single joint capsule: the tibiofemoral joint and the patellofemoral joint. At the tibiofemoral joint, the proximal joint surfaces are the convex medial and the lateral condyles of the distal femur (Fig. 9.1). Posteriorly and inferiorly, the longer medial condyle is separated from the lateral condyle by a deep groove called the intercondylar notch. Anteriorly, the condyles are separated by a shallow area of bone called the femoral patellar surface. The distal articulating surfaces are the two shallow concave medial and lateral condyles on the proximal end of the tibia. Two bony spines called the intercondylar tubercles separate the medial condyle from the lateral condyle. Two joint discs called menisci are attached to the articulating surfaces on the tibial condyles (Fig. 9.2). At the patellofemoral joint, the articulating surfaces are the posterior surface of the patella and the femoral patellar surface (Fig. 9.3).

The joint capsule that encloses both joints is large, loose, and reinforced by tendons and expansions from the surrounding muscles and ligaments. The quadriceps tendon, patellar ligament, and expansions from the extensor muscles provide anterior stability (see Fig. 9.3). The lateral and medial

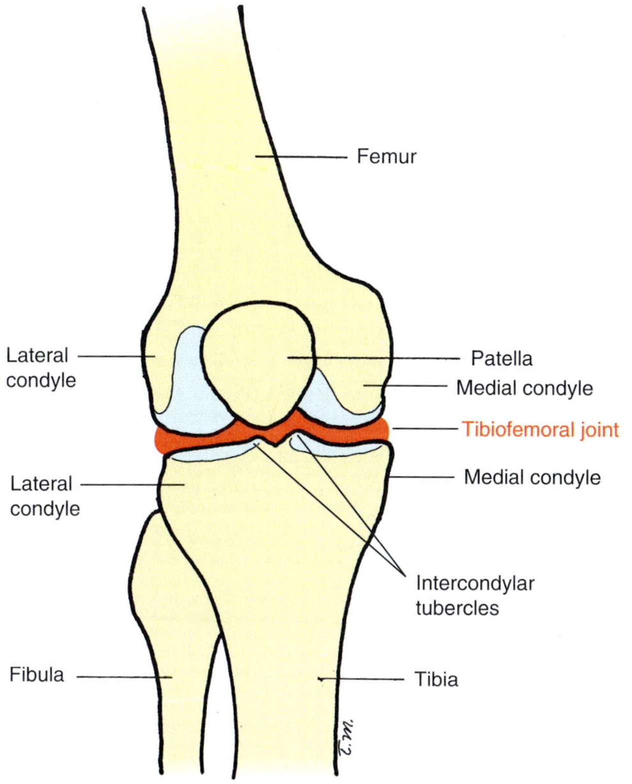

FIGURE 9.1 An anterior view of a right knee showing the tibiofemoral joint.

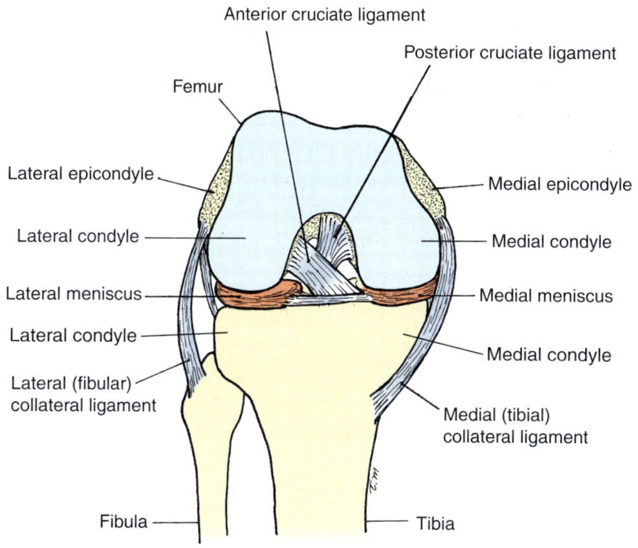

FIGURE 9.2 An anterior view of a right knee in the flexed position showing femoral and tibial condyles, medial and lateral menisci, and cruciate and collateral ligaments.

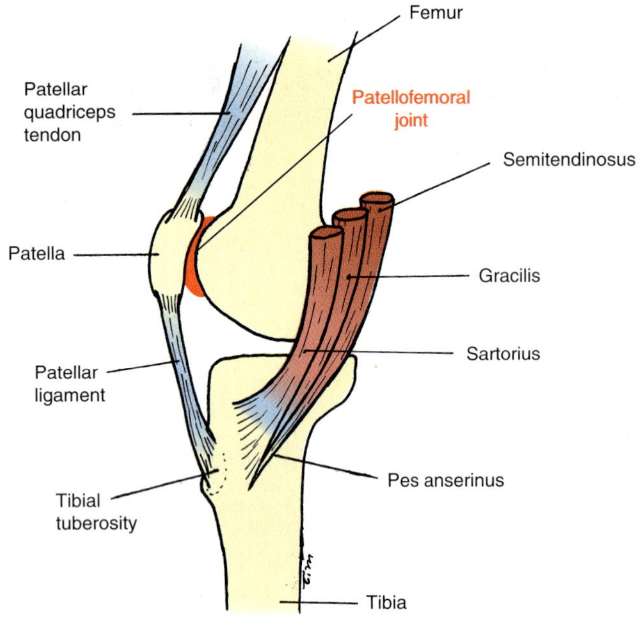

FIGURE 9.3 A view of a right knee showing the medial aspect, where the cut tendons of the three muscles that insert into the anteromedial aspect of the tibia make up the pes anserinus. Also included are the patellofemoral joint, the patellar ligament, and the patellar tendon.

collateral ligaments, iliotibial band, and pes anserinus help to provide medial–lateral stability, and the knee flexors help to provide posterior stability. In addition, the tibiofemoral joint is reinforced by the anterior and posterior cruciate ligaments, which are located within the joint (see Fig. 9.2).

Osteokinematics

The tibiofemoral joint is a double condyloid joint with 2 degrees of freedom. Flexion–extension occurs in the sagittal plane around a medial–lateral axis and rotation occurs in the transverse plane around a vertical (longitudinal) axis.[1] The incongruence and asymmetry of the tibiofemoral joint surfaces combined with muscle activity and ligamentous restraints produce an automatic rotation. This automatic rotation is involuntary and occurs primarily toward the end of extension when motion stops on the shorter lateral femoral condyle but continues on the longer medial condylar surface. During the last portion of the active extension range of motion (ROM) automatic rotation produces what is referred to as the screw-home mechanism, or "locking," of the knee. For example, during non-weight-bearing active knee extension with the tibia moving on the femur, the tibia laterally rotates during the last 10 to 15 degrees of extension to lock the knee.[2] Therefore, in the fully extended position of the knee, the tibia is laterally rotated in relation to the femur. To unlock the knee, either the tibia has to rotate medially or the femur has to rotate laterally.

This automatic rotation is not under voluntary control and should not be confused with the voluntary rotation that is possible when the knee is flexed. At 90 degrees of flexion the greatest range of tibial rotation is possible.[3,4] In a study by Almquist and colleagues of 120 healthy individuals (60 males and 60 females), about 40% of the total voluntary knee rotation was estimated as being internal rotation and 60% as external rotation.[5]

Arthrokinematics

In non-weight-bearing active motion, the concave tibial articulating surfaces slide on the convex femoral condyles in the same direction as the movement of the shaft of the tibia. The tibial condyles slide posteriorly on the femoral condyles during flexion and the tibial condyles slide anteriorly on the femoral condyles during extension.

In a weight-bearing situation the larger articulating surfaces of the convex femoral condyles must roll and slide in opposite directions to remain on the smaller tibial surfaces. During weight-bearing flexion, the femoral condyles roll posteriorly and slide anteriorly. The menisci follow the roll of the condyles by distorting posteriorly in flexion. In extension, the femoral condyles roll anteriorly and slide posteriorly.[1] In the last portion of extension, motion stops at the lateral femoral condyle, but sliding continues on the medial femoral condyle to produce locking of the knee.

The patella slides superiorly in extension and inferiorly in flexion. Some patellar rotation and tilting accompany the sliding during flexion and extension.

Capsular Pattern

The capsular pattern at the knee is characterized by a smaller limitation of extension than of flexion and no restriction of rotations.[6,7] Fritz and associates[8] found that patients with a capsular pattern, defined as a ratio of extension loss to flexion loss between 0.03 and 0.50, were 3.2 times more likely to have arthritis or arthroses of the knee.

RANGE OF MOTION TESTING PROCEDURES: Knee

Landmarks for Testing Procedures

Figure 9.4 provides a red dot at the center of the knee joint where the body of a goniometer should be centered. The red dots at the hip and ankle indicate sites where the arms of the goniometer should be aligned. In Figure 9.5, the anatomical landmarks are identified, that is, the lateral femoral epicondyle where the body of the goniometer should be placed and the goniometer arm placements at the greater trochanter at the hip and the lateral malleolus at the fibula.

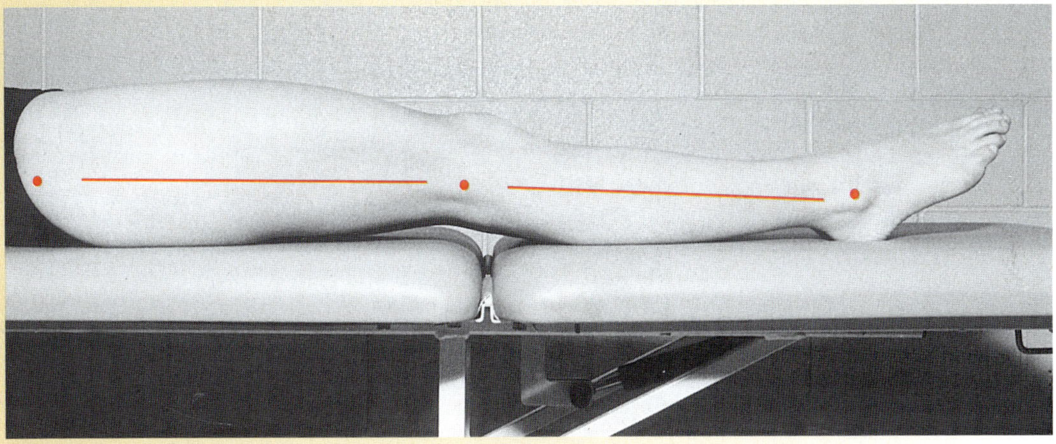

FIGURE 9.4 A lateral view of the right lower extremity showing surface anatomy landmarks for goniometer alignment.

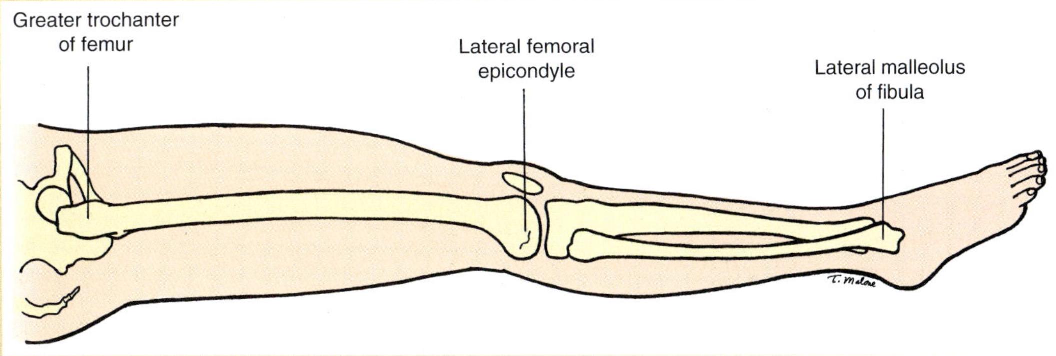

FIGURE 9.5 A lateral view of the right lower extremity showing bony anatomical landmarks for goniometer alignment for measuring knee flexion ROM.

KNEE FLEXION

Motion occurs in the sagittal plane around a medial–lateral axis. The normal range of flexion for adults varies from 130 to 140 degrees.[9,10] However, according to the sixth edition of the AMA's *Guides to the Evaluation of Permanent Impairment,* a knee flexion range of greater than 110 degrees is considered normal;[11] this definition of a normal range of motion is quite broad and not in agreement with other investigators. Please refer to Tables 9.1 through 9.3 in the Research Findings section for additional normal ROM values by age and gender.

Testing Position

Place the individual supine, with the knee in extension. Position the hip in 0 degrees of extension, abduction, and adduction. Place a towel roll under the ankle to allow the knee to extend as much as possible.

Stabilization

Stabilize the femur to prevent rotation, abduction, and adduction of the hip.

Testing Motion

Hold the ankle in one hand and the anterior thigh with the other hand. Move the individual's thigh to approximately 90 degrees of hip flexion and move the knee into flexion (Fig. 9.6). Stabilize the thigh to prevent further hip motion and guide the lower leg into knee flexion. The end of the range of knee flexion occurs when resistance is felt and attempts to overcome the resistance cause additional hip flexion.

Normal End-Feel

Usually, the end-feel is soft because of contact between the muscle bulk of the posterior calf and the thigh or between the heel and the buttocks. The end-feel may be firm because of tension in the vastus medialis, vastus lateralis, and vastus intermedialis muscles.

Goniometer Alignment

See Figures 9.7 and 9.8.

1. Center **fulcrum** of the goniometer over the lateral epicondyle of the femur.
2. Align **proximal arm** with the lateral midline of the femur, using the greater trochanter for reference.
3. Align **distal arm** with the lateral midline of the fibula, using the lateral malleolus and fibular head for reference.

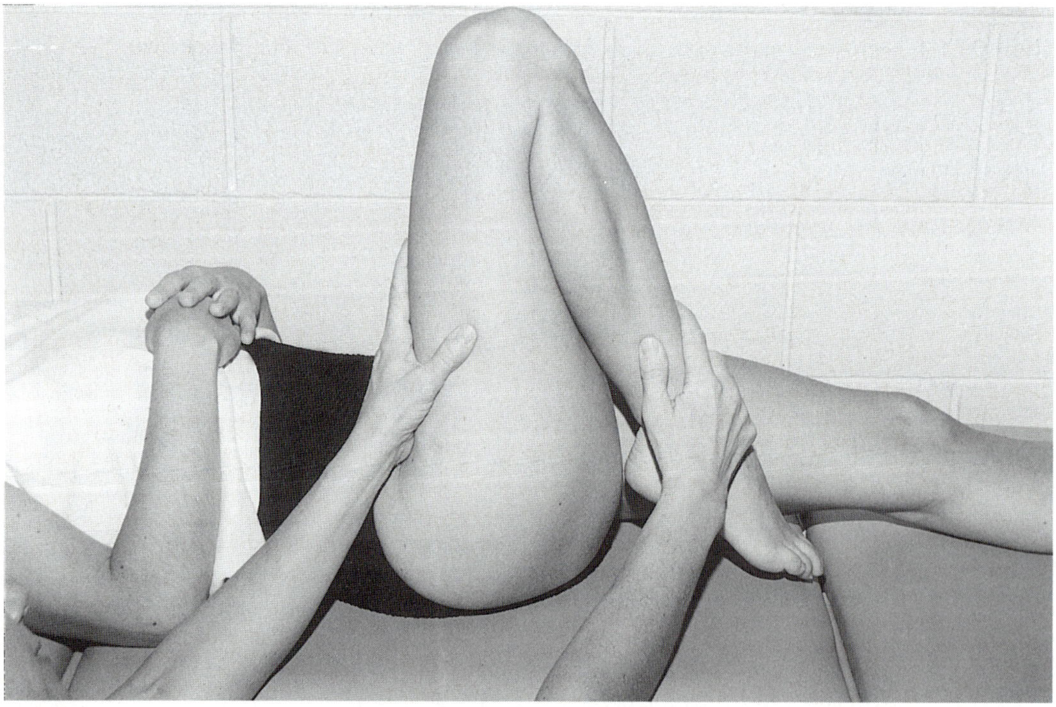

FIGURE 9.6 The right lower extremity at the end of knee flexion ROM. The examiner uses one hand to move the individual's thigh to approximately 90 degrees of hip flexion and then stabilizes the femur to prevent further flexion. The examiner's other hand guides the lower leg through full knee flexion ROM.

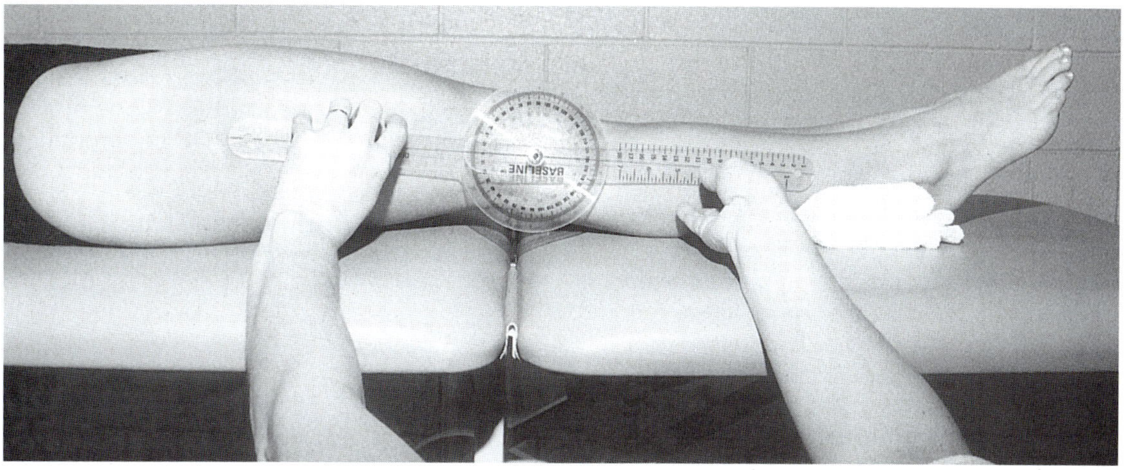

FIGURE 9.7 In the starting position for measuring knee flexion ROM, the individual is supine with the upper thigh exposed so that the greater trochanter can be visualized and palpated. A towel roll is placed under the ankle to elevate the lower leg so that the full beginning ROM can be measured. The examiner either kneels or sits on a stool to align and read the goniometer at eye level.

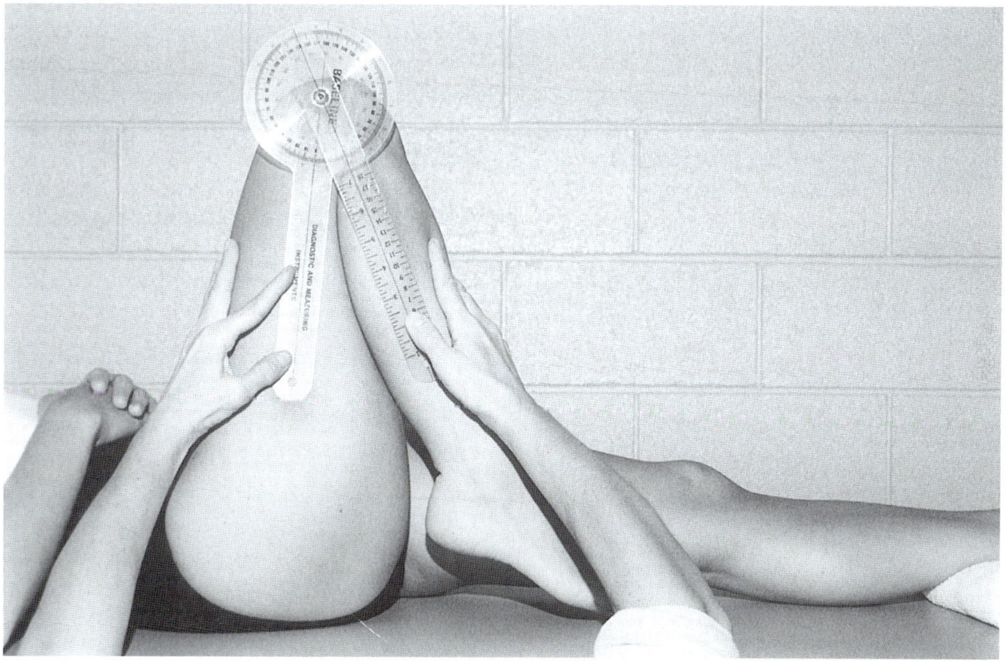

FIGURE 9.8 At the end of the knee flexion ROM, the examiner uses one hand to maintain knee flexion and also to align the distal arm of the goniometer with the lateral midline of the leg.

Measurements of knee flexion taken in a squatting position have been found to be greater than measurements taken in the supine position; therefore, it has been suggested by some researchers that perhaps measurements should be made in a squatting position for individuals who are capable of assuming that position.[12] However, caution should be used when asking individuals to assume a squatting position. If strength, balance, and joint integrity issues are present, there is a risk of falling and joint injury. The supine, non-weight-bearing position is considered a safer position for many individuals.

KNEE EXTENSION

Knee extension occurs in the sagittal plane around a medial-lateral axis and is usually recorded as the starting position for knee flexion ROM. Normal knee extension ROM values for adults are about 0 degrees. An extension limitation is present when the starting position for flexion ROM does not begin at 0 degrees but is in some amount of flexion. When extension goes beyond the 0 starting position, it may be within the normal limits of 5 to 10 degrees in children, but when it exceeds 5 or more degrees in adults,[1,2] it is called hyperextension or genu recurvatum. See Research Findings and Tables 9.1 to 9.4 for more information by age groups from neonates to older adults.

Testing Position

Place the individual supine in the 0 starting position for measuring knee flexion. Place a folded towel under the ankle to ensure that the knee is in full extension.

Stabilization

Stabilize the femur to keep the hip in neutral abduction, adduction, and rotation.

Testing Motion

To determine whether hyperextension is present, the examiner should place one hand on top of the lower thigh and exert a slight downward pressure.

Normal End-Feel

The end-feel is firm because of tension in the posterior joint capsule, the oblique and arcuate popliteal ligaments, the collateral ligaments, and the anterior and posterior cruciate ligaments.

Goniometer Alignment

1. Center **fulcrum** of the goniometer over the lateral epicondyle of the femur.
2. Align **proximal arm** with the lateral midline of the femur, using the greater trochanter for reference.
3. Align **distal arm** with the lateral midline of the fibula, using the lateral malleolus and fibular head for reference.

See Appendix B for a summary guide for measurement of knee ROM using a universal goniometer.

KNEE ROTATION

At this time, we are not able to recommend measuring voluntary knee rotation in the clinical setting because most methods for measuring rotational laxity are still in various stages of development.[13–16] Three of these methods have been tested for reliability with acceptable results.[13,15,16]

The only practical method that could be used in the clinical setting is the one used by Clarkson,[17] who measured total active tibial rotation ROM with the individual in a sitting position with the knee flexed to 90 degrees. An OB Myrin compass inclinometer was strapped on the tibia and the mean total ROM was given as 40 degrees in women and 58 degrees in men. However, the reliability and validity of this testing method were not reported.

MUSCLE LENGTH TESTING PROCEDURES: Knee

Landmarks for Testing Procedures

See Figures 9.4 and 9.5.

Knowledge of gross anatomy and physiology is essential for the identification of the structures that may be responsible for impaired ROM. Muscle length testing can help to differentiate ROM limitations caused by one-joint muscle from limitations caused by two-joint muscles. Isolated ROM testing of one joint at a time is necessary to determine whether a particular motion is being limited by joint structures and muscles that cross only one joint. To determine whether a muscle or muscles that cross more than one joint are causing the limitation, muscles must be stretched over all joints crossed.

KNEE EXTENSORS

The major knee extensor is the quadriceps femoris, which consists of the following four muscles: rectus femoris, vastus medialis, vastus lateralis, and vastus intermedius. The **rectus femoris** is the only one of the four muscles that crosses both the hip and the knee joints. It arises proximally from two tendons: an anterior tendon from the anterior inferior iliac spine and a posterior tendon from a groove superior to the brim of the acetabulum. The three **vastus muscles** originate on the femur and merge with the rectus femoris in a thick, flat common tendon called the quadriceps tendon, which inserts into the proximal aspect of the patella. The quadriceps tendon continues distally over the patella to attach to the apex of the patella. The part of the quadriceps tendon that continues distal to the patella to attach to the tibial tuberosity is known as the patella tendon or ligament (Fig. 9.9).

When the rectus femoris muscle contracts, it flexes the hip and extends the knee. If the rectus femoris muscle is short and knee flexion is attempted, the hip passively moves into flexion to accommodate the shortened muscle. The three vastus muscles also produce active knee extension but cross only the knee joint. These three muscles are all passively lengthened by knee flexion regardless of the position of the hip. The length of these muscles is automatically tested along with other joint structures during the measurement of knee flexion (in which the hip is flexed); therefore, a separate test has not been included.

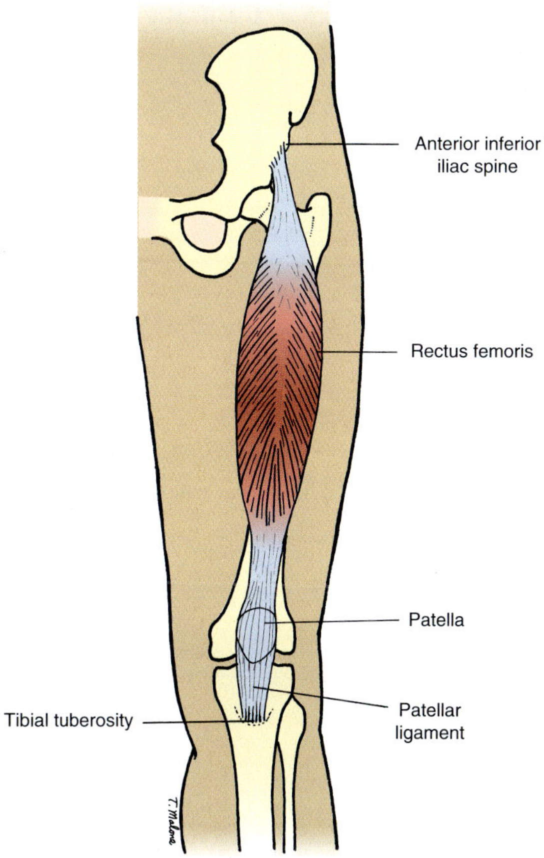

FIGURE 9.9 An anterior view of the left lower extremity showing the attachments of the rectus femoris muscle.

ELY TEST

The Ely test is used to evaluate the length of the rectus femoris muscle by positioning the hip in 0 degrees of flexion and then flexing the knee.

Testing Position

Place the individual prone, with both feet off the end of the examining table. Extend the knees and position the hips in 0 degrees of flexion, extension, abduction, adduction, and rotation (Fig. 9.10). If pain is present from pressure on the patella, a small towel roll may be placed under the distal femur to slightly elevate the thigh, thus reducing contact between the patella and the examining table.

Stabilization

Stabilize the hip to maintain the neutral position. Do not allow the hip to flex.

Testing Motion

Flex the knee by lifting the lower leg off the table (Figs. 9.11 and 9.12). The end of the ROM occurs when resistance is felt from tension in the anterior thigh and further knee flexion causes the hip to flex.

Normal End-Feel

The end-feel is firm owing to tension in the rectus femoris muscle.

Goniometer Alignment

See Figure 9.13.

1. Center **fulcrum** of the goniometer over the lateral epicondyle of the femur.
2. Align **proximal arm** with the lateral midline of the femur, using the greater trochanter as a reference.
3. Align **distal arm** with the lateral midline of the fibula, using the lateral malleolus and the fibular head for reference.

Interpretation

If the knee can be flexed to at least 90 degrees with the hip in the neutral position, the length of the rectus femoris is considered normal. In a study by Gnat and colleagues,[18] 14 students were selected from a healthy university student group of 30. Passive knee flexion positioning was prone on a table with a goniometer fastened to the lower leg at a point halfway between the apex of the patella and the line joining the two malleoli. A force gauge was fastened around the ankle. Extrapolating from the graph created by Gnat et al, it appears that ROM was between 125 and 132 degrees.

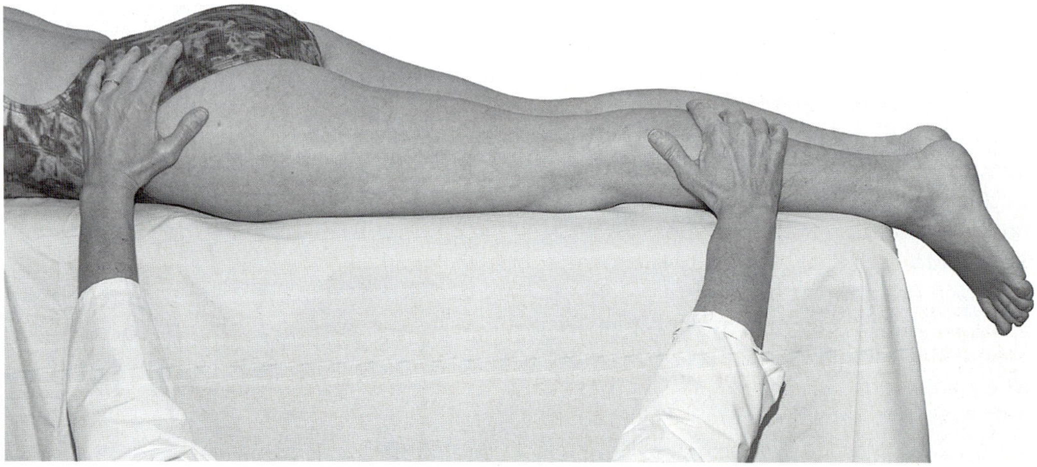

FIGURE 9.10 The individual is in the prone starting position for testing the length of the rectus femoris muscle.

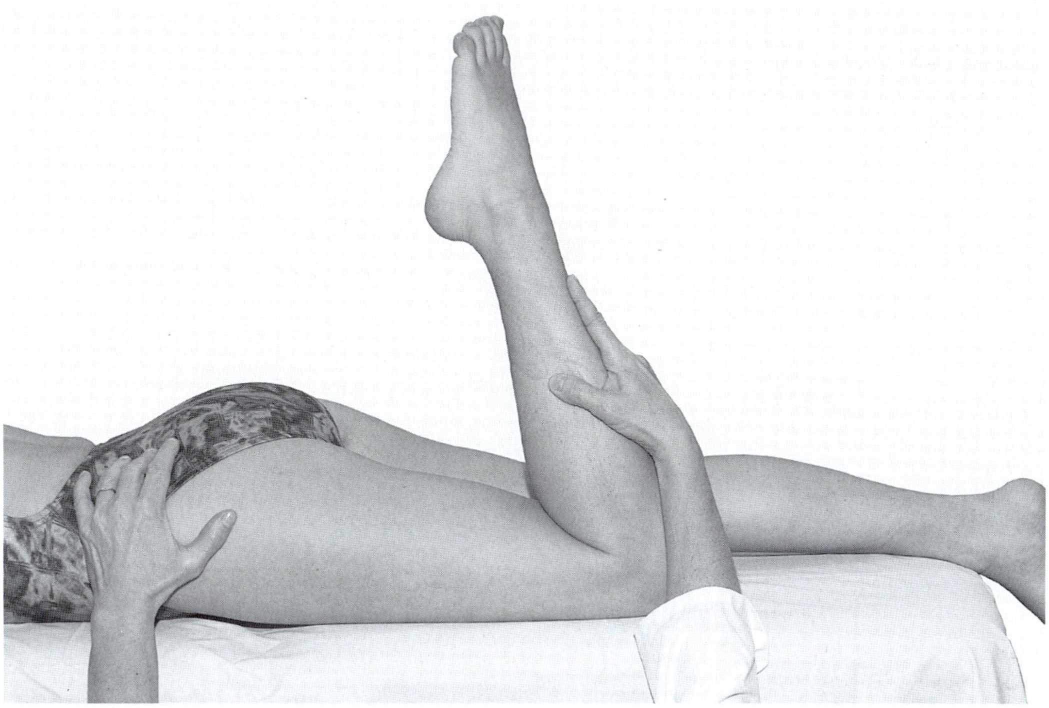

FIGURE 9.11 A lateral view of the individual at the end of the testing motion for the length of the left rectus femoris muscle.

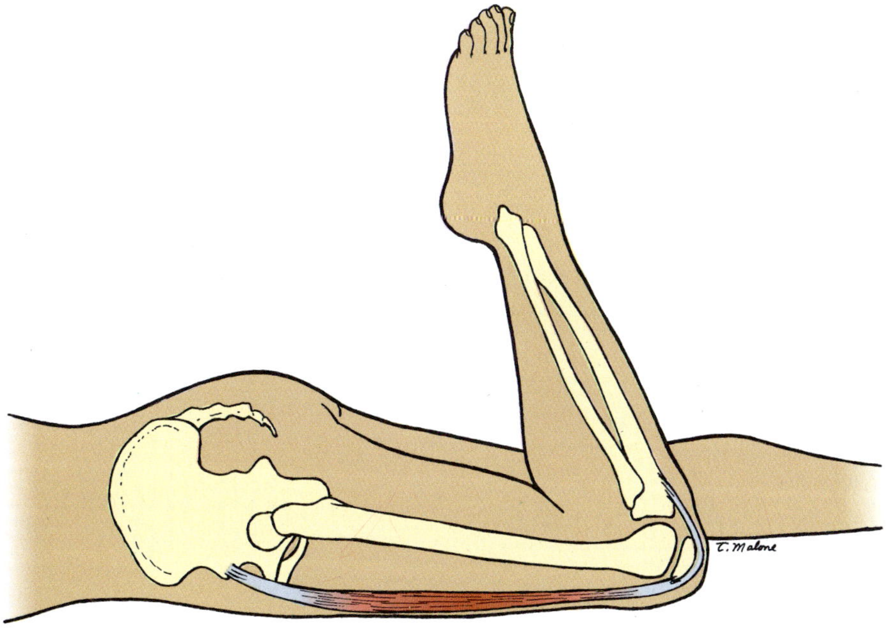

FIGURE 9.12 A lateral view of the left rectus femoris muscle being stretched over the hip and knee joints at the end of the testing motion.

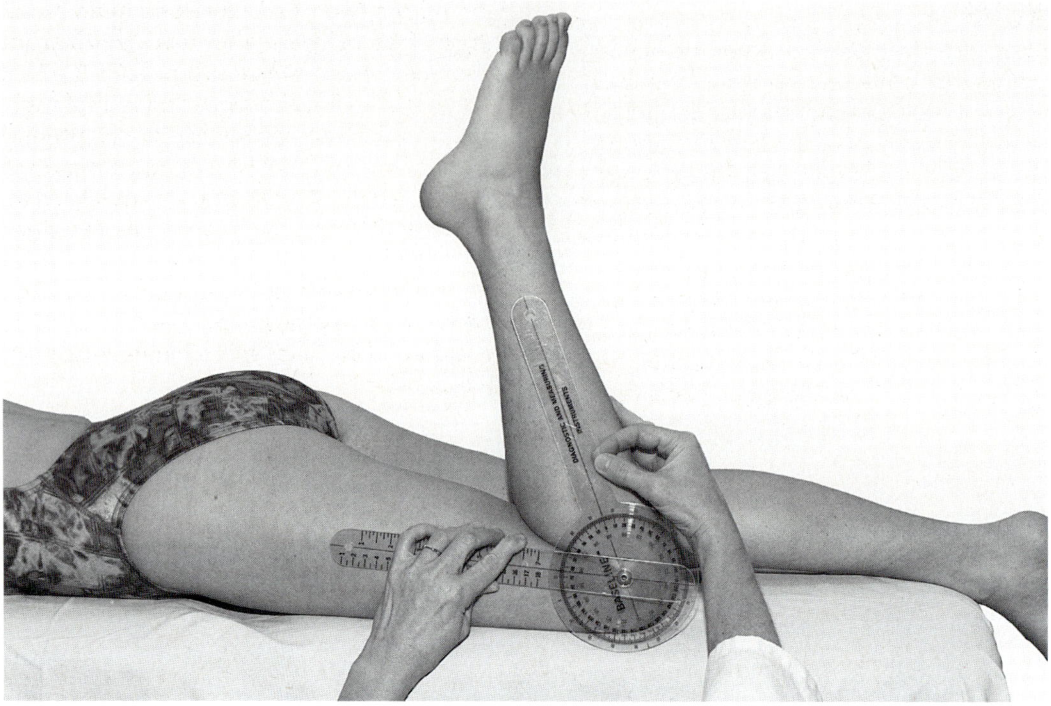

FIGURE 9.13 Goniometer alignment for measuring the position of the knee at the end of the Ely Test.

KNEE FLEXORS

The hamstring muscles are composed of the semitendinosus, semimembranosus, and biceps femoris (long and short heads). The semitendinosus, semimembranous, and long head of the biceps femoris, cross both the hip and the knee joints. The proximal attachment of the **semitendinosus** is on the ischial tuberosity, and the distal attachment is on the proximal aspect of the medial surface of the tibia (Fig. 9.14A). The proximal attachment of the **semimembranosus** is also on the ischial tuberosity, and the distal attachment is on the medial aspect of the medial tibial condyle (Fig. 9.14B). The **biceps femoris** muscle arises from two heads; the long head attaches to the ischial tuberosity and the sacrotuberous ligament, whereas the short head attaches to the femur along the lateral lip linear aspera and lateral supracondylar line, and the lateral intermuscular septum. The distal attachments of the biceps femoris are on the head of the fibula, with a small portion attaching to the lateral tibial condyle and the lateral collateral ligament (see Fig. 9.14A).

When the hamstring muscles contract, they extend the hip and flex the knee. These muscles are passively lengthened by placing the hip in flexion and the knee in extension.

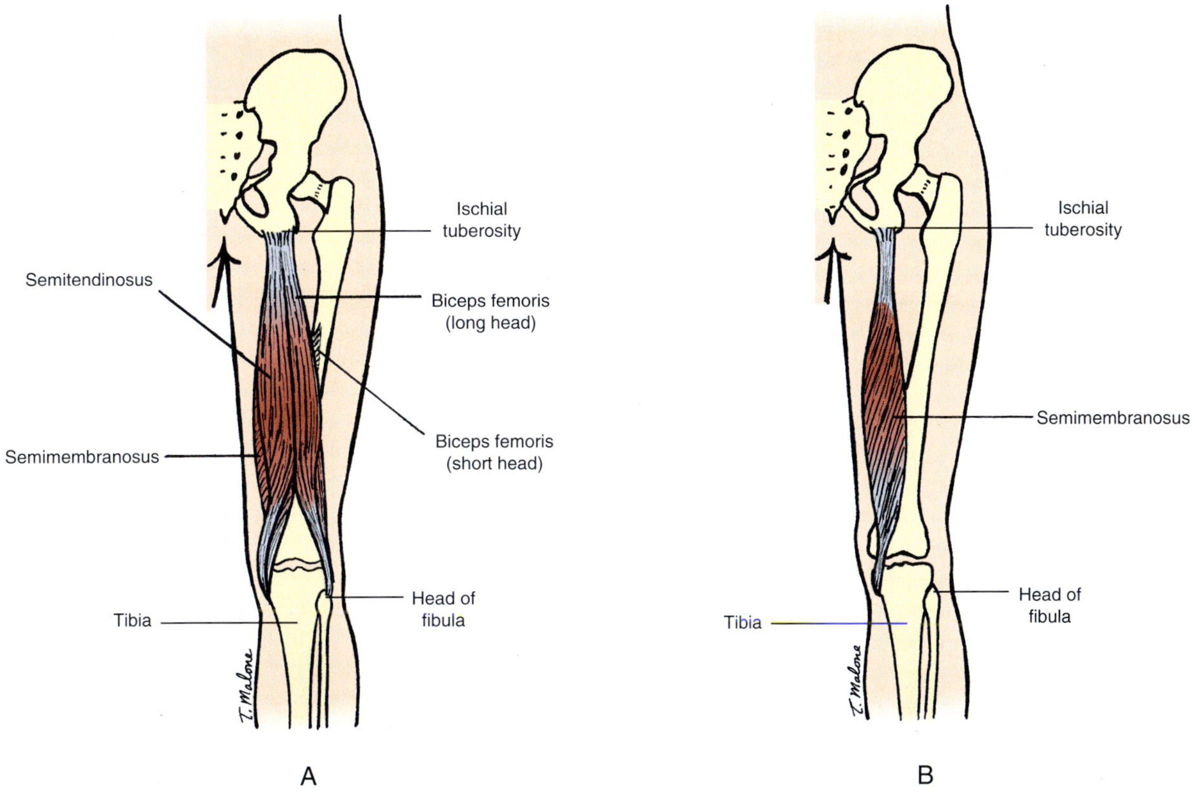

FIGURE 9.14 (A) A posterior view of the thigh showing the attachments of the semitendinosus and the biceps femoris muscles. (B) A posterior view of the thigh showing the attachments of the semimembranosus muscle, which lies under the two hamstring muscles shown in part A.

DISTAL HAMSTRING LENGTH TEST

The distal hamstring length test or hamstring passive knee extension (PKE) test is also called the popliteal angle (PA) test because the angle that is being measured is the popliteal angle between the femur and the lower leg.

Testing Position

Position the individual supine with the hip on the side being tested in 90 degrees of flexion and 0 degrees of abduction, adduction, and rotation (Fig. 9.15). Initially, the knee being tested is allowed to relax in flexion. The lower extremity that is not being tested rests on the examining table with the knee fully extended and the hip in 0 degrees of flexion, extension, abduction, adduction, and rotation.

Stabilization

Stabilize the femur to prevent rotation, abduction, and adduction at the hip and to maintain the hip in 90 degrees of flexion.

Testing Motion

Extend the knee to the end of the ROM. The end of the testing motion occurs when resistance is felt from tension in the posterior thigh and further knee extension causes the hip to move toward extension (Figs. 9.16 and 9.17).

Normal End-Feel

The end-feel is firm owing to tension in the semimembranosus, semitendinosus, and biceps femoris muscles.

Goniometer Alignment

See Figure 9.18.

1. Center **fulcrum** of the goniometer over the lateral epicondyle of the femur.
2. Align **proximal arm** with the lateral midline of the femur, using the greater trochanter for a reference.
3. Align **distal arm** with the lateral midline of the fibula, using the lateral malleolus and fibular head for reference.

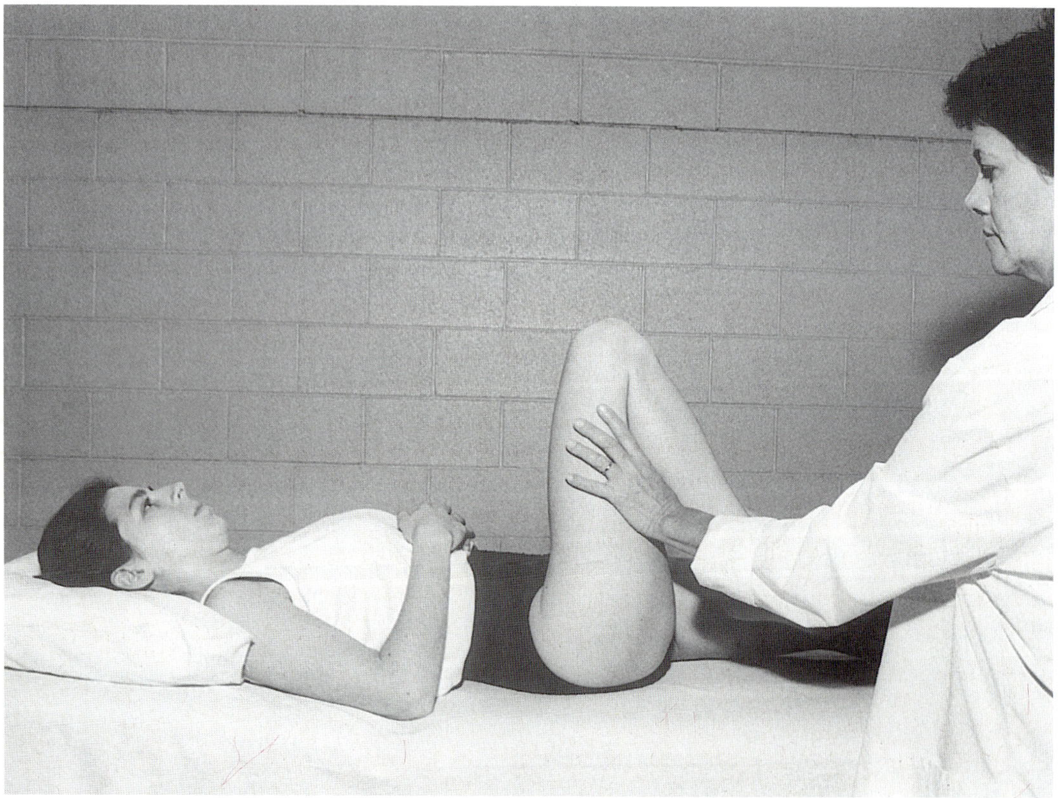

FIGURE 9.15 Starting position for measuring the length of the hamstring muscles.

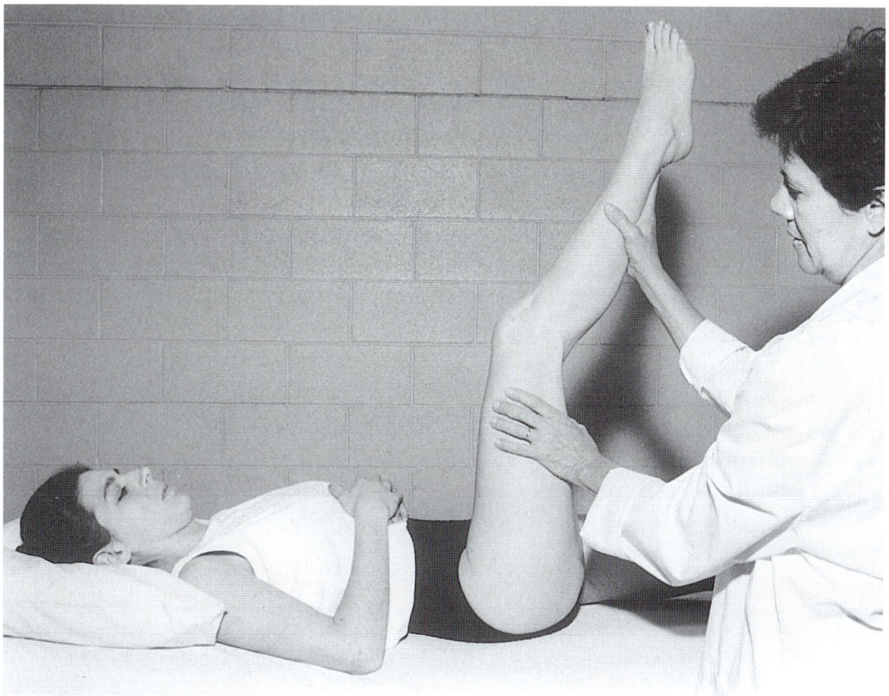

FIGURE 9.16 End of the testing motion for the length of the right hamstring muscles.

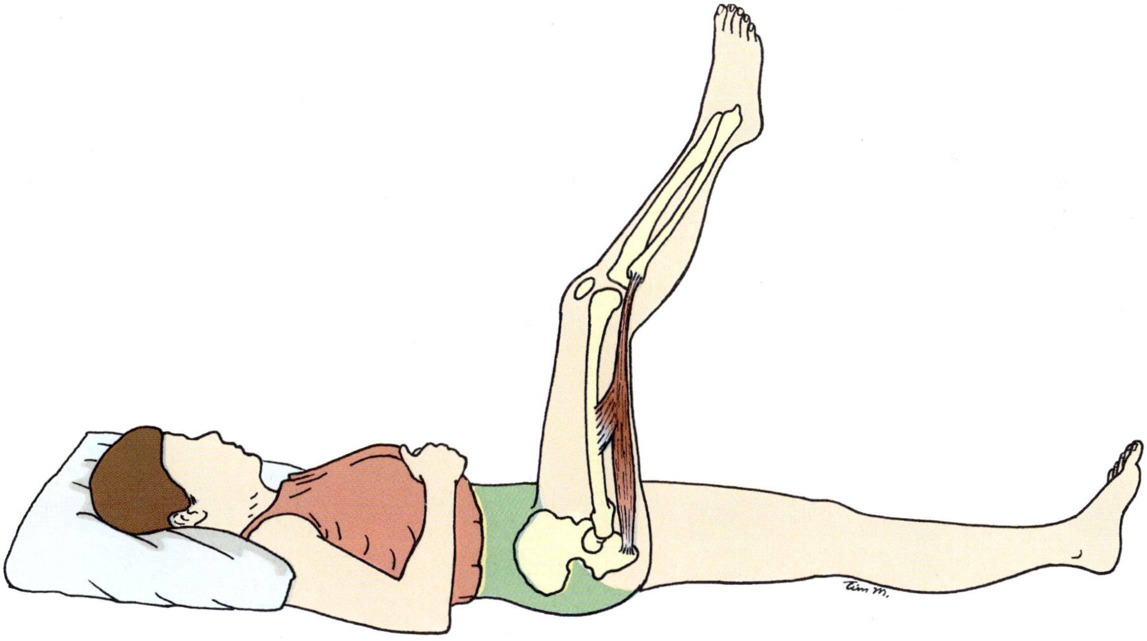

FIGURE 9.17 A lateral view of the right lower extremity shows the hamstring muscles being stretched over the hip and knee joints at the end of the testing motion.

Interpretation

Gajdosik and associates,[19] in a study of 30 healthy males aged 18 to 40 years, found a mean value of 31 degrees (standard deviation [SD] = 7.5 degrees). Some researchers have reported the supplementary angles to those noted by Gajdosik and associates. Youdas and colleagues[20] used a 360-degree universal goniometer to measure the popliteal angle (PA) in 214 individuals (108 women and 106 men) between the ages of 20 and 79 years. The mean value for the women of 152.0 degrees (SD = 10.6 degrees) was greater than the mean value for men of 141.4 degrees (SD = 8.1 degrees). The supplementary angles of these values for women and men are 28.0 and 38.6 degrees, respectively, which is generally consistent with the values noted by Gajdosik and associates.[19]

Gnat and associates[18] investigated the interrater and test-retest reliability of a modified version of the passive knee extension (PKE) test used to evaluate muscle length. Passive knee extension positioning was supine, with a belt securing the pelvis and the goniometer fastened to the lower leg at a point halfway between the apex of the patella and a line joining the two malleoli. A force gauge was fastened at the ankle.

Two testers in a study by Fredriksen and colleagues[21] found that PKE angle measurements for a single female subject tested 16 times per side ranged from 153 to 159 degrees for the left leg and from 154 to 165 degrees for the right leg. A standardized force using a dynamometer was used to extend the knee and the hip was positioned in 120 degrees of flexion, which is considerably larger than the 90 degrees of hip flexion used by both Youdas[20] and Gadjosik.[19]

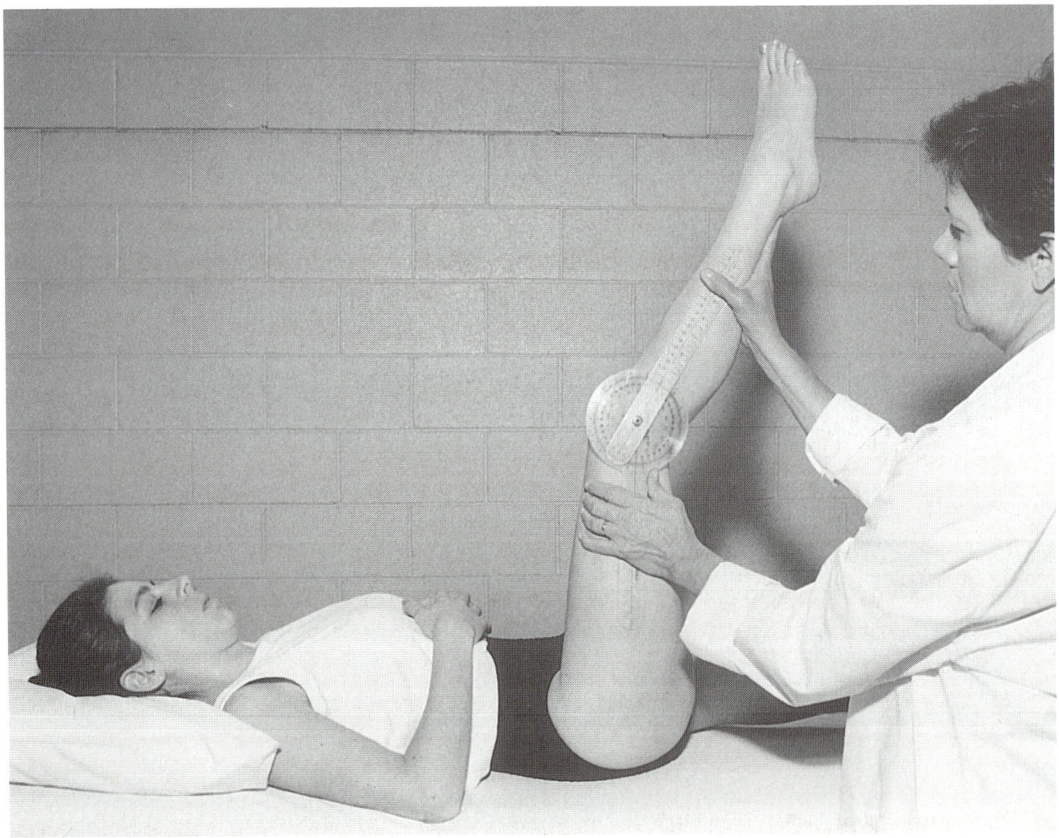

FIGURE 9.18 Goniometer alignment for measuring knee position at the end of the Distal Hamstring Length Test. This test is also called the Popliteal Angle Test.

Research Findings

This section of the chapter includes not only age and gender effects on knee ROM but also the effects of body mass. In addition, functional knee ROM required for stairs and other activities of daily living is followed by a sampling of reliability and validity studies in normal and patient populations. Table 9.1 provides knee flexion ROM values for adults from selected sources. Tables 9.2 through 9.4 provide information on neonates, normative values for infants and young children, and age effects on knee flexion ROM.

Effects of Age, Gender, and Other Factors

Age

Knee extension limitations of 15 to 20 degrees at birth are normal and similar to extension limitations found at the hip joint at birth. The term "extension limitation" is used rather than "flexion contracture" because contracture refers to an abnormal condition caused by fixed muscle shortness, which may be permanent.[22] Knee extension limitations in the neonate gradually disappear by about 12 or 13 years of age and extension, instead of being limited, may become excessive in the toddler. More details of research studies are provided below and in Tables 9.2 through 9.4.

Waugh and colleagues[23] and Drews and coworkers[24] found that newborns lacked approximately 15 to 20 degrees of knee extension. Schwarze and Denton,[25] in a study of 1,000 neonates (527 girls and 473 boys) in the first 3 days of life, found a mean extension limitation of 15 degrees. These findings agree with the findings of Wanatabe and associates,[26] who found that newborns lacked 14 degrees of knee extension. The extension limitation gradually disappears with increasing age, as shown by comparing Tables 9.2 and 9.3.

Broughton, Wright, and Menelaus[27] measured extension limitations in normal neonates at birth and again at 3 months and 6 months. At birth, 53 of the 57 (93%) neonates had extension limitations of 15 degrees or greater, whereas only 30 of 57 (53%) infants had extension limitations at 6 months of age. The mean reduction in extension limitations was 3.5 degrees per month from birth to 3 months and 2.8 degrees between 3 and 6 months (see Tables 9.2 and 9.3). The 2-year-olds in the study conducted by Wanatabe and associates[26] had no evidence of a knee extension limitation (see Table 9.3)

Knee extension beyond 0 degrees (often referred to as hyperextension) is considered a normal finding in young children but is not usually observed in adults,[3] who may have slightly less than full knee extension. Wanatabe and associates[26] found that the 2-year-olds had up to 5 degrees of extension beyond 0. This finding is similar to the mean of 5.4 degrees of extension beyond 0 noted by Boone[28] for a group of children between 1 and 5 years of age. Beighton, Solomon, and Soskolne,[29] in a study of joint laxity in 1,081 males and females, found that joint laxity decreased rapidly throughout childhood in both genders and decreased at a slower rate during adulthood. The authors used a ROM of greater than

TABLE 9.1 Knee Flexion ROM in Adults: Normal Values in Degrees

	Boone[9]	Roach and Miles[10]		Soucie[32]			
Gender, Age Range, Sample	Males 20–54 yr n = 56	Males and females 40–59 yr n = 727	Males and females 60–74 yr n = 523	Females 20–44 yr n = 143	Males 20–44 yr n = 114	Females 45–69 yr n = 123	Males 45–69 yr n = 96
Motion	**Mean (SD)**	**Mean (SD)**	**Mean (SD)**	**Mean (SD)**	**Mean (SD)**	**Mean (SD)**	**Mean (SD)**
Flexion	141.0 (5.4)	132.0 (11.0)	131.0 (11.0)	141.9 (6.3)	137.7 (6.5)	137.8 (7.4)	132.9 (6.3)

SD = Standard deviation.

TABLE 9.2 Knee Extension Limitations in Neonates 6 Hours to 7 Days of Age: Normal Values in Degrees

	Waugh et al[23]	Drews et al[24]	Schwarze and Denton[25]	Broughton et al[27]
Age Range Sample	6–65 hr n = 40	12 hr–6 days n = 54	1–3 days n = 1,000	1–7 days n = 57
Motion	**Mean (SD)**	**Mean (SD)**	**Mean**	**Mean (SD)**
Extension limitation	15.3 (9.9)	20.4 (6.7)	15.0	21.4 (7.7)

SD = standard deviation.

All values were obtained from passive ROM measurements with use of a universal goniometer.

TABLE 9.3 Knee Range of Motion in Infants and Young Children 0 to 12 Years of Age: Normal Values in Degrees

	Broughton et al[27]		Wanatabe et al[26]	Boone[28]	
Age	3 mo	6 mo	0–2 yr	1–5 yr	6–12 yr
Sample	*n* = 57	*n* = 57	*n* = 109	*n* = 19	*n* = 17
Motion	**Mean (SD)**	**Mean (SD)**	**Range of Means**	**Mean (SD)**	**Mean (SD)**
Flexion	145.5 (5.3)	141.7 (6.3)	148–159	141.7 (6.2)	147.1 (3.5)
Extension	10.7 (5.1)*	3.3 (4.3)*	5.0†	5.4 (3.1)†	0.4 (0.9)

SD = standard deviation.

*Indicates extension limitations.

†Indicates extension beyond 0 degrees.

10 degrees of knee extension beyond 0 as one of the criteria of joint laxity. Cheng, Chan, and Hui,[30] in a study of 2,360 Chinese children, found that the average of 16 degrees of knee extension beyond 0 in children of 3 years of age decreased to 7 degrees by the time the children reached 9 years of age.

Steinberg and colleagues,[31] in a study of 1,320 female dancers between the ages of 8 and 16 years of age and a control group of 226 nondancers of similar age, found that knee flexion ROM showed a small but significant decrease with increasing age in both groups. The authors suggested that the decreases in ROM might be related to a general increase in circumference in thigh and leg muscles that developed as the group matured and as subcutaneous fat was deposited. However, the decrease in ROM in nondancers appeared to be larger (15 degrees) than in dancers, which might be accounted for by the fact that the dancers were probably more active than the nondancers.

Soucie and colleagues[32] obtained bilateral passive knee ROM measurements on males and females in each of seven age-groups for a total of 674 healthy male and female individuals with a mean age of 33 years. Subjects were predominately white and included slightly more females than males. The authors found that joint ROM tended to decline with advancing age with the greatest difference between children (aged 2 to 8 years) and all other age-groups. The largest age-related difference between young and old was a 15-degree difference in mean knee flexion ROM between the 2-year-old group and the group aged 45 to 69.[32]

Also, a comparison of knee extension beyond 0 mean values for the group aged 13 to 19 years can be found in Table 9.4. Table 9.3 has extension values for the group aged 1 to 5 years, which demonstrates the decrease in knee extension beyond 0 that occurs in childhood.

Walker and colleagues[33] studied active ROM of the extremity joints in 30 men and 30 women (ranging in age from 60 to 84 years) from recreational centers. No differences were found in knee ROM between subjects aged 60 to 69 years and subjects aged 75 to 84 years. However, average values indicated that the subjects had an extension limitation (inability to attain a neutral 0-degree starting position). This finding was similar to the loss of extension noted at the hip, elbow, and first metatarsophalangeal joints. The 2-degree extension limitation found at the knee was much smaller than that found at the hip joint. According to the American Association of Orthopaedic Surgeons (AAOS) handbook,[34] extension limitations of 2 degrees are considered normal in adults. Extension limitations greater than 5 degrees in adults may be considered as knee flexion contractures. These contractures often occur in the elderly because of disease, sedentary lifestyles, and the effects of the aging process on connective tissues.

TABLE 9.4 Age Effects on Knee Flexion in Individuals 2 to 74 Years of Age: Mean Values in Degrees

	Soucie[32]*	Boone[28]		Roach and Miles[10]	
Age	2–8 yr	13–19 yr	20–29 yr	40–59 yr	60–74 yr
Sample	*n* = 39	*n* = 17	*n* = 19	*n* = 727	*n* = 523
Motion	**Mean (SD)**	**Mean (SD)**	**Mean (SD)**	**Mean (SD)**	**Mean (SD)**
Flexion	152.6 (4.5)	142.9 (3.7)	140.2 (5.2)	132.0 (11.0)	131.0 (11.0)
Extension	5.4 (4.9)	0.0 (0.0)	0.4 (0.9)		

SD = Standard deviation.

*Females.

Mollinger and Steffan[35] used a universal goniometer (UG) to assess knee ROM among 112 nursing home residents with an average age of 83 years. The authors found that only 13% of the subjects had full (0-degree) passive knee extension bilaterally. Thirty-seven of the 112 subjects (33%) had bilateral knee extension limitations of 5 degrees or less, which the AAOS considers normal in older adults. Forty-seven subjects (42%) had greater than 10 degrees of limitations in extension (flexion contractures). Residents with a 30-degree loss of knee extension had an increase in resistance to passive motion and a loss of ambulation.

Steultjens and coworkers[36] found knee flexion contractures in 31.5% of 198 patients with osteoarthritis of the knee or hip. (It should be noted that these authors considered knee flexion contractures as an inability to attain the horizontal 0 starting position for measuring flexion.) Flexion contractures of the knee or hip or both were found in 73% of patients. Generally, a decrease in active assistive ROM was associated with an increase in disability but was motion specific. The motions that had the strongest relationship with disability were knee flexion, hip extension, and lateral rotation. Ersoz and Ergun[37] found that in a group of 44- to 76-year-old patients with primary knee osteoarthritis, 33 out of the 40 knees tested (82.5%) had extension limitations ranging from 1 to 14 degrees.

Despite the knee flexion contractures found in the elderly by Mollinger and Steffan,[35] many elderly individuals appear to have at least a functional flexion ROM. Escalante and coworkers[38] used a UG to measure knee flexion passive ROM in 687 community-dwelling elderly subjects between the ages of 65 and 79 years. More than 90 degrees of knee flexion was found in 619 (90.1%) of the subjects. The authors used a cut-off value of 124 degrees of flexion as being within normal limits. Subjects who failed to reach 124 degrees of flexion were classified as having an abnormal ROM. Using this criterion, 76 (11%) right knees and 63 (9%) left knees were below this value and thus had abnormal (limited) passive ROM in flexion. Nonaka and colleagues[39] examined age-related changes at the hip and knee in 77 healthy male volunteers aged 15 to 73 years. The authors found that passive ROM of the hip joint decreased with increasing age but knee joint passive ROM remained unchanged. However, interactive motion of the hip and knee showed an age-related reduction, which the authors attributed to shortening of muscle and connective tissue.

Macedo and Magee[40] took goniometric passive ROM measurements of the ankle, knee, hip, shoulder, elbow, and wrist joints in 90 healthy Caucasian women ages 18 to 59. These authors found that only 11 of the tested motions, including knee flexion, showed that increasing age was associated with statistically significant decreases in passive ROM but that the decreases were small.

Gender

In general, it appears that females have greater knee ROM and more knee joint laxity than their male counterparts. Soucie and colleagues[32] found that in addition to age differences, the following gender difference was present: Females had greater joint mobility in all age-groups in nearly all joints compared with males. The authors also found some evidence to support the finding that the joint mobility index increases in females after they enter puberty.

Beighton, Solomon, and Soskolne[29] defined more than 10 degrees of knee extension beyond 0 as hyperextension and included this criterion in a study of joint laxity in 1,081 males and females. Females in the study had more joint laxity than males at any age. Loudon, Goist, and Loudon[41] operationally defined knee hyperextension (genu recurvatum) as more than 5 degrees of extension beyond the 0 position. Clinically, the authors had observed that not only was hyperextension more common in females than in males, but also that the condition might be associated with functional deficits in muscle strength, instability, and poor proprioceptive control of terminal knee extension. The authors cautioned that the female athlete with hyperextended knees may be at risk for anterior cruciate ligament injury. Hall and colleagues[42] found that 10 female patients diagnosed with hypermobility syndrome had alterations in proprioceptive acuity at the knee compared with an age-matched and gender-matched control group.

Almquist and colleagues[5] measured knee rotation in 60 healthy women and 60 healthy male volunteers aged 15 to older than 60 years. Measurements of total knee rotation were taken in both knees at 90, 60, and 30 degrees of knee flexion using applied torques of 6 and 9 Nm (newton meters). No significant differences were found in the total internal–external ROM between the right and left knees at any age or gender. However, the women in the study showed a significantly larger knee rotation ROM than the men at all tested degrees of knee flexion and at all applied torques. The women had a 10% to 20% larger range of total knee rotation than did the men.

James and Parker[43] studied knee flexion ROM in 80 men and women who ranged in age from 70 years to older than 85 years. Women had greater ROM in both active and passive knee flexion than men. Overall, knee flexion values were lower than expected for both genders, possibly owing to the fact that subjects were measured in the prone position, where the two-joint rectus femoris muscle may have limited the ROM.

In contrast to the findings of James and Parker,[43] Escalante and coworkers[38] found that female subjects had reduced passive knee flexion ROM compared with males of the same age. However, the women had on average only 2 degrees less knee flexion than did the men. The women also had a higher body mass index than did the men, which may have contributed to their reduced knee flexion.

Schwarze and Denton[25] observed no differences owing to gender in a study of 527 girls and 473 boys aged 1 to 3 days. However, it is possible that at this early stage of development gender differences had not yet had time to become manifest. Conversely, Cleffken and colleagues[44] also found no gender differences in active and passive knee flexion and extension ROM in 23 male and 19 female healthy volunteers aged 19 to 27 years.

Body Mass Index

Body mass index (BMI) is a simple index of weight-for-height that is used to classify overweight and obesity in both male and female adults. It is defined as a person's weight in kilograms divided by the square of height in meters (kg/m^2). According to the most recent fact sheet by the World Health Organization (WHO), a person is overweight if he or she has a BMI greater than or equal to 25. If the person has a BMI greater than or equal to 30, then that person is considered obese.[45] Lichtenstein and associates[46] found that among 647 community-dwelling elderly subjects (aged 64 to 78 years), those with high BMI had lower knee ROM than did their counterparts with low BMI. Elderly subjects who were severely obese had an average loss of 13 degrees of knee flexion ROM compared with their counterparts who were not obese. The authors determined that a loss of knee ROM of at least 1 degree occurred for each unit increase in BMI. Escalante and coworkers[38] found that obesity was significantly associated with a decreased passive knee flexion ROM. Subjects who were overweight had a knee flexion ROM that was 5 degrees less than subjects who were not obese. Sobti and colleagues[47] found that obesity was significantly associated with the risk of pain or stiffness at the knee or hip in a survey of 5,042 post office pensioners. Knees of subjects who were overweight had flexion ROM that was 5 degrees less than subjects who were not obese.

Park and associates[48] compared 30 ROM measurements including the shoulder, elbow, knee, and ankle joints between 20 obese males (BMI = 44) with a mean age of 26 years and 20 nonobese males (BMI = 22) with a mean age of 22 years. Obesity significantly reduced ROM for 9 of the 30 motions with the smallest reduction (11.1%) occurring for knee flexion. The nonobese group had a mean ROM for the right knee of 128.7 compared with a mean of the obese group's right knee ROM of 112.9. The nonobese group's mean left knee ROM was 129 compared with a mean of 114.7 for the obese group.

Ten studies found a strong association between a high BMI, certain occupational activities, and the development of knee osteoarthritis (OA).[49–58]

McCarthy and colleagues[59] used a sensor system to analyze gait in the knees of 39 individuals with OA and 42 healthy individuals. The authors found that knee flexion ROM during the stance phase of gait was able to discriminate between patients with knee OA and healthy matched controls even in cases where gait velocity is similar. Patients with knee OA showed a decrease of 39.7% in knee flexion ROM during the stance phase of gait compared with healthy controls. The authors suggested that the differences might be caused by each individual's attempt to avoid pain by reducing the quadriceps output at peak flexion in stance, which coincides with the peak flexion moment.

Functional Range of Motion

Walking, going up and down stairs, and various activities of daily living such as getting up and sitting down, getting in and out of a bath, squatting, and kneeling are included in the following section. Walking appears to require the least knee ROM, whereas going up and down stairs, getting in and out of a chair and a bath, kneeling, and squatting require the most ROM.

Table 9.5 provides knee ROM values required for various functional activities including gait and going up and down stairs. Figures 9.19 to 9.21 show functional activities requiring different amounts of knee flexion. Of the activities measured by Jevsevar and coworkers[60] (stair ascent and descent, gait, and rising from a chair), stair ascent required the greatest range of knee motion.

Oberg, Karsznia, and Oberg[61] used electrogoniometers to measure knee joint motion in midstance and swing phases of gait in 233 healthy males and females aged 10 to 79 years. Only minor changes were attributable to age, and the authors determined that an increase in knee angle of about 0.5 degrees per decade occurred at midstance and a decrease of 0.5 to 0.8 degrees in knee angle occurred in the swing phase.

Rowe and associates[62] found that walking required the least amount of knee flexion for the 20 elderly subjects (aged 54 to 90 years) in their study, whereas getting in and out of a bath required the most knee flexion (135 degrees). The authors suggested that a clinical guideline of at least 110 degrees of flexion is necessary to allow patients to be able to walk, negotiate stairs, and get in and out of chairs. A goal of 90 degrees of knee flexion is not adequate to allow patients to carry out normal activities.

Livingston, Stevenson, and Olney[63] used three testing staircases with different dimensions. Shorter subjects had a greater maximum mean knee flexion range (92 to 105 degrees) for stair ascent in comparison with taller subjects (83 to 96 degrees). Laubenthal, Smidt, and Kettlekamp[64] used an electrogoniometric method to measure knee motion in three planes (sagittal, coronal, and transverse). Eighty-three degrees of knee motion were required for both going up and down stairs for the 30 healthy young (mean age 25 years) males in the study.

Desloovere and colleagues[65] conducted a study to analyze a set of motor tasks (walking with sidestep and crossover turns, ascent onto and descent of a step, descent with a sidestep and crossover turns, chair rise, mid- and deep squats, and lunge). These activities were performed by 10 volunteers (9 males and 1 female) with a mean age of 29 years. Three motion analysis sessions were held on different days using a standard gait analysis system and protocol. Sidestep turns had a range of axial rotation significantly larger than in walking while maintaining similar levels of repeatability. Ascent was the most repeatable among chair rises, squats, and lunges, which all showed a larger range of flexion than walking.

TABLE 9.5 Knee Flexion Range of Motion Necessary for Functional Activities: Normal Values in Degrees

	Jevsevar et al*[60]	Livingston et al[63]	Laubenthal et al[64]	Deslooval et al[65]	Rowe et al[62]
Status, Gender, Age, and Sample	Healthy (6 males, 5 females) Mean = 53 yr *n* = 11	Healthy Women Range 19–26 yr *n* = 15	Healthy Men Mean = 25 yr *n* = 30	Healthy (9 males, 1 female) Mean = 29 yr *n* = 10	Healthy Elderly Mean = 67 yr *n* = 20
Activity	***Mean (SD)***	***Means***	***Mean (SD)***	***Mean (SD)***	***Mean (SD)***
Walk level surface	63.1 (7.7)			61.1 (5.0)	64.5 (5.9)
Walk with crossover turn				57.7 (4.2)	
Walk with sidestep				57.5 (8.0)	
Ascend stairs	92.9 (9.4), 99 young 88 old	83–105	83 (8.4)	83.6 (5.3)	80.3 (8.1)
Descend stairs	86.9 (5.7), 90 young 84 old	86–107	83 (8.2)	56.1 (3.7)	77.8 (8.3)
Rise from chair	90.1 (9.8), 97 young 84 old			81 (6.6)	89.8 (9.4)
Sit in chair			93 (10.3)		91.0 (11.8)
Tie shoes			106 (9.3)		
Squat (deep)				95.4 (25)	

SD = Standard deviation.

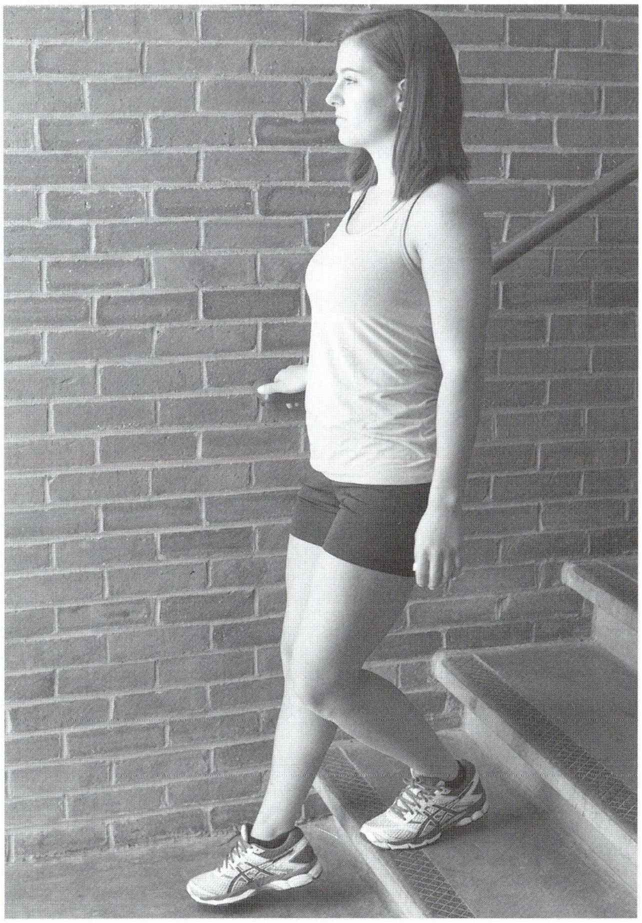

FIGURE 9.19 Descending stairs requires between 86 degrees and 107 degrees[67] of knee flexion depending on the stair dimensions.

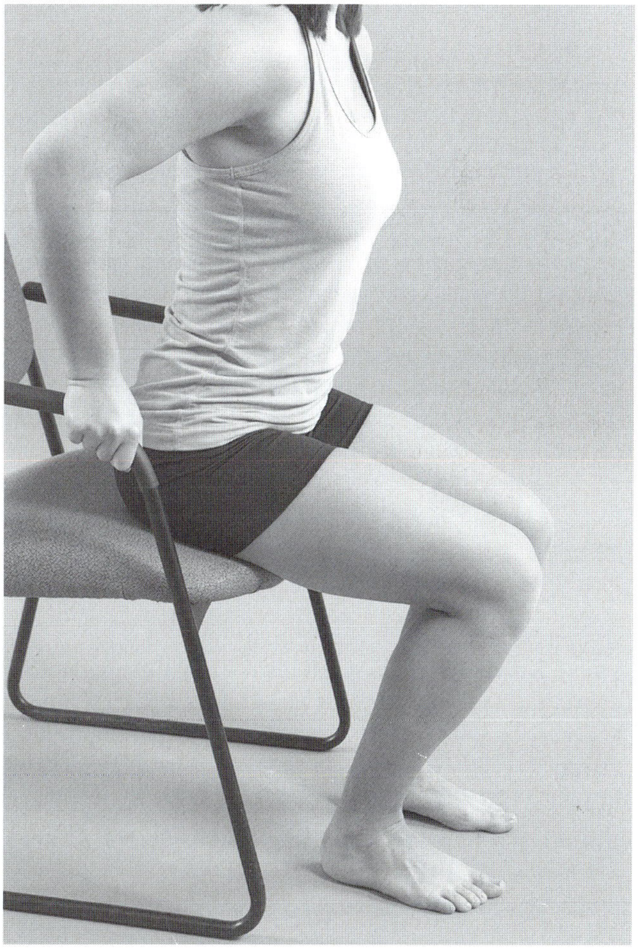

FIGURE 9.20 Rising from a chair requires a mean range of knee flexion of 90 degrees[60] to 95 degrees.[67]

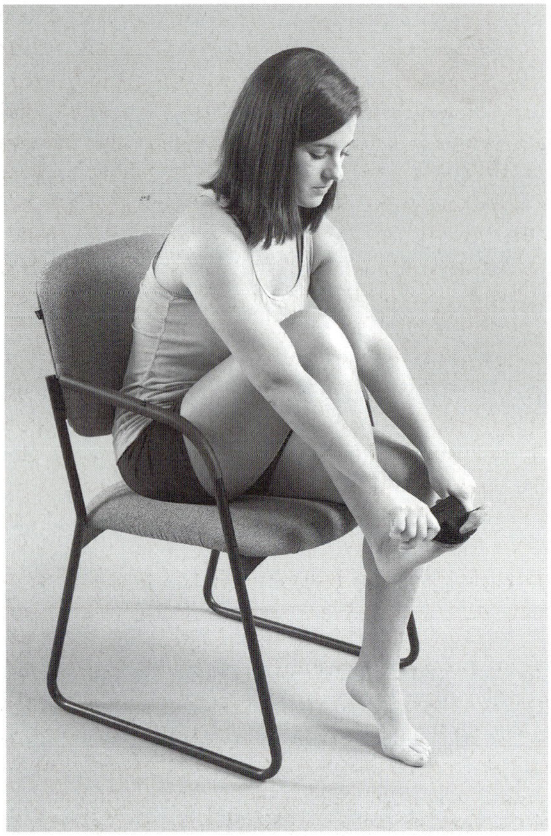

FIGURE 9.21 Putting on socks requires approximately 117 degrees of knee flexion.[64]

McFayden and Winter[66] used stair dimensions of 22 centimeters for stair height and 28 centimeters for stair tread to determine the knee flexion ROM necessary to ascend and descend stairs. The ROM needed for ascending stairs ranged from 10 to 100 degrees and the ROM for descending stairs ranged from 20 to 100 degrees. Similar dimension stairs were used by Protopapadaki and associates,[67] who used a rise height of 18 centimeters and a stair tread length of 28.5 centimeters to determine the knee motion during stair ascent and descent of 33 young healthy male and female subjects ranging in age from 18 to 39 years. The mean knee flexion angles were 93.9 degrees for stair ascent and 90.5 degrees for stair descent.

Lark and colleagues[68] compared knee ROM in stair descent in six healthy elderly males (mean age = 64 years) and six height- and weight-matched young males (mean age = 25 years). Knee flexion ROM was 12% less in the elderly group than it was in the younger group, but there was no difference between the groups in knee extension. However, the elderly group used 80% to 100% of their passive knee ROM, whereas the younger males used only 70% to 80%.

Functional Knee Motions in Non-Western Cultures

Mullholland and Wyss[69] reviewed the literature on the functional range of knee motions that are required in non-Western cultures for normal activities of daily living. The review revealed that in many parts of Asia, chairs were not commonly used and floor sitting, squatting, kneeling, or sitting cross-legged were the preferred positions (Figs. 9.22, 9.23, and 9.24). Hemmerich and colleagues[70] used an electrogoniometer motion-tracking device to determine the range of motion needed to perform squatting with the heels up and down, cross-legged sitting, and kneeling with ankles dorsiflexed and plantarflexed in 30 healthy Indian subjects (10 women and 20 men) with an average age of 48 years. Mean maximum knee flexion angles reached values greater than 150 degrees for both types of squatting and for kneeling with the ankles dorsiflexed. The mean maximal angle of knee flexion needed for kneeling with ankles plantarflexed was 144 degrees, whereas for squatting with the heels up was 157 degrees. Medial rotation at the knee accompanied hip flexion in all activities and was the greatest (33 degrees) during sitting cross-legged. The ranges of motion found in this study are far greater than can be accommodated by any existing prostheses and are many degrees more than the

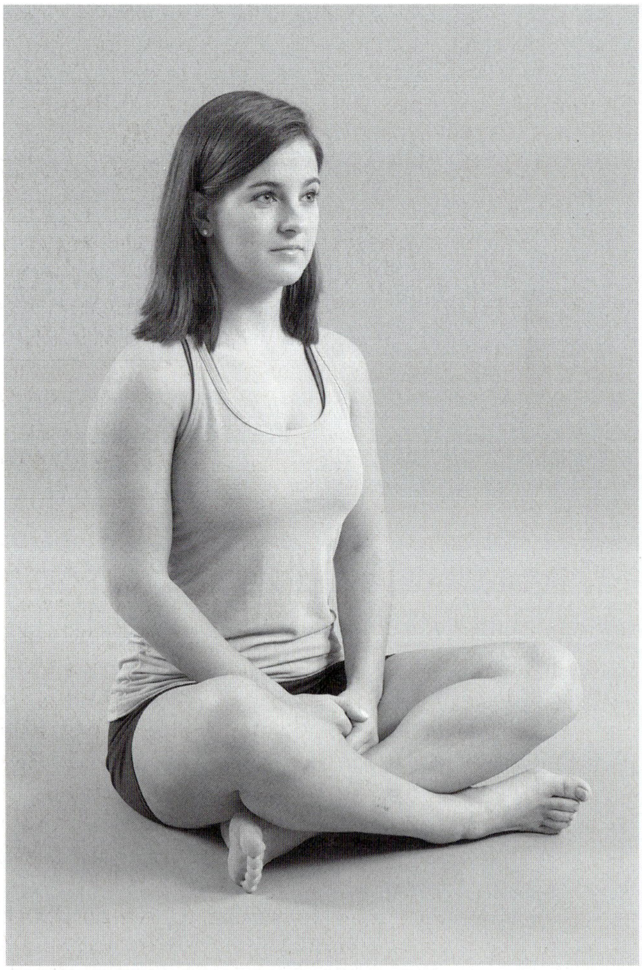

FIGURE 9.22 Cross-legged sitting requires about 33 degrees of medial knee rotation and about 37 degrees of lateral hip rotation.[70]

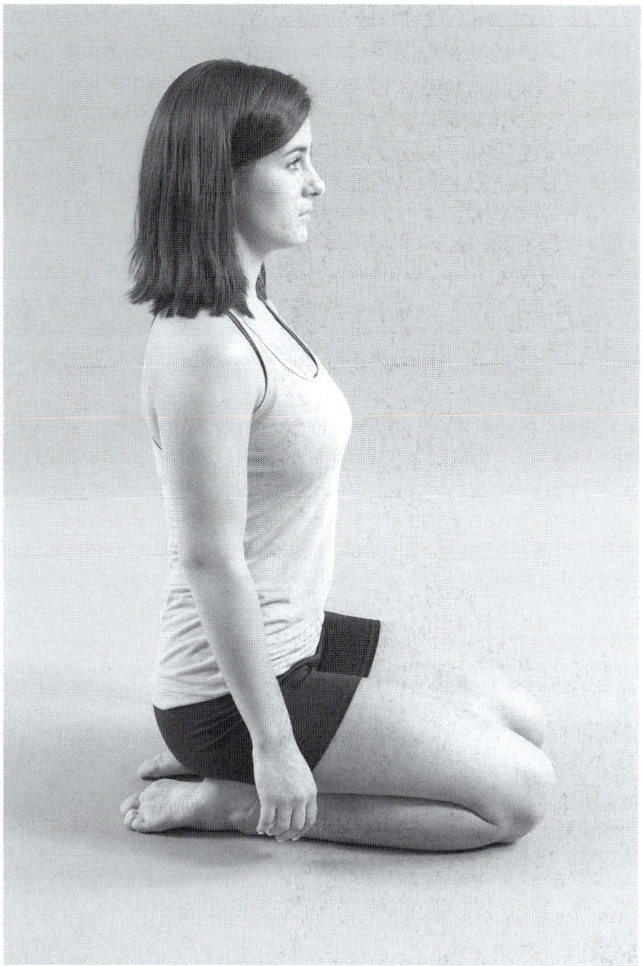

FIGURE 9.23 Kneeling with ankles plantarflexed requires knee flexion of approximately 144 degrees.[70]

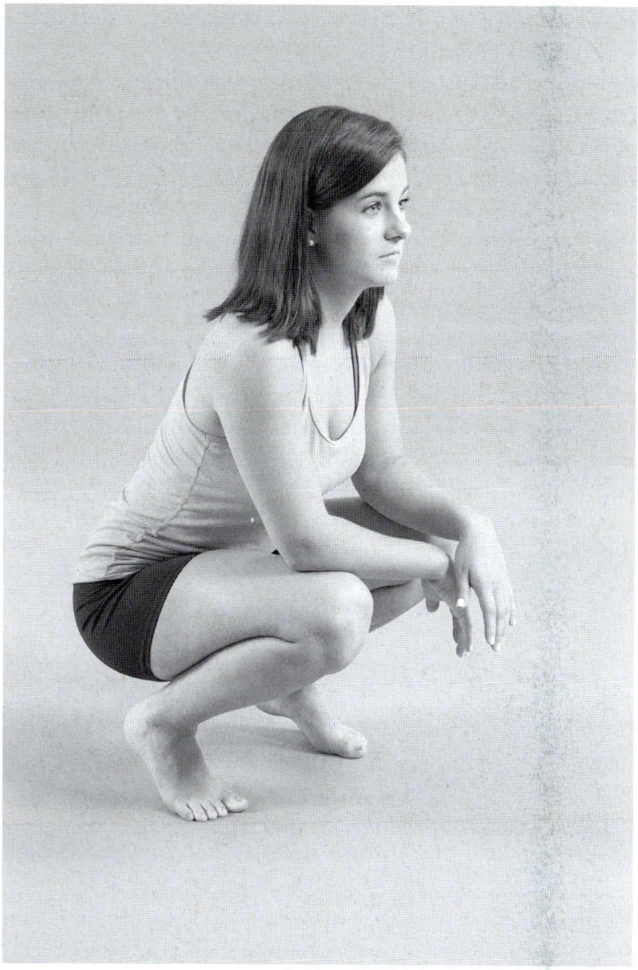

FIGURE 9.24 Squatting with heels up may require as much as 157 degrees of knee flexion.[70]

clinical guideline of 110 degrees of knee flexion suggested by both Rowe and associates[62] and the AMA.[11]

Smith and colleagues[71] identified an individual peak contact force of 49.7 N/kg during squatting at 149.9 degrees knee flexion. In comparison with stair climbing, the maximum average joint contact forces during squatting activities occurred at significantly higher flexion angles.

Zhou and associates[72] used an Optotrack Certus 3020 (three-dimensional) tracking system to measure the hip, knee, and ankle ROM during a typical kneeling posture assumed by healthy Chinese subjects. Fifteen males and 15 females with an average age of 24 years and 10 males and 10 females with an average age 64 years participated in the study. No differences were found between the two age groups in the ROM required during kneeling (mean knee flexion was 140 and 141 degrees for the younger and older groups, respectively.

Kapoor and associates[73] investigated the ROM required for cross-legged sitting, a posture essential to activities of daily living in Eastern and Asian cultures. Movements of the right hip, knee, and ankle joints were measured in 44 healthy volunteers from the Indian population. Maximum knee flexion ranged from 126 degrees to 142 degrees with a mean of 135 degrees, which, like Zhou's[72] findings, was a ROM in excess of present clinical guidelines for knee arthroplasty.

Reliability and Validity of Range of Motion Measurement

Reliability studies of active and passive range of knee motion have been conducted in healthy subjects[74–79] and in patient populations. Similar to findings at other joints, the results of knee studies show that usually intratester reliability is higher than intertester reliability. Reliability and ROM values also appear to be affected by measurement instruments and testing positions and by the type of motion (active or passive) tested. Factors that have been shown to improve reliability include training of testers, marking of landmarks, careful patient positioning, use of more than one person to assist with stabilization (especially in the presence of spasticity), and assistance in holding of heavy extremities.

Reliability of the Universal Goniometer in Healthy Populations

Boone and associates[74] had four testers use universal goniometers (UG) to measure active knee flexion and extension ROM at four weekly sessions. Intratester reliability was higher than intertester reliability, and the total intratester SD for measurements at the knee was 4 degrees, whereas the intertester SD was 5.9 degrees. The authors recommended that when more than one tester measures the range of knee motion, changes in ROM should exceed 6 degrees to show that a real change has occurred.

Rheault and coworkers[76] found good intertester reliability for the UG (Table 9.6) and the fluid-based inclinometer (r = 0.83) for measurements of active knee flexion. However, significant differences in the ROM values were found between the instruments. Therefore, the authors concluded that although the universal and fluid-based goniometers each appeared to have good reliability, they should not be used interchangeably in the clinical setting.

Bartholomy, Chandler, and Kaplan[77] had similar findings. These authors compared measurements of passive knee flexion ROM taken with a UG with measurements taken with a fluid-based inclinometer and an Optotrak motion-analysis system. Eighty healthy subjects aged 22 to 43 years were measured. Individually, the UG and the inclinometer were found to be reliable instruments for measuring passive knee flexion. Intraclass correlation coefficients (ICCs) for the UG were 0.97, and ICCs for the fluid inclinometer were 0.98. However, there were significant differences in the ROM values obtained among the three devices used, and the authors caution that these instruments should not be used interchangeably.

Mollinger and Steffan[35] collected intratester reliability data on measurement of knee extension made by two testers using a UG. Intraclass correlation coefficients for repeated measurements of knee extension were high (see Table 9.6), with differences between measurements averaging 1 degree.

TABLE 9.6 Intratester and Intertester Reliability: Knee Flexion Range of Motion Measured With a Universal Goniometer

Author	N	Sample	Motion	Intratester ICC	Intertester ICC	Intratester r	Intertester r
Boone et al[30]	12	Healthy adult males (25–54 yr)	AROM flexion	.87	.50		
Brosseau et al[78]	60	Healthy adults (mean age 20.6 yr)	Flexion fixed angles	.86–.97	.91–.94		
Rheault et al[76]	20	Healthy adults (mean age 24.8 yr)	AROM flexion				.87
Gogia et al[75]	30	Healthy adults (20–60 yr)	PROM flexion		.99		.98
Drews et al[24]	9	Healthy infants (12 hr–6 days)	PROM flexion				.69 left .89 right
Rothstein et al[80]	12	Patients (ages not reported)	PROM flexion extension	 .97–.99 .91–.97	 .84–.99 .59–.80	 .97–.99 .91–.96	 .83–.92 .57–.79
Watkins et al[81]	43	Patients (mean age 39.5 yr)	PROM flexion extension	 .99 .98	 .90 .86		
Pandya et al[82]	150* 21†	Duchenne muscular dystrophy (<1 yr–20 yr)	PROM extension	.93	.73		
Mollinger and Steffan[35]	10	Nursing home residents	Extension	.99	.97		

AROM = Active range of motion; ICC = Intraclass correlation coefficient; PROM = Passive range of motion; r = Pearson product-moment correlation coefficient.

*150 subjects were used to calculate intratester ICC.

†21 subjects were used to calculate intertester ICC.

Brosseau and associates[78] used a UG and a parallel goniometer (PG) to measure two flexion-angle positions in the right knees of 60 healthy subjects (44 females and 16 males). Intratester reliability of the smaller-angle (about 20 degrees) and larger-angle (about 100 degrees) positions were good to excellent for the UG and good for the PG. Intertester reliability was lower than intratester reliability for both positions and goniometers; however, the smaller angle had lower intertester reliability compared with the large angle (see Table 9.6).

Peters and colleagues[12] compared the use of a UG by two physical therapists to measure knee flexion and extension ROM with visual estimation (VE) by three physicians and with radiographic goniometry (RG) measurements. Radiographic measurements involved using a picture archive communication system for electronic medical imaging. Angles were determined using the long axis of the femur and tibia and estimated to the nearest degree through electronic goniometry. Twenty-one healthy male volunteers were randomly assigned to have either the right or left knee evaluated. Knee ROM examinations were repeated on 13 of the patients by three physicians and two physical therapists during separate sessions to allow for intrarater reliability evaluations. Radiographs of all 21 healthy volunteers were available for evaluation of agreement. All ICCs of intrarater reliability (VE, UG, and RG) for extension, flexion, and squat flexion (RG only) were acceptable. However, there was no agreement across methods. The authors attributed the lack of agreement to differences in the training of orthopedists and physical therapists. The mean radiographic squat flexion ROM was 158 degrees, which is 14 more degrees than supine flexion and raises the question of whether supine flexion is an accurate measure of maximum range of motion.

Reliability of the Universal Goniometer in Patient Populations

Rothstein, Miller, and Roettger[80] investigated intratester, intertester, and interdevice reliability in a study involving 12 patients referred to physical therapy for knee problems. Intratester reliability for passive ROM measurements for knee flexion and extension was high. Intertester reliability also was high among the 12 testers for passive ROM measurements for flexion but was lower for knee extension measurements (see Table 9.6). Intertester reliability was not improved by repeated measurements but was improved when testers used the same patient positioning. Interdevice reliability was high for all measurements. Neither the composition of the UG (metal or plastic) nor the size (large or small) had a significant effect on the measurements.

Watkins and associates[81] compared passive ROM measurements of the knees of 43 patients made by 14 physical therapists who used a UG and VE. These authors found that intratester reliability with the UG was high for both knee flexion and knee extension. Intertester reliability for goniometric measurements also was high for knee flexion but only good for knee extension (see Table 9.6). Both intratester and intertester reliability were lower for VE than for goniometric measurement. The authors suggested that therapists should not substitute VEs for goniometric measurements when assessing a patient's range of knee motion because of the additional error that is introduced with use of visual estimation.

Pandya and colleagues[82] studied intratester and intertester reliability of passive knee extension measurements in 150 children aged 1 to 20 years who had a diagnosis of Duchenne muscular dystrophy. Intratester reliability with use of the UG was high, but intertester reliability was only fair (see Table 9.6).

McWhirk and Glanzman[83] had two physical therapists measure the knee ROM and the popliteal angle in 46 knees in 25 children (aged 2 to 18 years) with spastic cerebral palsy. The intertester reliability of knee extension measurements was an ICC of 0.78 with a 95% confidence interval (CI) = ±1.75, and the popliteal angle measurement had an ICC of 0.93 with a 95% CI = ±1.47. The therapists helped each other during the measurements by having one or the other either provide support for the test leg or stabilize the other extremity.

In a study by Lessen and associates,[84] two physical therapists used a long-arm UG to measure active and passive knee flexion and extension in 30 patients within the first 4 days after total knee arthoplasty. Measurements were taken with the patients supine in a hospital bed and in the sitting position on an examination table. The highest levels of agreement between the testers were found for passive flexion and extension in the sitting position. The lowest level of agreement was found for passive flexion in the supine position with 16.2 to 19.0 degrees difference between the two testers. Intraclass correlation coefficient values for intertester reliability were highest for active and passive flexion while sitting.

Kilgour, McNair, and Stott[85] had three pediatric physical therapists measure bilateral knee extension in 25 children with spastic cerebral palsy ranging in age from 6 to 17 years and 25 age- and sex-matched controls. Intrasessional absolute differences ranged from 0 to 2.7 degrees in the control group and 0 to 2.4 degrees in the cerebral palsy (CP) group. Intrasessional ICCs were good in the control group (ICC = 0.79–0.87) and excellent in the CP group (ICC = 0.97–0.99). Intersessional ICCs were lower for both the control and CP groups, but only the control group had unacceptable ICCs (0.34–0.67) compared with an ICC of 0.89 to 0.92 for the CP group. The authors concluded that sagittal plane ROM measures have similar levels of reliability in children with spastic CP compared with healthy controls both within and between sessions.

Reliability of the Inclinometer

The mean knee flexion ROM for the Ely test was 138.5 degrees for four testers using an inclinometer in a study by Piva and associates.[86] Measurements were taken of 30 patients with patellofemoral pain syndrome ranging in age from 14 to 47 years. The intertester reliability ICC was 0.91.

In a study by Gnat and colleagues,[18] three physical therapists used a pleurimeter attached to the lower leg at a point halfway between the apex of the patella and the line joining the two malleoli to measure knee ROM. A force gauge attached to the ankle was used to measure the amount of force needed to produce passive extension/flexion of the knees of 26 students. Interrater reliability for knee flexion had ICCs ranging from 0.85 to 0.95 with the standard error of measurements (SEMs) ranging from 2.3 to 3.8 and smallest detectable differences (SDDs) ranging from 6.4 to 10.5. Interrater reliability for knee extension had ICCs ranging from 0.88 to 0.97 and SEMs ranging from 2.4 to 3.8, with SDDs ranging from 6.4 to 10.4.

Rheault and coworkers[76] investigated the concurrent validity of a UG and an inclinometer for measurements of active knee flexion. Each instrument had good validity, but instruments could not be used interchangeably.

Reliability of the Electronic Digital Inclinometer and Electrogoniometer

Cleffken and associates[44] conducted a study to determine both intratester and intertester reproducibility for measurements of active and passive knee flexion and extension in 42 healthy male volunteers. Each motion was measured by two testers three times in four measurement sessions using the CYBEX ED1320, an electronic digital inclinometer. Measurements of passive maximum flexion of the knee resulted in a smaller detectable difference than active knee flexion for intertester comparisons. Intratester reliability showed better reproducibility with SDDs reduced by 0.4 to 1.9 degrees over intertester values.

Piriyaprasarth and colleagues[87] assessed intratester and intertester reliability of knee measurements using a flexible electrogoniometer at two different fixed flexion angles (45 and 75 degrees) in sitting, supine, and standing positions. Thirty-seven healthy adults (mean age 31 years) participated in the intratester study, and 35 healthy adults (mean age 30 years) participated in the intertester reliability study. Ten repetitions of joint angles were taken by two testers. Intratester reliability of measurements ranged from fair for supine (ICC = 0.75–0.76), to good in sitting (ICC = 0.86–0.87), and in standing (ICC = 0.87–0.88). Intertester reliability was poor to fair for supine (ICC = 0.58–0.71), and for sitting (ICC = 0.68–0.79), and poor to good for standing (ICC = 0.57–0.80). The sitting position had higher ICCs and lower standard errors of measurement (SEMs) for both intratester and intertester reliability compared with the supine position. The SEM for repeated measures for the same tester was less than 1.7 degrees when the same tester repeated the measurements. One drawback of the study was that only angles less than 90 degrees were measured.

Reliability and Validity of Digital Imaging and Photography

Bennett and colleagues[88] recorded four digital images of each of 10 subjects' limbs in the following four positions: active extension, passive maximum extension, active flexion, and passive maximum flexion. A physical therapist and an orthopedic registrar independently measured each of the 40 images for interobserver reliability and the results were analyzed using Pearson product moment correlation coefficients ($r = 0.993 - 0.995$). Intraclass correlation coefficients ranged from 0.91 to 0.99 with SDs of 0.9 to 1.9 degrees. According to the authors, the advantages of using this technique are that it does not rely on skin marks over bony landmarks, which are often only visualized and not marked. It also eliminates the need for the repositioning of the goniometer and repalpation of bony landmarks that may be required when the overlying skin moves and alters the marking of the bony landmarks. Another advantage is that serial digital images can be made and rechecked. The major disadvantage is that it is relatively time consuming and both examiners were measuring from the same photograph, which is not typical in a clinical setting.

Naylor and associates[89] evaluated the validity and reliability of measuring knee ROM using a goniometer in conjunction with radiographs and photographs. Thirty-one volunteers (13 with arthritis and 18 healthy participants) were examined by three examiners using the following two methods of goniometer alignment: (1) the marker method using a skin marker on the greater trochanter, and (2) the line of femur method using estimation of the line of the femur. Day-to-day intrarater reliability for flexion and extension yielded high concordance correlation coefficients (CCCs) for all three examiners for both marker and line of femur methods, with slightly greater CCCs for flexion. Interrater reliability of goniometer measurements of photographs had slightly higher coefficients for flexion compared with extension and for the marker method compared with the line of femur method. For both intra- and interreliability, the mean differences were within 2 degrees and 95% limits of agreement were generally acceptable (within 5 degrees) for both methods. The authors concluded that photography offers a superior method of measurement over standard goniometry including a permanent record, which provides greater transparency and opportunities to confer.

Verhagen and associates[90] compared digital photographs with a plastic 360-degree UG with 20-centimeter arms to measure knee motion in maximal flexion and extension in 49 patients. Results showed higher intraobserver reliability for the photographic method in flexion and extension compared with traditional goniometry. For both methods, intraobserver reliability for extension was lower compared with flexion. Intraobserver SEM of the digital method was smaller than the UG method. The authors concluded that measuring maximum flexion and extension on digital photographs was more reliable than standard goniometry.

Krause and colleagues[91] examined the reliability of the Coaches Eye, a two-dimensional motion-analysis tablet computer application (app), for goniometric assessment of sagittal plane hip, knee, and ankle motion during the FMS (Functional Movement System) deep squat. (FMS is a battery of seven fundamental movement tests used to evaluate and categorize functional movement patterns.) A secondary objective was to compare ROM values obtained with the 3D Vicon motion-analysis program. Twenty-six healthy individuals aged 21 to 26 years participated in the study. Reliability of measurement ranged from 0.62 to 0.88 for the motion-analysis system and from 0.79 to 0.098 for the app. The MDC using the app was 6 degrees at the knee. The mean knee angle was 114 degrees and the ICC was 0.96. The authors concluded that the Coaches Eye app provides a reliable means of assessing sagittal plane kinematics during a deep squat maneuver.

Reliability of the Rotameter and Rottameter

A limited number of studies and instruments exist to measure voluntary knee rotation. Tsai and colleagues[15] at the University of Pittsburgh developed a device called the Rotameter to measure passive internal and external rotation at the knee. The device consists of a foam walker boot with a force/moment sensor affixed to the sole of the boot, which is used in conjunction with a magnetic tracking system. The device was tested on 11 subjects. Intratester reliability within one testing session with knee angles of 30 and 90 degrees of knee flexion found that the ICCs were both greater than 0.95 with associated SEMs less than 1 degree and a 95% confidence interval less than 2.0 degrees. Intertester reliability at 90 degrees of flexion had average ICCs and SEMs of 0.88 and 1.6, respectively.

Almquist and colleagues[16] examined the within-day and 1 week apart intratester reliability of an external device called the Rottameter. The ICCs ranged from 0.50 to 0.94 at all three flexion angles (90, 60, and 30 degrees) with 6 and 9 Nm of applied torque. A physiotherapist measured both knees in 10 healthy adults (6 females and 4 males), once in the morning and once in the afternoon of the same day. Another group of 10 females and males were tested 1 week apart at the same time of day. The highest within-day ICC was calculated at 0.94 Nm of applied torque at a 30-degree flexion angle. Intertester reliability was measured by two independent physiotherapists and the highest ICC was 0.87 at 90 degrees and 0.61 to 0.70 at 30 degrees at 6 Nm of applied torque. The Rottameter was judged by the authors to be a good (ICC = 0.75) to excellent (ICC above 0.75) device concerning reliability for measuring knee rotation with 6 and 9 Nm of applied torque at the three knee angles. The ROM for total rotations at 9 Nm of applied torque was 70 degrees to 79 degrees as measured by the Rottameter. The main drawback of this device is that it is not easily transported because it is a heavy wooden box-like structure and is a prototype.

Desloovere and colleagues[65] measured knee joint motion in three anatomical planes in 10 volunteers during 11 motor tasks using a gait-analysis technique. The authors found that the sidestep turn and descending a step showed that knee joint rotations were significantly larger by 8 to 9 degrees than during standard walking but still very repeatable. The results also showed that turning increases knee axial rotation significantly. Axial ROM in the range of 18 to 24 degrees was observed in the present study for 90-degree turning tasks, which was significantly greater than for normal walking.

Reliability and Validity of Smartphone Applications

Jenny[92] used a smartphone application to measure knee flexion angles taken during 10 total knee arthroplasties that were being performed on 4 men and 6 women (mean age of 69 years) with end-stage knee osteoarthritis. The smartphone was encased in a sterile plastic bag and placed as follows: one on the anterior surface of the thigh proximal to the skin incision and the other on the anterior surface of the distal tibia slightly distal to the incision. The knee was positioned according to the navigated system at six positions starting at full extension and ending at maximal flexion. Therefore, six navigated and six smartphone measurements were obtained for each patient giving a total of 60 navigated and 60 smartphone measurements. Results showed that there was a significant correlation between the navigated and smartphone measurements of all individual patients (r^2 = 0.88–0.99) that were operated on and the mean paired difference between the application and the navigation system was not significant (−1.1 degrees, ±6.8 degrees). Results showed that the coherence between both measurements was good. See Table 9.7.

Ockendon and Gilbert[93] compared a smartphone accelerometer-based knee goniometer with a long-armed conventional goniometer for the assessment of a fixed knee deformity. Five healthy males aged 30 to 40 years were studied. The smartphone goniometer had an intraobserver correlation of $r = 0.98$ compared with $r = 0.95$ for the UG. The smartphone goniometer had an interobserver correlation of $r = 0.98$ compared with $r = 0.93$ for the UG. The authors concluded that the smartphone goniometer is a reliable device for measurement of knee flexion in the clinic.

Ferriereo and colleagues[94] assessed the reliability of a smartphone-based application (Dr. Goniometer) developed for photographic-based goniometry by comparing the smartphone application's measurements of knee joint angles with measurements taken with a UG. In Part I, four raters performed repeated measurements with both the smartphone app and the UG at different fixed knee angles. The intrarater ICC was 0.95 and the interrater ICC was 0.99. In Part II, 10 other raters measured photographs of the knee at different flexion angles ranging from 20 to 145 degrees on a battery of 35 photographs. The results showed that inter- and intrarater correlations were always more than 0.96. However, according to the authors both UG and photographic angle goniometry are more reliable with greater degrees of knee flexion. Agreement between Dr. Goniometer and the UG showed a width of 18.2 degrees (95% limits of agreement [LOA]) (LOA = −7.5/+10.7 degrees) and 14.1 degrees (LOA = −6.6/+7.5). The authors concluded that because the smartphone app appears to be a reliable method for measuring knee ROM, it could be used as an alternative or additional method of knee joint measurement. It is easier to use than other photographic-based joint ROM assessments.

Validity of the Universal Goniometer

Validity of knee measurements in the following studies has been determined by comparison of UG measurements with radiographs. Gogia and colleagues[75] measured knee joint angles between 0 and 120 degrees of flexion. These measurements were immediately followed by radiographs. Intertester reliability was high (Table 9.6). The ICC for validity also was

TABLE 9.7 Intratester and Intertester Reliability of a Digital Inclinometer, Universal Goniometer, Digital Photography Imaging, and Smartphone Applications

Study	*N*	Raters	Methods	Motions	Intrarater ICC	Interrater ICC
Bennett et al[88]	10 patients (7 females, 3 males)	2 raters; PT, and orthopedic registrar	Gravity digital inclinometer Digital imaging	AROM extension PROM extension AROM flexion PROM flexion	.90 .95 .99 .99	.99 .95 .99 .99
Cleffken et al[44]	42 healthy males Mean age 22.1	2 raters	Electronic gravity digital inclinometer, in supine position with hip flexed to 20 degrees	AROM flexion PROM flexion AROM extension	r = .83 .87 .94	r = .83 .83 .94
Ferriero[93]		4 raters: 2 PTs, 2 student PTs, plus 10 additional raters	Smartphone app (Dr. Goniometer)	Fixed knee positions	.96	.99
			Universal goniometer	Battery of 32 photos with fixed knee positions 20–145 degrees	.99	.99
Jenny[91]	10 (4 males, 6 females) patients aged 57–81 yr having total knee arthroplasty	Operating surgeon and assistant surgeon	Smartphone app (Angle, Smudge) Navigation System (OrthoPilot, Aesculap, Tuttlingen)	Fixed knee flexion positions	.81	.79
Peters et al[12]	21 healthy male volunteers Mean age 29.6 yr	3 MDs	Visual estimation	Flexion Extension	.96 .95	.80 .80
		2 PTs	Universal goniometry	Flexion Extension	.97 .85	.88 .21
		3 MDs	Radiographic goniometry	Flexion Extension	.94 .87	.99
Naylor[89]	31 (13 arthritic, 18 healthy) Mean age: 33.8 yr	3 raters using 2 methods	Line of femur method	Flexion Extension	.99 .99	.99 .89
			Marker method	Flexion Extension	.99 .98	.99 .98
Okendon[92]	5 healthy males 30–40 yrs	2 experienced raters	Smartphone application Universal goniometer	Fixed knee flexion positions	r = 0.98 .94	.99 .95
Verhagen[90]	49 patients with various medical histories	4 raters	Digital photographs and goniometric measurements	Goniometry flexion Digital flexion Goniometry extension Digital extension	.95 .99 .82 .84	.92 .96 .64 .65

ICC = Intraclass correlation coefficient; r = Pearson product-moment correlation coefficient; AROM = Active range of motion; PROM = Passive range of motion; PT = physical therapist or physiotherapist; MD = medical doctor.

high (0.99). The authors concluded that the knee angle measurements taken with a UG were both reliable and valid.

Enwemeka[79] compared the measurements of six knee joint positions (0, 15, 30, 45, 60, and 90 degrees) taken with a UG with bone angle measurements provided by radiographs. The measurements were taken on 10 healthy adult volunteers (4 women and 6 men) between 21 and 35 years of age. The mean differences ranged from 0.52 to 3.81 degrees between goniometric and radiographic measurements taken between 30 and 90 degrees of flexion. However, mean differences were higher (4.59 degrees) between goniometric and radiographic measurements of the smaller knee joint angles between 0 and 15 degrees.

Ersoz and Ergun[37] used a UG with 25-centimeter arms and 1-degree increments to measure the ROM in both knees of 20 patients with bilateral knee osteoarthritis. Radiographs were taken of tibiofemoral, lateral tibiofemoral, and patellofemoral compartments of the same knees. The authors found a clear relationship between knee ROM measurements of flexion, extension, and medial and lateral rotation taken with a UG and radiographs. For example, limitations in internal rotation ROM provided a prediction of advanced disease in the lateral knee compartment. The authors concluded that measurements of joint ROM were helpful in the determination of the compartment or compartments that were affected by the disease process.

Brousseau and associates[78] measured active knee flexion in two positions in 60 healthy university students (44 females and 16 males) with a mean age of 21 years. Two trained testers alternately used either a universal (UG) or a parallelogram (PG) goniometer for the measurements. Eight measurements were taken with the knee flexed in the supine position and eight with the knee in the first 20 degrees of flexion in the supine position. A radiograph was taken of each subject in each knee position. Criterion validity was determined by calculating Pearson product moment correlation coefficients between each goniometric and radiologic measurement. Results showed that both the PGs and UGs had higher validity when measuring the larger fixed knee flexion angle compared with the smaller angle when using radiographs as the gold standard. Naylor and associates[89] found that validity of photographs referenced to radiographs showed that for each of the following (line of the femur and marker methods) all three examiners yielded very high CCCs for flexion (0.98–0.99) and moderate to substantial CCCs for extension (0.48–0.68). Mean differences and 95% limits of agreement were narrower for flexion than for extension. The authors concluded that measuring ROM from a photograph has excellent validity for flexion, whereas the validity for extension was less impressive.

Reliability and Validity of Muscle Length Testing

Gajdosik and associates,[19] in a study of 30 healthy males aged 18 to 40 years, found that intrarater reliability intraclass correlation coefficients (ICCs) for the knee extension test were 0.86 when knee extension was performed actively and 0.90 when performed passively. Youdas and colleagues[20] conducted a study to examine the effects of age and gender on hamstring muscle length (HML) as measured by passive straight leg raise and popliteal angle. The study consisted of 214 adults (108 women and 106 men) between the ages of 20 and 79 years. The trunk–thigh angle (PSLR) and the PA (thigh–leg angle) were estimated with a goniometer. Results showed that HML differed significantly between genders, with females demonstrating greater flexibility than their male counterparts. According to the data, the mean value of PSLR for women of 76.3 was closer to 80 degrees than the value for men of 68.5 degrees. The PSLR angle in men was significantly less than that in women.

Gnat and colleagues[18] calculated correlation coefficients, standard errors of measurement, and smallest detectable difference to evaluate reliability of the passive knee extension (PKE) test for length of the hamstring muscles. The results showed excellent reliability. The mean interrater ICC for the PKE test was 0.93.

REFERENCES

1. Levangie, PK, and Norkin, CC: Joint Structure and Function: A Comprehensive Analysis, ed 5. FA Davis, Philadelphia, 2011.
2. Williams, PL (ed): Gray's Anatomy, ed 38. Churchill Livingstone, New York, 1995.
3. Mossberg, KA, and Smith, LK: Axial rotation of the knee in women. J Orthop Sports Phys Ther 4:27, 1983.
4. Zarins, B, et al: Rotational motion of the knee. Am J Sports Med 11:152, 1983.
5. Almquist, PO, et al: Knee rotation in healthy individuals related to age and gender. J Orthop Res 31(1):23, 2013.
6. Kaltenborn, FM: Mobilization of the Extremity Joints, ed 5. Olaf Norlis Bokhandel, Oslo, Norway, 1999.
7. Cyriax, JH, and Cyriax, PJ: Illustrated Manual of Orthopaedic Medicine. Butterworths, London, 1983.
8. Fritz, JM, et al: An examination of the selective tissue tension scheme, with evidence for the concept of a capsular pattern of the knee. Phys Ther 78:1046, 1998.
9. Boone, DC, and Azen, SP: Normal range of motion of joints in male subjects. J Bone Joint Surg Am 61:756, 1979.
10. Roach, KE, and Miles, TP: Normal hip and knee active range of motion: The relationship to age. Phys Ther 71:656, 1991.
11. Rondinell, RD (ed): Guides to the Evaluation of Permanent Impairment, ed 6. American Medical Association, Chicago, 2009.
12. Peters, PG, et al: Knee range of motion: Reliability and agreement of 3 measurement methods. Am J Orthop 40(12):E249, 2011.
13. Alam, M, et al: A clinical device for measuring internal-external rotational laxity of the knee. Am J Sports Med 41(1):87, 2013.
14. Ahrens, P, et al: A novel tool for objective assessment of femorotibial rotation: A cadaver study. Int Orthop 35 (11):1611, 2011.
15. Tsai, AG, et al: Rotational knee laxity: Reliability of a simple measurement device in vivo. BMC Musculoskelet Disord 9:35, 2008.
16. Almquist, PO, et al: Measurements of knee rotation-reliability of an external device in vivo. BMC Musculoskelet Disord 12:291, 2011.
17. Clarkson, HM: Musculoskeletal Assessment Joint Motion and Muscle Testing, ed 3. Walters Klower Lippincott William and Wilkins, Philadelphia, 2013.
18. Gnat, R, et al: Reliability of the passive knee flexion and extension tests in healthy subjects. J Manipulative Physiol Ther 33:659, 2010.
19. Gajdosik, RL, et al: Comparison of four clinical tests for assessing hamstring muscle length. J Orthop Sport Phys Ther 18:614, 1993.
20. Youdas, JW, et al: The influence of gender and age on hamstring muscle length in healthy adults. J Orthop Sports Phys Ther 35:246, 2005.
21. Fredriksen, H, et al: Passive knee extension test to measure hamstring muscle tightness. Scand J Med Sci Sports 7:279, 1997.
22. Rothstein, JM, Roy, SH, and Wolf, SL: The Rehabilitation Specialist's Handbook, ed 2. FA Davis, Philadelphia, 1998
23. Waugh, KG, et al: Measurement of selected hip, knee, and ankle joint motions in newborns. Phys Ther 63:1616, 1983.
24. Drews, JE, Vraciu, JK, and Pellino, G: Range of motion of the lower extremities of newborns. Phys Occup Ther Pediatr 4:49, 1984.
25. Schwarze, DJ, and Denton, JR: Normal values of neonatal limbs: An evaluation of 1000 neonates. J Pediatr Orthop 13:758, 1993.
26. Wanatabe, H, et al: The range of joint motions of the extremities in healthy Japanese people: The difference according to age. Nippon Seikeigeka Gakkai Zasshi 53:275, 1979. (Cited by Walker, JM: Musculoskeletal development: A review. Phys Ther 71:878, 1991.)
27. Broughton, NS, Wright, J, and Menelaus, MB: Range of knee motion in normal neonates. J Pediatr Orthop 13:263, 1993.
28. Boone, DC: Techniques of measurement of joint motion. (Unpublished supplement to Boone, DC, and Azen, SP: Normal range of motion in male subjects. J Bone Joint Surg Am 61:756, 1979.)
29. Beighton, P, Solomon, L, and Soskolne, CL: Articular mobility in an African population. Ann Rheum Dis 32:23, 1973.
30. Cheng, JC, Chan, PS, and Hui, PW: Joint laxity in children. J Pediatr Orthop 11:752, 1991.
31. Steinberg, N, et al: Range of joint movement in female dancers and non-dancers aged 8–16 years. Am J Sports Med 34(5):814, 2006.
32. Soucie, JM, et al: Range of motion measurements reference values and a database for comparison studies. Haemophilia, 17(3):500, 2011.
33. Walker, JM, et al: Active mobility of the extremities in older subjects. Phys Ther 64:919, 1984.
34. Greene, WB, and Heckman, JD (eds): The Clinical Measurement of Joint Motion. American Academy of Orthopaedic Surgeons, Chicago, 1994.
35. Mollinger, LA, and Steffan, TM: Knee flexion contractures in institutionalized elderly: Prevalence, severity, stability and related variables. Phys Ther 73:437, 1993.
36. Steultjens, MPM, et al: Range of motion and disability in patients with osteoarthritis of the knee or hip. Rheumatology 39:955, 2000.
37. Ersoz, M, and Ergun, S: Relationship between knee range of motion and Kellgren-Lawrence radiographic scores in knee osteoarthritis. Am J Phys Med Rehabil 82:110, 2003.
38. Escalante, A, et al: Determinants of hip and knee flexion range: Results from the San Antonio Longitudinal Study of Aging. Arthritis Care Res 12:8, 1999.
39. Nonaka, H, et al: Age-related changes in the interactive mobility of the hip and knee joints: A geometrical analysis. Gait Posture 15:236, 2002.
40. Macedo, LG, and Magee, DJ: Effects of age on passive range of motion of selected peripheral joints in healthy adult females. Physiother Theory Pract 25(2):146, 200.
41. Loudon, JK, Goist, HL, and Loudon, KL: Genu recurvatum syndrome. J Orthop Sports Phys Ther 27:361, 1998.
42. Hall, MG, et al: The effect of hypermobility syndrome on knee joint proprioception. Br J Rheumatol 34:121, 1995.
43. James, B, and Parker, AW: Active and passive mobility of the lower limb joints in elderly men and women. Am J Phys Med Rehabil 68:162, 1989.
44. Cleffken, B, et al: Digital goniometric measurement of knee joint motion. Evaluation of usefulness for research settings and clinical practice. Knee 14:385, 2007.
45. Jasmuheen.com (http://www.who.int/mediacentre/factsheets/fs311/en/index .html).
46. Lichtenstein, MJ, et al: Modeling impairment: Using the disablement process as a framework to evaluate determinants of hip and knee flexion. Aging (Milano) 12:208, 2000.
47. Sobti, A, et al: Occupational physical activity and long term risk of musculoskeletal symptoms: A national survey of post office pensioners. Am J Indust Med 32:76, 1997.
48. Park,W, et al: Obesity effect on male active joint range of motion. Ergonomics 53(1):102, 2010.
49. Grotle, M, Hagen, KB, and Natvig, B: Obesity and osteoarthritis in knee, hip and hand. An epidemiological study in the general population with ten years follow up. BMC Musculoskelet Disord 9:132, 2008.
50. Richmond, SA, et al: Are joint injury, sport activity, physical activity, obesity or occupational activities predictors for osteoarthritis? A systematic review. J Orthop Sports Phys Ther 43(8):515, 2013.
51. Widmyer, MR, et al: High body mass index is associated with increased diurnal stains in articular cartilage of the knee. Arthritis Rheum 65(10):2615, 2013.
52. Vrezas, J, et al: Case control study of knee osteoarthritis and lifestyle factors considering their interaction with physical workload. Arch Occup Environ Health 83(3):291, 2010.
53. Jensen, LK, Rytter, S, and Bonde, JP: Symptomatic knee disorders in floor layers and graphic designers. A cross-sectional study. BMC Musculoskelet Disord 113:188, 2012.
54. Amin, S, et al: Occupation-related squatting, kneeling, and heavy lifting and the knee joint: A magnetic resonance imaging-based study in men. J Rheumatol 35(8), 2008.
55. Sowers, MF, et al: BMI versus body composition and radiographically defined osteoarthritis of the knee in women: A 4-year follow-up study. Osteoarthritis Cartilage 16:367, 2008.
56. Seidler, A, et al: The role of cumulative physical work load in symptomatic knee osteoarthritis—a case control study. J Occup Med Toxicol 14, 2008.
57. Teichtahl, AJ, et al: Occupational activity is associated with knee cartilage morphology in females. Maturitas 66(1):72, 2010.
58. Palmu, SA, et al: Childhood femoral fracture can lead to premature knee joint arthritis. Acta Orthop 84(1):71, 2013.
59. McCarthy, I, et al: Analysis of knee flexion characteristics and how they alter with the onset of knee osteoarthritis. A case control study. BMC Musculoskelet Disord 14: 169, 2013.
60. Jevsevar, DS, et al: Knee kinematics and kinetics during locomotor activities of daily living in subjects with knee arthroplasty and in healthy control subjects. Phys Ther 73:229, 1993.
61. Oberg, T, Karsznia, A, and Oberg, K: Joint angle parameters in gait: Reference data for normal subjects, 10–79 years of age. J Rehabil Res Dev 31:199, 1994.
62. Rowe, PJ, et al: Knee kinematics in gait and other functional activities measured using flexible electrogoniometry: How much knee motion is sufficient for a normal daily life? Gait Posture 12:143, 2000.

63. Livingston, LA, Stevenson, JM, and Olney, SJ: Stairclimbing kinematics on stairs of differing dimensions. Arch Phys Med Rehabil 72:398, 1991.
64. Laubenthal, KN, Smidt, GL, and Kettlekamp, DB: A quantitative analysis of knee motion during activities of daily living. Phys Ther 52:34, 1972.
65. Desloovere, K, et al: Range of motion and repeatability of knee kinematics for 11 clinically relevant motor tasks. Gait Posture 32(4):597, 2010.
66. McFayden, BJ, and Winter, DA: An integrated biomechanical analysis of normal stair ascent and descent. J Biomech 21:733, 1988.
67. Protopapadaki, A, et al: Hip, knee and ankle kinematics and kinetics during stair ascent and descent in healthy young individuals. Clin Biomech 22:203, 2007.
68. Lark, SD, et al: Knee and ankle range of motion during stepping down in elderly compared to young men. Eur J Appl Physiol 9:287, 2004.
69. Mulholland, SJ, and Wyss, UP: Activities of daily living in non-Western cultures: Range of motion requirements for hip and knee joints. Int J Rehabil Res 24:191, 2001.
70. Hemmerich, A, et al: Hip, knee and ankle kinematics of high range of motion activities of daily living. J Orthop Res 24:770, 2006.
71. Smith, SM, et al: Tibiofemoral contact forces and knee kinematics during squatting. Gait Posture 27(3):376, 2008.
72. Zhou, H, et al: Kinematics of the hip, knee, ankle of the young and elderly Chinese people during kneeling activity. J Zhejiang Univ Sci B 13(10):831, 2012.
73. Kapoor, A, et al: Range of movements of lower limb joints in cross-legged sitting. J Arthroplasty 23(3):451, 2008.
74. Boone, DC, et al: Reliability of goniometric measurements. Phys Ther 58:1355, 1978.
75. Gogia, PP, et al: Reliability and validity of goniometric measurements at the knee. Phys Ther 67:192, 1987.
76. Rheault, W, et al: Intertester reliability and concurrent validity of fluid based and universal goniometers for active knee flexion. Phys Ther 68:1676, 1988.
77. Bartholomy, JK, Chandler, RF, and Kaplan, SE: Validity analysis of fluid goniometer measurements of knee flexion [abstract]. Phys Ther 80:S46, 2000.
78. Brosseau, L, et al: Intratester and intertester reliability and criterion validity of the parallelogram and universal goniometers or active knee flexion in healthy adults. Physiother Res Int 2:150, 1997.
79. Enwemeka, CS: Radiographic verification of knee goniometry. Scand J Rehabil Med 18:47, 1986.
80. Rothstein, JM, Miller, PJ, and Roettger, RF: Goniometric reliability in a clinical setting. Phys Ther 63:1611, 1983.
81. Watkins, MA, et al: Reliability of goniometric measurements and visual estimates of knee range of motion obtained in clinical settings. Phys Ther 71:90, 1991.
82. Pandya, S, et al: Reliability of goniometric measurements in patients with Duchenne muscular dystrophy. Phys Ther 65:1339, 1985.
83. McWhirk, LB, and Glanzman, AM: Within-session inter-rater reliability of goniometric measures in patients with spastic cerebral palsy. Pediatr Phys Ther 18:262, 2006.
84. Lessen, AF, et al: Reproducibility of goniometric measurement of the knee in the in-hospital phase following total knee arthroplasty. BMC Musculoskelet Disord 8:83, 2007.
85. Kilgour, G, McNair, PM, and Stott, NS: Intrarater reliability of lower limb sagittal range-of-motion measures in children with spastic diplegia. Dev Med Child Neurol 45:391, 2003.
86. Piva, SR, et al: Reliability of measures of impairments associated with patellofemoral pain syndrome. BMC Musculoskelet Disord 7:33, 2006.
87. Piriyaprasarth, P, et al: The reliability of knee joint position testing using electrogoniometry. BMC Musculoskelet Disord 9:6, 2008.
88. Bennett, D, et al: Measurement of joint motion using digital imaging. Int Orthop 33(6):1627, 2009.
89. Naylor, JM, et al: Validity and reliability of using photography for measuring knee range of motion: A methodological study. BMC Musculoskelet Disord 12:77, 2011.
90. Verhagen, F, et al: Are clinical photographs appropriate to determine the maximal range of motion of the knee range of motion? Acta Orthop Belg 76(6), 2010.
91. Krause, D, et al: The reliability and accuracy of a goniometer mobile device application for video measurement of the functional movement screen deep squat test. Int J Sports Phys Ther 10:37, 2015.
92. Jenny, J-Y: Measurement of knee flexion angle with a smartphone application is precise and accurate. J Arthroplasty 28:784, 2013.
93. Ockendon, M, and Gilbert, RE: Validation of a novel smartphone accelerometer-based knee goniometer. J Knee Surg 25(4):341, 2012.
94. Ferreiro, G, et al: Reliability of a smartphone-based goniometer for knee goniometry. Int J Rehabil Res 36(2), 2013.

CHAPTER 10

The Ankle and Foot

D. Joyce White, PT, DSc

Structure and Function

Proximal and Distal Tibiofibular Joints

The proximal tibiofibular joint is typically composed of a slightly convex tibial facet and a slightly concave fibular facet, although the joint surfaces can vary in configuration in between individuals (Fig. 10.1A).[1,2] This synovial joint is surrounded by a joint capsule that is reinforced by anterior and posterior ligaments (Fig. 10.1B, C), as well as the tendon of the popliteus muscle.[1–3]

The distal tibiofibular joint is formed by a fibrous union between a concave facet on the lateral aspect of the distal tibia and a convex facet on the distal fibula (Fig. 10.1A). Both joints are supported by the interosseous membrane, which is located between the tibia and the fibula (Fig. 10.1B). The distal joint does not have a joint capsule but is supported by anterior and posterior ligaments and the crural interosseous tibiofibular ligament (Fig. 10.1B, C).[1–3]

Osteokinematics

The proximal and distal tibiofibular joints are anatomically distinct from the talocrural joint but function to serve the ankle. The proximal tibiofibular joint is a plane synovial joint that allows a small amount of superior and inferior sliding of the fibula on the tibia and a slight amount of rotation. The distal joint is a syndesmosis, or fibrous union, but it also allows a small amount of motion.[1–3]

Arthrokinematics

During dorsiflexion of the ankle, the fibula moves proximally and slightly posteriorly (lateral rotation) away from the tibia. During plantarflexion, the fibula glides distally and slightly anteriorly (medial rotation) toward the tibia. The fibular glides distally and slightly posteriorly during inversion, while gliding proximally and slightly ventrally during eversion.[4] These small motions of the fibula appear to be related to the asymmetrical shape of the dome of the talus (wider anteriorly), as well as the asymmetry in size and orientation of the lateral and medial facets of the talus that articulate with the fibula and tibia.[1]

Capsular Pattern

The capsular pattern is not defined for the tibiofibular joints.

Talocrural Joint

The talocrural joint comprises the articulations between the talus and the distal tibia and fibula. Proximally, the joint is formed by the concave surfaces of the distal tibia and the tibial and fibular malleoli. Distally, the joint surface is the convex dome of the talus.[1–3] The joint capsule is thin and weak especially anteriorly and posteriorly, and the joint is reinforced by lateral and medial ligaments.[1] Anterior and posterior talofibular ligaments and the calcaneofibular ligament provide lateral support for the capsule and joint (Fig. 10.2A, B). The deltoid ligament provides medial support (Fig. 10.3). The ligaments that connect the distal tibia and fibula are important for stability of the mortise and thus the talocrural joint as well.[1,3] These ligaments include the crural tibiofibular interosseous ligament, tibiofibular interosseous membrane, and the anterior and posterior tibiofibular ligaments (Fig. 10.1B, C).

Osteokinematics

The talocrural joint is a synovial hinge joint with 1 degree of freedom. The motions available are dorsiflexion and plantarflexion. Because the lateral malleolus is more distal and posterior than the medial malleolus, the axis for movement is oblique and thus motions do not occur purely in the sagittal plane.[2] Dorsiflexion of the ankle brings the foot up with slight abduction and pronation/eversion, whereas plantarflexion brings the foot down with slight adduction and supination/inversion. The ankle is considered to be in the 0-degree neutral position when the foot is at a right angle to the tibia.

Arthrokinematics

During dorsiflexion in the non-weight-bearing position, the talus rolls anteriorly and slides posteriorly. During plantarflexion, the talus rolls posteriorly and slides anteriorly.[2,4] During dorsiflexion, in the weight-bearing position with the

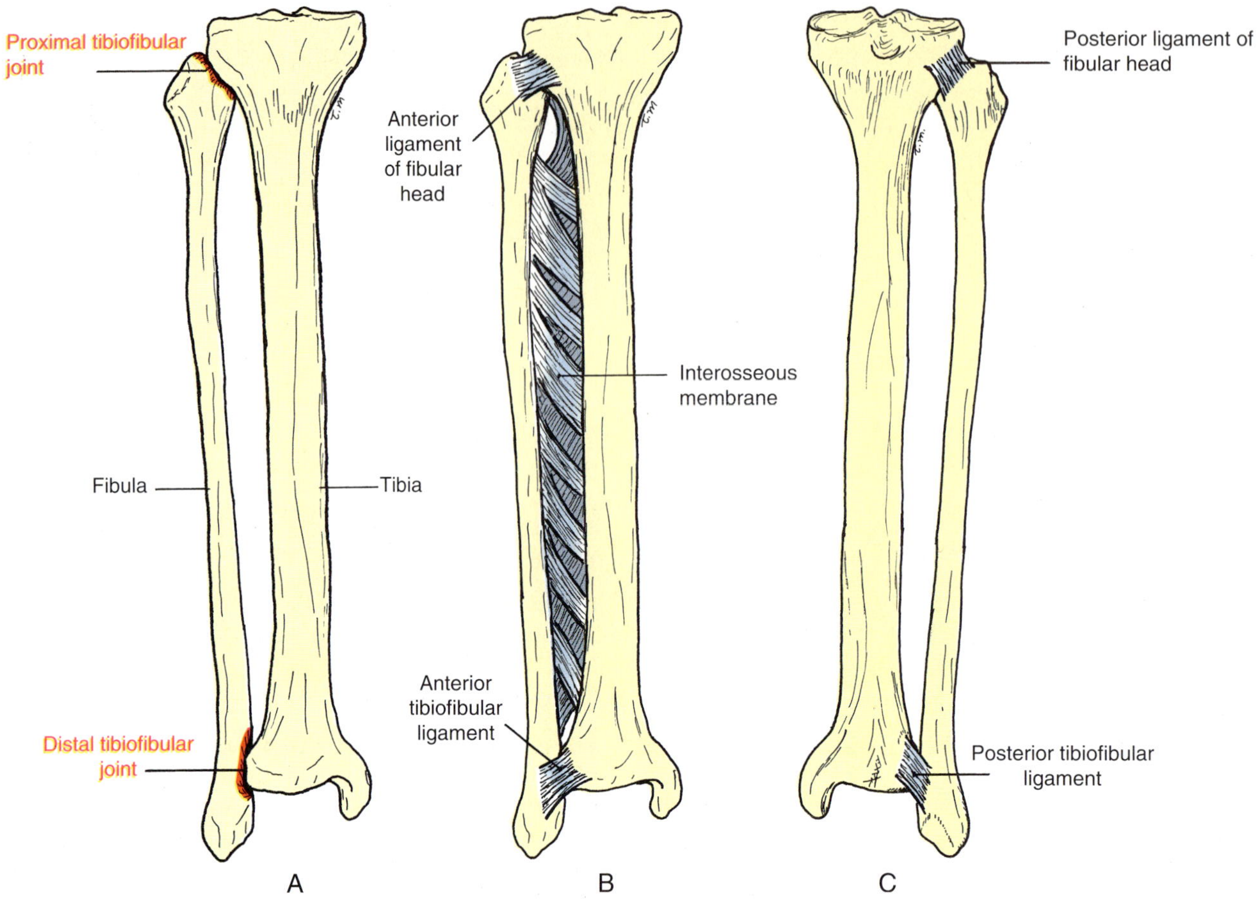

FIGURE 10.1 (A) The anterior aspect of the proximal and distal tibiofibular joints of a right lower extremity. (B) The anterior tibiofibular ligaments and the interosseous membrane. (C) The posterior aspect of the tibiofibular joints and the posterior tibiofibular ligaments of a right lower extremity.

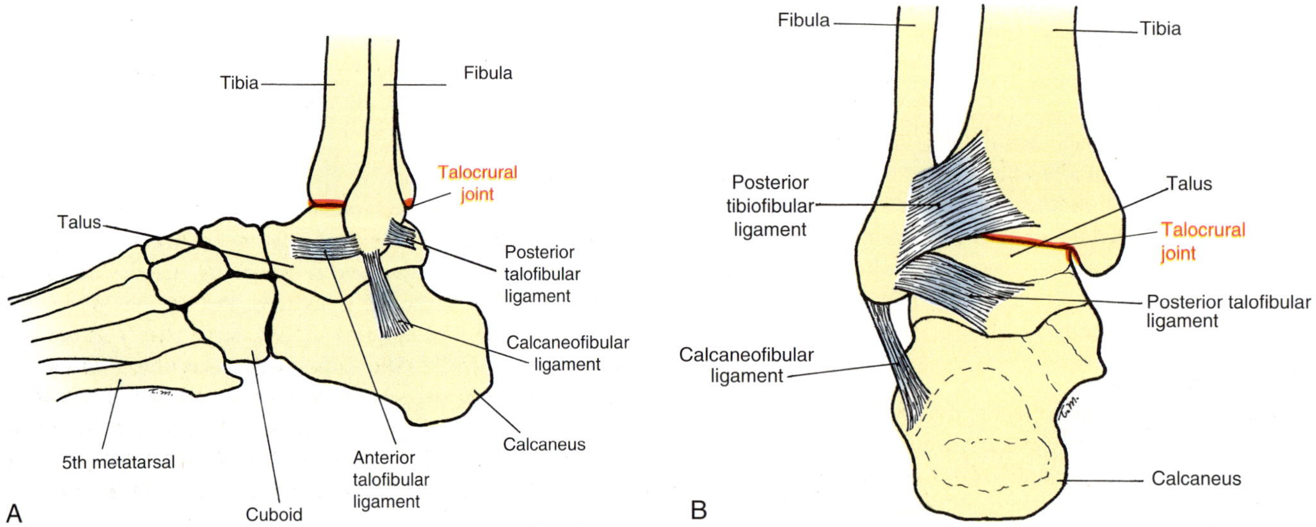

FIGURE 10.2 (A) A lateral view of a left talocrural joint with the anterior and posterior talofibular ligaments and the calcaneofibular ligament. (B) A posterior view of a left talocrural joint shows the posterior talofibular ligament and the calcaneofibular ligament.

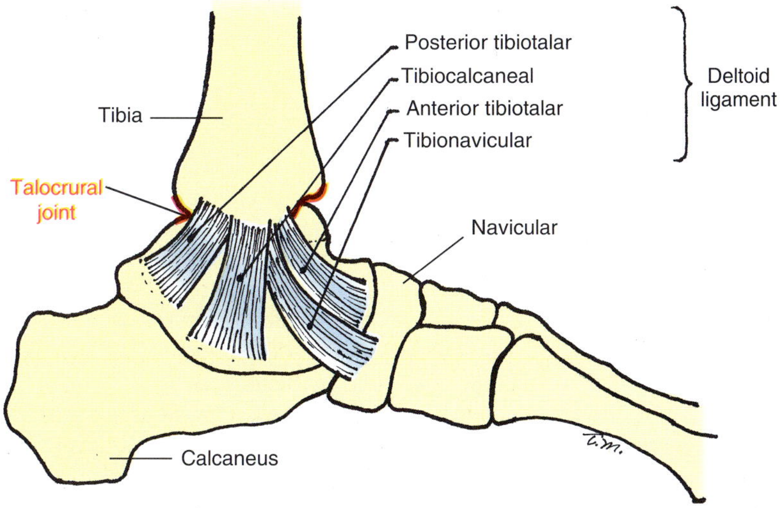

FIGURE 10.3 The deltoid ligament in a medial view of a left talocrural joint.

talus fixed, the tibia moves anteriorly. During plantarflexion in a weight-bearing position the tibia moves posteriorly.

Capsular Pattern

The pattern is a greater limitation in plantarflexion than in dorsiflexion.[4,5]

Subtalar Joint

The subtalar (talocalcaneal) joint is composed of three separate plane articulations: the posterior, anterior, and middle articulations between the talus and the calcaneus. The posterior articulation, which is the largest, includes a concave facet on the inferior surface of the talus and a convex facet on the body of the calcaneus.[1–3] The anterior and middle articulations are formed by two convex facets on the talus and two concave facets on the calcaneus. The posterior articulation has its own capsule, whereas the anterior and middle articulations share a joint capsule with the talonavicular joint. The subtalar joint is reinforced by anterior, posterior, lateral, and medial talocalcaneal ligaments and the interosseus talocalcaneal ligament (Figs. 10.4 and 10.5).

Osteokinematics

The motions permitted at the joint are inversion and eversion, which occur around an oblique axis that can be visualized as running from the lateral–posterior heel through the subtalar joint in an anterior, medial, and superior direction.[2] Inversion and eversion are composite motions consisting of a coupling of adduction–abduction, supination–pronation, and to a lesser extent flexion–extension. During non-weight-bearing inversion, the calcaneus adducts, supinates, and plantarflexes. During eversion, the calcaneus abducts, pronates, and dorsiflexes. The terms "supination" and "pronation" have also been used to describe the composite motions instead of "inversion" and "eversion," respectively.

Arthrokinematics

The alternating convex and concave facets limit mobility and create a twisting motion of the calcaneus on the talus.[1] The

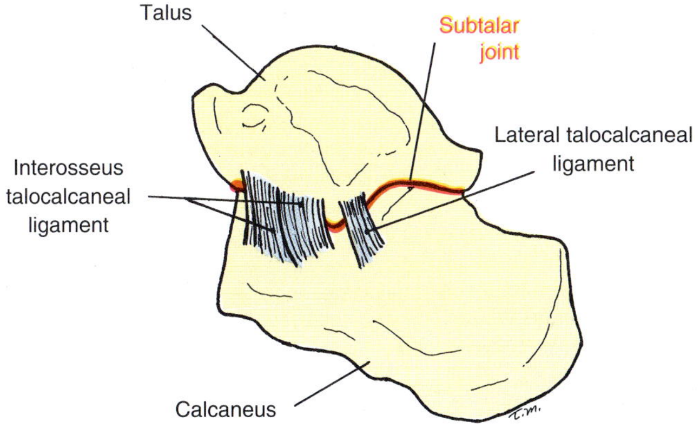

FIGURE 10.4 The interosseus talocalcaneal and lateral talocalcaneal ligaments in a lateral view of a left subtalar joint.

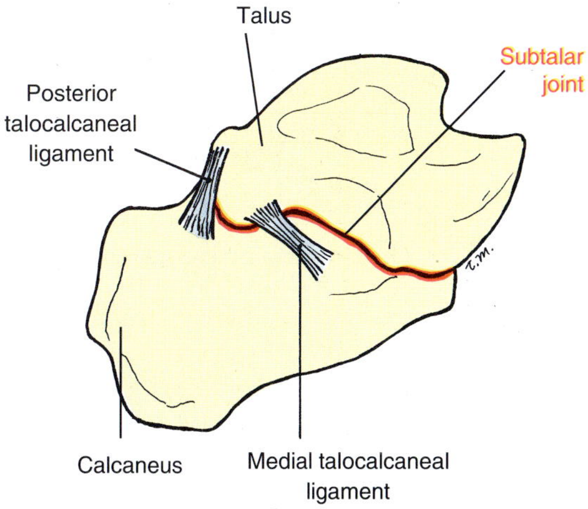

FIGURE 10.5 The medial and posterior talocalcaneal ligaments in a medial view of a left subtalar joint.

larger posterior part of the subtalar joint in which the talus is concave and calcaneus is convex defines the arthrokinematic motions. During inversion of the foot, the calcaneus rolls medially and slides laterally on a fixed talus. During eversion, the calcaneus rolls laterally and slides medially on the talus.[2,4]

Capsular Pattern

The capsular pattern consists of a greater limitation in varus (inversion) than valgus (eversion).[5]

Transverse Tarsal (Midtarsal) Joint

The transverse tarsal, or midtarsal, joint is a compound joint formed by the talonavicular and calcaneocuboid joints (Fig. 10.6A). The talonavicular joint is composed of the large convex head of the talus and the concave posterior portion of the navicular bone.[1–3] The concavity is enlarged by the plantar calcaneonavicular ligament (spring ligament). The joint shares a capsule with the anterior and middle portions of the subtalar joint and is reinforced by the spring, bifurcate (calcaneocuboid and calcaneonavicular), and dorsal talonavicular ligaments (Fig. 10.6B).

The calcaneocuboid joint is a saddle joint with shallow convex–concave surfaces on the anterior calcaneus and corresponding convex–concave surfaces on the posterior cuboid.[3,4] The joint is enclosed in a capsule that is reinforced by the bifurcate (calcaneocuboid and calcaneonavicular), dorsal calcaneocuboid, plantar calcaneocuboid, and long plantar ligaments (Fig. 10.6C).

Osteokinematics

The joint is considered to have two axes, one longitudinal and one oblique. Motions around both axes are triplanar and consist of inversion and eversion.[1,2] The transverse tarsal joint is the transitional link between the hindfoot and the forefoot.

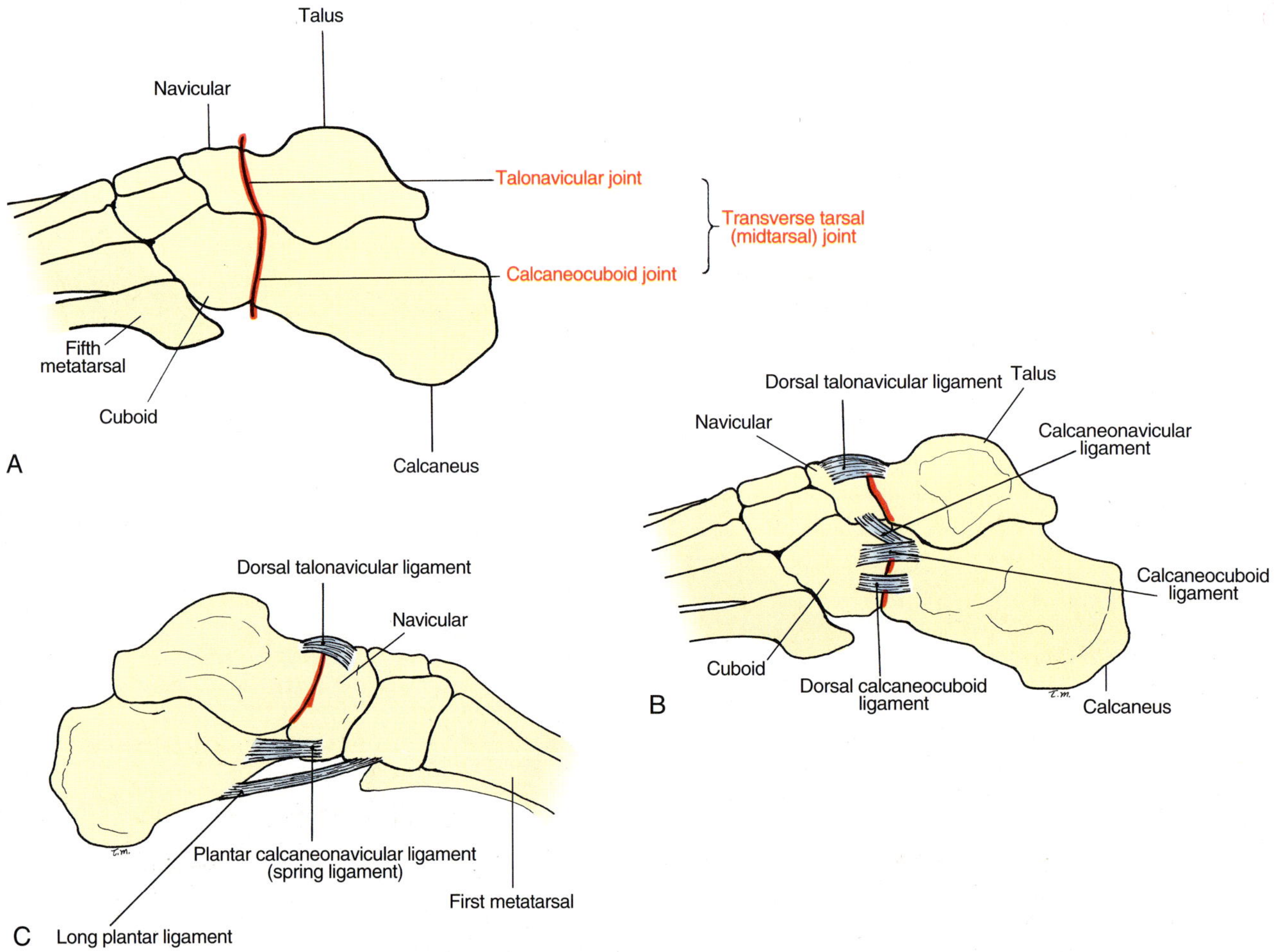

FIGURE 10.6 (A) The two joints that make up the transverse tarsal joint are shown in a lateral view of a left ankle. (B) The dorsal talonavicular ligament, the bifurcate ligament (calcaneonavicular and calcaneocuboid ligaments), and the dorsal calcaneocuboid ligament in a lateral view of a left ankle. (C) The long plantar ligament, the plantar calcaneonavicular ligament, and the dorsal talonavicular ligament in a medial view of a left ankle.

Arthrokinematics

During inversion in a non-weight-bearing position, the concave navicular slides medially and dorsally on the convex talus. The cuboid slides medially and toward the plantar surface on the calcaneus. In this manner, the medial side of the foot is raised.[2] During eversion, the navicular slides laterally and toward the plantar surface; the cuboid slides laterally and toward the dorsal surface. These motions result in the lateral side of the foot being raised.

Capsular Pattern

The capsular pattern consists of a limitation in adduction and medial rotation (inversion). Other motions are full.[5]

Tarsometatarsal Joints

The five tarsometatarsal (TMT) joints link the distal tarsals with the bases of the five metatarsals (Fig. 10.7). The concave base of the first metatarsal articulates with the convex surface of the medial cuneiform. The base of the second metatarsal articulates with the mortise formed by the intermediate cuneiform and the sides of the medial and lateral cuneiforms. The base of the third metatarsal articulates with the lateral cuneiform, and the base of the fourth metatarsal articulates with the lateral cuneiform and the cuboid. The fifth metatarsal articulates with the cuboid. The first joint has its own capsule, whereas the second and third joints and the fourth and fifth joints share capsules.[1–3] Each joint is reinforced by numerous dorsal, plantar, and interosseous ligaments.

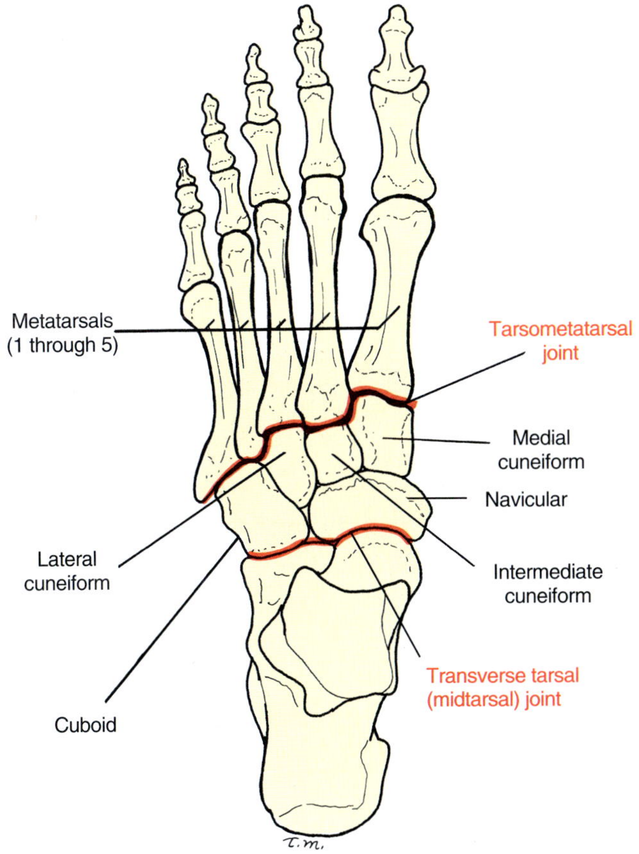

FIGURE 10.7 The tarsometatarsal joints and transverse tarsal joint in a dorsal view of a left foot.

Osteokinematics

The TMT joints are plane synovial joints that permit some motion, including flexion–extension, a minimal amount of abduction–adduction, and rotation. The type and amount of motion vary at each joint. For example, the second TMT joint has the most restricted motion and functions as the pillar of the foot, whereas the peripheral TMT joints have more mobility.[2] The combination of motions at the various joints contributes to the hollowing and flattening of the foot, which helps the foot conform to a supporting surface.

Arthrokinematics

The distal joint surfaces roll and glide in the same direction as the shafts of the metatarsals.

Metatarsophalangeal Joints

The five metatarsophalangeal (MTP) joints are formed proximally by the convex heads of the five metatarsals and distally by the concave bases of the proximal phalanges (Fig. 10.8A).[1–3] The first MTP joint has two sesamoid bones within the flexor hallucis brevis that lie in two grooves on the plantar surface of the distal metatarsal. The joint capsule of each of the MTP joints is reinforced by a medial and lateral collateral ligament. The plantar aponeurosis blends with the plantar part of each capsule to form a fibrous palmar plate (also called the palmar ligament), which helps to provide stability and limits extension. The four lesser toes are interconnected on the plantar surface by the deep transverse metatarsal ligament (Fig. 10.8B).

Osteokinematics

The five MTP joints are condyloid synovial joints with 2 degrees of freedom, permitting flexion–extension and abduction–adduction. The axis for flexion–extension is oblique and is referred to as the metatarsal break.[1] The range of motion (ROM) in extension is greater than it is in flexion, but the total ROM varies according to the relative lengths of the metatarsals and the weight-bearing status.

Arthrokinematics

In flexion, the concave bases of the phalanges roll and slide in a plantar direction on the heads of the metatarsals. In abduction, the concave bases of the phalanges roll and slide on the convex heads of the metatarsals in a lateral direction away from the second toe. In adduction, the bases of the phalanges roll and slide in a medial direction toward the second toe.

Capsular Pattern

The pattern at the first MTP joint is a gross limitation of extension and slight limitation of flexion.[5] Other sources report restrictions in all directions with more limitation in flexion[4] or a limitation pattern that is variable[6] in the second to fifth MTP joints.

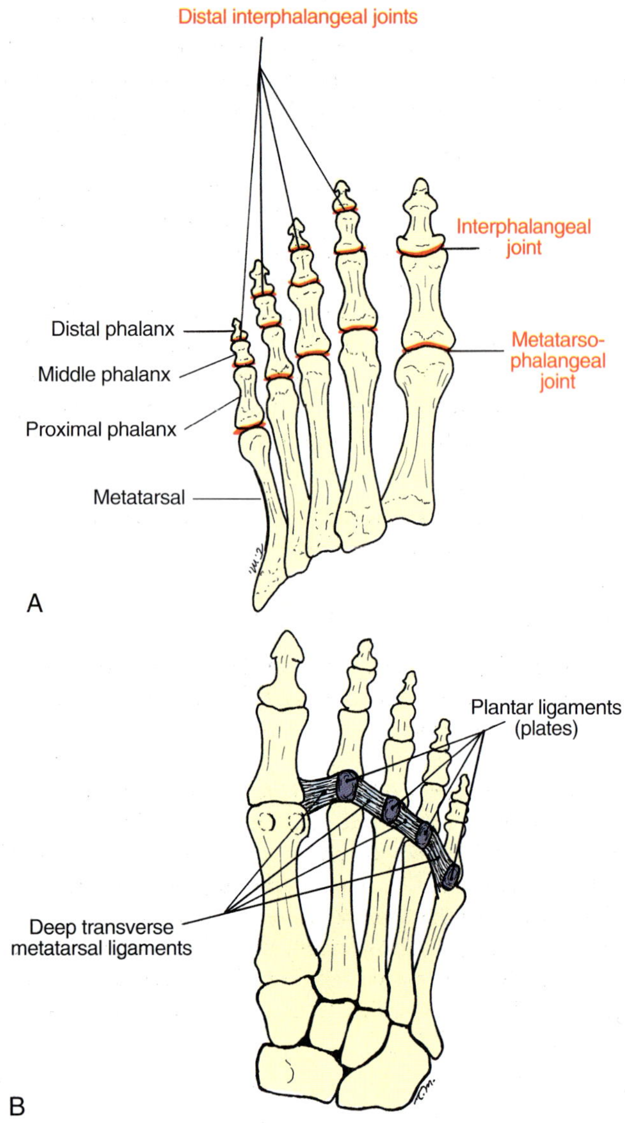

FIGURE 10.8 (A) The metatarsophalangeal, interphalangeal, and distal interphalangeal joints in a dorsal view of a left foot. (B) The deep transverse metatarsal ligaments and the plantar plates in a plantar view of a left foot.

Interphalangeal Joints

The structure of the interphalangeal (IP) joints of the feet is identical to that of the IP joints of the fingers. Each IP joint is composed of the concave base of a distal phalanx and the convex head of a proximal phalanx (see Fig. 10.8A).

Osteokinematics

The IP joints are synovial hinge joints with 1 degree of freedom. The motions permitted are flexion and extension in the sagittal plane. Each joint is enclosed in a capsule with a thickened palmar plate that is also called a palmar ligament. The capsule is reinforced with collateral ligaments.[1–3]

Arthrokinematics

The concave base of the distal phalanx rolls and slides on the convex head of the proximal phalanx in the same direction as the shaft of the distal bone. The concave base rolls and slides toward the plantar surface of the foot during flexion and toward the dorsum of the foot during extension.[4]

Capsular Pattern

The pattern is restriction in all direction, with distal interphalangeal (DIP) and proximal interphalangeal (PIP) joints reported to be more limited in extension[4] or flexion.[6]

RANGE OF MOTION TESTING PROCEDURES: Ankle and Foot

Landmarks for Testing Procedures: Talocrural Joint

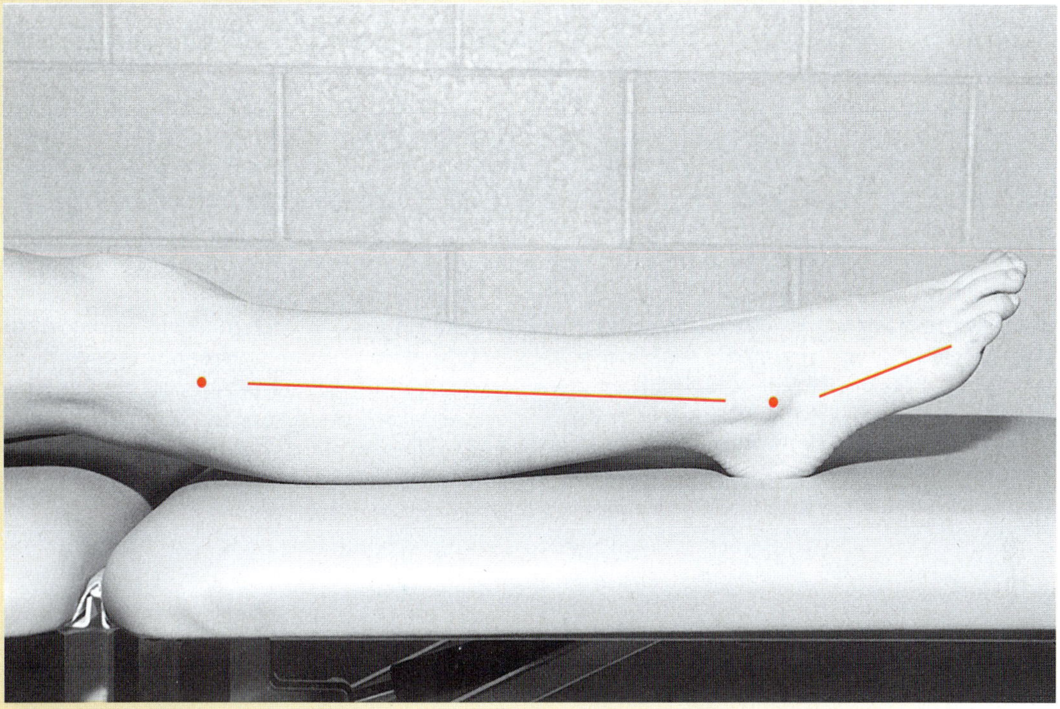

FIGURE 10.9 A lateral view of the right lower extremity showing the surface anatomy landmarks for goniometer alignment for measurement of dorsiflexion and plantarflexion range of motion.

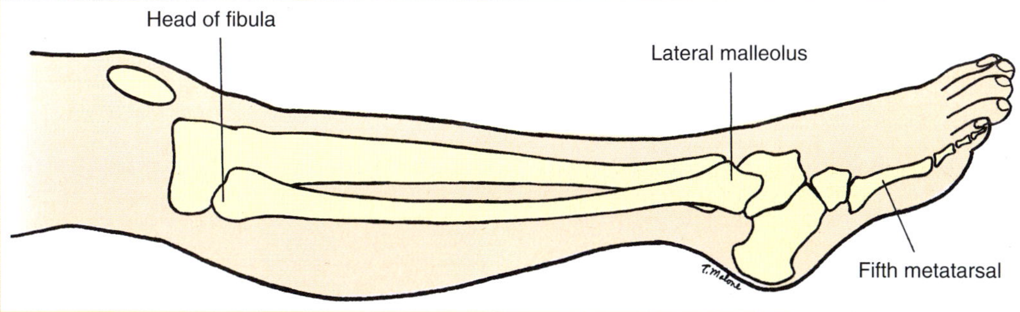

FIGURE 10.10 Bony anatomical landmarks for measuring dorsiflexion and plantarflexion range of motion.

TALOCRURAL JOINT: DORSIFLEXION

Motion occurs in the sagittal plane around a medial–lateral axis. Normal dorsiflexion ROM values for adults vary from about 15 to 20 degrees in non-weight-bearing positions. See Research Findings and Tables 10.1 and 10.3 to 10.5 for more detailed normal ROM values by age and gender.

Dorsiflexion ROM is affected by the testing position (knee flexed or extended) and by whether the measurement is taken in either a weight-bearing or non-weight-bearing position. Dorsiflexion ROM measured with the knee flexed is usually greater than that measured with the knee extended. Knee flexion slackens the gastrocnemius muscles, so passive tension in the muscle does not limit dorsiflexion ROM. Knee extension stretches the gastrocnemius muscle, and ROM measured in this position represents the length of the muscle. Weight-bearing dorsiflexion ROM in standing is usually greater than non-weight-bearing measurements in supine or prone; therefore, these positions should not be used interchangeably (see Research Findings and Table 10.7).

Testing Position

Place the individual sitting, with the knee flexed to 90 degrees. The foot should be in 0 degrees of inversion and eversion.

Stabilization

Stabilize the tibia and fibula to prevent knee motion and hip rotation.

Testing Motion

Use one hand to move the foot into dorsiflexion by pushing on the bottom of the foot (Fig. 10.11). Avoid pressure on the lateral border of the foot under the fifth metatarsal and the toes. A considerable amount of force is necessary to overcome the passive tension in the soleus and Achilles musculotendinous unit. Often, a comparison of the active and passive ROMs for a particular individual helps to determine the amount of upward force necessary to complete the passive ROM in dorsiflexion. The end of the ROM occurs when resistance to further motion is felt and attempts to produce additional motion cause knee extension.

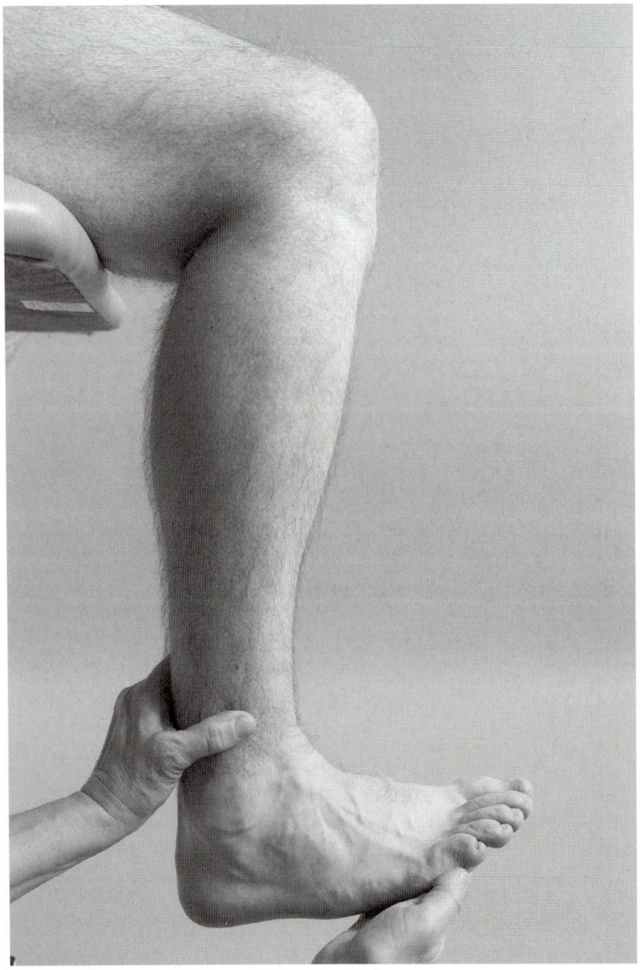

FIGURE 10.11 The right ankle at the end of dorsiflexion range of motion. The examiner holds the distal portion of the lower leg with one hand to prevent knee motion and uses her other hand to push on the palmar surface of the foot to achieve dorsiflexion.

Normal End-Feel

The end-feel is firm because of tension in the posterior joint capsule, the soleus muscle, the Achilles tendon, the posterior portion of the deltoid ligament, the posterior talofibular ligament, and the calcaneofibular ligament.

Goniometer Alignment

See Figures 10.12 and 10.13.

1. Center **fulcrum** of the goniometer over the lateral aspect of the lateral malleolus.
2. Align **proximal arm** with the lateral midline of the fibula, using the head of the fibula for reference.
3. Align **distal arm** parallel to the lateral aspect of the fifth metatarsal. Although it is usually easier to palpate and align the distal arm parallel to the fifth metatarsal, alternative methods have been proposed including the alignment of the distal arm parallel to the inferior aspect of the foot or parallel to the calcaneus. If these alternative landmarks are used, then ROM values for dorsiflexion and plantarflexion will differ considerably from the preferred technique,[7] but full cycle ROM in the sagittal plane (dorsiflexion plus plantarflexion) may be similar (see Research Findings: Effects of Age, Gender and Other Factors—Testing Landmarks for Goniometer Alignment). Most research studies on the reliability of ankle dorsiflexion and plantarflexion ROM have aligned the distal arm of the goniometer parallel with the fifth metatarsal.

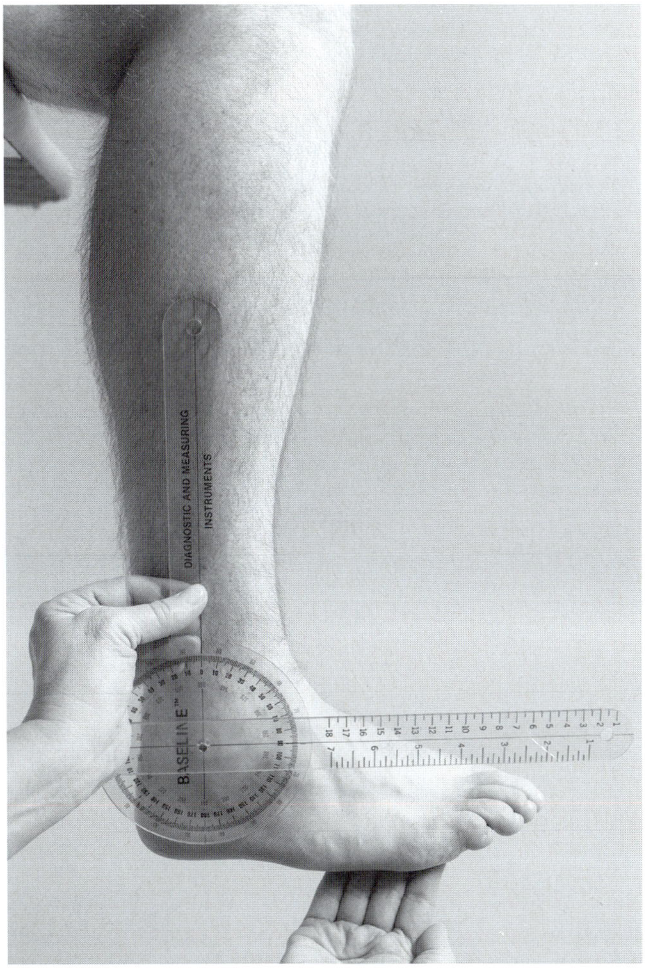

FIGURE 10.12 In the starting position for measuring dorsiflexion range of motion the ankle is positioned so that the goniometer is at 90 degrees. This goniometer reading is transposed and recorded as 0 degrees. The examiner sits on a stool or kneels in order to align the goniometer and perform the readings at eye level.

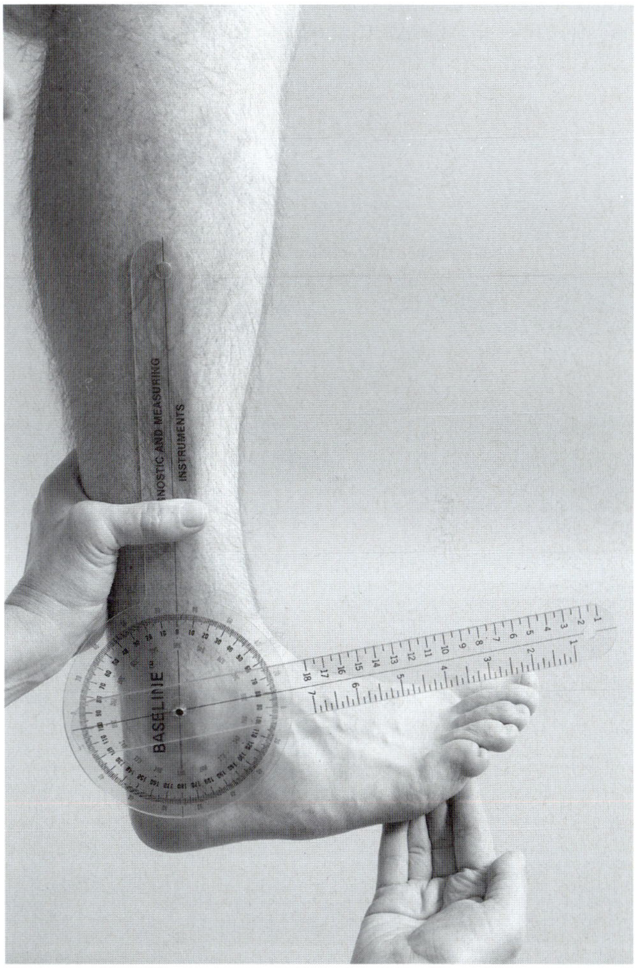

FIGURE 10.13 At the end of dorsiflexion range of motion, the examiner uses one hand to align the proximal goniometer arm while the other hand maintains dorsiflexion and aligns the distal goniometer arm. In this photograph the examiner has removed her hand from the distal goniometer arm so that the goniometer alignment that is parallel to the fifth metatarsal can be seen.

Alternative Testing Positions

Supine Non-Weight-Bearing

Place the individual supine with the knee flexed to 45 degrees and supported by a pillow. The foot should be in 0 degrees of inversion and eversion. Stabilization, Testing Motion, Normal End-Feel, and Goniometer Alignment are the same as that for the seated position.

Prone Non-Weight-Bearing

Position the individual prone with the knee flexed to 90 degrees (Fig. 10.14). The foot should be in 0 degrees of inversion and eversion. Stabilization, Testing Motion, Normal End-feel, and Goniometer Alignment are the same as that for the seated position.

Standing Weight-Bearing

Usually ROM measurements taken in the standing position are larger than measurements taken in non-weight-bearing positions; therefore, the two positions should not be used interchangeably. Weight-bearing measurements may be able to provide the examiner with information that is relevant to the performance of functional activities such as walking. However, it may be difficult to control substitute motions of the hindfoot and forefoot in the weight-bearing position. Some individuals may not have the strength and balance necessary to assume the weight-bearing position.

Position the individual standing with weight on the leg to be tested. The foot should be in 0 degrees of inversion and eversion. The knee of the test leg should be flexed as far as possible while maintaining the foot flat on the floor. The end of the motion occurs when additional motion causes the heel to rise from the floor (Fig. 10.15). Goniometer alignment is the same as that for the seated position.

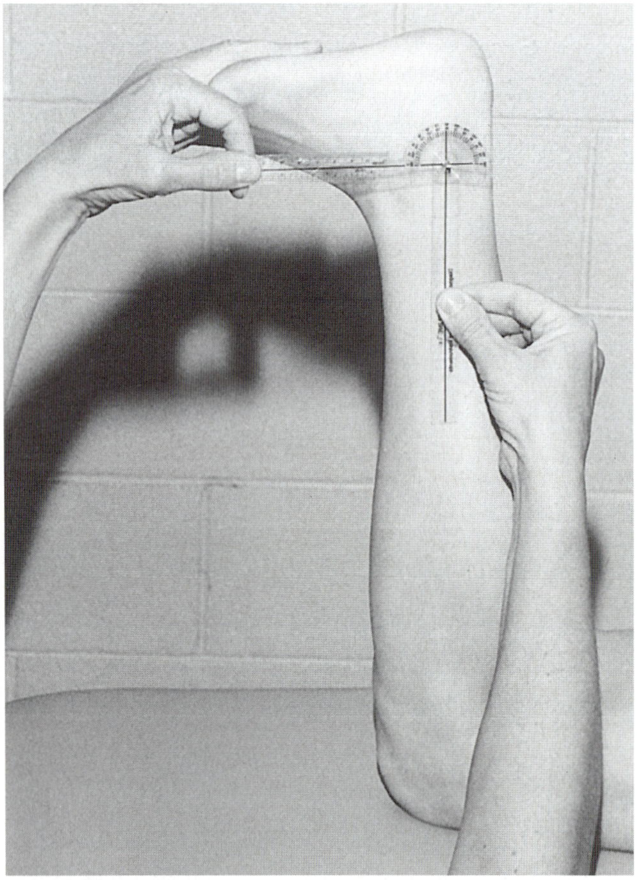

FIGURE 10.14 Goniometer alignment at the end of dorsiflexion range of motion. An alternative prone position with the knee flexed to 90 degrees is being used.

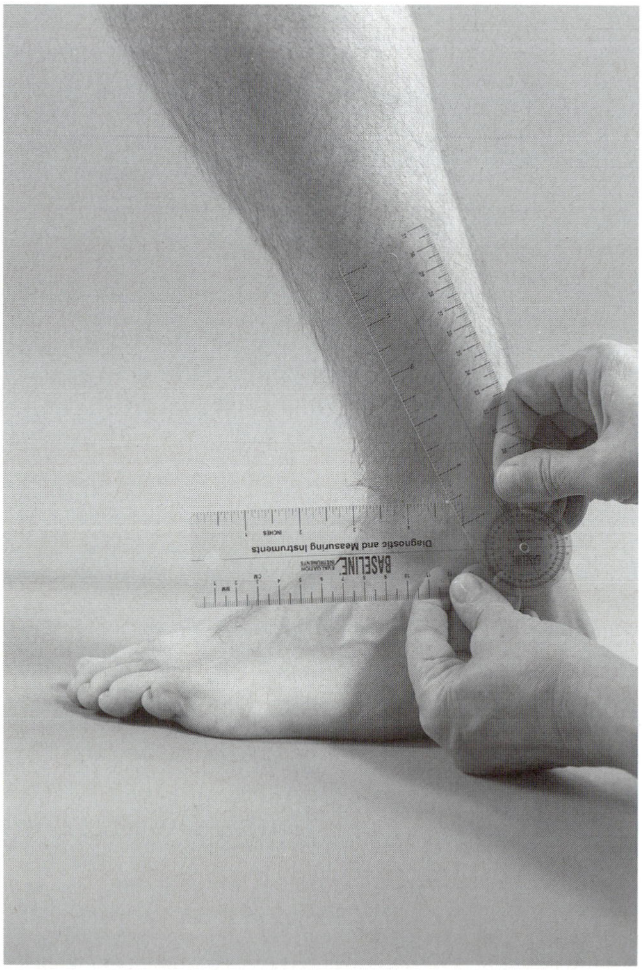

FIGURE 10.15 Goniometer alignment at the end of dorsiflexion range of motion using an alternative weight-bearing position. The knee is flexed so that ankle dorsiflexion ROM, rather than gastrocnemius muscle length, is being tested.

TALOCRURAL JOINT: PLANTARFLEXION

Motion occurs in the sagittal plane around a medial–lateral axis. Normal plantarflexion ROM values for adults vary from about 45 to 55 degrees. See Research Findings and Tables 10.1 and 10.3 to 10.5 for more detailed normal ROM values by age and gender.

Testing Position

Place the individual sitting with the knee flexed to 90 degrees. Position the foot in 0 degrees of inversion and eversion. Alternatively, it is possible to place the individual in the supine position.

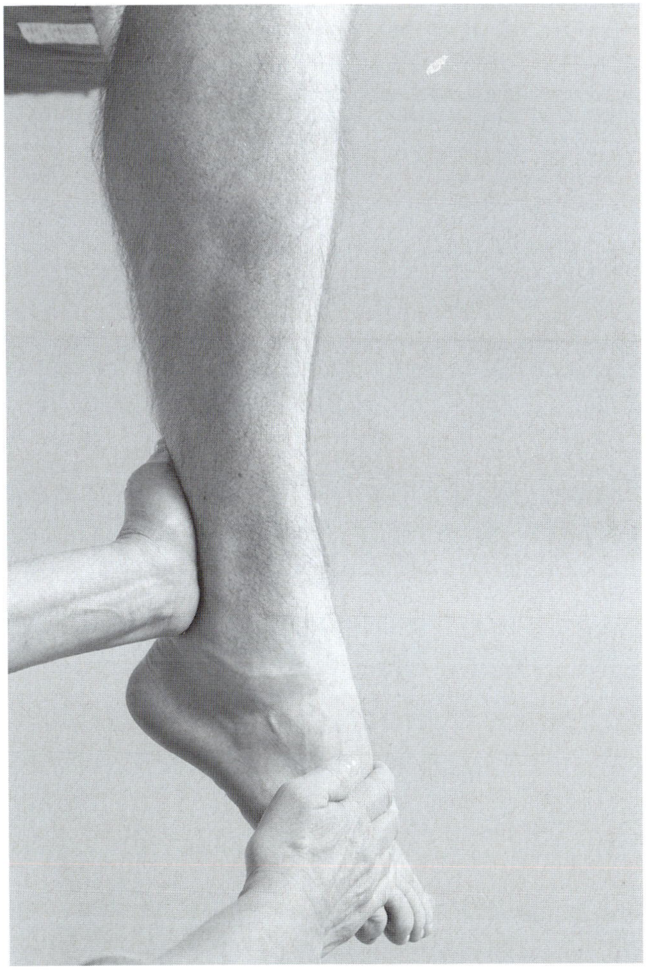

FIGURE 10.16 The right ankle at the end of plantarflexion range of motion (ROM). The examiner determines the end-feel and visually estimates the ROM.

Stabilization

Stabilize the tibia and fibula to prevent knee flexion and hip rotation.

Testing Motion

Push downward with one hand on the dorsum of the individual's foot to produce plantarflexion (Fig. 10.16). Do not exert any force on the individual's toes, and be careful to avoid pushing the ankle into inversion or eversion. The end of the ROM is reached when resistance is felt and attempts to produce additional plantarflexion result in knee flexion.

Normal End-Feel

Usually the end-feel is firm because of tension in the anterior joint capsule; the anterior portion of the deltoid ligament; the anterior talofibular ligament; and the tibialis anterior, extensor hallucis longus, and extensor digitorum longus muscles. The end-feel may be hard because of contact between the posterior tubercles of the talus and the posterior margin of the tibia.

Goniometer Alignment

See Figures 10.17 and 10.18.

1. Center **fulcrum** of the goniometer over the lateral aspect of the lateral malleolus.
2. Align **proximal arm** with the lateral midline of the fibula, using the head of the fibula for reference.
3. Align **distal arm** parallel to the lateral aspect of the fifth metatarsal. Although it is more common and usually easier to palpate and align the distal arm parallel to the fifth metatarsal, as an alternative the distal arm can be aligned parallel to the inferior aspect of the foot of the calcaneus. If the alternative landmarks are used, full cycle ROM in the sagittal plane (dorsiflexion plus plantarflexion) may be similar to full cycle ROM measurement using the fifth metatarsal as a landmark, but the single cycle ROM values for dorsiflexion and plantarflexion will differ considerably. Measurements taken with the alternative landmarks should not be used interchangeably with those taken using the fifth metatarsal landmark.

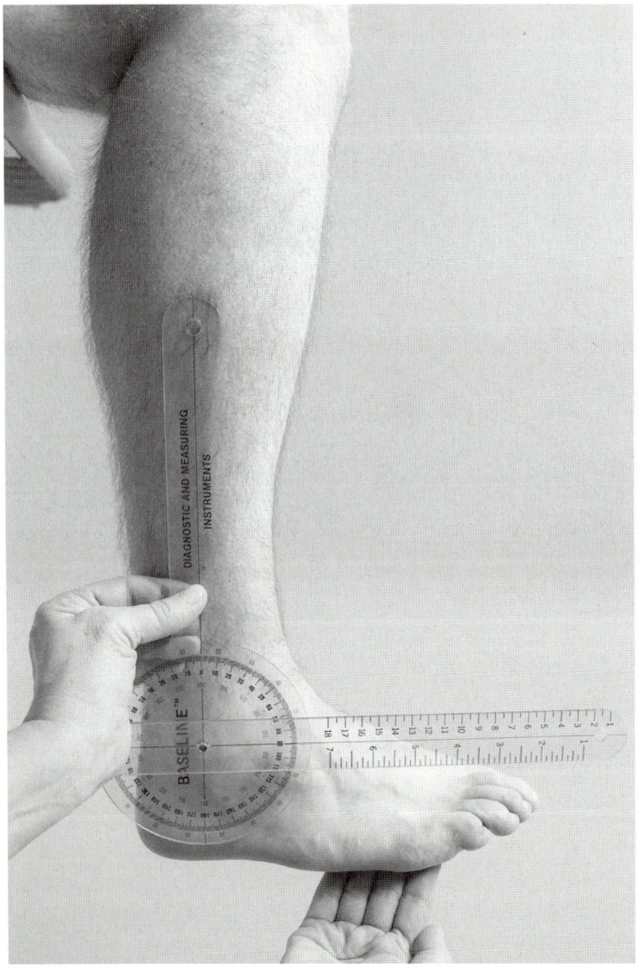

FIGURE 10.17 Goniometer alignment in the starting position for measuring plantarflexion range of motion. Note that the ankle is positioned so that the goniometer is at 90 degrees. This goniometer reading is transposed and recorded as 0 degrees.

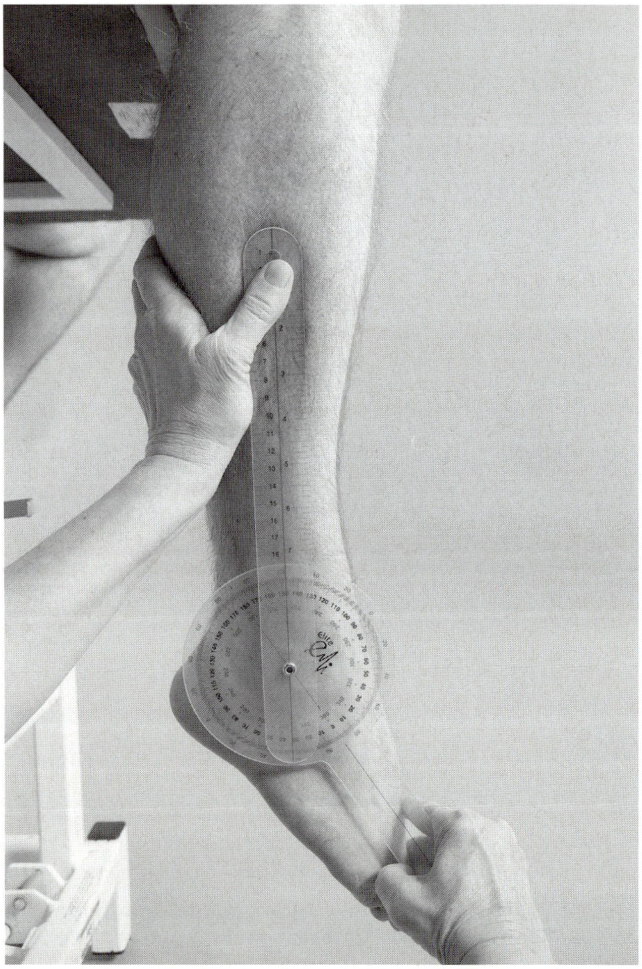

FIGURE 10.18 At the end of the plantarflexion range of motion, the examiner uses one hand to maintain plantarflexion and to align the distal goniometer arm. The examiner holds the dorsum of the individual's foot to avoid exerting pressure on the toes. She uses her other hand to stabilize the tibia and align the proximal arm of the goniometer.

Landmarks for Testing Procedures: Tarsal Joints

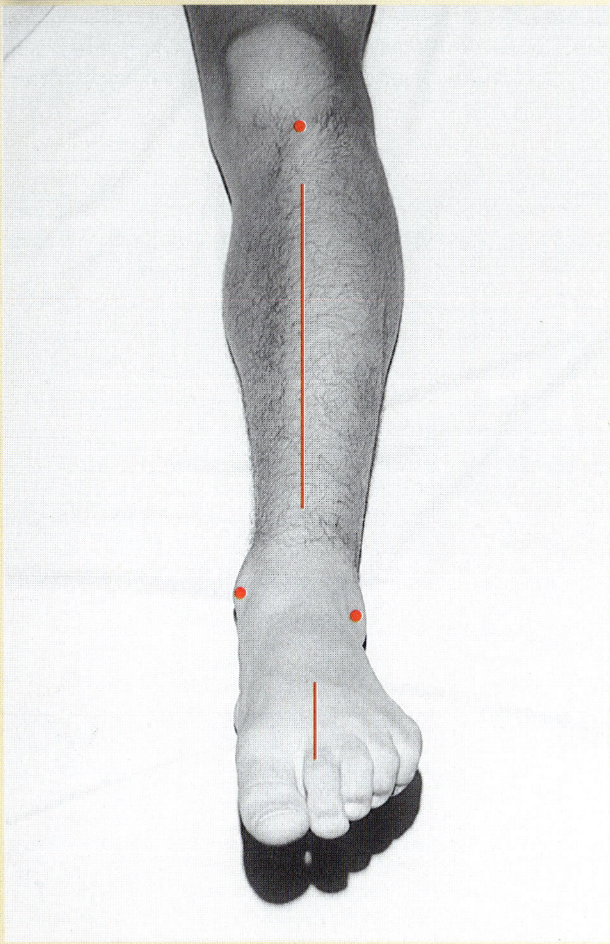

FIGURE 10.19 An anterior view of the left lower leg and foot with surface anatomy landmarks to indicate goniometer alignment for measuring inversion and eversion range of motion.

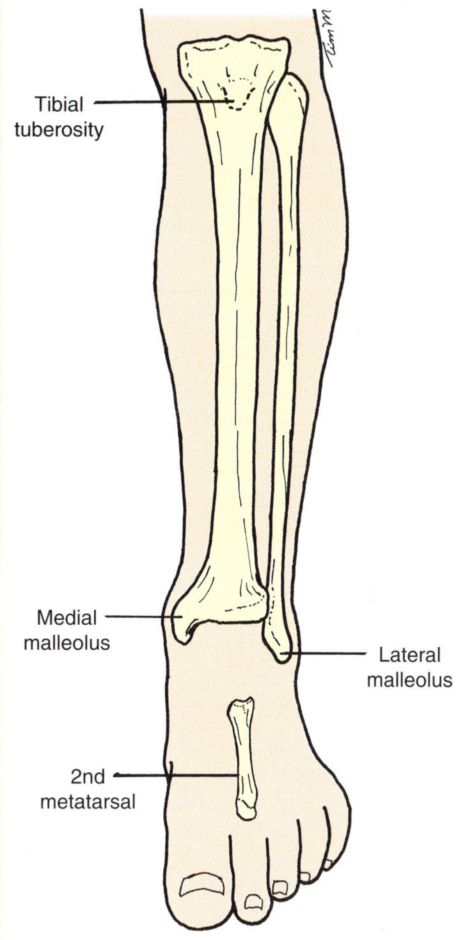

FIGURE 10.20 Bony anatomical landmarks for measuring inversion and eversion range of motion.

TARSAL JOINTS: INVERSION

Inversion is a combination of supination, adduction, and plantarflexion occurring in varying degrees at the subtalar, transverse tarsal (talocalcaneonavicular and calcaneocuboid), cuboideonavicular, cuneonavicular, intercuneiform, cuneocuboid, tarsometatarsal (TMT), and intermetatarsal joints. Because of the uniaxial limitations of the goniometer, inversion of the foot is measured in the frontal plane around an anterior–posterior axis. Normal tarsal inversion ROM values for adults vary from about 30 to 35 degrees. See Research Findings and Tables 10.1 and 10.3 to 10.5 for more information.

Testing Position

Place the individual in the sitting position, with the knee flexed to 90 degrees and the lower leg over the edge of the supporting surface. Position the hip in 0 degrees of rotation, adduction, and abduction. Alternatively, it is possible to place the individual in the supine position, with the foot over the edge of the supporting surface.

Stabilization

Stabilize the tibia and the fibula to prevent medial rotation and extension of the knee and lateral rotation and abduction of the hip.

Testing Motion

Push the forefoot medially into adduction and downward into plantarflexion, turning the sole of the foot medially into supination so that the medial side of the foot is higher than the lateral side to produce inversion (Fig. 10.21). The end of the ROM occurs when resistance is felt and attempts at further motion produce medial rotation of the knee and/or lateral rotation and abduction at the hip.

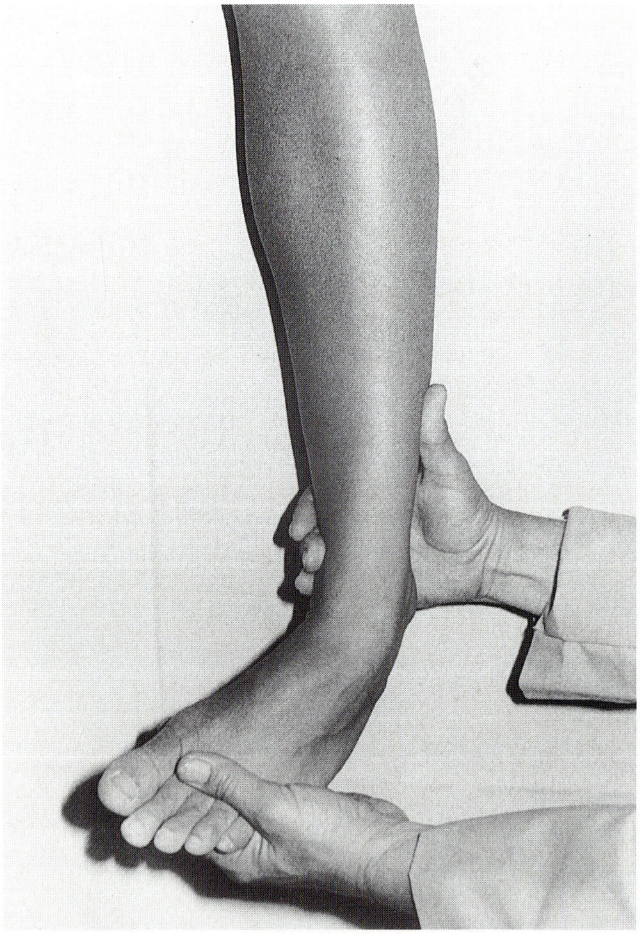

FIGURE 10.21 The left foot and ankle at the end of inversion range of motion. The examiner uses one hand on the distal lower leg to prevent knee and hip motion, while her other hand moves the foot into inversion.

Normal End-Feel

The end-feel is firm because of tension in the joint capsules; the anterior and posterior talofibular ligament; the calcaneofibular ligament; the anterior, posterior, lateral, and interosseous talocalcaneal ligaments; the dorsal calcaneal ligaments; the dorsal calcaneocuboid ligament; the dorsal talonavicular ligament; the lateral band of the bifurcate ligament; the transverse metatarsal ligament; various dorsal, plantar, and interosseous ligaments of the cuboideonavicular, cuneonavicular, intercuneiform, cuneocuboid, TMT, and intermetatarsal joints; and the peroneus longus and brevis muscles.

Goniometer Alignment

See Figures 10.22 and 10.23.

1. Center **fulcrum** of the goniometer over the anterior aspect of the ankle midway between the malleoli. (The flexibility of a plastic goniometer makes this instrument easier to use for measuring inversion than a metal goniometer.)
2. Align **proximal arm** of the goniometer with the anterior midline of the lower leg, using the tibial tuberosity for reference.
3. Align **distal arm** with the anterior midline of the second metatarsal.

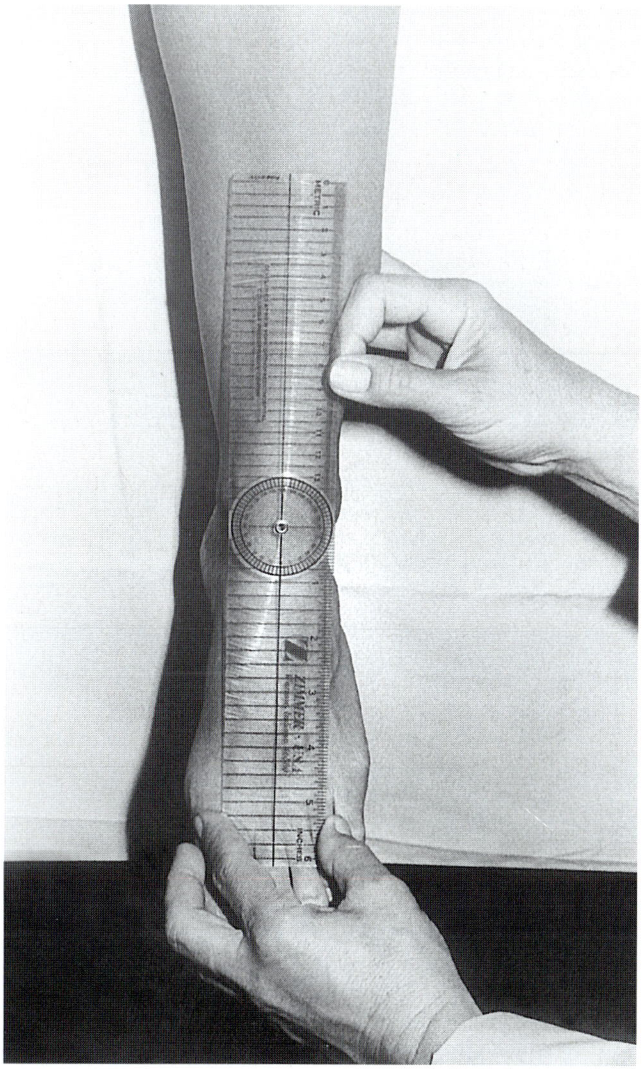

FIGURE 10.22 Goniometer alignment in the starting position for measuring inversion range of motion.

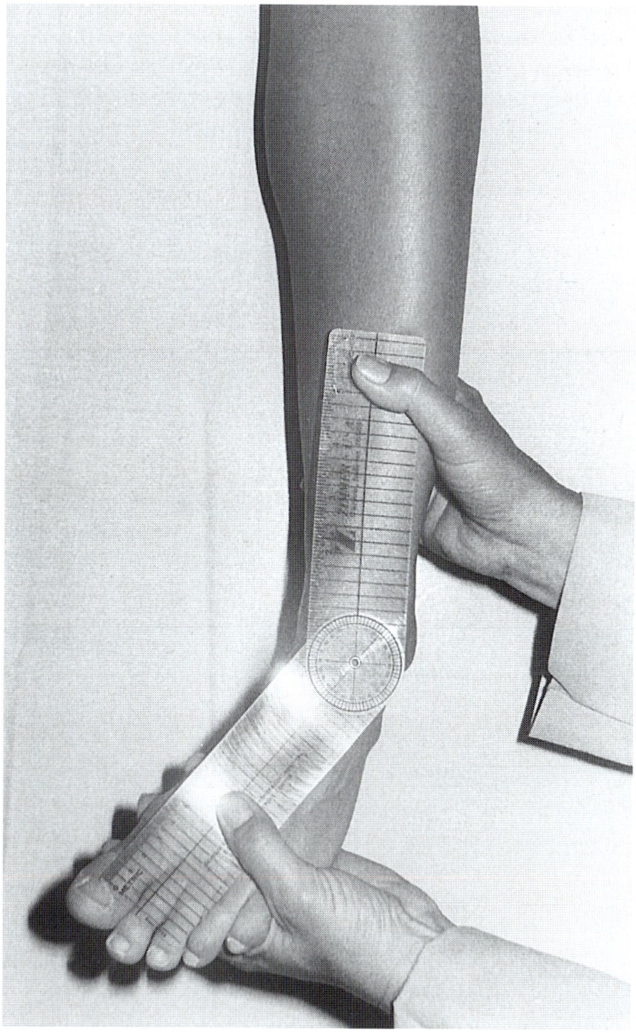

FIGURE 10.23 At the end of the range of motion, the examiner uses one hand to maintain inversion and to align the distal goniometer arm. The examiner's other hand, which had been stabilizing the lower leg during the motion, is now used to align the proximal goniometer arm.

TARSAL JOINTS: EVERSION

Eversion is a combination of pronation, abduction, and dorsiflexion occurring in varying degrees at the subtalar, transverse tarsal (talocalcaneonavicular and calcaneocuboid), cuboideonavicular, cuneonavicular, intercuneiform, cuneocuboid, TMT, and intermetatarsal joints. Because of the uniaxial limitations of the goniometer, eversion of the foot is measured in the frontal plane around an anterior–posterior axis. Normal tarsal eversion ROM values for adults vary from about 15 to 20 degrees. See Research Findings and Tables 10.1 and 10.3 to 10.5 for more detailed information.

Testing Position

Place the individual in the sitting position, with the knee flexed to 90 degrees and the lower leg over the edge of the supporting surface. Position the hip in 0 degrees of rotation, adduction, and abduction. Alternatively, it is possible to place the individual in the supine position, with the foot over the edge of the supporting surface.

Stabilization

Stabilize the tibia and fibula to prevent lateral rotation and flexion of the knee and medial rotation and adduction of the hip.

Testing Motion

Pull the forefoot laterally into abduction and upward into dorsiflexion, turning the forefoot into pronation so that the lateral side of the foot is higher than the medial side to produce eversion (Fig. 10.24). The

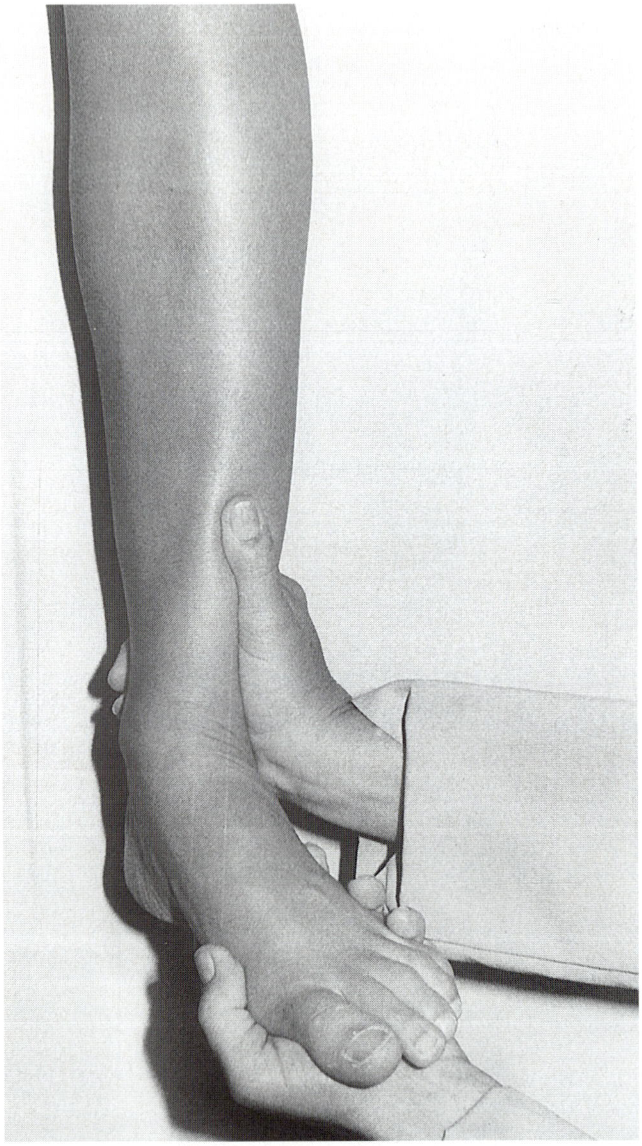

FIGURE 10.24 The left ankle and foot at the end of the range of motion (ROM) in eversion. The examiner uses one hand on the distal lower leg to prevent knee flexion and lateral rotation. The examiner's other hand moves the foot into eversion. The end-feel is determined and a visual estimate is made of the ROM.

end of the ROM occurs when resistance is felt and attempts at further motion cause lateral rotation at the knee and/or medial rotation and adduction at the hip.

Normal End-Feel

The end-feel may be hard because of contact between the calcaneus and the floor of the sinus tarsi. In some cases, the end-feel may be firm because of tension in the joint capsules; the deltoid ligament; the medial talocalcaneal ligament; the plantar calcaneonavicular and calcaneocuboid ligaments; the dorsal talonavicular ligament; the medial band of the bifurcated ligament; the transverse metatarsal ligament; various dorsal, plantar, and interosseous ligaments of the cuboideonavicular, cuneonavicular, intercuneiform, cuneocuboid, TMT, and intermetatarsal joints; and the tibialis posterior muscle.

Goniometer Alignment

See Figures 10.25 and 10.26.

1. Center the **fulcrum** of the goniometer over the anterior aspect of the ankle midway between the malleoli. (The flexibility of a plastic goniometer makes this instrument easier to use than a metal goniometer for measuring inversion.)
2. Align **proximal arm** of the goniometer with the anterior midline of the lower leg, using the tibial tuberosity for reference.
3. Align **distal arm** with the anterior midline of the second metatarsal.

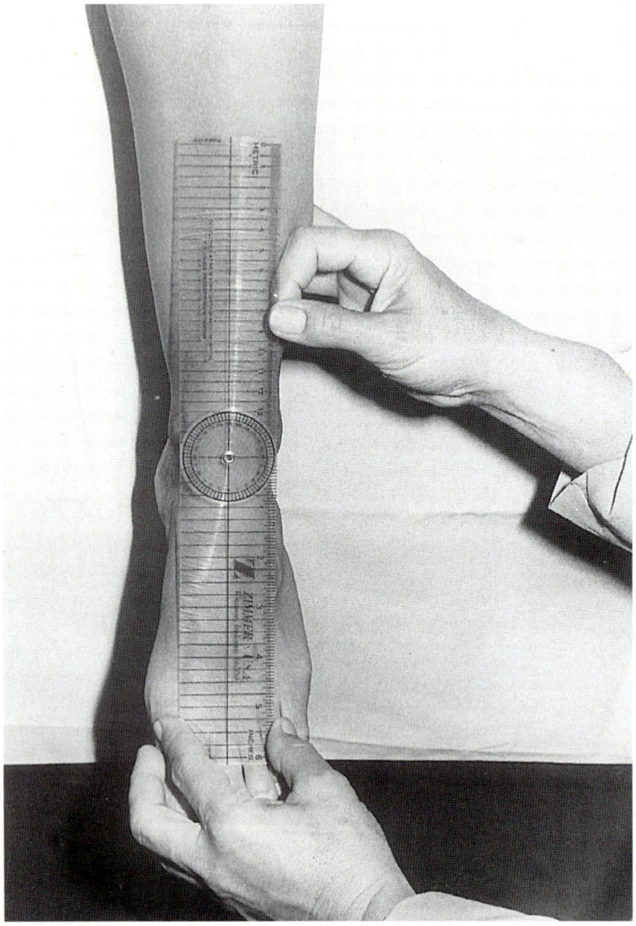

FIGURE 10.25 Goniometer alignment in the starting position for measuring eversion range of motion.

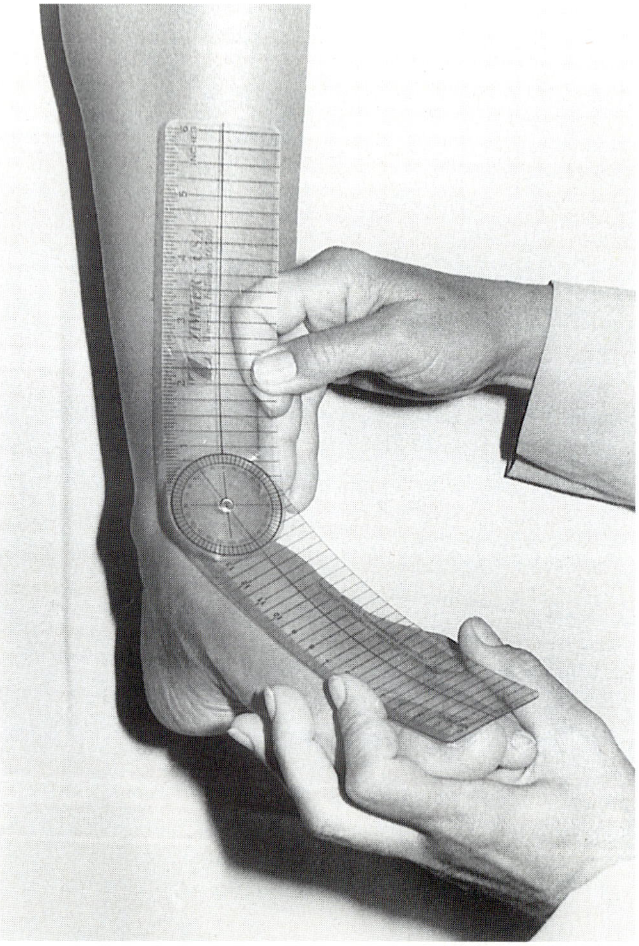

FIGURE 10.26 At the end of the eversion range of motion, the examiner's left hand maintains eversion and aligns the distal goniometer arm with the second metatarsal. The examiner's right hand, which had provided stabilization during the motion, is now used to align the proximal goniometer arm.

Landmarks for Testing Procedures: Subtalar Joint (Rearfoot)

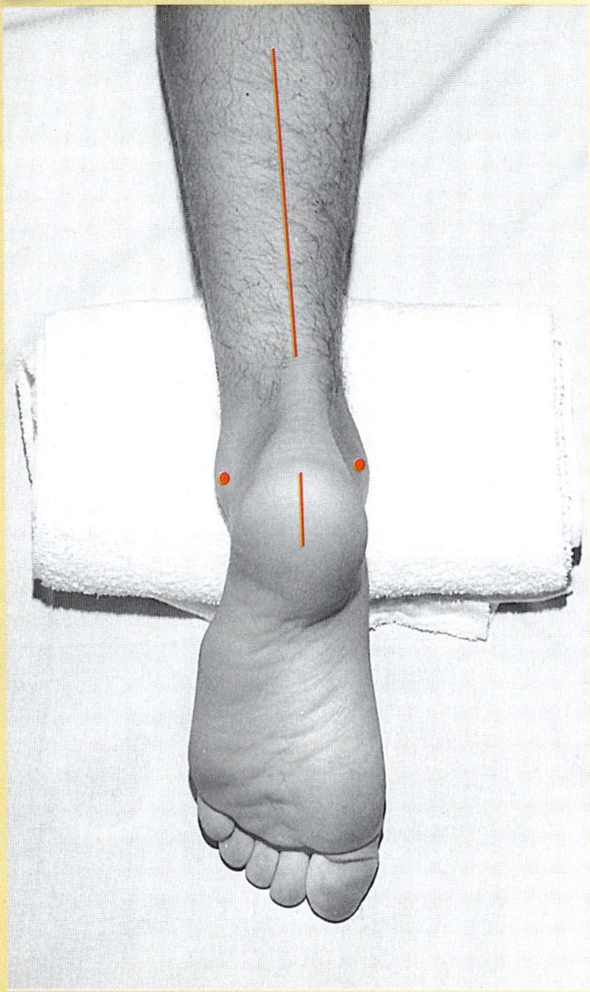

FIGURE 10.27 Posterior view of the left lower leg and foot showing the surface anatomy landmarks used in goniometer alignment for measuring subtalar (rearfoot) inversion and eversion range of motion.

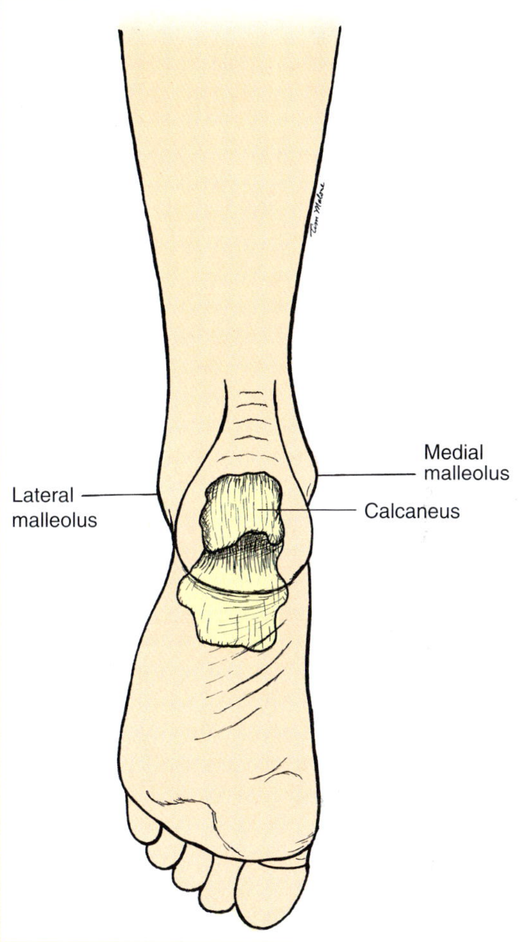

FIGURE 10.28 Bony anatomical landmarks for measuring subtalar inversion and eversion range of motion in a posterior view of the left lower leg and foot.

SUBTALAR JOINT (REARFOOT): INVERSION

Inversion is a combination of supination, adduction, and plantarflexion. Because of the uniaxial limitations of the goniometer, inversion of the subtalar joint is measured in the frontal plane around an anterior–posterior axis. Normal subtalar inversion ROM values for adults vary widely, including 5 degrees according to the American Academy of Orthopaedic Surgeons (AAOS),[8] 15 degrees of active ROM reported by Menadue et al,[9] and about 25 degrees of passive ROM as noted by Astrom and Arvidon.[10] See Research Findings and Table 10.1 for more information.

Testing Position

Place the individual in the prone position, with the hip in 0 degrees of flexion, extension, abduction, adduction, and rotation. Position the knee in 0 degrees of flexion and extension. Position the foot over the edge of the supporting surface.

Stabilization

Stabilize the tibia and fibula to prevent lateral hip and knee rotation and hip adduction.

Testing Motion

Hold the individual's lower leg with one hand and use the other hand to pull the calcaneus medially into adduction and to rotate it into supination, thereby producing rearfoot subtalar inversion (Fig. 10.29). Avoid pushing on the forefoot. The end of the ROM is reached when resistance to further motion is felt and attempts at overcoming the resistance produce lateral rotation at the hip or knee.

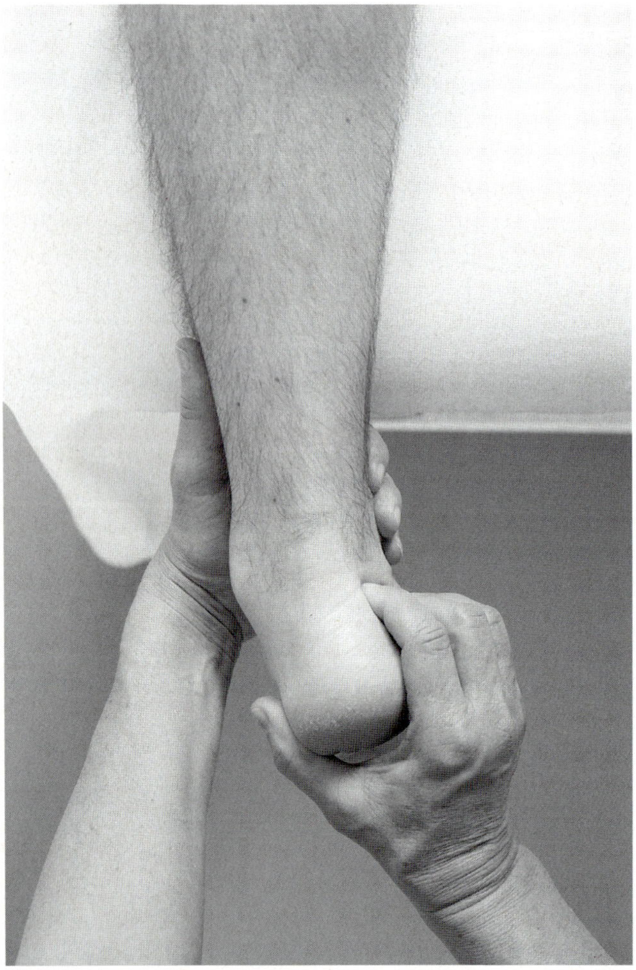

FIGURE 10.29 The left lower extremity at the end of subtalar inversion range of motion.

Normal End-Feel

The end-feel is firm because of tension in the lateral joint capsule; the anterior and posterior talofibular ligaments; the calcaneofibular ligament; and the lateral, posterior, anterior, and interosseous talocalcaneal ligaments.

Goniometer Alignment

See Figures 10.30 and 10.31.

1. Center **fulcrum** of the goniometer over the posterior aspect of the ankle midway between the malleoli.
2. Align **proximal arm** with the posterior midline of the lower leg.
3. Align **distal arm** with the posterior midline of the calcaneus.

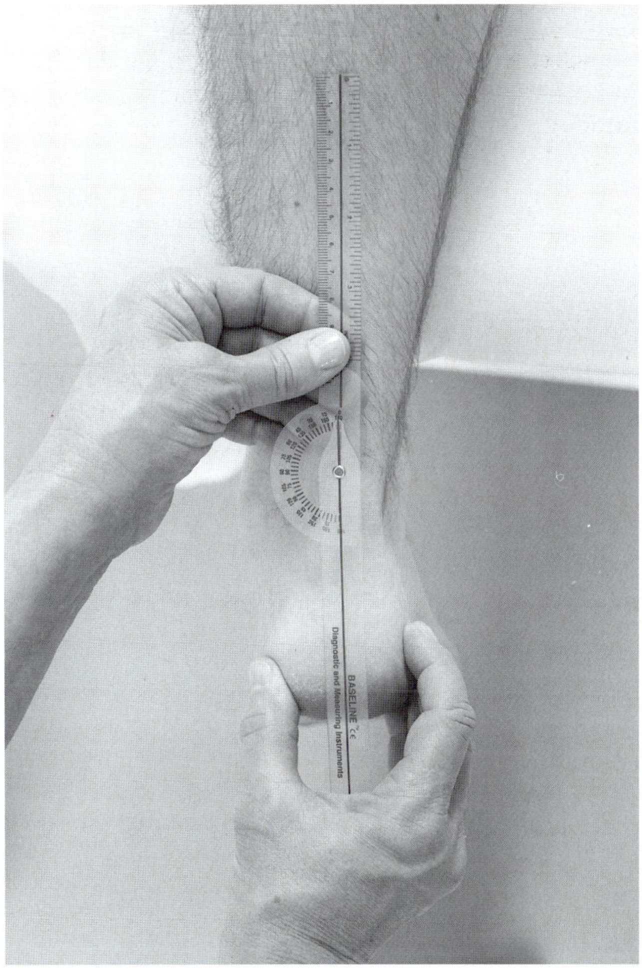

FIGURE 10.30 Goniometer alignment in the starting position for measuring subtalar inversion range of motion.

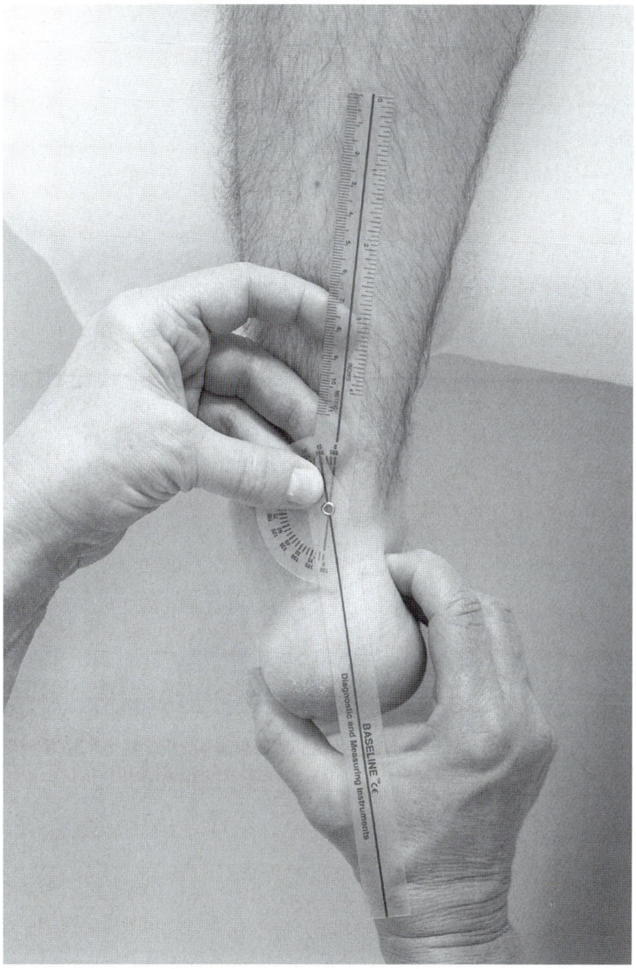

FIGURE 10.31 At the end of subtalar inversion, the examiner's hand maintains inversion. The examiner's other hand, which provided stabilization during the motion, is now used to align the arms of the goniometer.

SUBTALAR JOINT (REARFOOT): EVERSION

Eversion is a combination of pronation, abduction, and dorsiflexion. Because of the uniaxial limitations of the goniometer, eversion of the subtalar joint is measured in the frontal plane around an anterior–posterior axis. Normal subtalar eversion ROM values for adults vary from about 5 to 12 degrees. Values of between 8 and 9 degrees were reported during active ROM,[9] whereas slightly greater values of 12 degrees were noted during passive ROM.[10] See Research Findings and Table 10.1 for more information.

Testing Position

Place the individual prone, with the hip in 0 degrees of flexion, extension, abduction, adduction, and rotation.

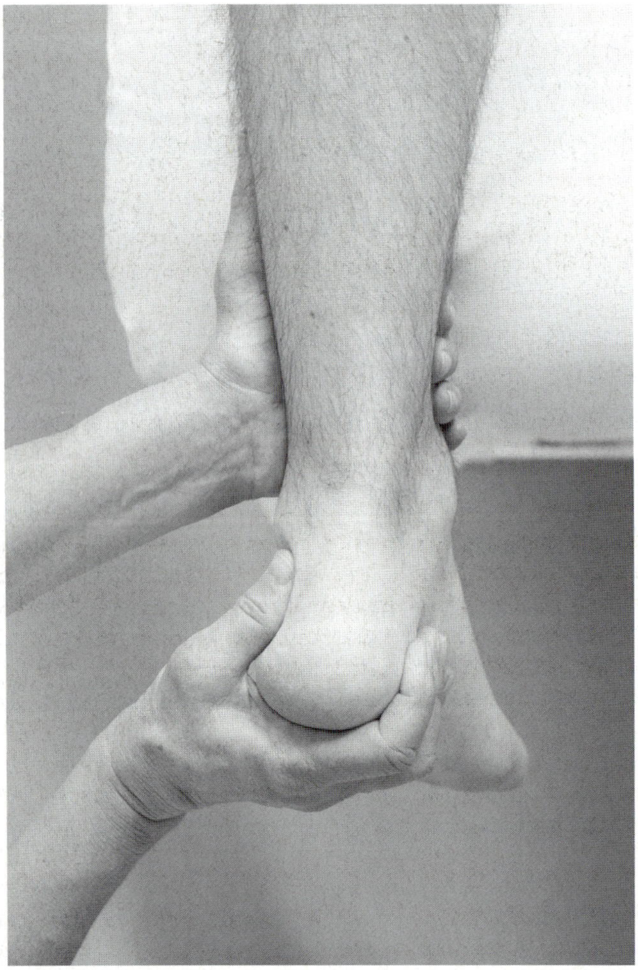

FIGURE 10.32 The left lower extremity at the end of subtalar eversion range of motion. The examiner's hand achieves subtalar eversion by pulling the calcaneus laterally.

Position the knee in 0 degrees of flexion and extension. Place the foot over the edge of the supporting surface.

Stabilization

Stabilize the tibia and fibula to prevent medial hip and knee rotation and hip abduction.

Testing Motion

Pull the calcaneus laterally into abduction and rotate it into pronation to produce subtalar eversion (Fig. 10.32). The end of the ROM occurs when resistance to further movement is felt and additional attempts to move the calcaneus result in medial hip or knee rotation.

Normal End-Feel

The end-feel may be hard because of contact between the calcaneus and the floor of the sinus tarsi, or it may be firm because of tension in the deltoid ligament, the medial talocalcaneal ligament, and the tibialis posterior muscle.

Goniometer Alignment

See Figures 10.33 and 10.34.

1. Center **fulcrum** of the goniometer over the posterior aspect of the ankle midway between the malleoli.
2. Align **proximal arm** with the posterior midline of the lower leg.
3. Align **distal arm** with the posterior midline of the calcaneus.

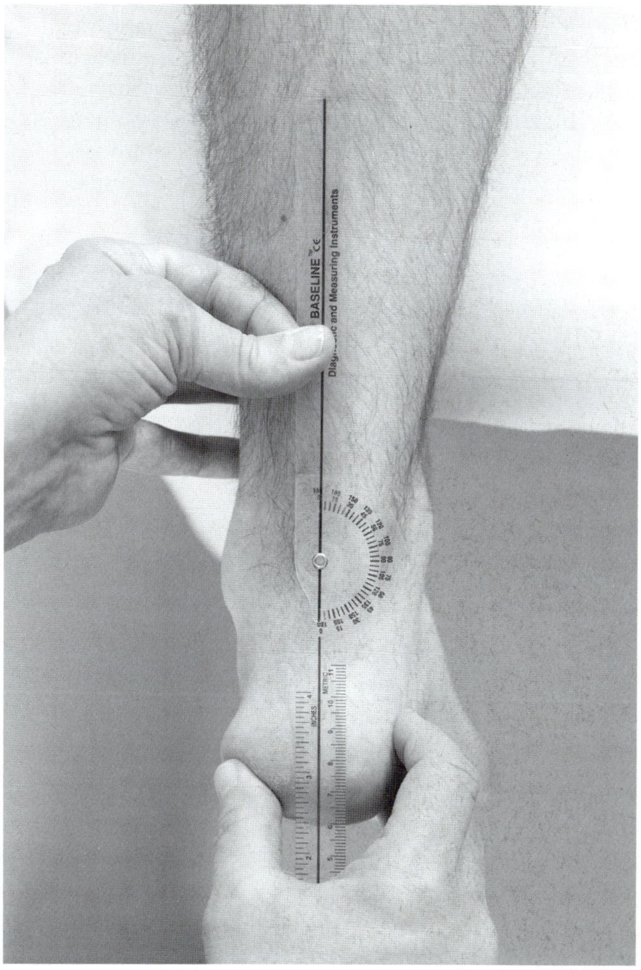

FIGURE 10.33 Goniometer alignment in the starting position for measuring subtalar eversion.

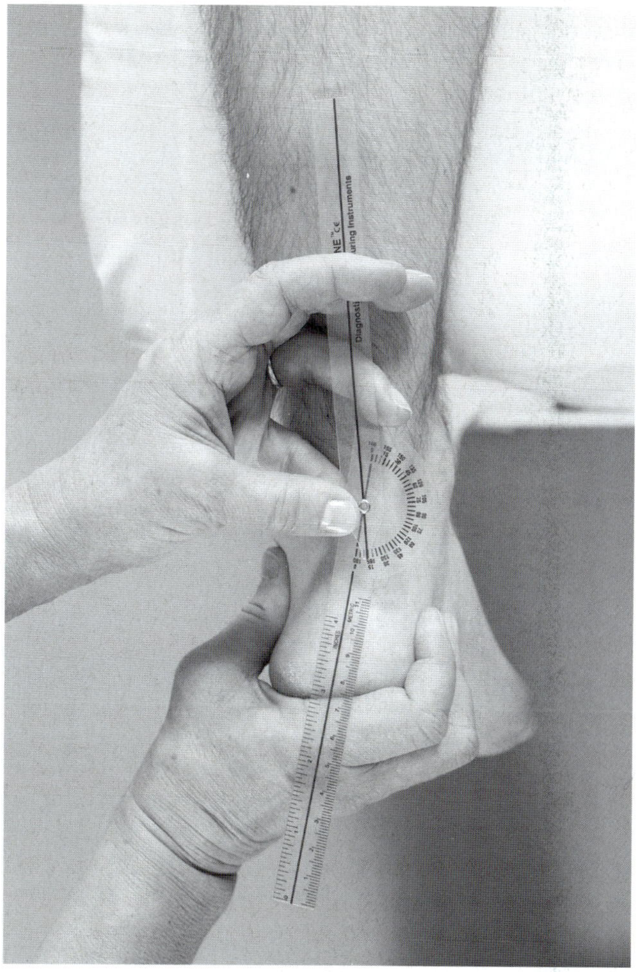

FIGURE 10.34 At the end of subtalar eversion, the examiner's hand maintains eversion. The examiner's other hand, which provided stabilization during the motion, is now used to align the arms of the goniometer.

TRANSVERSE TARSAL (MIDTARSAL) JOINT: INVERSION

Most of the motion in the forefoot occurs at the transverse tarsal joint, which comprises the talonavicular and calcaneocuboid joints. Some additional motion occurs at the cuboideonavicular, cuneonavicular, intercuneiform, cuneocuboid, and TMT joints.

Inversion is a combination of supination, adduction, and plantarflexion. Because of the uniaxial limitation of the goniometer, inversion of the transverse tarsal joint is measured in the frontal plane around an anterior–posterior axis. Normal ROM values for forefoot motions have not been established, but will be less than ROM values that include all of the tarsal joints.

Testing Position

Place the individual sitting, with the knee flexed to 90 degrees and the lower leg over the edge of the supporting surface. The hip is in 0 degrees of rotation, adduction, and abduction. The subtalar joint is placed and held in the 0 starting position so that the calcaneus is parallel to the midline of the lower leg. Alternatively, it is possible to place the individual supine, with the foot over the edge of the supporting surface.

Stabilization

Stabilize the calcaneus to prevent inversion of the subtalar joint and dorsiflexion of the ankle.

Testing Motion

Grasp the metatarsals rather than the toes and push the forefoot medially into adduction and slightly into plantarflexion. Turn the sole of the foot medially into supination, being careful not to dorsiflex the ankle (Fig. 10.35). The end of the ROM occurs when resistance is felt and attempts at further motion cause subtalar inversion and/or dorsiflexion.

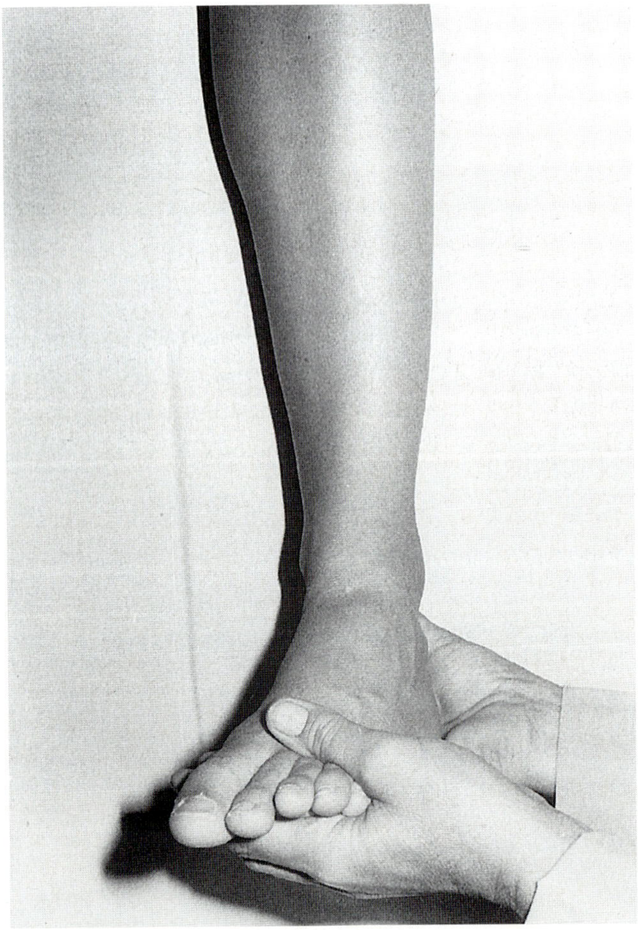

FIGURE 10.35 The left lower extremity at the end of transverse tarsal inversion range of motion (ROM). The examiner's hand stabilizes the calcaneus so that it is parallel to the midline of the lower leg and in anatomical neutral. Notice that the ROM for the transverse tarsal joint is less than the ROM for all of the tarsal joints combined.

Normal End-Feel

The end-feel is firm because of tension in the joint capsules; the dorsal calcaneocuboid ligament; the dorsal talonavicular ligament; the lateral band of the bifurcated ligament; the transverse metatarsal ligament; various dorsal, plantar, and interosseous ligaments of the cuboideonavicular, cuneonavicular, intercuneiform, cuneocuboid, TMT, and intermetatarsal joints; and the peroneus longus and brevis muscles.

Goniometer Alignment

See Figures 10.36 and 10.37.

1. Center **fulcrum** of the goniometer over the anterior aspect of the ankle slightly distal to a point midway between the malleoli.
2. Align **proximal arm** with the anterior midline of the lower leg, using the tibial tuberosity for reference.
3. Align **distal arm** with the anterior midline of the second metatarsal.

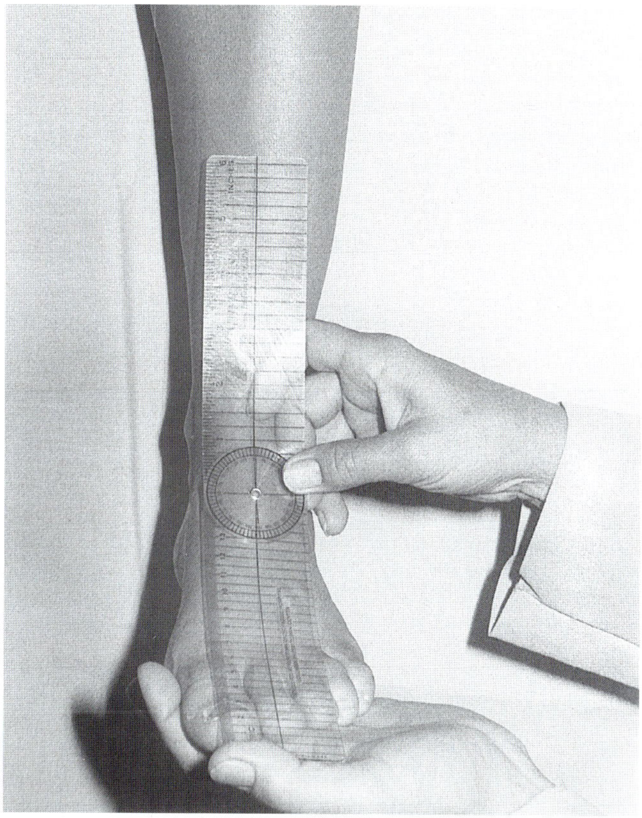

FIGURE 10.36 Goniometer alignment in the starting position for measuring transverse tarsal inversion.

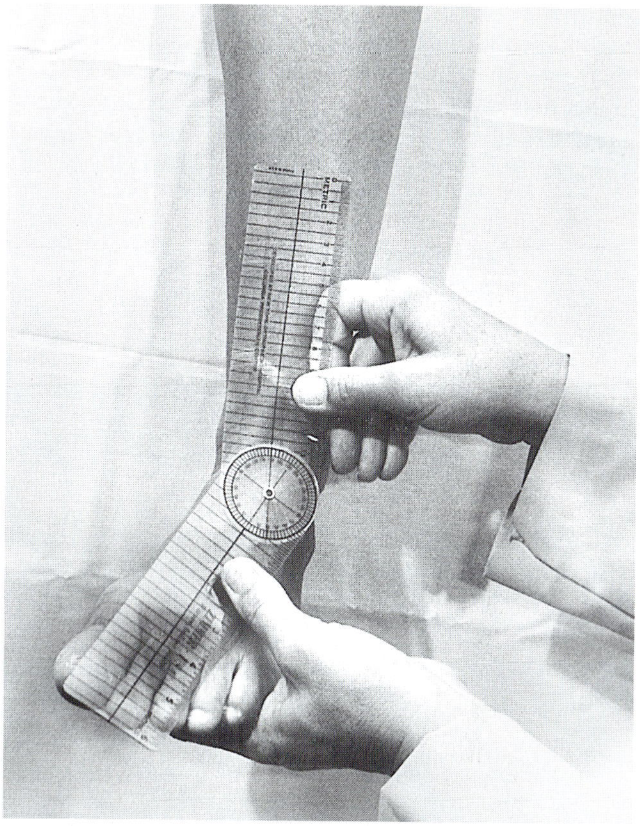

FIGURE 10.37 At the end of transverse tarsal inversion, one of the examiner's hands releases the calcaneus and aligns the proximal goniometer arm with the lower leg. The examiner's other hand maintains inversion and holds the distal goniometer arm aligned with the second metatarsal.

TRANSVERSE TARSAL (MIDTARSAL) JOINT: EVERSION

Eversion is a combination of pronation, abduction, and dorsiflexion. Because of the uniaxial limitations of the goniometer, eversion of the transverse tarsal joint is measured in the frontal plane around an anterior–posterior axis. Normal ROM values for forefoot motions have not been established, but will be less than ROM values that include all of the tarsal joints.

Testing Position

Place the individual sitting, with the knee flexed to 90 degrees and the lower leg over the edge of the supporting surface. Position the hip in 0 degrees of rotation, adduction, and abduction. The subtalar joint is placed and held in the 0 starting position so that the calcaneus is parallel to the midline of the lower leg. Alternatively, it is possible to place the individual supine, with the foot over the edge of the supporting surface.

Stabilization

Stabilize the calcaneus and talus to prevent eversion of the subtalar joint and plantarflexion of the ankle.

Testing Motion

Pull the forefoot laterally into abduction and slightly upward into dorsiflexion. Turn the forefoot into pronation so that the lateral side of the foot is higher than the medial side (Fig. 10.38). The end of the ROM occurs when resistance is felt and attempts to produce additional motion cause subtalar eversion and/or plantarflexion.

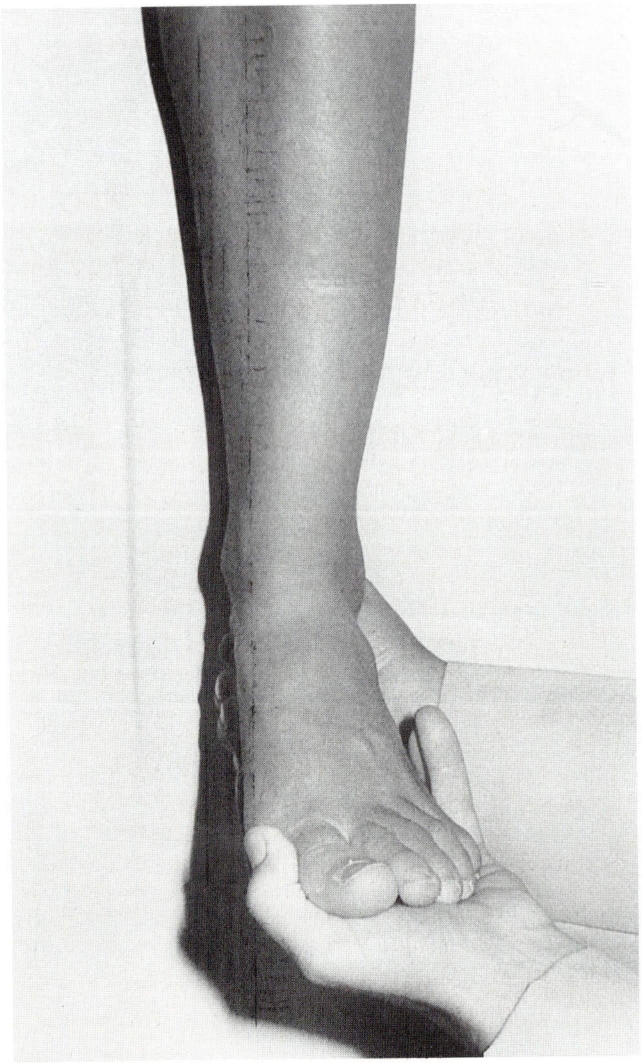

FIGURE 10.38 The end of transverse tarsal eversion range of motion. The examiner's hand stabilizes the calcaneus to prevent subtalar eversion. As can be seen in the photograph, only a small amount of motion is available at the transverse tarsal joint in this individual.

Normal End-Feel

The end-feel is firm because of tension in the joint capsules; the deltoid ligament; the plantar calcaneonavicular and calcaneocuboid ligaments; the dorsal talonavicular ligament; the medial band of the bifurcated ligament; the transverse metatarsal ligament; various dorsal, plantar, and interosseous ligaments of the cuboideonavicular, cuneonavicular, intercuneiform, cuneocuboid, TMT, and intermetatarsal joints; and the tibialis posterior muscle.

Goniometer Alignment

See Figures 10.39 and 10.40.

1. Center **fulcrum** of the goniometer over the anterior aspect of the ankle slightly distal to a point midway between the malleoli.
2. Align **proximal arm** with the anterior midline of the lower leg, using the tibial tuberosity for reference.
3. Align **distal arm** with the anterior midline of the second metatarsal.

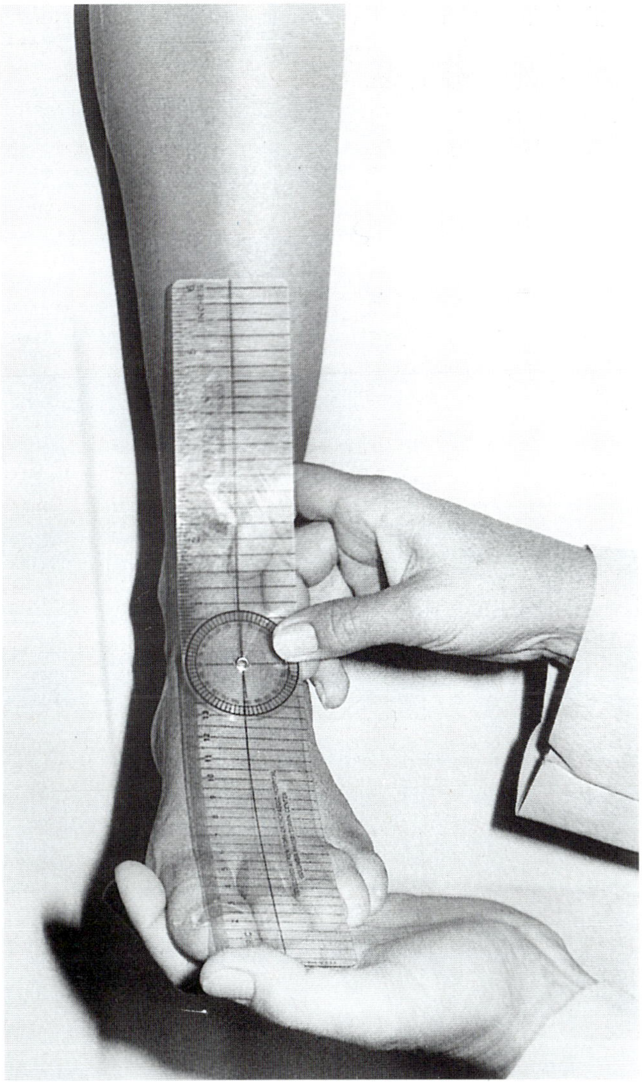

FIGURE 10.39 Goniometer alignment in the starting position for measuring transverse tarsal eversion range of motion.

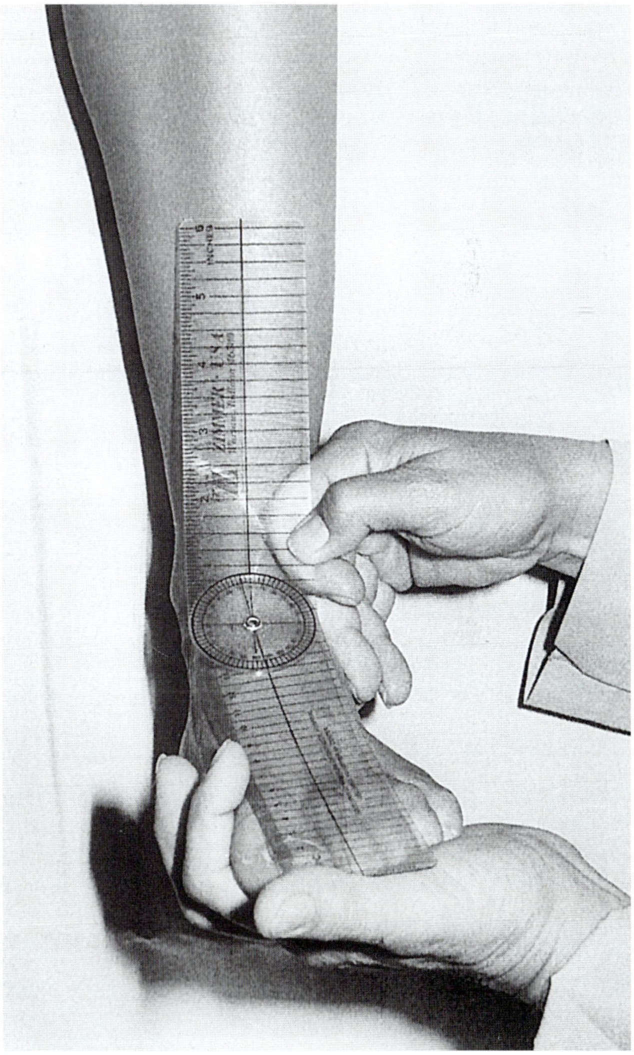

FIGURE 10.40 At the end of the transverse tarsal eversion range of motion, one of the examiner's hands releases the calcaneus and aligns the proximal goniometer arm with the lower leg. The examiner's other hand maintains eversion and alignment of the distal goniometer arm.

Landmarks for Testing Procedures: Metatarsophalangeal and Interphalangeal Joints

See Figures 10.41A and B, and 10.42A and B.

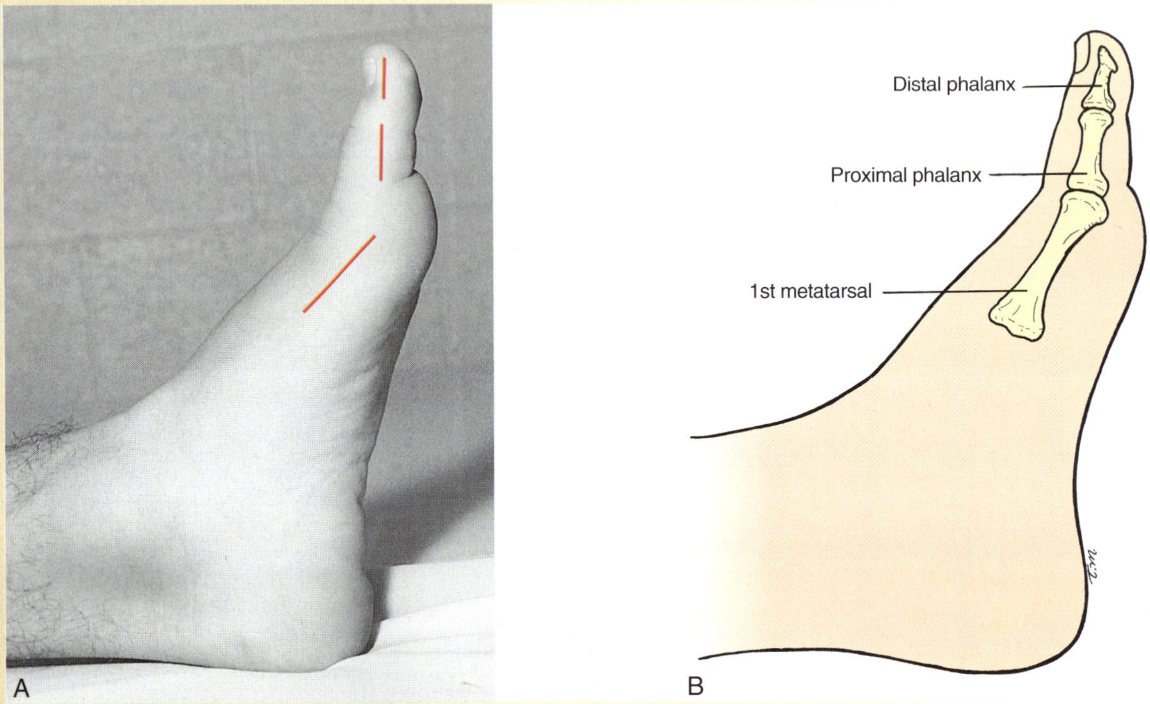

FIGURE 10.41 (A) A medial view of the left foot showing medial surface anatomy landmarks for measuring flexion and extension at the first metatarsophalangeal (MTP) joint and first interphalangeal (IP) joint. (B) Bony anatomical landmarks for measuring flexion and extension at the first MTP and IP joints.

Landmarks for Testing Procedures: Metatarsophalangeal and Interphalangeal Joints (continued)

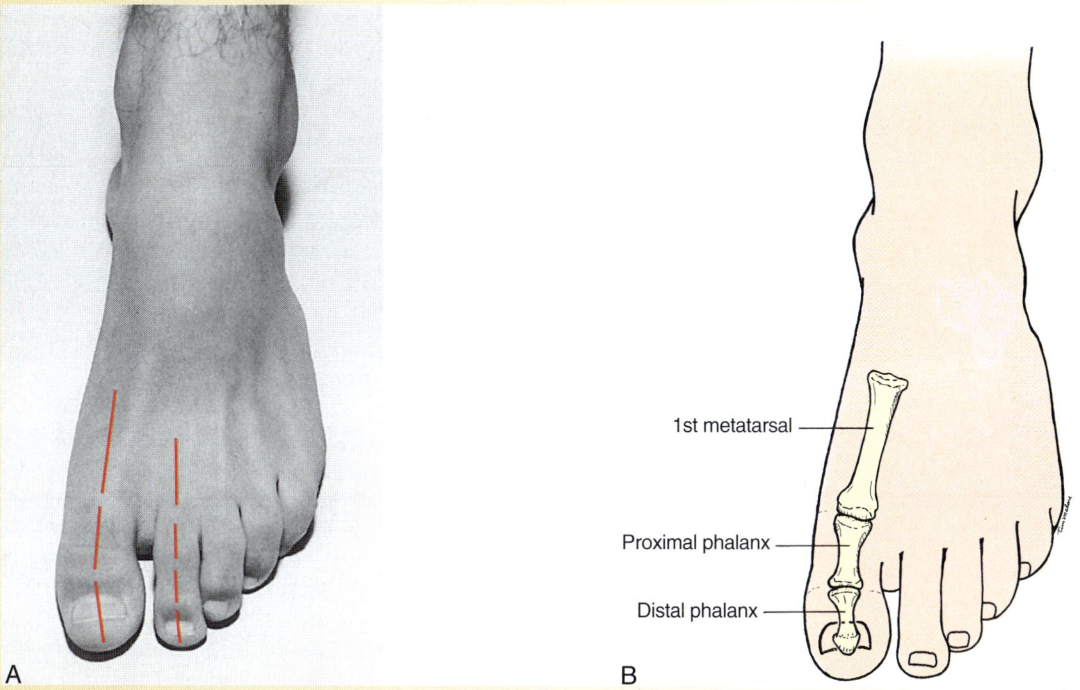

FIGURE 10.42 (A) Surface anatomy landmarks for the dorsal goniometer alignment for measuring flexion and extension range of motion at the first and second MTP and IP joints, and abduction and adduction at the first MTP joint. (B) Bony anatomical landmarks for flexion and extension at the first and second MTP and IP joints, and abduction and adduction at the first MTP joint. This individual has a slight valgus deformity at the IP joint of the first toe.

METATARSOPHALANGEAL JOINT: FLEXION

Motion occurs in the sagittal plane around a medial–lateral axis. Normal flexion ROM values at the first MTP joint vary from about 30 to 45 degrees. Using the straight-line position of the metatarsal and proximal phalanx as zero is strongly recommended because it provides more consistent and valid ROM measurements than using the position of the metatarsal and proximal phalanx in standing or a relaxed hanging position in sitting.[11] See Research Findings and Table 10.2 for more detailed information.

Testing Position

Place the individual supine or sitting, with the ankle and foot in 0 degrees of dorsiflexion, plantarflexion, inversion, and eversion. Position the MTP joint in 0 degrees of abduction and adduction and the IP joints in 0 degrees of flexion and extension. (If the ankle is plantarflexed and the IP joints of the toe being tested are flexed, tension in the extensor hallucis longus or extensor digitorum longus muscle will restrict the motion.)

Stabilization

Stabilize the metatarsal to prevent plantarflexion of the ankle and inversion or eversion of the foot. Do not hold the MTP joints of the other toes in extension because tension in the transverse metatarsal ligament will restrict the motion.

Testing Motion

Move the great toe downward toward the plantar surface into flexion (Fig. 10.43) by pushing on the proximal phalange. Avoid pushing on the distal phalanx and causing interphalangeal flexion. The end of the ROM is reached when resistance is felt and attempts at further motion cause plantarflexion at the ankle.

Normal End-Feel

The end-feel is firm because of tension in the dorsal joint capsule and the collateral ligaments. Tension in the extensor digitorum brevis muscle may contribute to the firm end-feel.

Goniometer Alignment

See Figures 10.44 and 10.45.

1. Center **fulcrum** of the goniometer over the dorsal aspect of the MTP joint.
2. Align **proximal arm** over the dorsal midline of the metatarsal.
3. Align **distal arm** over the dorsal midline of the proximal phalanx.

Alternative Goniometer Alignment for First Metatarsophalangeal Joint

1. Center **fulcrum** of the goniometer over the medial aspect of the first MTP joint.
2. Align **proximal arm** with the medial midline of the first metatarsal.
3. Align **distal arm** with the medial midline of the proximal phalanx of the first toe.

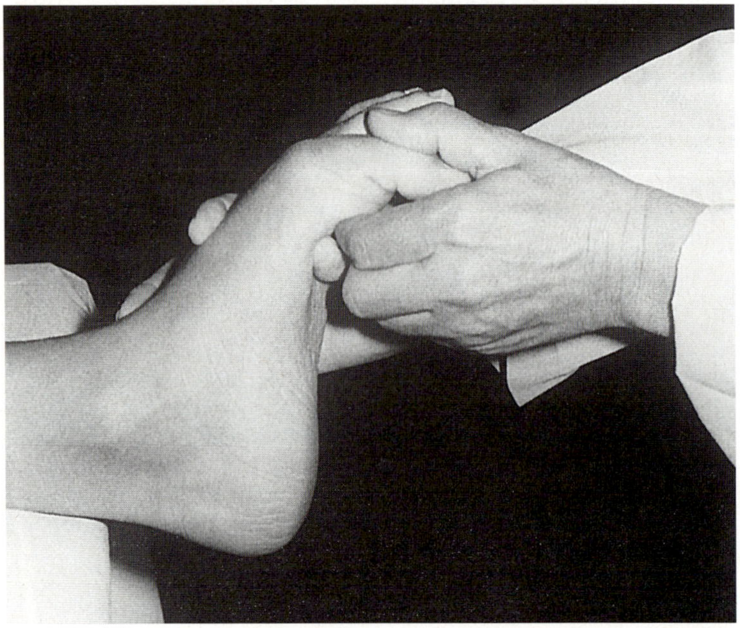

FIGURE 10.43 The left first metatarsophalangeal (MTP) joint at the end of the flexion range of motion. The individual is supine, with the foot and ankle placed over the edge of the supporting surface. However, the foot could rest on the supporting surface. The examiner uses her thumb across the metatarsals to prevent ankle plantarflexion. The examiner's other hand pushes on the proximal phalange to flex the first MTP joint.

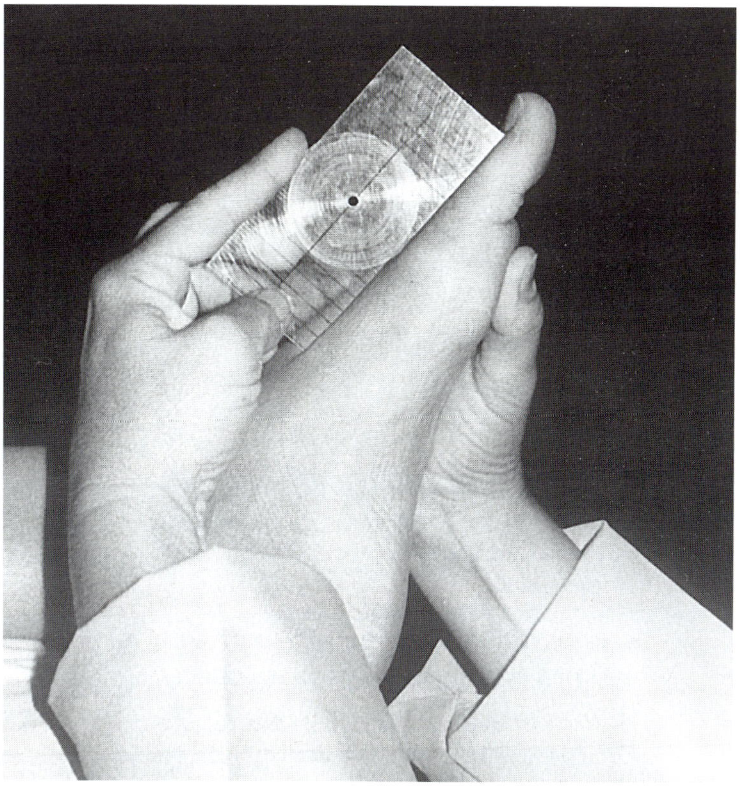

FIGURE 10.44 Goniometer alignment in the starting position for measuring metatarsophalangeal flexion range of motion. Note that the proximal phalanx is positioned in line with the metatarsal so that the goniometer reads 0 degrees. The arms of a 360-degree goniometer have been cut short to accommodate the length of the metatarsal and proximal phalanx.

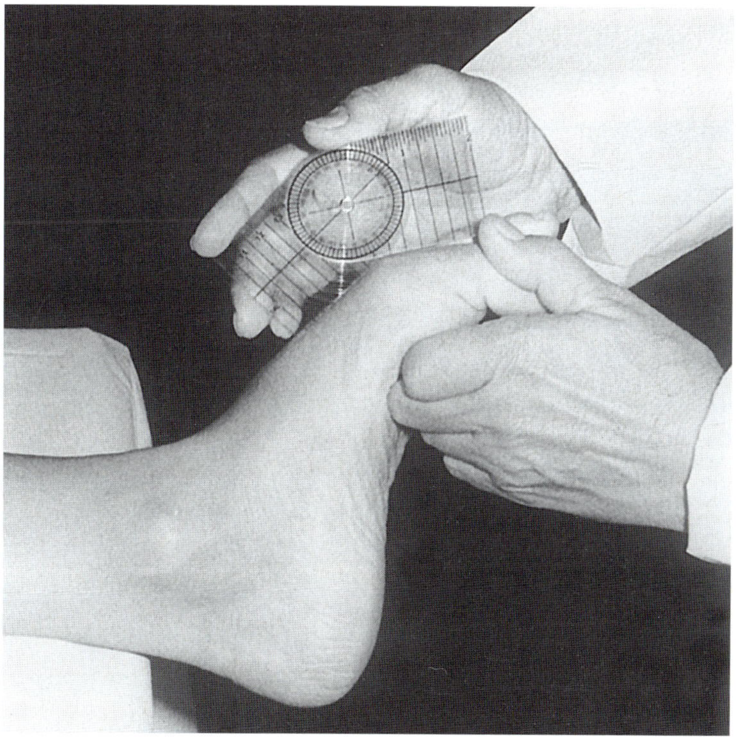

FIGURE 10.45 At the end of the range of motion, the examiner releases her stabilization of the metatarsals and uses that hand to align the goniometer, while her other hand maintains metatarsophalangeal flexion.

METATARSOPHALANGEAL JOINT: EXTENSION

Motion occurs in the sagittal plane around a medial–lateral axis. Normal extension ROM values at the first MTP joint in adults vary from about 70 to 80 degrees. See Research Findings and Table 10.2 for more detailed information.

Testing Position

The testing position is the same as that for measuring flexion of the MTP joint. (If the ankle is dorsiflexed and the IP joints of the toe being tested are extended, tension in the flexor hallucis longus or flexor digitorum longus muscle will restrict the motion. If the IP joints of the toe being tested are in extreme flexion, tension in the lumbricalis and interosseus muscles may restrict the motion.)

Stabilization

Stabilize the metatarsal to prevent dorsiflexion of the ankle and inversion or eversion of the foot. Do not hold the MTP joints of the other toes in extreme flexion because tension in the transverse metatarsal ligament will restrict the motion.

Testing Motion

Push the proximal phalanx upward toward the dorsum of the foot, moving the MTP joint into extension (Fig. 10.46). Avoid pushing on the distal phalanx, which causes IP extension. The end of the motion occurs when resistance is felt and attempts at further motion cause dorsiflexion at the ankle.

Normal End-Feel

The end-feel is firm because of tension in the plantar joint capsule; the plantar pad (plantar fibrocartilaginous plate); and the flexor hallucis brevis, flexor digitorum brevis, and flexor digiti minimi muscles.

Goniometer Alignment

See Figures 10.47 and 10.48.

1. Center **fulcrum** of the goniometer over the dorsal aspect of the MTP joint.
2. Align **proximal arm** over the dorsal midline of the metatarsal.
3. Align **distal arm** over the dorsal midline of the proximal phalanx.

Alternative Goniometer Alignment for First Metatarsophalangeal Joint

1. Center **fulcrum** of the goniometer over the medial aspect of the first MTP joint.
2. Align **proximal arm** with the medial midline of the first metatarsal.
3. Align **distal arm** with the medial midline of the proximal phalanx of the first toe.

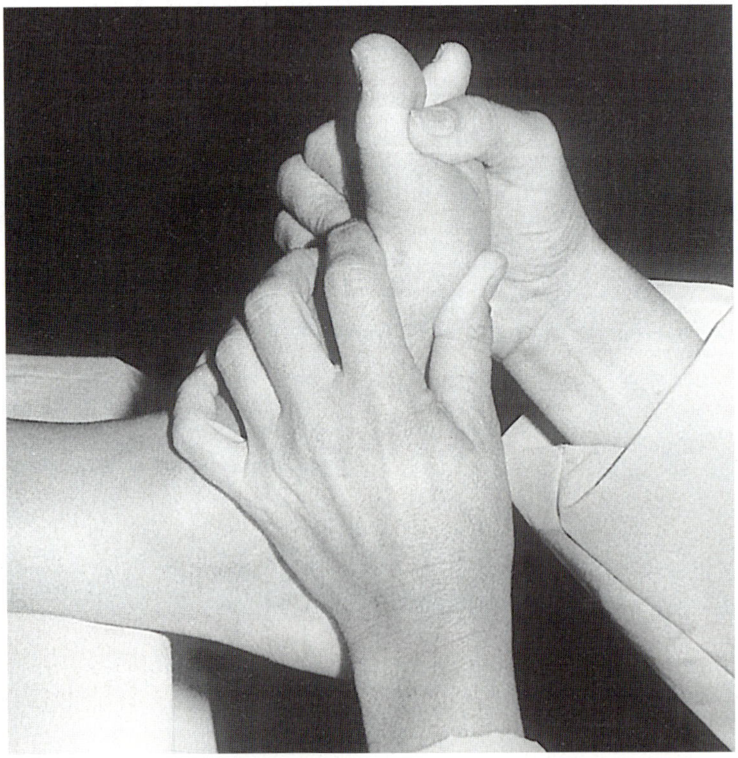

FIGURE 10.46 The left first metatarsophalangeal joint at the end of extension range of motion. The examiner places her digits on the dorsum of the individual's foot to prevent dorsiflexion and uses the thumb on her other hand to push the proximal phalanx into extension.

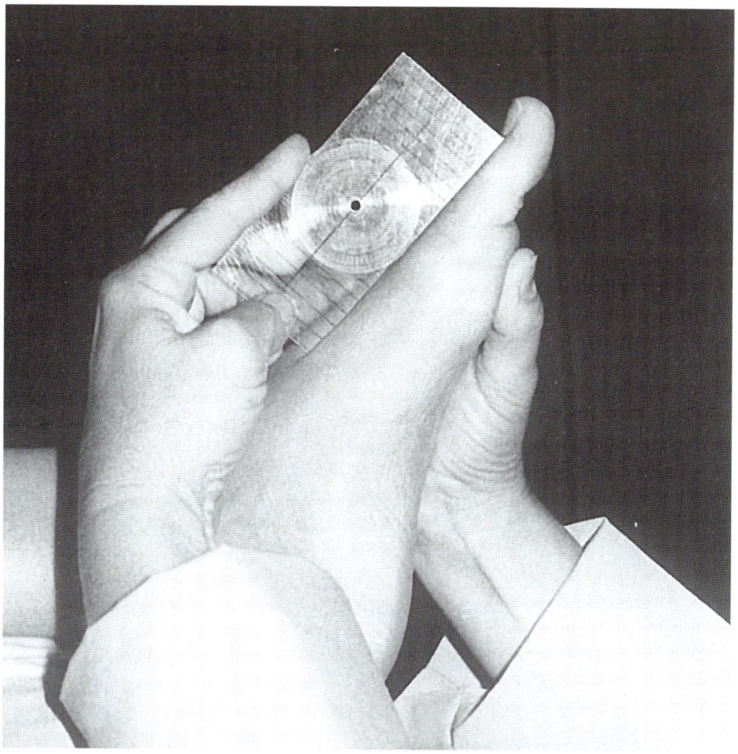

FIGURE 10.47 Goniometer alignment in the starting position for measuring extension at the first metatarsophalangeal joint.

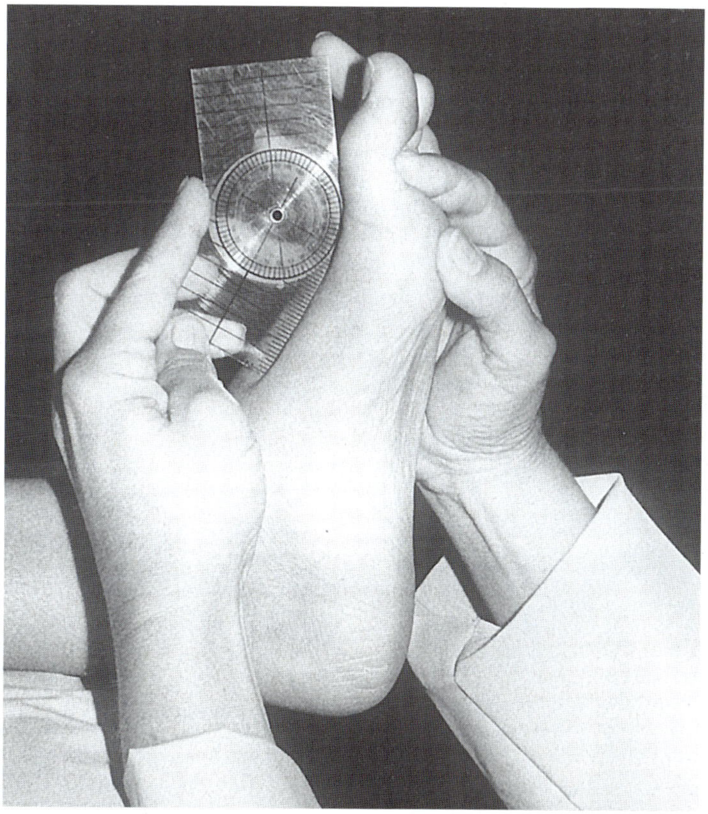

FIGURE 10.48 At the end of metatarsophalangeal (MTP) extension, the examiner releases the stabilization of the metatarsals and uses that hand to align the goniometer. The fingers of the examiner's other hand maintain extension.

METATARSOPHALANGEAL JOINT: ABDUCTION

Motion occurs in the transverse plane around a vertical axis when the individual is in anatomical position.

Testing Position

Place the individual supine or sitting, with the foot in 0 degrees of inversion and eversion. Position the MTP and IP joints in 0 degrees of flexion and extension. Stabilize the metatarsal to prevent inversion or eversion of the foot.

Stabilization

Stabilize the metatarsal to prevent inversion or eversion of the foot.

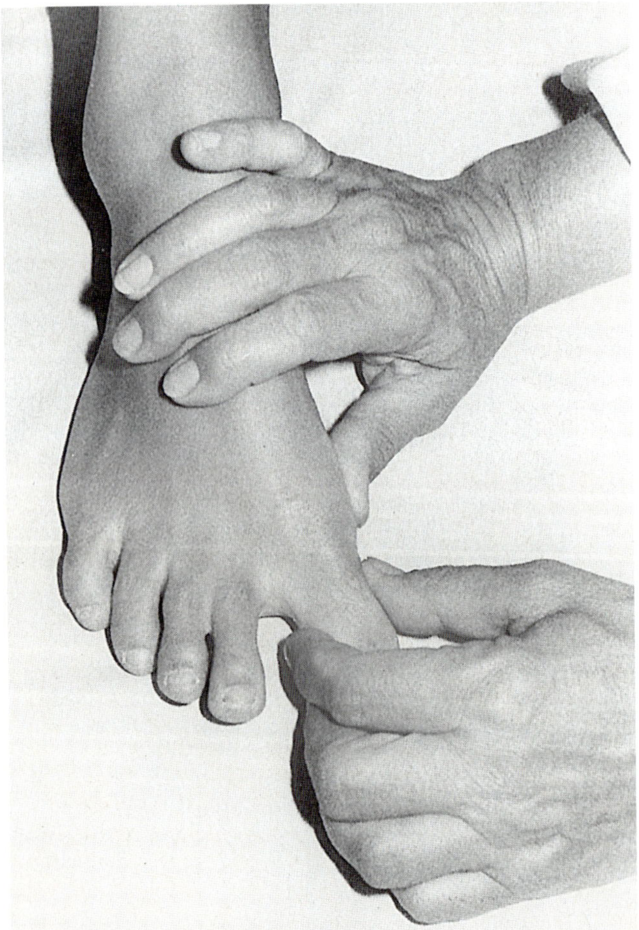

FIGURE 10.49 The right first toe at the end of abduction range of motion. The examiner uses one thumb to stabilize the metatarsal to prevent transverse tarsal inversion. She uses the index finger and thumb of her other hand to pull the proximal phalanx into abduction.

Testing Motion

Pull the proximal phalanx of the toe laterally away from the midline of the foot into abduction (Fig. 10.49). Avoid pushing on the distal phalanx, which places a strain on the IP joint. The end of the ROM occurs when resistance is felt and attempts at further motion cause either inversion or eversion of the foot.

Normal End-Feel

The end-feel is firm because of tension in the joint capsule, the collateral ligaments, the fascia of the web space between the toes, and the adductor hallucis and plantar interosseus muscles.

Goniometer Alignment

See Figures 10.50 and 10.51.

1. Center **fulcrum** of the goniometer over the dorsal aspect of the MTP joint.
2. Align **proximal arm** with the dorsal midline of the metatarsal.
3. Align **distal arm** with the dorsal midline of the proximal phalanx.

METATARSOPHALANGEAL JOINT: ADDUCTION

Motion occurs in the transverse plane around a vertical axis when the individual is in anatomical position. Adduction is the return from abduction to the 0 starting position and is not usually measured.

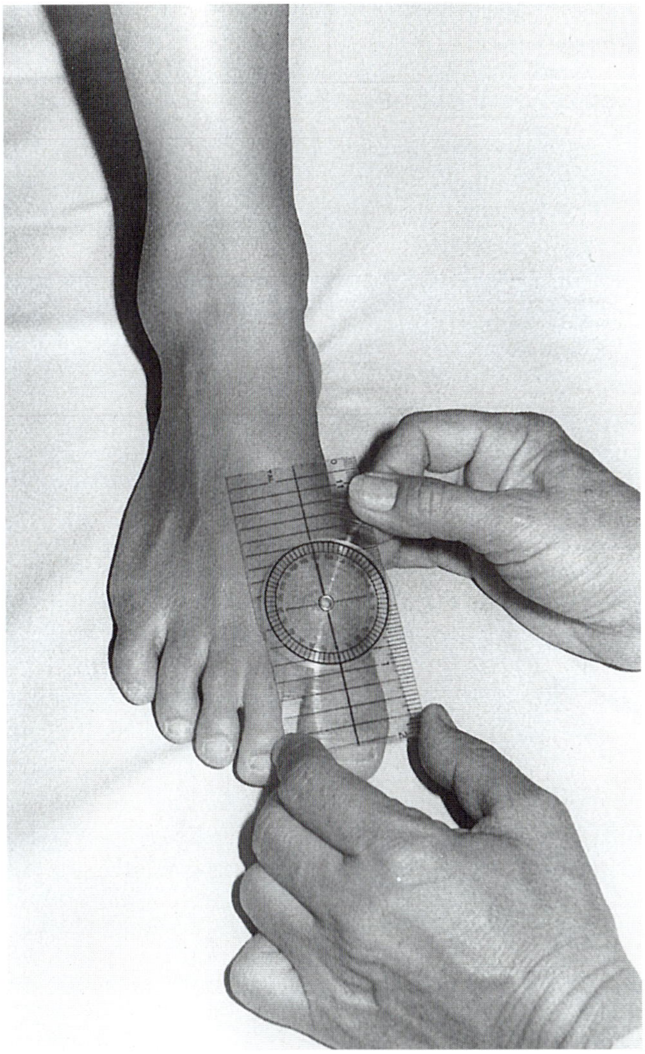

FIGURE 10.50 Goniometer alignment in the starting position for measuring metatarsophalangeal abduction range of motion. The metatarsal and proximal phalanx are in a straight line.

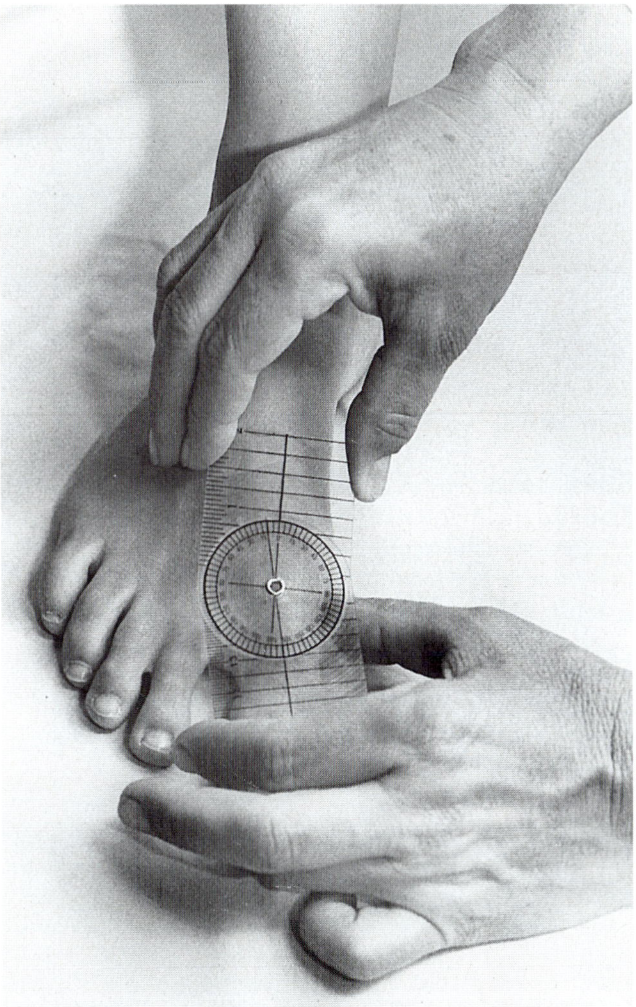

FIGURE 10.51 At the end of metatarsophalangeal (MTP) abduction, the examiner's hand is used to align the distal goniometer arm while keeping the MTP joint in abduction.

INTERPHALANGEAL JOINT OF THE FIRST TOE AND PROXIMAL INTERPHALANGEAL JOINTS OF THE FOUR LESSER TOES: FLEXION

Motion occurs in the sagittal plane around a medial–lateral axis. Reported normal IP flexion ROM values for the first toe vary widely from 30 degrees[12] to 90 degrees.[8] Normal PIP flexion ROM values for the lesser toes are reported to be 35 degrees.[8] See Research Findings and Table 10.2 for normal ROM values from several sources.

Testing Position

Place the individual supine or sitting, with the ankle and foot in 0 degrees of dorsiflexion, plantarflexion, inversion, and eversion. Position the MTP joint in 0 degrees of flexion, extension, abduction, and adduction. (If the ankle is positioned in plantarflexion and the MTP joint is flexed, tension in the extensor hallucis longus or extensor digitorum longus muscles will restrict the motion. If the MTP joint is positioned in full extension, tension in the lumbricalis and interosseus muscles may restrict the motion.)

Stabilization

Stabilize the metatarsal and proximal phalanx to prevent dorsiflexion or plantarflexion of the ankle and inversion or eversion of the foot. Avoid flexion and extension of the MTP joint.

Testing Motion

Push the distal phalanx of the first toe or the middle phalanx of the lesser toes down toward the plantar surface of the foot. The end of the ROM occurs when resistance is felt and attempts at further flexion cause plantarflexion of the ankle or flexion at the MTP joint.

Normal End-Feel

The end-feel for flexion of the IP joint of the big toe and the proximal interphalangeal (PIP) joints of the smaller toes may be soft because of compression of soft tissues between the plantar surfaces of the phalanges. Sometimes the end-feel is firm because of tension in the dorsal joint capsule and the collateral ligaments.

Goniometer Alignment

1. Center **fulcrum** of the goniometer over the dorsal aspect of the interphalangeal joint being tested.
2. Align **proximal arm** over the dorsal midline of the proximal phalanx.
3. Align **distal arm** over the dorsal midline of the phalanx distal to the joint being tested.

INTERPHALANGEAL JOINT OF THE FIRST TOE AND PROXIMAL INTERPHALANGEAL JOINTS OF THE FOUR LESSER TOES: EXTENSION

Motion occurs in the sagittal plane around a medial–lateral axis. Usually this motion is not measured because it is a return from flexion to the 0 starting position.

DISTAL INTERPHALANGEAL JOINTS OF THE FOUR LESSER TOES: FLEXION

Motion occurs in the sagittal plane around a medial–lateral axis. Normal flexion ROM in adults is reported to be about 50 to 60 degrees.[8]

Testing Position

Place the individual supine or sitting, with the ankle and foot in 0 degrees of dorsiflexion, plantarflexion, inversion, and eversion. Position the MTP and PIP joints in 0 degrees of flexion, extension, abduction, and adduction.

Stabilization

Stabilize the metatarsal, proximal, and middle phalanx to prevent dorsiflexion or plantarflexion of the ankle and inversion or eversion of the foot. Avoid flexion and extension of the MTP and PIP joints of the toe being tested.

Testing Motion

Push the distal phalanx toward the plantar surface of the foot. The end of the motion occurs when resistance is felt and attempts to produce further flexion cause flexion at the MTP and PIP joints and/or plantarflexion of the ankle.

Normal End-Feel

The end-feel is firm because of tension in the dorsal joint capsule, the collateral ligaments, and the oblique retinacular ligament.

Goniometer Alignment

1. Center **fulcrum** of the goniometer over the dorsal aspect of the distal interphalangeal (DIP) joint.
2. Align **proximal arm** over the dorsal midline of the middle phalanx.
3. Align **distal arm** over the dorsal midline of the distal phalanx.

DISTAL INTERPHALANGEAL JOINTS OF THE FOUR LESSER TOES: EXTENSION

Motion occurs in the sagittal plane around a medial–lateral axis. Usually this motion is not measured because it is a return from flexion to the 0 starting position.

Landmarks for Testing Procedures

See Figures 10.9 and 10.10.

MUSCLE LENGTH TESTING PROCEDURES: Ankle Plantarflexors

ANKLE PLANTARFLEXORS

Two muscles have the primary function of performing ankle plantarflexion and will limit ankle dorsiflexion if they are short in length. The **gastrocnemius** muscle is a two-joint muscle that crosses both the ankle and knee. The medial head of the gastrocnemius originates proximally from the posterior aspect of the medial condyle of the femur, whereas the lateral head of the gastrocnemius originates from the posterior lateral aspect of the lateral condyle (Fig. 10.52).[3] Both heads join with the tendon of the soleus muscle to form the tendocalcaneus (Achilles) tendon, which inserts distally into the posterior surface of the calcaneus. When the gastrocnemius contracts, it plantarflexes the ankle and flexes the knee. The gastrocnemius is passively lengthened by placing the knee in extension and the ankle in dorsiflexion.

In contrast to the gastrocnemius, the **soleus** crosses only the ankle joint. The soleus originates proximally from the posterior aspect of the head and proximal surfaces of the fibula, the middle third of the tibia, and the aponeurosis between the tibia and fibula.[3] It joins with the gastrocnemius to form the Achilles tendon, which inserts distally into the posterior surface of the calcaneus. The soleus is passively lengthened by dorsiflexing the ankle regardless of the position of the knee. The length of the soleus is automatically tested along with other joint structures during the measurement of ankle dorsiflexion ROM; therefore, we do not include a separate test of the length of the soleus.

GASTROCNEMIUS MUSCLE LENGTH TEST: SUPINE NON-WEIGHT-BEARING

This test is used to evaluate the length of the gastrocnemius by carefully positioning the knee in extension and then dorsiflexing the ankle.

Testing Position

Place the individual supine, with the knee extended and the foot in 0 degrees of inversion and eversion.

Stabilization

Hold the knee in full extension. Usually the weight of the limb and hand pressure on the anterior leg can maintain an extended knee position.

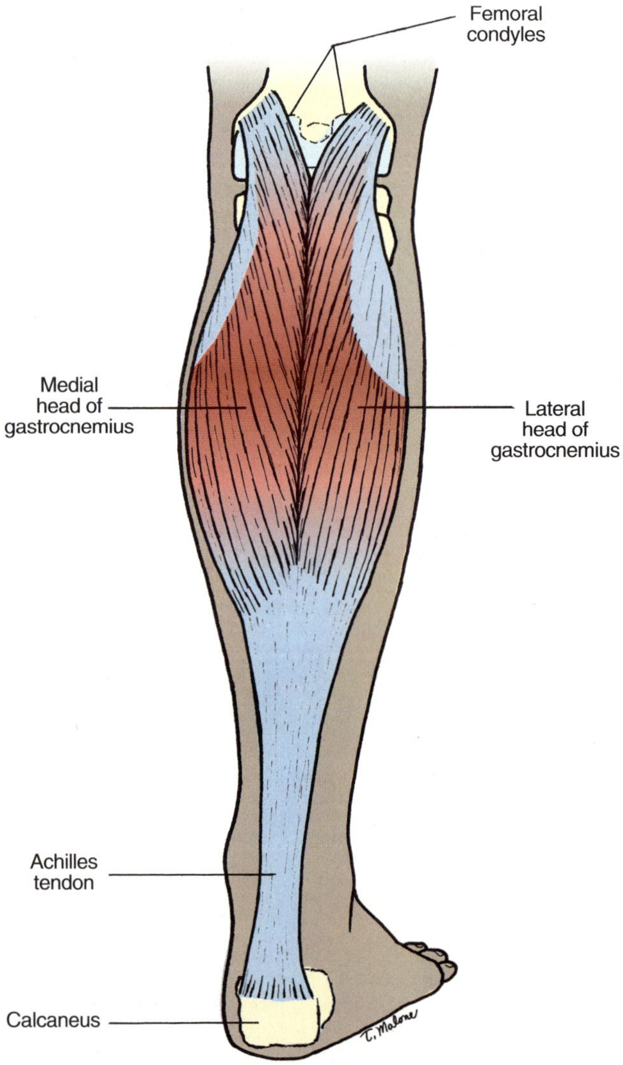

FIGURE 10.52 A posterior view of a right lower extremity shows the attachments of the gastrocnemius muscle.

Testing Motion

Dorsiflex the ankle to the end of the ROM by pushing upward across the plantar surface of the metatarsal heads (Figs. 10.53 and 10.54). Do not allow the foot to rotate and move into inversion or eversion. The end of the testing motion occurs when considerable resistance is felt from tension in the posterior calf and knee, and further ankle dorsiflexion causes the knee to flex.

Normal End-Feel

The end-feel is firm owing to tension in the gastrocnemius muscle.

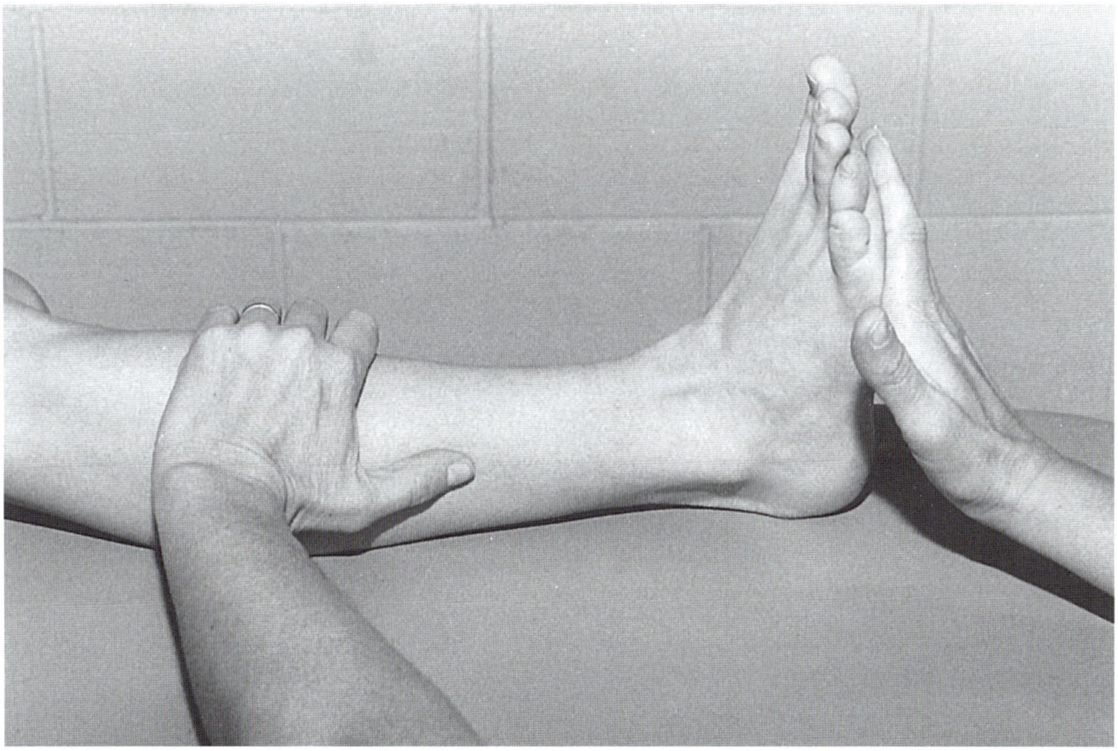

FIGURE 10.53 The right ankle at the end of the testing motion for the length of the gastrocnemius muscle. This individual has minimal dorsiflexion with the knee extended.

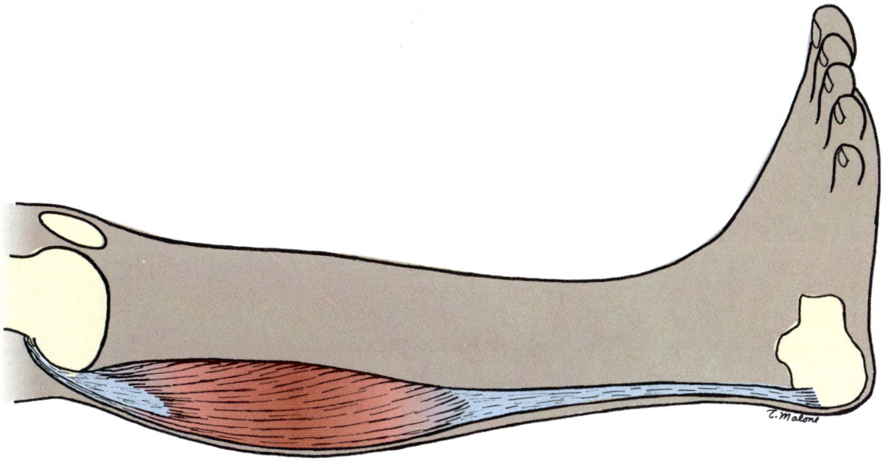

FIGURE 10.54 The gastrocnemius muscle is stretched over the extended knee and dorsiflexed ankle.

Goniometer Alignment

See Figure 10.55.

1. Center **fulcrum** of the goniometer over the lateral aspect of the lateral malleolus.
2. Align **proximal arm** with the lateral midline of the fibula, using the head of the fibula for reference.
3. Align **distal arm** parallel to the lateral aspect of the fifth metatarsal.

Interpretation

If the gastrocnemius is short, it limits ankle dorsiflexion when the knee is in extension. If dorsiflexion is limited regardless of whether the knee is flexed or extended, the limitation is due to abnormalities of the ankle joint surfaces; by shortening of the joint capsule, ligaments such as the posterior portion of the deltoid ligament, the posterior talofibular ligament, and calcaneofibular ligament; or by shortening of the soleus.

Normal dorsiflexion ROM values for adults with the knee extended in non-weight-bearing positions such as supine or prone vary from about 10 to 20 degrees. In some cases, these values are greater than those reported by other investigators of dorsiflexion ROM values with the knee flexed—most likely due to variations in measurement landmarks, devices, and active versus passive motion. In studies that compared dorsiflexion ROM with the knee flexed and extended in the same subjects, ROM values with the knee extended decreased by about 3 to 7 degrees. See Research Findings and Tables 10.6 and 10.7 for more information by ages.

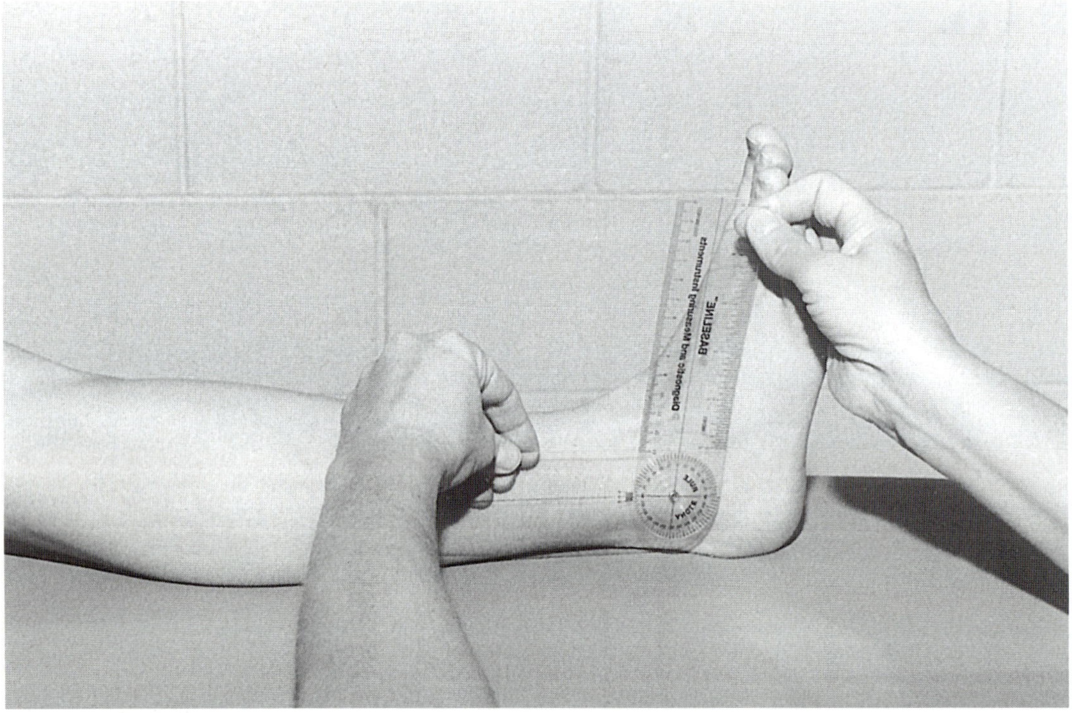

FIGURE 10.55 Goniometer alignment at the end of the non-weight-bearing test for the length of the gastrocnemius muscle. The proximal goniometer arm is aligned with the fibula, the axis is over the lateral malleolus, and the distal goniometer arm is aligned parallel to the fifth metatarsal.

GASTROCNEMIUS MUSCLE LENGTH TEST: STANDING WEIGHT-BEARING

This test is used to evaluate the length of the gastrocnemius in weight-bearing by positioning the knee in extension, and then dorsiflexing the ankle.

Testing Position

Place the individual standing, with the knee extended and the foot in 0 degrees of inversion and eversion. The foot is in line (sagittal plane) with the lower leg and knee. The individual stands facing a wall or examining table, which can be used for balance and support.

Stabilization

Maintain the knee in full extension, and ensure the heel remains in total contact with the floor. The examiner may assist by holding the heel in contact with the floor.

Testing Motion

The individual dorsiflexes the ankle by leaning the body forward (Fig. 10.56). The end of the testing motion occurs when the individual feels tension in the posterior calf and knee, and further ankle dorsiflexion causes the knee to flex and the heel to lift off the floor.

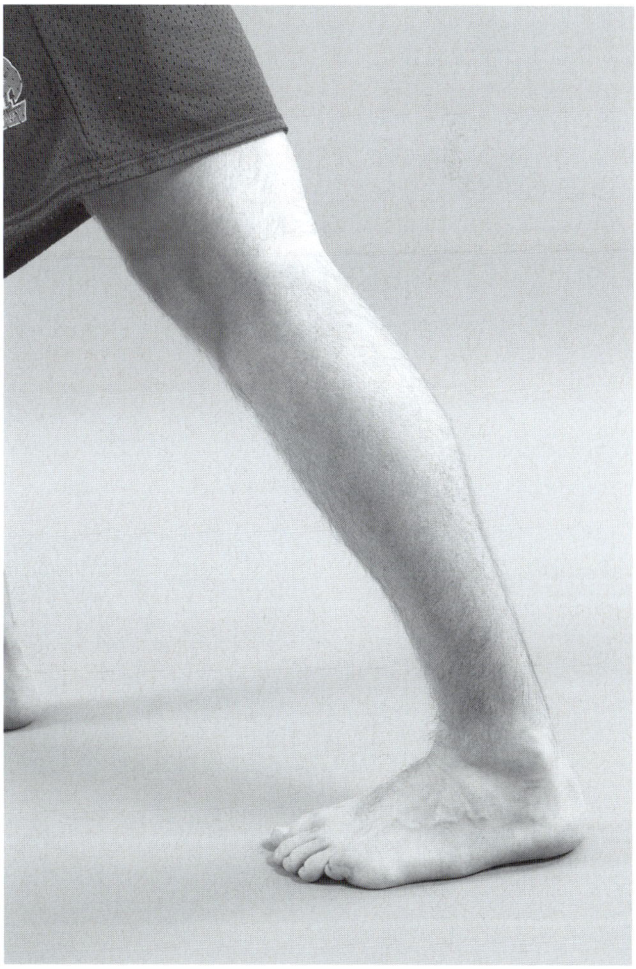

FIGURE 10.56 The left ankle at the end of the weight-bearing test for the length of the gastrocnemius muscle. The knee must be maintained in extension during the test. The foot must be in line with the lower leg and not allowed to rotate.

Goniometer Alignment

See Figure 10.57.

1. Center **fulcrum** of the goniometer over the lateral aspect of the lateral malleolus.
2. Align **proximal arm** with the lateral midline of the fibula, using the head of the fibula for reference.
3. Align **distal arm** parallel to the lateral aspect of the fifth metatarsal.

Interpretation

If the gastrocnemius is short, it limits ankle dorsiflexion when the knee is in extension. If dorsiflexion is limited regardless of whether the knee is flexed or extended, the limitation is due to abnormalities of the ankle joint surfaces; by shortening of the joint capsule, ligaments such as the posterior portion of the deltoid ligament, the posterior talofibular ligament, and calcaneofibular ligament; or by the soleus.

Normal dorsiflexion ROM values for adults with the knee extended in weight-bearing positions vary from about 22 to 25 degrees. These measurements in weight-bearing are greater than measurements in non-weight-bearing such as supine or prone. See Research Findings and Table 10.7 for more information.

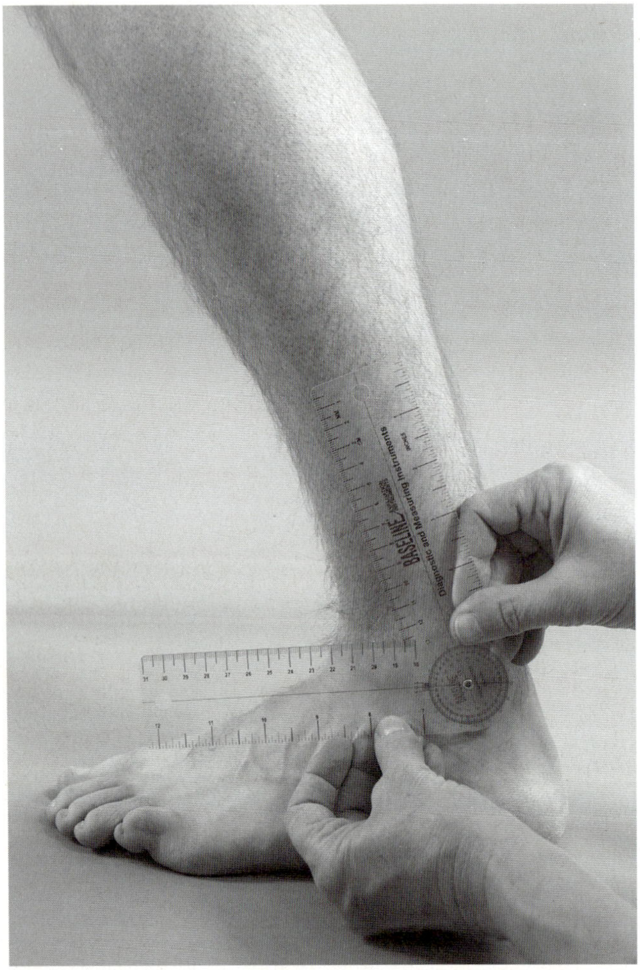

FIGURE 10.57 Goniometer alignment in the weight-bearing testing position.

Research Findings

Effects of Age, Gender, and Other Factors

Tables 10.1 and 10.2 provide ankle and toe ROM values for adults from various sources. Dorsiflexion ROM values vary from about 15 to 20 degrees, and plantarflexion varies from 40 to 60 degrees. Inversion ROM is consistently greater than eversion ROM when measuring combined midfoot and rearfoot motions, as well as isolated rearfoot (subtalar) motions. This relationship of inversion to eversion ROM in as much as a 2:1 ratio has also been noted by other researchers, as well those included in Table 10.1.[10,13] Although the AAOS[8] and the American Medical Association (AMA)[12] do not report measurement methods and study samples, all other sources in the tables took measurements with a universal goniometer in non-weight-bearing positions with defined study populations. The publication by the AAOS in 1994[14] also sites some of these same sources. Dorsiflexion values were taken with the knee in flexion to reflect ankle joint motion rather than gastrocnemius muscle length.

Most research studies of toe ROM focus only on the MTP joint of the first toe, but the AAOS[8] and AMA[12] also provide ROM values for the lesser toes[2–5] and some interphalangeal joints. In general, flexion and extension of the first toe is greater than flexion and extension of the lesser toes. All sources in Table 10.2 considered the MTP joint to be at 0 degrees when the metacarpal and proximal phalanx are in a straight line. Measurements of the MTP joint varied as to whether the goniometer was aligned on the dorsal or medial aspect, but it is unclear whether this difference in alignment has an important effect. Hopson, McPoil, and Cornwall[18] found that MTP extension ROM of the first toe was greater when measured medially than dorsally with mean values of 95.9 and 85.0, respectively. However, Buell and colleagues[11] reported a mean of 82 degrees of MTP extension measured medially, which is similar to the dorsally measured value reported by Hopson, McPoil, and Cornwall. In any case, MTP flexion and extension of the 2–4 toes would be difficult to measure on the medial or lateral surfaces and require a dorsal placement of the goniometer. One study by Kwon and associates[19] found that the dorsal placement of the goniometer resulted in an 8- to 10-degree underestimation of MTP extension of the 2–4 toes as compared with computed tomography (CT) scans, but that the measurements were highly correlated.

Age

As shown in Table 10.3, newborns and infants have a larger dorsiflexion and smaller plantarflexion ROM than older children and adults. The mean values for dorsiflexion in these youngest age-groups are more than double the average adult values presented in Tables 10.1, 10.4, and 10.5. However, between 1 and 5 years of age, dorsiflexion values show a decrease. This substantial decrease in dorsiflexion in older children as compared to infants less than 1 year of age was also noted by Kumar and associates[20] in a study of an Asian Indian population in which lifestyle activities often included squatting and sitting cross-legged. Plantarflexion ROM in newborns is smaller than for adults, but newborns attain adult

TABLE 10.1 Normal Ankle ROM Values for Adults in Degrees From Selected Sources

	AAOS[8]	AMA[12]	Boone and Azen*[15]	Roass and Andersson†[16]	Macedo and Magee**[17]	Menadue et al‡[9]
			20–54 yr n = 56 Males	34–40 yr n = 96 Males	18–59 yr n = 90 Females	21–59 yr n = 11 Males, 20 Females
Motion			**Mean (SD)**	**Mean (SD)**	**Mean (SD)**	**Mean (SD)**
Dorsiflexion	20	20	12.2 (4.1)	15.3 (5.8)	13 (9)	—
Plantarflexion	50	40	54.3 (5.9)	39.7 (7.5)	60 (13)	—
Inversion	35	30	36.2 (4.2)	27.7 (6.9)	47 (9)	31.5 (8.8)
Eversion	15	20	19.2 (4.9)	27.7 (4.6)	33 (10)	11.1 (7.4)
Subtalar inversion	5	—	—	—	—	15.0 (6.1)
Subtalar eversion	5	—	—	—	—	8.3 (3.6)

AMA = American Medical Association; AAOS = American Association of Orthopaedic Surgeons; SD = Standard deviation.

* Values are for active ROM measured with universal goniometer.

† Values are for passive ROM of right ankle measured with a universal goniometer, in supine with knee flexed.

** Values are for passive ROM with a universal goniometer; dorsiflexion and plantarflexion measured with universal goniometer in sitting with the knee flexed; inversion and eversion measured in supine with knee extended.

‡ Values are for active ROM with a universal goniometer; inversion and eversion measured sitting, subtalar ROM measured prone using methods from the first edition of this text.

TABLE 10.2 Normal Toe ROM Values for Adults in Degrees From Selected Sources

Joint	Extension				Flexion		
	AMA[12]	AAOS[8]	Buell et al*[11] 19–75 yr *n* = 33 Females, 17 Males	Hopson et al†[18] 21–43 yr *n* = 10 Males, 10 Females	AMA[12]	AAOS[8]	Buell et al*[11] 19–75 yr *n* = 33 Females, 17 Males
			Mean	*Mean (SD)*			*Mean*
MTP 1	50	70	82	85.0 (10.7)	30	45	17
2	40	40			30	40	
3	30	40			20	40	
4	20	40			10	40	
5	10	40			10	40	
IP 1	—	—			30	90	
PIP 2–5	—	—			—	35	
DIP 2–5	—	—			—	60	

AMA = American Medical Association; AAOS = American Association of Orthopaedic Surgeons; SD = Standard deviation; DIP = Distal interphalangeal; IP = Interphalangeal; MTP = Metatarsophalangeal; PIP = Proximal interphalangeal.

* Measurements were taken from lateral aspect. 0 degrees = metacarpal and proximal phalanx in straight line.

† Measurements were taken from dorsal aspect. 0 degrees = metacarpal and proximal phalanx in straight line. When measurements taken from lateral aspect: mean = 95.9 and SD = 9.7 degrees.

values in the first few weeks of life. According to Walker,[25] the persistence in infants of a limited ROM in plantarflexion may indicate pathology.

Tables 10.4 and 10.5 provide evidence that slight decreases in dorsiflexion and plantarflexion ROM occur with increases in age in children through adults. Soucie and coworkers[24] reported a decrease in dorsiflexion for both males and females, and a decrease in plantarflexion for males, with the greatest age-related differences between the children (aged 2–8 years) and all other groups. Statistically significant differences were generally noted between adolescents (aged 9–19) and older adults (aged 45–69) but not between adolescents and younger adults (aged 20–44). The investigators suggested that the differences may be due to loss in the resilience of cartilage, reduced elasticity of ligaments, fat redistribution, and decreased strength of muscle in the case of active ROM.[24,29] Kumar and associates[20] likewise found a decrease in dorsiflexion and plantarflexion with increasing age in an Asian Indian population, but mean differences were less than 5 degrees between children aged 3 to 10 years versus adults aged

TABLE 10.3 Effects of Age on Ankle ROM in Newborns and Children: Normal Values in Degrees

	Waugh et al[21]	Wanatabe et al[22]	Boone[23]		Soucie et al[24]		Kumar et al[20]		
	6–72 hr	2 wk–2 yr	1–5 yr	6–12 yr	2–8 yr		<1 yr	1–3 yr	3–10 yr
	n = 40	Males and Females *n* = 45	Males *n* = 19	Males *n* = 17	Males *n* = 55	Females *n* = 39	Males and Females *n* = 32	Males and Females *n* = 25	Males and Females *n* = 43
Motion	*Mean (SD)*	*Range of means*	*Mean (SD)*	*Mean (SD)*	*Mean (SD)*	*Mean (SD)*	*Mean (SD)*	*Mean (SD)*	*Mean (SD)*
Dorsiflexion	58.9 (7.9)	53 to 41	14.5 (5.0)	13.8 (4.4)	22.8 (5.6)	24.8 (7.2)	48.0 (9.6)	32.8 (4.1)	27.0 (4.9)
Plantarflexion	25.7 (6.3)	58 to 62	59.7 (5.4)	59.6 (4.7)	55.8 (5.2)	67.1 (7.4)	43.3 (6.0)	46.4 (5.5)	38.6 (5.9)
Inversion			40.4 (2.5)	37.2 (4.5)					
Eversion			25.0 (3.2)	23.5 (3.3)					

SD = Standard deviation.

TABLE 10.4 Effects of Age and Gender on Ankle ROM in Adolescents and Younger Adults: Normal Values in Degrees

	Boone[23]			Soucie et al[24]				Kumar et al[20]	
	13–19 yr	20–29 yr	30–39 yr	9–19 yr		20–44 yr		10–15 yr	15–25 yr
	Males *n* = 17	Males *n* = 19	Males *n* = 18	Males *n* = 48	Females *n* = 56	Males *n* = 114	Females *n* = 143	Males and Females *n* = 65	Males and Females *n* = 57
Motion	**Mean (SD)**	**Mean (SD)**	**Mean (SD)**	**Mean (SD)**	**Mean (SD)**	**Mean (SD)**	**Mean (SD)**	**Mean (SD)**	**Mean (SD)**
Dorsiflexion	10.6 (3.7)	12.1 (3.4)	12.2 (4.3)	16.3 (5.1)	17.3 (6.4)	12.7 (5.9)	13.8 (5.5)	29.8 (4.8)	24.3 (5.9)
Plantarflexion	55.5 (5.7)	55.4 (3.6)	54.6 (6.0)	52.8 (7.0)	57.3 (9.4)	54.6(7.8)	62.1 (9.3)	36.2 (5.0)	40.0 (8.5)
Inversion	34.7 (5.1)	35.9 (5.2)	36.4 (3.1)						
Eversion	18.1 (4.2)	17.6 (4.5)	18.9 (4.1)						

SD = Standard deviation.

TABLE 10.5 Effects of Age and Gender on Ankle ROM in Older Adults: Normal Values in Degrees

	Boone[23]	Boone[26]	Soucie et al[24]		Nigg et al*[27]		Nigg et al*[27]		Mecagni et al[28]
	40–54 yr	61–69 yr	45–69 yr		40–59 yr		70–79 yr		64–87 yr
	Males *n* = 19	Males *n* = 10	Males *n* = 96	Female *n* = 123	Males *n* = 15	Female *n* = 15	Males *n* = 15	Female *n* = 15	Females *n* = 34
Motion	**Mean (SD)**	**Mean (SD)**	**Mean (SD)**	**Mean (SD)**	**Mean (SD)**	**Mean (SD)**	**Mean (SD)**	**Mean (SD)**	**Mean (SD)**
Dorsiflexion	12.4 (4.7)	8.2 (4.6)	11.9 (5.0)	11.6 (5.5)	27.1 (5.9)	23.7 (5.7)	26.4 (4.7)	18.5 (4.8)	10.9 (4.2)
Plantarflexion	52.9 (7.6)	46.2 (7.7)	49.4 (8.4)	56.5 (8.7)	40.0 (6.2)	40.6 (9.4)	33.7 (6.9)	40.5 (5.9)	60.8 (8.7)
Inversion	36.2 (4.3)	37.9 (4.8)							29.1 (5.5)
Eversion	20.9 (5.5)	20.3 (5.7)							18.2 (4.0)

SD = Standard deviation.

* A laboratory coordinate system ROM instrument using shoe and footplate was used to measure active ROM in subjects sitting with the knee flexed. (Other studies used a universal goniometer to take ROM measurements.)

25 to 75 years. Boone and Azen[15] found that males less than 19 years of age had less plantarflexion, inversion, and eversion than males 19 to 54 years of age, with mean differences of 3.9, 1.3, and 2.1 degrees, respectively. Nigg and associates[27] found age-related changes in ankle ROM that were motion specific and differed between males and females. For the entire group of 121 subjects between the ages of 20 and 79 years, decreases in active ROM with increases in age occurred in plantarflexion, inversion (supination), abduction, and adduction, but not in eversion (pronation) and dorsiflexion. Plantarflexion decreased about 8 degrees from the youngest to the oldest group. Measurements were taken in the sitting position with the knee flexed using a laboratory coordinate system and footplate.

Decreases in ankle ROM have also been noted in older adults. James and Parker[30] found a consistent reduction in both active and passive ROM with increasing age in all ankle joint motions in a group of 80 active men and women ranging in age from 70 to 92 years. The most rapid reduction in ROM occurred for individuals in the ninth decade. Ankle dorsiflexion measured with the knee extended (a test of the length of the gastrocnemius muscle) showed the most marked change. The investigators suggested that the decrease in extensibility of the plantarflexor muscle–tendon unit was due to connective tissue changes associated with the aging process. In another study that examined the effects of aging on dorsiflexion ROM with the knee extended (gastrocnemius muscle length), Gajdosik, VanderLinden, and Williams[31] used an isokinetic dynamometer to passively stretch the calf muscles in 74 females (aged 20–84 years). The older women (aged 60–84 years) had a significantly smaller mean dorsiflexion angle of 15.4 degrees than the younger women (aged 20–39 years), who had a mean of 25.8 degrees, and the middle-aged women, who had a mean of 22.8 degrees (Table 10.6). The decrease in dorsiflexion in

TABLE 10.6 Effect of Age on Gastrocnemius Muscle Length (Dorsiflexion ROM Measured With the Knee Extended) in Non-Weight-Bearing Positions: Normal Values in Degrees

Gajdosik et al*[31]			Moseley et al†[33]	Jonson and Gross‡[34]	Vandervoort et al§[35]	
20–24 yr $n = 24$ Females	40–59 yr $n = 24$ Females	60–84 yr $n = 33$ Females	15–34 yr $n = 298$ Males and Females	18–30 yr $n = 57$ Males and Females	55–60 yr $n = 36$ Males and Females	80–85 yr $n = 35$ Males and Females
Mean (SD)	***Mean (SD)***	***Mean (SD)***	***Mean (SD)***	***Mean (SD)***	***Mean (SD)***	***Mean (SD)***
25.83 (5.5)	22.8 (4.4)	15.4 (5.8)	18.1 (6.9)	16.2 (3.7)	20.3 (4.6)	11.8 (5.2)

SD = Standard deviation.

* Measurements are of passive ROM taken in the supine position with a universal goniometer.

† Measurements are of passive ROM taken in the prone position with use of a protractor and the application of 12.0 Newton meter (Nm) of torque.

‡ Measurements are of active assistive ROM in the prone position with a universal goniometer.

§ Measurements are of active ROM in the prone position with use of a footplate and a potentiometer.

the older women was associated with a decrease in plantarflexor muscle–tendon unit extensibility.

In a subsequent study, Gajdosik and colleagues[32] compared the passive stretch and release characteristics of the calf muscles of 15 healthy older women with a mean age of 79 years with that of 15 healthy young women with a mean age of 24 years. The right ankles were stretched from plantarflexion to maximal dorsiflexion and then released into plantarflexion. Older women had less calf muscle length extensibility, less passive resistive force, less stored passive-elastic energy, and less mean maximum passive dorsiflexion ROM (10.3 degrees), compared with younger women (28.0 degrees).

Diminishing motion of the MTP joint of the first toe has also been associated with increasing age. Buell and colleagues,[11] in a study of 33 females and 17 males ranging in age from 19 to 75 years, found a substantial decrease with age for MTP extension (dorsiflexion) and less of a difference for flexion (plantarflexion). The youngest age-group (19–29 years) had mean extension values of 95 degrees versus 82 degrees in the middle age-group (30–45 years) and 65 degrees in the oldest age-group (over 45 years). Flexion values for the three age-groups were 20, 17, and 14 degrees, respectively.

Gender

Gender effects on ROM are joint and motion specific and are often related to age. In general, studies suggest that women have more plantarflexion than men, whereas men may have more dorsiflexion than women. Soucie and coinvestigators[24] found that female subjects had greater joint mobility in nearly all joints and age-groups studied, but most obviously for ankle plantarflexion. Nigg and associates[27] found gender differences in ankle motion but determined that the differences changed with increasing age. Only in the oldest group did women have more (8 degrees) plantarflexion than men. The only gender differences noted by Boone, Walker, and Perry[26] were that females in the 1- to 9-year-old group and those in the 61- to 69-year-old group had significantly more ROM in plantarflexion than their male counterparts. Four other studies also found that females had more plantarflexion than males.[13,30,36,37] Alanen and colleagues,[13] in a study of ankle joint mobility in 245 children aged 7 to 14 years (mean age 10 years), found that girls had a significantly greater range of passive plantarflexion compared with the boys in the study. However, according to the authors, the differences were small and probably not of clinical importance. Walker and colleagues[37] studied active ROM in 30 men and 30 women ranging in age from 60 to 84 years. Women had 11 degrees more ankle plantarflexion than men. James and Parker[30] found that the only motion that showed a significant difference between the genders was plantarflexion. Women and men had similar mean values in the group between 70 and 74 years of age, but the reduction in active and passive plantarflexion ROM over the entire age range was greater for men (25.2%) than for women (11.3%). Wearing high-heeled shoes has been proposed by Nigg and associates[27] as one reason why women have a greater ROM in plantarflexion than men.

In addition to the findings that women have greater ROM in plantarflexion than men, some investigators have found that males have greater active and passive dorsiflexion ROM than females.[27,35,37] In a study of 121 subjects by Nigg and associates,[27] males in the oldest group had a greater active ROM in dorsiflexion (8 degrees) measured with the knee flexed than females in the same age-group (Table 10.5). Females showed a significant decrease in active dorsiflexion ROM with increasing age, from a mean of 26.0 degrees in the youngest group to 18.5 degrees in the oldest group. Females also showed a significant decrease in eversion of 5.8 degrees with increasing age. Males, however, had little or no change in either active dorsiflexion or eversion ROM from the youngest to the oldest group. Vandervoort and coworkers[35] experienced similar findings in a study measuring passive dorsiflexion ROM with the knee flexed using a footplate. Females in the study showed a decrease in passive dorsiflexion ROM, from a high of 19.3 degrees in the youngest group (aged 55–60 years) to a low of 12.1 degrees in the oldest group (aged 81 to 85 years). In comparison, male subjects showed a decrease of only 2.3 degrees in dorsiflexion from the youngest group (mean = 15.4 degrees) to the oldest group (mean = 13.1 degrees). Males had greater passive elastic stiffness than females in 10 degrees of dorsiflexion.

A study by Baggett and Young[38] of 10 male and 20 female subjects aged 18 to 66 years found males had less dorsiflexion ROM in non-weight-bearing and a greater ROM in weight-bearing than females. However, the differences in ROM were small between the genders and believed to be of little clinical significance.

Several studies have reported that females have greater ROM in both plantarflexion and dorsiflexion than males. Bell and Hoshizaki[36] studied 17 joint motions in 124 females and 66 males ranging in age from 18 to 88 years. Females between 17 and 30 years of age had a greater plantarflexion–dorsiflexion ROM (about 10 degrees difference) than males in the same age-groups. Grimston and associates[39] measured active ROM in 120 subjects (58 males and 62 females) ranging in age from 9 to 20 years. These authors found that females generally had a greater ROM in all ankle motions than males. Both males and females showed a consistent trend toward decreasing ROM with increasing age, but females had a larger decrease than males.

In contrast to the gender-related findings of the previously mentioned studies, Kumar et al[20] found no significant differences between males and females in the same age-groups for ankle dorsiflexion and plantarflexion ROM in 326 Asian Indian subjects ranging in age from 1 month to 75 years. Saxena and Kim[40] also found no differences in dorsiflexion ROM values in a relatively small study between 24 male and 16 female adolescents aged 14 to 17 years. Van der Worp and associates[41] found no gender difference in dorsiflexion ROM measured with knee extended in standing in 22 male and 20 female recreational runners. Female runners did have greater first toe MTP extension ROM than males, with values of 79 and 70 degrees, respectively. MTP extension was measured by lifting the heel while in standing position with the knee extended.

Body Mass Index

Increases in body mass index (BMI) have not been associated with changes in ankle ROM. Park and colleagues[42] found nonsignificant increases of 1 to 2 degrees in dorsiflexion and plantarflexion in adult males whose BMI was greater than 30 kg/m^2 compared with nonobese males in a study of 40 subjects.

Right Versus Left Sides

Studies that have compared right and left ankle ROM have generally found no significant difference between sides or between dominant and nondominant legs. These findings support the use of setting ROM rehabilitative goals based on results taken from a healthy contralateral ankle.

Soucie and coworkers,[24] in a study of 674 subjects ranging in age from 2 to 69 years (54.6% female), found no significant difference in ankle dorsiflexion and plantarflexion ROM between sides. Moseley, Crosbie, and Adams[33] reported no flexibility or dorsiflexion ROM differences between right and left sides nor between the dominant and nondominant legs in 300 healthy male and female subjects between 15 and 34 years. Likewise, no differences due to side or dominance were reported for ankle dorsiflexion, plantarflexion, eversion, and inversion ROM by Roaas and Andersson[16] in a study that included 192 ankles in male Swedish subjects between the ages of 30 and 40 years.

Several studies have found minimal differences between sides for particular motions that most likely are of little clinical relevance. No difference between sides was found for various measures of dorsiflexion, plantarflexion, inversion, and eversion in a study of 121 male and female subjects conducted by Alstrom and Arvidson.[10] A statistical difference between sides was found for calcaneal (subtalar) eversion; however, that difference was only 1 degree and was disregarded by the investigators because it was small and close to observer error. Macedo and Magee[43] found no differences between dominant and nondominant sides for active and passive eversion, inversion, and active dorsiflexion, but did find differences for passive ankle dorsiflexion and plantarflexion and active plantarflexion in a study of 90 females aged 18 to 59 years. Mean differences were less than 3.5 degrees and were considered clinically insignificant. The investigators concluded that their results supported the use of the opposite side of the body as an indicator of preinjury or normal. Small mean differences of 1 to 3 degrees were noted between the left and right sides for eversion, dorsiflexion, and plantarflexion motions in a study by Alanen et al[13] of 245 children aged 7 to 14 years. The investigators considered these differences to be clinically and practically small. However, 5% of the children had differences of greater than 10 degrees, which led the investigators to be cautious about using the "healthy ankle" as a reference for ROM in children.

Testing Position

A variety of positions are used to measure dorsiflexion ROM, including sitting with the knee flexed, supine with the knee either flexed or extended, prone with the knee either flexed or extended, and standing with the knee either flexed or extended. Positions in which the knee is flexed bring the distal and proximal attachments of the gastrocnemius muscle closer together and result in relaxing the muscle so that its effect on dorsiflexion ROM is reduced. Positions in which the knee is extended generally are used for testing the length of the gastrocnemius muscle and result in less dorsiflexion ROM than when the knee is flexed (see Tables 10.6 and 10.7). Dorsiflexion measurements taken in weight-bearing positions are usually greater than measurements taken in non-weight-bearing positions. Plantarflexion ROM values are reported to be less in weight-bearing (tiptoe) than in non-weight-bearing supine position.[20]

Several studies have directly compared dorsiflexion ROM measurements taken with the knee flexed with measurements taken with the knee extended in the same subjects (Table 10.7). As might be expected, in a study of 27 healthy

TABLE 10.7 Comparison Between Dorsiflexion Range of Motion Measurements Taken With the Knee Flexed and Extended (Gastrocnemius Muscle Length Test): Normal Values in Degrees

	Bennell et al*[44]	Ekstrand et al†[45]		McPoil and Cornwall‡[46]	Mecagni et al§[28]
	8–11 yr *n* **= 49 Females**	**20–25 yr** *n* **= 10 Males**	**22–30 yr** *n* **= 12 Males**	**Mean 26.1 yr** *n* **= 56 Feet**	**64–87 yr** *n* **= 34 Females**
	Mean (SD)	***Mean (SD)***	***Mean (SD)***	***Mean (SD)***	***Mean (SD)***
Knee flexed	29.9 (6.4)	26.6 (2.5)	24.9 (0.8)	16.2 (3.2)	10.9 (4.2)
Knee extended	26.1 (9.0)	22.9 (2.5)	22.5 (0.7)	10.1 (2.2)	8.4 (3.7)

SD = Standard deviation.

* Measurements were taken in weight-bearing positions with use of an inclinometer.

† Measurements were taken in weight-bearing positions with use of a Leighton Flexometer (a type of inclinometer).

‡ Measurements were taken with a universal goniometer in 18 females and 9 males. The testing position was not reported.

§ Active-assistive ROM measurements were taken in non-weight-bearing positions with a universal goniometer and reported on the right foot.

young adults McPoil and Cornwall[46] found the mean dorsiflexion ROM (16.2 degrees) with the knee flexed to be about 6 degrees greater than the mean (10.1 degrees) with the knee extended. Alanen and colleagues,[13] in a study of 7- to 14-year-olds, found that dorsiflexion measurements taken with the knee flexed to 90 degrees were 10 to 19 degrees greater than measurements taken with the knee extended. Similar findings of less dorsiflexion ROM with the knee extended than flexed have also been reported by Mecagni et al,[28] Bennell et al,[44] and Ekstrand et al,[45] with mean differences ranging from about 2.5 to 7 degrees.

Riemann and coworkers[47] measured the resistance to passive dorsiflexion from 23 degrees of plantarflexion to 13 degrees of dorsiflexion in 12 physically active men and 12 women (mean age 21 years). Passive movements at a constant angular velocity were applied using an isokinetic dynamometer in passive mode. Significantly higher stiffness values were found in the knee-extended position compared with the knee-flexed position. The stiffness values in the gastrocnemius increased significantly as the ankle moved from plantarflexion toward dorsiflexion. Stiffness was defined by the authors as representing the amount of deformation proportional to the load applied.

Dorsiflexion ROM values reported by studies in which the subjects were in non-weight-bearing positions such as supine or prone are generally less than studies in which the subjects were standing in weight-bearing. Baggett and Young[38] directly compared measurements of dorsiflexion ROM taken in the non-weight-bearing supine position with those taken in the standing weight-bearing position in 10 males and 20 female patients aged 18 to 66 years. Both supine and standing measurements were taken with the knees extended. The average dorsiflexion ROM in the supine position was 8.3 degrees, whereas the average dorsiflexion ROM in the standing position was 20.9 degrees. Little correlation was found between measurements taken in the non-weight-bearing position with those taken in the weight-bearing position. Consequently, the authors recommended to examiners that the non-weight-bearing and weight-bearing positions should not be used interchangeably and that the weight-bearing position might be more clinically relevant. Kumar and associates[20] found that mean dorsiflexion ROM was greater in a weight-bearing squat position as compared with non-weight-bearing supine position with the knees flexed to 45 degrees, with dorsiflexion values of 40.5 and 24.3 degrees, respectively, in 104 Asian Indian subjects aged 25 to 75 years. Similar differences in dorsiflexion were found in the younger age-groups. In contrast, mean plantarflexion ROM was slightly less in weight-bearing tiptoe (33.4 degrees) as compared with supine (37.0 degrees) position in the 25- to 75-year-old age-group.

The effect of testing position on inversion and eversion ROM has also been studied. Lattanza, Gray, and Kanter[48] measured subtalar joint eversion in weight-bearing and non-weight-bearing postures in 15 females and 2 males. Measurements of subtalar joint eversion in a weight-bearing posture were found to be significantly greater than those in a non-weight-bearing posture. The authors advocated measurement in both positions.

Nawoczenski, Baumhauer, and Umberger[49] measured active and passive extension ROM of the MTP joint of the first toe in different positions in 14 women and 19 men between the ages of 20 and 54 years. Active and passive toe extension measurements were taken with the subject standing on a platform with toes extending over the edge. Passive measurements were taken in the non-weight-bearing seated position and during heel rise in standing. Mean values in the weight-bearing position were 37.0 degrees for passive MTP extension and 44.0 degrees for active MTP extension, compared with a mean value of 57.0 degrees obtained in the non-weight-bearing seated position and 58 degrees during heel rise in the standing position. Similar to the effects of different testing positions on ankle ROM, the results showed that the positions could not be used interchangeably when measuring MTP extension, with the exception of the heel rise in standing and seated non-weight-bearing positions.

Testing Landmarks for Goniometer Alignment

The choice of landmarks used to determine the angle of dorsiflexion also has been shown to affect ROM measurement values. Bohannon, Tiberio, and Zito,[7] in a study of 36 females aged 20 to 36 years, measured ankle dorsiflexion ROM supine with the knee straight from photographs using a protractor and three sets of landmarks. In all three situations, the proximal landmark was parallel with the fibula, whereas the distal landmarks varied between the heel, fifth metatarsal, or plantar surface of the foot. Dorsiflexion ROM values differed significantly according to which landmarks were used but were correlated. The use of the heel resulted in the greatest dorsiflexion angle, whereas using the fifth metatarsal resulted in the least angle. The amount of passive force applied by the examiner and active assistance provided by the subjects also affected the results.

Injury/Disease

Ankle ROM has been studied as a risk factor for various injuries. Kaufman and associates[50] tracked 449 trainees at a Naval Special Warfare Training Center to determine whether an association existed between foot structure and the development of musculoskeletal overuse injuries of the lower extremities. Restricted dorsiflexion ROM was one of the five risk factors associated with overuse injury.

Morrison and Kaminski[51] reviewed the literature for the years 1965 to 2005 for information that identified the risk factors for acute and chronic ankle inversion injuries and for the role that the foot played in these types of injuries. The authors found that the most commonly identified risk factors were a high longitudinal arch; large foot width; cavovarus foot deformity; large calcaneal eversion ROM measured in an open-chain position in women; subtalar joint instability; and a large ROM in MTP extension. However, the authors suggested that a great deal of research was necessary to adequately evaluate these risk factors.

Wilson and Gansneder[52] measured physical impairments (loss of passive ankle dorsiflexion, plantarflexion ROM, and swelling), functional limitations, and disability duration in 21 athletes with acute ankle sprains. The authors found that the combination of ROM loss and swelling predicted an acceptable estimate of disability duration, accounting for one-third of the variance. Functional limitation measures alone provided a better estimate of disability duration, accounting for 67% of the variance in the number of days the athletes were unable to work after the acute ankle sprain.

Reduced dorsiflexion ROM has been noted following ankle fractures. Chesworth and Vandervoort[53] measured dorsiflexion ROM after ankle fractures resulting from snowboarding accidents. They found that large differences occurred in the maximum passive dorsiflexion ROM between fractured ankles and the contralateral uninvolved ankles. Maximum passive dorsiflexion was defined as that point just prior to the initiation of muscle activity in the plantarflexor muscles. The authors hypothesized that the reflex length–tension relationship was altered in the fractured ankles and that this reflex activity acted as a protective mechanism to prevent overstretching of the fragile plantarflexors after a period of immobilization. Other investigators, using animal models, noted a significant (70%) loss of dorsiflexion ROM following 6 weeks of immobilization of a healthy limb in rats. The authors suggested that the loss of extensibility of the musculotendinous unit was probably caused by tissue remodeling that occurred during extended immobilization.[54]

Diabetes mellitus also appears to affect ankle motion. Salsich, Mueller, and Sahrmann[55] found that patients with diabetes mellitus and peripheral neuropathy demonstrated less dorsiflexion ROM (extensibility of the musculotendinous unit) than a group of age-matched control subjects. Rao and colleagues[56] compared ankle ROM and stiffness in 25 individuals with diabetes mellitus and 64 people without diabetes who were similar in age and gender. Peak dorsiflexion ROM with the knee extended was 13 degrees in the group with diabetes and 21 degrees in the controls. Peak dorsiflexion with the knee flexed was 20 degrees in the group with diabetes and 28 degrees in the controls. The authors suggested that the resistance to passive elongation may be attributed to change in the properties of the contractile and elastic elements of the plantarflexors in people with diabetes. Hastings and coworkers[57] identified limited dorsiflexion ROM as a risk factor for increased plantar pressures during walking and decreased functional performance in patients with diabetes mellitus.

Functional Range of Motion

An adequate ROM at the ankle, foot, and toes is necessary for normal gait on level surfaces. Table 10.8 provides a summary of mean maximal ankle ROM during gait and common functional tasks as reported by various sources. At least 10 degrees[58,59] to 15 degrees[60] of dorsiflexion are necessary in the stance phase of gait so that the tibia can advance over the foot. Approximately 15 to 30 degrees of plantarflexion occur in the preswing phase of gait.[58–60] Five degrees of eversion are necessary at loading response to unlock the midtarsal joint for shock absorption.[58] When the midtarsal joint is unlocked, the foot is able to accommodate to various surfaces by tilting medially and laterally. A small amount of inversion occurs in terminal stance and preswing phases of gait to enable a more rigid foot for push-off. In normal walking, about 30 degrees of extension are required at the MTP joints in the terminal stance phase of gait. In preswing, extension at the MTP joints reaches a maximum of approximately 60 to 65 degrees when the toes maintain contact with the floor after heel rise.[18,58] The individual standing on her toes in Figure 10.58 has an adequate extension ROM at the MTP joints for normal gait. If the ROM at the MTP joints is limited, it will interfere with forward progression, and the step length of the contralateral leg will be decreased.[58]

Running requires 0 to 20 degrees of dorsiflexion and 0 to 30 degrees of plantarflexion.[61] These ROMs are similar to the amount of motion required for stair ascent and descent, as shown in Table 10.8. Ascending stairs generally requires a maximum of between 10 and 25 degrees of dorsiflexion, whereas descending stairs (Fig. 10.59) requires a maximum

TABLE 10.8 Ankle Motion During Functional Activities: Mean Maximal Values in Degrees

Activity	Study						
	First author	*N*	*Measurement*	*Dorsiflexion*	*Plantarflexion*	*Inversion*	*Eversion*
Gait on level surface	Begg[62]	24	3D video system	22 (young) 17 (older)	31 (young) 17 (older)		
	Hageman[63]	39	2D high-speed cinematography system		31(young)* 24 (older)*		
	Locke[64]	20	2 electrogoniometers	10 (young) 13 (older)	25 (young) 17 (older)	4 (young) 4 (older) (calcaneus varus)	7 (young) 6 (older) (calcaneus valgus)
	Murray[59]			10	15–30		
	Ostrosky[60]	60	2D video system	12 (young) 14 (older)	28 (young) 24 (older)		
	Rancho Los Amigos[58]			10	15		
Stair ascent	Livingston[65]	15	Cinematography system, 20.3 cm rise height, 30.5 tread depth	22–27†	24†		
	Livingston	15	Cinematography system, 20.3 cm rise height, 21 tread depth	20–24	24–30		
	Livingston	15	Cinematography system, 12.7 cm rise height, 41.9 tread depth	14–19	24–28		
	Protopapadaki[66]	33	3D optical system, 18 cm rise height	11	31		
Stair descent	Lark[67]	12	2D single camera optoelectric system	~20 (young) ~25 (older)			
	Livingston	15	Cinematography system, 20.3 cm rise height, 30.5 tread depth	21–32†	28–30†		
	Livingston	15	Cinematography system, 20.3 cm rise height, 21 tread depth	26–36	26–31		
	Livingston	15	Cinematography system, 12.7 cm rise height, 41.9 tread depth	29–32	24–28		
	Protopapadaki	33	3D optical system, 18 cm rise height, 28.5 cm tread depth	21	40		
Rise from a chair	Ikeda[68]	18	3D optoelectric system, chair seat height 80% of knee height	27 (young) 29 (older)			

TABLE 10.8 Ankle Motion During Functional Activities: Mean Maximal Values in Degrees (continued)

Activity	Study						
	First author	*N*	*Measurement*	*Dorsiflexion*	*Plantarflexion*	*Inversion*	*Eversion*
	Rodosky[69]	10	3D optoelectric system, chair seat height 80% knee height	23 (right) 29 (left)			
	Rodosky	10	3D optoelectric system, chair seat height 115% knee height	13 (right) 20 (left)			
	Rodosky	10	3D optoelectric system, chair seat height 65% knee height	27 (right) 31 (left)			
Kneeling	Hemmerich[70]	26	3D electromagnetic system, ankle dorsiflexed**	40	–3	13	9
	Hemmerich	6	3D electromagnetic system, ankle plantarflexed**	33	24	12	12
Squatting	Hemmerich	26	3D electromagnetic system, heels down**	39	–3	0	18
	Hemmerich	26	3D electromagnetic system, heels up**	38	–4	10	7
	Kumar[20]	104	Universal goniometer, heels down	40			
Sitting cross-legged	Hemmerich	26	3D electromagnetic system**	32	26	25	17
	Kapoor[71]	44	Universal goniometer		29		
Standing on tiptoe	Kumar	104	Universal goniometer		33		

Generally, young age-groups were between 20 and 40 years and older age-groups were 60 years and older. cm = centimeter.

*Values reported as ankle ROM with no distinction as to dorsiflexion or plantarflexion.

†Range of mean maximal angles for the three groups of females with varying heights: shorter, medium, taller.

**Values reported included getting into and out of the position.

of between 20 and 35 degrees of dorsiflexion and between 25 and 40 degrees of plantarflexion.[65–67] The height and depth of the stair risers and the height of the individual will affect the amount of ROM required.[65]

Age appears to have some influence on gait parameters while walking on level surfaces and stairs. Several studies found that older subjects during free-speed gait had a slower velocity, significantly shorter stride and step lengths, increased double-support stance period, a more flat-footed landing, and less ankle motion—all of which contributed toward a more stable and safer gait pattern.[63,72,73] Lark and associates[67] noted that the elderly had 30% greater maximum dorsiflexion angle during stair descent than the young subjects. Young subjects rose more quickly up onto the ball of the foot as they stepped down, whereas older subjects spent more time with the foot flat in single leg support, which increased their stability.

Activities of daily living vary according to culture. In Western cultures, activities of daily living often include getting into and out of a chair or bed. Rising from a typical chair (Fig. 10.60) in which the seat is about 80% of an individual's knee height requires about 25 to 30 degrees of ankle dorsiflexion.[68,69] Increases in chair seat height have been shown to require less dorsiflexion during rising, while decreases in chair seat height require more dorsiflexion.[69,74] Rodosky and associates[69] also found asymmetries during rising from a

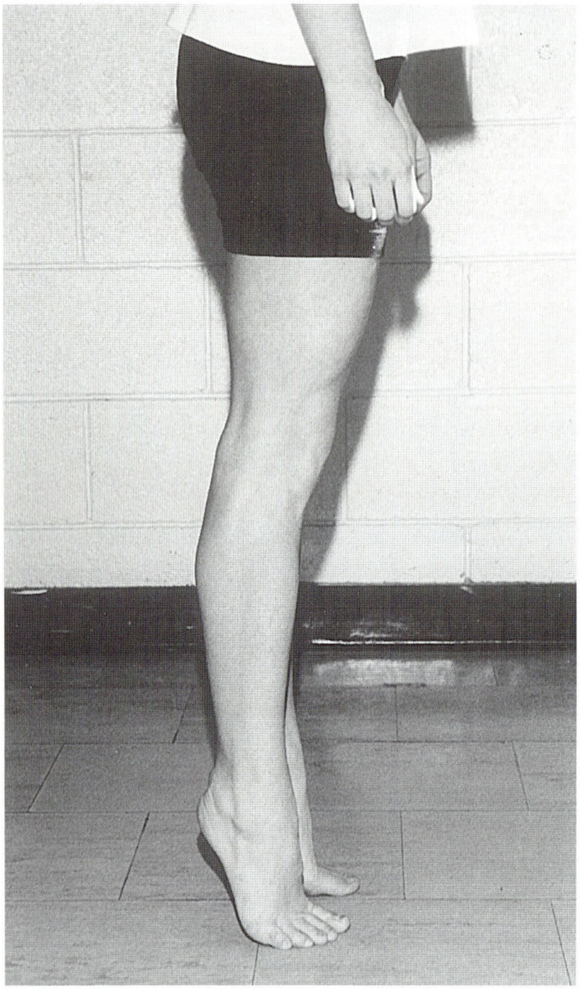

FIGURE 10.58 Standing on tiptoe requires a full range of motion in ankle plantarflexion and 58 to 60 degrees of extension[49] at the first metatarsophalangeal joint.

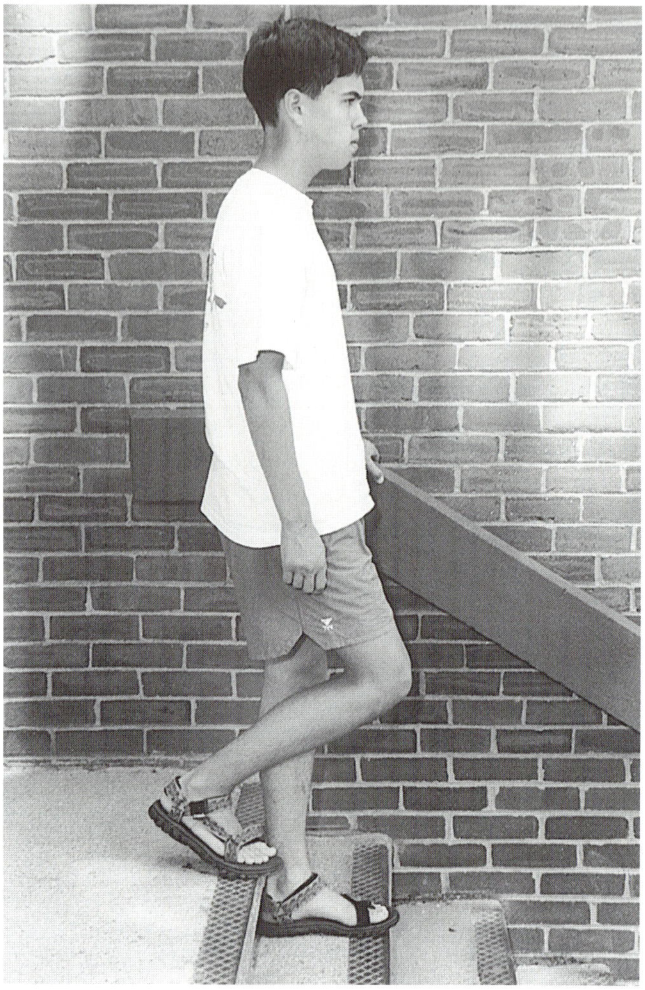

FIGURE 10.59 Descending stairs requires an average of 21 to 36 degrees of ankle dorsiflexion depending on the rise height of the stairs.[65]

chair, with great dorsiflexion ROM occurring in the left ankle than the right ankle. (See Table 10.8.)

In countries outside of North America and Europe, activities of daily living often involve positions of kneeling, squatting, or sitting cross-legged. These positions may require larger amounts of dorsiflexion ROM than positions needed for typical activities of daily living in Western cultures (see Table 10.8). Hemmerich and associates,[70] in a study of 30 Asian Indians, found that about 40 degrees of dorsiflexion were required for kneeling with the ankles dorsiflexed, and squatting with the heels up or down. Cross-legged sitting on the floor was found to require a maximum angle of about 25 to 30 degrees of plantarflexion[71] and 25 degrees of inversion.[70] Health-care workers need to recognize that people from various cultures may require different ROM goals for rehabilitation.

Adequate ROM of the ankle and foot ROM also appears to be necessary for balance during gait. Mecagni and colleagues,[28] in a study of 34 healthy community-dwelling older women aged 64 to 87 years, found that decreases in ankle ROM were correlated to measures of decreased balance and may be a risk factor for falls. Correlations between the Performance Oriented Mobility Assessment (POMA) gait subtest indicated that all ankle motions contributed to the maintenance of balance during gait: inversion (Pearson correlation coefficients [r] = 0.50), dorsiflexion with knee flexed ($r = 0.44$), plantarflexion ($r = 0.42$), and eversion ($r = 0.32$). Active assistive ROM had higher correlations compared with passive ROM. The highest correlation was between total active assistive ROM and the POMA gait subtest ($r = 0.63$). Bilateral ankle ROM correlated higher than unilateral ankle ROM with balance tests, suggesting that the impact of two restricted ankles on balance is greater than the impact of one restricted ankle.

Reliability and Validity

Reliability studies for measuring ROM and muscle length at the ankle have been conducted on healthy populations and on patient populations. These studies have used universal

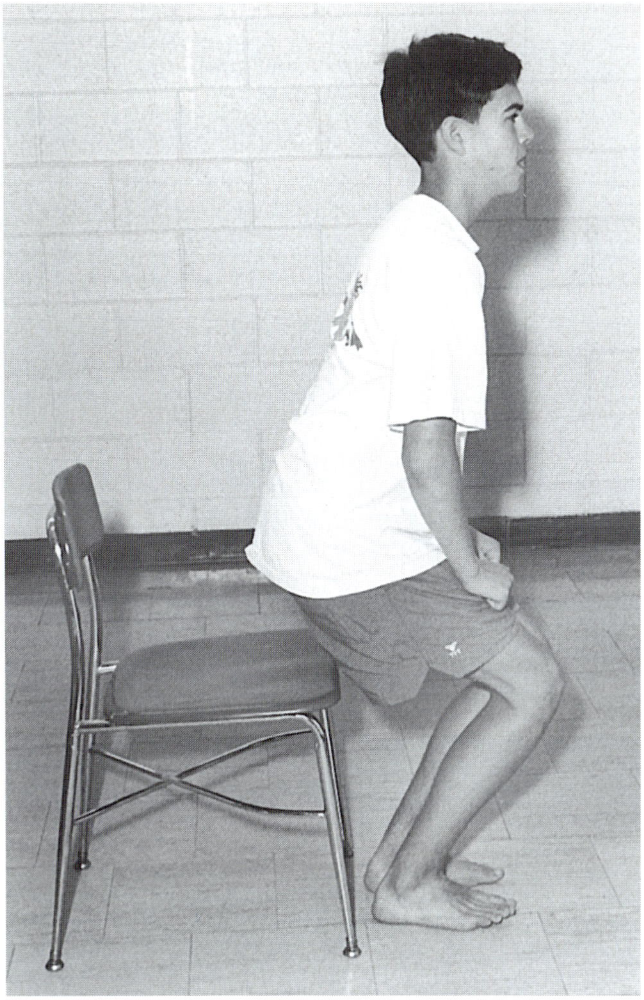

FIGURE 10.60 Getting out of a chair may require a full dorsiflexion range of motion (ROM), depending on the height of the chair seat. The lower the seat, the greater the dorsiflexion ROM required.

goniometers, inclinometers, and specialized measurement equipment and techniques. In addition, the reliability of measuring ROM of the foot combining motion at midtarsal and subtalar joints, ROM at the subtalar joint, the subtalar joint neutral position, and the forefoot position have been investigated. The results of some of these studies are presented in Tables 10.9 and 10.10 and are briefly summarized below. Few studies have explored the reliability of measuring the ROM of the toes or the validity of measuring ankle, foot, and toe ROM.

Reliability of Measuring Ankle and Foot Motions With Universal Goniometers

In 2004, Martin and McPoil[75] reviewed the existing literature on goniometric measurement of ankle dorsiflexion and plantarflexion ROM. Ample evidence was found supporting good to excellent intratester reliability for dorsiflexion and plantarflexion ROM, some evidence for intertester reliability of dorsiflexion, but little current evidence of intertester reliability for plantarflexion ROM. The authors also determined that subject diagnosis, with the exception of cerebral palsy, did not appear to affect intratester reliability. Training sessions prior to measurement appeared to have a positive effect on intrarater reliability. However, the authors concluded that on the basis of the literature review, the responsiveness of ankle measurements to detect change was uncertain and needs additional studies using patient populations.

Healthy Populations

A number of studies have focused on the reliability of ankle and foot ROM measurements taken with universal goniometers in healthy populations. Selected studies are included in Tables 10.9 and 10.10 and discussed below. As in other regions of the body, intratester reliability has been shown to be better than intertester reliability for measuring dorsiflexion, plantarflexion, inversion, and eversion ROM, thus providing evidence that it is better for the same examiner to take repeated ankle and foot ROM measurements on a patient during follow-up care than for another examiner to do so. The use of well-defined landmarks and consistent methods has been shown to be helpful in improving reliability. No individual ankle or foot motions were consistently found in multiple studies to have better reliability than other motions. Given the small range of some ankle and foot motions such as dorsiflexion and inversion, intraclass correlation coefficients (ICCs) and Pearson correlation coefficients (r) may be affected by this limited variability and be lower than expected.[76,77] Absolute measures of reliability such as the standard error of measurement (SEM) and minimal detectable change (MDC) may be more accurate and helpful to the clinician in determining the expected error in ROM measurements at these joints. The reader is urged to refer to Chapter 3 for more information on statistical methods used to evaluate reliability.

Bovens and associates,[79] in a study of the reliability of measuring nine joint motions throughout the body, used a universal goniometer to examine dorsiflexion, plantarflexion, and inversion and eversion of the foot. Three physician testers and eight healthy subjects participated. Inversion and plantarflexion in particular were considered by the investigators to have excellent intratester reliability as indicated by ICC values. Standard deviations for the repeated measurements made by the same tester ranged from 2.1 degrees for dorsiflexion to 5.6 degrees for eversion. Standard deviations for repeated measurements made by different testers were slightly larger and ranged from 3.3 degrees for dorsiflexion to 6.0 degrees for inversion (see Tables 10.9 and 10.10).

Boone and coworkers[78] examined the reliability of measuring six active motions of extremity joints that included inversion of the foot. Four physical therapists used universal goniometers to measure these motions in 12 healthy males once a week for 4 weeks. The investigators found that some joints and motions can be measured more reliably than others. Intratester reliability (ICC = 0.80) for foot inversion was better than that obtained for hip and wrist motions, but it was not as good as that obtained for selected motions at the shoulder, elbow, and knee. As with most motions and

Text continued on page 402

TABLE 10.9 Intratester Reliability of Ankle and Foot ROM Measurements Using Goniometers for Healthy and Patient Populations

Study	N	Sample	Methods	Motion	r	ICC	Absolute Reliability (degrees)
Healthy Populations							
Boone et al[78]	12	Healthy males	AROM, 4 testers (PT), universal goniometer aligned with anterior tibia and second metatarsal	Inversion of foot		.80	SD for tester = 0.6 SD total = 3.8
Bovens et al[79]	8	Healthy adults	AROM, 3 testers (physicians), supine, knee position not defined, universal goniometer	 Dorsiflexion Plantarflexion Inversion of foot Eversion of foot	(tester 1, 2, 3) .64, .74, .75 .82, .86, .87 .83, .91, .93 .57, .66, .75		Repeated measures SD: 2.1, 2.4, 3.0 3.5, 3.7, 3.9 4.4, 4.4, 5.0 3.2, 3.2, 5.6
Clapper and Wolfe[80]	20	Healthy adults	AROM, 1 tester (PT), supine, knee extended, 2 devices: universal goniometer and Ortho Ranger inclinometer	Goniometer: Dorsiflexion Plantarflexion Ortho Ranger: Dorsiflexion Plantarflexion		 .92 .96 .80 .93	
Jonson and Gross[34]	18	Healthy adults	AAROM, 2 testers (PT), prone, knee extended, universal goniometer	Dorsiflexion		.74	Mean absolute difference = 1.7
Kilgour et al[81]	25	Healthy children (9–17 yr)	PROM, 1 tester (PT), supine with knee flexed and extended, universal goniometer with 10-cm arms, intrasession measurements	Dorsiflexion: Knee flexed Knee extended		 .97–.98 .95–.98	Mean absolute difference: 2.7 2.2
Macedo and Magee[17]	12	Healthy adults	PROM, 1 tester, dorsiflexion and plantarflexion sitting with knee flexed, inversion and eversion supine knee extended, universal goniometer	Dorsiflexion Plantarflexion Inversion Eversion		.77 .90 .68 .69	SEM = 2.5, MDC_{95} = 6.8 SEM = 4.6, MDC_{95} = 12.8 SEM = 3.9, MDC_{95} = 10.7 SEM = 6.2, MDC_{95} = 17.2
McPoil and Cornwall[46]	27	Healthy adults	1 tester (PT), universal goniometer knee flexed to 90° and knee extended, universal goniometer	Dorsiflexion: knee flexed knee extended Subtalar inversion Subtalar eversion		 .97 .98 .95 .96	
Mecagni et al[28]	8	Healthy older women (64 to 87 yr)	1 tester (PT), universal goniometer, Norkin and White method	Dorsiflexion Plantarflexion Inversion Eversion		.97 .99 .93 .94	
Menadue et al[9]	30	No ankle injury within 4 weeks (60 ankles)	AROM, 3 testers (exercise scientist, PT, PT student), inversion and eversion in sitting, subtalar inversion and eversion in prone, universal goniometer, within session reported	 Inversion Eversion Subtalar inversion Subtalar eversion sitting		(tester 1, 2, 3) .92, .91, .96 .90, .82, .93 .94, .94, .94 .94, .83, .88	 SEM = 2.1, 2.6, 1.9 SEM = 2.1, 2.9, 2.2 SEM = 1.4, 1.6, 1.2 SEM = 1 .0, 1.4, 1.2
van Gheluwe et al[82]	30	Healthy adults	5 testers (podiatrists), prone with knee extended, protractor, Root method, left leg reported	Dorsiflexion Subtalar inversion Subtalar eversion		.86–.98 .90–.95 .89–.97	SEM = 0.7–1.6 SEM = 1.3–1.9 SEM = 1.1–2.2

Patient Populations							
Allington et al[83]	24	Children with spastic cerebral palsy (3–14 yr)	PROM, 2 testers (PT), universal goniometer, supine with strict protocol	Dorsiflexion: knee flexed knee straight Plantarflexion Inversion Eversion	(tester 1, 2) .93, .95 .94, .95 .85, .86 .76, .78 .84, .90		Mean measurement error: 4, 4 4, 4 5, 5 6, 6 7, 9
Diamond et al[84]	25	Adults with diabetes mellitus	PROM, 2 testers (PT), prone with knee extended in STJN for dorsiflexion, anatomical neutral for inversion and eversion, universal goniometer	 Dorsiflexion Subtalar inversion Subtalar eversion		(L, R) .96, .89 .96, .92 .96, .96	SEM: 1, 3 2, 2 1, 1
Elveru et al[85]	43	Patients with orthopedic or neurological disorders (12–81 yr)	PROM, 14 testers (PT), positions for dorsiflexion and plantarflexion not standardized, inversion and eversion prone with knee extended measured from anatomical neutral and STJN, universal goniometer with 5-inch arms.	Dorsiflexion Plantarflexion Subtalar Inversion Subtalar Eversion		.90 .86 .74, .62* .75, .59*	
Kilgour et al[81]	25	Children with spastic diplegia (9–17 yr)	PROM and AROM, 1 tester (PT), supine with knee flexed and extended, universal goniometer with 10-cm arms, intrasession measurements	Dorsiflexion (PROM): Knee flexed Knee extended Dorsiflexion (AROM): Knee extended		 .98–.99 .96–.99 .96–.98	Mean absolute difference: 3.3 2.0 3.3
Mutlu et al[86]	38	Children with spastic cerebral palsy (1–9 yr)	PROM, 2 testers (PT), supine, universal goniometer	Dorsiflexion		.81, .83, .90	
Pandya et al[87]	150	Children with Duchenne muscular dystrophy	PROM, 5 testers (PT), universal goniometer, supine, AAOS method, measured 3 times over 1 month	Dorsiflexion		.90	
Salsich et al[55]	34	17 adults with diabetes mellitus and 17 healthy adults	AROM, 1 tester, prone knee extended, universal goniometer	Dorsiflexion		.95	
Youdas et al[88]	38	Patients with orthopedic disorders (13–71 yr)	AROM, 10 testers (PT), no standard positions but knee extended 87.7% of tests, universal goniometer	Dorsiflexion: single measure mean of 2 measures Plantarflexion: single measure mean of 2 measures		 .64–.92 .78–.96 .47–.96 .64–.98	

ICC = Intraclass correlation coefficient; AAOS = American Academy of Orthopaedic Surgeons; AROM = Active range of motion; AAROM = Active assistive range of motion; PROM = Passive range of motion; *r* = Pearson product moment correlation coefficient; SEM = Standard error of measurement; L = left; R = right; PT = Physical therapist(s); STJN = Subtalar joint neutral; cm = Centimeter.

TABLE 10.10 Intertester Reliability of Ankle and Foot ROM Measurements Using Goniometers for Healthy and Patient Populations

Study	N	Sample	Methods	Motion	r	ICC	Absolute Reliability (degrees)
			Healthy Populations				
Boone et al[78]	12	Healthy males	AROM, 4 testers (PT), universal goniometer aligned with anterior tibia and second metatarsal	Inversion		.69	Tester SD = 2.4 Total SD = 4.4
Bovens et al[79]	8	Healthy adults	AROM, 3 testers (physicians), supine, knee position not defined, universal goniometer	 Dorsiflexion Plantarflexion Inversion Eversion	 .63 .76 .80 .56		Repeated measures SD: 3.3 4.4 6.0 4.4
Jonson and Gross[34]	18	Healthy adults	AAROM, 2 testers (PT), prone, knee extended, universal goniometer	Dorsiflexion		.65	Mean absolute difference = 2.4
Leard et al[89]	18	Healthy adults	2 testers (PT students), universal goniometer	Dorsiflexion: knee flexed knee extended		 .71 .45	 SEM = 12.1 SEM = 12.4
Menadue et al[9]	30	No ankle injury within 4 weeks (60 ankles)	AROM, 3 testers (exercise scientist, PT, PT student), inversion and eversion in sitting, subtalar inversion and eversion in prone, universal goniometer, within session reported	Inversion Eversion Subtalar inversion Subtalar eversion sitting		.73 .62 .54 .41	SEM = 4.6 SEM = 4.5 SEM = 4.1 SEM = 2.8
van Gheluwe et al[82]	30	Healthy adults	5 testers (podiatrists), prone with knee extended, protractor, left leg reported	Dorsiflexion Subtalar inversion Subtalar eversion		.26 .28 .46	SEM = 3.7 SEM = 4.9 SEM = 2.8
			Patient Populations				
Allington et al[83]	24	Children with spastic cerebral palsy (3–14 yr)	PROM, 2 testers (PT), universal goniometer, supine with strict protocol	Dorsiflexion: knee flexed knee straight Plantarflexion Subtalar inversion Subtalar eversion	 .95 .94 .84 .80 .93		Mean measurement error: 4 5 5 6 5
Diamond et al[84]	25	Adults with diabetes mellitus	PROM, 2 testers (PT), prone with knee extended in STJN for dorsiflexion, anatomical neutral for inversion and eversion, universal goniometer	 Dorsiflexion Subtalar inversion Subtalar eversion		(L, R) .87, .74 .89, .86 .78, .79	SEM: 2, 3 3, 3 4, 2

Elveru et al[85]	43	Patients with orthopedic or neurological disorders (12–81 yr)	PROM, 14 testers (PT), positions for dorsiflexion and plantarflexion not standardized, inversion and eversion prone measured from anatomical neutral and STJN, universal goniometer with 5-inch arms	Dorsiflexion Plantarflexion Subtalar inversion Subtalar eversion	.50 .72 .32, .15* .17, .12*	
McWhirk and Glanzman[90]	25	Children with spastic cerebral palsy (2–18 yr)	PROM, 2 testers (PT), universal goniometer, methods described by Norkin and White	Dorsiflexion	.87	Mean absolute difference = 3.6 (95% CI = 1.2)
Mutlu et al[86]	38	Children with spastic cerebral palsy (1–9 yr)	PROM, 2 testers (PT), supine, universal goniometer	Dorsiflexion	.88	
Pandya et al[87]	150	Children with Duchenne muscular dystrophy	PROM, 5 testers, universal goniometer, supine, AAOS method, measured 3 times over 1 month	Dorsiflexion	.73	
Smith-Oricchio and Harris[91]	20	Adults with recent ankle pathology (bone or soft tissue)	PROM, 3 testers (PT), prone, universal goniometer	Subtalar inversion Subtalar eversion	.42 .25	
Youdas et al[88]	38	Patients with orthopedic disorders (13–71 yr)	AROM, 10 testers (PT), no standard positions, universal goniometer, mean of 2 measures used	Dorsiflexion Plantarflexion	.28 .25	

ICC = Intraclass correlation coefficient; AROM = Active range of motion; AAROM = Active assistive range of motion; PROM = Passive range of motion; *r* = Pearson product moment correlation coefficient; SEM = Standard error of measurement; L = left; R = right; PT = Physical therapist(s); STJN = Subtalar joint neutral.

joints, the intertester reliability of measuring inversion of the foot was lower than intratester reliability (see Tables 10.9 and 10.10).

Macedo and Magee,[17] in a preliminary study of 12 healthy females, examined the intratester reliability of measuring 30 different movements throughout the body, including passive ROM of ankle dorsiflexion and plantarflexion in sitting with the knee flexed and inversion and eversion in supine with the knee extended. One physical therapist took repeated measurements with a masked universal goniometer, while another read and recorded the ROM values. Reliability as indicated by ICC values was fair to excellent, with values ranging from 0.68 to 0.90 (see Table 10.9). Standard error of measurement values were the best (lowest) for dorsiflexion (2.5 degrees), followed by inversion (3.9 degrees), plantarflexion (4.6 degrees), and eversion (6.2 degrees).

In a study of 27 healthy young adults, McPoil and Cornwall[46] examined the intratester reliability of goniometric measurements of ankle dorsiflexion ROM with the knee flexed and extended and subtalar inversion and eversion ROM. Measurements were taken twice in one session by an experienced physical therapist using a masked goniometer; another examiner read and recorded the results. Intratester reliability was excellent, with ICC values greater than 0.95 for all four of these motions. A total of 17 static measures were included in an effort to predict dynamic rearfoot motion during walking (see Table 10.9).

Mecagni and associates[28] conducted a preliminary pilot study of the reliability of measuring dorsiflexion, plantarflexion, inversion, and eversion ROM with a universal goniometer in eight healthy community-dwelling older women (mean age 74.7 years). Intratester reliability was excellent, with all ICC values greater than 0.93, with the calibrated side of the goniometer shielded from the tester's view. Methods used in the study were those described in the 2003 edition of this textbook (see Table 10.9).

Menadue and colleagues[9] assessed active inversion and eversion ROM in sitting for motions that included the subtalar and midtarsal joints and prone for motions of the subtalar joint. The methods referenced were from the 1985 edition of this text. The 30 healthy adults in the study had both ankles measured by three testers using a blinded universal goniometer. Three repeated measurements for each motion were made in two sessions between 1 and 2 weeks apart. Within-session intratester reliability was good to excellent, with ICC values ranging from 0.83 to 0.94 and SEM values ranging from 1.0 to 2.9 degrees (see Table 10.9). Intertester reliability ranged from poor (ICC = 0.41) to fair (ICC = 0.73), with SEM values from 2.8 to 4.6 degrees (see Table 10.10). The reliability of between-sessions measurements was lower, with intratester ICC values ranging from 0.42 to 0.80 and SEM increased to between 2.1 to 5.4 degrees. The investigators suggested that difficulty identifying bony landmarks, especially for subtalar motions, as well as difference in subjects' effort during the active ROM could have contributed to measurement error.

Clapper and Wolf[80] found that both the universal goniometer and a type of electronic inclinometer, the Ortho Ranger (Orthotronics, Daytona Beach, FL), were reliable instruments for measuring dorsiflexion and plantarflexion in 20 healthy adults by one tester. However, intraclass correlation coefficients (ICCs) were higher for the universal goniometer. The ICC for measurements of active dorsiflexion for the universal goniometer was 0.92 in comparison with 0.80 for the Ortho Ranger. The ICC for measuring plantarflexion with the universal goniometer was 0.96 and 0.93 for the Ortho Ranger. (See Table 10.9.)

Van Gheluwe and associates[82] assessed intratester and intertester reliability of biomechanical measurements commonly used in podiatric practice. Ankle dorsiflexion, subtalar inversion (supination), and eversion (pronation) were measured with a protractor. Five podiatrists took two repeated measurements of each motion within one session. Intratester reliability was considered excellent, with all ICC values greater than 0.86 and SEM less than 2.2 degrees. Intertester reliability was considered poor because ICC values ranged from 0.21 to 0.46, although SEM values were 3.7 degrees for dorsiflexion, 2.8 degrees for eversion, and 4.9 degrees for inversion. (See Tables 10.9 and 10.10.)

Alanen and colleagues[13] used a universal goniometer to assess the ROM of the ankle in 245 healthy children aged 7 to 14 years. Twenty-seven children were also measured again 3 to 6 days later by the same physician tester to assess reliability. Passive dorsiflexion was measured directly from anatomical landmarks in the prone position with the knee flexed and extended. Plantarflexion was measured in the supine position. Inversion and eversion were also measured in prone, but used a method of tracing the landmarks and then measuring the angle with a goniometer. Dorsiflexion in the weight-bearing position was measured from photographs. The range of ICCs varied from a low of 0.51 for right eversion to 0.88 for weight-bearing dorsiflexion measurements in both ankles.

Patient Populations

A number of studies have examined the reliability of passive ROM measurements on children with cerebral palsy. Four studies that focused on this population are included in Tables 10.9 and 10.10 and are briefly summarized below. Based on the findings of most of these studies, it appears possible to obtain reliable goniometric measurements of ankle dorsiflexion ROM by the same and different physical therapists in children with spastic cerebral palsy, especially if positions and landmarks for goniometer alignment are well defined. The assistance of another person to maintain the patient's position during measurement seems helpful in producing more reliable ROM measurements. More experienced examiners appear to produce more reliable results than less experienced examiners.

Allington, Leroy, and Doneux[83] had two testers follow a strict protocol to assess intratester and intertester reliability and reproducibility of ankle ROM in 24 children aged 3 to 14 years with spastic cerebral palsy. Pearson's correlation coefficients for intratester and intertester reliability for both the universal goniometer and visual estimates were excellent ($r > 0.90$) for dorsiflexion with the knee flexed and extended. The coefficients for intratester and intertester reliability for plantarflexion for both goniometric and visual estimates were good ($r > 0.80$) and fair to good for inversion and eversion. The SEM for dorsiflexion and plantarflexion was 4 to 5 degrees; the SEM for eversion was 6 to 9 degrees; and the SEM for inversion was 5 to 9 degrees. According to the investigators, even though both goniometric and visual estimates were reliable, the mean measurement error of 5 degrees and standard deviation (SD) of the error of 5 degrees produced a 0- to 10-degree error that would have to be taken into account in clinical decision-making. (See Tables 10.9 and 10.10.)

Kilgour and associates[81] determined intratester reliability of passive ankle dorsiflexion with the knee flexed and extended in 25 children aged 6 to 17 years with spastic diplegic cerebral palsy and in 25 healthy age- and sex-matched controls. Children with cerebral palsy also had measurements taken of active dorsiflexion with the knee extended. Repeated measurements using a universal goniometer with 10-centimeter arms were taken by one physiotherapist with the assistance of two others during the same session and then again 7 days later. All measurements repeated during the same session (intrasession measurements) were highly reliable, with ICC values above 0.95 and mean absolute difference ranging from 2.2 to 3.3 degrees. Comparisons of dorsiflexion measurements taken 7 days apart (intersession measurements) were less reliable, with ICC values ranging from 0.70 to 0.90 with the knee flexed to lower values of 0.51 to 0.74 with the knee extended. Mean absolute difference also showed less reliability and increased to between 4.3 to 6.0 degrees. Averaging two measurements did not improve intersession reliability compared with the use of one measurement. (See Table 10.9.)

McWhirk and Glanzman[90] assessed intertester reliability of measurements of ankle dorsiflexion in 25 children (aged 2 to 18 years) with spastic cerebral palsy. The two therapists who took the measurements successively on the same day helped each other hold the limbs at end range. Intertester reliability was very good, with an ICC of 0.87 and a mean absolute difference of 3.6 degrees. The 95% confidence interval around the mean absolute difference was ±1.2 degrees. (See Table 10.10.)

Mutlu, Livanelioglu, and Gunel[86] assessed the intratester and intertester reliability of goniometric measurements of ankle dorsiflexion that were taken by three physiotherapists in 38 children (ages 18 to 108 months) with spastic cerebral palsy. The therapists used a 360-degree universal goniometer to measure dorsiflexion once in two sessions a week apart. Intratester reliability was good to excellent, with ICC values of 0.83, 0.81, and 0.90, with the most experienced tester obtaining the highest reliability. Intertester reliability was very good, with ICC values of 0.88. Each examiner was assisted by another therapist to maintain the positions of the subjects and to record the results. Based on the findings of this study and the previous study, it appears to be possible to obtain reliable goniometric measurements in this population of children with spastic cerebral palsy. (See Tables 10.9 and 10.10.)

Patients with orthopedic conditions have been included in several reliability studies of ankle and foot ROM measurements (see Tables 10.9 and 10.10). Elveru and associates[85] recruited 14 physical therapists using universal goniometers to measure the passive ankle and subtalar ROM in 43 patients with either neurological or orthopedic disorders. The ICC values for intratester reliability for plantarflexion and dorsiflexion were considered good to excellent; intertester reliability was poor for dorsiflexion (ICC = 0.50) and fair for plantarflexion (ICC = 0.72). Intratester reliability for inversion and eversion was fair, with ICC values of 0.74 and 0.75, respectively, whereas intertester reliability was poor, with ICC values of 0.32 and 0.17, respectively. Patient diagnosis affected the measurement of some motions such that patients with neurological conditions sometimes had slightly lower measurement reliability than those with orthopedic conditions. Sources of error were identified as variable amounts of force being exerted by the therapist, resistance to movement in neurological patients, and difficulties encountered by a single examiner in maintaining the foot and ankle in the desired position while holding the goniometer.

Youdas, Bogard, and Suman[88] used 10 examiners to determine the intratester and intertester reliability for active ROM in dorsiflexion and plantarflexion in 38 patients with orthopedic problems. The authors compared measurements made by a universal goniometer with visual estimates. Fair to excellent reliability was noted when repeated measurements were made by the same therapist using a goniometer. Reliability was higher using the mean of two repeated measurements than it was using one measurement. A considerable measurement error was found when different therapists made repeated goniometric or visual estimates of the ankle ROM on the same patient (see Tables 10.9 and 10.10). Therapists used various patient positions and goniometer alignment methods because methods were not standardized. The authors suggested that the same therapist should make two goniometric measurements and record the average value when making repeated measurements of ankle ROM.

Twenty adults with recent orthopedic ankle pathology (fracture, soft tissue condition, or bone aberration,) were studied by Smith-Oricchio and Harris[91] to determine the intertester reliability of calcaneal motion and static position. Passive subtalar inversion and eversion ROM measurements taken in prone by three physical therapists had poor intertester reliability, with ICC values of 0.42 and 0.25, respectively. The intertester reliability of measuring static calcaneus position in bilateral and single-leg standing, 0.91 and 0.75, respectively, was better than ROM measurements.

People with diabetes mellitus are another patient population that has been included in several ROM reliability studies of the ankle and foot. As with healthy individuals and other patient populations, intratester reliability was excellent, whereas intertester reliability was fair to good. Diamond and associates[84] measured the reliability of measuring ankle dorsiflexion and subtalar inversion and eversion ROM in adults with diabetes mellitus. Two physical therapists measured 31 subjects for intertester reliability, and one of the physical therapists measured 25 subjects again to determine intratester reliability. Both examiners participated in extensive training prior to data collection; specific measurement protocols were followed. Dorsiflexion measurements were taken prone in a subtalar joint neutral position as described by McPoil and Brocato.[92] Subtalar inversion and eversion ROM was measured from anatomical neutral. Intratester reliability was excellent, with ICC values ranging from 0.89 to 0.96 and SEM values ranging from 1 to 3 degrees. Intertester reliability was fair to good, with ICC values ranging from 0.74 to 0.89 and SEM values ranging from 1 to 4 degrees. Salsich and colleagues[55] also found excellent intratester reliability (ICC = 0.95) when measuring active dorsiflexion ROM in a group of adults in which 17 had diabetes mellitus and peripheral neuropathy and 17 were healthy age-matched controls. Subjects were positioned prone with the knee extended. (See Tables 10.9 and 10.10.)

Reliability of Measuring Ankle Motion With Inclinometers

Some studies have focused on the reliability of measuring ankle and foot ROM with an inclinometer. Typically, inclinometers have been used to measure ROM in weight-bearing positions. Bennell and colleagues[93] determined intertester and intratester reliability using a weight-bearing lunge position with the knee flexed for measuring dorsiflexion in 13 healthy young adults. Four examiners used an inclinometer to measure the angle of the anterior border of the tibia to vertical, and they used a tape measure to determine the maximal distance of the lunging first toe from the wall with the knee maintaining contact with the wall. Intratester and intertester reliability was very high (ICC = 0.97–0.99) for the four examiners with both methods of assessment.

Konor and associates[94] included 20 healthy young adults in a study of three methods of measuring ankle dorsiflexion in a weight-bearing lunge position with the knee flexed. A trained exercise science student took three measurements using each method. Intratester reliability was good to excellent for the digital inclinometer, 7-inch universal goniometer, and tape measure, with ICC values of 0.96, 0.85, and 0.98, respectively, for the right side, and 0.97, 0.96, and 0.99, respectively, for the left side. The SEM values for the inclinometer were 1.4 and 1.3 degrees; for the goniometer, 2.8 and 1.8 degrees; and for the tape measure, 0.6 and 0.4 centimeters. The inclinometer, which measured the angle between vertical and the tibial tuberosity, had a mean of 38.8 degrees, and the goniometer, which measured the angle between the floor and lateral midline of the fibula, had a mean of 43.2 degrees. The tape measure was used to record the maximal distance between the first toe and the wall in a manner similar to that used by Bennell et al.[93]

Van der Worp and associates[41] enrolled 42 healthy recreational runners (22 males and 20 females) in a study that examined the reliability of measuring weight-bearing dorsiflexion of the posterior leg in a lunge position with the knee straight. An inclinometer measured the angle between the middle of the anterior tibia and vertical. Two physical therapists took two measurements within one session. Intratester and intertester reliability was high, with ICC values of 0.86 and 0.88. Interestingly, intertester measurement error (SEM = 2.4 degrees) was less than intratester measurement error (SEM = 8.7 degrees), which the researchers noted might reflect the experience of the testers, the efficacy of pretraining, the standardized measurement protocol, and the inclusion of all healthy subjects.

Reliability of Measuring the Subtalar Joint Neutral Position

The subtalar joint neutral position, which has been the focus of numerous studies, is not the same as the 0 starting position for the subtalar joint as used in this book and many others, including those of the AAOS,[8,14] the AMA,[12] and Clarkson.[95] The subtalar joint neutral position is defined as one in which the calcaneus inverts twice as many degrees as it everts. According to Elveru and associates,[96] this position can be found when the head of the talus either cannot be palpated or is equally extended at the medial and lateral borders of the talonavicular joint. This is the position usually used in the casting of foot orthotics, but it also has been used for measurement of joint motion. However, Elveru, Rothstein, and Lamb[85] found that referencing passive ROM measurements for inversion and eversion to the subtalar joint neutral position consistently reduced reliability (see Tables 10.9 and 10.10). Based on the study by Elveru, Rothstein, and Lamb[85] and information from the following studies, we decided not to use the subtalar neutral position in this text.

Bailey, Perillo, and Forman[97] used tomography to study the subtalar joint neutral position in 2 female and 13 male volunteers aged 20 to 30 years. These authors found that the neutral subtalar joint position was quite variable in relation to the total ROM and that it was not always found at one-third of the total ROM from the maximally everted position. Furthermore, the neutral position varied not only from subject to subject but also between right and left sides of each subject.

Picciano, Rowlands, and Worrell[98] conducted a study to determine the intratester and intertester reliability of measurements of open-chain and closed-chain subtalar joint neutral positions. Both ankles of 15 healthy subjects were measured by two inexperienced physical therapy students. The students had a 2-hour training session using a universal goniometer prior to data collection. The method of taking measurements was based on the work of Elveru and associates.[96] Intratester reliability of open-chain measurements of the subtalar joint neutral position was an ICC of 0.27 for one tester and ICC of 0.06 for the other tester. Intertester reliability was 0.00. Intratester and intertester reliability also were poor for closed-kinematic-chain measurements. The authors concluded that subtalar joint neutral measurements taken by inexperienced testers were unreliable; they recommended that clinicians practice taking measurements and performing repeated measurements to determine their own reliability for these measurements. However, Torburn, Perry, and Gronley[99] suggested that inaccuracy of measurement technique with use of a universal goniometer, rather than the ability of examiners to position the subtalar joint in the neutral position, might be responsible for poor reliability findings for subtalar joint neutral positioning. The ICC for intertester reliability for three examiners was an ICC of 0.76 for positioning the subtalar joint in the neutral position. In this study, the examiners palpated the head of the talus in 10 subjects lying in the prone position while an electrogoniometer was used to record the position.

Keenan and Bach[100] used the prone measurement position system to assess the non-weight-bearing subtalar neutral position and subtalar inversion and eversion in 24 healthy subjects. Static and dynamic measurements were made on two different occasions by four experienced clinicians using a universal goniometer. Intertester reliability was poor and so was test-retest reliability for static measurements. Reliability was also poor for visual assessments of dynamic measurements. The most experienced clinician had the highest overall reliability, whereas the clinician with only a year's experience had the lowest reliability. However, the same trend was not evident in static measurements.

In contrast to the low reliability found in the aforementioned studies, McPoil and Cornwall[46] found high intratester reliability for measuring subtalar joint neutral position with a universal goniometer. The mean ICC value was 0.97 for one experienced physical therapist in repeated measurement of 27 healthy young adults. The measurement of the subtalar joint neutral position was one of 17 static tests that was included in the study. Smith-Oricchi and Harris,[91] in a study of 20 patients with recent ankle pathology, measured subtalar joint neutral position with a universal goniometer and reported lower intertester reliability (ICC = 0.60). Subtalar joint neutral position was determined by palpating and moving the subtalar joint until the medial and lateral sides of the talus were equal. Three physical therapists took the measurements.

Reliability of Measuring Metatarsophalangeal (MTP) Motion With Universal Goniometers

Hopson[18] used four clinical methods to measure extension ROM of the first MTP joint in 20 healthy adult subjects between 21 and 45 years of age. A universal goniometer with 2-inch arms was used to measure passive ROM for each method three times and the average was used for analysis. Two non-weight-bearing methods were used with subjects supine and the goniometer aligned over the medial or dorsal surface of the first metatarsal and proximal phalanx. The partial weight-bearing method was conducted in sitting by raising the heel and plantarflexing the ankle as much as possible. The full weight-bearing method used a standing position at the end of step length. All measurement techniques were found to be reliable ($r > 0.91$) but not interchangeable (see Table 10.11). The investigators concluded that all ROM values were at least 24% greater than the amount of first MTP extension required for walking, so that any of these four methods would be adequate for determining whether a patient had enough ROM at that joint for gait.

McPoil and Cornwall[46] included first MTP extension ROM in a study of 27 healthy adults. The intratester reliability of measuring first MTP extension ROM with a universal goniometer was highly reliable (ICC = 0.99).

Validity of Measuring Ankle, Foot, and MTP Joint Motions With Universal Goniometers

We are unaware of any studies that have investigated the concurrent validity of goniometric measurements of ankle and foot ROM values by comparing these measurements with the gold standard of radiographs.

The concurrent validity of goniometric measurements compared with radiographs or computed tomography (CT) scans at the first MTP joint has been examined. A study by Buell and associates[11] compared clinical methods of

TABLE 10.11 Intratester Reliability of First Metacarpophalangeal ROM Measurements With Goniometers for Healthy and Patient Populations

Study	N	Sample	Methods	Motion	r	ICC	Absolute Reliability (degrees)
			Healthy Populations				
Hopson et al[18]	20	Healthy adults	PROM, 1 tester, 2 positions: partial and full WB, universal goniometer: 2 alignments on medial and dorsal foot	Extension:			
				Medial alignment		.95	
				Dorsal alignment		.91	
				Partial WB		.95	
				Full WB		.98	
McPoil and Cornwall[46]	27	Healthy adults	1 tester (PT), universal goniometer, non-WB	Extension		.99	

ICC = Intraclass correlation coefficient; PROM = Passive range of motion; r = Pearson product moment correlation coefficient; SEM = Standard error of measurement; WB = Weight-bearing; PT = Physical therapist.

measuring flexion and extension ROM of the first MTP joint with radiographs in the 20 feet of 10 healthy subjects who were part of a larger study establishing normative ROM values. The clinical method aligned the goniometer with the medial longitudinal axis of the first metatarsal and proximal phalanx, in a manner similar to the method of determining joint angle from the radiographs. The mean difference between the radiographs and clinical goniometric measures of MTP motions ranged from 1 degree for active extension and active-assisted flexion, to 5 degrees for active-assisted extension and active flexion. The investigators stated that clinical and radiographic values for active and active-assisted MTP extension correlated very closely and validated this clinical methodology. There were differences in the stabilization of the foot and application of assisting pressure between the clinical and radiographic measures that may have contributed to some of the differences. Using the straight-line position of the proximal phalanx and metatarsal as zero was strongly recommended for consistency rather than using the angle between these bones in relaxed stance position or a relaxed hanging position in sitting as zero.

Kwon and associates[19] compared the static angular position of the 2–4 MTP joints taken with CT scans with angles taken with a goniometer applied to the dorsal midlines of the metatarsal and proximal phalanx. Ankles were stabilized in 30 degrees of plantarflexion with a board while the toes remained relaxed in the 29 subjects (27 hammer toes and 31 non–hammer toes). The concurrent validity of MTP angles taken with the two devices was good to excellent, with ICC values ranging from 0.84 to 0.90. However, the angle measurements taken by CT scan were 8.6 to 10.4 degrees greater than the angles determined with the goniometer. The underestimation of goniometric measurements was believed to be due to soft tissue over the dorsum of the foot. The investigators concluded that the results suggest that dorsal goniometric measures of MTP joint angle are good indicators of true MTP joint angle in the second to fourth toes, but goniometric measures are not interchangeable with the gold standard CT measures.

REFERENCES

1. Martin, RL: The Ankle and Foot Complex. In Levangie, PK, and Norkin, CC: Joint Structure and Function: A Comprehensive Analysis, ed 5. FA Davis, Philadelphia, 2011.
2. Neumann, DA: Kinesiology of the Musculoskeletal System, ed 2. Mosby, St. Louis, MO, 2009.
3. Standring, S (ed): Gray's Anatomy, ed 41. Elsevier, New York, 2016.
4. Kaltenborn, FM: Manual Mobilization of the Extremity Joints, ed 7. Olaf Norlis Bokhandel, Oslo, 2011.
5. Cyriax, JM, and Cyriax, PJ: Illustrated Manual of Orthopaedic Medicine. Butterworths, London, 1983.
6. Magee, DJ: Orthopedic Physical Assessment, ed 4. Elsevier, Philadelphia, 2006.
7. Bohannon, RW, Tiberio, D, and Zito, M: Selected measures of ankle dorsiflexion range of motion: Differences and intercorrelations. Foot Ankle 10:99, 1989.
8. American Academy of Orthopaedic Surgeons: Joint Motion: Method of Measuring and Recording. AAOS, Chicago, 1965.
9. Menadue, C, et al: Reliability of two goniometric methods of measuring active inversion and eversion range of motion at the ankle. BMC Musculoskelet Disord 7:60, 2006.
10. Astrom, M, and Arvidson, T: Alignment and joint motion in the normal foot. J Orthop Sports Phys Ther 22:216, 1995.
11. Buell, T, Green, DR, and Risser, J: Measurement of the first metatarsophalangeal joint range of motion. J Am Podiatr Med Assoc 78(9):439, 1988.
12. American Medical Association: Guides to the Evaluation of Permanent Impairment, ed 3 (revised). AMA, Chicago, 1988.
13. Alanen, JT, et al: Ankle joint complex mobility of children 7–14 years old. J Pediatr Orthop 21:731, 2001.
14. Greene, WB, and Heckman, JD (eds): The Clinical Measurement of Joint Motion: American Academy of Orthopaedic Surgeons, Chicago, 1994.
15. Boone, DC, and Azen, SP: Normal range of motion of joints in male subjects. J Bone Joint Surg Am 61:756, 1979.
16. Roass, A, and Andersson, GB: Normal range of motion of the hip, knee, and ankle joints in male subjects, 30–40 years of age. Acta Orthop Scand 53:205, 1982.
17. Macedo, LG, and Magee, DJ: Effects of age on passive range of motion of selected peripheral joints in healthy adult females. Physiother Theory Pract 25(2):145, 2009.
18. Hopson, M, McPoil, TG, and Cornwall, MW: Motion of the first metatarsophalangeal joint: Reliability and validity of four measurement techniques. J Am Podiatr Med Assoc 85(4):199, 1995.
19. Kwon, OY, et al: Reliability and validity of measures of hammer toe deformity angle and tibial torsion. Foot (Edinb) 19(3):149, 2009.
20. Kumar, S, et al: Normal range of motion of hip and ankle in Indian population. Acta Orthop Traumatiol Turc 45(6):421, 2011.
21. Waugh, KG, et al: Measurement of selected hip, knee and ankle joint motions in newborns. Phys Ther 63:1616, 1983.
22. Wanatabe, H, et al: The range of joint motion of the extremities in healthy Japanese people: The differences according to age. Nippon Seikeigeka Gakkai Zasshi 53:275, 1979. (Cited in Walker, JM: Musculoskeletal development: A review. Phys Ther 71:878, 1991.)
23. Boone, DC: Techniques of measurement of joint motion. (Supplement to Boone, DC, and Azen, SP: Normal range of motion in male subjects. J Bone Joint Surg Am 61:756, 1979.)
24. Soucie, JM, et al: Range of motion measurements: Reference values and a database for comparison studies. Haemophilia 17:500, 2011.
25. Walker, JM: Musculoskeletal development: A review. Phys Ther 71:878, 1991.
26. Boone, DC, Walker, JM, and Perry, J: Age and sex differences in lower extremity joint motion. Presented at the National Conference, American Physical Therapy Association, Washington, DC, 1981.
27. Nigg, BM, et al: Range of motion of the foot as a function of age. Foot Ankle 613:336, 1992.
28. Mecagni, C, et al: Balance and ankle range of motion in community-dwelling women aged 64–87 years: A correlational study. Phys Ther 80:1004, 2000.
29. Freemont, AJ, and Hoyland, JA: Morphology, mechanisms and pathology of musculoskeletal ageing. J Pathol 211:252, 2007.
30. James, B, and Parker, AW: Active and passive mobility of lower limb joints in elderly men and women. Am J Phys Med Rehabil 68:162, 1989.
31. Gajdosik, RL, VanderLinden, DW, and Williams, AK: Influence of age on length and passive elastic stiffness: Characteristics of the calf muscle-tendon unit of women. Phys Ther 79:827, 1999.
32. Gajdosik, RL, et al: Slow passive stretch and release characteristics of the calf muscles of older women with limited dorsiflexion range of motion. Clin Biomech 19:398, 2004.
33. Moseley, AN, Crosbie, J, and Adams, R: Normative data for passive plantarflexion-dorsiflexion flexibility. Clin Biomech (Bristol, Avon) 16:514, 2001.
34. Jonson, SR, and Gross, MT: Intraexaminer reliability, interexaminer reliability and mean values for nine lower extremity skeletal measures in healthy midshipmen. J Orthop Sports Phys Ther 25:253, 1997.
35. Vandervoort, AA, et al: Age and sex effects on the mobility of the human ankle. J Gerontol 476:M17, 1992.
36. Bell, RD, and Hoshizaki, TB: Relationships of age and sex with range of motion of seventeen joint actions in humans. Can J Appl Sport Sci 6:202, 1981.
37. Walker, JM, et al: Active mobility of the extremities of older subjects. Phys Ther 64:919, 1984.
38. Baggett, BD, and Young, G: Ankle joint dorsiflexion: Establishment of a normal range. J Am Podiatr Med Assoc 83:251, 1993.
39. Grimston, SK, et al: Differences in ankle joint complex range of motion as a function of age. Foot Ankle 14:215, 1993.
40. Saxena, A, and Kim, W: Ankle dorsiflexion in the adolescent. J Am Podiatr Med Assoc 93:312, 2003.
41. van der Worp, MP, et al: Reproducibility of and sex differences in common orthopaedic ankle and foot tests in runners. BMC Musculoskelet Disord 15:171, 2014.
42. Park, W, et al: Obesity effect on male active joint range of motion. Ergonomics 53:102, 2010.
43. Macedo, LG, and Magee, DJ: Differences in range of motion between dominant and nondominant sides of upper and lower extremities. J Manipulative Physiol Ther 31:577, 2008.
44. Bennell, K, et al: Hip and ankle range of motion and hip muscle strength in young female ballet dancers and controls. Br J Sports Med 33:340, 1999.
45. Ekstrand, MD, et al: Lower extremity goniometric measurements: A study to determine their reliability. Arch Phys Med Rehabil 63:171, 1982.
46. McPoil, TG, and Cornwall, MW: The relationship between static lower extremity measurements and rearfoot motion during walking. J Orthop Sports Phys Ther 24:309, 1996.
47. Riemann, BL, et al: The effects of sex, joint angle, and the gastrocnemius muscle on passive ankle joint complex stiffness. J Athl Train 93:312, 2003.
48. Lattanza, L, Gray, GW, and Kanter, RM: Closed versus open kinematic chain measurements of subtalar joint eversion: Implications for clinical practice. J Orthop Sports Phys Ther 9:310, 1988.
49. Nawoczenski, DA, Baumhauer, JF, and Umberger, BR: Relationship between clinical measurements and motion of the first metatarsophalangeal joint during gait. J Bone Joint Surg 81:370, 1999.
50. Kaufman, KR, et al: The effect of foot structure and range of motion on musculoskeletal overuse injuries. Am J Sports Med 27:585, 1999.
51. Morrison, KE, and Kaminski, TW: Foot characteristics in association with inversion ankle injury. J Athl Train 42:135, 2007.
52. Wilson, RW, and Gansneder, BM: Measures of functional limitation as predictors of disablement in athletes with acute ankle sprains. J Orthop Sports Phys Ther 30:528, 2000.
53. Chesworth, BM, and Vandervoort, AA: Comparison of passive stiffness variables and range of motion in uninvolved and involved ankle joints of patients following ankle fractures. Phys Ther 75:253, 1995.
54. Reynolds, CA, et al: The effect of nontraumatic immobilization on ankle dorsiflexion stiffness in rats. J Orthop Sports Phys Ther 23:27, 1996.
55. Salsich, GB, Mueller, MJ, and Sahrmann, SA: Passive ankle stiffness in subjects with diabetes and peripheral neuropathy versus an age matched comparison group. Phys Ther 80:352, 2000.
56. Rao, SR, et al: Increased passive ankle stiffness and reduced dorsiflexion range of motion in individuals with diabetes mellitus. Foot Ankle Int 27:617, 2006.
57. Hastings, MK, et al: Effects of a tendo-Achilles lengthening procedure on muscle function and gait characteristics in a patient with diabetes mellitus. J Orthop Sports Phys Ther 30:85, 2000.
58. Pathokinesiology Service and Physical Therapy Dept: Observational Gait Analysis, ed 4. LAREI, Ranchos Los Amigos National Rehabilitation Center, Downey, CA, 2001.
59. Murray, MP: Gait as a total pattern of movement. Am J Phys Med Rehabil 46:290, 1967.
60. Ostrosky, KM: A comparison of gait characteristics in young and old subjects. Phys Ther 74:637, 1994.

61. McPoil, TG, and Cornwall, MW: Applied Sports Biomechanics in Rehabilitation Running. In Zachazeweski, JE, Magee, DJ, and Quillen, WS (eds): Athletic Injuries and Rehabilitation. WB Saunders, Philadelphia, 1996.
62. Begg, RK, and Sparrow, WA: Ageing effects on knee and ankle joint angles at key events and phases of the gait cycle. J Med Eng Tech 30(6):382, 2006.
63. Hageman, PA, and Blanke, DJ: Comparison of gait of young women and elderly women. Phys Ther 66(9):1382, 1986.
64. Locke, M, et al: Ankle and subtalar motion during gait in arthritic patients. Phys Ther 64:504, 1984.
65. Livingston, LA, Stevenson, JM, and Olney, SJ: Stairclimbing kinematics on stairs of differing dimensions. Arch Phys Med Rehabil 72:398, 1991.
66. Protopapadaki, A, et al: Hip, knee, ankle kinematics and kinetics during stair ascent and descent in healthy young individuals. Clin Biomech 22:203, 2007.
67. Lark, SD, et al: Knee and ankle range of motion during stepping down in elderly compared to young men. Eur J Appl Physiol 91:287, 2004.
68. Ikeda, ER, Schenkman, ML, and O'Riley, P: Influence of age on dynamics of rising from a chair. Phys Ther 71:473, 1991.
69. Rodosky, MW, Andriacchi, TP, and Andersson, GB; The influence of chair height on lower limb mechanics during rising. J Orthop Res 7:266, 1989.
70. Hemmerich, A, Brown, H, and Smith, S: Hip, knee and ankle kinematics of high range of motion activities of daily living. J Orthop Res 24:770, 2006.
71. Kapoor, A, et al: Range of movements of lower limb joints in cross-legged sitting posture. J Arthroplasty 23(3):451, 2008.
72. Winter, DA, et al: Biomechanical walking pattern changes in the fit and healthy elderly. Phys Ther 70:340, 1990.
73. Murray, MP, Kory, RC, and Clarkson, BH: Walking patterns in healthy old men. J Gerontol 24:169, 1969.
74. Janssen, WGM, Bussmann, HBJ, and Stam, HJ: Determinants of the sit-to-stand movement: A review. Phys Ther 82(9):866, 2002.
75. Martin, RL, and McPoil, TG: Reliability of ankle goniometric measurements: A literature review. J Am Podiatr Med Assoc 95:564, 2005.
76. Portney, LG, and Watkins, MP: Foundations of Clinical Research: Applications to Practice, ed. 3. Pearson Prentice Hall, Upper Saddle River, NJ, 2009.
77. Eliasziw, M, et al: Statistical methodology for the concurrent assessment of interrater and intrarater reliability: Using goniometric measurement as an example. Phys Ther 74:777, 1994.
78. Boone, DC, et al: Reliability of goniometric measurements. Phys Ther 68:1355, 1978
79. Bovens, AMPM, et al: Variability and reliability of joint measurements. Am J Sports Med 18(1):58, 1990.
80. Clapper, MP, and Wolf, SL: Comparison of the reliability of the Orthoranger and the standard goniometer for assessing active lower extremity range of motion. Phys Ther 68:214, 1988.
81. Kilgour, G, McNair, P, and Stott, NS: Intrarater reliability of lower limb sagittal range-of-motion measures in children with spastic diplegia. Dev Med Child Neurol 45:391, 2003.
82. van Gheluwe, B, et al: Reliability and accuracy of biomechanical measurements of the lower extremity. J Am Podiatric Med Assoc 92(6):317, 2002.
83. Allington, NJ, Leroy, N, and Doneux, C: Ankle joint range of motion measurements in spastic cerebral palsy children: Intraobserver and interobserver reliability and reproducibility of goniometry and visual estimation. J Pediatr Orthop 11:2236, 2002.
84. Diamond, J, et al: Reliability of a diabetic foot evaluation. Phys Ther 69(10):797, 1989.
85. Elveru, RA, Rothstein, J, and Lamb, RL: Goniometric reliability in a clinical setting: Subtalar and ankle joint measurements. Phys Ther 68:672, 1988.
86. Mutlu, A, Livanelioglu, A, and Gunel, MK: Reliability of goniometric measurements in children with spastic cerebral palsy. Med Sci Monit 23:CR323, 2007.
87. Pandya, S, et al: Reliability of goniometric measurements in patients with Duchenne muscular dystrophy. Phys Ther 65(9):1339, 1985.
88. Youdas, JW, Bogard, CL, and Suman, VJ: Reliability of goniometric measurements and visual estimates of ankle joint range of motion obtained in a clinical setting. Arch Phys Med Rehabil 74:1113, 1993.
89. Leard, JS, Crane, BA, and Ball, KA: Intrarater and interrater reliability of 22 clinical measures associated with lower quarter malalignment. J Manipulative Physiol Ther 32(4):270, 2009.
90. McWhirk, LB, and Glanzman, AM: Within-session inter-rater reliability of goniometric measures in patients with spastic cerebral palsy. Pediatr Phys Ther 18:262, 2006.
91. Smith-Oricchio, K, and Harris, BA: Interrater reliability of subtalar neutral, calcaneal inversion and eversion. J Orthop Sports Phys Ther 12(1):10, 1990.
92. McPoil, TG, and Brocato, RS: The Foot and Ankle: Biomechanical Evaluation and Treatment. In Gould, JA, and Davies, GJ (eds): Orthopaedic and Sports Physical Therapy. CV Mosby, St. Louis, 1985.
93. Bennell, K, et al: Interrater and intrarater reliability of a weight-bearing lunge measure of ankle dorsiflexion. Aust Physiother 44:175, 1998.
94. Konor, MM, et al: Reliability of three measures of ankle dorsiflexion range of motion. Int J Sports Phys Ther 7(3):279, 2012.
95. Clarkson, HM: Musculoskeletal Assessment: Joint Range of Motion and Manual Muscle Strength, ed. 3. Lippincott Williams & Wilkins, Philadelphia, 2005.
96. Elveru, RA, et al: Methods for taking subtalar joint measurements: A clinical report. Phys Ther 68:678, 1988.
97. Bailey, DS, Perillo, JT, and Forman, M: Subtalar joint neutral: A study using tomography. J Am Podiatry Assoc 74:59, 1984.
98. Picciano, AM, Rowlands, MS, and Worrell, T: Reliability of open and closed kinetic chain subtalar joint neutral positions and navicular drop test. J Orthop Sports Phys Ther 18:553, 1993.
99. Torburn, L, Perry, J, and Gronley, JAK: Assessment of rearfoot motion: Passive positioning, one-legged standing, gait. Foot Ankle Int 19:688, 1998.
100. Keenan, A-M, and Bach, TM: Clinician's assessment of the hindfoot: A study of reliability. Foot Ankle Int 27:451, 2006.

PART IV

TESTING OF THE SPINE AND TEMPOROMANDIBULAR JOINT

OBJECTIVES

On completion of Part IV, you will be able to:

1. **Identify:**
   - appropriate planes and axes for each spinal and jaw motion
   - normal ranges of motion for cervical, thoracolumbar, and lumbar spine and temporomandibular joint
   - expected normal end-feels
   - structures (contractile and noncontractile) that have the potential to limit the end of the range of motion (ROM)
2. **Describe:**
   - testing positions for measuring motions of the cervical, thoracolumbar, and lumbar spine and the temporomandibular joint
   - goniometer, tape measure, the cervical range of motion (CROM) device, and inclinometer alignments
   - capsular patterns of restricted motion
   - range of motion necessary for selected functional activities
3. **Explain:**
   - how age, gender, and other factors may affect the range of motion
   - how sources of error in measurement such as a lack of adequate stabilization or inappropriate positioning may affect testing results
4. **Perform a range of motion assessment of the cervical spine using the universal goniometer, tape measure, inclinometers (double and single), and the CROM device.**
5. **Perform a ROM assessment of the thoracolumbar and lumbar spine using the universal goniometer, tape measure, and inclinometers.**
6. **Perform a ROM assessment of the temporomandibular joint using a ruler.**
7. **Assess the intratester and intertester reliability of measurements of the spine and temporomandibular joint.**
8. **Discuss the reliability and validity of ROM measurements using the universal goniometer, tape measure, double and single inclinometers, CROM device, and ruler.**

Chapters 11 through 13 present common clinical techniques for measuring gross motions of the cervical, thoracolumbar, and lumbar spine and the temporomandibular joint. Evaluation of the ROM and end-feels of individual facet joints of the spine are not included.

CHAPTER 11

The Cervical Spine

Cynthia C. Norkin, PT, EdD

Structure and Function

Atlanto-Occipital and Atlantoaxial Joints

The atlanto-occipital joint is composed of the right and left deep concave superior facets of the atlas (C1) that articulate with the right and left convex occipital condyles of the skull (Fig. 11.1).

The atlantoaxial joint is composed of three separate articulations: the median atlantoaxial and two lateral joints. The median atlantoaxial joint consists of an anterior facet on the dens (the odontoid process of C2) that articulates with a facet on the internal surface of the atlas (C1). The two lateral joints are composed of the right and left superior facets of the axis (C2) that articulate with the right and left slightly convex inferior facets on the atlas (C1) (Fig. 11.2).

The atlanto-occipital and atlantoaxial joints are reinforced anteriorly by the anterior–occipital and atlantoaxial membranes (Fig. 11.3A) and posteriorly by the posterior atlanto-occipital, atlantoaxial, and tectorial membranes (Fig. 11.3B).

Osteokinematics

The atlanto-occipital joint, which is composed of the atlas (C1) and occipital condyles (Oc), is a condylar synovial joint that permits active flexion–extension as a nodding motion.[1] A limited amount of axial rotation and lateral flexion may also be produced. Flexion–extension takes place in the sagittal plane around a medial–lateral axis. Extremes of flexion are limited by osseous contact of the anterior ring of the foramen magnum with the dens. Normally, flexion is limited by tension in the posterior neck muscles and tectorial membrane and by impaction of the submandibular tissues against the throat. Extension is limited by the occiput compressing the

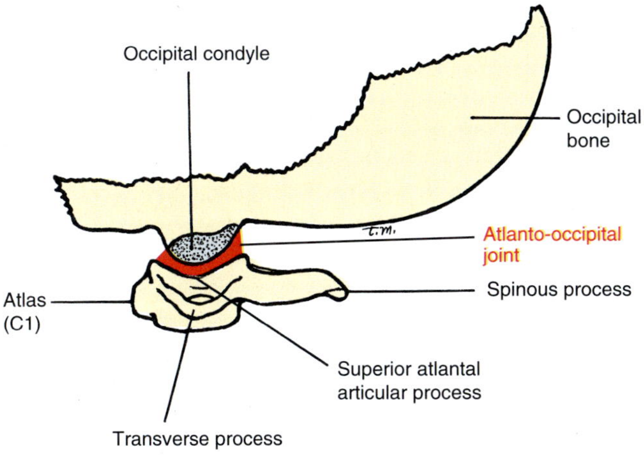

FIGURE 11.1 A lateral view of a portion of the atlanto-occipital joint shows the superior atlantal articular process of the atlas (C1) and the corresponding occipital condyle. The joint space has been widened to show the articular processes.

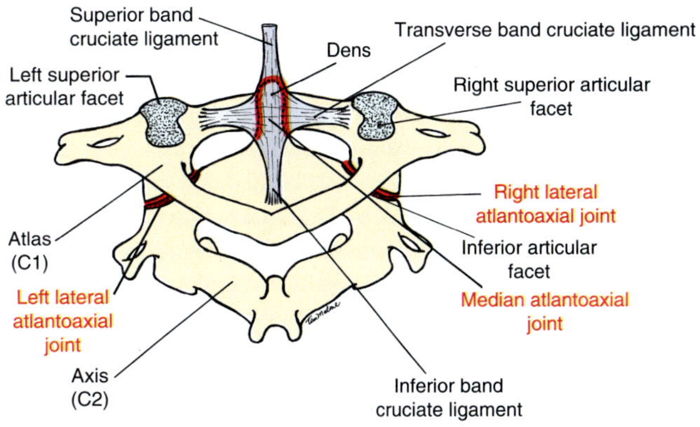

FIGURE 11.2 A posterior view of the atlantoaxial joint showing its three separate articulations: the median atlantoaxial joint and two lateral joints. The median joint is composed of an anterior facet on the dens that articulates with a facet on the internal surface of the atlas (C1). The two lateral joints are composed of the right and left superior facets of the axis (C2) that articulate with the right and left inferior facets on the atlas (C1). (Also shown are the superior, inferior, and transverse bands of the cruciate ligament.)

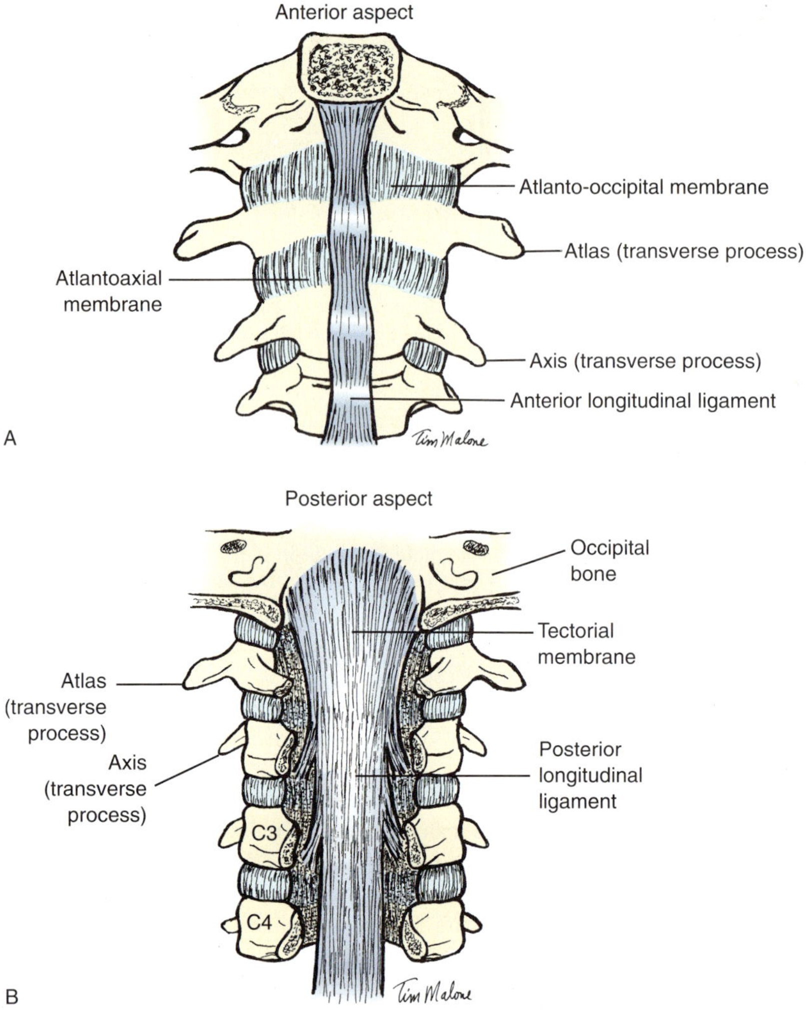

FIGURE 11.3 (A) The anterior atlanto-occipital and atlantoaxial membranes help to support the anterior aspect of the atlanto-occipital and atlantoaxial joints. (B) The posterior atlanto-occipital, atlantoaxial, and tectorial membrane help to support the posterior aspect of the atlanto-occipital and atlantoaxial joints.

suboccipital muscles. Combined flexion–extension is reported to be between 20 degrees[2] and 30 degrees[3] and is usually described as the amount of motion that occurs during nodding of the head. However, according to Cailliet,[4] the range of motion (ROM) in flexion is 10 degrees and the range in extension is 30 degrees. Maximum rotation at the atlanto-occipital joint is between approximately 2.5% and 5% of the total cervical spine rotation.[5] In a three-dimensional MRI study, a mean of about 2 degrees of rotation and lateral flexion to each side was reported at the Oc-C1 joint.[6,7] Others note that lateral flexion is approximately 10 degrees.[2]

The two lateral atlantoaxial joints are plane synovial joints that allow flexion–extension, lateral flexion, and rotation. The median atlantoaxial joint is a synovial trochoid (pivot) joint that permits rotation. Rotation at the median atlantoaxial joint is limited primarily by the two alar ligaments, with minor restraint being provided by the capsules of the lateral atlantoaxial joints.[1] Motions permitted at the three atlantoaxial articulations are flexion–extension, lateral flexion, and rotation.[8] Approximately 55% of the axial rotation of the craniocervical range of rotation occurs at the atlantoaxial joint, whereas the remaining rotation occurs from C2 to C7.[9] An average 36 degrees of rotation to each side has been noted at the atlantoaxial joint during in vivo studies using three-dimensional magnetic resonance imaging (MRI).[6] Others report about 45 degrees of rotation to the right and left sides.

Some motions in the vertebral column are coupled with other motions; this coupling varies from region to region. A coupled motion is one in which one motion around one axis is consistently associated with another motion or motions around a different axis or axes. Coupled lateral flexion has been observed in the direction opposite to axial rotation at both the atlanto-occipital (Oc–C1) and atlantoaxial joints (C1–C2). Extension coupled with axial rotation was present at both joints as well.[6]

Arthrokinematics

At the atlanto-occipital joint when the head moves on the atlas (convex surfaces moving on concave surfaces), the occipital condyles roll in the same direction as the top of the head and glide in the direction opposite to the movement of the top of the head. For example, in flexion, the occipital condyles roll anteriorly and glide posteriorly on the concave articular surfaces of the atlas. In extension, the occipital condyles roll posteriorly and glide anteriorly on the atlas and the back of the head moves posteriorly.[1]

At the lateral atlantoaxial joints the inferior zygapophyseal articular facets of the atlas are convex and articulate with the superior concave articular facets of the axis. At the median joint the atlas forms a ring with the transverse ligament (band) of the cruciate ligament, and this ring rotates around the dens (odontoid process), which serves as a pivot for rotation. The dens articulates with a small facet in the central area of the anterior arch of the atlas.

Capsular Pattern

The capsular pattern for the atlanto-occipital joint is an equal restriction of extension and lateral flexion. Rotation and flexion are not affected.[2]

Intervertebral and Zygapophyseal (Facet) Joints

The intervertebral joints are composed of the superior and inferior surfaces of the vertebral bodies and the adjacent intervertebral discs (Fig. 11.4). The joints are reinforced anteriorly by the anterior longitudinal ligament, which limits extension (Fig. 11.5), and posteriorly by the posterior longitudinal ligament (Fig. 11.6), ligamentum nuchae, ligamentum flavum, supraspinous and interspinous ligaments, and the back extensors, which help to limit flexion.

The zygapophyseal joints (also called facet joints) are formed by the right and left superior articular facets (processes) of one vertebra, and the right and left inferior articular facets of an adjacent superior vertebra (Fig. 11.7). Each joint has its own capsule and capsular ligaments, which are lax and permit a relatively large ROM. The ligamentum flavum helps to reinforce the joint capsules.

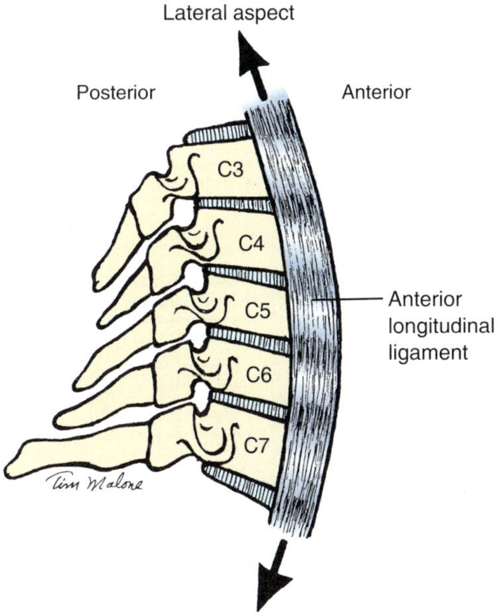

FIGURE 11.5 The anterior longitudinal ligament reinforces the anterior aspect of the intervertebral discs and helps to prevent extremes of extension ROM.

Osteokinematics

According to White and Panjabi,[8] one vertebra can move in relation to an adjacent vertebra in six different directions (three translations and three rotations) along and around three axes. The compound effects of sliding and tilting (rolling) at a series of vertebrae produce a large ROM for the column as a whole, including flexion–extension, lateral flexion, and rotation.

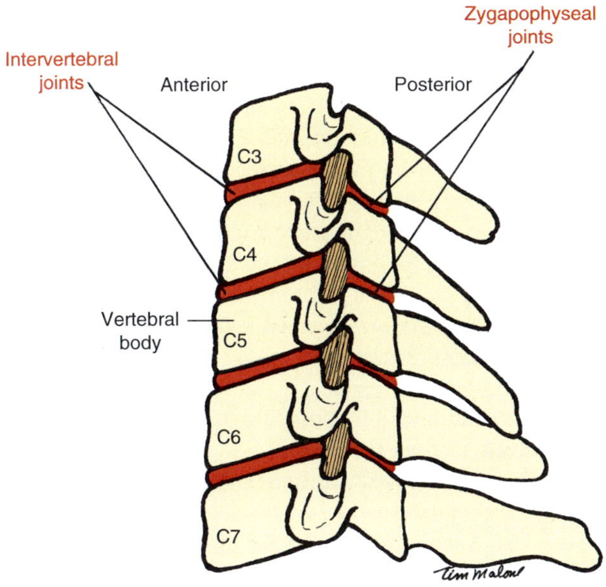

FIGURE 11.4 A lateral view of the cervical spine shows the intervertebral and zygapophyseal joints from C3 to C7. An intervertebral disc is located within each of these intervertebral joints.

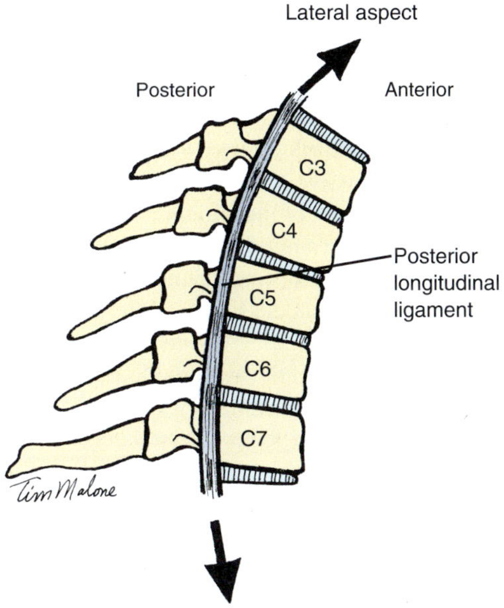

FIGURE 11.6 The posterior longitudinal ligament reinforces the posterior aspect of the intervertebral discs and helps to prevent extremes of flexion ROM.

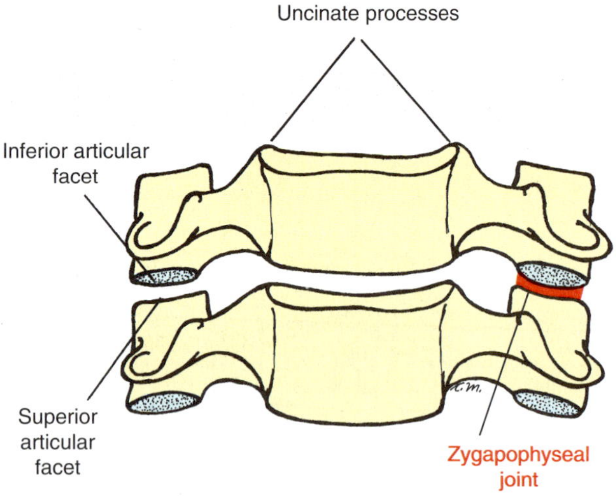

FIGURE 11.7 An anterior view of the right and left zygapophyseal joints between two cervical vertebrae. The vertebrae have been separated to provide a clear view of the inferior articular facets of the superior vertebra and the superior articular facets of the adjacent inferior vertebra.

The intervertebral joints are cartilaginous joints of the symphysis type. The zygapophyseal joints are synovial plane joints. In the cervical region, the facets are oriented at 45 degrees to the transverse plane. The inferior facets of the superior vertebrae face anteriorly and inferiorly. The superior facets of the inferior vertebrae face posteriorly and superiorly. The orientation of the articular facets, which varies from region to region, determines the direction of the tilting and sliding of the vertebra, whereas the size of the disc determines the amount of motion. In addition, passive tension in a number of soft tissues and bony contacts controls and limits motions of the vertebral column. In general, although regional variations exist, the soft tissues that control and limit extremes of motion in forward flexion include the supraspinous and interspinous ligaments, zygapophyseal joint capsules, ligamentum flavum, posterior longitudinal ligament, posterior fibers of the annulus fibrosus of the intervertebral disc, and back extensors.

Extension is limited by bony contact of the spinous processes and by passive tension in the zygapophyseal joint capsules, anterior fibers of the annulus fibrosus, anterior longitudinal ligament, and anterior trunk muscles. Lateral flexion is limited by the intertransverse ligaments, by passive tension in the annulus fibrosus on the side opposite the motion on the convexity of the curve, and by the uncinate processes. Rotation is limited by fibers of the annulus fibrosus.

Coupling of secondary motions with primary motions also occurs in the middle and lower cervical regions. For example, left lateral flexion as the primary motion from C2 to C6 is accompanied by (coupled with) axial rotation to the same (left) side (spinous processes move to the right).[7] Coupled lateral flexion with axial rotation occurs in the same direction as axial rotation and is present from all levels from C2 to T1.[10] Ishii et al[10] found that coupled extension with axial rotation was present in the middle cervical region C2 to C5, whereas in the lower cervical spine C5 to T1, flexion was coupled with axial rotation.

In a large study of 232 healthy volunteers, Demaille-Wlodka and colleagues not only determined the degrees of the principal motion in each of six age-groups but also the percentages of coupled motions associated with the principal motion within different age-groups.[11] The minimal amounts of coupled motion found in the spine were 13.42% of lateral flexion associated with the principal motion of extension, whereas the maximum amount of coupled motion was 142% of axial rotation associated with the principal motion of right lateral flexion. Similar to Crisco,[5] the authors found that lateral flexion and axial rotation were always coupled. Therefore, when we measure cervical ROM we need to be aware of the coupled motions that accompany the principal motion.

Arthrokinematics

The intervertebral joints permit a small amount of sliding and tilting (rolling) of one vertebra on another. In all of the motions at the intervertebral joints, the nucleus pulposus of the intervertebral disc acts as a pivot for the tilting and sliding motions of the vertebrae. Flexion is a result of anterior sliding and tilting of a superior vertebra on the interposed disc of an adjacent inferior vertebra. Extension is the result of posterior sliding and tilting.

The zygapophyseal joints permit small amounts of sliding of the right and left inferior facets on the right and left superior facets of an adjacent inferior vertebra. In flexion, the inferior facets of the superior vertebrae slide anteriorly and superiorly on the superior facets of the inferior vertebrae. In extension, the inferior facets of the superior vertebrae slide posteriorly and inferiorly on the superior facets of the inferior vertebrae. In lateral flexion and rotation, one inferior facet of the superior vertebra slides inferiorly and posteriorly on the superior facet of the inferior vertebra on the side to which the spine is laterally flexed. The opposite inferior facet of the superior vertebra slides superiorly and anteriorly on the superior facet of the adjacent inferior vertebra.

Capsular Pattern

The capsular pattern for C2 to C7 is recognizable by pain and equal limitation of all motions except flexion, which is usually minimally restricted. The capsular pattern for unilateral facet involvement is a greater restriction of movement in lateral flexion to the opposite side and in rotation to the same side. For example, if the right articular facet joint capsule is involved, lateral flexion to the left and rotation to the right are the motions most restricted.

Measurement of cervical spine ROM is complicated by the region's multiple joint structure, lack of well-defined and standardized landmarks, lack of an accurate and workable definition of the neutral position, and lack of a standardized method of stabilization to isolate cervical motion from thoracic spine motion. The search for instruments and methods that are capable of providing accurate and affordable measurements of the cervical spine ROM is ongoing. Tables 11.1 through 11.8 in the Research Findings section provide normal cervical spine ROM values from various sources and ROM values by age and gender.

RANGE OF MOTION TESTING PROCEDURES: Cervical Spine

Landmarks for Testing Procedures

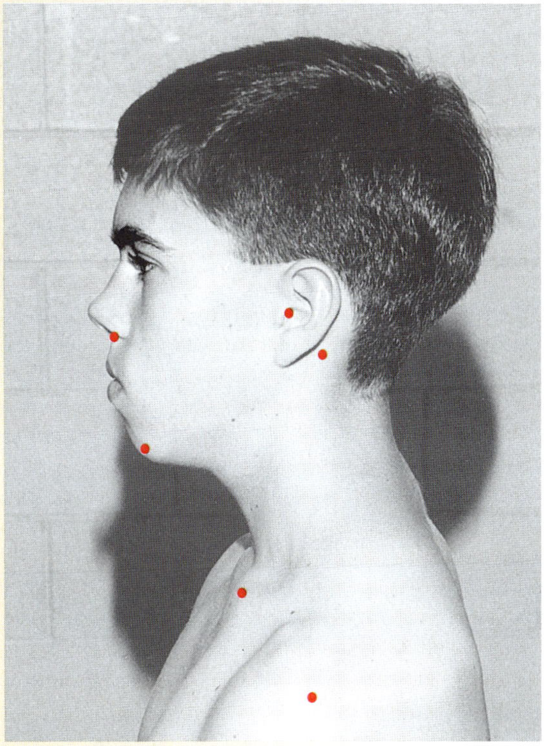

FIGURE 11.8 Surface anatomy landmarks for the universal goniometer and tape measure for measuring cervical ROM. Please refer to Figure 11.9 for landmark labeling.

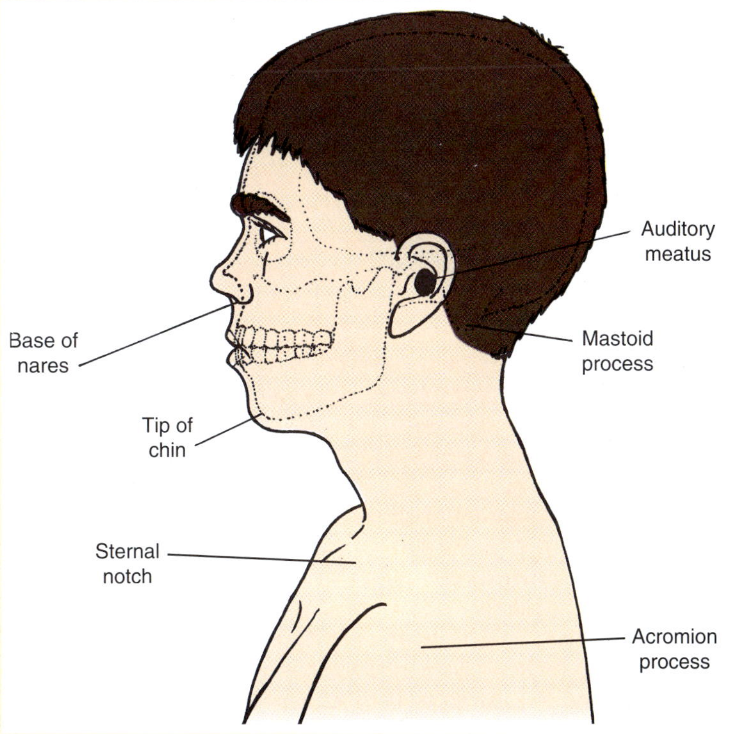

FIGURE 11.9 Bony anatomical landmarks for universal goniometer alignment for measuring cervical flexion and extension.

Landmarks for Testing Procedures (continued)

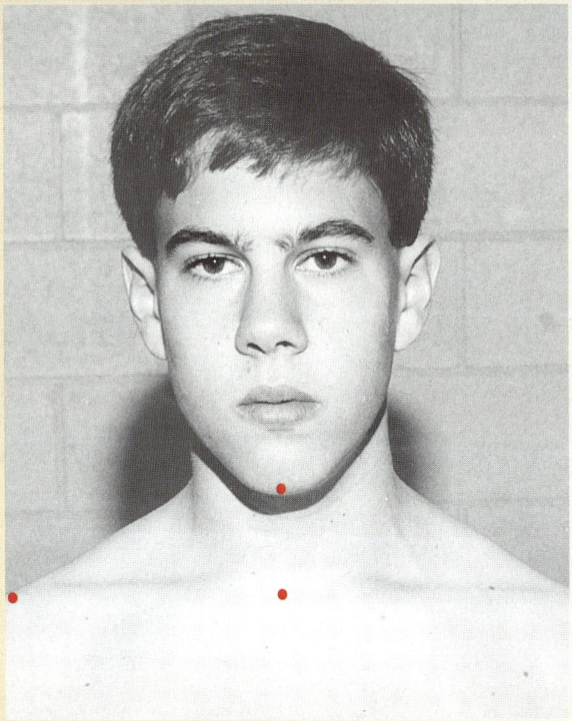

FIGURE 11.10 Surface anatomy landmarks used to measure cervical motion with a tape measure: tip of the chin, sternal notch, and acromial process. The mastoid process, which is used to measure lateral flexion, is shown in Figures 11.8 and 11.9.

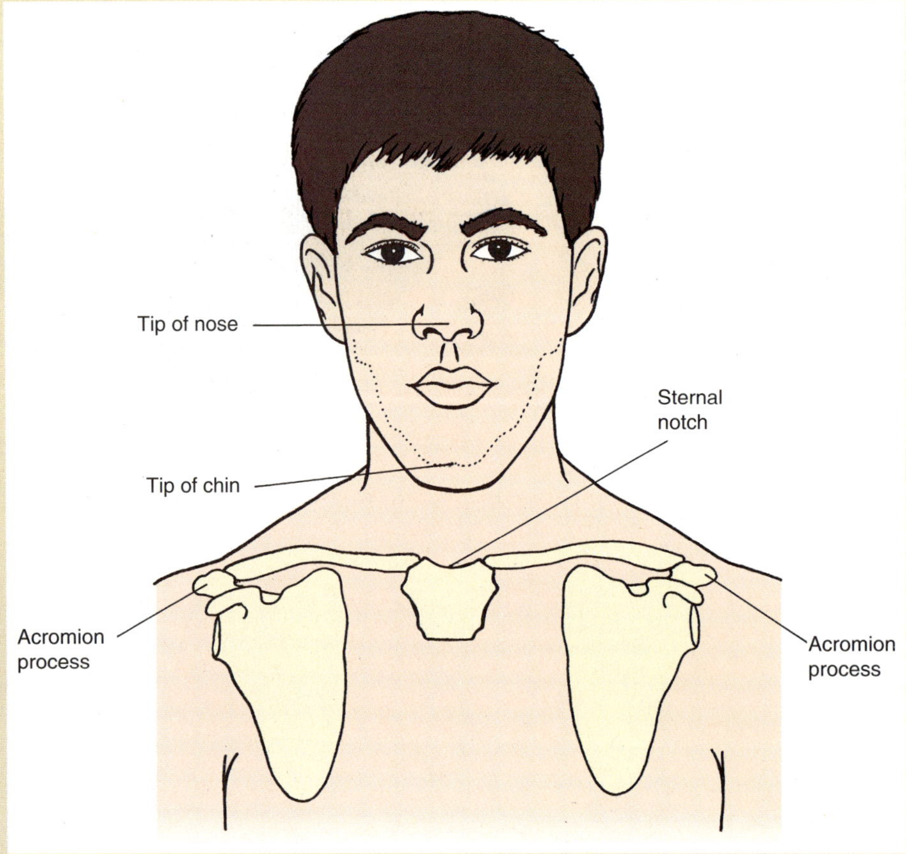

FIGURE 11.11 Bony anatomical landmarks for measuring cervical ROM with the universal goniometer and the tape measure.

Landmarks for Testing Procedures (continued)

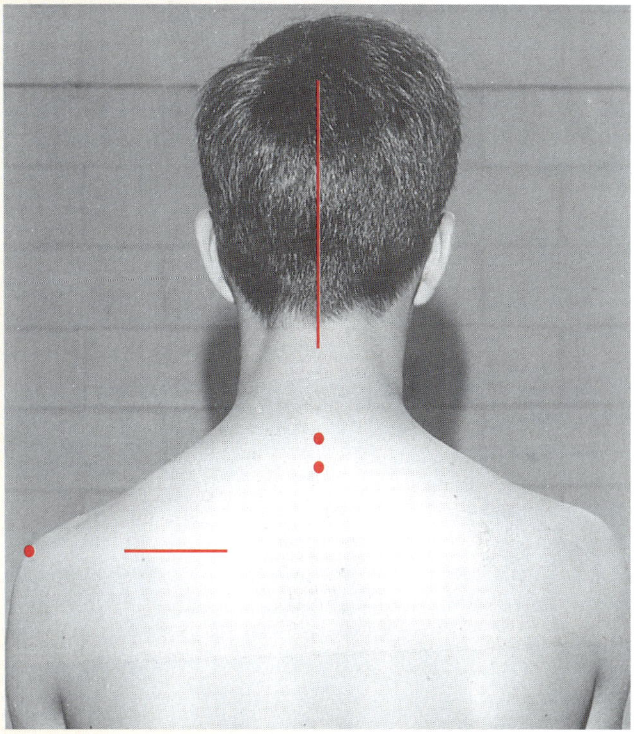

FIGURE 11.12 A posterior view of the individual's head and cervical spine shows the surface anatomy landmarks for measuring lateral flexion with a universal goniometer and flexion and extension with inclinometers.

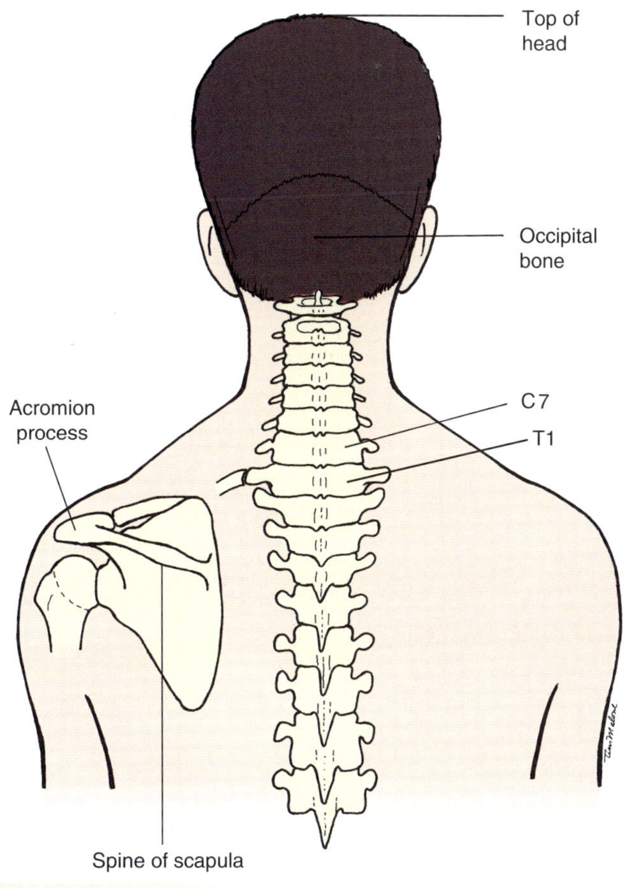

FIGURE 11.13 Bony anatomical landmarks used to align the universal goniometer with C7 and the inclinometers with the spinous process of the T1 vertebra.

CERVICAL FLEXION: UNIVERSAL GONIOMETER

Motion occurs in the sagittal plane around a medial–lateral axis. The mean cervical flexion ROM measured with a universal goniometer is about 40 degrees in adults.[12] See Youdas et al[12] in Table 11.3 in the Research Findings section for additional information on normal values.

Testing Position

Place the individual in the sitting position, with the thoracic and lumbar spine well supported against the back of a chair. Feet should be flat on the floor and shoulders should be relaxed with hands resting on the thighs. Position the head in 0 degrees of rotation and lateral flexion.

Stabilization

The testing position helps to provide stabilization. During active ROM the examiner may be able to use a free hand to stabilize the shoulder girdle or sternum to prevent forward flexion of the thoracic spine. During passive ROM the examiner's hands are involved with the measurement, so if additional stabilization is needed a strap can be placed around the chest and the back of the chair.

Testing Motion: Passive ROM

Put one hand on the back of the individual's head and with the other hand hold the individual's chin. Push gently but firmly on the back of the individual's head to move the head anteriorly. Pull the individual's chin in toward the chest to move the head through flexion ROM (Fig. 11.14). The end of the ROM occurs when resistance to further motion is felt and further attempts at flexion cause forward flexion of the trunk.

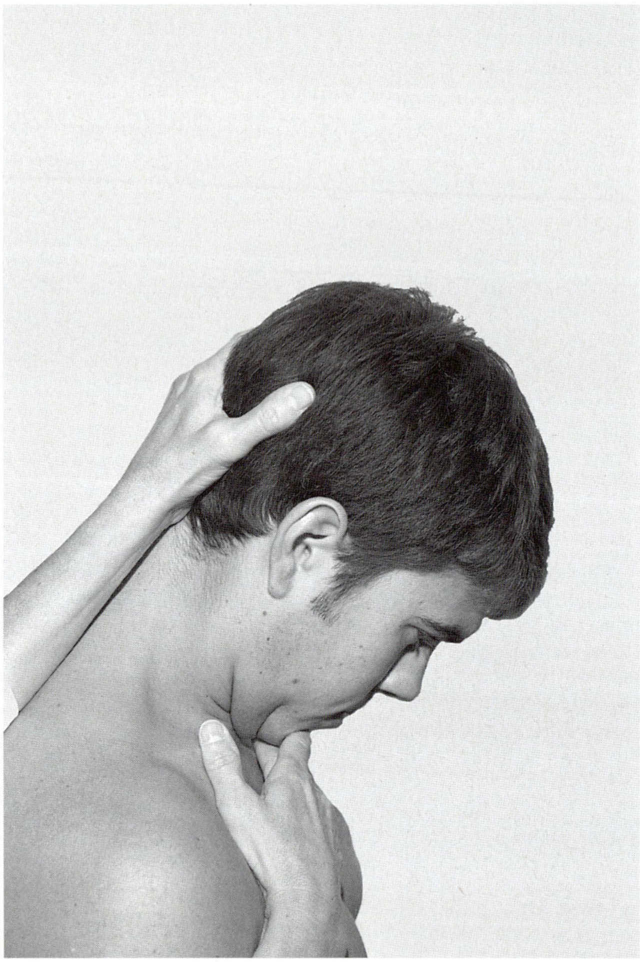

FIGURE 11.14 The individual at the end of the cervical flexion range of motion.

Testing Motion: Active ROM

Ask the individual to tuck the chin in toward the chest and bend the head forward until resistance to further motion is felt or the trunk begins to flex forward.

Normal End-Feel

The normal end-feel is firm owing to stretching of the posterior ligaments (supraspinous, infraspinous, ligamentum flavum, and ligamentum nuchae), posterior fibers of the annulus fibrosus in the intervertebral disks, and the zygapophyseal joint capsules and because of impaction of the submandibular tissues against the throat and passive tension in the following muscles: iliocostalis cervicis, longissimus capitis, longissimus cervicis, obliquus capitis superior, rectus capitis posterior major, rectus capitis posterior minor, semispinalis capitis, semispinalis cervicis, splenius cervicis, splenius capitis, spinalis capitis, spinalis cervicis, and upper trapezius.

Goniometer Alignment

See Figures 11.15 and 11.16.

1. Center **fulcrum** of the goniometer over the external auditory meatus.
2. Align **proximal arm** so that it is either perpendicular or parallel to the ground.
3. Align **distal arm** with the base of the nares.

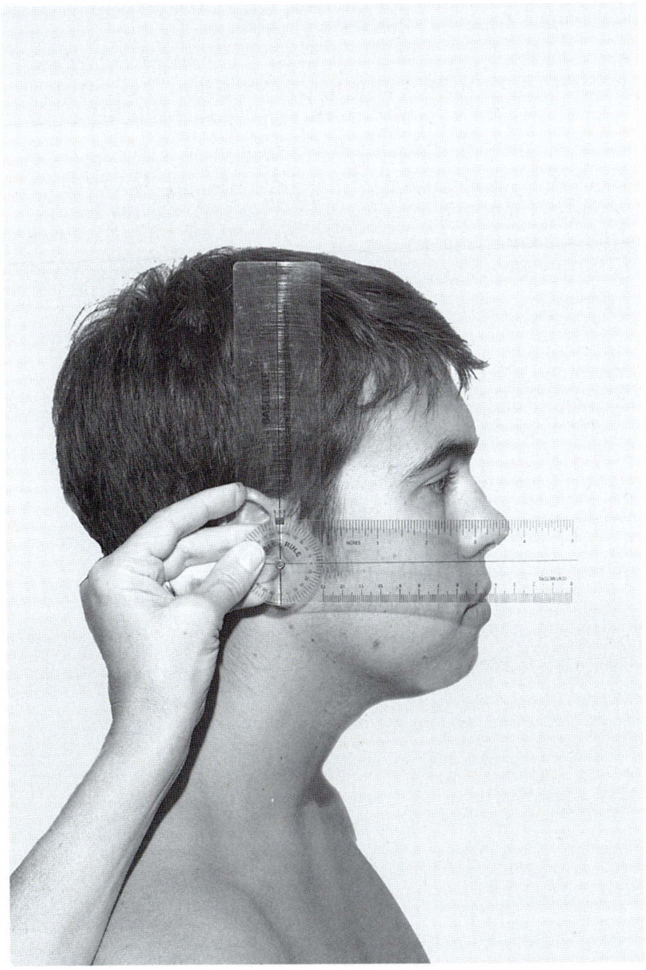

FIGURE 11.15 The proximal arm of the goniometer is perpendicular to the ground and the distal arm is aligned with the base of the nares. In this zero starting position for measuring cervical flexion ROM, the goniometer reads 90 degrees but this reading should be transposed and recorded as 0.

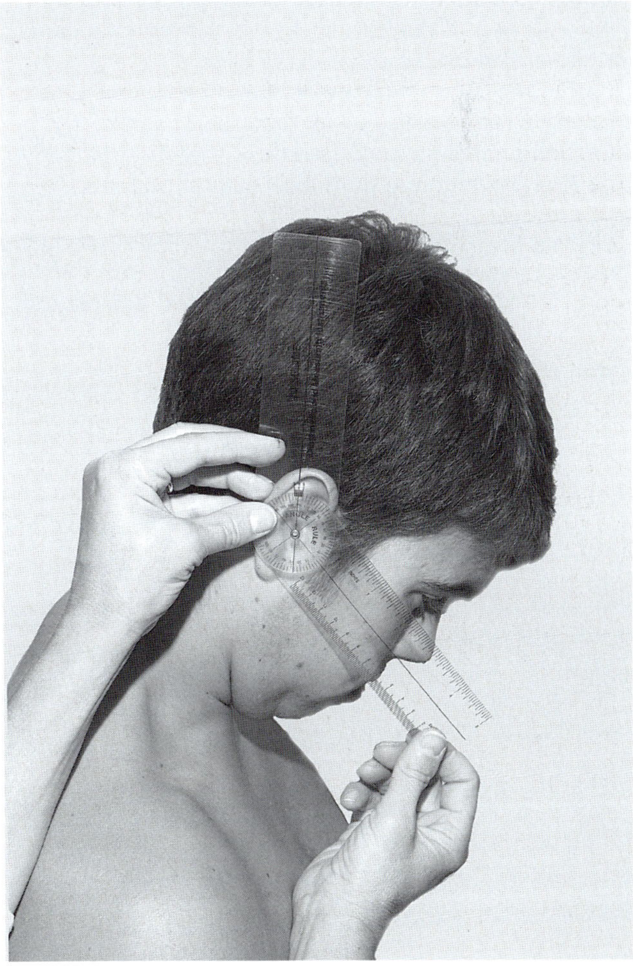

FIGURE 11.16 The goniometer reads 135 degrees at the end of the ROM, but it should be recorded as 0–45 degrees.

CERVICAL FLEXION: TAPE MEASURE

The mean cervical flexion ROM obtained with a tape measure ranges from 1.0 to 4.3 centimeters for those aged 14 to 31 years.[13,14] See Table 11.2 in the Research Findings section for normal values, but remember that you need to check to see whether the landmarks that are being used by the researchers are the same as the ones that you are using.

Several investigators have questioned the accuracy and reproducibility of measuring cervical motions with a tape measure in the clinical setting, whereas other investigators, Malmström et al[15] and Alaranta et al,[16] continue to use this method. Note that this method of measurement has been deemed doubtful for reproducibility by de Koning et al[17] and as being inaccurate and not to be used in clinical practice by Whitcroft et al.[18] We have included the tape measure in this section because not every clinician has access to other means of measurement. An important aspect of using a tape measure is to mark and use exactly the same landmarks for each repetitive measurement so that changes in range of motion can be obtained.

Testing Position

Place the individual in the sitting position, with the thoracic and lumbar spine well supported against the back of a chair. Feet should be flat on the floor and shoulders should be relaxed with hands resting on the thighs. Position the head in 0 degrees of rotation and lateral flexion.

Stabilization

The testing position helps provide stabilization. During active ROM the examiner may be able to use a free hand to stabilize the shoulder girdle or sternum to prevent forward flexion of the thoracic spine. During passive ROM the examiner's hands are involved with the measurement, so if additional stabilization is needed, a strap placed around the chest and the back of the chair may be used.

Testing Motion: Passive ROM

Put one hand on the back of the individual's head and with the other hand hold the individual's chin. Push gently but firmly on the back of the individual's head to move the head anteriorly. Pull the individual's chin in toward the chest to move head through flexion ROM (see Fig. 11.14). The end of the ROM occurs when resistance to further motion is felt and further attempts at flexion cause forward flexion of the trunk.

Testing Motion: Active ROM

Ask individual to tuck chin in toward the chest and bend the head forward until resistance to further motion is felt or the trunk begins to flex forward.

Tape Measure Alignment

1. In the starting testing position, use a skin marking pencil to place marks on the following landmarks: the lower edge of the sternal notch and the middle of the tip of the chin.
2. At the end of the ROM measure the distance between the mark on the **tip of the chin** and the mark at the lower edge of the **sternal notch.** Make sure that the individual's mouth remains closed during the motion (Fig. 11.17).

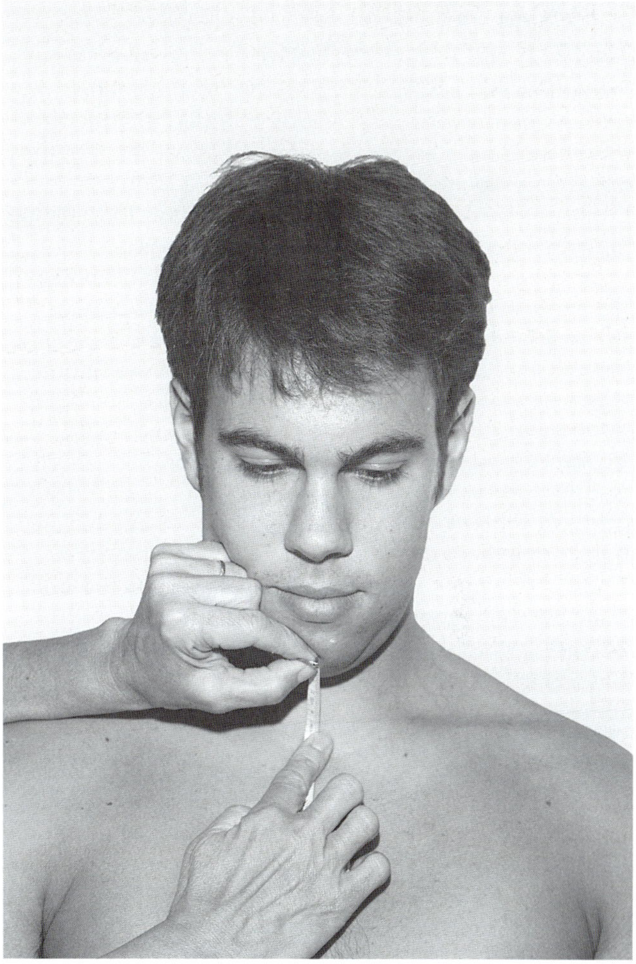

FIGURE 11.17 The examiner uses a tape measure for cervical flexion by determining the distance from the tip of the chin to the sternal notch.

CERVICAL FLEXION: DOUBLE INCLINOMETERS

The AMA's fifth edition of the *Guides to Evaluation of Permanent Impairment*[19] recommended the use of double inclinometers for determining impairment of the spine. However, the most recent (2008) edition of the *Guides* no longer uses ROM as a basis for defining impairment but does support its use to monitor clinical progress in individuals.[20] Double and single inclinometers are relatively easy to use. The single inclinometer, discussed in the next section, has shown good reliability and validity (see Research Findings section). Additional research needs to be performed using double inclinometers. Normal ROM values for adults measured with double inclinometers are about 50 degrees.[14,19]

Testing Position

Place the individual in the sitting position, with the thoracic and lumbar spine well supported by the back of a chair. Feet should be flat on the floor and arms relaxed on thighs. Position the head in 0 degrees of rotation and lateral flexion.

Stabilization

The testing position helps provide stabilization. During active ROM the examiner may be able to use a free hand to stabilize the shoulder girdle or sternum to prevent forward flexion of the thoracic spine. During passive ROM the examiner's hands are involved with the measurement, so if additional stabilization is needed a strap placed around the chest and the back of the chair may be used.

Testing Motion: Active ROM

Instruct the individual to tuck in chin and then bring the head forward into flexion while keeping the trunk straight.

Normal End-Feel

Refer to Cervical Flexion: Universal Goniometer.

Double Inclinometer Alignment

Both inclinometers must be zeroed after they are positioned on the individual and prior to the beginning of the measurement. To zero the inclinometer, adjust the rotating dial so the bubble or pointer is at 0 degrees on the scale.

1. Place **one inclinometer** directly over the spinous process of the T1 vertebra, making sure that the inclinometer is adjusted to 0 degrees (Fig. 11.18). The examiner should maintain firm contact between the inclinometer and the vertebra throughout the motion.
2. Place the **second inclinometer** firmly on the top of the head, making sure that the inclinometer is adjusted to 0 degrees. The examiner should maintain firm contact between the inclinometer and the head throughout the motion.
3. At the end of the motion, read the degrees on the dials of each inclinometer. The ROM is the difference between the readings of the two inclinometers (Fig. 11.19).

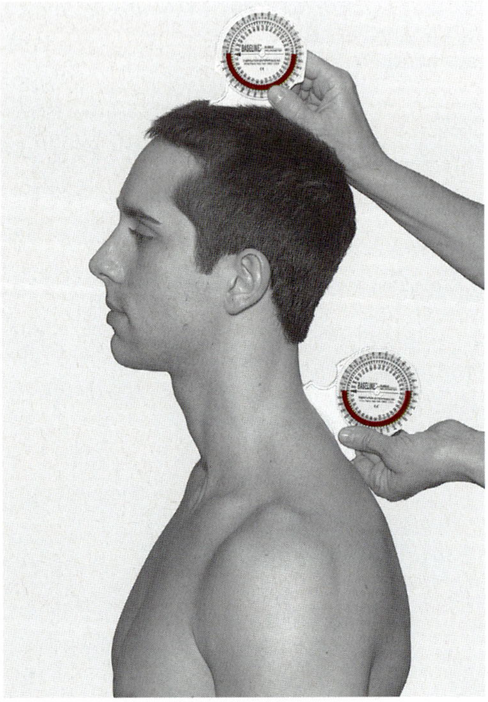

FIGURE 11.18 Dual inclinometer alignment in the starting position for measuring cervical flexion ROM. Note that the lower inclinometer is positioned over the T1 vertebra. Red coloring has been added to the photograph to call attention to the liquid in the fluid inclinometer.

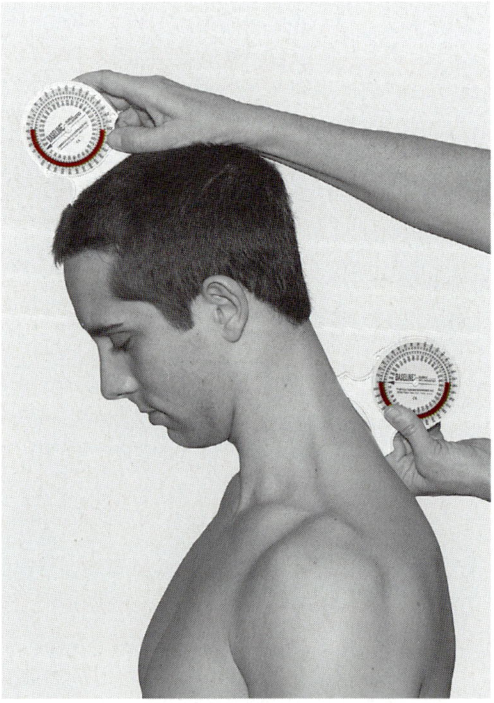

FIGURE 11.19 Double inclinometer alignment at the end of the cervical range of motion.

CERVICAL FLEXION: SINGLE INCLINOMETER

Flexion ROM measurements from various sources using a single inclinometer range from 57 degrees[21] to 90 degrees.[22] See Table 11.3 in the Research Findings section for additional normal values, including measurements taken with a Myrin single inclinometer that is attached with a strap to the head.

Testing Position

Place the individual in the sitting position, with the thoracic and lumbar spine well supported by the back of a chair. Feet should be flat on the floor and shoulders relaxed with hands on the thighs. Position the head in 0 degrees of rotation and lateral flexion.

Stabilization

The testing position helps provide stabilization. During active ROM the examiner may be able to use a free hand to stabilize the shoulder girdle or sternum to prevent forward flexion of the thoracic spine. During passive ROM the examiner's hands are involved with the measurement, so if additional stabilization is needed a strap can be placed around the chest and the back of the chair.

Testing Motion: Active ROM

Instruct the individual to tuck chin in and bring the head forward into flexion while keeping the trunk straight.

Normal End-Feel

Refer to Cervical Flexion: Universal Goniometer.

Single Inclinometer Alignment

1. Place the inclinometer on the top of the individual's head, making sure that the dial is adjusted to 0 degrees. The examiner should maintain firm contact between the inclinometer and the individual's head throughout the motion (Fig. 11.20).
2. At the end of the motion, read and record the degrees on the dial of the inclinometer (Fig. 11.21).

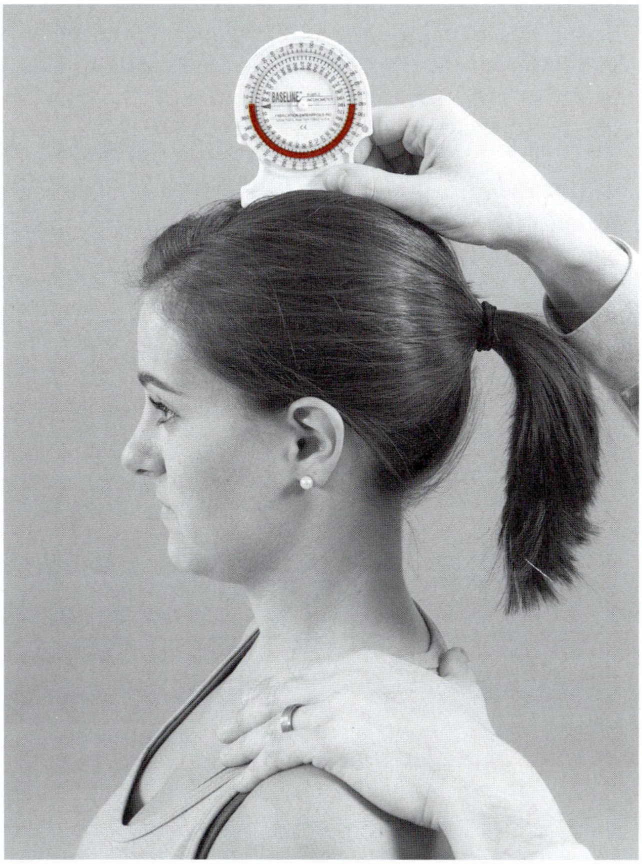

FIGURE 11.20 Single inclinometer alignment in the 0 starting position for measuring cervical flexion ROM. Position individual in the seated position. Place the inclinometer on vertex of the head and rotate the dial so that the fluid is aligned with zero.

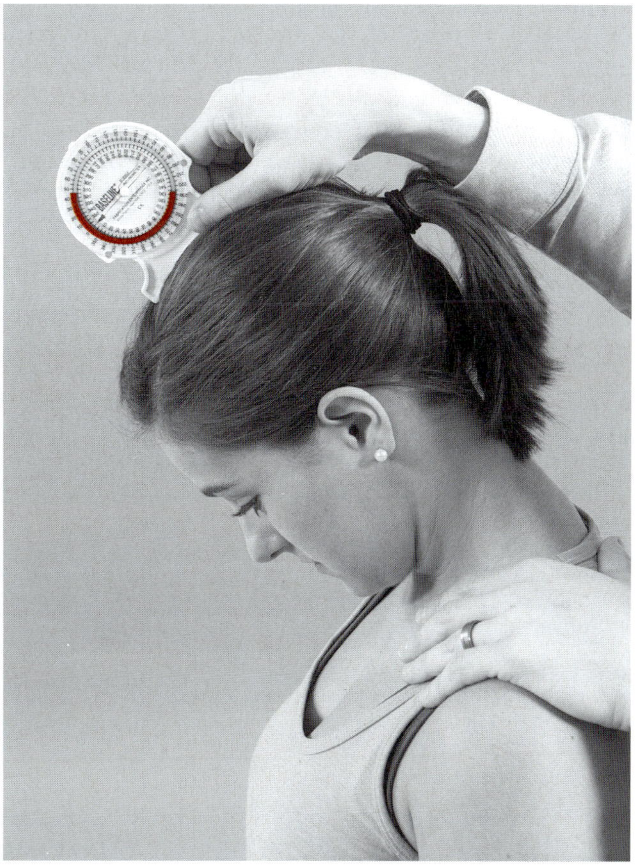

FIGURE 11.21 Ask individual to bend neck forward toward the chest, keeping the chin as close to the chest as possible. Make sure that the spine and trunk are stabilized during the motion. Hold inclinometer firmly on the head throughout the ROM.

CERVICAL FLEXION: CERVICAL RANGE OF MOTION DEVICE

The mean flexion ROM using the cervical range of motion (CROM) device ranges from 64 degrees in subjects aged 11 to 19 years, to 40 degrees in older adults aged 80 to 89 years.[12] For additional flexion ROM values by age and gender, refer to Tousignant et al[23] in Table 11.1 in the Research Findings section; to Youdas et al[12] in Table 11.3; and to Nilsson et al[24] for full cycle flexion-extension ROM in Table 11.6.

Familiarize yourself with the CROM device prior to beginning the measurement. The CROM device consists of a headpiece that supports two gravity inclinometers and a compass inclinometer. One gravity inclinometer is located on the side of the head in the sagittal plane and is used to measure flexion and extension. The other gravity inclinometer is located over the forehead in the frontal plane and is used to measure lateral flexion. The compass inclinometer has a gravity needle and is situated over the top of the head in the transverse plane and is used to measure rotation. A neckpiece containing two strong magnets is placed around the individual's neck when using the compass inclinometer to ensure accuracy.

Testing Position

The individual should be carefully positioned by being seated in a straight back chair with midback region in contact with the back of the chair. Feet should be flat on the floor and shoulders should be relaxed with hands resting on thighs.

Stabilization

The testing position helps provide stabilization. During active ROM the examiner may be able to use a free hand to stabilize the shoulder girdle or sternum to prevent forward flexion of the thoracic spine. During passive ROM the examiner's hands are involved with the measurement, so if additional stabilization is needed, a strap can be placed around the chest and the back of the chair to stabilize the thoracic spine and prevent it from contributing to the motion.

CROM Device Alignment

1. Place the CROM device carefully on the individual's head so that the nosepiece is on the bridge of the nose and the Velcro strap fits snugly across the back of the head (Fig. 11.22). One size instrument fits all, and it is relatively easy for an examiner to obtain a good fit.[25]
2. Position the head so that the inclinometer on the side of the head reads 0 degrees and check to see that the ears, earlobes, and nares are horizontal and mouth and chin are vertically aligned.
3. At the end of the motion, read the dial on the inclinometer on the side of the head and record the reading.

Testing Motion: Passive ROM

Push gently but firmly on the back of the individual's head to move it anteriorly and inferiorly through flexion ROM (Fig. 11.23). At the end of the motion, read the dial on the inclinometer on the side of the head and record the reading.

Testing Motion: Active ROM

Instruct the individual to bring the head forward into flexion while keeping the trunk straight.

Normal End-Feel

Refer to Cervical Flexion: Universal Goniometer.

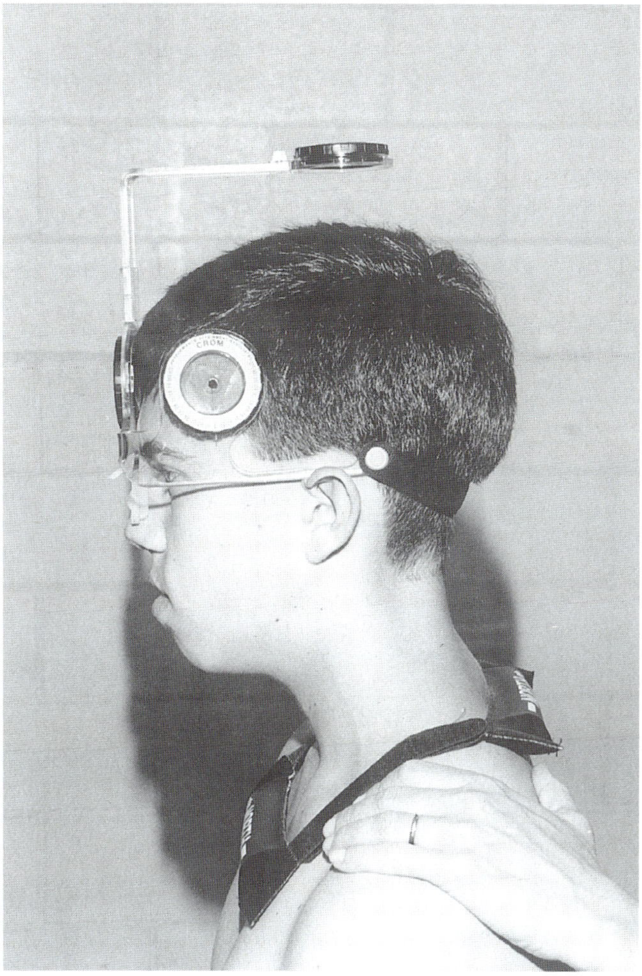

FIGURE 11.22 The CROM device is positioned on the individual's head in the starting position for measuring cervical flexion ROM. The neck piece containing two strong magnets is placed around the individual's neck. The dial on the gravity inclinometer located on the side of the head is at 0 degrees.

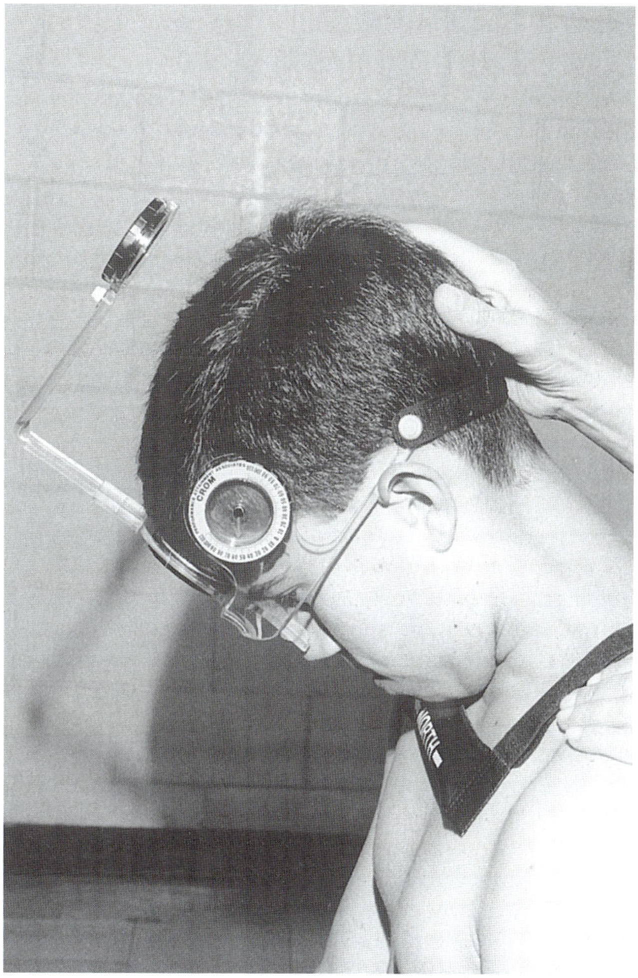

FIGURE 11.23 The examiner is shown stabilizing the trunk with one hand and maintaining the end of the flexion ROM with her other hand.

CERVICAL EXTENSION: UNIVERSAL GONIOMETER

Motion occurs in the sagittal plane around a medial–lateral axis. Mean cervical extension ROM measured with a universal goniometer is about 50 degrees[25] to 70 degrees[2,22] in adults. Refer to Youdas et al[12] in Table 11.1 in the Research Findings section for additional normal extension ROM values.

Testing Position

Place the individual in the sitting position, with the thoracic and lumbar spine well supported by the back of a chair. Position the cervical spine in 0 degrees of rotation and lateral flexion.

Stabilization

Stabilize the shoulder girdle and chest to prevent extension of the thoracic and lumbar spine. Usually, the stabilization is achieved through the cooperation of the individual and support from the back of the chair. A strap placed around the chest and the back of the chair also may be used.

Testing Motion: Passive ROM

Put one hand on the back of the individual's head and with the other hand hold the chin. Push gently but firmly upward and posteriorly on the chin to move the head through the ROM in extension (Fig. 11.24). The end of the ROM occurs when resistance to further motion is felt and further attempts at extension cause extension of the trunk.

Testing Motion: Active ROM

Start in the neutral head position and ask the individual to tuck in the chin and then look up and back as far as possible without moving trunk. The individual should not move shoulders or change the amount of pressure being exerted on the back of the chair.

Normal End-Feel

The normal end-feel is firm owing to the passive tension developed by stretching of the anterior longitudinal ligament, anterior fibers of the annulus fibrosus, zygapophyseal joint capsules, and the following muscles: sternocleidomastoid, longus capitis, longus colli, rectus capitis anterior, and scalenus anterior. Extremes of extension may be limited by contact between the spinous processes.

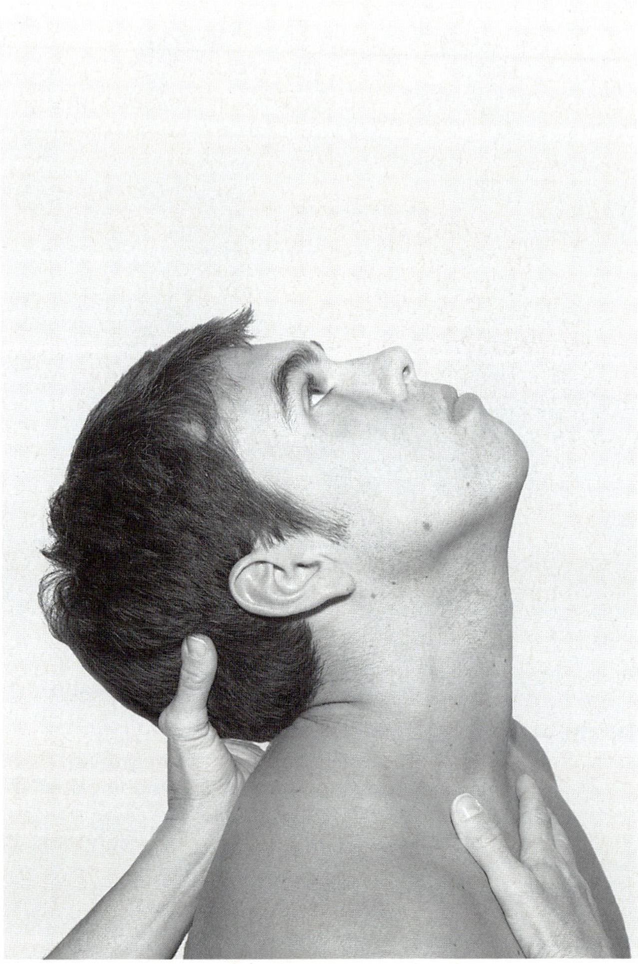

FIGURE 11.24 The end of cervical extension ROM. The examiner helps to prevent cervical rotation and lateral flexion by holding the back of the individual's head.

Goniometer Alignment

See Figures 11.25 and 11.26.

1. Center **fulcrum** of the goniometer over the external auditory meatus.
2. Align **proximal arm** so that it is either perpendicular or parallel to the ground.
3. Align **distal arm** with the base of the nares.

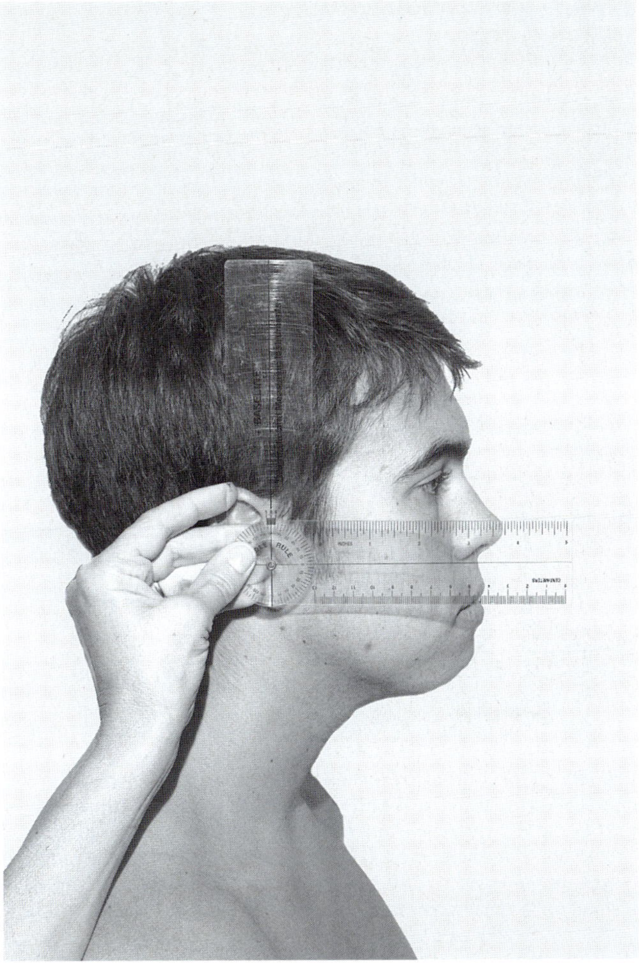

FIGURE 11.25 In the 0 starting position for measuring cervical extension ROM, the goniometer reads 90 degrees. This reading should be transposed and recorded as 0 degrees.

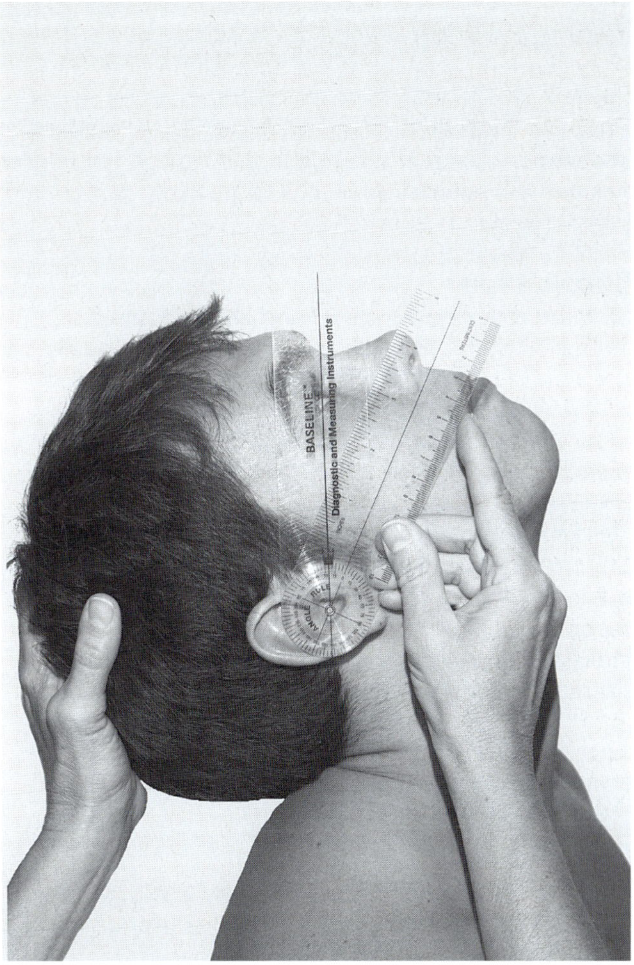

FIGURE 11.26 At the end of the cervical extension, the examiner maintains the perpendicular alignment of the proximal goniometer arm and keeps the distal arm aligned with the base of the nares.

CERVICAL EXTENSION: TAPE MEASURE

The mean cervical extension ROM measured with a tape measure ranges from 18.5 to 22.4 centimeters in adults.[13,14] See Table 11.2 in the Research Findings section for additional information.

Testing Position

Place the individual in the sitting position, with the thoracic and lumbar spine well supported by the back of a chair. Feet should be flat on the floor, shoulders should be relaxed and hands should rest on the thighs. Position the cervical spine in 0 degrees of rotation and lateral flexion.

Stabilization

Stabilize the shoulder girdle and chest to prevent extension of the thoracic and lumbar spine. Usually, the stabilization is achieved through the cooperation of the individual and support from the back of the chair. A strap may be placed around the chest and the back of the chair.

Testing Motion: Active ROM

Start in the neutral head position and ask the individual to tuck in the chin and then look up and back as far as possible without moving trunk. The individual should not move shoulders or change the amount of pressure being exerted on the back of the chair.

Normal End-Feel

Refer to Cervical Extension: Universal Goniometer.

Tape Measure Alignment

1. In the starting testing position, use a skin marking pencil to place marks on the following landmarks: the lower edge of the sternal notch and the middle of the tip of the chin.
2. At the end of the ROM measure the distance between the mark on the **tip of the chin** and the mark at the lower edge of the **sternal notch.** Make sure that the individual's mouth remains closed during the motion (Fig. 11.27).

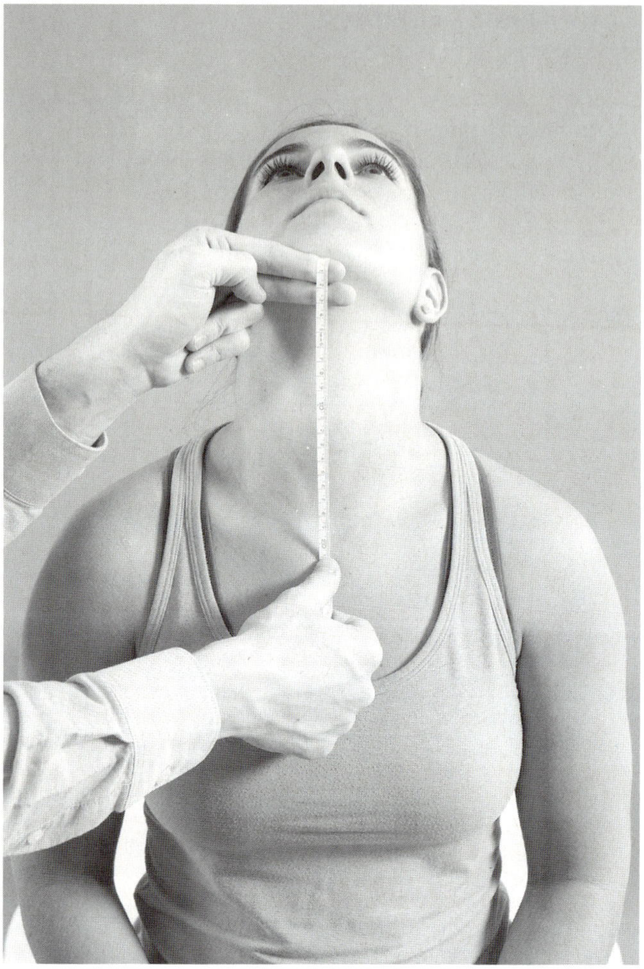

FIGURE 11.27 In the tape measure method for measuring cervical extension, one end of the tape measure is placed on the tip of the individual's chin; the other end is placed at the sternal notch. The distance between the two points of reference is recorded in centimeters. Be sure that the individual's mouth remains closed during the measurement.

CERVICAL EXTENSION: DOUBLE INCLINOMETERS

Testing Position

Place the individual in the sitting position, with the thoracic and lumbar spine well supported by the back of a chair. Hands should be placed on thighs and shoulders should be relaxed. Position the cervical spine in 0 degrees of rotation and lateral flexion.

Stabilization

Stabilize the shoulder girdle and chest to prevent extension of the thoracic and lumbar spine. Usually, the stabilization is achieved through the cooperation of the individual and support from the back of the chair. A strap may be placed around the chest and the back of the chair.

Testing Motion Active ROM

Instruct the individual to move head into extension while keeping the trunk straight.

Normal End-Feel

Refer to Cervical Extension: Universal Goniometer.

Double Inclinometer Alignment

1. Place **one inclinometer** directly over the spine of the scapula or lateral to the T1 vertebra. Adjust the dial of the inclinometer so that it reads 0 degrees. (If the inclinometer is placed over the first thoracic vertebra, it may contact the back of the head in full extension.)
2. Place the **second inclinometer** firmly on the top of the head, making sure that the inclinometer reads 0 degrees (Fig. 11.28).
3. At the end of the motion, read and record the information on the dials of each inclinometer. The ROM is the difference between the readings of the two inclinometers (Fig. 11.29).

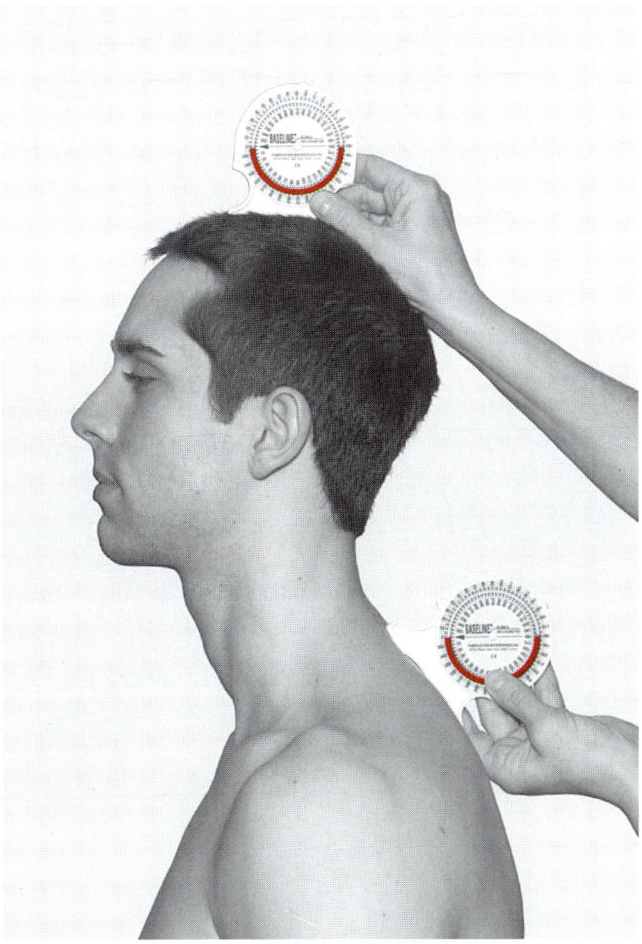

FIGURE 11.28 Double inclinometer alignment in the starting position for measuring cervical ROM. The examiner has zeroed both inclinometers prior to beginning the motion.

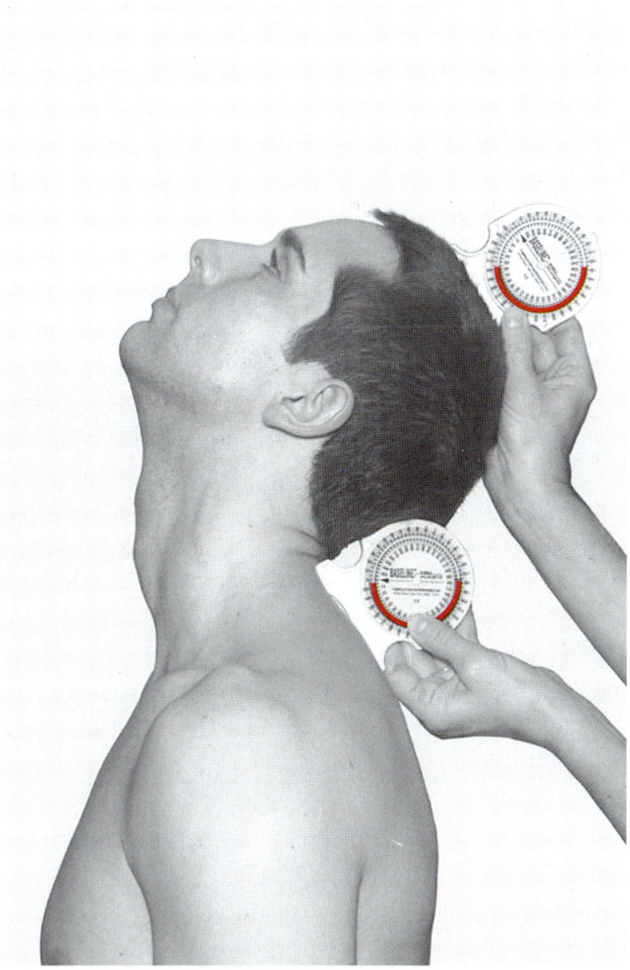

FIGURE 11.29 Double inclinometer at the end of the cervical extension ROM.

CERVICAL EXTENSION: SINGLE INCLINOMETER

The mean normal range of motion value for adults using a single inclinometer is 51 degrees as reported by Pringle.[21] Balogen[14] and Malmström[15] measured cervical extension using the Myrin Single Inclinometer and found means ranging from 64 to 67 degrees. Additional information may be found in Table 11.1 in the Research Findings section.

Testing Position

Place the individual in the sitting position, with the thoracic and lumbar spine well supported by the back of a chair. Hands should rest on thighs and shoulders should be relaxed. The cervical spine should be in 0 degrees of rotation and lateral flexion.

Stabilization

Stabilize the shoulder girdle and chest to prevent extension of the thoracic and lumbar spine. Usually, the stabilization is achieved through the cooperation of the individual and support from the back of the chair. A strap placed around the chest and the back of the chair also may be used.

Testing Motion: Active ROM

Instruct the individual to move head into extension while keeping the trunk straight.

Normal End-Feel

Refer to Cervical Extension: Universal Goniometer.

Single Inclinometer Alignment

1. Place the inclinometer on the top of the individual's head, making sure that the dial is adjusted to 0 degrees. Hold the inclinometer firmly on the individual's head throughout the motion (Fig. 11.30).
2. Instruct the individual to raise chin first and then move head backward as far as possible without moving the trunk (Fig. 11.31).
3. When the individual has reached the end of the motion record the information on the dial of the inclinometer.

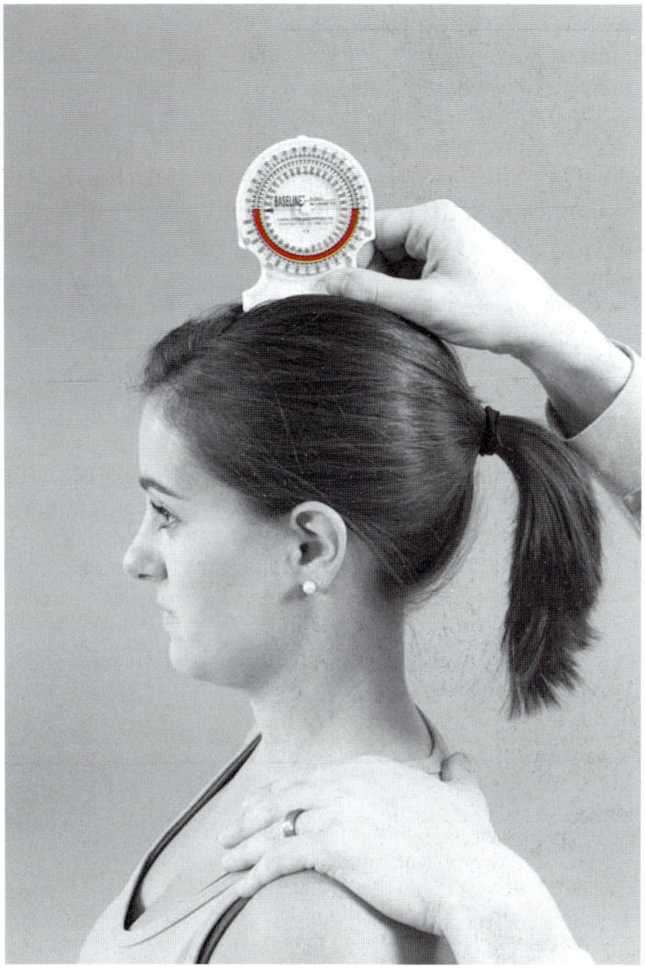

FIGURE 11.30 Single inclinometer in the starting position for measuring cervical extension ROM. Place individual in a seated position and situate single inclinometer on vertex of the head. Move rotating dial so that the fluid is aligned with the point of the arrow and the zero on the dial.

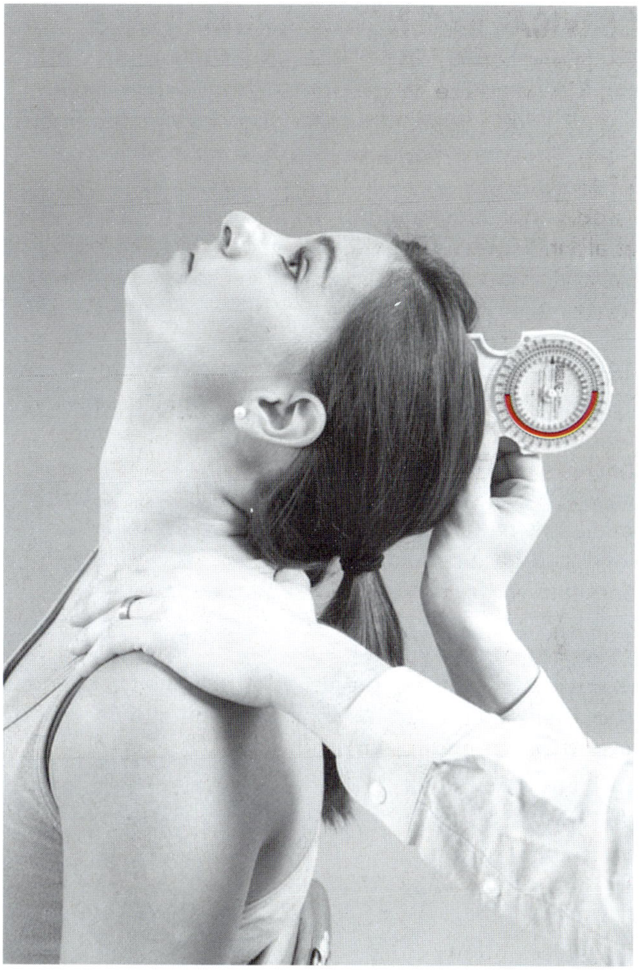

FIGURE 11.31 Hold the inclinometer firmly while individual is asked to move head posteriorly so that the back of the head is as close to the upper back as possible. Read the degrees indicated by the fluid in the inclinometer.

CERVICAL EXTENSION: CROM DEVICE

The mean cervical ROM in extension measured with the CROM device ranges from 86 degrees in males aged 11 to 19 years and to 49 degrees in males aged 80 to 89 years.[12] For additional normal extension ROM values by age and gender, refer to ROM values listed under Tousignant et al[23] in Table 11.1; to Youdas et al[12] in Tables 11.4 and 11.5; and Nilsson et al[24] for full cycle flexion-extension ROM in Table 11.6 in the Research Findings section.

Testing Position

The individual also should be carefully positioned by being seated in a straight back chair with the mid-back region in contact with the back of the chair. Feet should be flat on the floor and shoulders should be relaxed with hands on thighs. The head should be level and gaze should be straight ahead with mouth and chin vertically aligned and eyes horizontal.

Stabilization

A strap or straps may be placed across the chest and shoulders to stabilize the thoracic spine and prevent it from contributing to the motion.

Testing Motion: Passive ROM

Guide the individual's head posteriorly and inferiorly through extension ROM.

Testing Motion: Active ROM

Ask the individual to raise the chin and then move head backward as far as possible until resistance is felt.

Normal End-Feel

Refer to Cervical Extension: Universal Goniometer.

CROM Device Alignment

1. Place the CROM device carefully on the individual's head so that the nosepiece is on the bridge of the nose and the Velcro strap fits snugly across the back of the head (Fig. 11.32).
2. Position the individual's head so that the gravity inclinometer on the side of the head reads 0 degrees.
3. At the end of the motion read the dial on the inclinometer on the side of the head (Fig. 11.33).

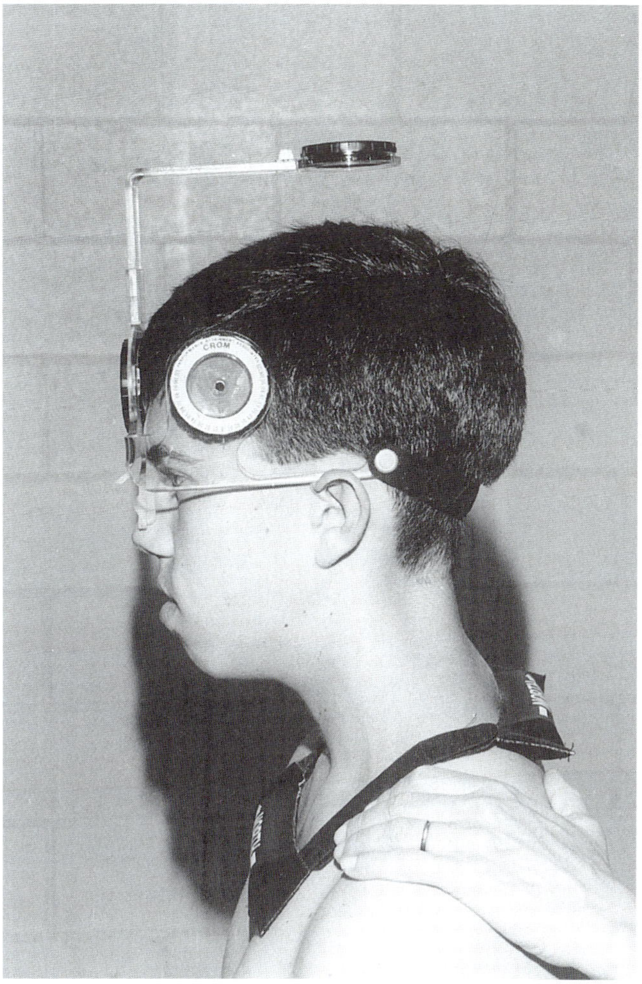

FIGURE 11.32 The individual is positioned in the starting position with the CROM device in place. The gravity inclinometer located at the side of the individual's head is at 0 degrees prior to beginning the motion.

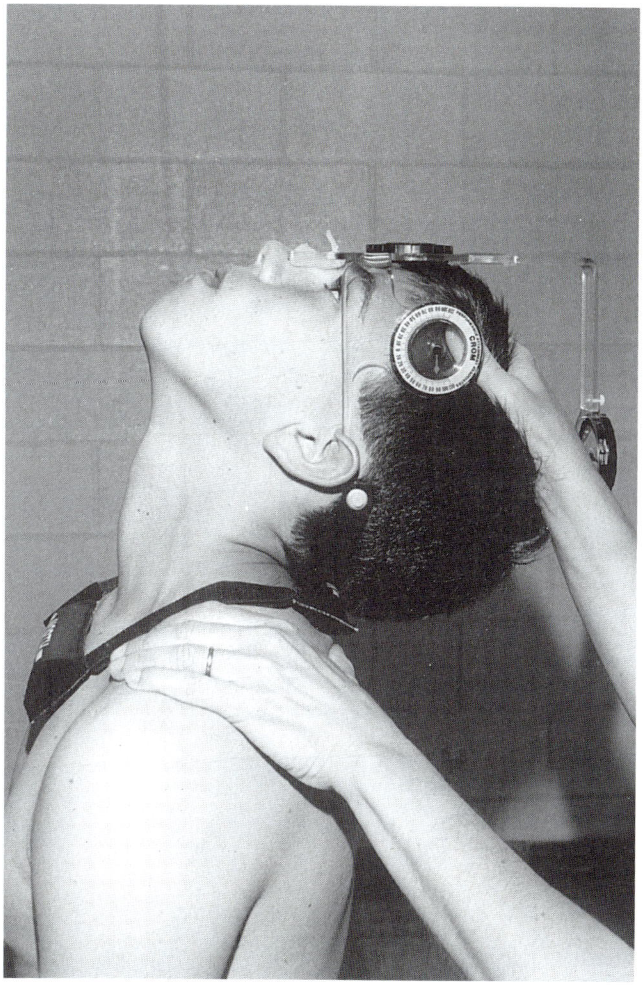

FIGURE 11.33 At the end of the cervical extension ROM, the examiner is stabilizing the trunk with one hand and maintaining the end of the ROM with her other hand on top of the individual's head.

CERVICAL LATERAL FLEXION: UNIVERSAL GONIOMETER

Motion occurs in the frontal plane around an anterior–posterior axis. The mean cervical lateral flexion ROM to one side, measured with a universal goniometer, is about 22 degrees in adults.[26] See Youdas et al[26] in Table 11.1 in the Research Findings section for additional normal ROM values.

Testing Position

The individual also should be carefully positioned by being seated in a straight back chair with the mid-back region in contact with the back of the chair. Feet should be flat on the floor and shoulders should be relaxed with hands on thighs. The cervical spine should be in 0 degrees of flexion, extension, and rotation.

Stabilization

Stabilize the shoulder girdle and chest to prevent lateral flexion of the thoracic and lumbar spine.

Testing Motion: Passive ROM

Hold the individual's head at the top and side (opposite to the direction of the motion). Move the head toward the shoulder. Do not allow the head to rotate, forward flex, or extend during the motion (Fig. 11.34). The end of the motion occurs when resistance to motion is felt and attempts to produce additional motion cause lateral trunk flexion.

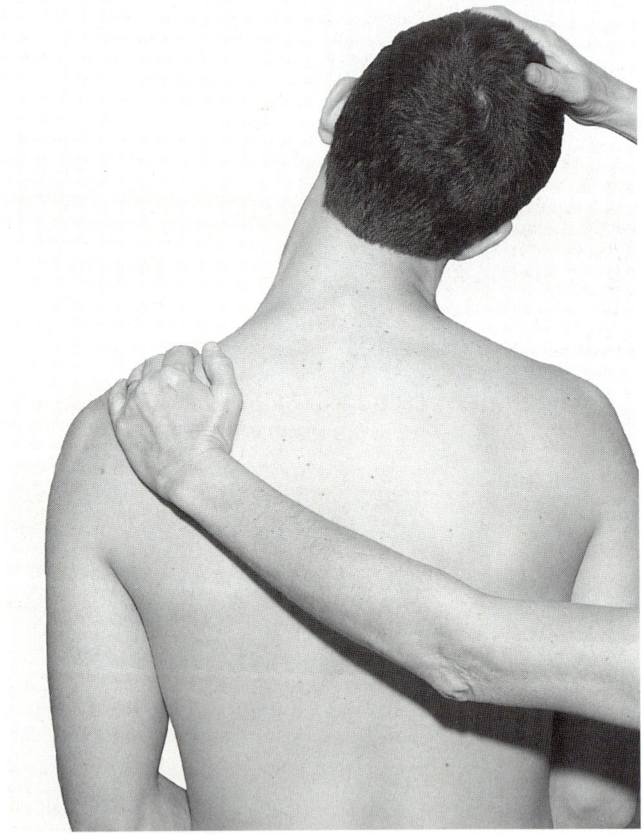

FIGURE 11.34 The end of the cervical spine lateral flexion ROM. The examiner's hand holds the individual's left shoulder to prevent lateral flexion of the thoracic and lumbar spine. The examiner's other hand maintains cervical lateral flexion by pulling the individual's head laterally.

Testing Motion: Active ROM

Direct the individual to try to touch the ear to the shoulder without moving the head forward, rotating, or extending it during the motion.

Normal End-Feel

The normal end-feel is firm owing to the passive tension developed in the intertransverse ligaments, the lateral annulus fibrosus fibers, and the following contralateral muscles: longus capitis, longus colli, scalenus anterior, and sternocleidomastoid.

Goniometer Alignment

See Figures 11.35 and 11.36.

1. Center **fulcrum** of the goniometer over the spinous process of the C7 vertebra.
2. Align **proximal arm** with the spinous processes of the thoracic vertebrae so that the arm is perpendicular to the ground.
3. Align **distal arm** with the dorsal midline of the head, using the occipital protuberance for reference.

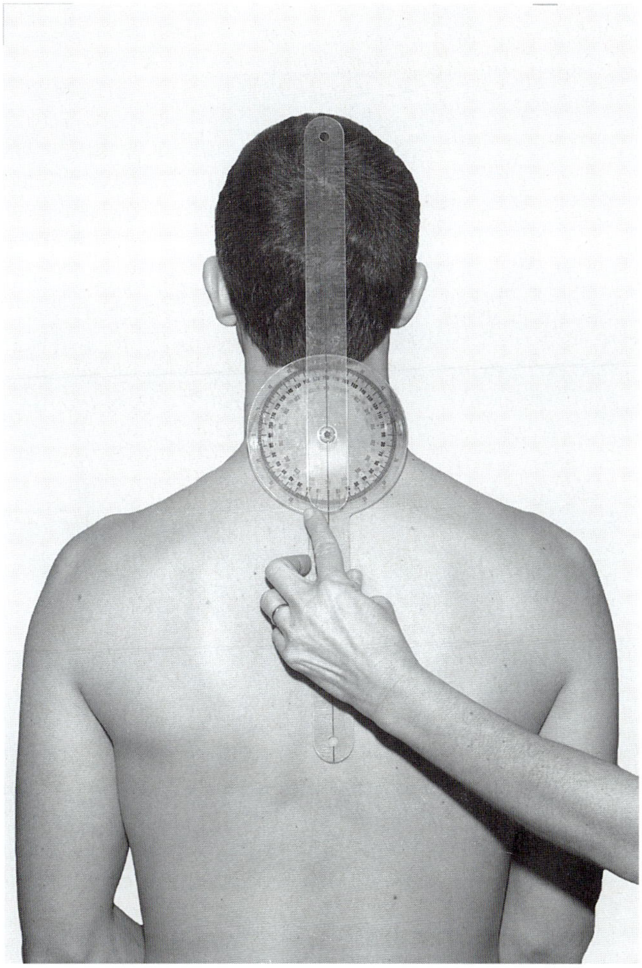

FIGURE 11.35 In the starting position for measuring cervical lateral flexion ROM, the proximal goniometer arm is perpendicular to the floor.

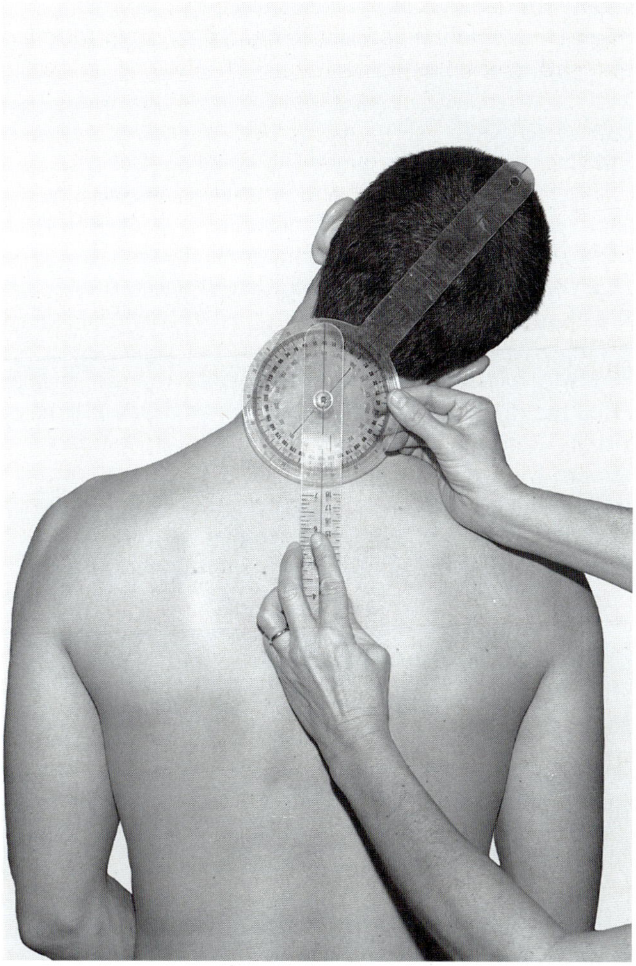

FIGURE 11.36 At the end of the cervical lateral flexion ROM, the examiner maintains alignment of the proximal goniometer arm.

CERVICAL LATERAL FLEXION: TAPE MEASURE

The mean cervical lateral flexion ROM measured with a tape measure ranges from about 11 to 13 centimeters for subjects 14 to 31 years of age. Refer to Table 11.2 in the Research Findings section for additional information on normal ROM values.

Testing Position

Place the individual in the sitting position, with the thoracic and lumbar spine well supported by the back of a chair. Feet should be flat on the floor, shoulders should be relaxed, and hands should rest on the thighs. Position the cervical spine in 0 degrees of rotation and lateral flexion.

Stabilization

Stabilize the shoulder girdle and chest to prevent extension of the thoracic and lumbar spine. Usually, the stabilization is achieved through the cooperation of the individual and support from the back of the chair. A strap placed around the chest and the back of the chair also may be used.

Testing Motion: Passive Motion

Hold the individual's head at the top and side (opposite to the direction of the motion). Move the head toward the shoulder. Do not allow the head to rotate, forward flex, or extend during the motion. The end of the motion occurs when resistance to motion is felt and attempts to produce additional motion cause lateral flexion.

Testing Motion: Active ROM

Direct the individual to try to touch the ear to the shoulder without moving the head forward, rotating, or extending it during the motion.

Normal End-Feel

Refer to Cervical Lateral Flexion: Universal Goniometer.

Tape Measure Alignment

Use a skin marking pencil to place marks on the individual's mastoid process and on the lateral tip of the acromial process. Measure the distance between the two marks at the end of cervical lateral flexion ROM (Fig. 11.37).

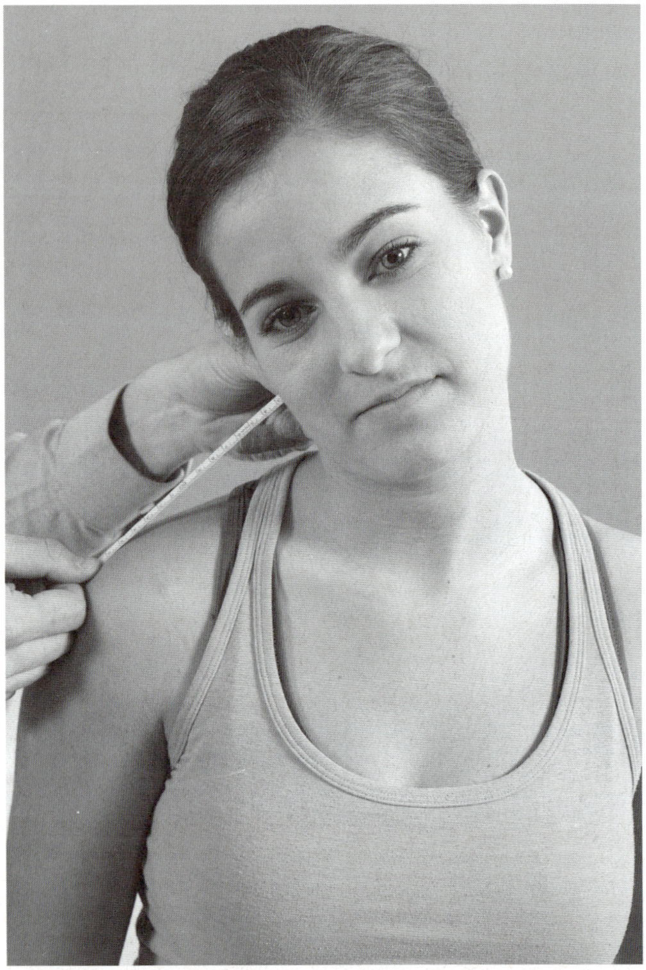

FIGURE 11.37 A tape measure is being used to measure the distance between the mastoid process and tip of the acromion process at the end cervical lateral flexion ROM.

CERVICAL LATERAL FLEXION: DOUBLE INCLINOMETERS

Testing Position

Position the individual in a sitting position with feet flat on the floor and shoulders relaxed with hands on thighs. Clothing should be arranged to expose the T1 vertebra so that the inclinometer can be positioned directly over the vertebra.

Stabilization

Stabilize the shoulder girdle and chest to prevent extension of the thoracic and lumbar spine. Usually, the stabilization is achieved through the cooperation of the individual and support from the back of the chair. A strap placed around the chest and the back of the chair also may be used.

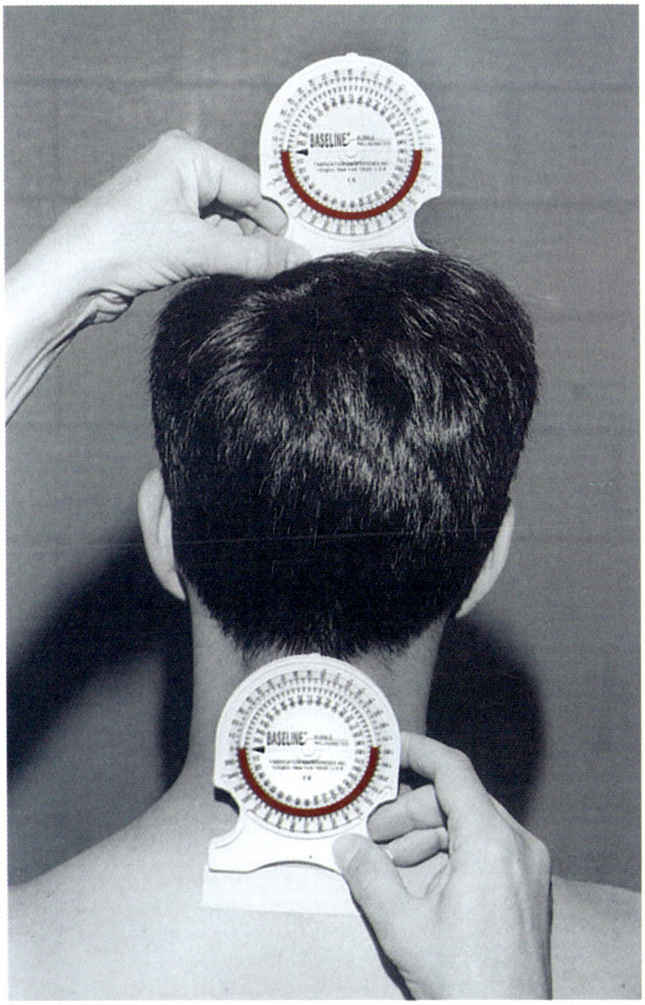

FIGURE 11.38 In the starting position for measuring cervical lateral flexion ROM with dual inclinometers, one inclinometer is positioned at the level of the spinous process of the T1 vertebra. A piece of tape has been placed at that level to help align the inclinometer. The examiner has zeroed both the inclinometers prior to beginning the motion.

Testing Motion: Active Motion

Instruct the individual to try to touch the ear to the shoulder while keeping the trunk straight and shoulders relaxed. The end of the motion occurs when resistance to motion is felt and attempts to produce additional motion cause lateral flexion of the trunk.

Normal End-Feel

Refer to Cervical Lateral Flexion: Universal Goniometer.

Double Inclinometer Alignment

1. Position **one inclinometer** directly over the spinous process of the T1 vertebra. Adjust the rotating dial so that the bubble is at 0 on the scale (Fig. 11.38).
2. Place the **second inclinometer** firmly on the top of the individual's head and adjust the dial so that it reads 0.
3. At the end of the motion, read and record the information on the dials of each inclinometer. The ROM is the difference between the two inclinometers (Fig. 11.39).

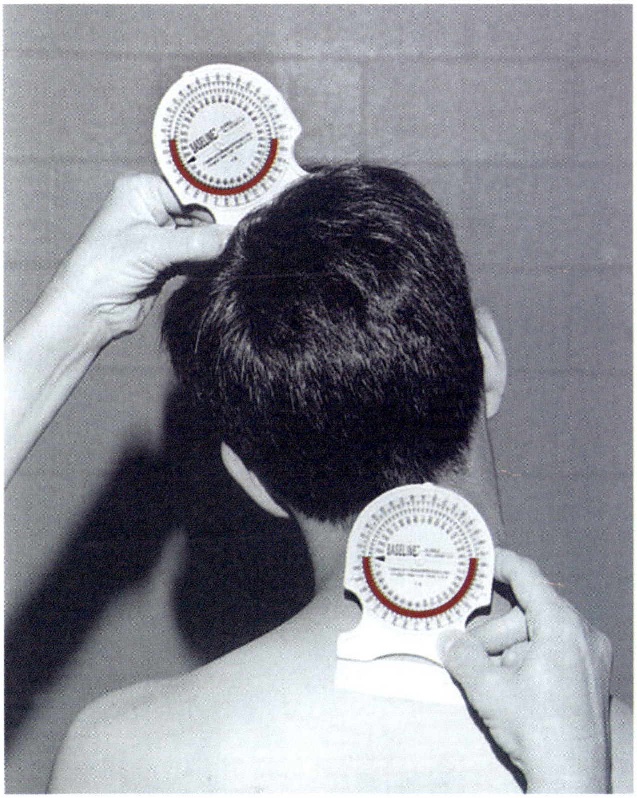

FIGURE 11.39 Hold the inclinometer firmly on the head while the individual is directed to tilt the head to the left by bringing the ear as close as possible to the top of the left shoulder. Repeat motion to the right. Both shoulders should be relaxed during the motion.

CERVICAL LATERAL FLEXION: SINGLE INCLINOMETER

Lateral flexion ROM for adults measured with a single inclinometer is about 48 degrees as described by Pringle.[20] Lateral flexion measured by Balogen et al[14] and Malmström et al[15] with a Myrin Single Inclinometer was 41 to 42 degrees. See Table 11.1 for additional information for ROM values using a Myrin Single Inclinometer.

Testing Position

Position the individual in a sitting position with feet flat on the floor and shoulders relaxed with hands on the thighs.

Testing Motion: Active ROM

Instruct the individual to tilt the head sidewise as if the person were going to touch the ear to the shoulder while keeping the trunk straight. The end of the motion occurs when resistance to motion is felt and attempts to produce additional motion cause lateral flexion of the trunk.

Inclinometer Alignment

1. Position the inclinometer on the top of the individual's head. Adjust the dial so that the bubble is on zero (Fig. 11.40).
2. Hold the inclinometer firmly throughout the motion.
3. At the end of the motion read the dial on the inclinometer and record the number of degrees (Fig. 11.41).

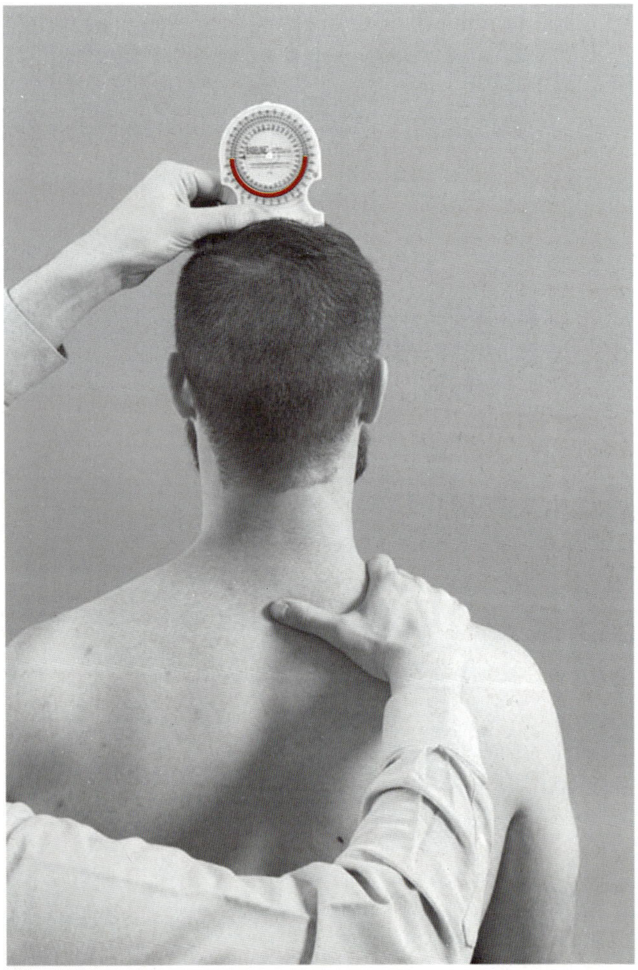

FIGURE 11.40 The starting position for measuring cervical lateral flexion ROM with a single inclinometer. Place individual in a seated position and situate inclinometer on the vertex of the head. Move rotating dial so that the fluid is aligned with the point of the arrow and the zero on the dial.

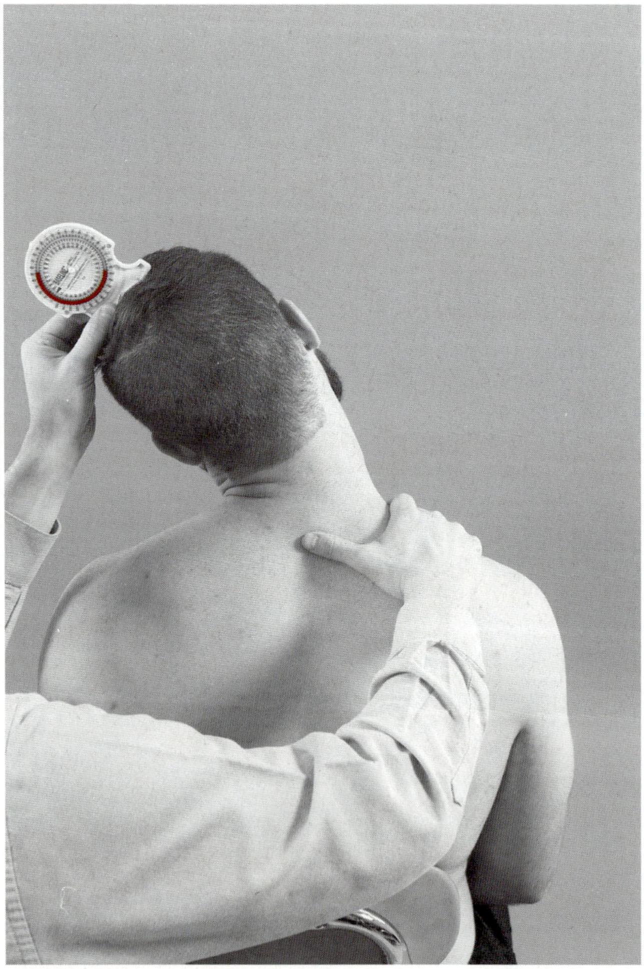

FIGURE 11.41 Hold the inclinometer firmly on the head while the individual is directed to tilt the head to the left by bringing the ear as close as possible to the top of the left shoulder. Repeat motion to the right. Both shoulders should be relaxed during the motion.

CERVICAL LATERAL FLEXION: CROM DEVICE

The ROM in lateral flexion using the CROM device varies from a mean of 45 degrees in individuals aged 11 to 19 years, to a mean of 24 degrees in male subjects and 26 degrees in female subjects aged 80 to 89 years.[12] For additional normal lateral flexion ROM values by age and gender, see Tousignant et al[23] in Table 11.1; Youdas et al[12] in Tables 11.4 and 11.5; and Nilsson et al[24] for full cycle lateral flexion ROM in Table 11.7 in the Research Findings section.

Testing Position

The individual should be carefully positioned by being seated in a straight back chair with the midback region in contact with the back of the chair. Feet should be flat on the floor and shoulders should be relaxed with hands on thighs or knees. The head should be level with gaze straight ahead, mouth and chin vertically aligned, and eyes horizontal. A strap or straps should be placed across the chest and shoulders to stabilize the thoracic spine and prevent it from contributing to the motion.

CROM Device Alignment[27]

1. Place the CROM device on the individual's head so that the nosepiece is on the bridge of the nose and the band fits snugly across the back of the subject's head.
2. Position the individual in the testing position as described above and be sure that the gravity inclinometer on the front of the CROM device reads 0 degrees (Fig. 11.42).

Testing Motion: Passive ROM

Guide the individual's head into lateral flexion (Fig. 11.43). At the end of the motion, read the dial located in front of the forehead and record the number of degrees.

Testing Motion: Active ROM

Ask the individual to tilt the head to the side without moving the head forward, rotating it, or extending it. At the end of the motion, read the dial located in front of the forehead and record the number of degrees.

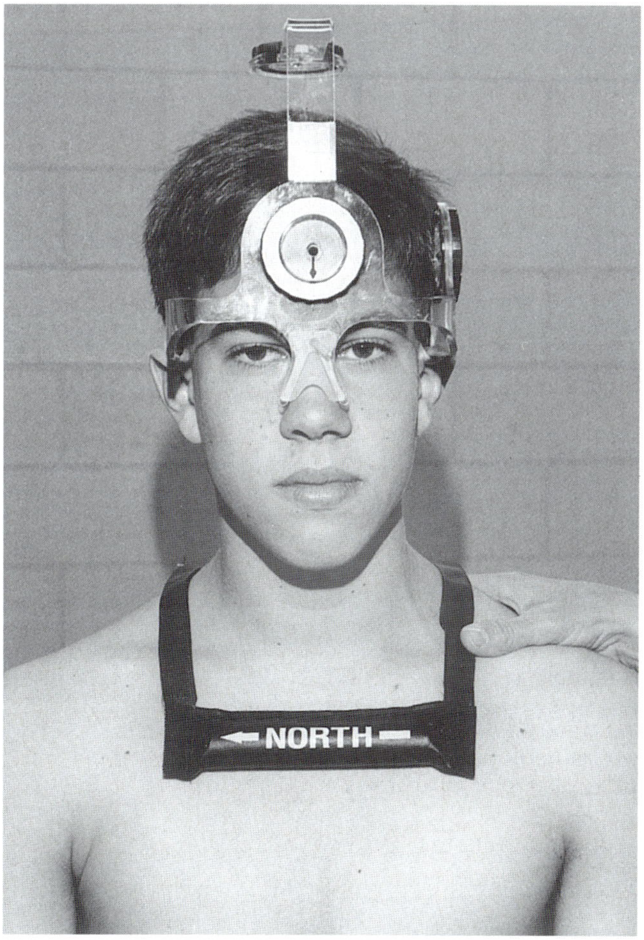

FIGURE 11.42 The individual is placed in the starting position for measuring cervical lateral flexion ROM with the CROM device. The inclinometer is located in front of the individual's forehead and is zeroed before starting the motion.

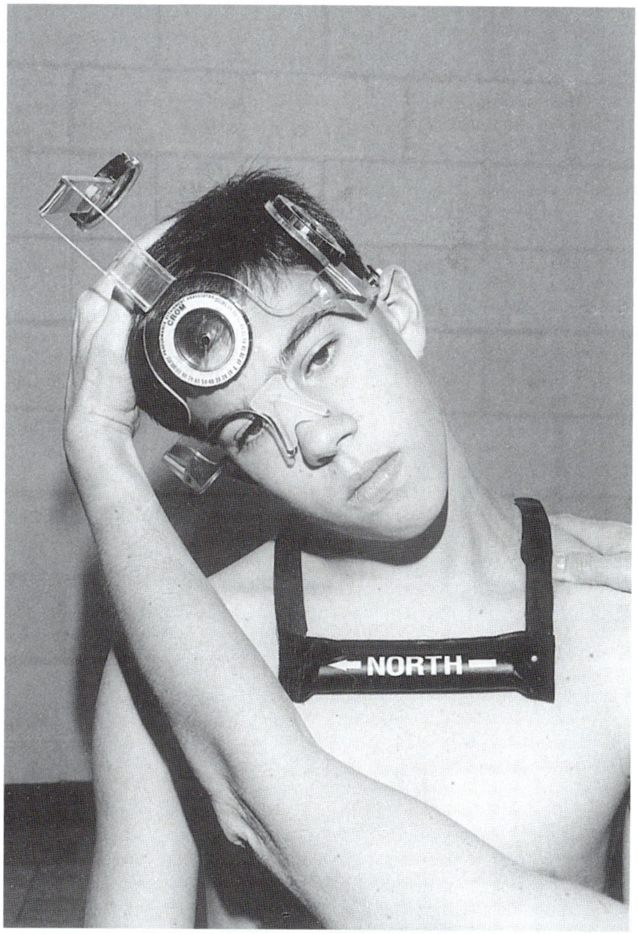

FIGURE 11.43 At the end of lateral flexion ROM with the CROM device, the examiner is stabilizing the individual's shoulder with one hand and maintaining the end of the ROM with her other hand on the individual's head.

CERVICAL ROTATION: UNIVERSAL GONIOMETER

Motion occurs in the transverse plane around a vertical axis. The mean cervical ROM in rotation measured with a universal goniometer is about 50 degrees in adults.[26] See Youdas et al.[26] in Table 11.1 in the Research Findings section for additional information. Magee[2] reports that the ROM in rotation is between 70 and 90 degrees but cautions that cervical rotation past 50 degrees may lead to kinking of the contralateral vertebral artery. The ipsilateral artery may kink at 45 degrees of rotation.[2]

Testing Position

Place the individual sitting, with the thoracic and lumbar spine well supported by the back of the chair. Position the cervical spine in 0 degrees of flexion, extension, and lateral flexion.

Stabilization

Stabilize the shoulder girdle and chest to prevent rotation of the thoracic and lumbar spine. A strap across the chest may be used to keep the trunk from rotating.

Testing Motion: Passive ROM

Grasp the individual's chin and rotate the head by turning the chin toward the shoulder, as shown in Figure 11.44. The end of the ROM occurs when resistance to movement is felt and further movement causes rotation of the trunk.

Testing Motion: Active ROM

Ask the individual to rotate the head by turning the chin toward the shoulder without moving the trunk. Stabilize as directed above.

Normal End-Feel

The normal end-feel is firm owing to stretching of the alar ligament, the fibers of the zygapophyseal joint capsules, and the following contralateral muscles: longus capitis, longus colli, and scalenus anterior. Passive tension in the ipsilateral sternocleidomastoid may limit extremes of rotation.

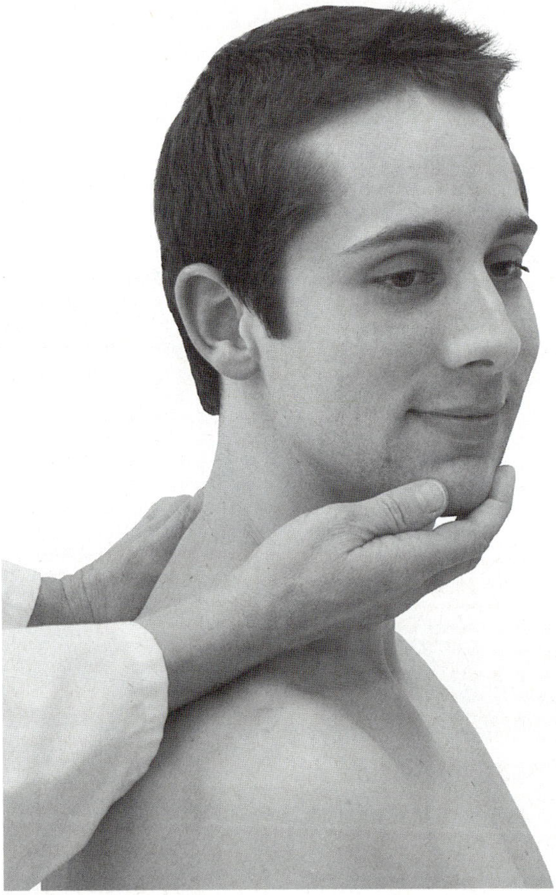

FIGURE 11.44 The end of the cervical rotation ROM. One of the examiner's hands maintains rotation and prevents cervical flexion and extension. The examiner's other hand is placed on the individual's left shoulder to prevent rotation of the thoracic and lumbar spine.

Goniometer Alignment

See Figures 11.45 and 11.46.

1. Center **fulcrum** of the goniometer over the center of the cranial aspect of the head.
2. Align **proximal arm** parallel to an imaginary line between the left and right acromial processes.
3. Align **distal arm** with the tip of the nose.

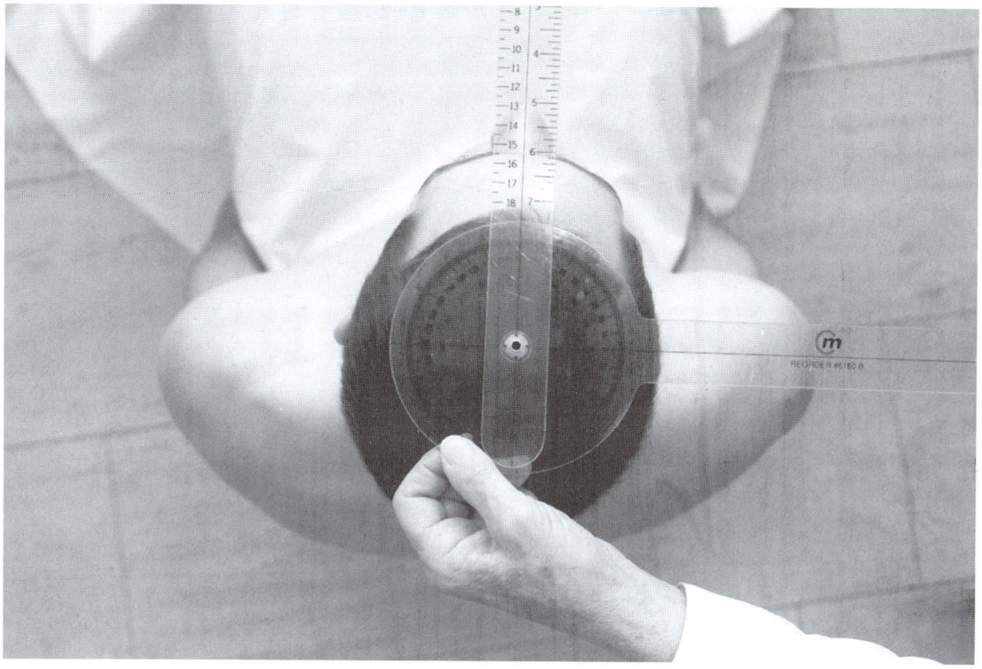

FIGURE 11.45 To align the goniometer at the starting position for measuring cervical rotation ROM with a goniometer, the examiner stands in back of the individual who is seated in a low chair.

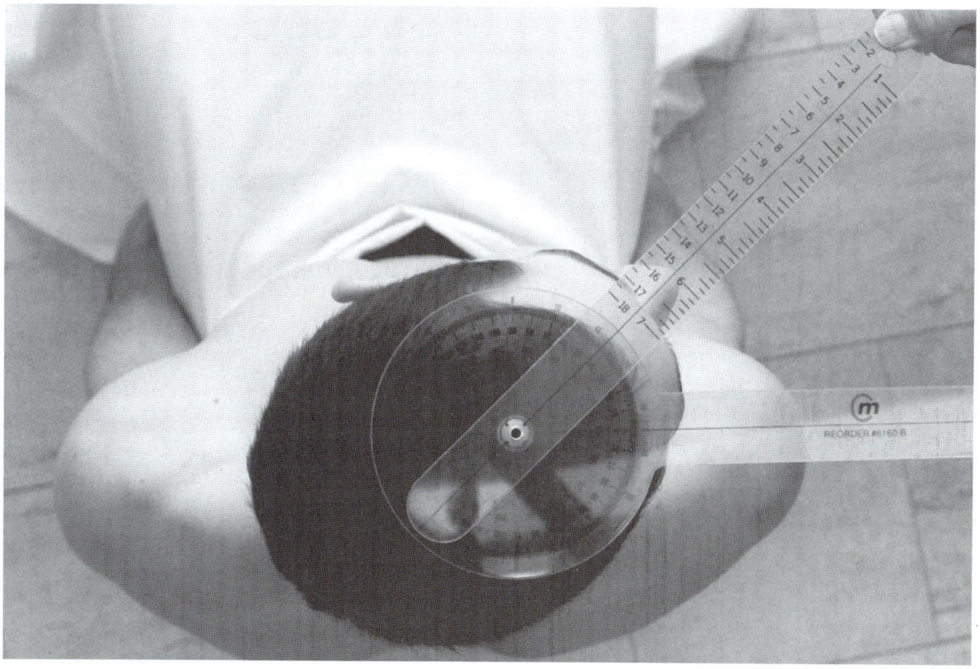

FIGURE 11.46 At the end of the range of right cervical rotation, one of the examiner's hands maintains alignment of the distal goniometer arm with the tip of the individual's nose. The examiner's other hand keeps the proximal arm aligned parallel to the imaginary line between the acromial processes.

CERVICAL ROTATION: TAPE MEASURE

The mean cervical rotation ROM to the left measured with a tape measure ranges from 11.0 to 13.2 centimeters in 14- to 31-year-olds.[13,14] See Table 11.2 in the Research Section for more information.

Use a skin marking pencil to place marks on the tip of the chin and the acromial process. Have the individual look straight ahead and then turn the head to the right as far as possible without rotating the trunk. Measure the distance between the two marks at the end of the motion (Fig. 11.47). Have the individual return the head to the neutral starting position and then turn the head as far to the left as possible without rotating the trunk.

CERVICAL ROTATION: SINGLE INCLINOMETER

According to the AMA,[19] the normal ROM for rotation using a single inclinometer is 80 degrees to each side. Malmström et al[15] found that left and right rotation in a group of 60 males and females aged 22 to 58 years was 76 degrees, and Alaranta et al[16] obtained 75 degrees as the average for a group of 508 white- and blue-collar workers aged 35 to 54 years.

Testing Position

Place the individual supine with the head in neutral rotation, lateral flexion, flexion, and extension.

Inclinometer Alignment

1. Place the inclinometer in the middle of the individual's forehead, and zero the inclinometer (Fig. 11.48).
2. Hold the inclinometer firmly while the head moves through rotation ROM (Fig. 11.49).

Testing Motion

Instruct the individual to roll his or her head into rotation without tilting the head forward, backward, or lateral. The ROM can be read on the inclinometer at the end of the ROM.

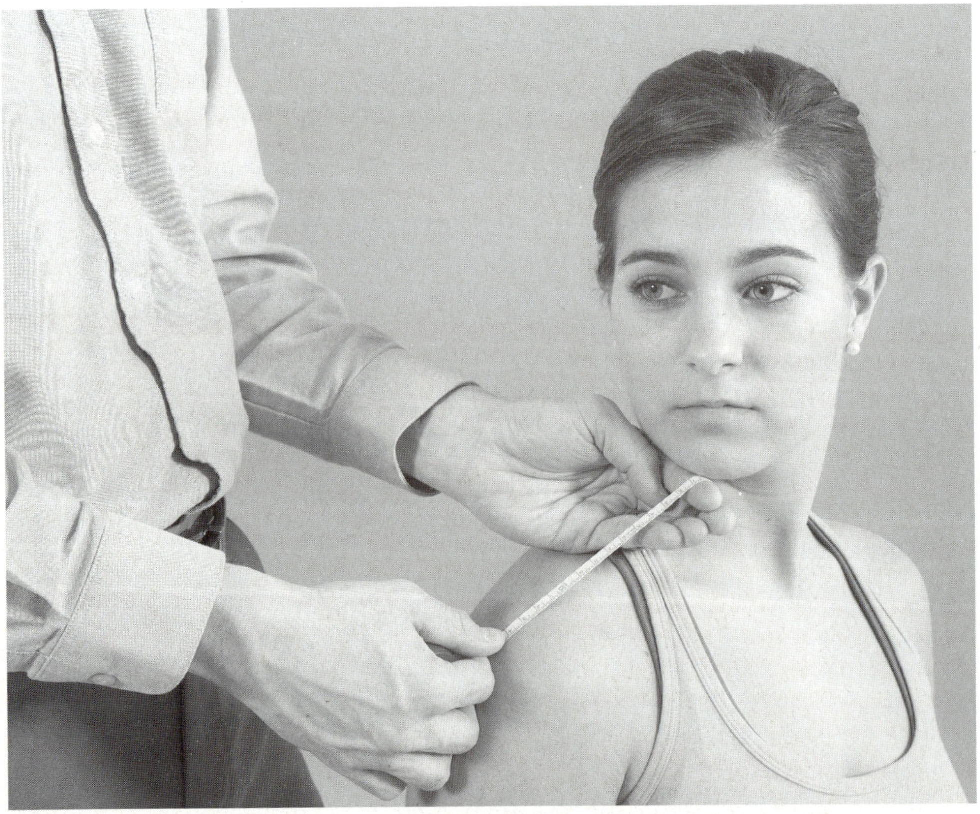

FIGURE 11.47 At the end of the right cervical ROM, the examiner is using a tape measure to determine the distance between the tip of the individual's chin and her right acromial process.

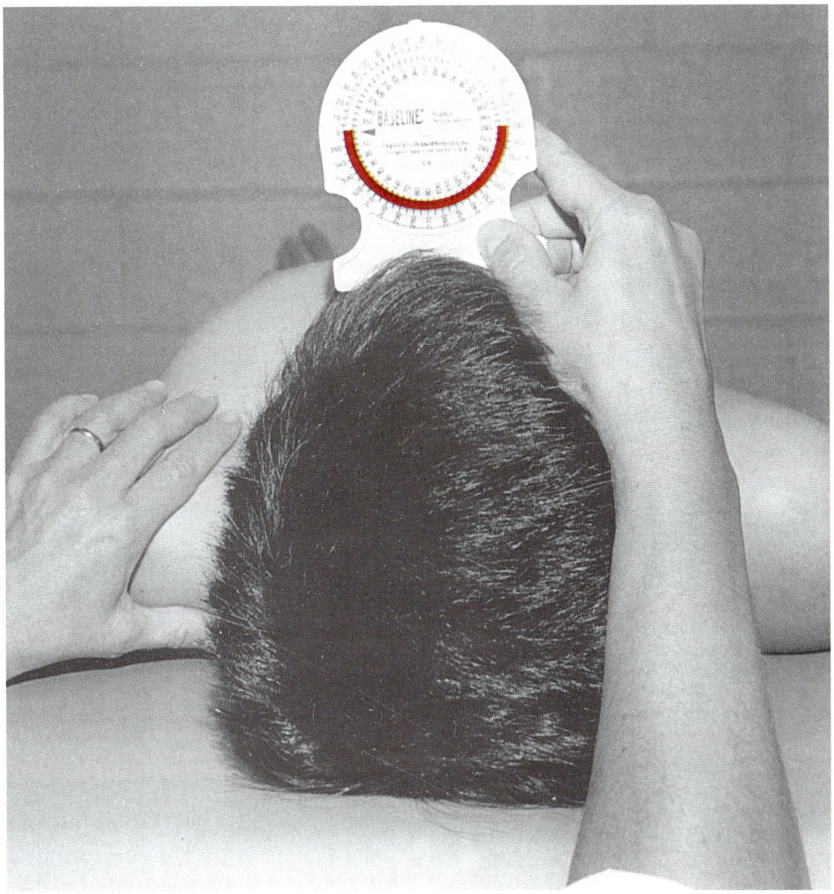

FIGURE 11.48 Inclinometer alignment in the starting position for measuring cervical rotation ROM. Only one inclinometer is used for this measurement.

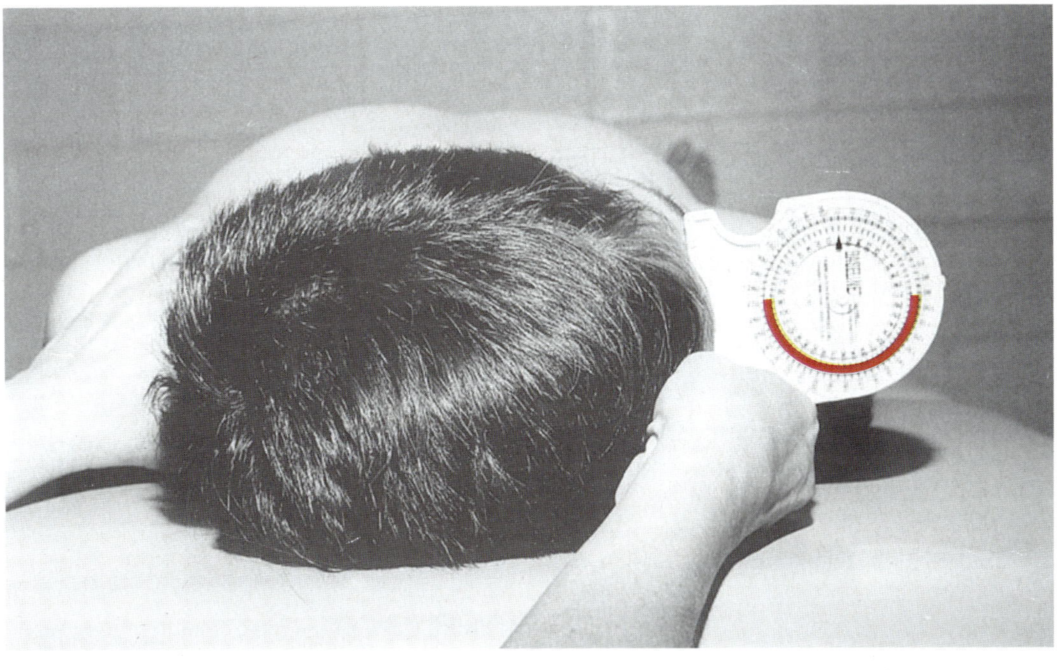

FIGURE 11.49 Inclinometer alignment at the end of the cervical ROM. The number of degrees on the dial of the inclinometer equals the ROM in rotation.

CERVICAL ROTATION: CROM DEVICE

The mean ROM in right rotation with use of the CROM device varies from 75 degrees in female subjects aged 11 to 19 years to 46 degrees in male subjects aged 80 years.[12] For additional rotation ROM values by age and gender, refer to Tousignant et al[23] in Table 11.1; Youdas et al[12] in Tables 11.4 and 11.5; and Nilsson et al[24] for full cycle rotation ROM in Table 11.8 in the Research Findings section.

Testing Position

The individual should be carefully positioned by being seated in a straight back chair with the midback region in contact with the back of the chair. Feet should be flat on the floor and shoulders should be relaxed with hands on thighs or knees. The head should be level with gaze straight ahead, mouth and chin vertically aligned, and eyes horizontal. A strap or straps should be placed across the chest and shoulders to stabilize the thoracic spine and prevent it from contributing to the motion.

CROM Device Alignment[27]

1. Place the CROM device on the individual's head so that the nosepiece is on the bridge of the nose and the band fits snugly across the back of the head.
2. Place the magnetic yoke over the individual's shoulders so that the arrow on the magnetic yoke is pointing north (Fig. 11.50).
3. To ensure that the compass inclinometer is level, adjust the position of the individual's head so that both gravity inclinometers read 0 degrees.
4. After leveling the compass inclinometer, turn the rotation meter on the compass inclinometer until the pointer is at 0 degrees.

Testing Motion: Passive ROM

Guide the individual's head into rotation and read the inclinometer on top of the head at the end of the ROM (Fig. 11.51).

Testing Motion: Active ROM

Instruct the individual to stare straight ahead and turn the chin toward the shoulder as far as possible without tilting it forward, backward, or lateral. Keep shoulders relaxed.

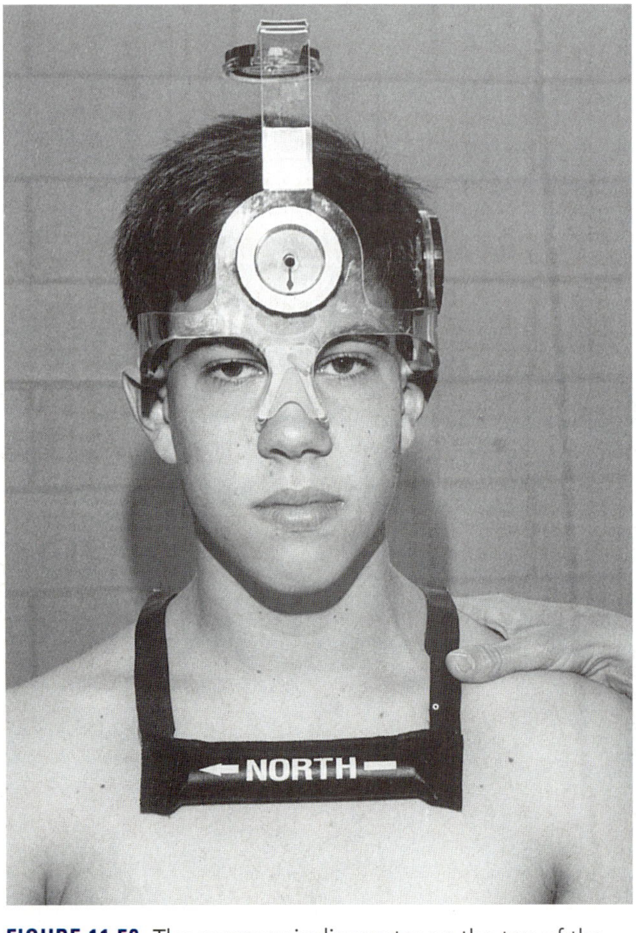

FIGURE 11.50 The compass inclinometer on the top of the CROM device has been leveled so that the examiner is able to zero it prior to the beginning of the motion.

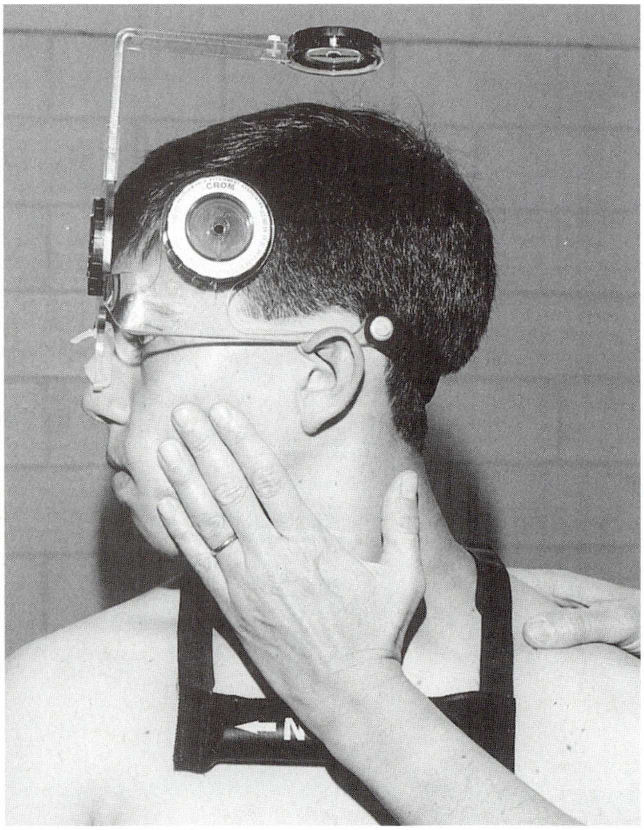

FIGURE 11.51 At the end of the right rotation ROM, the examiner is stabilizing the individual's shoulder with one hand and maintaining the end of rotation ROM with the other hand. The examiner will read the dial of the inclinometer on the top of the CROM device. Rotation ROM will be the number of degrees on the dial at the end of the ROM.

Research Findings

Measurement of the cervical spine ROM is complicated by the region's multiple joint structure and lack of well-defined landmarks, a workable definition of the neutral position, and a standardized method of stabilization to isolate cervical motion from thoracic motion. The search for instruments and methods capable of providing accurate and affordable measurements of the cervical spine is ongoing. At this time the universal goniometer appears to be the most commonly used instrument in the clinic, although relatively few research studies are available to provide normative data and to attest to the goniometer's reliability and validity values. Normative ROM values using a universal goniometer from a study by Youdas et al[26] are presented in Table 11.1, along with values from studies using different measurement methods.

The tape measure and single inclinometer also may be used in clinical settings. Although both methods of measuring ROM have had good reviews by some investigators, they have not been recommended by others. Range of motion values using a tape measure can be found in Table 11.2.

The CROM device has gained considerable popularity because it has received good intra- and interrater reliability ratings and a positive validity rating.[13,17,24,28–33] In reviews by Audette et al[28] and Williams et al,[29] the CROM device had the best ratings for reproducibility, responsiveness, and validity in comparison with radiographs. Normative ROM values for cervical motions using a CROM device are presented in Tables 11.3, 11.4, and 11.5.

Effects of Age, Gender, and Other Factors

Age

A large number of researchers have investigated the effects of age on cervical ROM,[12,24,25,34–53] including coupled motion, but differences between the populations tested and the wide variety of instruments and procedures employed in these studies can make it difficult to compare results. However, most researchers agree that in adults a tendency exists for cervical ROM to decrease with increasing age (Tables 11.3 to 11.8). The only exception found by two studies is that axial rotation (occurring primarily at the atlantoaxial joint) has been shown either to stay the same or to increase with increasing age to compensate for an age-related decrease in rotation in the lower cervical spine.[35,41] Age appears to have a stronger effect on cervical ROM than does gender. A brief review of studies which focuses on the effect of age effect on ROM is included below.

O'Driscoll and Tomenson[34] studied cervical ROM across age-groups using a type of inclinometer. They measured 79 females and 80 males ranging in age from 0 to 79 years and found that ROM decreased with increasing age and differences existed between males and females. In another study that included a relatively large number of subjects (250) and a large age range (from 14 to 70 years), Feipel and colleagues[40] found a significant decrease in all cervical motions with increasing age. Kuhlman[42] compared the range of motion of 42 subjects aged 70 to 90 years and 31 subjects aged 20 to 30 years and found that the elderly group had significantly less motion than did the younger group for all motions measured, including rotation. Sforza and coworkers,[46] who studied the effects of age on ROM in 20 male adolescents (mean age 16 years), 30 young adult males (mean age 23 years), and 20 middle-aged men (mean age 37 years), also found that all cervical active ROMs decreased between the youngest group and the oldest group.

Youdas and associates[12] measured active cervical motions in 337 subjects using the CROM device in nine groups of males and females ranging from 11 years to 89 years (see Tables 11.3 to 11.5). The authors found that both males and females lose about 5 degrees of active extension and 3 degrees of active flexion, lateral flexion, and rotation with each 10-year increase in age. For example, the two oldest groups of males

TABLE 11.1 Cervical Spine Range of Motion: Normal Values in Degrees

	Youdas et al[26]	Balogun et al[14]	Malmström et al[15]	Tousignant et al[23]
	Universal Goniometer Mean age = 59 yr *n* = 20	Myrin Single Inclinometer Mean age = 22 yr *n* = 21	Myrin Single Inclinometer 22–58 yr *n* = 60	CROM Device Mean age = 51 yr *n* = 55
Motion	***Mean (SD)***	***Mean (SD)***	***Mean (SD)***	***Mean (SD)***
Flexion	40 (12)	32 (13)	65 (8)	47 (11)
Extension	50 (14)	64 (17)	67 (12)	50 (14)
Right lateral flexion	22 (8)	41 (9)	41 (7)	30 (9)
Left lateral flexion	22 (7)	42 (9)	42 (7)	33 (9)
Right rotation	51 (11)	64 (17)	76 (9)	56 (10)
Left rotation	49 (9)	68 (15)	76 (8)	56 (12)

CROM = Cervical range of motion device; SD = Standard deviation.

TABLE 11.2 Cervical Spine Range of Motion Measured With a Tape Measure: Normal Values in Centimeters

	Hsieh and Yeung*[13] 14–31 yr		Balogun et al†[14] 18–26 yr
	Tester 1 *n* = 17	Tester 2 *n* = 17	*n* = 21
Motion	***Mean (SD)***	***Mean (SD)***	***Mean (SD)***
Flexion	1.6 (1.7)	1.8	4.3 (2.0)
Extension	22.4 (1.6)	20.8 (2.4)	18.5 (2.0)
Right lateral flexion	11.0 (1.9)	11.5 (2.1)	12.9 (2.4)
Left lateral flexion	10.7 (1.9)	11.1 (2.1)	12.8 (2.5)
Right rotation	11.6 (1.7)	12.6 (2.5)	11.0 (2.5)
Left rotation	11.2 (1.9)	13.2 (2.4)	11.0 (2.5)

SD = Standard deviation.

* 99% confidence interval (CI) of measurement error ranged from 1.4 to 2.6 centimeters for tester 1 (experienced). CI ranged from 1.9 to 3.3 centimeters for tester 2 (inexperienced).

† Pearson product moment correlation coefficient *r* values ranged from 0.26 to 0.88 for intratester reliability and from 0.30 to 0.92 for intertester reliability.

and females, aged 80 to 89 years, had about 20 degrees less cervical flexion than the youngest group of 11- to 19-year-olds. In addition, the authors found a significant gender effect for all motions except flexion with females having about 2 to 5 degrees more ROM than males.

Bible and colleagues[54] used an electrogoniometer and torsimeter to evaluate active cervical motion during functional tasks performed by 60 healthy individuals (30 males and 30 females) aged 20 to 75 years. As part of the study, a multivariate analysis was conducted that determined that age was a highly significant predictor of decreased active ROM in each of the three motion planes.

The purpose of a study by Swinkels and Swinkels-Meewisse was to generate normal values for active ROM of the cervical spine using the CROM device and to examine the effects of age and gender on cervical ROM.[55] A group of 400 healthy persons was divided into subgroups of 100 (50 males and 50 females) for each decade from 20 to 60 years. Active ROM decreased significantly in all directions in the decade from 50 to 60 years when compared with persons younger than 40 years. In a comparison between persons older than 50 years with persons aged 40 to 50 years, ROM was shown to decrease significantly except for extension and lateral flexion. In addition, there was a significant difference in lateral flexion and extension between the 20- and 29-year-olds and other decades. Because the authors did not stabilize the thoracic spine either through the use of straps or by having a supporting back to the stool, some of the ROM findings could have been compromised by movement of the upper thoracic spine. However, a linear regression analysis showed that age had an overall effect on active ROM in all directions.

Salo and colleagues used a device similar to the CROM device called a Cervical Measurement System (CMS) to measure the ROM of 220 healthy women aged 20 to 59 years.[49] These authors found that passive ROM decreased linearly with increasing age in all planes and for all motions except flexion.

Simpson et al,[51] Park et al,[52] and Yukawa et al[53] used radiographs to evaluate the effects of aging on the cervical ROM. Simpson and colleagues conducted a multivariate analysis of cervical segmental ROM using flexion–extension radiographs of 195 patients (133 females and 62 males ranging in age from

TABLE 11.3 Age Effects on Half Cycle Active Cervical Flexion ROM in Males and Females Aged 11 to 89 Years: Normal Values in Degrees Using the CROM Device

11–19 yr *n* = 40	20–29 yr *n* = 42	30–39 yr *n* = 41	40–49 yr *n* = 42	50–59 yr *n* = 40	60–69 yr *n* = 40	70–79 yr *n* = 40	80–89 yr *n* = 38
Mean (SD)	***Mean (SD)***	***Mean (SD)***	***Mean (SD)***	***Mean (SD)***	***Mean (SD)***	***Mean (SD)***	***Mean (SD)***
64 (9)	54 (9)	47 (10)	50 (11)	46 (9)	41 (8)	39 (9)	40 (9)

SD = Standard deviation; CROM = Cervical range of motion device.

Adapted from Youdas, JW, et al.[12] Reprinted from Physical Therapy with the permission of the American Physical Therapy Association.

TABLE 11.4 Age and Gender Effects on Half Cycle Active Cervical Spine ROM in Males and Females Aged 11 to 49 Years: Normal Values in Degrees Using the CROM Device

	11–19 yr		20–29 yr		30–39 yr		40–49 yr	
	Males *n* = 20	Females *n* = 20	Males *n* = 20	Females *n* = 20	Males *n* = 20	Females *n* = 21	Males *n* = 20	Females *n* = 22
Motion	***Mean (SD)***	***Mean (SD)***	***Mean (SD)***	***Mean (SD)***	***Mean (SD)***	***Mean (SD)***	***Mean (SD)***	***Mean (SD)***
Extension	86 (12)	84 (15)	77 (13)	86 (11)	68 (13)	78 (14)	63 (12)	78 (13)
Right lateral flexion	45 (8)	49 (7)	45 (7)	46 (7)	43 (9)	47 (8)	38 (11)	42 (9)
Left lateral flexion	46 (7)	47 (7)	41 (7)	43 (5)	41 (10)	44 (8)	36 (8)	41 (9)
Right rotation	74 (8)	75 (10)	70 (6)	75 (6)	67 (7)	72 (6)	65 (10)	70 (7)
Left rotation	72 (7)	71 (10)	69 (7)	72 (6)	65 (9)	66 (8)	62 (8)	64 (8)

SD = Standard deviation; CROM = Cervical range of motion device.

Adapted from Youdas, JW, et al.[12] Reprinted from *Physical Therapy* with the permission of the American Physical Therapy Association.

15 to 93 years. Age had a significant negative association with ROM at each level from C2–C6, which was independent of degeneration and amounted to a 5-degree decrease in subaxial ROM every 10 years.

Park and coworkers compared cervical ROM in young (20 to 29 years) versus middle-aged (50 to 59 years) adults.[52] A total of 104 asymptomatic adults were randomly selected out of 791 individuals who underwent lateral cervical radiographs in neutral, flexion, and extension positions. There was no significant difference between the two age-groups in the ROM of the upper cervical and lower cervicothoracic regions during flexion and extension but there was a difference between the two groups in the midcervical spine in which the ROM in the older group decreased significantly. This change in ROM in the older group is consistent with findings that the midcervical levels are most likely to develop both symptomatic and asymptomatic degenerative changes.

Yukawa et al[53] studied the anteroposterior, lateral, flexion, and extension radiography of the cervical spine performed on 1,230 healthy Japanese volunteers (616 men and 614 women). Flexion and extension x-rays were taken with the neck in maximum flexion and extension. The C2–C7 ROM was about 68 degrees in the third decade and decreased to 45 degrees in the eighth decade. Extension ROM decreased more than flexion ROM with increasing age and this decrease appeared to be compensated by an increase in C2–C7 lordotic alignment.

Pellecchia and Bohannon[38] found that the mean values for lateral flexion in subjects younger than 30 years of age exceeded 42 degrees, whereas mean values for lateral flexion in subjects older than 79 years of age were less than 25 degrees. Nilsson, Hartvigsen, and Christensen,[24] in a study of 90 healthy men and women aged 20 to 60 years, concluded that the decrease in half cycle cervical passive ROM with increasing age could be explained by using a simple linear regression of ROM as a function of age. Chen and colleagues,[39] in a detailed review of the literature regarding the effects of aging on cervical spine ROM, concluded that active cervical ROM decreased by 4 degrees per decade. This finding is very close

TABLE 11.5 Age and Gender Effects on Half Cycle Active Cervical Spine ROM in Males and Females Aged 50 to 89 Years: Mean Values in Degrees Using the CROM Device

	Ages 50–59 yr		Ages 60–69 yr		Ages 70–79 yr		Ages 80–89 yr	
	Males *n* = 20	Females *n* = 20	Males *n* = 20	Females *n* = 20	Males *n* = 20	Females *n* = 20	Males *n* = 20	Females *n* = 18
Motion	***Mean (SD)***	***Mean (SD)***	***Mean (SD)***	***Mean (SD)***	***Mean (SD)***	***Mean (SD)***	***Mean (SD)***	***Mean (SD)***
Extension	60 (10)	65 (16)	57 (11)	65 (13)	54 (14)	55 (10)	49 (11)	50 (15)
Right lateral flexion	36 (5)	37 (7)	30 (5)	33 (10)	26 (7)	28 (7)	24 (6)	26 (6)
Left lateral flexion	35 (7)	35 (6)	30 (5)	34 (8)	25 (8)	27 (7)	24 (7)	23 (7)
Right rotation	61 (8)	61 (9)	54 (7)	65 (10)	50 (10)	53 (9)	46 (8)	53 (11)
Left rotation	58 (9)	63 (8)	57 (7)	60 (9)	50 (9)	53 (9)	47 (9)	51 (11)

SD = Standard deviation; CROM = Cervical range of motion device.

Adapted from Youdas, JW, et al.[12] Reprinted from *Physical Therapy* with the permission of the American Physical Therapy Association.

TABLE 11.6 Age and Gender Effects on Full Cycle Cervical Flexion–Extension ROM: Normal Values in Degrees*

	Nilsson et al†[24]	Dvorak et al‡[35]	Castro et al§[41]	Nilsson et al[24]	Dvorak et al[35]	Castro et al[41]
	Males *n* = 31	**Males** *n* = 86	**Males** *n* = 71	**Females** *n* = 59	**Females** *n* = 64	**Females** *n* = 86
Age Groups (in years)	***Mean (SD)***	***Mean (SD)***	***Mean (SD)***	***Mean (SD)***	***Mean (SD)***	***Mean (SD)***
20–29	129 (6)	153 (20)	149 (18)	128 (12)	149 (12)	152 (15)
30–39	120 (8)	141 (11)	135 (26)	120 (12)	156 (23)	141 (12)
40–49	110 (6)	131 (19)	129 (21)	114 (10)	140 (13)	125 (13)
50–59	111 (8)	136 (16)	116 (14)	117 (19)	127 (15)	124 (24)
60–69	—	116 (19)	110 (16)	—	133 (8)	117 (15)
70–79	—	—	102 (13)	—	—	121 (21)
80+	—	—	—	—	—	98 (11)

SD = Standard deviation.

* The values in this table represent the combined total of flexion and extension range of motion.

† Nilsson et al used the cervical range of motion device (CROM) to measure passive range of motion.

‡ Dvorak et al used the CA-6000 Spine Motion Analyzer to measure passive ROM.

§ Castro et al used an ultrasound-based coordinate measuring system, the CMS 50, to measure active range of motion.

to the 3- to 5-degree decrease per decade found by Simpson and colleagues[51] and by Youdas and associates.[12]

Three groups of females, 22 of whom were aged 15 to 19 years; 25 of whom were aged 20 to 30 years; and 16 of whom were aged 35 to 45 years, participated in a study by Tommasi et al.[56] All active cervical ranges of motion were obtained with an optoelectronic motion analysis system. The study authors found that all primary motions were always associated with coupled movements. For example, lateral flexion was performed with axial rotation and flexion–extension, whereas during axial rotation large components of extension and lateral flexion were observed. The total motion of flexion–extension decreased about 10 degrees with increasing age but the difference was not statistically significant. However,

TABLE 11.7 Age and Gender Effects on Full Cycle Cervical Lateral Flexion ROM: Normal Values in Degrees*

	Nilsson et al†[24]	Dvorak et al‡[35]	Castro et al§[41]	Nilsson et al[24]	Dvorak et al[35]	Castro et al[41]
	Males *n* = 31	**Males** *n* = 86	**Males** *n* = 71	**Females** *n* = 59	**Females** *n* = 64	**Females** *n* = 86
Age Groups (in years)	***Mean (SD)***	***Mean (SD)***	***Mean (SD)***	***Mean (SD)***	***Mean (SD)***	***Mean (SD)***
20–29	122 (4)	101 (13)	92 (14)	116 (18)	100 (9)	90 (13)
30–39	111 (12)	95 (10)	89 (23)	108 (14)	106 (18)	86 (18)
40–49	102 (15)	84 (14)	74 (15)	99 (11)	88 (16)	77 (12)
50–59	104 (12)	88 (29)	70 (12)	97 (7)	76 (10)	69 (15)
60–69	—	74 (14)	65 (14)	—	80 (18)	68 (12)
70–79	—	—	47 (12)	—	—	70 (14)
80+	—	—	—	—	—	50 (18)

SD = Standard deviation.

* The values in this table represent the combined total of right and left lateral flexion range of motion.

† Nilsson et al used the cervical range of motion (CROM) device to measure passive range of motion.

‡ Dvorak et al used the CA-6000 Spine Motion Analyzer to measure passive range of motion.

§ Castro et al used an ultrasound-based coordinate measuring system, the CMS 50, to measure active range of motion.

TABLE 11.8 Age and Gender Effects on Full Cycle Cervical Rotation ROM: Normal Values in Degrees*

	Nilsson et al†[24]	Dvorak et al‡[35]	Castro et al§[41]	Nilsson et al[24]	Dvorak et al[35]	Castro et al[41]
	Males $n = 31$	Males $n = 86$	Males $n = 71$	Females $n = 59$	Females $n = 64$	Females $n = 86$
Age Groups (in years)	*Mean (SD)*	*Mean (SD)*	*Mean (SD)*	*Mean (SD)*	*Mean (SD)*	*Mean (SD)*
20–29	174 (13)	184 (12)	161 (16)	174 (13)	182 (10)	160 (14)
30–39	166 (12)	175 (10)	156 (32)	167 (13)	186 (10)	150 (15)
40–49	161 (21)	157 (20)	141 (15)	170 (10)	169 (14)	142 (15)
50–59	158 (10)	166 (14)	145 (11)	163 (12)	152 (16)	139 (19)
60–69	—	146 (13)	136 (18)	—	154 (15)	126 (14)
70–79	—	—	121 (14)	—	—	135 (16)
80+	—	—	—	—	—	113 (21)

SD = Standard deviation.

* The values in this table represent the combined total of right and left rotation range of motion.

† Nilsson et al used the cervical range of motion device (CROM) to measure passive range of motion.

‡ Dvorak et al used the CA-6000 Spine Motion Analyzer to measure passive ROM.

§ Castro et al used an ultrasound-based coordinate measuring system, the CMS 50, to measure active ROM.

a general trend for age-related reductions was observed. The largest decrement was found for head and neck extension, approximately 4 degrees for each age-group.

Hole, Cook, and Bolton[44] determined that the loss of cervical mobility equals to approximately 4% per decade in flexion and lateral flexion and 6% to 7% for extension. The decrease in extension, lateral flexion, and rotation occurred between 20- and 29-year-olds and 30- and 39-year-olds in their study of 84 asymptomatic men and women. Demaille-Wlodyka and colleagues,[11] in a study of 232 healthy volunteers ranging in age from 15 to 65 years or older, found that all cervical motions decreased after age 25 and that the age effect was significant. Nilsson and associates[24] measured passive ROM using the CROM device in 90 healthy men and women ranging in age from 21 to 60 years. The authors determined that the decrease in passive ROM as age increases could be described by a simple linear regression.

Other investigators have postulated that the effects of age on ROM and coupled motions may be motion specific and age specific; however, the evidence appears to be somewhat controversial. Trott and colleagues[37] found a significant decrease in the means of all motions (flexion–extension, lateral flexion, and axial rotation) with increasing age, but they determined that most coupled motions were not affected by age. In contrast to Trott's findings, Demaille-Wlodyka et al[11] found that coupled motions showed a tendency to decrease with age. Tommasi et al determined that the rotation coupled with the primary motion of lateral flexion decreased significantly with increasing age.[56]

Lantz, Chen, and Buch,[45] in a study of 52 matched males and females, found a significant age effect, with subjects in the third decade having greater ROM in rotation and flexion–extension than subjects in the fourth decade. Dvorak and associates[35] determined that the most dramatic decrease in ROM in 150 healthy men and women (aged 20 to 60 years and older) occurred between the 30-year-old group and the 40-year-old group. A somewhat similar result was found by Peolsson and colleagues,[47] who investigated the age effects on cervical motion in 51 men and 50 women aged 25 to 63 years. These authors found that active ROM in all planes decreased by about 30 degrees from the 25- to 34-year-old group to the 55- to 64-year-old group. The decrease in active ROM was statistically significant in all planes but was most pronounced in extension and least evident in flexion (0.3 degrees/year).

In contrast to the findings of Dvorak and associates[35] and Peolsson and colleagues,[47] Trott and colleagues[37] found that the greatest decrease in flexion–extension ROM in 60 healthy men and women (aged 20 to 59 years) occurred between the 20-year-old group and the 30-year-old group.

Pearson and Walmsley[36] and Walmsley, Kimber, and Culham[25] were the only authors to include the cervical spine motions of retraction and protraction in their studies. Pearson and Walmsley[36] found that the older age-groups had less ROM in retraction but that they showed no age difference in the neutral resting position. In contrast to Pearson and Walmsley's[36] findings, Walmsley, Kimber, and Culham[25] found age-related decreases in both protraction and retraction.

Quek and colleagues investigated the relationship between thoracic kyphosis and forward head posture in 51 older adult patients with cervical spine dysfunction.[50] Increased kyphosis found in the older women was associated with greater forward head posture and greater forward head posture was associated with decreased cervical flexion and rotation ROM.

The decrease in ROM one sees in aging adults appears to be different in young children as they get older. Arbogast et al[43] found that in 67 young children active ROM in cervical flexion and right and left rotation measured by the CROM device actually increased slightly between 3 and 12 years of age. Öhman and Beckung measured passive ROM in rotation and lateral flexion in a group of 23 infants (10 females, 13 males) and again when the children were 3.5 to 5 years of age.[57] The present passive ROM (mean = 100 degrees in rotation and 70 degrees in lateral flexion) was compared with the passive ROM when the children were infants. In contrast to Arbogast's findings, Öhman and Beckung found no change in lateral flexion passive ROM during the first 5 years of life but a significant decrease in rotation was noted. The difference in age range between the two studies may have contributed to the difference in findings regarding rotation.

Seacrist et al quantified cervical motion using an eight-camera motion-capture system with reflective markers that captured passive neck flexion angles of the head relative to the thoracic spine.[48] Participants in the study were 10 healthy pediatric females (6–12 years), 9 pediatric males (6–12 years), 10 female adults (21–40 years), and 9 adult males (20–36 years). Passive cervical flexion was 111 degrees for pediatric males, 103 degrees for adult females, 104 degrees for pediatric males, and 94 degrees for adult males. In general, the authors found that passive cervical spine flexion decreased significantly with increasing age in both genders and that females exhibited significantly greater flexion than did males.

Lynch-Caris et al used the CROM device to measure active range of motion for 106 subjects aged 8 to 10 years.[58] Active range of motion for flexion was 66 degrees (SD = 13), extension 85 degrees (SD = 14), lateral flexion 58 degrees (SD = 8), and rotation 77 degrees (SD = 7). The observed data differed from the American Medical Association guidelines for adults, but it fell within the range of reference values for 10-year-olds.

Gender

Many of the same researchers who looked at the effects of age on cervical ROM also studied the effects of gender, but the results of these studies appear to be more inconsistent and controversial than the results of the age studies. In some studies, the trend for women to have a greater ROM than men was apparent, although differences were small and generally not significant. In some instances, the effects of gender appeared to be motion specific and age specific in that some motions at some ages were affected more than others.

Castro et al[41] was one of the authors who found significant gender differences in cervical ROM, but noted that the differences occurred primarily in the motions of lateral flexion and flexion–extension in subjects between the ages of 70 and 79 years (see Tables 11.6 and 11.7). Women older than 70 years of age were on the average more mobile in flexion–extension than were men of the same age. Nilsson, Hartvigsen, and Christensen[24] found a significant difference between genders in lateral flexion ROM, but in this study males were more mobile than females, as seen in Table 11.7. Lantz, Chen, and Buch[45] studied a total of 56 healthy men and women aged 20 to 39 years. The authors found no difference between genders in total combined left and right lateral flexion, but women had greater ranges of active and passive axial rotation and flexion–extension than did men of the same age. Women had an average of 12.7 degrees more active flexion–extension and an average of 6.5 degrees more active axial rotation than did men of the same age. Women also had greater passive ROM in all cervical motions. Dvorak and associates[35] found that women between 40 and 49 years of age had greater ROM in all motions than did men in the same age-group. However, within each of the other age-groups—20 to 29 years, 60 to 69 years, 70 to 79 years, and 80 to 89 years—no differences in cervical ROM were found between genders.

Ferrario and associates[59] used a digital optoelectronic instrument to measure cervical motion in 30 women and 30 men and found that the women had greater ROM in all motions than men. More support for a gender difference comes from Demaille-Wlodyka et al,[11] who found that of 232 healthy subjects aged 15 to 79 years, females had greater range of motion in flexion–extension and lateral flexion than did males but this was not the case in axial rotation.

Abelin-Genevois and colleagues randomly selected 150 full spine standing views to examine upper cervical angle, inferior cervical angle, and tilt at C7.[60] Cervical spine alignment was found to be significantly different between the two groups (mean of 8.8 years and 14.2 years) except for the global cervical lordosis (C1–C7), which remained stable. A significant gender difference was found for all cervical angles.

Simpson and colleagues, in a multivariate study of 133 patients including 68% women and 32% men, found that a patient's gender was a significant predictor of ROM only in the upper cervical spine, where the authors found an average decrease in cervical ROM for males of about 1.3 degrees at C2–C3 level compared with females.[51] Otherwise, gender appeared to have little influence on ROM.

Yukawa and coworkers, in a study of 1,200 healthy Japanese volunteers (616 men and 614) women, found that there was a significant difference in C2–C7 alignment and ROM between men and women.[53] The axis of total ROM based on the neutral position did not change with increasing age in males but shifted toward the extension position in females.

Seacrist et al,[48] whose study was described earlier, found that females exhibited consistently greater flexion (on average 8 to 9 degrees) than males across all ages.

In contrast to the preceding studies, a number of investigators concluded that gender had no effect on cervical ROM.[25,37,39,40,44] Ordway and associates[61] found a nonsignificant gender effect, and Pellecchia and Bohannon,[38] in a study of 135 subjects aged 15 to 95 years with a history of neck pain, concluded that neither neck pain nor gender had any effect on ROM. Arbogast and coworkers[43] also found no effects of gender in the 67 children tested between the ages of 3 and 12 years. Hole, Cook, and Bolton[44] determined that gender had no significant effect on cervical range of motion in a group of 84 healthy men and women 20 to 69 years of age. Mannion et al[62] also found no effects of gender in a small study of 10 men and women whose active ROM was measured in all cervical motions. In agreement with the above authors, Swinkels and Swinkels-Meewisse, in an age and gender study of cervical active ROM in 400 healthy participants aged 20 to 60 years, also found no significant effect of gender.[55] Prushansky, Deryi, and Jabarreen found that higher cervical range of motion values were recorded in 15 women compared with 15 men, which reached significance only in right and left lateral flexion.[63]

Active Versus Passive ROM

The AMA's fifth and sixth editions of the *Guides to the Evaluation of Permanent Impairment* recommend that active ROM be performed.[19] The authors of the *Guides* are aware that a number of factors may affect a person's performance of active ROM, such as pain, fear of injury, and motivation; therefore, they stress that a patient must be encouraged to put forth a maximal effort. If a patient can perform a full ROM actively, then there is no reason to perform passive ROM.[19]

Other reasons for using active ROM rather than passive ROM have been investigated by the following researchers, who have found that active ROM is more reliably measured than passive ROM and has less variability. Assink and coworkers[64] determined that the intraclass correlation coefficients (ICCs) of active ROM measurements were higher than the ICCs of passive ROM measurements in 30 symptomatic and 30 asymptomatic volunteers. In asymptomatic subjects, passive ROM was generally larger than in active ROM. In symptomatic subjects, the percentage of paired observations within 5 degrees varied from a low of 17% for passive ROM in extension to a high of 60% for active ROM in rotation.

Nilsson[24] used the CROM device to measure half cycle passive ROM in 14 asymptomatic volunteers (7 men and 7 women between the ages of 23 and 45 years). All motions were measured by two testers from neutral 0, and intratester reliability was found to be acceptable to the author, ranging from an r of 0.61 for right lateral flexion to an r of 0.85 for extension. Intertester reliability was unacceptable because the correlation coefficients fell below 0.60 in four out of the six directions, ranging from an r of 0.29 for left rotation to an r of 0.71 for flexion.

Nilsson, Christensen, and Hartvigsen[65] conducted a study to correct any problems in the previous study. More extensive training was arranged for the testers, and the number of subjects was increased from 14 to 35 (17 men and 18 women) who ranged in age from 20 to 28 years. Intertester reliability still was unacceptable for half cycle passive ROM because three out of six measurements fell below an r of 0.60. Intertester reliability for full cycle passive ROM was much better, with r values in three planes ranging from 0.61 to 0.88. It appears as if the half cycle motions may be contributing more than the passive ROM to the poor intertester reliability.

Bergman and associates[66] found that the highest variation in both the 58 subjects in the symptomatic group and the 48 men and women in the asymptomatic group occurred in passive ROM testing versus active ROM testing. The variation over a 12-week period ranged from 20.4 degrees for passive lateral flexion in the asymptomatic group to 85.2 degrees for passive rotation in the symptomatic group. The fact that a substantial amount of variation occurred in passive ROM measurement prompted the authors to question whether passive ROM should be used as an outcome measure in intervention studies. Demaille-Wlodyka and colleagues[11] recommended that passive ROM should not be used because it overestimates a subject's mobility.

Testing Position

The lack of a well-defined neutral cervical spine position is thought to be responsible for the lower reliability of cervical spine motions starting in the neutral position compared with those starting at the end of one ROM and continuing to the end of another ROM (full cycle motions). Examples of full cycle motions are flexion–extension and right rotation to left rotation.

Studies that have attempted to better define the neutral position have used either radiographs[61,67] or motion-analysis systems.[68,69] In the radiographic study conducted by Ordway and associates,[61] the authors determined that when the cervical spine is in the neutral position, the upper segments are in flexion and the lower segments are in progressively less flexion; therefore, at C6–C7, the spine is in a considerable amount of extension. Miller, Polissar, and Haas,[67] in the other radiographic study, found that the cervical spine is in the neutral position when the hard palate is in the horizontal plane. Although these findings are of considerable interest, they provide little help to the average clinician, who does not have access to radiographs for patient positioning.

Two studies that are more clinically relevant used the CA-6000 Spine Motion Analyzer.[68,69] This motion-analysis system is capable of giving the location of neutral 0 position as coordinates in three dimensions corresponding to the three planes of motion. Christensen and Nilsson[68] found that the ability of 38 young (20 to 30 years of age) subjects to reproduce the neutral spine position with eyes and mouth closed was very good. The mean difference from neutral 0 in three motion planes was 2.7 degrees in the sagittal plane, 1.0 degrees in the horizontal plane, and 0.65 degrees in the frontal plane. It is possible that patients may be able to find the neutral position on their own, but the subjects in this study were healthy individuals and the ability of patients to reproduce the neutral position is unknown.

In 2013, Wibault et al used the CROM device to compare head repositioning accuracy between 71 individuals with cervical radiculopathy related to cervical disc disease (CDD) and 173 healthy individuals and to assess the criterion validity between the CROM device and a laser in neck-healthy individuals.[70] The test-retest reliability of the CROM device in individuals with CDD showed ICCs of 0.79 to 0.85, and SEMs of 1.4 to 2 degrees. The criterion validity between the laser in neck-healthy individuals showed ICCs of 0.43 to 0.91 and SEMs of 0.8 to 1.3 degrees. The results appear to support the use of the CROM device for quantifying head repositioning accuracy in individuals with CDD.

Solinger, Chen, and Lantz[69] attempted to standardize a neutral head position when measuring cervical motion in 20 subjects. For flexion and extension, the authors described a neutral position as one in which the corner of the eye was aligned with the upper angle of the ear, at the point where it meets the scalp. For lateral flexion, neutral was defined as the point at which the axis of the head was perceived to be vertically aligned. Compared with data collected using a less stringent head positioning, Solinger, Chen, and Lantz[69] demonstrated that by standardizing head position they obtained increases in reliability of 3% to 15% for rotation and lateral flexion but showed a decrease in reliability of up to 14% for flexion–extension.

Demaille-Wlodyka and colleagues[11] determined that neither age nor gender affected the 232 healthy volunteers' ability to return their heads to a self-defined neutral position after performing a cervical ROM. However, Owens,[71] who used a computer interface electrogoniometer to measure head position in 48 students (36 males and 12 females) with a mean age of 28 years, found that active contractions of the posterior neck muscles caused subjects to undershoot their target neutral position by 2.1 degrees. This finding demonstrated that a recent history of cervical paraspinal muscle contraction can influence head repositioning in flexion–extension. Likewise, in a study using the 3Space Isotrak system, Pearson and Walmsley[36] found a significant difference in the neutral resting position (it became more retracted) after repeated neck retractions performed by 30 healthy subjects, but no statistically significant difference was found in the neck retraction ROM.

Another potential positional problem that testers need to be aware of has been identified by Lantz, Chen, and Buch.[45] These authors found that ROM measurements of the cervical spine taken in the seated position were consistently about 2.6 degrees greater than measurements taken in the standing position in all planes of motion. Greater differences occurred between seated and standing positions when flexion and extension were measured starting in the neutral 0 position as opposed to measurement of full cycle motions. For axial rotation, there was no significant difference between sitting and standing positions.

In a study by Dunleavy and Goldberg, the influence of habitual self-selected unsupported seated posture (HAB) on cervical ROM was compared with erect seated posture (ER) in adults 50 years or older with chronic cervical pain.[72] Testing of 36 adults was conducted by five examiners with three trials of cervical ROM in each of the two seated postural conditions. Extension, total rotation, total lateral flexion, and right lateral flexion ROM increased significantly when measured in the ER posture compared with the HAB posture, whereas flexion decreased. Extension increased by 3.6 degrees in the ER posture, whereas flexion decreased by 7.4 degrees. Total lateral flexion increased by 3.3 degrees and right lateral flexion increased by 2.7 degrees in the ER posture. Measurement reliability was similar in both postures. The results of this study indicate not only the need to document the seated posture used when testing cervical ROM but also the importance of taking measurements in a consistent erect seated posture rather than in a self-selected seated posture.

Body Size

Castro et al[41] found that patients who were obese were not as mobile as patients who were not obese. Mean values for cervical motions in all planes decreased with increasing body weight. Chibnall, Duckro, and Baumer,[73] in a study of 42 male and female subjects, found that body size reflected by distances between specific anatomical landmarks (e.g., between the chin and the acromial process) influenced ROM measurements taken with a tape measure. Any variation in body size among subjects resulted in an underestimation of ROM for subjects with large distances between landmarks and an overestimation of ROM for subjects with small distances between landmarks. The authors concluded that the use of **proportion of distance** (POD) should be used when comparing testing results among subjects. The use of POD (calculated by dividing the distance between the at-rest value and the end-of-range value by the at-rest value) helps to eliminate the effect of body size on ROM values obtained with a tape measure. Obviously, calculation of POD is not necessary if the progress of only one subject is measured. Peolsson and colleagues[47] found no significant correlation between body mass index (BMI) and active ROM, with the exception of extension for both men and women, and flexion for men.

A combination of increased head flexion, neck flexion, and trunk flexion was significantly associated with increased weight and BMI in a study by Brink and colleagues of 194 students aged 15 to 17 years enrolled in a computer application technology course.[74] A three-dimensional posture analysis tool captured five postural angles (head flexion, neck flexion, lateral head bend, craniocervical angle, and trunk flexion) while the students were working on desktop computers. Trunk flexion was the most variable angle because students in the study sat with greater range of trunk flexion (leaning forward or reclining) when using the classroom computer.

Functional Range of Motion

Motion of the cervical spine accompanies most activities of daily living (ADLs) and most recreational and occupational activities. Bennett, Schenk, and Simmons[75] used the CROM device to determine the range of cervical motion required for 13 ADLs performed by 28 college students. The greatest amount of motion was required for the following activities: backing up a car, tying shoes, and crossing the street. Star gazing or simply looking up at the ceiling required a full range of motion in cervical extension (Fig. 11.52) and drinking required more cervical extension than did eating. Using a telephone required lateral flexion and rotation, and bathing and grooming also required a considerable amount of motion.[75] Relatively small amounts of flexion, extension, and rotation were required for eating, reading, writing, and using a computer.

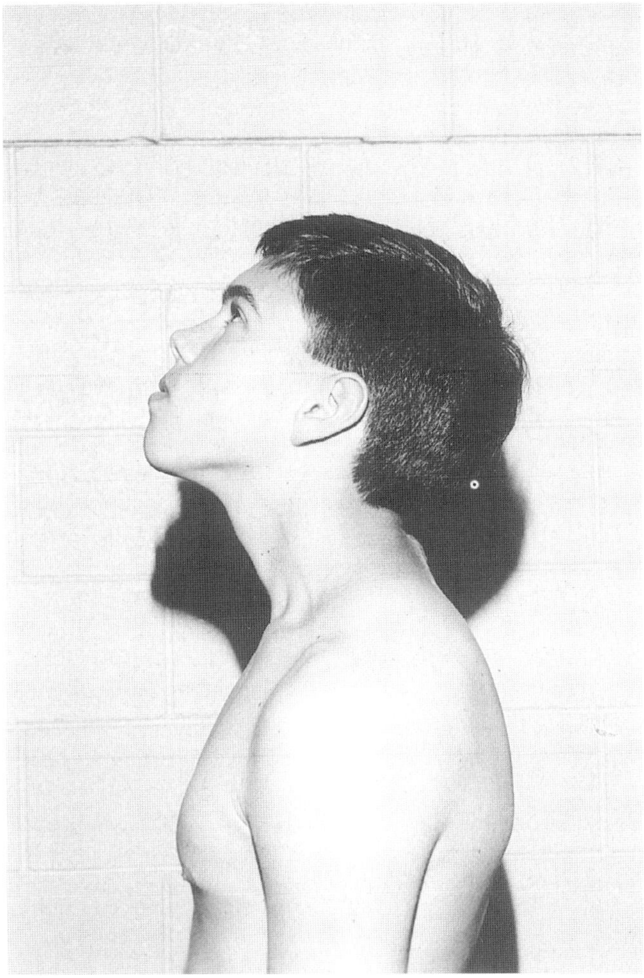

FIGURE 11.52 One needs at least 40 to 50 degrees of cervical extension ROM to look up at the ceiling. If cervical extension ROM is limited, the person must extend the entire spine in an effort to place the head in a position whereby the eyes can look up at the ceiling.

Bible and colleagues used a noninvasive electrogoniometer and torsimeter to measure the ROM of the cervical spines of 60 healthy individuals (30 females and 30 males aged 20 to 73 years) during 15 simulated functional tasks.[54] The active cervical ROM used during the ADLs was 13 to 32 degrees of flexion-extension, 13 to 21 degrees of lateral flexion, and 13 to 57 degrees of rotation. Similar to the findings of Bennett,[75] backing up a car required the most ROM of all the ADLs and involved 32 degrees (32%) of flexion–extension, 20 degrees (26%) of lateral flexion, and 57 degrees (92%) of rotation. Descending stairs required significantly more sagittal and rotational motion than ascending stairs, whereas squatting to pick up an object from the floor required significantly less lateral flexion and rotation than bending at the waist. Going from a standing to sitting position required significantly more lateral flexion than going from a sitting to standing position.

Cobian and coinvestigators also conducted a study to characterize the maximum, cumulative, and average cervical motion required to perform common ADLs.[76] Ten healthy young adults (5 males and 5 females with a mean age of 22.8 years) performed 16 ADLs while three-dimensional kinematics were recorded using an eight-camera optical motion-capture system. The majority of activities used 20% to 40% of available cervical motion. Similar to the findings of both Bible and Bennett, backing up a car was found to require one of the largest amounts of cervical motion (93% of rotation). Looking for traffic (which was not included in either the Bennett or Bible study) used the largest amount of rotation (113 degrees) in this study.

In another study by Cobian and colleagues, 10 healthy young adults were fitted with a portable motion measurement system called the Wisconsin Analysis of Spine Motion Performance system that recorded movement around each primary axis of motion.[77] The participants wore the apparatus continuously for 5 days to record their daily activities with corresponding times. The majority of athletic activity (92%) and work activity (90%) required less than 25 degrees of lateral flexion, whereas a greater range of movements occurred in flexion–extension and rotation. However, none of these motions exceeded 50 degrees. The activity that produced the lowest median range of motion was driving a car, with 8, 9, and 10 degrees of motion for lateral flexion, flexion–extension, and rotation, respectively.

Shugg, Jackson, and Dickey conducted a study to determine the amount of time spent by drivers outside of a neutral cervical spine position and to obtain information on the peak cervical axial rotation angles used by drivers during various driving conditions.[78] According to research, more severe injuries occur when the cervical spine is rotated during a car crash than when the spine is in neutral position. Ten female drivers aged 28 years and one male driver aged 43 years were monitored by the 3Space Isotrak II (Polhemus Inc., Colchester, VT) using sensors secured to their foreheads and on the manubrium; the drivers' postures and hand positions were videotaped. The results showed that these drivers spent significantly more time outside the neutral neck position during residential driving than during highway driving, but overall the cervical range of motion was highly variable.

Cote et al obtained physical performance measures including ROM for 736 middle-aged manufacturing workers (221 women and 515 men) from six participating facilities in Connecticut.[79] Cervical range of motion testing was performed using a CROM inclinometer with participants seated in a straight back chair. Cervical and spine mobility measures were markedly different in this cohort compared with other working populations—the male workers did not have the age-expected reductions in cervical flexibility and the female workers had a progressive increase in spinal flexibility with increasing age. The authors concluded that the healthy worker effect (preservation of strength and mobility) might have played a role in the findings from this selective group of subjects.

Sports activities such as serving a tennis ball, catching or batting a baseball, canoeing, and kayaking may require a full

ROM in all planes. Different types of sports activities may have effects on ROM. For example, Guth[80] compared cervical rotation ROM in a group of 40 swimmers with ROM in 40 nonathletes. The swimmers, aged 14 to 17 years, had a mean total rotation ROM that was 9 degrees greater than the ROM of those aged 14 to 17 years in the control group.

In contrast to the increase in cervical range of motion found in swimmers, rugby players have decreases in cervical ROM over a single season and ROM declines with the increased number of playing years. In a cross-sectional study of 22 rugby players from elite English Premiership clubs, Lark and McCarthy compared group means and changes over the playing season.[81] The percentage of change indicated a decrease in ROM, with most occurring in the second half of the season. Most of the relative change in cervical ROM occurred in right lateral flexion. Lark and McCarthy raised the possibility that the off-season period may not be long enough to allow cervical ROM to recover.[82] Rugby forwards have cervical ranges of motion similar to patients with acute whiplash injuries and need to have sufficient rehabilitation to recover.

Certain occupational activities such as house painting or wallpapering require a full range of cervical extension and, possibly, a full range of flexion. A full ROM in cervical rotation is essential for safe driving of cars or trucks (Fig. 11.53).

Reliability and Validity

An article by Jordan[83] provides an excellent review of reliability studies and the instruments and methods used to evaluate cervical range of motion. The author identifies a number of problems with studies including, among others, the lack of an adequate sample size, appropriate statistical methods, and standardized protocols for measurement and for performance of the motions. These deficits make it difficult to compare studies and to be able to use the data that they generate. The introduction of systematic reviews has provided a great deal of data regarding reliability and validity of cervical ROM measures.

Many different methods and instruments have been employed to assess motion of the head and neck. Similar to other areas of the body, intratester reliability generally is better than intertester reliability, no matter what instrument is used. Also, some motions seem to be more reliably measured than others. For example, the full cycle motions such as flexion–extension and right–left lateral flexion measured from one extreme of the range to the other appear to be more reliably measured than half cycle motions such as flexion measured from the neutral position.[11,15,31,64–66,83] This finding may be due to the variability of the neutral position and the lack of a standardized method that an examiner can use for placing an individual's head in the neutral position. However, the problem with only measuring full cycle motions is that full cycle measurements do not provide the clinician with information about where unilateral limitations in motion occur.

Nilsson[31] found that intratester reliability was good when measuring half cycle motions, but intertester reliability was poor. Nilsson, Christensen, and Hartvigsen[65] found that the intertester reliability of passive range of motion measurements

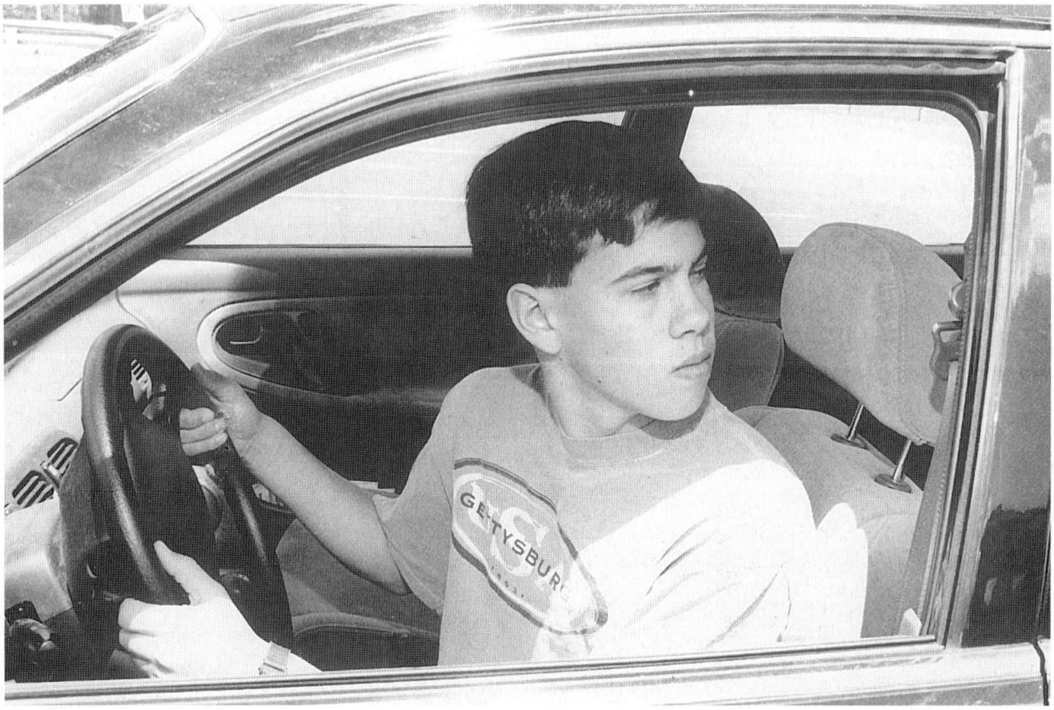

FIGURE 11.53 One needs a minimum of 60 to 70 degrees of cervical rotation to look over the shoulder. If cervical rotation ROM is limited, the person has to rotate the entire trunk to position the head to check for oncoming traffic.

of half cycle motions was poor ($r = 0.39–0.70$), but the intertester reliability of passive range of motion measurements of full cycle motions was acceptable ($r = 0.61–0.70$). Jordan and colleagues,[84] who used the three-dimensional Fastrak system to measure cervical ROM, also found that the intertester reliability of full cycle motions (intraclass correlation coefficients [ICCs] = 0.81–0.89) was better than the reliability of half cycle motions (ICCs = 0.61–0.80) in 40 healthy subjects with two testers. The same was true for intratester reliability in which the ICCs for full cycle motions ranged from 0.76 to 0.82, whereas the ICCs for half cycle motions ranged from 0.54 to 0.70 in 32 healthy subjects with one tester on three occasions.

Malmström and colleagues,[15] using both the Zebris ultrasonic system and the Myrin inclinometer, found that the full cycle motions showed less variability than the half cycle motions although the reliability of both cycles were considered good to excellent in 60 healthy adults (25 men and 35 women) 22 to 58 years of age. The ICCs ranged from 0.92 to 0.97 for full cycle motions and from 0.88 to 0.93 for half cycle motions. The full cycle motions also showed better concurrent validity with the Zebris than did half cycle measurements.

Demaille-Wlodyka,[11] in a study of 232 subjects, determined that full cycle motions had better validity than half cycle motions but half cycle motions allow for better assessment of unilateral limitations. Piva and associates,[85] using a single gravity goniometer to measure half cycle motions in 30 patients with neck pain, found that the standard error of measurement (SEM) ranged from 3.7 degrees for right lateral flexion to 5.6 degrees for extension. Intraclass correlation coefficients ranged from 0.78 for flexion to 0.91 for axial rotation, and intertester reliability was moderate to substantial for measuring active ROM in the sagittal and transverse planes of motion.

According to Chen and colleagues,[39] it is not possible to obtain a true validation of cervical ROM measurements because radiographic measurement has not been subjected to reliability and validity studies. Therefore, no valid gold standard exists. The only option available for investigators at the present time is to conduct concurrent validity studies to obtain agreement between instruments and procedures.[39] However, many researchers still consider radiographic measurement to be the gold standard.

Some of the studies that have been conducted to assess reliability or validity (or both) of the various instruments and methods are reviewed in the following section. The terms "high," "good," "fair," "poor," and "unacceptable" are used to designate different degrees of reliability:

- High reliability refers to ICCs of 0.90 to 0.99
- Good reliability refers to ICCs of 0.80 to 0.89
- Fair reliability refers to ICCs of 0.70 to 0.79
- Low or poor reliability is an ICC of 0.60 to 0.69
- Unacceptable reliability is an ICC of less than 0.60

These definitions of reliability appear to be the most commonly used terms in the following studies, although a few authors have used the interpretation by Portney and Watkins[86] in which correlation coefficients higher than 0.75 indicate good reliability and coefficients of less than 0.75 indicate poor to moderate reliability.

Reliability of the Universal Goniometer

Tucci and coworkers[87] found that the ICCs for intertester reliability of cervical spine motion ranged from –0.08 for flexion to 0.82 for extension for measurements taken with the universal goniometer by two experienced testers on 10 volunteer subjects.

Youdas, Carey, and Garrett[26] measured half cycle active ROM in 60 patients ranging in age from 21 to 84 years with orthopedic problems. The patients were divided into three groups of 20 people each. Each subject performed five repetitions of the motion in each plane to increase the compliance of the neck's soft tissues. In contrast to Tucci's findings, intratester reliability was good for flexion (ICC = 0.83), extension (ICC = 0.86), right lateral flexion (ICC = 0.85), left lateral flexion (ICC = 0.84), and right rotation (ICC = 0.90). Intratester reliability was fair for left rotation (ICC = 0.78). Intertester reliability was fair (ICC = 0.72–0.79) for extension, left lateral flexion, and right lateral flexion. Intertester reliability was poor (ICC = 0.54–0.62) for flexion and left and right rotation.

Pile and associates[88] used a universal goniometer to measure half cycle lateral flexion and flexion and extension in 10 patients with ankylosing spondylitis with minimal disease activity and ranging from 28 to 73 years of age. The testers included a rheumatologist, a rheumatology registrar, and three physical therapists. For intratester reliability each tester measured one patient four times. The authors did not present intratester reliability coefficients. The intertester reliability coefficient for right lateral flexion was 0.74; for left lateral flexion it was 0.68. The landmarks used for the lateral flexion measurement were the sternal notch as the axis and a line through the nose and forehead for the proximal arm. Flexion and extension were measured in the same way as the goniometer is used in this text. The intertester reliability coefficient for flexion was unacceptable (0.21), whereas the coefficient for extension was somewhat better (0.59), but still not considered good.

Maksymowych and colleagues[89] measured full cycle rotation active ROM using a plastic universal goniometer in 44 patients with a mean age of 42.7 years who had ankylosing spondylitis. All measurements were taken by two testers (a trained clinical nurse and a rheumatologist) in midmorning to avoid the effects of early morning stiffness. Intratester reliability was high for two testers (ICC = 0.98 and 0.97), and intertester reliability also was high (ICC = 0.95).

Twenty healthy volunteers, 16 females and 4 males between 20 and 30 years of age, participated in a study by Yankai and Manosan to compare the universal goniometer (UG) and an invented gravitation goniometer (GG).[90] Subjects sat upright on a straight back wooden chair with their midthoracic spine contacting the chair and a strap preventing trunk extension during cervical extension and preventing trunk flexion when performing cervical flexion. Measurements were made by two fourth-year physiotherapy students while a third student read and recorded all measurement values. In each of two sessions 2 weeks apart, each subject was measured twice by each of two raters and by each of two devices. Within-session intrarater reliability results were high for the UG (ICC = 0.80–0.99) and very high for the GG (ICC = 0.90–0.99). Between-session results were high to very high for both devices. Within-session interrater reliability ranged from high to very high for both devices, but only UG measurements for cervical extension had very high interrater reliability for both sessions.

Whitcroft and coworkers used the CROM device as the reference instrument when comparing the UG, tape measure, and visual estimation.[18] Spearman's coefficients were used to show the rank order of agreement with the CROM. When used with fixed landmarks instead of anatomical landmarks, the UG had correlation coefficients of 0.91 for both flexion and lateral flexion, compared with 0.29 for flexion with the tape measure and 0.35 for visual estimation for right lateral flexion. Visual estimation correlation coefficients were unacceptable for extension (0.11), flexion (0.10), and right rotation (0.32).

Validity of the Universal Goniometer

In a search of the literature, no validity studies were found for the universal goniometer in which radiographs were used as the gold standard.

Reliability of the Tape Measure

The fact that the landmarks used to obtain the measurements varied from study to study diminishes the usefulness of some of the following information. Landmarks and methods need to be standardized to make valid comparisons. The landmarks and results of studies by the authors[13,14] in Table 11.2 and by others are described in the following paragraphs.

Hsieh and Yeung[13] used two testers (one experienced and one inexperienced) to measure half cycle active ROM in 27 men and 7 women with an average age of 18 years. The landmarks used in the study for flexion and extension were the sternal notch and the chin. The landmarks for rotation were the acromial process and the chin, and the landmarks for lateral flexion were the acromial process and the lowest point of the earlobe. One tester measured 17 subjects, and the other tester measured a different group of 17 subjects. Intratester reliability coefficients (Pearson's r) ranged from 0.80 to 0.95 for the experienced tester and from 0.78 to 0.91 for the inexperienced tester. Measurement error for the experienced tester at the 99% confidence interval (CI) was approximately ±1 centimeter for sagittal motions and ±2 centimeters for other motions. The inexperienced tester had a higher measurement error of approximately ±2 to 3 centimeters for sagittal motions and ±3 centimeters for other motions.

Balogun and associates[14] employed three physical therapists to measure half cycle active ROM in 21 physical therapy students. The test-retest interval ranged from 4 to 110 days. The landmarks used to measure cervical flexion were the tip of the chin and the sternal notch. Landmarks for measuring lateral flexion were the anterior dimples in the shoulder to the lowest point of the earlobe. For rotation, the landmarks were the tip of the chin and the anterior dimples in the shoulder. Intratester reliability coefficients (r) for measuring neck flexion were poor for all three therapists. Intratester reliability for extension was very good for two therapists and fair for one therapist. The intratester values for left and right rotation ranged from an r of 0.58 to 0.86. The fact that the interval between the first and second sessions was so long may have had an adverse effect on the intratester values. Intertester values ranged from an r of 0.35 to 0.90 in Session I and from an r of 0.47 for left lateral flexion to an r of 0.92 for extension in Session II.

Haywood and associates[91] used a plastic tape measure for measuring half cycle active ROM in 159 patients with ankylosing spondylitis. The authors used the tip of the nose and the acromioclavicular joint as landmarks to measure right and left cervical rotation. The ROM was the difference between the tape measurement in the neutral position and the measurement in maximal ipsilateral rotation. Fifty-five patients participated in the reliability study. The intratester reliability (test-retest at 2-week interval) was high (ICC > 0.90), but intertester reliability was unacceptable for the neutral starting position.

Maksymowych and coworkers[89] measured full cycle rotation active ROM on 263 patients with ankylosing spondylitis from three different countries. Forty-four of the patients were involved in the reliability study. Landmarks used for measuring rotation were the tragus of the right ear and the suprasternal notch. Measurements were taken with a tape-based tool at full right rotation (D1) and at full left rotation (D2). Full cycle rotation was defined as the distance between the two measurements (D1–D2). Intratester reliability was good for the two testers (ICC = 0.80 and 0.89); intertester reliability also was good (ICC = 0.82).

Viitanen and associates[92] measured cervical lateral flexion and rotation in a series of 52 male patients with a mean age of 45 years with idiopathic ankylosing spondylitis. Testing was done by two physical therapists. Intratester and intertester reliability coefficients for tape measurements were excellent for cervical lateral flexion (ICC = 0.96 and ICC = 0.97, respectively) and for rotation (ICC = 0.98 and ICC = 0.97, respectively).

Validity of the Tape Measure

The authors recommended that the tape measure method be used more widely. Balogun and associates[14] compared measurements taken with a tape measure with measurements taken with a Myrin gravity-reference goniometer. The r values of each of the three testers were higher for the tape measuring method than for the inclinometer method. Therefore, Viitanen and associates[92] compared cervical rotation and lateral flexion tape measurements with radiologic changes such as changes in the apophyseal joints, calcification of discs, and ossification of spinal ligaments. Cervical rotation and lateral flexion measurements correlated significantly with cervical radiologic changes and, therefore, according to the authors, the tape measure was an appropriate method for assessing disease severity and progression.

Maksymowych and coworkers[89] compared measurements of cervical active ROM taken with a tape measure with measurements of cervical rotation active ROM taken with a plastic universal goniometer. The authors found that the tape measure approach was comparable to the universal goniometer, which the authors used as the gold standard.

Reliability of the Inclinometer

Viitanen and associates[92] used the Myrin gravity-reference goniometer (a single inclinometer attached to the head) to measure active ROM in 52 male patients with a mean age of 44.7 years with ankylosing spondylitis. Two physical therapists measured patients on successive days. Both intratester reliability and intertester reliability were high, with ICCs of 0.89 to 0.98. Balogun and coworkers[14] employed three testers to use the Myrin gravity-reference goniometer to measure the active ROM of half cycle motions. Twenty-one healthy students were measured over a period of several days (between 4 and 110). Intratester reliability coefficients (r) values for all motions ranged from unacceptable ($r = 0.31$) for flexion to good ($r = 0.86$) for extension. Intertester reliability coefficients across two testing sessions ranged from unacceptable ($r = 0.26$) for left rotation to good ($r = 0.84$) for extension.

Malmström and associates[15] used the single Myrin gravity-reference goniometer to measure both full and half cycle active ROM in 60 neck-healthy volunteers (35 women and 25 men) ranging in age from 22 to 58 years. Intratester reliability was high, with ICCs of 0.90 and higher for full cycle flexion–extension, lateral flexion, and rotation. Intratester reliability was lower for half cycle motions, with the ICCs ranging from 0.69 for left rotation to 0.89 for extension.

Alaranta and associates[16] used a liquid single inclinometer, the MIE (Medical Research Ltd, London), which they attached by Velcro to a cloth helmet on the top of the subject's head to measure half cycle active ROM flexion and extension and lateral flexion. A gravitational inclinometer was attached to the helmet, and the subject was placed in a supine position to measure rotation. Ninety-nine subjects participated in the intratester reliability part of the study in which one physiotherapist measured all subjects twice at an interval of 1 year. The correlation coefficient values for half cycle motions were an r of 0.68 for flexion and extension, r of 0.61 for lateral flexion, and unacceptable ($r = 0.37$) for rotation. Forty-eight subjects participated in the intertester reliability study in which two physiotherapists did the testing at a 1-week interval. The values for full cycle motions ranged from an r of 0.69 for flexion–extension to an r of 0.86 for left-right rotation.

Hole, Cook, and Bolton[44] also had two testers use an MIE single inclinometer to measure active ROM in 30 healthy volunteers aged 20 to 69 years. Intratester reliability for flexion–extension, right lateral flexion, and right rotation was high (ICC = 0.93–0.94) and intratester reliability for left lateral flexion and left rotation was good (ICC = 0.84–0.88). Intertester reliability was good (ICC = 0.81–0.86) for flexion–extension, both right and left lateral flexion and left rotation. However, intertester reliability was only fair for right rotation (ICC = 0.76).

Piva and coworkers[85] measured half cycle active ROM with the MIE single inclinometer in 30 patients aged 18 to 75 years who had symptoms in their neck, scapula, or head. Intraclass correlation coefficient values ranged from fair to high (ICC = 0.78–0.91). The minimal detectable change (MDC) the authors considered to be adequate for clinical use ranged from 9 degrees for left rotation in flexion to 16 degrees for the motions of flexion and extension.

Nineteen individuals with neck pain and 20 healthy controls were examined by two physical therapists on separate days.[93] A single gravity inclinometer (Medical Research Limited, Leeds, UK) was used to quantify the following motions: active cervical flexion, extension, and lateral flexion. Three trials were performed in each motion to assess intrarater reliability for within-session measurements and the average of three measurements from each rater was used to assess interrater reliability between sessions. Intrarater reliability coefficients (ICCs) for cervical ROM across all movement directions ranged from 0.95 to 0.98 in the healthy group and from 0.94 to 0.98 in the neck pain group. Interrater reliability ranged from moderate to substantial in both groups: healthy (ICC = 0.45–0.79) and neck pain (ICC = 0.47–0.78). Minimal detectable change values ranged from 5 to 15 degrees for the healthy group and from 9 to 21 for the neck pain group.

Hoving and associates[94] used a Cybex Electronic Digital Inclinometer-320 (EDI-320) to measure full cycle active ROM in 32 patients 18 to 70 years of age with neck pain, neck stiffness, or both. Intratester reliability was high for motions in three planes, with values ranging from an ICC of 0.93 for lateral flexion for both raters to an ICC of 0.97 for flexion–extension for one rater. Intertester reliability was good to high, with ICCs of 0.89 and higher. The smallest detectable differences (SDDs) based on intratester agreement results for one of the testers were 11.1 degrees for flexion–extension, 10.4 degrees for lateral flexion, and 13.5 degrees for rotation. Therefore, only changes greater than these values can be detected beyond measurement error when a single therapist performs the measurements. The SDD values were higher if two different raters performed the measurements.

In the search for relatively simple, inexpensive instruments for measuring active cervical motion, Prushanksy, Deryi, and Jabarreen tested a single digital inclinometer using the Zebris CMS 70P as the reference instrument.[63] Six primary motions were measured in two sessions spread over 7 days in 15 healthy women and 15 healthy men aged 24 years. In the first session measurements were taken with both a digital inclinometer (DI) and the Zebris CMS 70P, whereas in the second session only the DI was used. No significant differences were found between the two instruments in the sagittal and frontal planes but the measurement of rotation by the DI was significantly greater than rotation measurements taken with the Zebris. Interdevice interclass correlation coefficients

(ICCs) for the DI were 0.72 (right lateral flexion), 0.62 (left lateral flexion), 0.77 (flexion), and 0.83 (extension). Poor correlations were found for rotations. The investigators suggested that the poor results for rotations were probably due to the fact that the DI required a supine testing position for rotations whereas all of the Zebris measurements were taken in the sitting position. Intratester reproducibility of the test-retest DI measurements showed good to excellent reproducibility in all planes with ICCs ranging from 0.82 (left lateral flexion) to 0.94 (extension). The SEM ranged from 1.6 degrees for right rotation to 2.6 degrees for flexion. The authors concluded that the relatively inexpensive DI was reproducible and valid for measuring sagittal and frontal plane motions in healthy individuals.

Validity of the Inclinometer

Bredenkamp-Herrmann[95] took radiographic measurements of passive ROM of neck flexion–extension in 16 individuals aged 2 to 68 years. The radiographic measurements were compared with those obtained by means of a pendulum goniometer (inclinometer). Intraclass correlation coefficients of 0.98 indicated a good agreement between the two methods.

Bush and associates[96] compared three methods of inclinometry measurements of sagittal and frontal plane cervical motion with radiographic measurements. Transverse plane motion measurements were compared with computed tomography scan measurements. The authors defined validity as those inclinometry measurements that fell within ±5 degrees of radiographic measurements. Using this standard, only the single and double inclinometer methods were valid for measuring flexion; only the single inclinometer and single stabilization methods were valid for measuring extension. No methods were valid for measuring either lateral flexion or rotation. The single inclinometer method had the highest validity among the three methods.

Lantz, Chen, and Buch[45] compared the Dualer digital dual inclinometer and the CA-6000 electrogoniometer. Simultaneous measurements by the two instruments were performed twice over a 1-week interval. Concurrent validity of the two instruments showed almost identical mean values for flexion, extension, and lateral flexion. The ICC for between-instrument comparison in the same session was high.

Malmström and associates[15] compared the single Myrin gravity-reference goniometer with a three-dimensional ultrasound motion device—the Zebris CMS 30/70P system (Zebris Medizintechnik GmbH, Isny, Germany). Both instruments were used to measure full cycle active ROM in 60 healthy adults (35 women and 25 men) ranging in age from 22 to 58 years. The test and retest ICC was high, greater than 0.90 for intradevice reliability. The ICC was greater than 0.93 for concurrent validity. The authors concluded that their research supports the continued use of the Myrin in routine clinical work.

Reliability of the CROM Device

Capuano-Pucci and colleagues[97] in 1981 conducted one of the earliest studies on the CROM device in which two testers took measurements of each half cycle of active ROM performed by 20 subjects (16 women and 4 men) with a mean age of 23.5 years. The author found good intratester reliability for four out of six half cycle motions for one tester and for five out six motions for the second tester. All correlation coefficients were greater than 0.80 for intertester reliability, which was slightly higher than intratester reliability. This unusual finding was attributed to the fact that the time interval between testers was only minutes, whereas the time interval between the first and second trials by one tester was 2 days. More detailed information about this study and other studies in the section can be found in Tables 11.9 and 11.10.

In the 1991 study by Youdas, Carey, and Garrett,[26] 11 volunteer physical therapists were given a 1-hour training session on the CROM device prior to measuring half cycle active ROM in 60 patients (39 women and 21 men) with orthopedic disorders. The patients, ranging in age from 21 to 84 years, were divided into groups of 20 and were tested twice by two therapists. The results of the testing showed high intratester reliability and good intertester reliability for both flexion and extension. Intratester reliability was good for left neck lateral flexion (ICC = 0.84) and was high for right lateral flexion (ICC = 0.92). Intertester reliability was fair for left lateral flexion and good for right lateral flexion. Intratester reliability was high for both left and right rotation, and intertester reliability for rotation ranged from good for left rotation to high for right rotation.

Youdas and associates[12] used five testers to measure half cycle active ROM in 337 healthy subjects (171 women and 166 men) who were 11 to 97 years of age. Each subject performed three repetitions of each motion, and each subject was tested by three testers within minutes of each other. Intratester reliability was low for flexion (ICC = 0.76), high for extension (ICC = 0.94), and good for left and right lateral flexion. Intratester reliability for rotation also was good, with ICCs of 0.84 for left rotation and 0.80 for right rotation. The intertester reliability of all half cycle neck motion measurements was good except for left rotation, which was poor (ICC = 0.66).

Nilsson[31] measured half cycle passive ROM on 14 volunteers 23 to 45 years of age. Each subject was measured three times at 20-minute intervals. Intratester reliability was considered acceptable (r = 0.61–0.86). Intertester reliability was unacceptable (r = 0.29–0.66) based on the mean of five repeated measures and the fact that in four out of six motions the r was less than 0.60.

Hole, Cook, and Bolton[44] selected 30 of 84 asymptomatic subjects for the reliability portion of a study of full cycle active ROM. Intratester reliability was high (ICC = 0.96) for the full cycle combined motion of flexion and extension, and intertester reliability was good (ICC = 0.88). Intratester reliability was high (ICC = 0.96) for full cycle right-left lateral flexion, and intertester reliability was good (ICC = 0.84). Both intratester and intertester reliability were high (ICC = 0.92) for the full cycle motion of left–right rotation.

Nilsson, Christensen, and Hartvigsen[65] measured half and full cycle passive ROM on 17 males and 18 females 20 to

Text continued on page 463

TABLE 11.9 Intratester Reliability: Cervical ROM Using the CROM Device

Study	*N*	Sample	Testers	Motion	ICC [or *r*]	SEM (degrees)	LOA (degrees)	MDC (degrees)
Healthy Populations								
Audette et al[28]	20	Healthy 9 M, 11 F Mean age: 37 yr	Not identified	Flexion AROM	0.89	2.8		6.5
				Extension AROM	0.98	2.2		5.1
				R lateral flexion AROM	0.97	1.6		3.6
				L lateral flexion AROM	0.97	1.8		4.2
				R rotation AROM	0.92	2.6		6.1
				L rotation AROM	0.95	2.1		4.9
Capuano-Pucci et al[97]	20	Healthy Mean age: 23.5 yr	21	Flexion AROM				
				Tester 1	[0.63]			
				Tester 2	[0.91]			
				Extension AROM				
				Tester 1	[0.90]			
				Tester 2	[0.82]			
				R lateral flexion AROM				
				Tester 1	[0.79]			
				Tester 2	[0.89]			
				R rotation AROM				
				Tester 1	[0.85]			
				Tester 2	[0.62]			
Fletcher and Bandy[30]	25	Healthy 8 M, 17 F Mean age: 26.4 yr	1 physical therapist and 1 athletic trainer	Flexion AROM	0.87	2.8		6.5
				Extension AROM	0.90	4.0		9.3
				R lateral flexion AROM	0.92	2.5		5.9
				L lateral flexion AROM	0.92	2.5		5.9
				R rotation AROM	0.90	2.4		5.5
				L rotation AROM	0.94	2.3		5.4
Florêncio et al[108]	20	Healthy F Mean age: 22 yr	3	Flexion	0.70			
				Extension	0.81			
				R lateral flexion	0.88			
				L lateral flexion	0.81			
				R rotation	0.69			
				L rotation	0.79			
Nilsson[31]	14	Healthy Age range: 23–45 yr		Flexion PROM	[0.76]			6°*
				Extension PROM	[0.85]			5°
				R lateral flexion PROM	[0.61]			5°
				R Rotation PROM	[0.75]			6°

(table continues on page 460)

TABLE 11.9 Intratester Reliability: Cervical ROM Using the CROM Device (continued)

Study	*N*	Sample	Testers	Motion	ICC [or *r*]	SEM (degrees)	LOA (degrees)	MDC (degrees)
Healthy Populations								
Olson et al[109]	12	Healthy Age range: 21–47 yr	2	Flexion Extension R lateral flexion R rotation	0.88 0.99 0.98 0.99			
Peolsson et al[47]	30	Healthy Mean age: 32.3 yr	2 physiotherapists	Flexion-extension AROM R and L lateral flexion AROM R and L rotation AROM	0.94–0.96 0.88–0.95 0.93–0.95			
Youdas et al[12]	6	Healthy Mean age: 27.2 yr	5 physical therapists	Flexion Extension R lateral flexion R rotation	0.88 0.94 0.85 0.80			
Patient Populations								
Dunleavy and Goldberg[72]	32	Neck pain for more than 3 months Mean age: 59 yr		Habitual posture Erect posture	0.87–0.96 0.88–0.96	2.4–6.4 2.1–4.2	6.6–17.7 5.8–11.6	
Fletcher and Bandy[30]	22	Neck pain 7 M, 15 F Mean age: 33.6 yr	1 physical therapist and 1 athletic trainer	Flexion Extension R lateral flexion L lateral flexion R rotation L rotation	0.88 0.92 0.93 0.89 0.92 0.96	4.1 3.0 2.5 3.9 3.3 2.9		9.6 7.0 5.9 9.1 7.6 6.7
Williams et al[99]	38 19 M, 19 F	1-month post–whiplash injury Mean age: 38 yr	1 physiotherapist	Flexion AROM Extension AROM R rotation AROM R lateral flexion AROM Flexion PROM Extension PROM R rotation PROM R lateral flexion PROM	0.99 0.99 0.98 0.98 0.98 0.99 0.99 0.98	1.4 1.6 2.0 1.3 2.1 1.8 1.9 1.6	–4.3–2.9 –5.0–5.0 –6.4–4.5 –4.2–3.0 –6.5–4.6 4.3–4.4 –6.9–5.1 –4.4–4.0	
Youdas et al[26]	60, three groups of 20	Orthopedic disorders: Mean age: 55.9 yr Mean age: 60.7 yr Mean age: 60.8 yr	11 physical therapists	Flexion AROM Extension AROM R lateral flexion AROM R rotation AROM	0.95 0.90 0.92 0.93			

ICC = Interclass correlation coefficient *r* = Pearson product moment correlation coefficient; LOA = Limits of agreement; MDC = Minimal detectable change; SEM = Standard error of measurement; AROM = Active range of motion; PROM = Passive range of motion; R = Right; L = Left.

*95% confidence interval for single subject measurement

TABLE 11.10 Intertester Reliability: Cervical ROM Using the CROM Device

Study	*N*	Sample	Testers	Motion	ICC [or *r*]	SEM (degrees)	LOA (degrees)	MDC (degrees)
Healthy Populations								
Florêncio et al[108]	20	Healthy women Mean age: 22 yr	3	Flexion Extension R lateral flexion L lateral flexion R rotation L rotation	0.85 0.91 0.93 0.89 0.76 0.81			
Nilsson[31]	14	Healthy Age range: 23–45 yr		Flexion PROM Extension PROM R lateral flexion PROM R rotation PROM	[0.71] [0.55] [0.58] [0.66]			
Nilsson[65]	35	Healthy Age range: 20–28 yr	2	Flexion PROM Extension PROM R lateral flexion PROM R rotation PROM Flexion–extension PROM R and L lateral flexion PROM R and L rotation PROM	0.65 0.54 0.64 0.41 0.60 0.69 0.88			
Olson et al[109]	12	Healthy Age range: 21–47 yr	2	Flexion Extension R lateral flexion R rotation	0.58 0.97 0.96 0.96	4 3 2 3		
Peolsson et al[47]	30	Healthy Mean age: 32.3 yr	2 physiotherapists	Flexion–extension AROM R and L lateral flexion AROM R and L rotation AROM	0.90, 0.95 0.90, 0.90 0.75, 0.90			
Youdas et al[12]	20	Healthy Mean age: 33 yr	5 physical therapists	Flexion AROM Extension AROM R lateral flexion AROM R rotation AROM	0.83 0.90 0.87 0.82			

(table continues on page 462)

TABLE 11.10 Intertester Reliability: Cervical ROM Using the CROM Device (continued)

Study	*N*	Sample	Testers	Motion	ICC [or *r*]	SEM (degrees)	LOA (degrees)	MDC (degrees)
Patient Populations								
Williams et al[99]	196 M, 13 F	1-month post whiplash injury, Mean age: 41 yr	2 physiotherapists	Flexion AROM	0.83	6.5	–21.6–16.1	
				Extension AROM	0.88	6.3	–18.9–18.0	
				R rotation AROM	0.92	4.9	–13.5–15.5	
				R lateral flexion AROM	0.82	3.7	–12.0–10.0	
				Flexion PROM	0.90	5.4	–16.9–14.0	
				Extension PROM	0.96	3.9	–9.5–12.8	
				R rotation PROM	0.89	6.1	–10.3–19.9	
				R lateral flexion PROM	0.77	4.8	–16.6–7.9	
Youdas et al[26]	60, three groups of 20	Orthopedic disorders	11 physical therapists	Flexion AROM	0.86			
		Mean age: 55.9 yr		Extension AROM	0.86			
		Mean age: 60.7 yr		R lateral flexion AROM	0.88			
		Mean age: 60.8 yr		R rotation AROM	0.92			

ICC = Interclass correlation coefficient *r* = Pearson product moment correlation coefficient; LOA = Limits of agreement; MDC = Minimal detectable change; SEM = Standard error of measurement; R = Right; L = Left

*95% confidence interval for single subject measurement

28 years of age. Subjects were asked to close their eyes and position their heads in neutral while the dials on the CROM device were set to 0. Intertester reliability was acceptable ($r = 0.61–0.88$) for full cycle motions, but intertester reliability for measuring single cycle motions was an r of 0.39 to 0.70. Rheault and colleagues[32] found only small mean differences ranging from 0.5 degrees to 3.6 degrees between two testers who measured half cycle extension active ROM with the CROM device.

Lindell, Eriksson, and Strender[98] compared the performance of a medically untrained tester with an experienced physical therapist. The untrained tester received 4 hours of training and practice in 10 tests including measurements of half cycle cervical flexion and extension and rotation taken with the CROM device. The subjects in the study included 30 patients with neck and back pain and 20 healthy subjects. In the interrater reliability study, all 50 subjects were tested once by each tester. In the intertester study, each tester measured neck motions twice in 10 of the 20 healthy subjects. Intratester reliability for the therapist was good for flexion (ICC = 0.86) and high for extension (ICC = 0.98), with an SEM of 2 degrees for each measurement. The ICCs for intratester reliability for the other tester were 0.62 for flexion and 0.80 for extension. The ICC for the therapist for right rotation was high; for left rotation the ICC was good. The other tester had good ICCs for both right and left rotation and slightly higher SEMs compared with the therapist. Cervical flexion and extension had poor intertester reliability, which the authors attributed to the need for manual stabilization. Other tests that required manual stabilization also had poor intertester reliability, but overall, the medically untrained tester was able to perform acceptably in 7 out of 10 tests.

Audette and colleagues[28] examined the between-day test-retest reliability of the CROM device for measuring cervical range of motion, and concurrent validity with the Fastrak electromagnetic motion-analysis system. Nine healthy men and 11 women between 23 and 71 years of age participated in the study, and data were collected during two sessions separated by 48 hours to assess test-retest reliability of the CROM device. Test-retest reliability was good to excellent as ICC values for all cervical motions ranged from 0.89 for flexion to 0.98 for extension. Minimal detectable change values for a 90% confidence level ranged from 3.6 degrees for right lateral flexion to 6.5 degrees for flexion. The authors concluded that any change larger than 6.5 degrees in cervical ROM measurements in any direction would represent a true change.

The purpose of a study by Williams et al was to evaluate the reproducibility of the CROM device for measuring both active ROM and passive ROM in a group of individuals with subacute whiplash-associated disorders (WAD).[99] Two research physiotherapists with 5 and 10 years' experience, respectively, performed the measurements after participating in 2 hours of training and practice using the CROM device on healthy volunteers. Thirty-eight participants with moderate pain and disability levels were included in the intraobserver study but only 19 individuals were available for the interobserver study. The authors concluded that the CROM device produces substantially reliable ROM measurements for both active and passive ROM in a population of individuals with WAD.

Validity of the CROM Device

Ordway and coworkers[100] simultaneously measured full cycle active ROM of combined flexion–extension with the CROM device, 3Space system, and radiographs in 20 healthy volunteers (11 women and 9 men) between 20 and 49 years of age. The authors found no significant difference between CROM device measurements and the radiographic angle between the occipital line and the vertical body, nor between the 3Space system and radiographic angle between the occipital line and the C7 vertebral body. However, there was a significant difference between flexion and extension measurements taken with the CROM device and the 3Space system. Therefore, these methods could not be used interchangeably. The authors determined that full cycle flexion–extension could be reliably measured by all three methods but that standardization of positioning was required to minimize upper thoracic motion with the CROM device. Protraction and retraction measured with the 3Space system were in agreement with the radiographic measurements but differed significantly from the measurements taken with the CROM device. The CROM device's advantages over the 3Space system were lower cost and ease of use.

Tousignant et al[101] used radiographs to determine the criterion validity of the CROM device for measuring half cycle flexion and extension on 31 healthy adults 18 to 25 years of age. Measurements with the CROM device were highly correlated with measurements obtained by the radiographic method for extension ($r = 0.98$) and flexion ($r = 0.97$) so that the validity of the CROM device for measuring flexion and extension was supported.

In another study, Tousignant and associates[33] determined that the CROM measurements of half cycle active ROM of lateral flexion demonstrated a very good linear relationship with radiographic measurements. A physiotherapist who had received 4 hours of instruction in using the CROM device measured right and left lateral flexion in 24 patients with neck pain. The correlation between the CROM device and radiographic measurements was good for both left ($r = 0.82$) and right ($r = 0.84$) lateral flexion. Therefore, the criterion validity of the CROM device for measuring lateral flexion was supported.

Tousignant and associates,[23] in another criterion validity study, compared half cycle active ROM measurements taken with the CROM device with measurements taken with the Optotrak (an optoelectronic system). Subjects included 34 women (21 to 85 years of age) and 21 men (19 to 80 years of age) recruited from the community. The results showed a very strong linear relationship between cervical rotation measured with the CROM device and the values obtained with the Optotrak. Pearson correlation coefficients (r) between CROM values and Optotrak values were good to excellent for rotation and for all other cervical motions. Based on their findings, the authors concluded that the validity of the CROM device was supported for the measurement of half cycle rotation in healthy individuals.

Hole, Cook, and Bolton[44] compared measurements of full cycle active ROM taken with the CROM device with measurements taken with a single gravity inclinometer (MIE) to determine the reliability and concurrent validity of the two instruments for measuring cervical motion. Eighty-four asymptomatic subjects were included in the study. There was good agreement between the two instruments when measuring active ROM in the sagittal and coronal planes, and concurrent validity was supported for flexion–extension and for right–left lateral flexion, but there was no agreement when measuring rotation in the transverse plane because, according to the authors, motion was consistently overestimated by the MIE.

Audette and coworkers[28] examined the concurrent validity of the CROM device with the Fastrak electromagnetic three-dimensional system in 20 healthy adults. Pearson correlation coefficients (r) between measurements taken with the Fastrak and CROM ranged from 0.93 to 0.99 for all cervical motions. Mean differences ranged from 0.9 to 1.2 degrees except for flexion at 5.3 degrees. The authors concluded that there was good concurrent validity of the CROM device compared with the Fastrak.

Reliability of the CA-6000 Electrogoniometer

Lantz, Chen, and Buch[45] measured active and passive half cycle motions in healthy students with the CA-6000. Intratester reliability ICCs ranged from fair (0.76) to high (0.97) for active ROM for full cycle motions and from poor (0.58) to high (0.95) for passive ROM for full cycle motions. Intertester ICCs for full cycle active ROM were higher, ranging from good (0.84) to high (0.91), compared with ICCs for full cycle passive ROM, which were fair (0.74) to good (0.86).

Solinger, Chen, and Lantz[69] measured half and full cycle active ROM in 20 healthy subjects (9 men and 11 women) ranging in age from 20 to 40 years. Each subject's ROM was measured twice by two experienced testers. Intertester and intratester reliability for full cycle motions of rotation and lateral flexion had high ICCs, ranging from 0.93 to 0.97, whereas intertester and intratester reliability ICCs for half cycle motions ranged from good (0.83) to high (0.95). Reliability values were consistently lower for measurements beginning in the neutral position compared with full cycle motions. The ICCs indicated that the electrogoniometer performed very reliably for rotation and lateral flexion but only at an acceptable level for flexion–extension (0.75 to 0.93). Flexion from the neutral position was the least reliable measurement even when taken by a single tester.

Christensen and Nilsson[102] found good intratester and intertester reliability for measurements of active ROM in 40 individuals tested by two testers. Intratester reliability was also good for passive ROM, but intertester reliability was good only for full cycle motions.

Validity of the CA-6000 Spine Motion Analyzer Electrogoniometer

Mannion and associates[62] compared cervical CROM measurements taken with the CA-6000 Spine Motion Analyzer with measurements taken with a three-dimensional ultrasound motion device Zebris CMS system. Initial measurements by both systems were taken in 19 healthy volunteers, and the same measurements were taken 3 days later. Test-retest reliability was good for each instrument, but a small significant difference (1% to 10%) between the values obtained by each instrument occurred.

Petersen and coworkers[103] determined that there was a large difference between the measurements obtained with the CA-6000 Spine Motion Analyzer and radiographs.

A cross-sectional reliability study using the Electronic CROM Goniometer from ARCON TM Functional Capacity Evaluation Systems was conducted on 54 individuals (26 with neck pain and 26 without neck pain) aged 20 to 70 years.[104] All motions were measured in the sitting position except for rotation, which was measured in the supine position. Intratester and intertester reliability was high for both groups, with ICCs ranging from 0.75 to 0.92.

Reliability of Visual Estimation

The reliability of visual estimates has been studied by Viikari-Juntura[105] in a neurological patient population and by Youdas, Carey, and Garrett[26] in an orthopedic patient population. In the study by Viikari-Juntura,[105] the subjects were 52 male and female neurological patients ranging in age from 13 to 66 years who had been referred for cervical myelography. Intertester reliability between two testers of visual estimates of cervical ROM was determined by the authors to be fair. The weighted kappa reliability coefficient for intratester agreement in categories of normal, limited, or markedly limited ROM ranged from 0.50 to 0.56.

In the study by Youdas, Carey, and Garrett,[26] the subjects were 60 orthopedic patients ranging in age from 21 to 84 years. Intertester reliability for visual estimates of both active flexion and extension was poor (ICC = 0.42). Intertester reliability for visual estimates of active lateral flexion ROM was fair; ICC for left lateral flexion was 0.63; for right lateral flexion it was 0.70. The intertester reliability for visual estimates of rotation was poor for left rotation (ICC = 0.69) and good for right rotation (ICC = 0.82).

Whitcroft et al[18] used the CROM device as the reference instrument when comparing ROM measurements taken with the UG, with a tape measure, and by visual estimation. Spearman's coefficients were used to show the rank order of agreement with the CROM. Correlation coefficients were unacceptable for visual estimation: 0.11 for extension and 0.32 and 0.28 for right and left rotation.

Reliability and Validity of Smartphone Applications

We are pleased to include some information on using smartphones to assess ROM. Although additional research is needed to ensure that these instruments can provide reliable and valid data, most evaluators of human function will undoubtedly welcome these instruments that are used so commonly in our society.

Quek and colleagues used a three-dimensional motion analysis (3DMA) system as the gold standard to validate the use of the customized Android Phone Application.[106] Twenty-one healthy individuals (11 males and 10 females mean age of 31 years) were examined on the first day and 16 participants returned 1 to 7 days later so that intrarater reliability could be assessed. All motions were performed actively by the participants, who were seated in a straight back chair. Cervical flexion, extension, and right and lateral flexion had ICCs of 0.82 to 0.90, but results were poor for rotation.

Tousignant-Laflamme et al had two examiners measure cervical range of motion in 28 healthy participants twice, once using the iPhone and once with the CROM device, which served as the gold standard.[107] The highest ICCs were observed for examiner 1, and they varied from 0.66 to 0.84. The ICCs were 0.78 for flexion and 0.84 for extension. The authors concluded that they could not recommend the iPhone for measuring motion in all directions because even though the iPhone had good intrarater reliability and moderate to good validity for motions in the sagittal and frontal planes, it had poor validity for rotation.

Summary

Each of the techniques for measuring cervical ROM discussed in this chapter has certain advantages and disadvantages. The universal goniometer and single inclinometer are among the least expensive and easiest to obtain, transport, and use, and therefore may be more acceptable clinically than other instruments. Generally, for most instruments intratester reliability is better than intertester reliability. Therefore, if these methods are used to determine a patient's progress, repeated measurements should be taken by the same examiner (a single therapist) and at the same time of day whenever possible.

In consideration of the cost and availability of the various instruments for measuring cervical ROM, and because of the fact that the intratester reliability of the universal goniometer appears comparable with that of measurements taken with other instruments, we have retained the universal goniometer but added both the double and single inclinometers and the CROM device to this textbook. The latter has the most research to support its use but it is more expensive than the other devices. If the tape measure is being used to compare ROM among different subjects, calculation of proportion of distance (POD) should help to eliminate the effects of different body sizes on measurements (refer to Body Size in the Research Findings section).[73]

REFERENCES

1. Bogduk, N, and Mercer, S: Biomechanics of the cervical spine. I: Normal kinematics. Clin Biomech 15:633, 2000.
2. Magee, DJ: Orthopedic Physical Assessment, ed 4. WB Saunders, Elsevier Health Sciences USA, Philadelphia, 2006.
3. Goel, V, et al: Moment-rotation relationships of the ligamentous occipito-atlanto-axial complex. J Biomech 21:673, 1988.
4. Cailliet, R: Soft Tissue Pain and Disability, ed 3. FA Davis, Philadelphia, 1991.
5. Crisco, JJ, Panjabi, MM, and Dvorak, J: A model of the alar ligaments of the upper cervical spine in axial rotation. J Biomech 24:607, 1991.
6. Ishii, T, et al: Kinematics of the upper cervical spine in rotation: In vivo three-dimensional analysis. Spine 29:E139, 2004.
7. Ishii, T, et al: Kinematics of the cervical spine in lateral bending: In vivo three-dimensional analysis. Spine 31:155, 2006.
8. White, A, and Panjabi, M: Clinical Biomechanics of the Spine, ed 2. JB Lippincott, Philadelphia, 1990.
9. Neumann, DA: Kinesiology of the Musculoskeletal System: Foundations for Rehabilitation, ed 2. Mosby, St. Louis, 2010.
10. Ishii, T, et al: Kinematics of the subaxial cervical spine in rotation: In vivo three-dimensional analysis. Spine 29:2826, 2004.
11. Demaille-Wlodyka, S, et al: Cervical range of motion and cephalic kinesthesis: Ultrasonographic analysis by age and sex. Spine 32:E254, 2007.
12. Youdas, JW, et al: Normal range of motion of the cervical spine: An initial goniometric study. Phys Ther 72:770, 1992.
13. Hsieh, C-Y, and Yeung, BW: Active neck motion measurements with a tape measure. J Orthop Sports Phys Ther 8:88, 1986.
14. Balogun, JA, et al: Inter- and intratester reliability of measuring neck motions with tape measure and Myrin gravity-reference goniometer. J Orthop Sports Phys Ther 10:248.
15. Malmström, E-M, et al: Zebris versus Myrin: A comparative study between a three-dimensional ultrasound movement analysis and an inclinometer/compass method: Intradevice reliability, concurrent validity, intertester comparison, intratester reliability, and intraindividual variability. Spine 28:E433, 2003.
16. Alaranta, H, et al: Flexibility of the spine: Normative values of goniometric and tape measurements. Scand J Rehabil Med 26:147, 1994.
17. de Koning CH, et al: Clinimetric evaluation of active range of motion measures in patients with non-specific neck pain: A systematic review. Eur Spine J 17:905, 2008.
18. Whitcroft, KL, et al: Comparison of methods of measuring active cervical range of motion. Spine 35:E976, 2010.
19. American Medical Association: Guides to the Evaluation of Permanent Impairment, ed 5. AMA, Chicago, 2000.
20. Rondinelli, R: Guides to the Evaluation of Permanent Impairment, ed 6. American Medical Association, Chicago, 2008.
21. Pringle, RK: Intra-instrument reliability of 4 goniometers. J Chiropr Med 2:91, 2003.
22. American Occupational Medicine Association (AOMA): Range of Motion (ROM) Booklet, 2010. Retrieved from https://www.scribd.com/doc/281488439/ROM-Booklet
23. Tousignant, M, et al: Criterion validity study of the cervical range of motion (CROM) device for rotational range of motion on healthy adults. J Orthop Sports Phys Ther 36:242, 2006.
24. Nilsson, N, Hartvigsen, J, and Christensen, HW: Normal ranges of passive cervical motion for women and men 20-60 years old. J Manipulative Physiol Ther 19:306, 1996.
25. Walmsley, RP, Kimber, P, and Culham, E: The effect of initial head position on active cervical axial rotation range of motion in two age populations. Spine 21:2435, 1996.
26. Youdas, JW, Carey, JR, and Garrett, TR: Reliability of measurements of cervical spine range of motion—comparison of three methods. Phys Ther 71:98, 1991.
27. CROM Procedure Manual: Procedure for Measuring Neck Motion With the CROM. Performance Attainment Association, St Paul, MN, 1988. Retrieved from http://www.spineproducts.com/pdf/CROMManual.pdf
28. Audette, I, et al: Validity and between-day reliability of the cervical range of motion (CROM) device. J Orthop Sports Phys Ther 40:318, 2010.
29. Williams, MA, et al: A systematic review of reliability and validity studies of methods for measuring active and passive cervical range of motion. J Manipulative Physiol Ther 33:138, 2010.
30. Fletcher, JP, and Bandy, WD: Intrarater reliability of CROM measurement of cervical spine active range of motion in persons with and without neck pain. J Orthop Sports Phys Ther 38:640, 2008.
31. Nilsson, N: Measuring passive cervical motion: A study of reliability. J Manipulative Physiol Ther 18:293, 1995.
32. Rheault, W, et al: Intertester reliability of the flexible ruler for the cervical spine. J Orthop Sports Phys Ther 10:254, 1989.
33. Tousignant, M, et al: Validity study for the cervical range of motion device used for lateral flexion in patients with neck pain. Spine 27:812, 2002.
34. O'Driscoll, S, and Tomenson, J: The cervical spine. Clin Rheum Dis 8:617, 1982.
35. Dvorak, J, et al: Age and gender related normal motion of the cervical spine. Spine 17:S393, 1992.
36. Pearson, ND, and Walmsley, RP: Trial into the effects of repeated neck retractions in normal subjects. Spine 20:1245, 1995.
37. Trott, P, et al: Three-dimensional analysis of active cervical motion: The effect of age and gender. Clin Biomech 11:201, 1996.
38. Pellecchia, G, and Bohannon, R: Active lateral neck flexion range of motion measurements obtained with a modified goniometer: Reliability and estimates of normal. J Manipulative Physiol Ther 21:443, 1998.
39. Chen J, et al: Meta-analysis of normative cervical motion. Spine 24:1571, 1999.
40. Feipel, V, et al: Normal global motion of the cervical spine: An electrogoniometric study. Clin Biomech 14:462, 1999.
41. Castro, WH, et al: Noninvasive three-dimensional analysis of cervical spine motion in normal subjects in relation to age and sex: An experimental examination. Spine 25:443, 2000.
42. Kuhlman, KA: Cervical range of motion in the elderly. Arch Phys Med Rehabil 74:1071, 1993.
43. Arbogast, KB, et al: Normal cervical spine range of motion in children 3–12 years old. Spine 32:E309, 2007.
44. Hole, D, Cook, J, and Bolton, J: Reliability and concurrent validity of two instruments for measuring cervical range of motion: Effects of age and gender. Man Ther 1:36, 1995.
45. Lantz, CA, Chen, J, and Buch, D: Clinical validity and stability of active and passive cervical range of motion with regard to total and unilateral uniplanar motion. Spine 24:1082, 1999.
46. Sforza, C, et al: Three-dimensional analysis of active head and cervical spine range of motion: Effect of age in healthy male subjects. Clin Biomech 17:611, 2002.
47. Peolsson, A, et al: Intra- and inter-tester reliability and range of motion of the neck. Physiother Can 52:233, 2000.
48. Seacrist, T, et al: Passive cervical spine flexion: The effect of age and gender. Clin Biomech 27:326, 2012.
49. Salo, PK, et al: Quantifying the effect of age on passive range of motion of the cervical spine in healthy working-age women. J Orthop Sports Phys Ther 39:478, 2009.
50. Quek, J, et al: Effects of thoracic kyphosis and forward head posture on cervical range of motion in older adults. Man Ther 18:65, 2013.
51. Simpson, AK, et al: Quantifying the effects of age, gender, degeneration, and adjacent level degeneration on cervical spine range of motion using multivariate analyses. Spine 33:183, 2008.
52. Park, MS, et al: Age-related changes in cervical sagittal range of motion and alignment. Global Spine J 4:151, 2014.
53. Yukawa, Y, et al: Age-related changes in osseous anatomy, alignment, and range of motion of the cervical spine. Part I: Radiographic data from over 1,200 asymptomatic subjects. Eur Spine J 21:1492, 2012.
54. Bible, JE, et al: Normal functional range of motion of the cervical spine during 15 activities of daily living. J Spinal Disord Tech 23:15, 2010.
55. Swinkels, RA, and Swinkels-Meewisse, IE: Normal values for cervical range of motion. Spine 39:362, 2014.
56. Tommasi, DG, et al: Active head and cervical range of motion: Effect of age in healthy females. Spine 34:1910, 2009.
57. Öhman, AM, and Beckung, ER: A pilot study on changes in passive range of motion in the cervical spine, for children aged 0–5 years. Physiother Theory Pract 29:457, 2013.
58. Lynch-Caris, T, et al: Establishing reference values for cervical spine range of motion in pre-pubescent children. J Biomech 41:2714, 2008.
59. Ferrario, VF, et al: Active range of motion of the head and cervical spine: A three-dimensional investigation in healthy young adults. J Orthop Res 20:122, 2002.
60. Abelin-Genevois, K, et al: Cervical spine alignment in the pediatric population: A radiographic normative study of 150 asymptomatic patients. Eur Spine J 23:1442, 2014.
61. Ordway, NR, et al: Cervical flexion, extension, protrusion, and retraction: A radiographic segmental analysis. Spine 24:240, 1999.

62. Mannion, A, et al: Range of global motion of the cervical spine: Intraindividual reliability and the influence of measurement device. Eur Spine J 9:379, 2000.
63. Prushansky, T, Deryi, O, and Jabarreen, B: Reproducibility and validity of digital inclinometry for measuring cervical range of motion in normal subjects. Physiother Res Int 15:42, 2010.
64. Assink, N, et al: Interobserver reliability of neck-mobility measurement by means of the flock-of-birds electromagnetic tracking system. J Manipulative Physiol Ther 28:408, 2005.
65. Nilsson, N, Christensen, HW, and Hartvigsen, J: The interexaminer reliability of measuring passive cervical range of motion, revisited. J Manipulative Physiol Ther 19:302, 1996.
66. Bergman, GJ, et al: Variation in the cervical range of motion over time measured by the "flock of birds" electromagnetic tracking system. Spine 30:650, 2005.
67. Miller, JS, Polissar, NL, and Haas, M: A radiographic comparison of neutral cervical posture with cervical flexion and extension ranges of motion. J Manipulative Physiol Ther 19:296, 1996.
68. Christensen, HW, and Nilsson, N: The ability to reproduce the neutral zero position of the head. J Manipulative Physiol Ther 22:26, 1999.
69. Solinger, AB, Chen, J, and Lantz, CA: Standardized initial head position in cervical range-of-motion assessment: Reliability and error analysis. J Manipulative Physiol Ther 23:20, 2000.
70. Wibault, J, et al: Using the cervical range of motion (CROM) device to assess head repositioning accuracy in individuals with cervical radiculopathy in comparison to neck-healthy individuals. Man Ther 18:403, 2013.
71. Owens, EF, et al: Head repositioning errors in normal student volunteers: A possible tool to assess the neck's neuromuscular system. Chiropr Osteopat 14:5, 2006.
72. Dunleavy, K, and Goldberg, A: Comparison of cervical range of motion in two seated postural conditions in adults 50 or older with cervical pain. J Man Manip Ther 21:33, 2013.
73. Chibnall, JT, Duckro, PN, and Baumer, K: The influence of body size on linear measurements used to reflect cervical range of motion. Phys Ther 74:1134, 1994.
74. Brink, Y, et al: The spinal posture of computing adolescents in a real-life setting. BMC Musculoskelet Disord 15:212, 2014.
75. Bennett, SE, Schenk, RJ, and Simmons, ED: Active range of motion utilized in the cervical spine to perform daily functional tasks. J Spinal Disord Tech 15:307, 2002.
76. Cobian, DG, et al: Active cervical and lumbar range of motion during performance of activities of daily living in healthy young adults. Spine 38:1754, 2013.
77. Cobian, DG, et al: Task specific frequencies of neck motion measured in healthy young adults over a 5 day period. Spine 34:E202, 2009.
78. Shugg, JA, Jackson, CD, and Dickey, JP: Cervical spine rotation and range of motion: Pilot measurements during driving. Traffic Inj Prev 12:82, 2011.
79. Cote, M, et al: Reference values for physical performance measures in the aging working population. Hum Factors 56:228, 2014.
80. Guth, EH: A comparison of cervical rotation in age-matched adolescent competitive swimmers and healthy males. J Orthop Sports Phys Ther 21:21, 1995.
81. Lark, SD, and McCarthy, PW: The effects of a single game of rugby on active cervical range of motion. J Sports Sci 27:491, 2009.
82. Lark, S, and McCarthy, P: Active cervical range of motion recovery following the rugby off-season. J Sports Med Phys Fitness 50:318, 2010.
83. Jordan, K: Assessment of published reliability studies for cervical spine range-of-motion measurement tools. J Manipulative Physiol Ther 23:180, 2000.
84. Jordan, K, et al: The reliability of the three-dimensional FASTRAK measurement system in measuring cervical spine and shoulder range of motion in healthy subjects. Rheumatology 39:382, 2000.
85. Piva, SR, et al: Inter-tester reliability of passive intervertebral and active movements of the cervical spine. Man Ther 11:321, 2006.
86. Portney, L, and Watkins, M: Foundations of Clinical Research: Applications to Practice, ed 2. Prentice-Hall, Upper Saddle River, NJ, 2000.
87. Tucci, SM, et al: Cervical motion assessment: A new, simple and accurate method. Arch Phys Med Rehabil 67:225, 1986.
88. Pile, K, et al: Clinical assessment of ankylosing spondylitis: A study of observer variation in spinal measurements. Rheumatology 30:29, 1991.
89. Maksymowych, WP, et al: Development and validation of a simple tape-based measurement tool for recording cervical rotation in patients with ankylosing spondylitis: Comparison with a goniometer-based approach. J Rheumatol 33:2242, 2006.
90. Yankai, A, and Manosan, P: Reliability of the universal and invented gravity goniometers in measuring active cervical range of motion in normal healthy subjects. Int J Applied Biomedical Engineering 2:49, 2009.
91. Haywood, K, et al: Spinal mobility in ankylosing spondylitis: Reliability, validity and responsiveness. Rheumatology 43:750, 2004.
92. Viitanen, J, et al: Clinical assessment of spinal mobility measurements in ankylosing spondylitis: A compact set for follow-up and trials? Clin Rheumatol 19:131, 2000.
93. Shahidi, B, et al: Reliability and group differences in quantitative cervicothoracic measures among individuals with and without chronic neck pain. BMC Musculoskelet Disord 13:215, 2012.
94. Hoving, JL, et al: Reproducibility of cervical range of motion in patients with neck pain. BMC Musculoskelet Disord 6:59, 2005.
95. Bredenkamp-Herrmann, D: Validity study of head and neck flexion-extension motion comparing measurements of a pendulum goniometer and roentgenograms. J Orthop Sports Phys Ther 11:414, 1989.
96. Bush, KW, et al: Validity and intertester reliability of cervical range of motion using inclinometer measurements. J Man Manip Ther 8:52, 2000.
97. Capuano-Pucci, D, et al: Intratester and intertester reliability of the cervical range of motion device. Arch Phys Med Rehabil 72:338, 1991.
98. Lindell, O, Eriksson, L, and Strender, L-E: The reliability of a 10-test package for patients with prolonged back and neck pain: Could an examiner without formal medical education be used without loss of quality? A methodological study. BMC Musculoskelet Disord 8:31, 2007.
99. Williams, MA, et al: Reproducibility of the cervical range of motion (CROM) device for individuals with sub-acute whiplash associated disorders. Eur Spine J 21:872, 2012.
100. Ordway, NR, et al: Cervical sagittal range-of-motion analysis using three methods: Cervical range-of-motion device, 3Space, and radiography. Spine 22:501, 1997.
101. Tousignant, M, et al: Criterion validity of the cervical range of motion (CROM) goniometer for cervical flexion and extension. Spine 25:324, 2000.
102. Christensen, HW, and Nilsson, N: The reliability of measuring active and passive cervical range of motion: An observer-blinded and randomized repeated-measures design. J Manipulative Physiol Ther 21:341, 1998.
103. Petersen, CM, et al: Agreement of measures obtained radiographically and by the OSI CA-6000 Spine Motion Analyzer for cervical spinal motion. Man Ther 13:200, 2008.
104. Law, EYH, and Chiu, TT-W: Measurement of cervical range of motion (CROM) by electronic CROM goniometer: A test of reliability and validity. J Back Musculoskelet Rehabil 26:141, 2013.
105. Viikari-Juntura, E: Interexaminer reliability of observations in physical examinations of the neck. Phys Ther 67:1526, 1987.
106. Quek, J, et al: Validity and intra-rater reliability of an Android phone application to measure cervical range-of-motion. Measurements 5:6, 2014.
107. Tousignant-Laflamme, Y, et al: Reliability and criterion validity of two applications of the iPhone to measure cervical range of motion in healthy participants. J Neuroeng Rehabil 10:69, 2013.
108. Florêncio, LL, et al: Agreement and reliability of two non-invasive methods for assessing cervical range of motion among young adults. Rev Bras Fisioter 14(2):175, 2010. Epub 2010 May 14.
109. Olson, SL, et al: Tender point sensitivity, range of motion, and perceived disability in subjects with neck pain. J Orthop Sports Phys Ther 30:13, 2000.

CHAPTER 12

The Thoracic and Lumbar Spine

Cynthia C. Norkin, PT, EdD

Structure and Function

Thoracic Spine

The 12 vertebrae of the thoracic spine form a curve that is convex posteriorly (Fig. 12.1A). This sagittal plane curve is referred to as the thoracic kyphosis, which ranges from 20 to 50 degrees when assessed radiographically.[1] The vertebrae composing the curve have a number of unique features. Spinous processes slope inferiorly from T1 to T10 and overlap from T5 to T8, whereas the spinous processes of T11 and T12 take on the horizontal orientation of the lumbar region's spinous processes. The transverse processes from T1 to T10 are large, with thickened ends that support paired costal facets for articulation with the ribs. Paired demifacets (superior and inferior costovertebral facets), also for articulation with the ribs, are located on the posterolateral corners of the vertebral bodies from T2 to T9.

The intervertebral and zygapophyseal joints in the thoracic region have essentially the same structure as described for the cervical region, except that the superior articular zygapophyseal facets face posteriorly, somewhat laterally, and cranially. The superior articular facet surfaces are slightly convex, whereas the inferior articular facet surfaces are slightly concave. The inferior articular facets face anteriorly and slightly medially and caudally. In addition, the joint capsules are tighter than those in the cervical region.

The costovertebral joints are formed by slightly convex costal superior and inferior demifacets (costovertebral facets) on the head of a rib and corresponding demifacets on the vertebral bodies of a superior and an inferior vertebra (Fig. 12.1B). From T2 to T8, the costovertebral facets articulate with concave demifacets located on the inferior body of one vertebra and on the superior aspect of the adjacent inferior vertebral body. Some of the costovertebral facets also articulate with the interposed intervertebral disc, whereas the 1st, 11th, and 12th ribs articulate with only one vertebra. A thin, fibrous capsule, which is strengthened by radiate ligaments (see Fig. 12.1B) and the posterior longitudinal ligament, surround the costovertebral joints. An intra-articular ligament lies within the capsule and holds the head of the rib to the annulus pulposus.

The costotransverse joints are the articulations between the costal tubercles of the 1st to the 10th ribs and the costal facets on the transverse processes of the 1st to the 10th thoracic vertebrae. The costal tubercles of the 1st to the 7th ribs are slightly convex and the costal facets on the corresponding transverse processes are slightly concave. The articular surfaces of the costal and vertebral facets are quite flat from about T7 to T10. The costotransverse joint capsules are strengthened by the medial, lateral, and superior costotransverse ligaments.

Osteokinematics

The zygapophyseal articular facets lie in the frontal plane from T1 to T6 and therefore limit flexion and extension in this region. The articular facets in the lower thoracic region are oriented more in the sagittal plane and thus permit somewhat more flexion and extension. The ribs and costal joints restrict lateral flexion in the upper and middle thoracic region, but in the lower thoracic segments lateral flexion and rotation are relatively free because these segments are not limited by the ribs. In general, the thoracic region is less flexible than the cervical spine because of the limitations on movement imposed by the overlapping spinous processes, the tighter joint capsules, and the rib cage.

Arthrokinematics

In flexion, the body of the superior thoracic vertebra tilts anteriorly, translates anteriorly, and rotates slightly on the adjacent inferior vertebra. At the zygapophyseal joints, the inferior articular facets of the superior vertebra slide upward on the superior articular facets of the adjacent inferior vertebra. In extension, the opposite motions occur: The superior vertebra tilts and translates posteriorly and the inferior articular facets glide downward on the superior articular facets of the adjacent inferior vertebra.

In lateral flexion to the right, the right inferior articular facets of the superior vertebra glide downward on the right superior articular facets of the inferior vertebra. On the

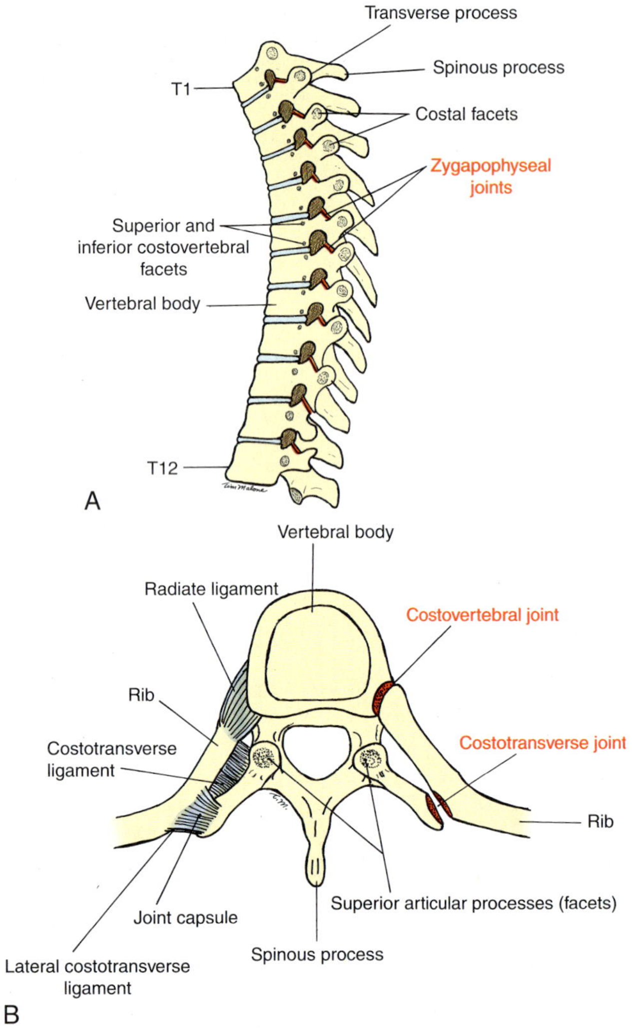

FIGURE 12.1 (A) A lateral view of the thoracic spine shows the spine's convex posterior sagittal plane curvature. The costal facets are visible on the enlarged ends of the transverse processes from T1 to T10 and the costovertebral facets can be seen on the lateral edges of the superior and inferior aspects of the vertebral bodies. The zygapophyseal joints are shown between the inferior articular facets of the superior vertebrae and the superior articular facets of the adjacent inferior vertebrae. (B) A superior view of a thoracic vertebra shows the articulations between the vertebra and the ribs: the left and right costovertebral joints, the costotransverse joints between the costal facets on the left and right transverse processes, and the costal tubercles on the corresponding ribs.

contralateral side, the left inferior articular facets of the superior vertebra glide upward on the left superior articular facets of the adjacent inferior vertebra.

In axial rotation, the superior vertebra rotates on the inferior vertebra, and the inferior articular surfaces of the superior vertebra impact on the superior articular surfaces of the adjacent inferior vertebra. For example, in rotation to the left, the right inferior articular facet impacts on the right superior articular facet of the adjacent inferior vertebra. Rotation and gliding motions occur between the ribs and the vertebral bodies at the costovertebral joints. A slight amount of rotation is possible between the joint surfaces of the ribs and the transverse processes at the upper costotransverse joints, and more rotation is allowed in the gliding that occurs at the lower joints (T7 to T10). The movements at the costal joints are primarily for ventilation of the lungs but also allow some flexibility of the thoracic region.

Capsular Pattern

The capsular pattern for the thoracic spine is a greater limitation of extension, lateral flexion, and rotation than of forward flexion.[2]

Lumbar Spine

The bodies of the five lumbar vertebrae are more massive than those in the other regions of the spine in order to support the weight of the trunk. Spinous processes are broad and thick and extend almost horizontally (Fig. 12.2A). The 5th lumbar vertebra differs from the other four vertebrae in having a wedge-shaped body, with the anterior height greater than the posterior height. The inferior articular facets of the 5th vertebra are widely spaced for articulation with the sacrum.

The surfaces of the superior articular facets at the zygapophyseal joints are concave and face medially and posteriorly. The inferior articular facet surfaces are convex and face laterally and anteriorly. Joint capsules are strong and ligaments of the region are essentially the same as those for the thoracic region, except for the addition of the iliolumbar ligament and thoracolumbar fascia and the fact that the posterior longitudinal ligament is not well developed in the lumbar area. The supraspinous ligament is well developed only in the upper lumbar spine. However, the intertransverse ligament is well developed in the lumbar area, and the anterior longitudinal ligament is strongest in this area (Fig.12.2B). The interspinous ligaments connect one spinous process to another, and the iliolumbar ligament helps to stabilize the lumbosacral joint and prevent anterior displacement.

Osteokinematics

The zygapophyseal articular facets of L1 to L4 lie primarily in the sagittal plane, which favors flexion and extension and limits lateral flexion and rotation. However, flexion is more limited than extension. During combined flexion and extension, the greatest mobility takes place between L4 and L5, whereas the greatest amount of flexion takes place at the lumbosacral joint, L5–S1. Lateral flexion and rotation are greatest in the upper lumbar region, and little or no lateral flexion is present at the lumbosacral joint because of the orientation of the facets.

Arthrokinematics

According to Bogduk,[3] flexion at the lumbar intervertebral joints consistently involves a combination of 8 to 13 degrees of anterior rotation (tilting), 1 to 3 millimeters of anterior translation (sliding), and some axial rotation. The superior vertebral body rotates, tilts, and translates (slides) anteriorly on the adjacent inferior vertebral body (Fig.12.3A). During

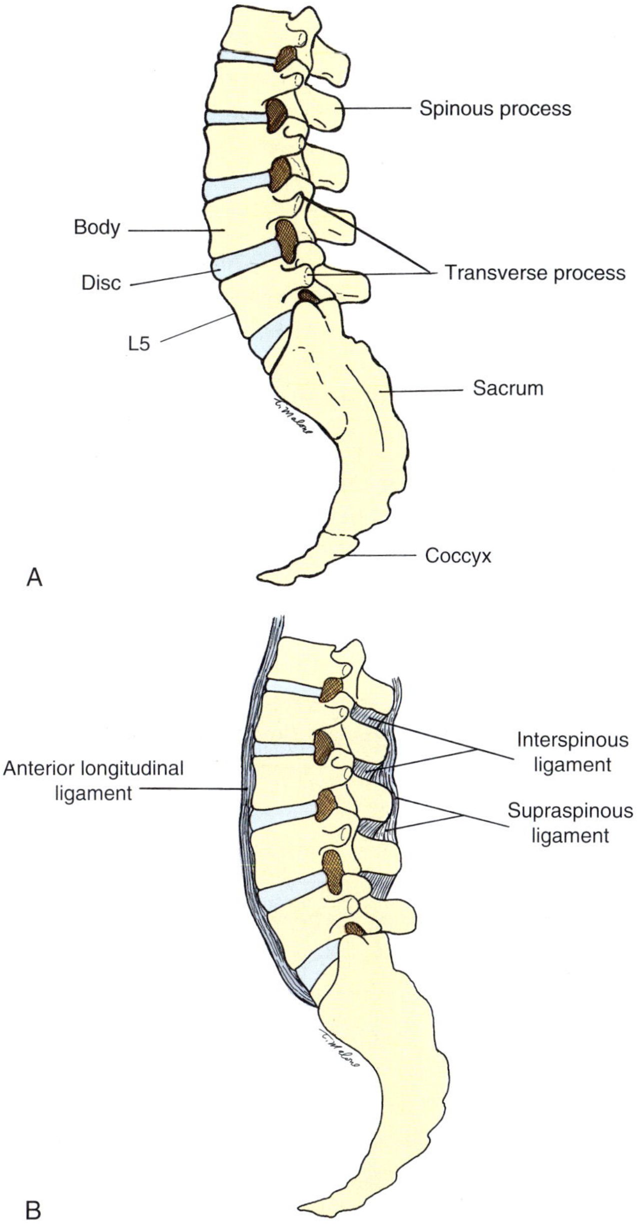

FIGURE 12.2 (A) A lateral view of the lumbar spine shows that the spine is convex anteriorly and that it has broad, thick, horizontally oriented spinous processes and large vertebral bodies. (B) The lateral view also shows the anterior longitudinal, supraspinous, and interspinous ligaments.

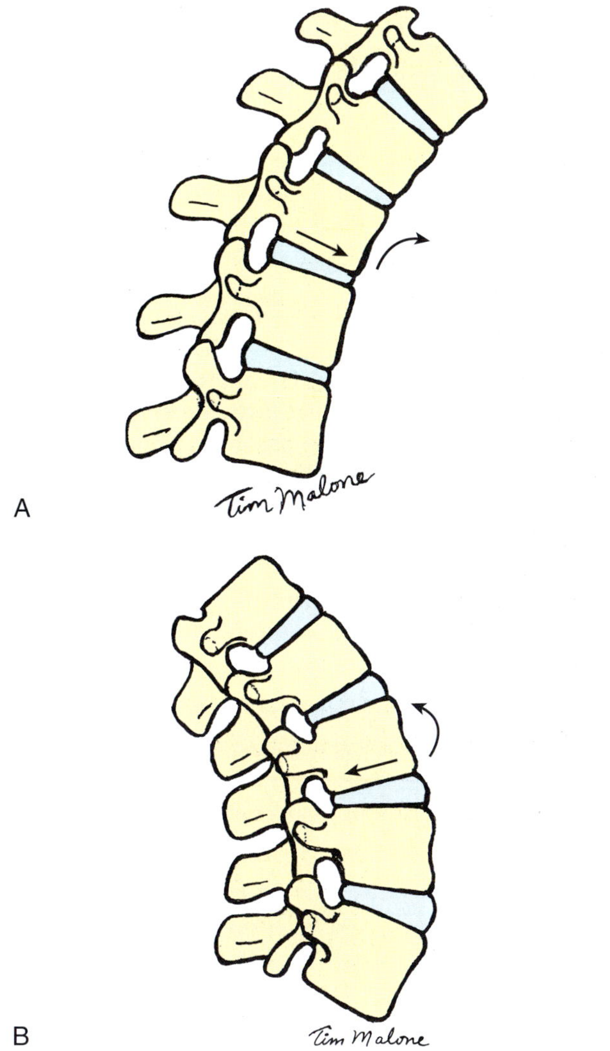

FIGURE 12.3 (A) Flexion involves anterior rotation, tilting, and sliding of the superior lumbar vertebral body on the adjacent inferior lumbar vertebral body. (B) Extension involves the opposite motions as the body of the superior vertebra rotates, tilts, and slides posteriorly on the adjacent inferior vertebra and the inferior facets of the superior vertebra slide downward on the superior articular facets of the adjacent inferior vertebra.

flexion at the zygapophyseal joints, the inferior articular facets of the superior vertebra slide upward on the superior articular facets of the adjacent inferior vertebra. In extension, the opposite motions occur: The vertebral body of the superior vertebra tilts and slides posteriorly on the adjacent inferior vertebra, and the inferior articular facets of the superior vertebra slide downward on the superior articular facets of the adjacent inferior vertebra (Fig.12.3B).

In lateral flexion, the superior vertebra tilts and translates laterally on the adjacent vertebra below. In lateral flexion to the right side, the right inferior articular facets of the superior vertebra slide downward on the right superior facets of the adjacent inferior vertebra. The left inferior articular facets of the superior vertebra slide upward on the left superior facets of the adjacent inferior vertebra.

In axial rotation, the superior vertebra rotates on the inferior vertebra, and the inferior articular surfaces of the superior vertebra impact on the superior articular facet surfaces of the adjacent inferior vertebra. In rotation to the left, the right inferior articular facet impacts on the right superior facet of the adjacent inferior vertebra.

Capsular Pattern

The capsular pattern for the lumbar spine is a marked and equal restriction of lateral flexion followed by restriction of flexion and extension.[2]

RANGE OF MOTION TESTING PROCEDURES: Thoracic and Lumbar Spine

Measurement of the thoracic and lumbar spine is complicated by the region's multiple joint structure, lack of well-defined landmarks, and difficulty separating thoracic and lumbar motion from hip motion. These difficulties have given rise to the variety of different methods used to measure range of motion (ROM) in the clinic including the following: tape measure method, the Modified-Modified Schober Test (MMST), the universal goniometer (UG) method, and the single and double inclinometer methods. These methods were selected because they are inexpensive, relatively easy to use, and generally have acceptable reliability. The double inclinometer method was included in the last edition of this book because the fifth edition of the American Medical Association's (AMA) *Guides to the Evaluation of Permanent Impairment*[4] required that this method be used to obtain spinal mobility measurements for disability determination. However, the sixth edition of the *Guides*[5] recommends that double inclinometers be used only for tracking patient progress and not for disability evaluation because insufficient evidence exists regarding the method's reliability and validity. We have included the double inclinometer method in our book because it appears to be useful for monitoring patient status.

Normal thoracic and lumbar spine ROM values using a variety of instruments are located in the Research Findings section, where Table 12.1 provides adult ROM values from various studies, and Tables 12.2 through 12.6 provide information about the effects of age and gender on thoracic and lumbar ROM. This information is followed by functional ranges of motion and a review of research studies on the reliability and validity of various instruments and testing methods. Note that in the following testing procedures active ROM is being measured.

Landmarks for Testing Procedures

Surface and bony landmarks of the thoracic and lumbar spine are shown in Figures 12.4 and 12.5.

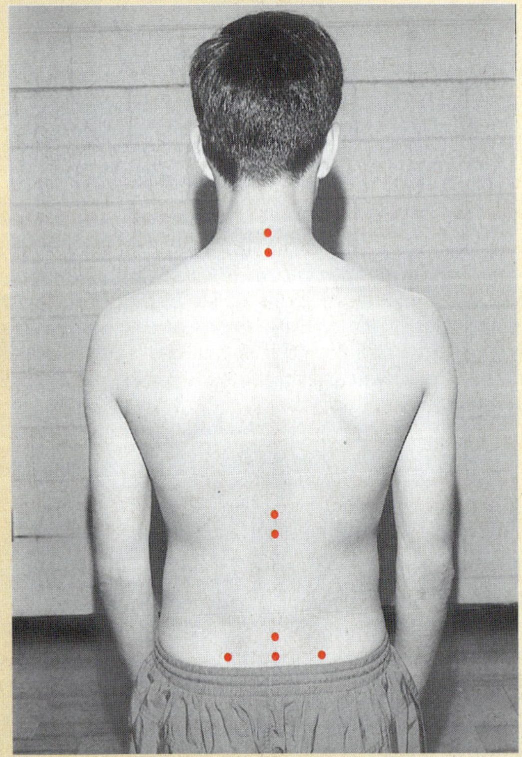

FIGURE 12.4 Surface anatomy landmarks for tape measure, universal goniometer, and inclinometer alignment for measuring thoracolumbar spine motion. The dots are located over spinous processes of C7, T1, T12, L1, L5, and S2 and over the right and left posterior superior iliac spines (PSIS).

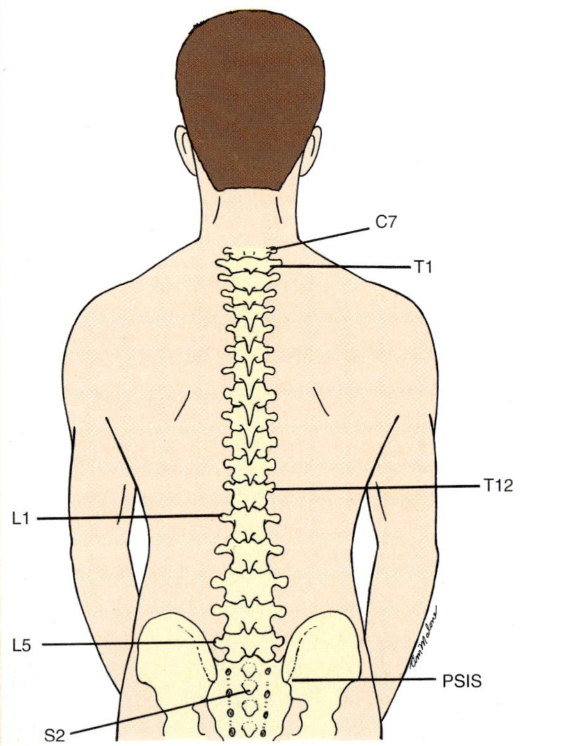

FIGURE 12.5 Bony anatomical landmarks for tape measure, universal goniometer, and inclinometer alignment for measuring thoracolumbar spine motion.

THORACOLUMBAR FLEXION

Motion occurs in the sagittal plane around a medial–lateral axis.

Testing Position

Ask the individual to assume a standing position with feet shoulder width apart and with the cervical, thoracic, and lumbar spine in 0 degrees of lateral flexion and rotation.

Stabilization

The examiner should stabilize the pelvis to prevent anterior tilting.

Testing Motion

Direct the individual to bend forward gradually while keeping the arms relaxed (Fig. 12.6) and the knees straight. The end of the motion occurs when resistance to additional flexion is experienced by the individual and the examiner feels the pelvis start to tilt anteriorly.

Normal End-Feel

The normal end-feel is firm owing to the stretching of the posterior longitudinal ligament (in the thoracic region), the ligamentum flavum, the supraspinous and interspinous ligaments, and the posterior fibers of the annulus pulposus of the intervertebral discs and the zygapophyseal joint capsules. Passive tension in the thoracolumbar fascia and the following muscles may contribute to the end-feel: spinalis thoracis, semispinalis thoracis, iliocostalis lumborum and iliocostalis thoracis, interspinales, intertransversarii, longissimus thoracis, and multifidus. The orientation of the zygapophyseal facets from T1 to T6 restricts flexion in the upper thoracic spine.

➧ **NOTE:** Use the same testing position, stabilization, testing motion, and normal end-feel described in the Thoracolumbar Flexion section for the following flexion measurement methods unless changes are noted.

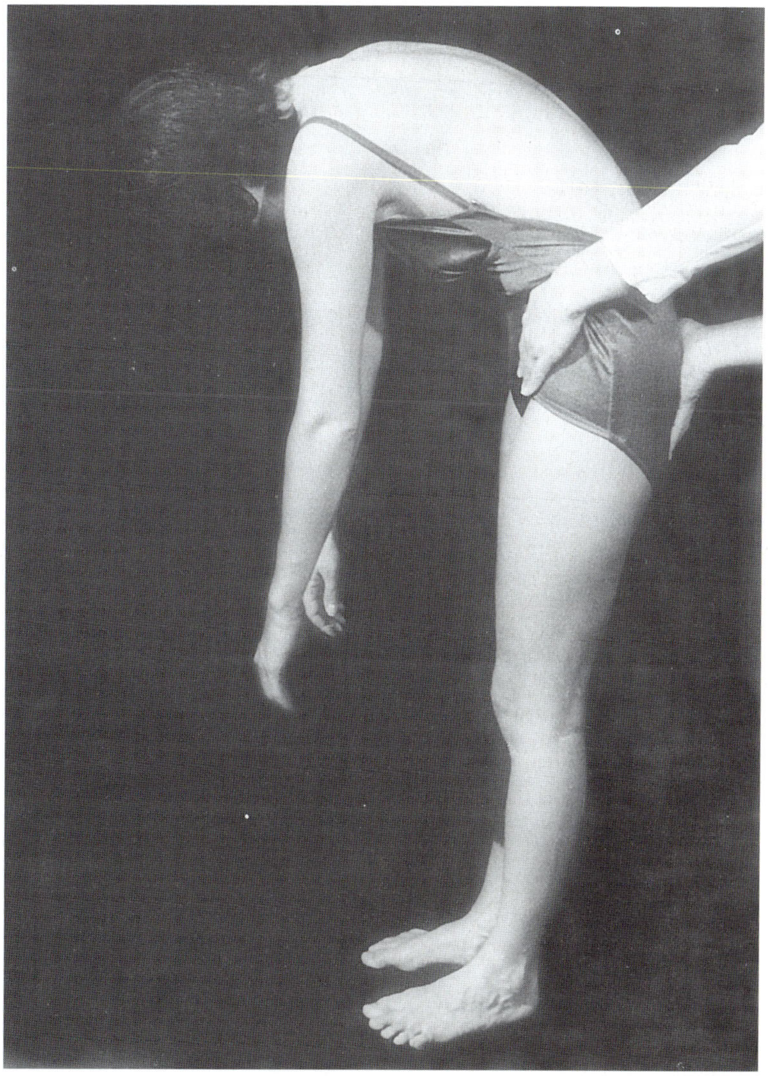

FIGURE 12.6 The individual is shown at the end of thoracolumbar flexion ROM. The examiner is shown stabilizing the pelvis to prevent anterior pelvic tilting.

THORACOLUMBAR FLEXION: TAPE MEASURE

Four inches (10 centimeters) between T1 and S1 is considered to be an average measurement for healthy adults.[6]

The following procedure for this measurement uses T1 and S2 instead of S1. The S2 vertebra can be identified more easily than the S1 vertebra and therefore may improve the reliability of the measurement. The spinous process of S2 is on a horizontal line with the posterior superior iliac spine (PSIS) and there is no motion between S1 and S2.

Procedure

1. With the individual in the standing position, mark the spinous processes of the T1 and S2 vertebrae using a skin marking pencil.
2. Align the tape measure between the two spinous processes (T1 and S2) and record the distance at the beginning of the ROM (Fig. 12.7).
3. Hold the tape measure in place as the individual performs flexion ROM. (Allow the tape measure to unwind and accommodate the motion.)
4. Record the distance at the end of the ROM (Fig. 12.8). The difference between the first and the second measurements indicates the amount of thoracolumbar flexion ROM.

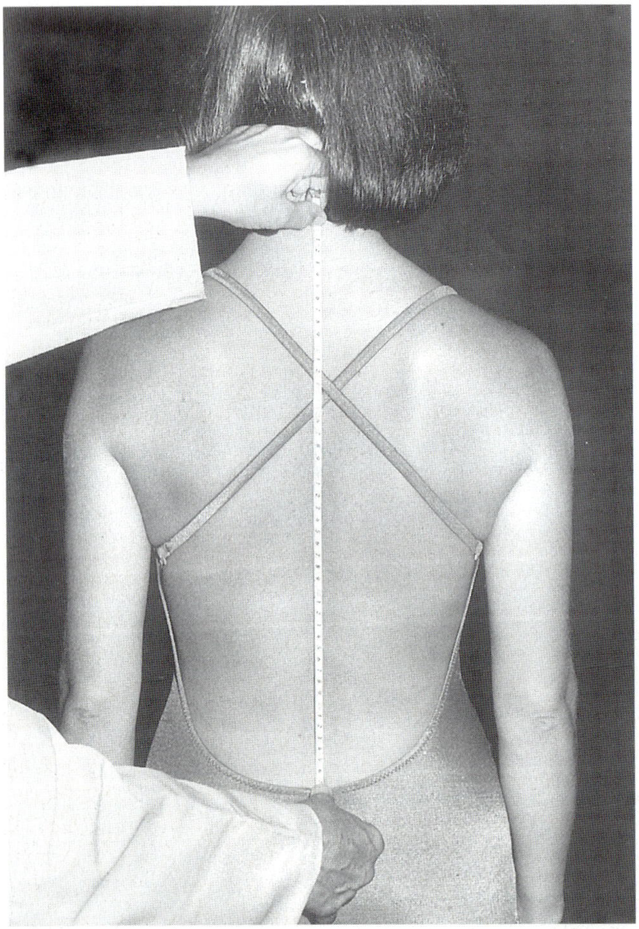

FIGURE 12.7 Tape measure alignment in the starting position for measuring thoracolumbar flexion ROM.

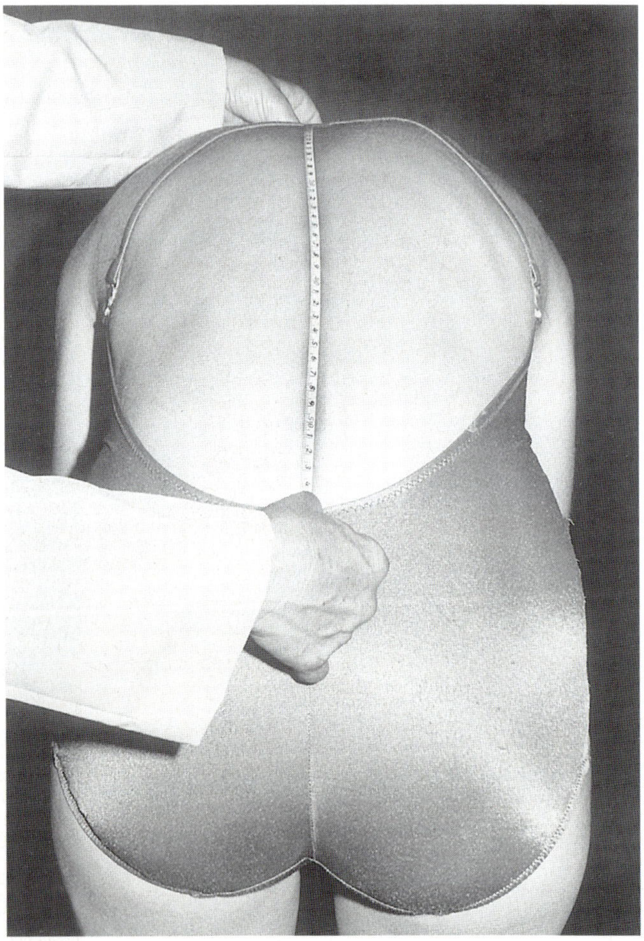

FIGURE 12.8 Tape measure alignment at the end of thoracolumbar flexion ROM. The metal tape measure case (not visible in the photo) is in the examiner's right hand.

THORACOLUMBAR FLEXION: FINGERTIP-TO-FLOOR

In a study by Quack and associates,[6] the fingertip-to-floor distance was 0.1 centimeters for 70 healthy females with a mean age of 53 years. In a study by Lindell and colleagues,[7] the ROM was 2.2 centimeters for 6 males and 14 females ranging in age from 22 to 55 years.

Procedure

1. Ask the individual to assume a standing position and then slowly bend forward as far as possible in an attempt to touch the floor while keeping the knees extended and feet together. No stabilization on the pelvis is provided by the examiner, thus allowing hip motions to occur.
2. At the end of the motion, measure the perpendicular distance between the tip of the individual's middle finger and the floor either with a tape measure or ruler (Fig. 12.9).

In a study by Artun and colleagues,[8] forward flexion fingertip-to-floor distance in adolescents had a clinically acceptable intraclass correlation coefficient (ICC) of 0.75 and a high interrater reliability ICC of 0.91.

Similar to Artun and colleagues, Perret and associates[9] determined that the forward flexion fingertip-to-floor test had excellent intratester and intertester reliability (ICC = 0.99) and validity. However, this test can be used only to assess general body flexibility because it combines spinal and hip flexion, making it impossible to isolate either motion.

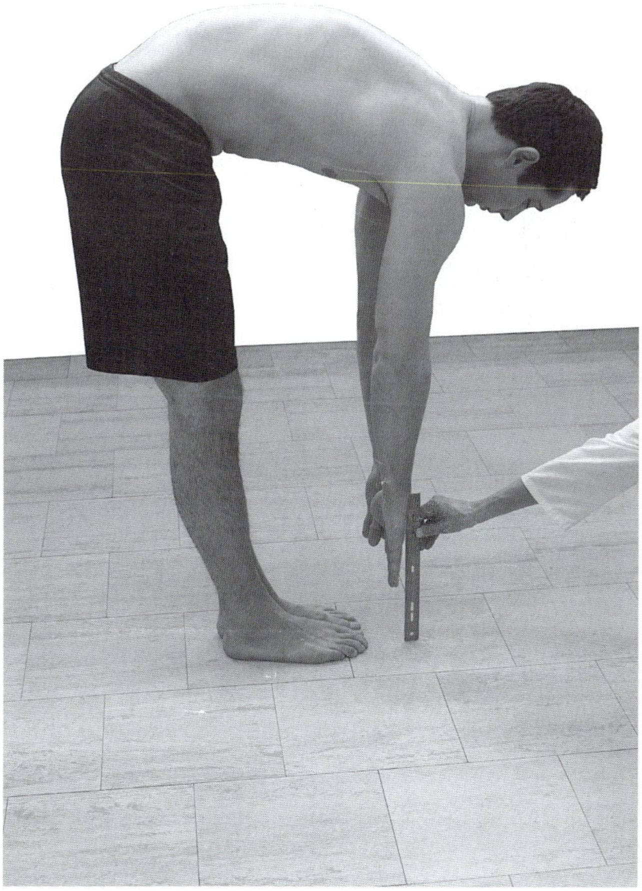

FIGURE 12.9 At the end of trunk and hip flexion the examiner measures the distance between the tip of the individual's middle finger and the floor with either a centimeter ruler or a tape measure. The individual in this photograph has been allowed to tilt the pelvis and flex the hip during this active motion.

THORACOLUMBAR FLEXION: DOUBLE INCLINOMETERS

According to the AMA,[10] normal ROM is 60 degrees for thoracolumbar flexion.

Procedure

1. Ask the individual to assume a standing position. Use a skin marking pencil to mark the spinous process of the T1 vertebra and the spinous process of the S2 vertebra.
2. Position one inclinometer over the spinous process of T1 and the second inclinometer over the sacrum at the level of S2. Then zero both inclinometers (Fig. 12.10).
3. At the end of the motion, read and record the values on both inclinometers (Fig. 12.11). The difference between the two inclinometers indicates the amount of thoracolumbar flexion ROM.

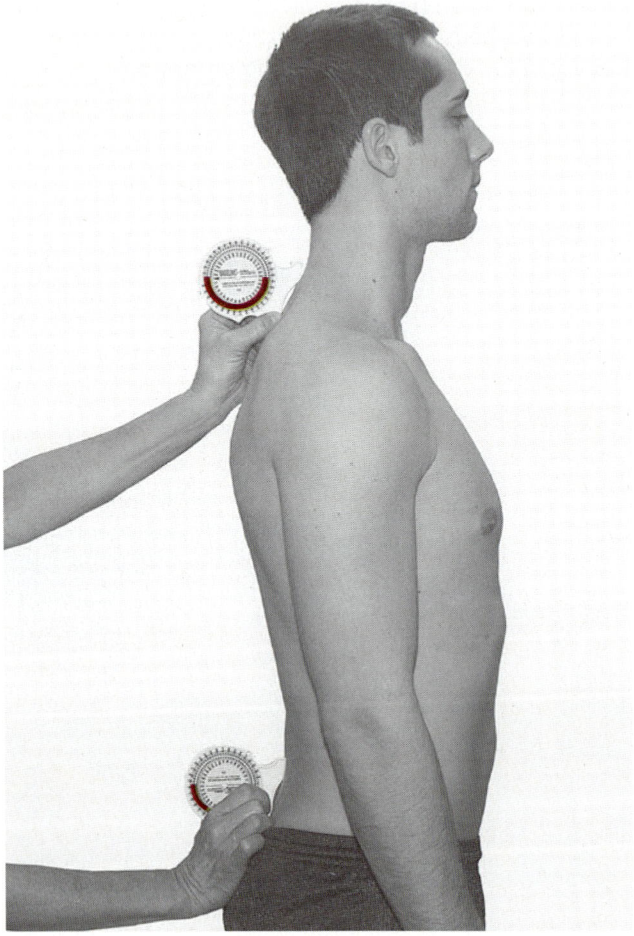

FIGURE 12.10 The starting position for measuring thoracolumbar flexion with both inclinometers aligned and zeroed.

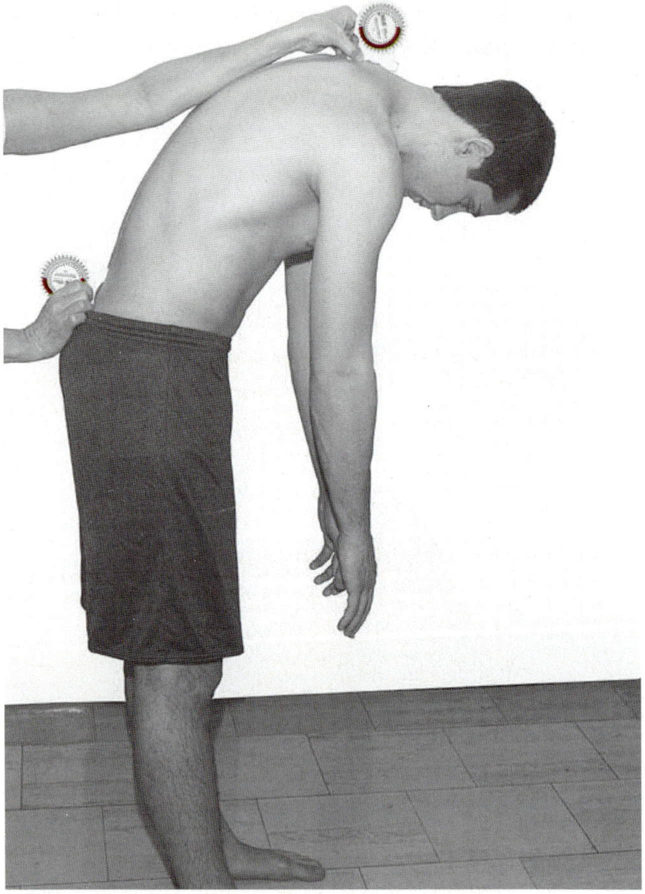

FIGURE 12.11 Inclinometer alignment at the end of thoracolumbar flexion ROM.

THORACOLUMBAR EXTENSION

Motion occurs in the sagittal plane around a medial–lateral axis.

Testing Position

Ask the individual to assume a standing position with feet shoulder width apart, knees extended, and with the cervical, thoracic, and lumbar spine in 0 degrees of lateral flexion and rotation.

Stabilization

Stabilize the pelvis to prevent posterior tilting.

Testing Motion

Ask the individual to extend the spine as far as possible (Fig. 12.12). The end of the extension ROM occurs when the pelvis begins to tilt posteriorly.

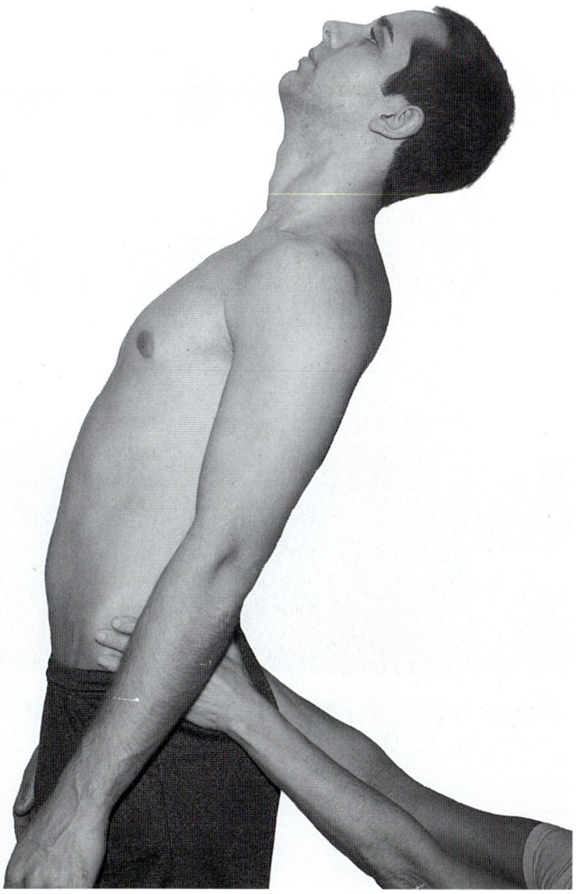

FIGURE 12.12 At the end of thoracolumbar extension ROM, the examiner uses her hands on the iliac crests to prevent posterior pelvic tilting. If the individual has balance problems or muscle weakness in the lower extremities, the measurement can be taken in either the prone or side-lying position.

Normal End-Feel

The end-feel is firm owing to stretching of the zygapophyseal joint capsules, anterior fibers of the annulus fibrosus, anterior longitudinal ligament, rectus abdominis, and external and internal oblique abdominals. The end-feel also may be hard owing to contact by the spinous processes and the zygapophyseal facets.

NOTE: Use the same testing position, stabilization, testing motion, and normal end-feel described in the Thoracolumbar Extension section above for the following extension measurement methods unless changes are noted.

THORACOLUMBAR EXTENSION: TAPE MEASURE

Procedure

1. Ask the individual to assume a standing position with feet shoulder width apart and knees extended. Mark the spinous processes of the T1 and S2 vertebrae using a skin marking pencil.
2. Align the tape measure between the two spinous processes and record the measurement (Fig. 12.13).
3. Ask the individual to bend backward. Keep the tape measure aligned during the motion and record the measurement at the end of the ROM (Fig. 12.14). The difference between the measurement taken at the beginning of the motion and that taken at the end indicates the amount of thoracolumbar extension.

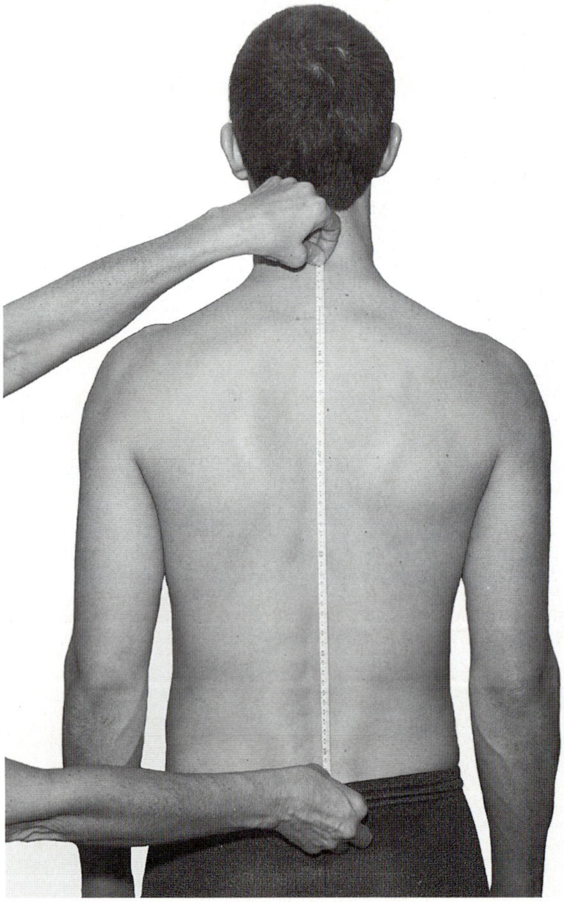

FIGURE 12.13 Tape measure alignment in the starting position for measurement of thoracolumbar extension. When the individual moves into extension, the tape slides into the tape measure case in the examiner's hand.

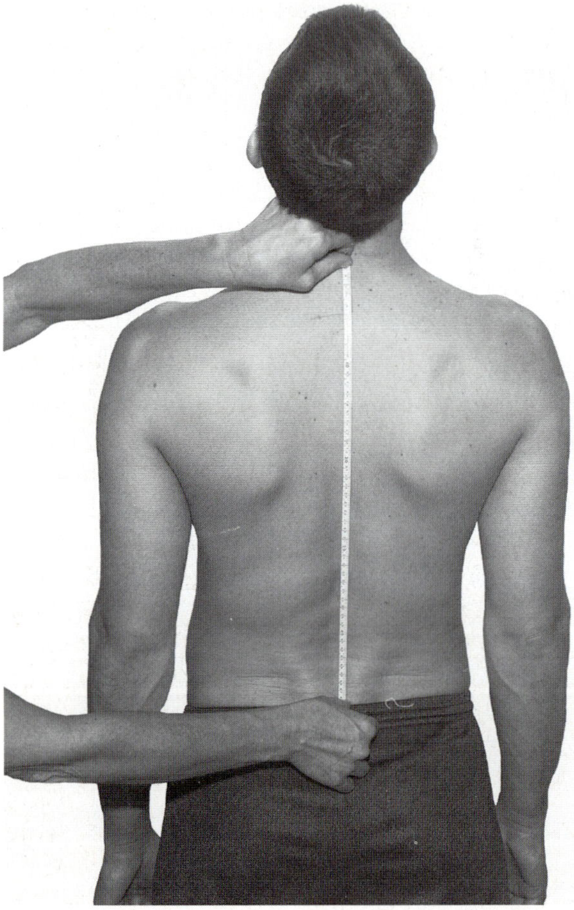

FIGURE 12.14 At the end of thoracolumbar extension ROM, the distance between the two landmarks is less than it was in the starting position.

THORACOLUMBAR EXTENSION: PRONE PUSH-UP

Procedure

1. Ask the individual to lie on the stomach on a table or plinth with the palms of hands positioned at shoulder level (Fig. 12.15).
2. Place a strap or belt over the pelvis to prevent it from lifting up off the support surface.
3. Direct the individual to extend elbows to raise the trunk up off the table and extend the thoracolumbar spine (Fig. 12.16).
4. Locate the individual's sternal notch and use the tape measure to measure the distance from the sternal notch to the supporting surface. Check to make sure the tape measure is vertical and record the measurement (Fig. 12.17).

This test can be used only in individuals who have good upper extremity strength and who can comfortably assume a prone lying position. If individuals have any muscle weakness in their upper extremities the test should not be attempted.

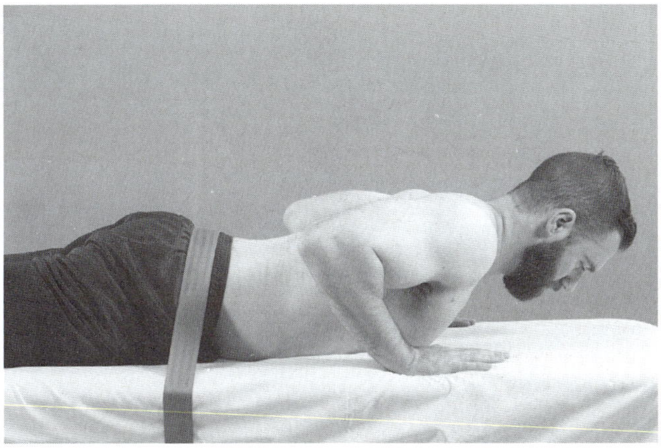

FIGURE 12.15 The individual assumes a prone lying position with palms of hands placed flat on the supporting surface at shoulder level.

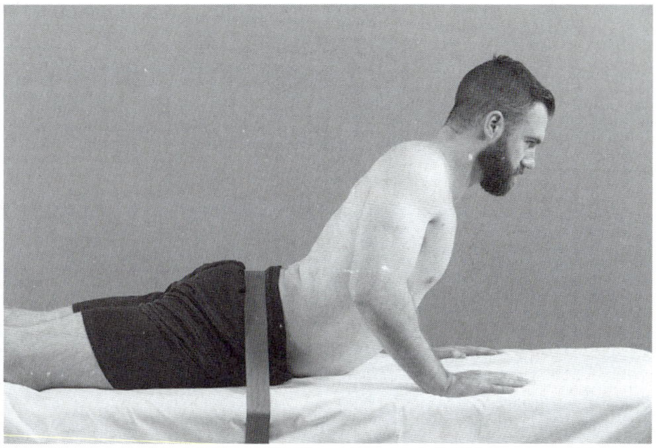

FIGURE 12.16 The individual extends elbows to push up the trunk as far as possible and to hold the position until a measurement can be taken.

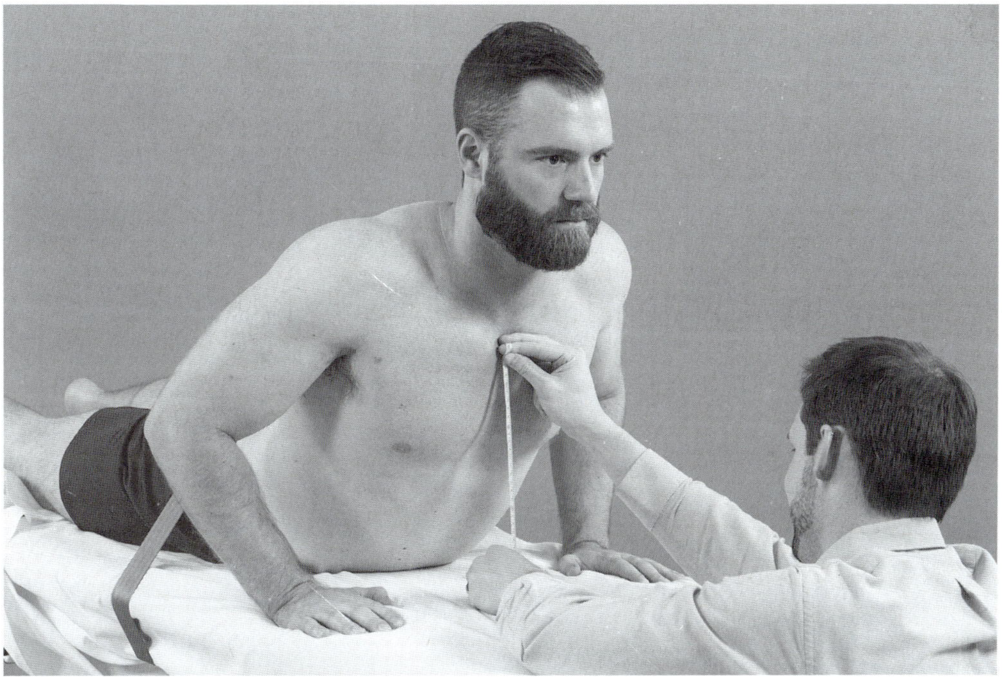

FIGURE 12.17 The examiner locates the individual's sternal notch and measures distance from the notch to the supporting surface using a tape measure, which must be kept vertical.

THORACOLUMBAR EXTENSION: DOUBLE INCLINOMETERS

According to the AMA,[10] normal ROM is 25 degrees for thoracolumbar extension.

Procedure

1. Ask the individual to assume a standing position. Mark the spinous processes of the T1 and S2 vertebrae using a skin marking pencil.
2. Position one inclinometer over the spinous process of T1 and the second inclinometer over the sacrum at the level of S2. Then zero both inclinometers (Fig. 12.18).
3. At the end of the motion, read and record the values on both inclinometers (Fig. 12.19). The difference between the two inclinometers indicates the amount of thoracolumbar extension.

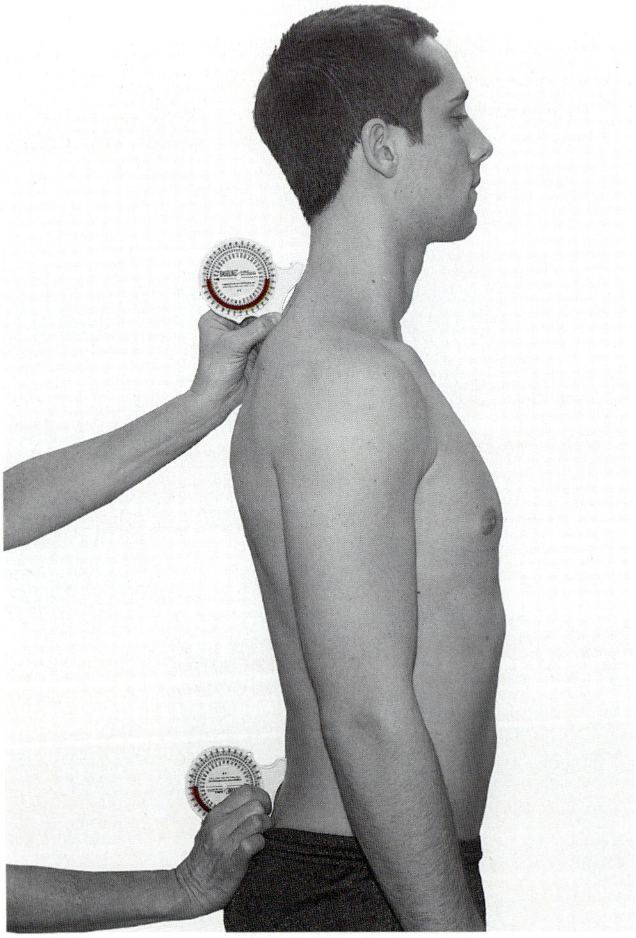

FIGURE 12.18 The starting position for measuring thoracolumbar extension with both inclinometers aligned and zeroed.

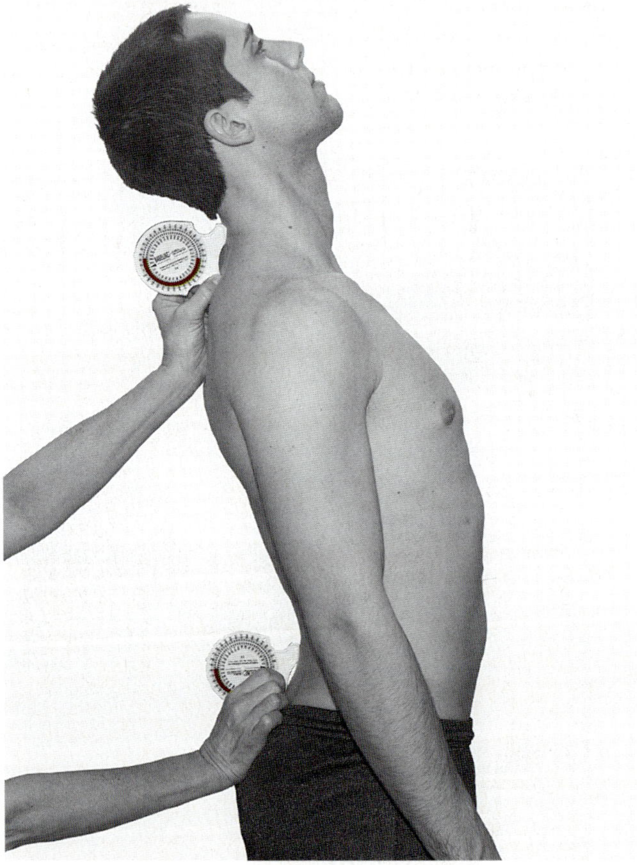

FIGURE 12.19 Inclinometer alignment at the end of thoracolumbar extension.

THORACOLUMBAR LATERAL FLEXION

Testing Position

Ask the individual to assume a standing position with the feet shoulder width apart and the cervical, thoracic, and lumbar spine in 0 degrees of flexion, extension, and rotation.

Stabilization

Stabilize the pelvis to prevent lateral tilting.

Testing Motion

Ask the individual to bend to one side while keeping the arms in a relaxed position at the sides of the body. Both feet should be kept flat on the floor with the knees extended (Fig. 12.20). The end of the motion occurs when the heel begins to rise on the foot opposite to the side of the motion and the pelvis begins to tilt laterally.

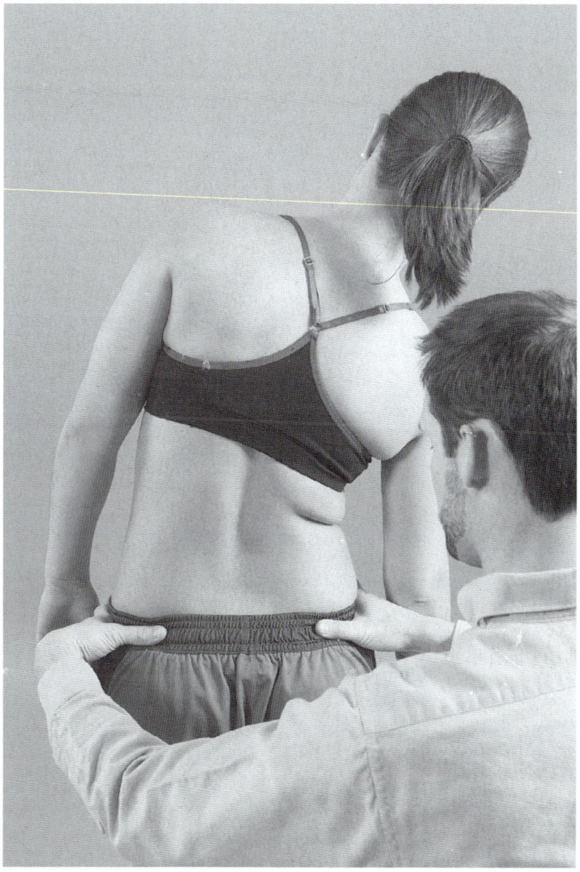

FIGURE 12.20 The end of thoracolumbar lateral flexion ROM. The examiner places both hands on the individual's pelvis to prevent lateral pelvic tilting.

Normal End-Feel

The end-feel is firm owing to the stretching of the contralateral fibers of the annulus fibrosus, zygapophyseal joint capsules, intertransverse ligaments, thoracolumbar fascia, and the following muscles: external and oblique abdominals, longissimus thoracis, iliocostalis lumborum and thoracis lumborum, quadratus lumborum, multifidus, spinalis thoracis, and serratus posterior inferior. The end-feel may also be hard owing to impact of the ipsilateral zygapophyseal facets (right facets when bending to the right) and the restrictions imposed by the ribs and costal joints in the upper thoracic spine.

NOTE: Use the same testing position, stabilization, testing motion, and normal end-feel described in the Thoracolumbar Lateral Flexion section above for the following lateral flexion measurement methods unless changes are noted.

THORACOLUMBAR LATERAL FLEXION: UNIVERSAL GONIOMETER

According to the American Academy of Orthopaedic Surgeons (AAOS),[11] the ROM is 35 degrees to each side for a young adult female and 38 degrees for a young adult male (see Table 12.1 in the Research Findings section). Fitzgerald and associates[12] found that normal values ranged from a mean of 37.6 degrees (in a group of 20- to 29-year-olds) to 18.0 degrees (in a group of 70- to 79-year-olds). See Table 12.2 in the Research Findings section for additional information. According to Sahrmann,[13] more than three-fourths of thoracic and lumbar lateral flexion ROM takes place in the thoracic spine.

Procedure

1. Ask the individual to assume a standing position. Mark the spinous processes of T1and S2 vertebrae using a skin marking pencil.
2. Center the fulcrum of the goniometer over the posterior aspect of the spinous process of S2 (Fig. 12.21).
3. Align proximal arm so that it is perpendicular to the ground.
4. Align distal arm with the posterior aspect of the spinous process of T1 (Fig. 12.22).
5. Read the goniometer, remove, and record the measurement.

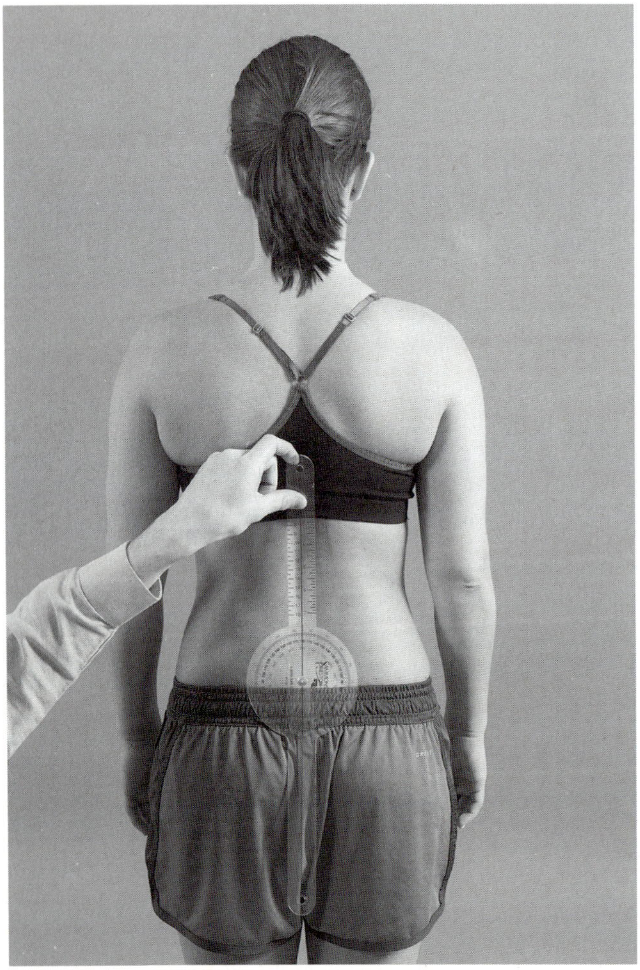

FIGURE 12.21 The individual is shown with the goniometer aligned in the starting position for measurement of thoracolumbar lateral flexion.

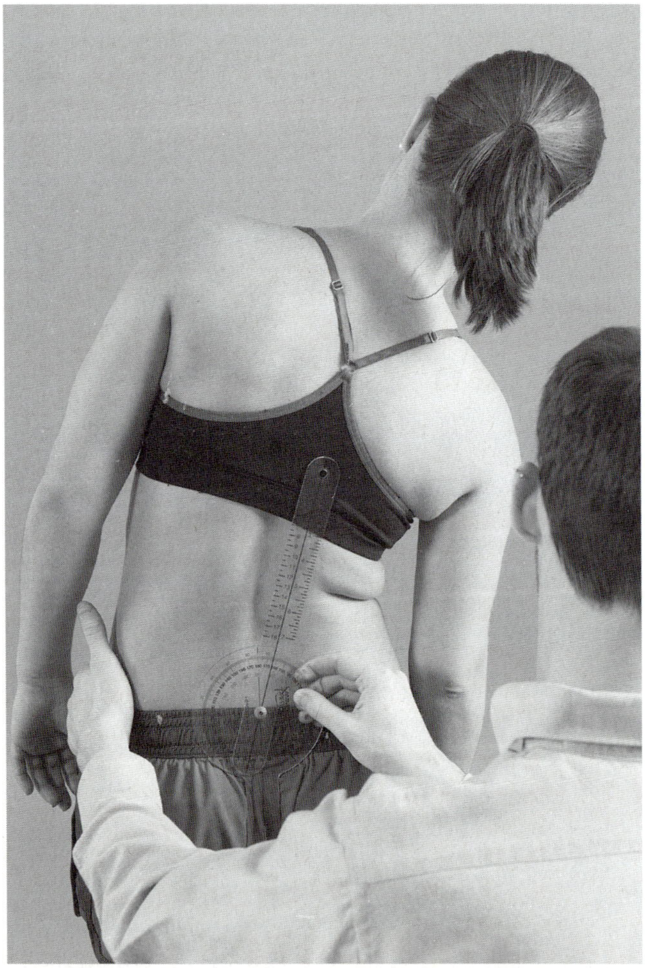

FIGURE 12.22 At the end of thoracolumbar lateral flexion, the examiner keeps the distal goniometer arm aligned with the individual's T1 vertebra. The examiner makes no attempt to align the distal arm with the individual's vertebral column. As can be seen in the photograph, the lower thoracic and upper lumbar spine become convex to the left during right lateral flexion.

THORACOLUMBAR LATERAL FLEXION: FINGERTIP-TO-FLOOR

The normal values for 39 asymptomatic individuals averaged 21.6 (5.6) centimeters.[14] One problem with this method is that it will be affected by the individual's body proportions. Therefore, it should be used only to compare repeated measurements for a single individual and not for comparing one individual with another.

Procedure

1. Ask the individual to assume a standing position with back flat against the wall, feet shoulder width apart, and arms hanging freely at the sides of the body.

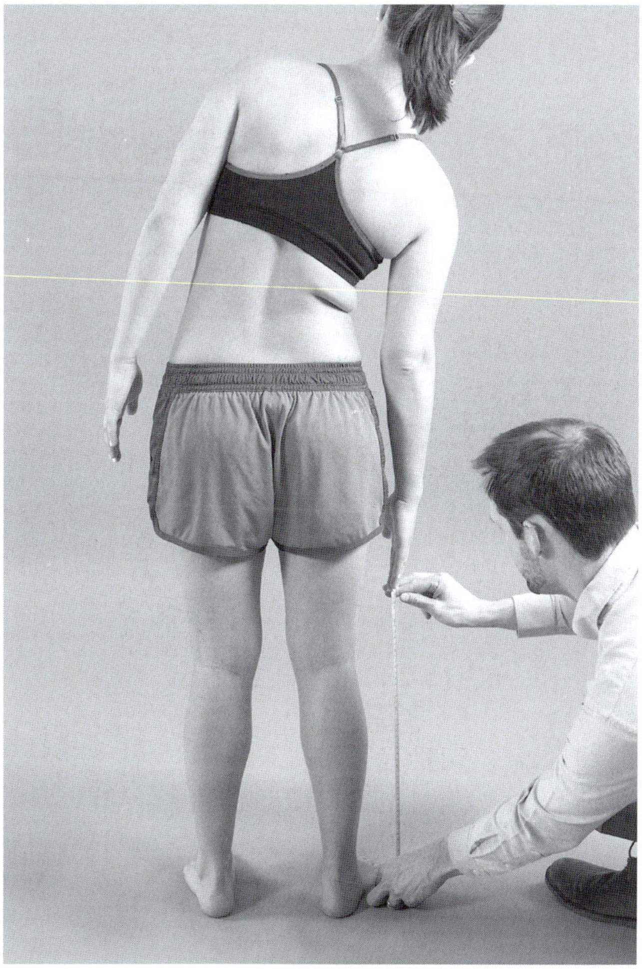

FIGURE 12.23 At the end of thoracolumbar lateral flexion range of motion, the examiner uses a tape measure to determine the distance from the tip of the individual's third finger to the floor. Lateral pelvic tilting should be avoided.

2. Direct the individual to bend to the side as far as possible while keeping back and shoulders against the wall and both feet flat on the ground with knees extended.
3. At the end of the ROM, make a mark on the leg level with the tip of the middle finger and use a tape measure or ruler to measure the distance between the mark on the leg and the floor. Alternately, the distance between the tip of the middle finger and the floor can be measured (Fig. 12.23).

THORACOLUMBAR LATERAL FLEXON: FINGERTIP-TO-THIGH

This method is a variation of the fingertip-to-floor method, designed to account for differences in body size. The normal ROM values for children aged 11 to 16 years were 21.0 centimeters for both right and left lateral flexion.[15] Range-of-motion values derived from 39 healthy adults[14] were 21.6 centimeters. Lindell and associates[7] found similar values for 20 healthy adults aged 22 to 55 years. Right lateral flexion was 21.2 centimeters and left lateral flexion was 21.0 centimeters. Alaranta and colleagues,[16] in a study of 119 blue- and white-collar workers aged 35 to 59 years, found a mean value of 19.1 centimeters. See Table 12.7 in the Research Findings section for reliability information on this procedure.

Procedure

1. Ask the individual to assume a standing position with the back against the wall, feet shoulder width apart, and arms hanging freely at the sides.
2. Place a mark on the thigh where the tip of the individual's third finger rests (Fig. 12.24).
3. Direct the individual to bend to the side as far as possible while keeping the back and shoulders against the wall and both feet flat on the ground with knees extended.
4. At the end of the ROM, make a second mark on the leg level with the tip of the middle finger (Fig. 12.25).
5. Use a tape measure or ruler to measure the distance between the first mark on the leg and the second mark on the leg (Fig. 12.26). The distance between the two marks is the value for thoracolumbar lateral flexion ROM.

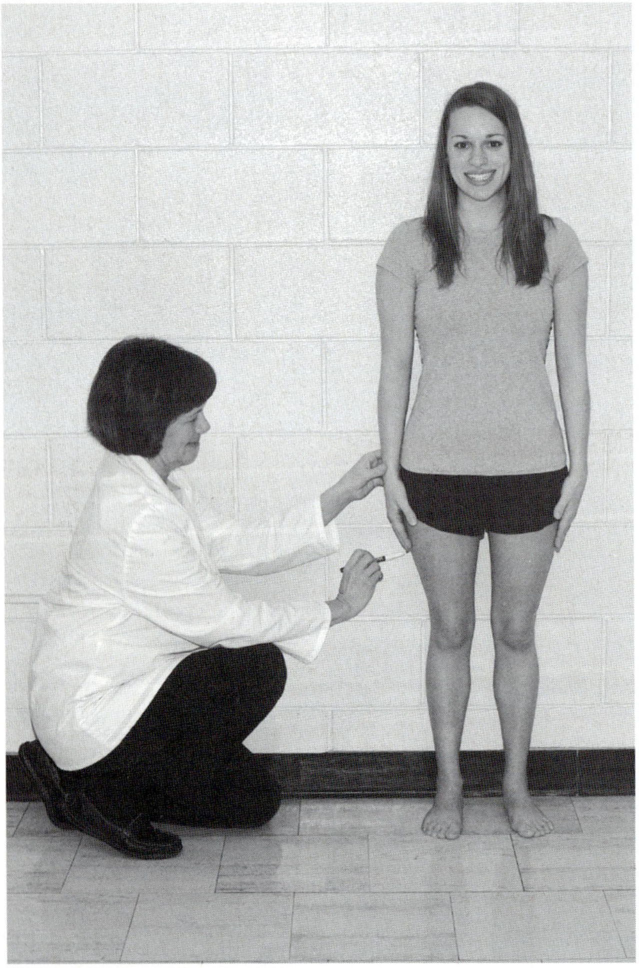

FIGURE 12.24 In the starting position for measuring thoracolumbar lateral flexion the examiner marks the thigh at the level of the tip of the individual's middle finger.

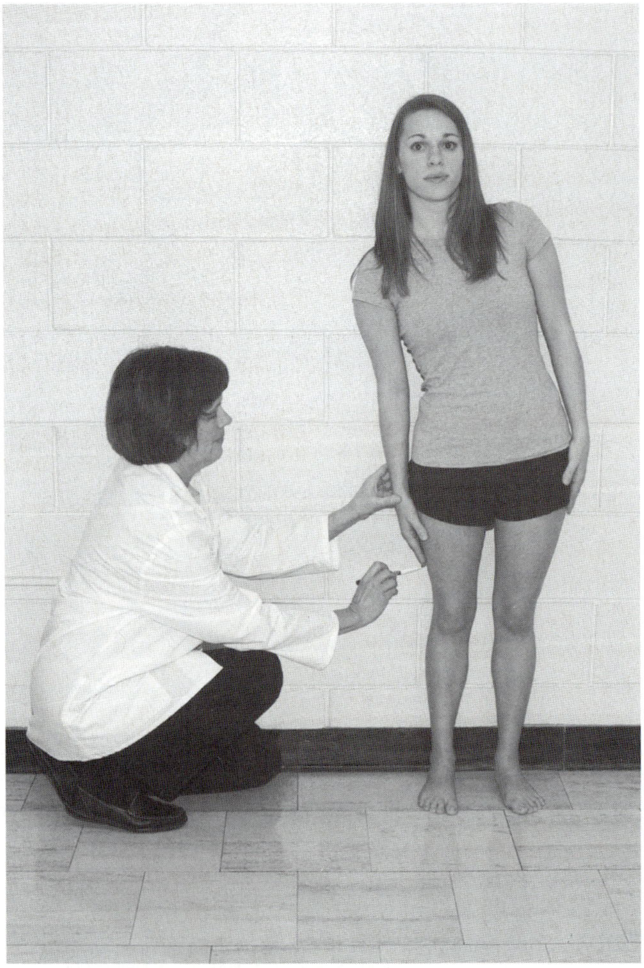

FIGURE 12.25 At the end of thoracolumbar lateral flexion the examiner places a second mark on the thigh on a level with the new position of the tip of the individual's middle finger.

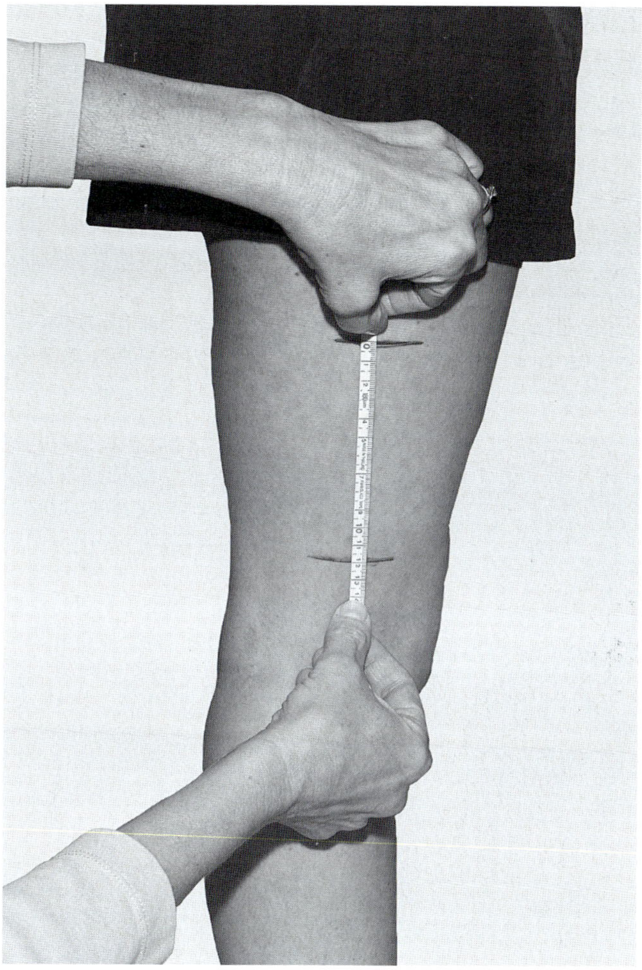

FIGURE 12.26 The examiner uses a tape measure or ruler to measure the distance between the two thigh marks to obtain the ROM.

THORACOLUMBAR LATERAL FLEXION: DOUBLE INCLINOMETERS

According to the AMA,[10] normal ROM is 25 degrees for thoracolumbar lateral flexion.

Procedure

1. Ask the individual to assume a standing position. Mark the spinous processes of the T1 and S2 vertebrae using a skin marking pencil.
2. Place one inclinometer over the T1 spinous process and the second inclinometer over the sacrum at the level of S2. Then zero both inclinometers (Fig. 12.27).
3. Ask the individual to bend to the side as far as possible while keeping both knees straight and both feet firmly on the ground (Fig. 12.28).
4. At the end of the ROM, read and record the information on both inclinometers. Subtract the degrees on the sacral inclinometer from the degrees on the thoracic inclinometer to obtain the lateral flexion ROM.
5. Repeat the measurement process to measure lateral flexion ROM on the other side.

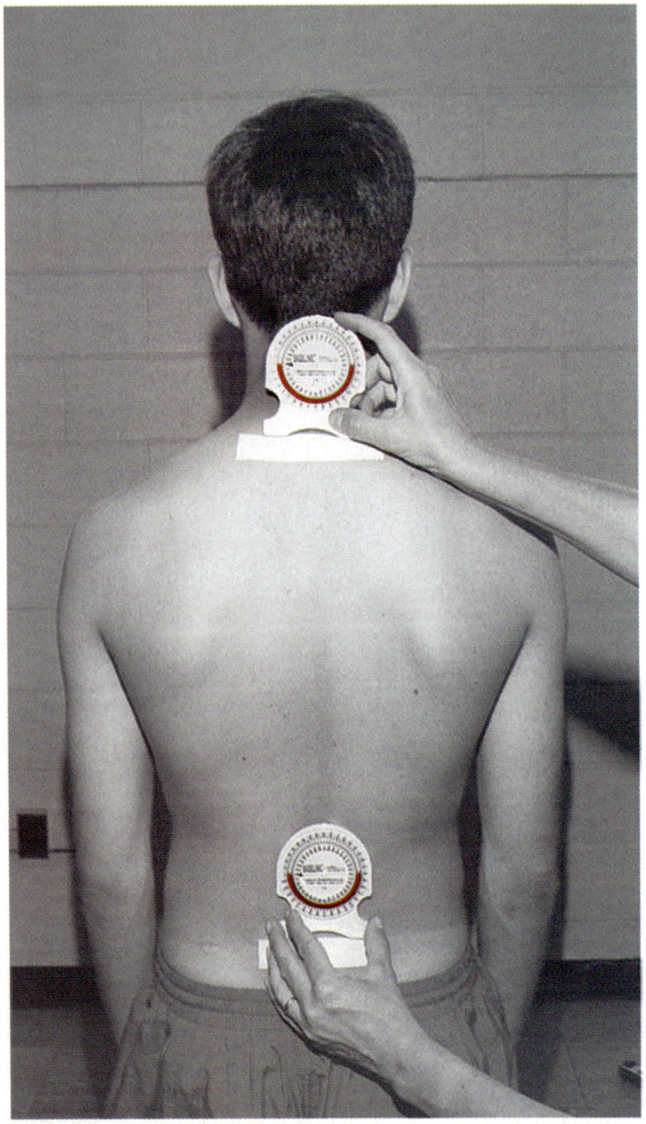

FIGURE 12.27 The individual is in the starting position for measurement of thoracolumbar lateral flexion with both inclinometers aligned and zeroed.

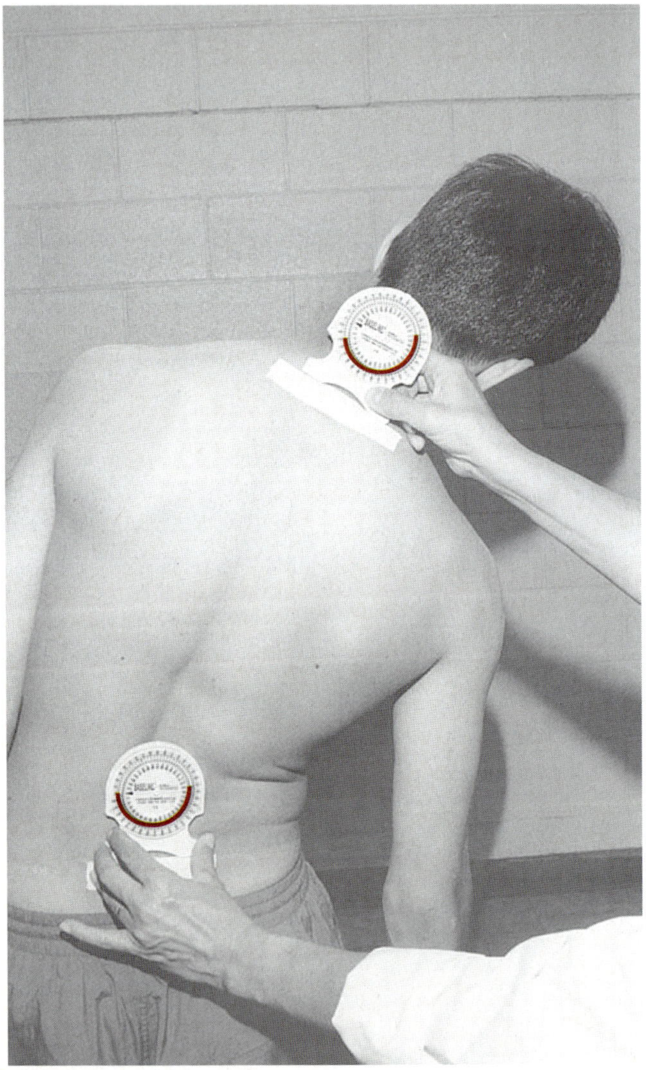

FIGURE 12.28 Inclinometer alignment at the end of thoracolumbar lateral flexion. The measurement at S2 is subtracted from the measurement at T1 to determine the ROM.

THORACOLUMBAR ROTATION

Motion occurs in the transverse plane around a vertical axis.

Testing Position

Place the individual sitting, with feet on the floor to help stabilize the pelvis. A seat without a back support is preferred so that rotation of the spine can occur freely. The cervical, thoracic, and lumbar spine are in 0 degrees of flexion, extension, and lateral flexion.

Stabilization

Stabilize the pelvis to prevent rotation. Avoid flexion, extension, and lateral flexion of the spine.

Testing Motion

Ask the individual to turn the body to one side as far as possible, keeping the trunk erect and feet flat on the floor (Fig. 12.29). The end of the motion occurs when the examiner feels the pelvis start to rotate.

Normal End-Feel

The end-feel is firm owing to stretching of the fibers of the contralateral annulus fibrosus and zygapophyseal joint capsules; costotransverse and costovertebral joint capsules; supraspinous, interspinous, and iliolumbar ligaments; and the following muscles: rectus abdominis, external and internal obliques and multifidus, and semispinalis thoracis and rotatores. The end-feel may also be hard owing to contact between the zygapophyseal facets.

NOTE: Use the same testing position, stabilization, testing motion, and normal end-feel described in the Thoracolumbar Rotation section above for the following rotation measurement methods unless changes are noted.

THORACOLUMBAR ROTATION: UNIVERSAL GONIOMETER

According to the AMA,[10] the normal ROM value for thoracolumbar rotation using the universal goniometer is 45 degrees. See Figures 12.30 and 12.31.

Procedure

1. Seat the individual in a chair without a back. Center fulcrum of the goniometer over the center of the cranial aspect of the individual's head.
2. Align proximal arm parallel to an imaginary line between the two prominent tubercles on the iliac crests.
3. Align distal arm with an imaginary line between the two acromial processes.
4. Ask the individual to turn the body to one side as far as possible, keeping the trunk erect and feet flat on the floor. The end of the motion occurs when the examiner feels the pelvis start to rotate.

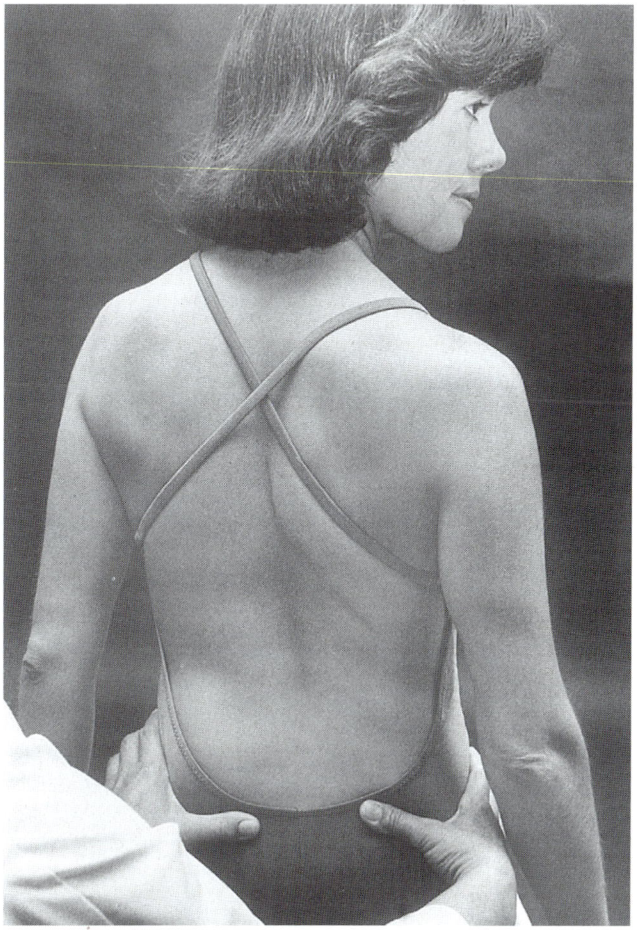

FIGURE 12.29 The individual is shown at the end of the thoracolumbar rotation ROM. The individual is seated on a low stool without a back rest so that spinal movement can occur without interference. The examiner positions her hands on the iliac crests to prevent pelvic rotation.

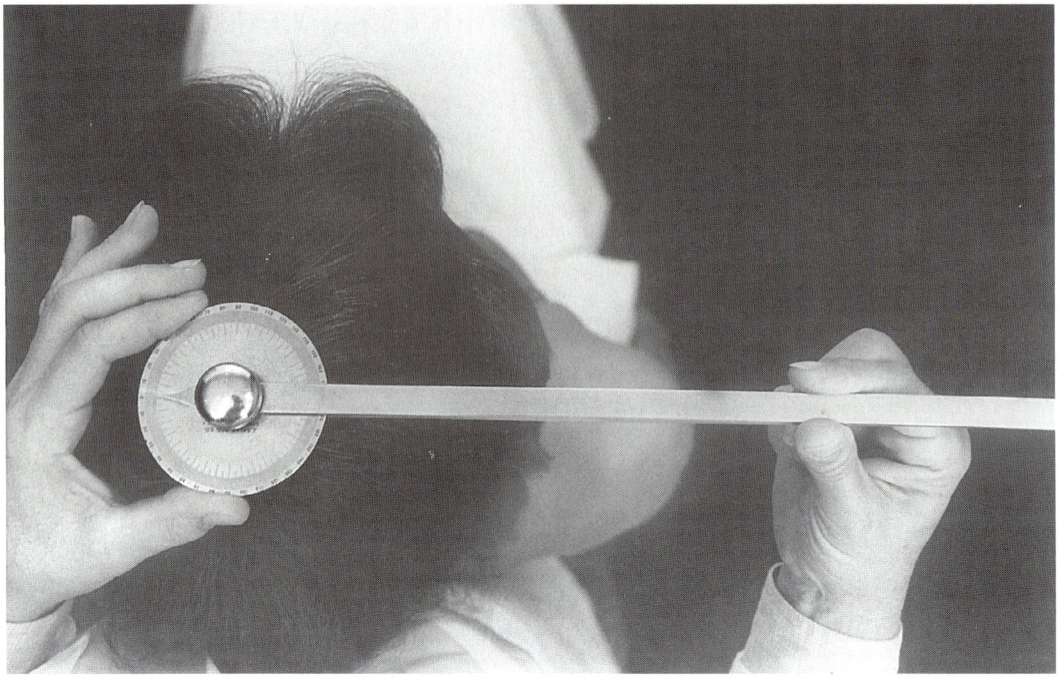

FIGURE 12.30 In the starting position for measurement of rotation range of motion, the examiner stands behind the seated individual. The examiner positions the fulcrum of the goniometer on the superior aspect of the individual's head. One of the examiner's hands is holding both arms of the goniometer aligned with the acromial processes. The individual should be positioned so that the acromial processes are aligned directly over the iliac tubercles.

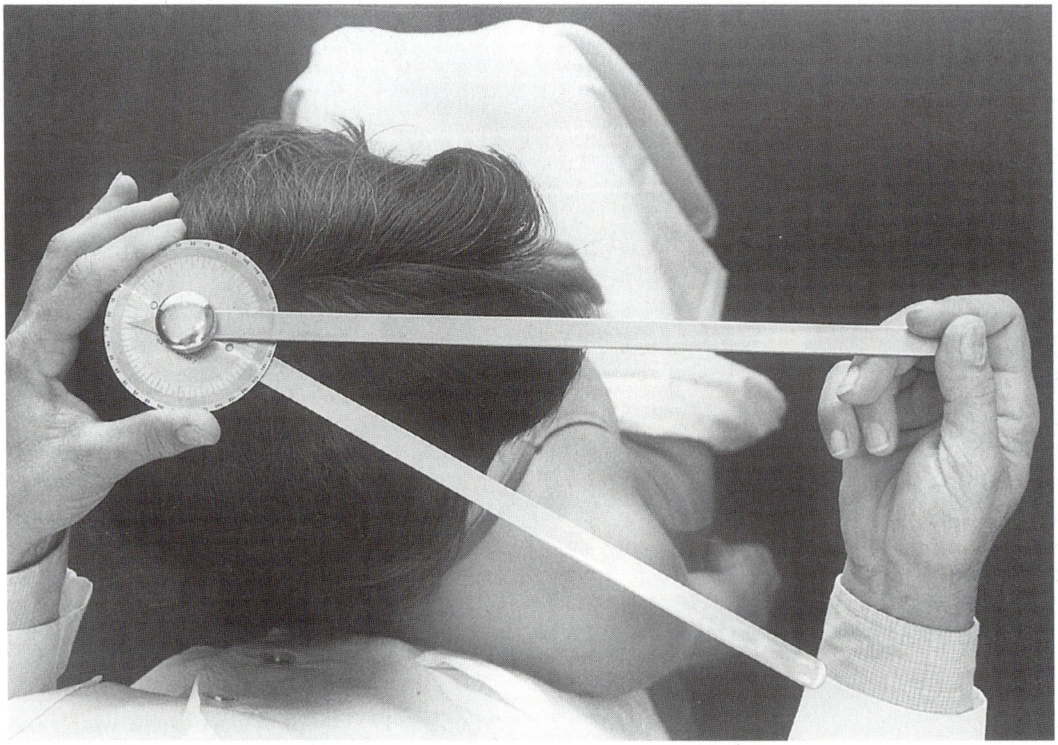

FIGURE 12.31 At the end of rotation, one of the examiner's hands keeps the proximal goniometer arm aligned with the individual's iliac tubercles while keeping the distal goniometer arm aligned with the right acromial process.

THORACOLUMBAR ROTATION: DOUBLE INCLINOMETERS

This test primarily measures thoracic motion. It should be used only in young people who are flexible and have good balance.

Procedure

1. Mark the spinous processes of the T1 and S2 vertebrae using a skin marking pencil.
2. Place the individual in a forward flexed standing position so that the individual's back is parallel to the floor.
3. Place one inclinometer over the spinous process of T1 and the second inclinometer over the sacrum at the level of S2. Then zero both inclinometers (Fig. 12.32).
4. Ask the individual to rotate the trunk as far as possible without moving into extension (Fig. 12.33). The examiner needs to hold the inclinometers firmly against the individual's back during the motion.
5. Note the degrees shown on the inclinometers at the end of the motion. The difference between inclinometer readings is the rotation ROM.

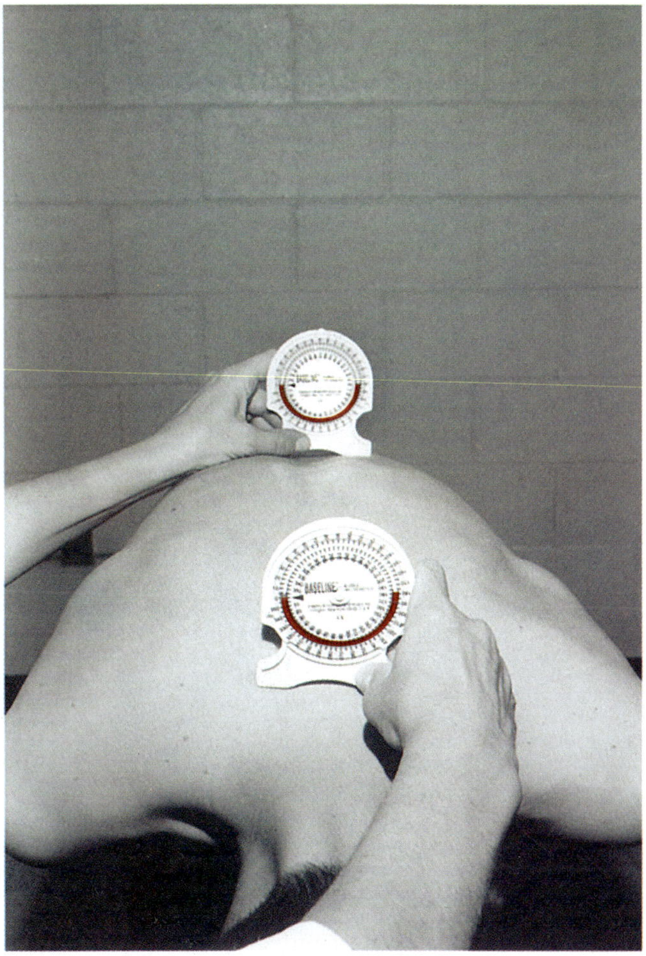

FIGURE 12.32 The individual is in the starting position for measurement of thoracolumbar rotation with inclinometers aligned and zeroed. This position may be stressful for many patients and should be avoided if it increases symptoms.

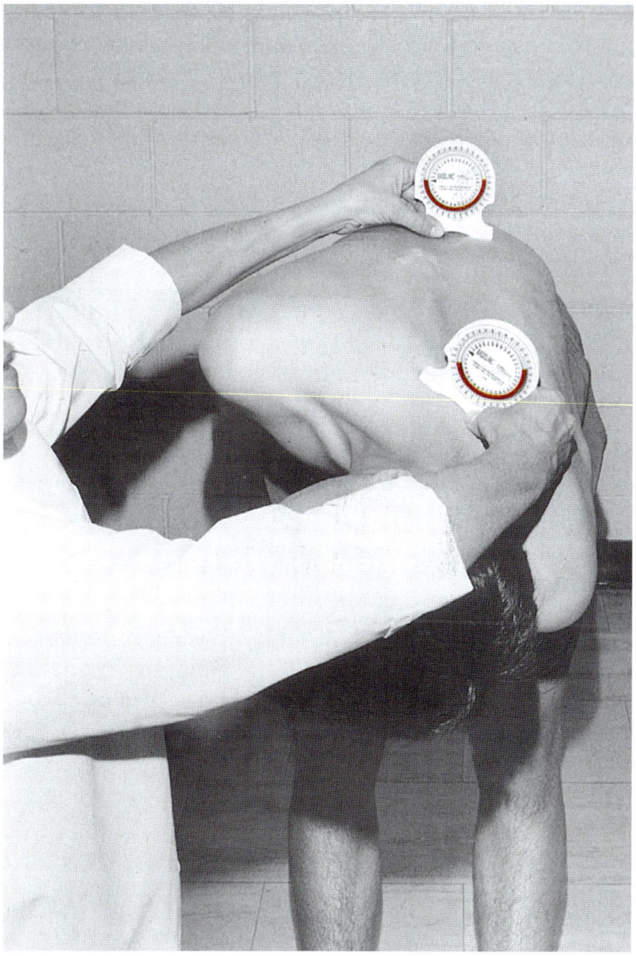

FIGURE 12.33 The individual is shown with the inclinometers aligned at the end of thoracolumbar rotation range of motion.

LUMBAR FLEXION

Testing Position

Place the individual standing, with the cervical, thoracic, and lumbar spine in 0 degrees of lateral flexion and rotation.

Stabilization

Stabilize the pelvis to prevent anterior tilting.

Testing Motion

Ask the individual to bend forward as far as possible while keeping the knees straight.

Normal End-Feel

The end-feel is firm owing to stretching of the ligamentum flavum; posterior fibers of the annulus fibrosus and zygapophyseal joint capsules; thoracolumbar fascia; illiolumbar ligaments; and the multifidus, quadratus lumborum, and iliocostalis lumborum muscles. The location of the following muscles suggests that they may limit flexion, but the actual actions of the interspinales and intertransversaii mediales and laterales are unknown.[2]

➧ **NOTE:** Use the same testing position, stabilization, testing motion, and normal end-feel described in the Lumbar Flexion section above for the following flexion measurement methods unless changes are noted.

LUMBAR FLEXION: MODIFIED-MODIFIED SCHOBER TEST (MMST) OR SIMPLIFIED SKIN DISTRACTION TEST[17,18,19]

Normal values for the MMST for individuals between 15 and 18 years of age are 6.7 centimeters for males and 5.8 centimeters for females in the same age-group.[17,18] Jones and associates[15] found a slightly larger normal value of 7.7 centimeters in a study of 89 healthy children between the ages of 11 and 16 years.

Procedure

1. Ask the individual to assume a standing position. Use a ruler to locate and place a first mark at a midline point on the sacrum that is level with the posterior superior iliac spines (this mark will be over the spinous process of S2). Make a second mark 15 centimeters above the midline sacral mark (Fig. 12.34).*
2. Align the tape measure between the superior and inferior marks (Fig. 12.35). Ask the individual to bend forward as far as possible while keeping the knees straight. Maintain the tape measure against the individual's back during the motion, but allow the tape measure to unwind to accommodate the motion.
3. At the end of flexion ROM, note the distance between the two marks (Fig. 12.36). The ROM is the difference between 15 centimeters and the length measured at the end of the motion.

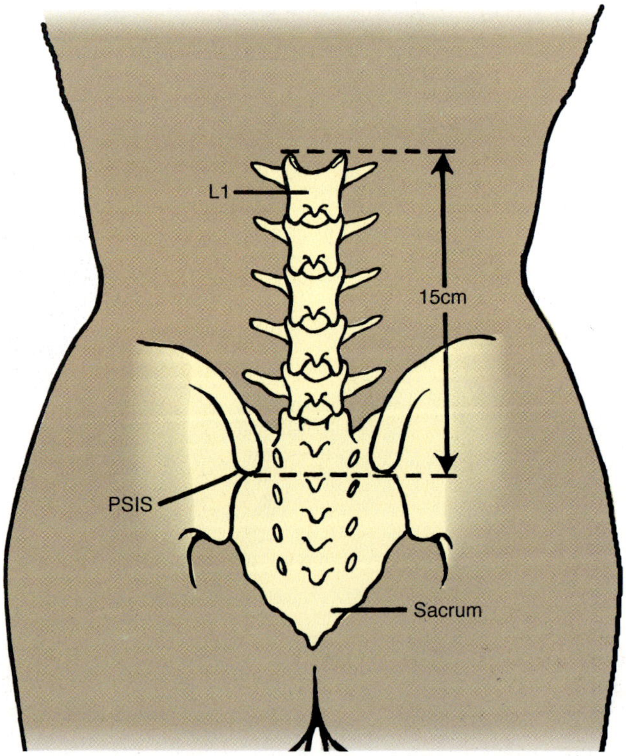

FIGURE 12.34 A dashed line is drawn between the two posterior superior iliac spines and the point at which the lower end of the tape measure should be positioned. The location of the 15-centimeter mark shows that all five of the lumbar vertebrae in this individual are included.

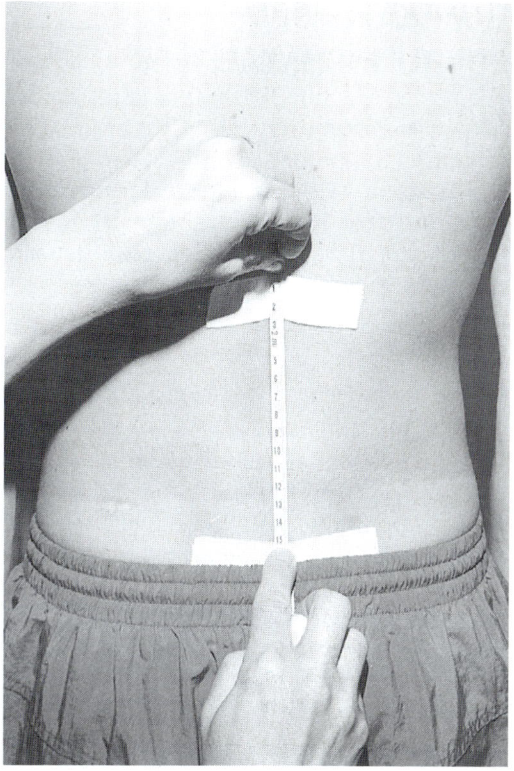

FIGURE 12.35 The tape measure is aligned between the upper and the lower landmarks at the beginning of lumbar flexion range of motion. Paper tape was placed over the skin marking pencil dots to improve visibility of landmarks for the photograph.

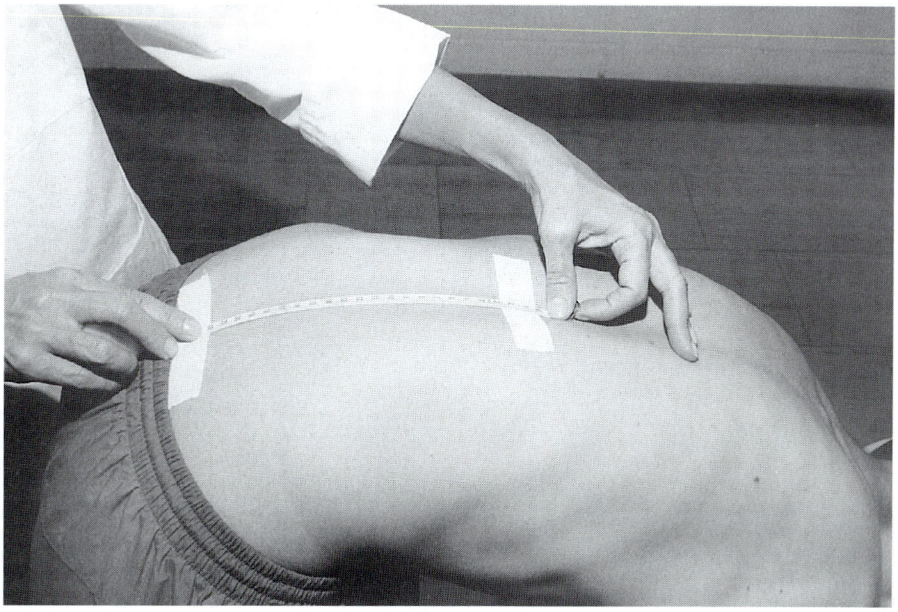

FIGURE 12.36 The tape measure is stretched between the upper and the lower landmarks at the end of lumbar flexion range of motion.

---

* In the original Schober method, the examiner made only two marks on the back. The first mark was made at the lumbosacral junction, and the second mark was made 10 centimeters above the first mark on the spine. Macrae and Wright[20] decided to modify the Schober method (Modified Schober Test) because they found that skin movement was a problem in the original method. They believed that the skin was more firmly attached in the region below the lumbosacral junction and therefore decided to use three marks—the first mark at the lumbosacral junction, the second mark 10 centimeters above the first mark, and the third mark 5 centimeters below the lumbosacral junction. The tape measure was placed between the most superior and the most inferior marks. However, difficulty in correctly identifying the lumbosacral junction led to another modification of the original Schober test, called the Modified-Modified Schober Test (or MMST), proposed by van Adrichem and van der Korst.[18] The MMST is also referred to as the simplified skin distraction test and is the test that we are using today.[19]

LUMBAR FLEXION: DOUBLE INCLINOMETERS

The normal adult ROM is 60 degrees according to the AMA.[10] Neumann states that the approximate range of motion for lumbar flexion is 40 to 50 degrees[21] and Loebl[22] found that lumbar flexion ROM was 66 degrees for 15 to 30 year olds. Ng[23] and associates found a mean value of 52 degrees for healthy men with a mean age of 29 years.

Procedure

1. Ask the individual to assume a standing position. Mark the spinous processes of the T12 and S2 vertebrae using a skin marking pencil.
2. Place one inclinometer over the spinous process of T12 and the second inclinometer over the sacrum at the level of S2. Zero both inclinometers (Fig. 12.37).
3. Ask the individual to bend forward as far as possible while keeping the knees straight. Maintain the inclinometers firmly against the spine during the motion.
4. Note the information on the inclinometers at the end of flexion ROM (Fig. 12.38). Calculate the ROM by subtracting the degrees on the sacral inclinometer from the degrees on T12 inclinometer. The degrees on the sacral inclinometer are supposed to represent hip flexion ROM, and that is why they are subtracted.[22]

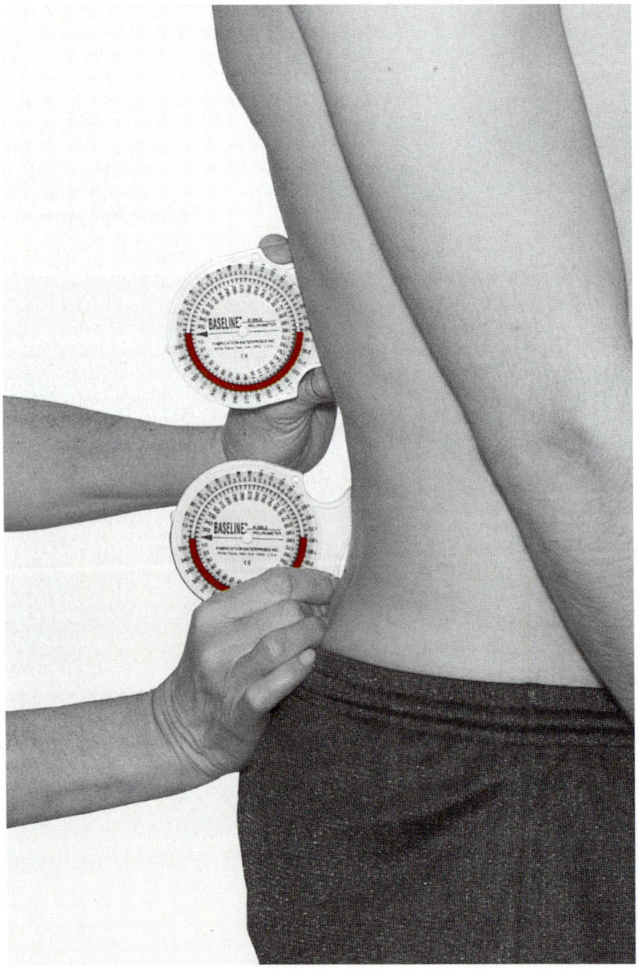

FIGURE 12.37 The starting position for measurement of lumbar flexion range of motion, with double inclinometers aligned and zeroed.

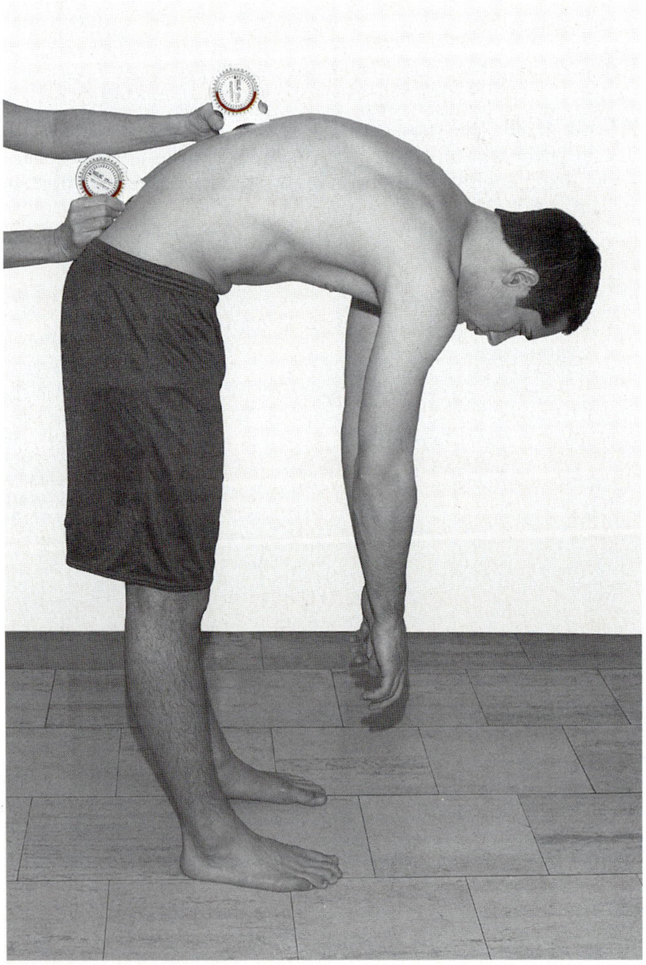

FIGURE 12.38 The end of lumbar flexion, with inclinometers aligned over the spinous processes of T12 and S2. Subtract the measurement taken at S2 from the measurement taken at T12 to obtain lumbar flexion ROM.

LUMBAR FLEXION: SINGLE INCLINOMETER

Procedure

1. Ask the individual to assume a standing position. Mark the spinous processes of the T12 and S2 vertebrae using a skin marking pencil. Place and zero the inclinometer on T12 (Fig. 12.39).
2. Ask the individual to bend forward through available flexion ROM while keeping knees straight and feet shoulder width apart. Maintain the inclinometer at T12 throughout the motion and take a measurement at T12 at the end of the motion (Fig. 12.40).

Text continued on page 494

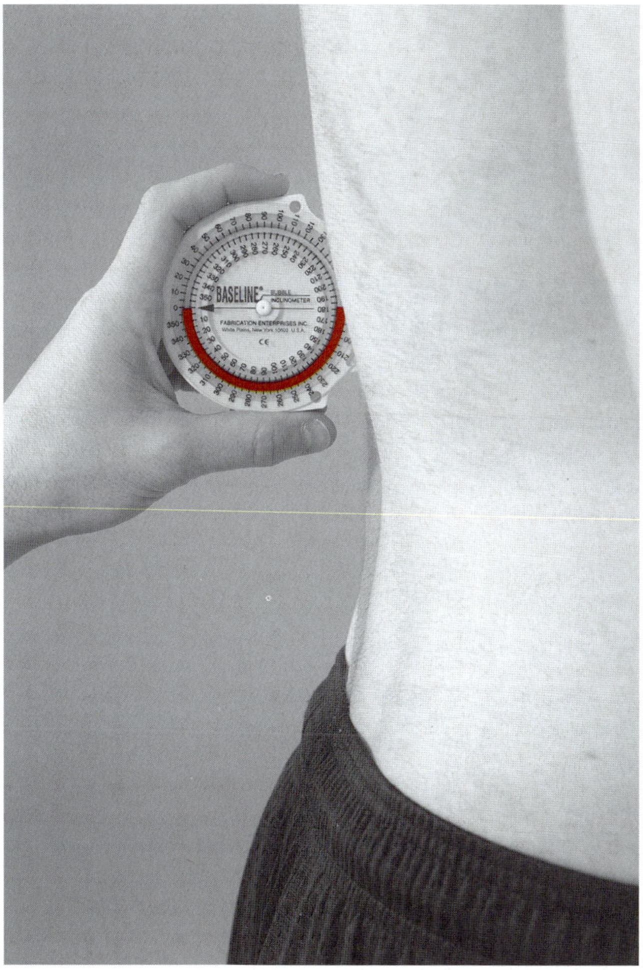

FIGURE 12.39 In the starting position for measuring lumbar flexion ROM using a single inclinometer, the inclinometer is placed at T12 and zeroed.

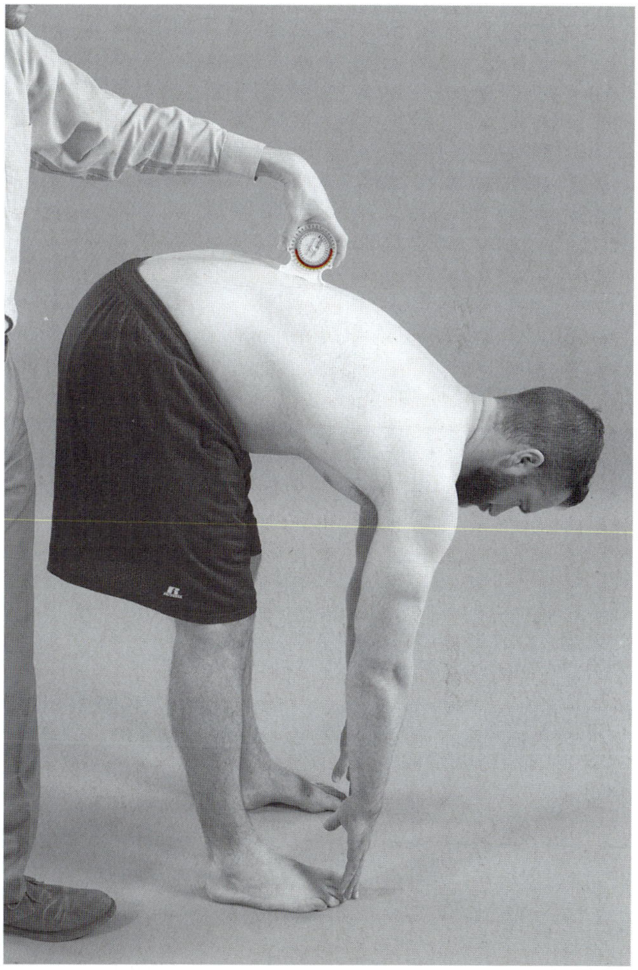

FIGURE 12.40 Inclinometer is maintained at T12 throughout flexion; a measurement is taken at T12 at the end of flexion and the individual returns to standing.

3. Have the individual stand upright. Place and zero the inclinometer at S2 (Fig. 12.41).
4. Ask the individual to bend forward again while the examiner maintains the S2 inclinometer on S2 until the end of the motion and then takes a measurement at S2 (Fig. 12.42).
5. Subtract S2 (hip motion) from TI2 measurement to obtain flexion ROM.

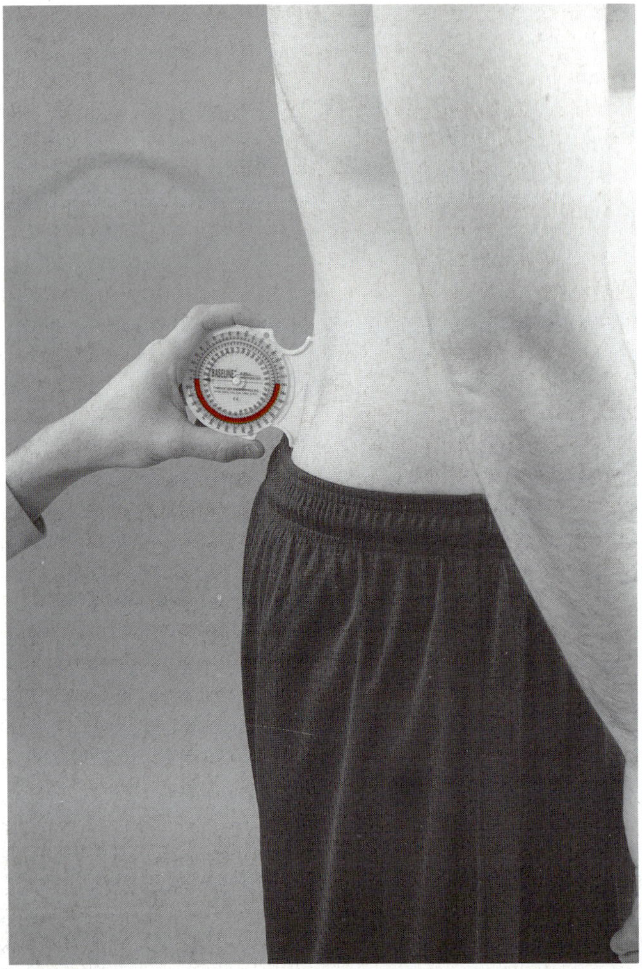

FIGURE 12.41 Inclinometer is placed at S2 and zeroed with the individual in the starting position again.

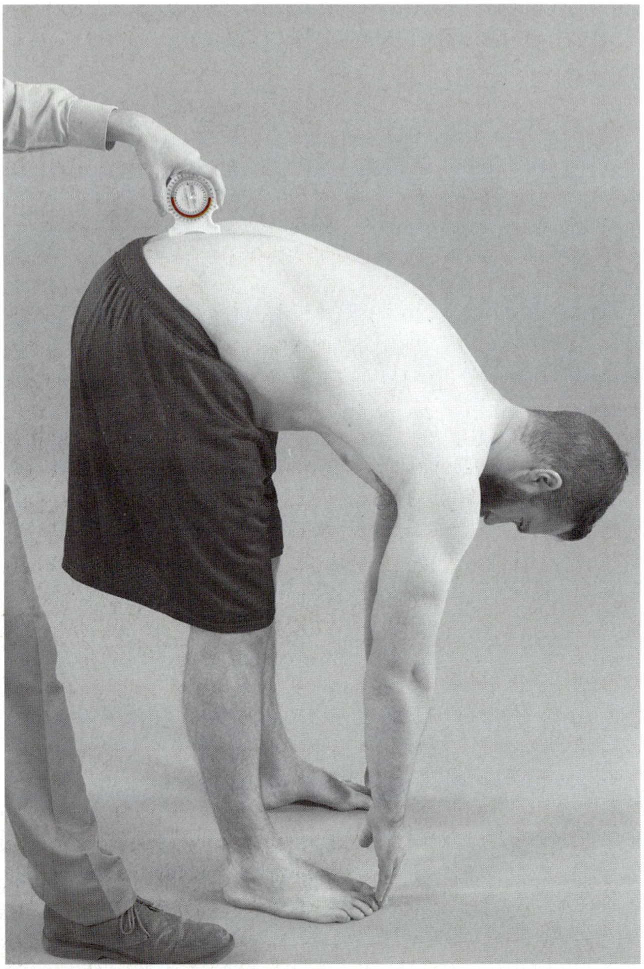

FIGURE 12.42 The individual repeats lumbar flexion. Inclinometer contact is maintained at S2 throughout flexion and read at the end of the motion. Subtract the S2 measurement from the T12 measurement to obtain lumbar flexion ROM.

LUMBAR EXTENSION

Neumann[21] lists the approximate range of lumbar extension as 15 to 20 degrees.

Testing Position

Ask the individual to assume a standing position with the cervical, thoracic, and lumbar spine in 0 degrees of lateral flexion and rotation.

Stabilization

Stabilize the pelvis to prevent posterior tilting.

Testing Motion

Ask the individual to extend the spine as far as possible. The end of the extension ROM occurs when the pelvis begins to tilt posteriorly.

Normal End-Feel

The end-feel is firm owing to stretching of the anterior longitudinal ligament, anterior fibers of the annulus fibrosus, zygapophyseal joint capsules, rectus abdominis, and external and internal oblique muscles. The end-feel may also be hard owing to contact between the spinous processes.

➧ **NOTE:** Use the same testing position, stabilization, testing motion, and normal end-feel described in the Lumbar Extension section above for the following extension measurement methods unless changes are noted.

LUMBAR EXTENSION: MODIFIED-MODIFIED SCHOBER TEST OR SIMPLIFIED SKIN ATTRACTION TEST

Procedure

1. Ask the individual to assume a standing position with the feet shoulder width apart and cervical, thoracic, and lumbar spine in 0 degrees of lateral flexion and rotation.
2. The examiner should hold a ruler between two posterior superior iliac spines (PSIS) and place a first mark on a midline point of the sacrum that is on a level with the PSIS; this will be over the spinous process of S2. A second mark should be made on the lumbar spine that is 15 centimeters above the first mark.
3. Align the tape measure between the first and second marks on the spine (Fig. 12.43), and ask the individual to bend backward as far as possible. As the individual extends the spine, the examiner allows the tape to retract into the tape measure case.
4. At the end of the ROM, record the distance between the superior and the inferior marks (Fig. 12.44). The ROM is the difference between 15 centimeters and the length measured at the end of the motion.

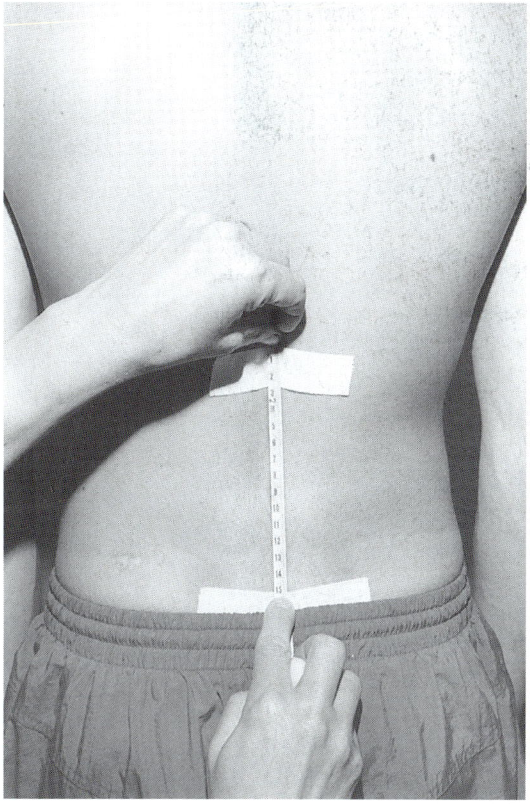

FIGURE 12.43 Tape measure alignment in the starting position for measurement of lumbar extension range of motion with the use of the simplified skin attraction method (Modified-Modified Schober Test).

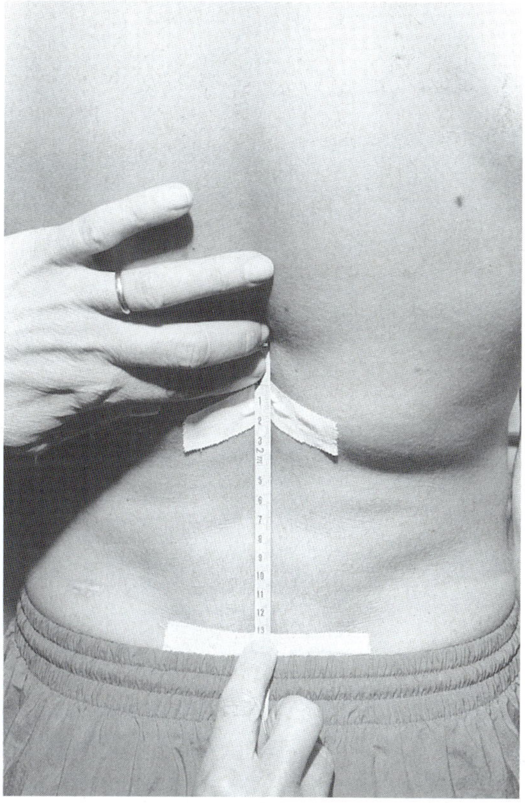

FIGURE 12.44 Tape measure alignment at the end of lumbar extension range of motion, with use of the simplified skin attraction method.

LUMBAR EXTENSION: DOUBLE INCLINOMETERS

The normal ROM values for young-adult males (15 to 30 years) is 38 degrees, whereas the value for middle-age males (31 to 60 years) is 35 degrees. In males older than age 60 years the ROM is 33 degrees. In young-adult females the ROM is 42 degrees, in middle-aged females the ROM is 40 degrees, and in females older than 60 years the ROM is 36 degrees.[22] According to the AMA,[10] the normal ROM for adults is from 20 to 25 degrees, which is considerably less than the values that were found by Loebl.[22]

Procedure

1. Ask the individual to assume a standing position with the feet shoulder width apart and the cervical, thoracic, and lumbar spine in 0 degrees of lateral flexion and rotation.
2. Mark the spinous processes of the T12 and S2 vertebrae using a skin marking pencil.
3. Place one inclinometer over the spinous process of T12 and the second inclinometer over the midline of the sacrum at S2. Then zero both inclinometers (Fig. 12.45).
4. Ask the individual to bend backward as far as possible. Maintain the inclinometers firmly against the spine during the motion (Fig. 12.46).
5. Read and record the degrees from both inclinometers at the end of the motion. Subtract the degrees on the sacral inclinometer from the degrees on the T12 inclinometer to obtain lumbar extension ROM.

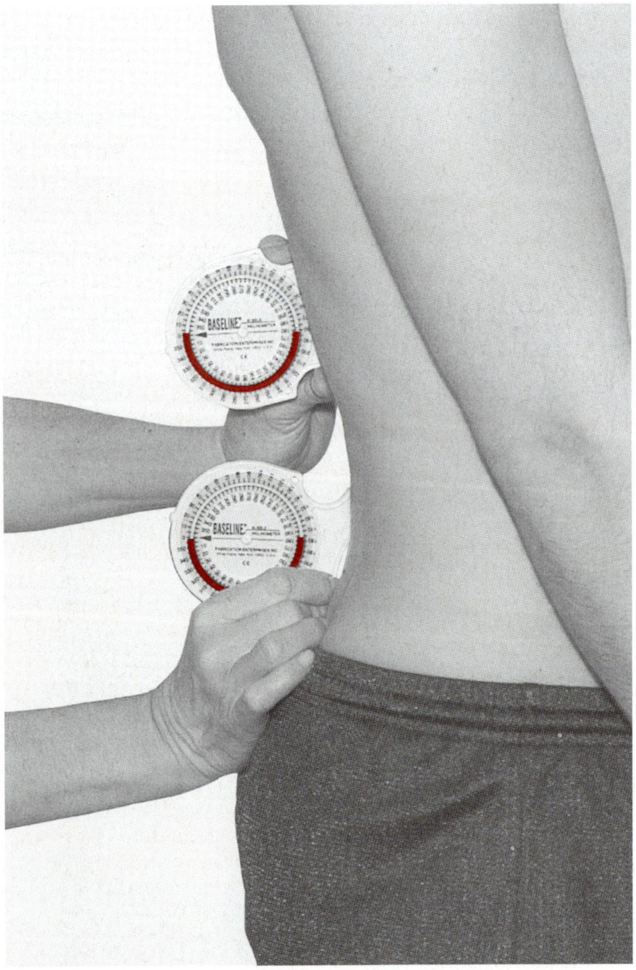

FIGURE 12.45 Starting position for measuring lumbar extension range of motion with double inclinometers placed over the T12 and S2 spinous processes.

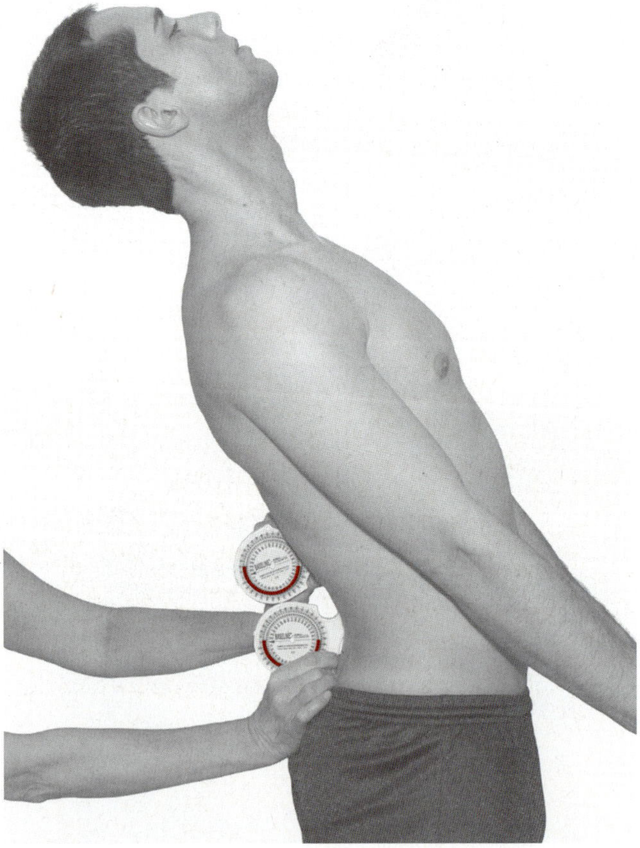

FIGURE 12.46 At the end of the lumbar extension range of motion (ROM), read and record the degrees on both inclinometers. Subtract the degrees on the sacral inclinometer from the T12 reading to obtain the ROM.

LUMBAR EXTENSION: SINGLE INCLINOMETER

Procedure

1. Ask the individual to assume a standing position with hands on hips. Mark the spinous processes of the T12 and S2 vertebrae using a skin marking pencil.
2. Place single inclinometer over the T12 vertebra and zero the inclinometer (Fig. 12.47).
3. Ask individual to bend backward as far as possible. Maintain the inclinometer at T12 throughout the motion and take a measurement at T12 at the end of the motion (Fig. 12.48).
4. Have the individual stand upright again and zero the inclinometer at S2 (Fig. 12.49).
5. Ask the individual to bend backward again. Maintain the inclinometer on S2 until the end of the motion and take another measurement at S2 (Fig. 12.50).
6. Subtract S2 (hip motion) from T12 measurement to obtain extension ROM.

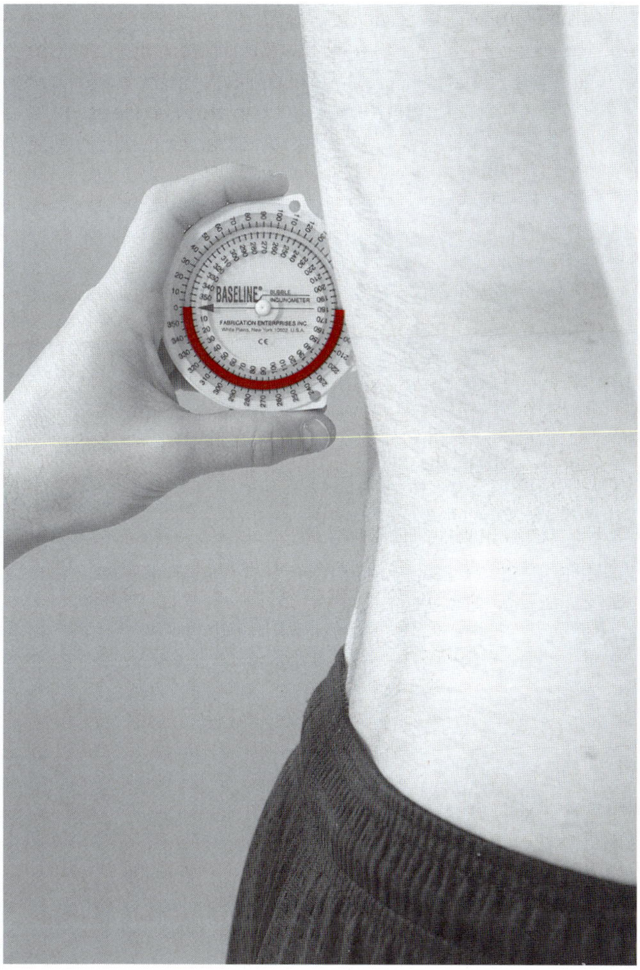

FIGURE 12.47 Starting position for measuring lumbar extension ROM uses a single inclinometer placed over the T12 spinous process and zeroed.

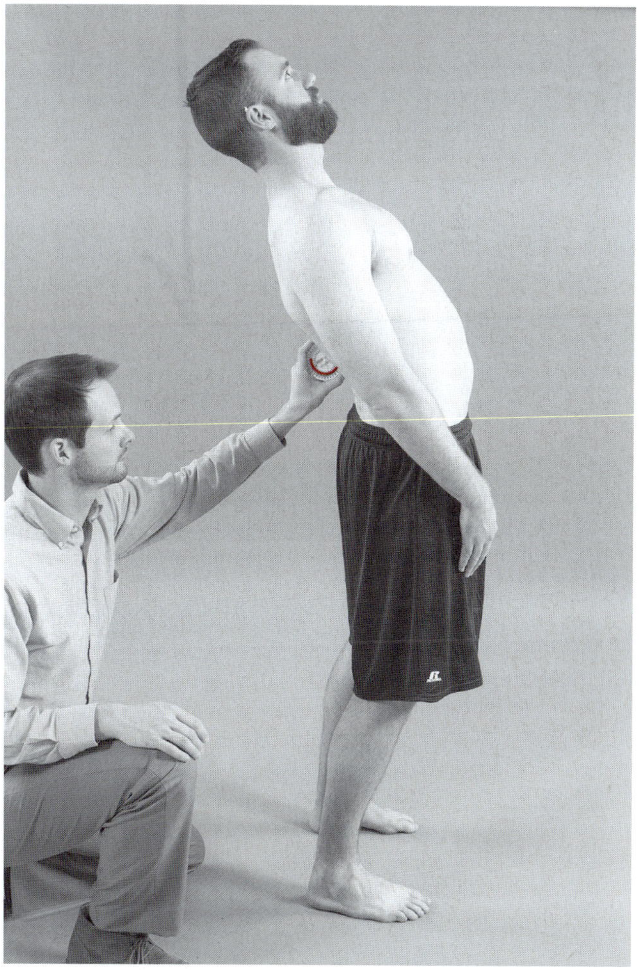

FIGURE 12.48 Maintain the inclinometer over T12 while the individual bends backward. Take another measurement at the end of the motion and have the individual return to a standing position. Repeat the backward bend with the inclinometer positioned over S2 and take a measurement at the end of the motion.

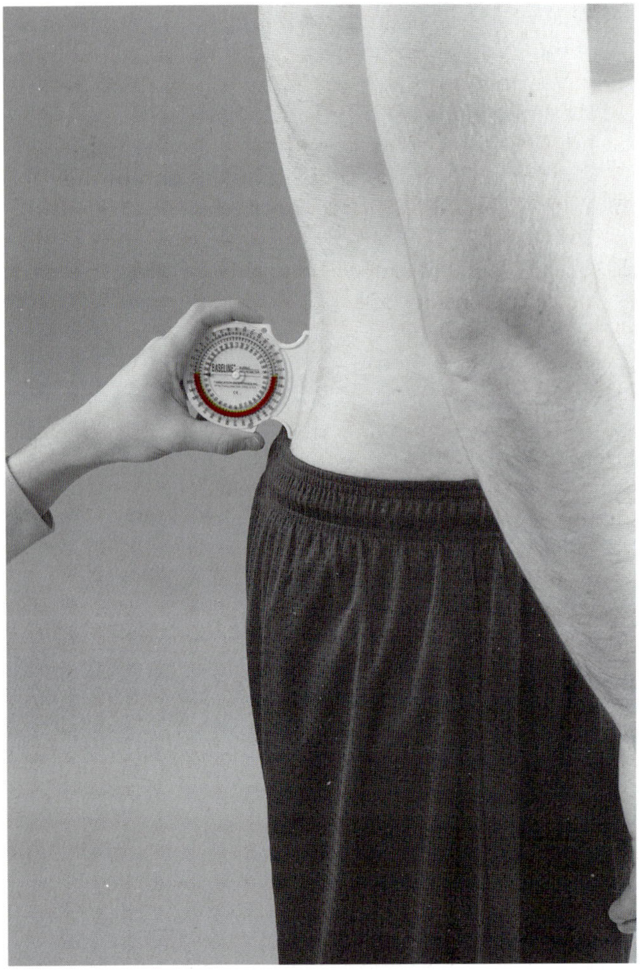

FIGURE 12.49 Inclinometer is placed at S2 and zeroed with the individual in the starting position again.

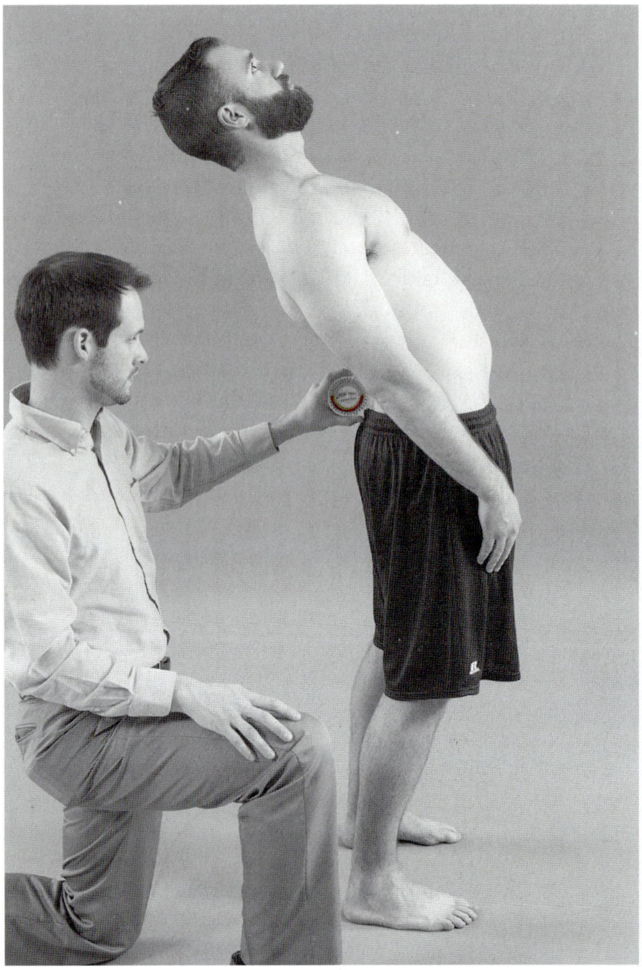

FIGURE 12.50 The individual repeats lumbar extension with the inclinometer maintained at S2. The inclinometer is read at the end of the motion. Subtract S2 measurement from T12 measurement to obtain lumbar extension ROM.

LUMBAR LATERAL FLEXION

Testing Position

Ask the individual to assume a standing position with the feet shoulder width apart and the cervical, thoracic, and lumbar spine in 0 degrees of lateral flexion and rotation.

Stabilization

Stabilize the pelvis to prevent lateral tilting.

Testing Motion

Ask the individual to bend to the side as far as possible. The end of the lateral flexion ROM occurs when the pelvis begins to tilt laterally and/or the heel of the foot begins to raise from the floor.

Normal End-Feel

The end-feel is firm owing to stretching of the contralateral band of the iliolumbar ligament, contralateral thoracolumbar fascia, contralateral fibers of the annulus fibrosus, and zygapophyseal joint capsules. The following contralateral muscles may contract eccentrically to control and resist lateral flexion when gravity begins to affect the motion: quadratus lumborum, interspinales, and iliocostales lumborum. The end-feel could be hard owing to contact of the ipsilateral apophyseal joints.

➧ **NOTE:** Use the same testing position, stabilization, testing motion, and normal end-feel described in the Lumbar Lateral Flexion section above for the following lateral flexion measurement methods unless changes are noted.

LUMBAR LATERAL FLEXION: DOUBLE INCLINOMETERS

The ROM value is 25 to 30 degrees to each side.

Procedure

1. Ask the individual to assume a standing position with the feet shoulder width apart and the cervical, thoracic, and lumbar spine in 0 degrees of lateral flexion and rotation.
2. Mark the spinous processes of the T12 and S2 vertebrae using a skin marking pencil.
3. Position one inclinometer over the T12 spinous process and the second inclinometer over the sacrum at the level of S2. Then, zero both inclinometers (Fig. 12.51).
4. Ask the individual to bend the trunk laterally while keeping both feet flat on the ground and the knees straight (Fig. 12.52).
5. Read and record the degrees on both inclinometers. Subtract the degrees on the sacral inclinometer from the degrees on the T12 inclinometer to obtain the lumbar lateral flexion ROM to one side.
6. Repeat the measurement process to measure lumbar lateral flexion ROM on the other side.

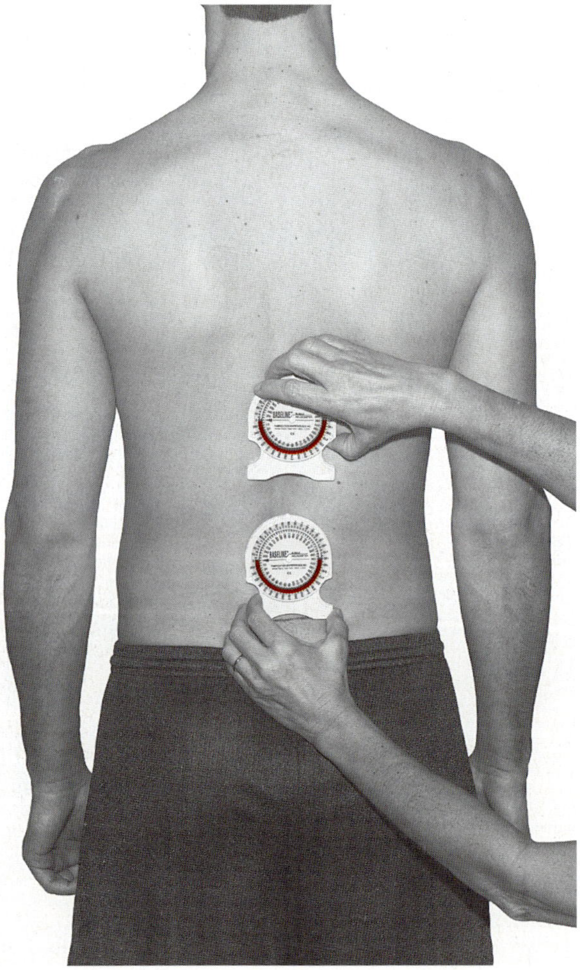

FIGURE 12.51 Measurement of lumbar lateral flexion ROM using double inclinometers requires placement of one inclinometer over the spinous process of T12 and the other over the spinous process of S2.

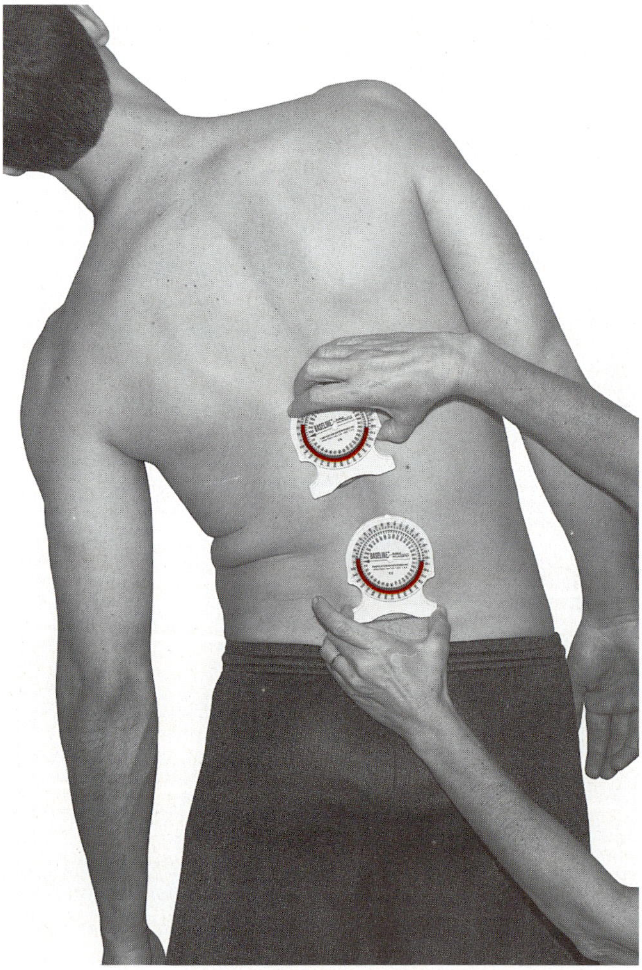

FIGURE 12.52 At the end of lumbar lateral flexion range of motion (ROM), read and record the degrees on each inclinometer. Subtract the degrees on the sacral inclinometer from the T12 reading to obtain the ROM.

LUMBAR LATERAL FLEXION: SINGLE INCLINOMETER

Procedure

1. Ask the individual to assume a standing position with hands on hips. Mark the spinous processes of the T12 and S2 vertebrae using a skin marking pencil.
2. Place single inclinometer over the T12 vertebra and zero the inclinometer (Fig. 12.53).
3. Ask the individual to bend to the side as far as possible without raising the heel of the foot from the ground.
4. Maintain the inclinometer at T12 throughout the motion and take another measurement at TI2 at the end of the motion (Fig. 12.54).
5. Have the individual stand upright again and zero the inclinometer at S2 (Fig. 12.55).
6. Ask the individual to bend sideways again.
7. Maintain the inclinometer on S2 until the end of the motion and take another measurement (Fig. 12.56).
8. Subtract S2 (hip motion) from TI2 measurement to obtain lateral flexion ROM.

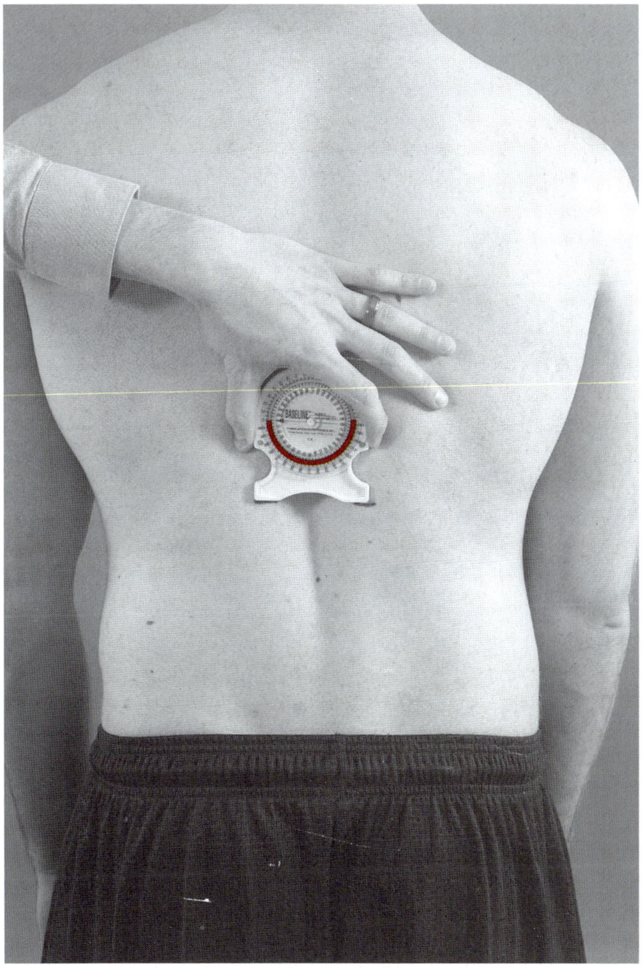

FIGURE 12.53 The starting position for measuring lumbar lateral flexion with a single inclinometer is standing erect. Place the inclinometer at T12 and zero the instrument.

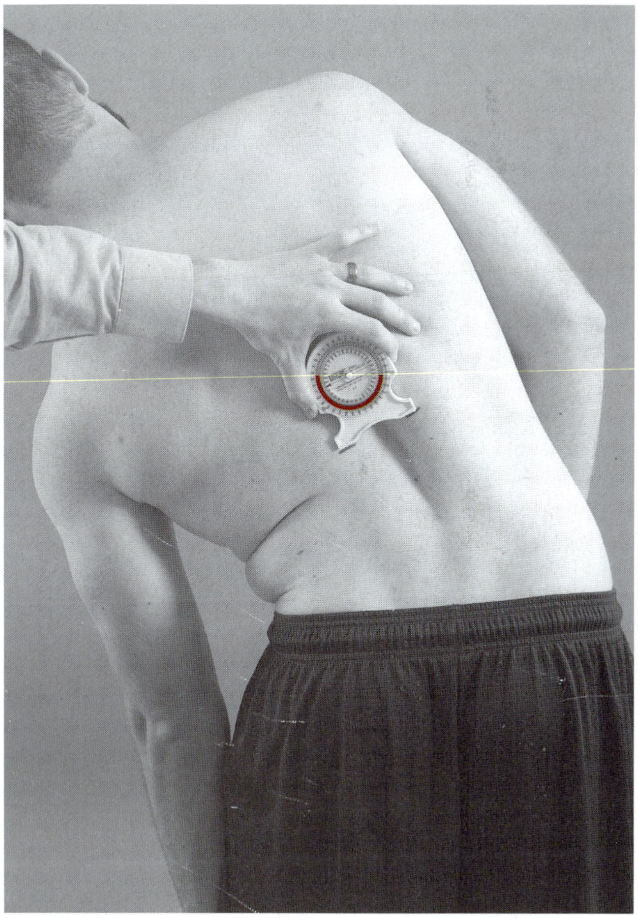

FIGURE 12.54 Maintain the inclinometer at T12 throughout the motion and take a measurement at T12 at the end of the motion.

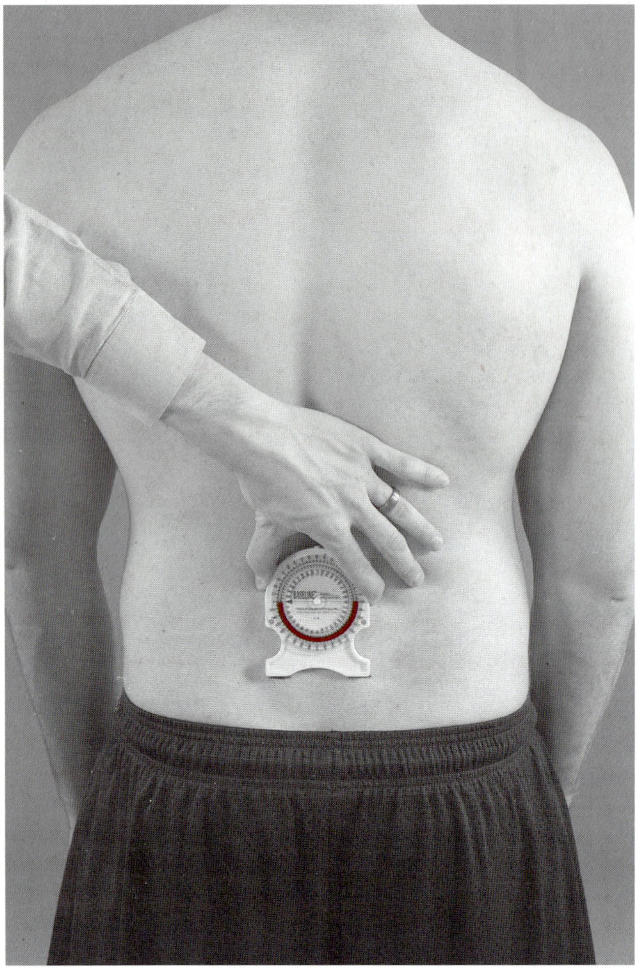

FIGURE 12.55 The individual returns to the starting position; the examiner then places and zeroes the inclinometer at S2.

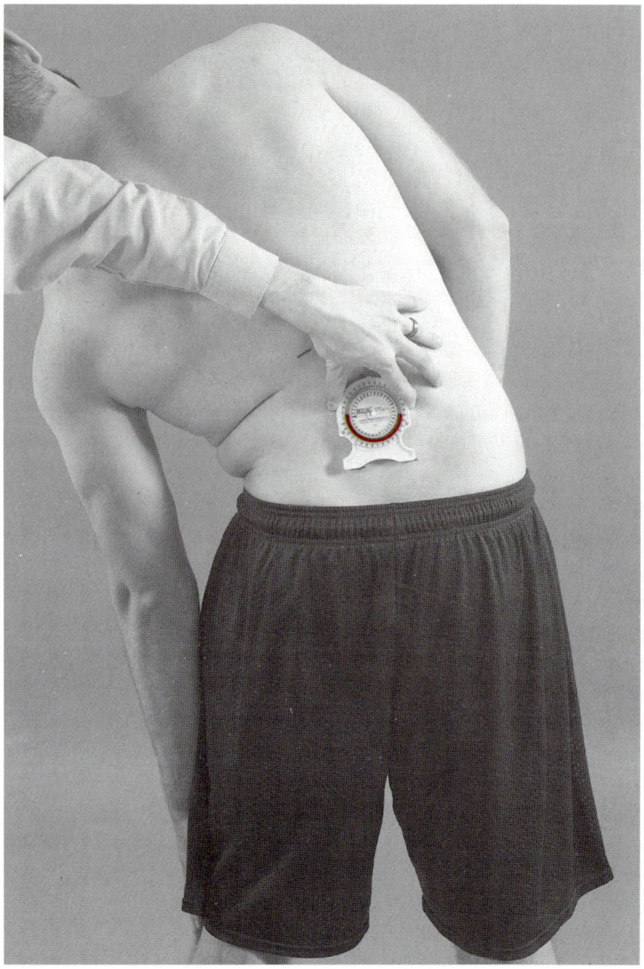

FIGURE 12.56 Ask the individual to bend sideways again while keeping the inclinometer on S2. At the end of the motion take a measurement at S2. Subtract the S2 measurement from the T12 measurement to obtain lateral flexion ROM.

Research Findings

Table 12.1 shows thoracolumbar spine ROM values from the AAOS and lumbar spine ROM values from the AMA and selected other studies.

Effects of Age, Gender, and Other Factors

Age

Many instruments and methods have been used to determine the range of thoracic, thoracolumbar, and lumbar motion. Therefore, comparisons between studies are difficult. As is true for other regions of the body, conflicting evidence exists regarding the effects of age on ROM. However, the majority of studies appear to indicate that age-related decreases in spinal ROM do occur and that these changes may affect certain motions more than others at the same joint or region.[22–33]

The following group of studies with relatively large numbers of subjects and extended age ranges arrived at similar conclusions regarding the motions that showed the greatest and least decrease in ROM with increasing age. Extension was identified as the one motion that showed the greatest decrease with increasing age and axial rotation was the motion that showed the least decrease in ROM. Lumbar flexion and lateral flexion each showed decreases but the data were more inconsistent and decreases seemed to be related to different age ranges.

McGregor, McCarthy, and Hughes[27] found that although age had a significant effect on all planes of motion, the effect varied for each motion, and age accounted for only a small portion of the variability seen in the 203 normal subjects studied. Maximum extension was the most affected motion, with significant decreases between each decade. Lateral flexion decreased after age 40 and each decade thereafter. Flexion decreased initially after age 30 but stayed the same until an additional decrease after age 50. No similar decreases or trends were found in axial rotation.

The findings of Troke and associates[29,30] were similar in that these authors found no change in lumbar axial rotation in 405 asymptomatic subjects (196 females and 209 males) aged 16 to 90 years. However, lumbar extension showed the greatest decline in ROM (approximately 76%). Male and female lumbar spine flexion range of motion declined considerably less, by about 40% over the age span, and right and left lateral flexion each declined about 43%. These authors used the CA-6000 Spine Motion Analyzer to measure half cycle motions at different times of the day to account for diurnal variations.

In another fairly large study, Moll and Wright[25] used skin markings and a plumbline to measure the range of lumbar extension in a study involving 237 subjects (119 men and 118 women) aged 20 to 90 years. These authors found a wide variation in normal values but detected a gradual decrease in lumbar extension in subjects between 35 and 90 years of age.

Van Herp and associates,[31] in a study of 100 healthy male and female subjects aged 20 to 77 years, used the 3Space System to measure lumbar ROM from T12 to S1. The authors found a constant decrease with increasing age in all lumbar motions except for flexion in 50- to 59-year-old males.

Fitzgerald and associates[12] determined that the oldest group had considerably less motion than the youngest group in all motions except for flexion. The coefficients of variation indicated that a greater amount of variability existed in the ROM in the oldest groups (Table 12.2).

Alaranta and coworkers[16] used both a tape measure and an inclinometer to assess lumbar ROM in 508 males and females 35 to 45 years of age. Some of these individuals had either

TABLE 12.1 Thoracolumbar and Lumbar Spine Motion: Normal Values for Adults in Inches and Degrees From Selected Sources

Instrument Spine Region Authors Sample	Tape measure and goniometer Thoracolumbar AAOS*[11]	Double inclinometers Lumbar AMA†[10]	BROM II Lumbar Breum et al[70] 18–38 yr	3Space Isotrak system Lumbar Van Herp et al[31] 20–29 yr	Inclinometer Lumbar Ng et al[23] 30 yr
Motion			***Mean (SD)***	***Mean (SD)***	***Mean (SD)***
Flexion	4 inches	60 degrees	56.3 (1.3) degrees	56.4 (7.1) degrees	52 (90) degrees
Extension	20–30 degrees	25 degrees	21.5 (8.2) degrees	22.5 (7.8) degrees	19 (9) degrees
Right lateral flexion	35 degrees	25 degrees	33.3 (5.9) degrees	26.2 (8.4) degrees	31 (6) degrees
Left lateral flexion	35 degrees	25 degrees	33.6 (6.2) degrees	25.8 (7.8) degrees	30 (6) degrees
Right rotation	45 degrees			14.4 (5.1) degrees	33 (9) degrees

SD = Standard deviation; AAOS = American Association of Orthopaedic Surgeons; AMA = American Medical Association.

* Flexion measurement in inches was obtained with a tape measure using the spinous processes of C7 and S1 as reference points. The remaining motions were measured with a universal goniometer and are in degrees.

† Lumbar motion was measured from sacrum (S1) to T12.

TABLE 12.2 Age Effects on Lumbar and Thoracolumbar Spine Motion in Individuals Aged 20 to 79 Years: Normal Values in Centimeters and Degrees

Sample	20–29 yr n = 31	30–39 yr n = 42	40–49 yr n = 16	50–59 yr n = 43	60–69 yr n = 26	70–79 yr n = 9
Motion	***Mean (SD)***	***Mean (SD)***	***Mean (SD)***	***Mean (SD)***	***Mean (SD)***	***Mean (SD)***
Flexion*	3.7 (0.7)	3.9 (1.0)	3.1 (0.8)	3.0 (1.1)	2.4 (0.7)	2.2 (0.6)
Extension	41.2 (9.6)	40.0 (8.8)	31.1 (8.9)	27.4 (8.0)	17.4 (7.5)	16.6 (8.8)
Right lateral flexion	37.6 (5.8)	35.3 (6.5)	27.1 (6.5)	25.3 (6.2)	20.2 (4.8)	18.0 (4.7)
Left lateral flexion	38.7 (5.7)	36.5 (6.0)	28.5 (5.2)	26.8 (6.4)	20.3 (5.3)	18.9 (6.0)

SD = Standard deviation.

* Flexion measurements were obtained with use of the Schober method and are reported in centimeters.

All other measurements were obtained with use of a universal goniometer and are reported in degrees.

Adapted from Fitzgerald, GK, et al: Objective assessment with establishment of normal values for lumbar spine range of motion. Phys Ther 63:1776, 1983.[12] With the permission of the American Physical Therapy Association.

neck or back pain, but all were actively employed. Lumbar flexion showed more than a 10% decrease when comparing the youngest with the oldest subjects, but lateral flexion showed an even greater decrease (19%) with increasing age. This decrease in lateral flexion is similar to the findings of McGregor, McCarthy, and Hughes,[27] who found that lateral flexion showed a slightly higher decrease in ROM (43%) than the decrease in forward flexion (40%).

Dreischarf and colleagues[32] used a novel noninvasive measuring system to assess lumbar shape and mobility in 323 asymptomatic volunteers (139 males and 184 females). The participants were aged 20 to 75 years, with a body mass index greater than 26. Lumbar lordosis was measured in three body positions: standing, maximal flexion, and extension of the upper body. A significant reduction of the total lordosis occurred in each consecutive age-group but there was only a small reduction in lordosis between 20 and 29 years and 30 and 39 years. The total lordosis was significantly reduced by approximately 20%, flexion ROM by 12%, and extension ROM by 31% in the oldest group (> 50 years) compared with the youngest age cohort (20–29 years). These decreases occurred mainly in the middle of the lordosis and less toward the lumbosacral and thoracolumbar transitions. The lower part of the lumbar spine retained its lordosis and mobility, whereas the middle part flattened and became less mobile. The authors concluded that aging is a crucial factor for a reduction in total ROM.

Lee and colleagues[33] took whole spine radiographs of the spine in standing, supine, and sitting positions in young 25-year-olds and elderly 66-year-olds. The results showed that when changing positions from sitting to standing, lumbar lordosis increased in the standing position for both young (52.8 degrees) and elderly (53.0 degrees). When going from standing to 90-degree sitting and from standing to supine, lumbar lordosis decreased. When changing sitting positions with the chair back inclined 30, 60, or 90 degrees, lumbar lordosis decreased regardless of age. The authors concluded that a decrease in spinal mobility in the older group could be due to aging because the upper lumbar spine is more flexible in individuals in their 20s compared with those in their 60s.

Saidu and colleagues[34] used the Modified Schober method and a 180-degree goniometer in a study of lumbar spinal mobility involving 135 normal male and female Nigerian adults ranging in age from 29 to 72 years. Spinal mobility was significantly different among all age-groups, and the ROM decreased in 18-year intervals, especially in trunk flexion and right lateral flexion, in both sexes. The most significant differences occurred between the two youngest and two oldest groups, with the middle age-group showing no significant differences. However, extension had the greatest decline in ROM with increasing age, which is similar to the findings in the studies by McGregor, McCarthy, and Hughes[27] and Troke et al.[29,30]

Bible and coinvestigators[35] analyzed radiographs of 250 patients including 137 females and 121 males whose ages ranged from 18 to 92 years. Multivariate regression analyses were performed for each level (L1–S1). Age had a significantly negative association with ROM from L1–L2 to L4–L5. Body mass index had a significantly negative association with ROM from L2–L3 to L4–L5. The Kellgren score of degeneration had a significant association with ROM only at L5–S1. In conclusion, age was the strongest statistical predictor of ROM and was associated with declining ROM of approximately a 3-degree decrease in total sagittal lumbar ROM in the upper four segments every 10 years.

Although it appears as if there is a great deal of evidence that lumbar extension decreases more with increasing age than lumbar flexion, the following studies reported that both flexion and extension ROM were found to decline with increasing age. However, in some of the studies the motions were full cycle motions, so it is difficult to tell whether the decrease was in flexion or in extension.

In one of the earlier studies, in 1967 Loebl[22] used an inclinometer to measure active sagittal plane ROM of the thoracic and lumbar spine of 126 males and females between 15 and 84 years of age. He found age-related effects for both males and females and concluded that both genders should expect a loss of about 8 degrees of spinal ROM per decade with increases in age.

Sullivan, Dickinson, and Troup[24] used double inclinometers to measure sagittal plane lumbar motion in 1,126 healthy male and female subjects. These authors found that when gender was controlled, both flexion and extension decreased with increasing age. The authors suggested that the ROM thresholds that determine impairment ratings should take age into consideration.

In 1969, Macrae and Wright[20] used a modification of the Schober technique to measure forward lumbar flexion in 195 women and 147 men (18 to 71 years of age). The authors concluded that active flexion ROM decreased with age.

The preceding studies are fairly consistent in concluding that both thoracolumbar and lumbar ROM including extension decreases with increasing age, and according to one study lateral flexion may be affected more than flexion. Axial rotation was not measured in the majority of studies, but when it was measured, no age-related changes in ROM were found

The following two studies investigated segmental mobility. Gracovetsky and associates[26] found a significant difference between young and old in a group of 40 subjects aged 19 to 64 years. Older subjects had decreased segmental mobility in the lower lumbar spine compared with younger subjects. To compensate for the decrease in mobility, the older subjects increased the contribution of the pelvis to flexion and extension.

Wong and colleagues[36] assessed intervertebral lumbar flexion and extension in 100 healthy volunteers (50 males and 50 females) aged 20 to 76 years. The results showed that all segmental lumbar spinal motion profiles within the ROM of 10 degrees of extension to 40 degrees of flexion did not change as age increased until subjects were 51 years of age or older. Subjects in the oldest age-group had a decrease in maximum flexion and extension ROM, and an increase in the slopes of the intervertebral flexion–extension curves at each lumbar segment.

Kondratek and coinvestigators[28] conducted a study to find normative values for active lumbar ROM in 116 girls and 109 boys (5, 7, 9, and 11 years of age). Measurements were taken with the back range of motion (BROM 11) device. In a comparison between 11-year-olds and 5-year-olds, flexion was found to be more variable in both boys and girls and an apparent age difference was observed in that flexion was less in 11-year-olds compared with 5-year-olds.

Genetic Influences

The results of genetic influences on lumbar range of motion were investigated in a study by Battie, Levalalti, and Videman[37] involving 300 male monozygotic and dizygotic twin pairs. The investigators found that the proportion of variance in lumbar ROM attributable to genetic influence (heritability estimate) was 47%. The extent of lumbar ROM in flexion was predominately determined by genetic influences (64%). One pathway of genetic effects on lumbar flexion ROM appeared to be through genetic influences on body weight. Lumbar ROM in extension, although being influenced by genes, was primarily influenced by environmental and behavioral factors. However, up to 18% of the variance in extension ROM could be explained by genetic influences shared by disc degeneration variables. Statistically significant age-adjusted genetic correlations were found between lumbar extension and disc degeneration and between lumbar flexion and body weight.

Gender

In the following studies, investigators used different instruments and methods, which makes comparisons between studies difficult. Investigations into the effects of gender on lumbar spine ROM indicate that the effects may be motion specific and possibly age specific, but controversy still exists concerning which motions are affected. However, the following five studies appear to agree that the ROM in flexion is greater in males than it is in females, at least in subjects 15 to 65 years of age. This difference in lumbar flexion ROM between males and females is apparent even in children between the ages of 5 and 11 years.[38] At the other end of the age spectrum, this difference between the genders in flexion ROM may have evened out by the time men and women were in their 80s.

Macrae and Wright[20] found that females had significantly less forward flexion than did males across all age-groups. Sullivan, Dickinson, and Troup[24] also found that when age was controlled, mean flexion ROM was greater in males. However, mean extension ROM and total ROM were significantly greater in females. Subjects in the study were 1,126 healthy male and female volunteers aged 15 to 65 years. The authors noted that although female total ROM was significantly greater than male total ROM, the difference of 1.5 degrees was not clinically relevant. Age and gender combined accounted for only 14% of the variance in flexion, 25% in extension, and 20% of the variance in total ROM (Table 12.3). Alaranta and associates,[16] in a study of 508 males and females aged 35 to 45 years, also determined that men had greater flexion ROM than did women. However, these authors found no difference between the sexes in extension ROM.

Kondratek and associates,[28] in a study of 116 girls and 109 boys aged 5 to 11 years, found a statistically significant difference between the youngest and oldest subjects in active lumbar flexion in girls and active lumbar lateral flexion and rotation in both girls and boys. The girls, aged 11 years, consistently demonstrated less motion in forward flexion and right and left lateral flexion than did the boys. Extension varied very little in either gender. Troke and colleagues[29,30] found that men had greater ROM in flexion at 16 years than did women, but in the final decade*s* (80 to 90 years) men and women were equal.

Moll and Wright's[25] findings are directly opposite to the findings of the previous three studies in that Moll and Wright determined that male mobility in extension significantly exceeded female mobility by 7%. Differences in findings between studies may have resulted from the fact that Moll and Wright[25] did not control for age. These authors measured the

TABLE 12.3 Age and Gender Effects on Lumbar Motion in Individuals Aged 15 to 65 Years: Normal Values in Degrees Using a Fluid-Filled Inclinometer

Sample	16–24 yr Male *n* = 122	15–24 yr Female *n* = 161	25–34 yr Male *n* = 295	25–34 yr Female *n* = 143	35–65 yr Male *n* = 269	35–65 yr Female *n* = 136
Motion	***Mean (SD)***	***Mean (SD)***	***Mean (SD)***	***Mean (SD)***	***Mean (SD)***	***Mean (SD)***
Flexion	33 (9)	26 (9)	31 (8)	24 (8)	27 (8)	22 (8)
Extension	54 (10)	63 (9)	52 (9)	60 (10)	47 (9)	53 (9)

SD = Standard deviation.

Adapted from Sullivan, MS, Dickinson, CE, and Troup, JDG: The influence of age and gender on lumbar spine sagittal plane range of motion: A study of 1126 healthy subjects. Spine 19:682, 1994.[24]

range of lumbar extension in a study involving 237 subjects (119 males and 118 females), aged 15 to 90 years, who were clinically and radiologically normal relatives of patients with psoriatic arthritis (Table 12.4).

Van Herp and associates,[31] in an investigation of lumbar range of motion in 100 subjects (50 male and 50 female) 20 to 77 years of age, found that females consistently showed greater flexibility than did males in lumbar flexion–extension, lateral flexion, and axial rotation throughout the age range. Because flexion was not separated from extension, it is difficult to know which motion was responsible for the increase.

Intolo and colleagues[38] conducted a systematic review in which 16 studies provided data from 109 females and 154 males. Gender-related reductions occurred in flexion, extension, and lateral flexion from 40 to 50 years and after 60 years. In males, extension ROM decreased by a mean of 8 degrees from 20 to 70 years and flexion decreased by a mean of 16.3 degrees. Females had a greater decrease than did males in extension from 20 to 70 years and a smaller decrease in flexion than did males. Extension ROM was reduced in each decade after 40 years for females and after 30 years for males. Flexion reduction was more pronounced after 40 years for females and after 50 years for males. Both genders showed little effect of age in rotation ROM.

Dreischarf and colleagues,[32] in a study of 323 asymptomatic males and females who performed flexion and extension in standing, found that the reduction in total lordosis was more evident in females, who showed a significant decrease of 7.9 degrees compared with males, who had a 6.7 degree reduction. In both sexes, there was only a small lordosis reduction between 20 and 29 years and 30 and 39 years. After 39 years, females showed a continuous decrease in lordosis, whereas the decrease in males occurred primarily between the ages of 30 and 39 years and 40 and 49 years. The smallest decrease in lordosis in males was found in the 40- to 49-year-old group and no statistical difference in lordosis occurred in males between 40 to 49 years whereas there was significant

TABLE 12.4 Age and Gender Effects on Lumbar and Thoracolumbar Motion in Individuals Aged 15 to 44 Years: Normal Values in Centimeters

Sample	15–24 yr		35–44 yr		35–44 yr	
	Male *n* = 21	Female *n* = 10	Male *n* = 13	Female *n* = 16	Male *n* = 14	Female *n* = 18
Motion	***Mean (SD)***	***Mean (SD)***	***Mean (SD)***	***Mean (SD)***	***Mean (SD)***	***Mean (SD)***
Flexion*	7.23 (0.92)	6.66 (1.03)	7.48 (0.82)	6.69 (1.09)	6.88 (0.88)	6.29 (1.04)
Extension*	4.21 (1.64)	4.34 (1.52)	5.05 (1.41)	4.76 (1.53)	3.73 (1.47)	3.09 (1.31)
Right lateral flexion†	5.43 (1.30)	6.85 (1.46)	5.34 (1.06)	6.32 (1.93)	4.83 (1.34)	5.30 (1.61)
Left lateral flexion†	5.06 (1.40)	7.20 (1.66)	5.93 (1.07)	6.13 (1.42)	4.83 (0.99)	5.48 (1.30)

SD = Standard deviation.

*Lumbar motion.

†Thoracolumbar motion.

Adapted from Moll, JMH, and Wright, V: Normal range of spinal mobility: An objective clinical study. Ann Rheum Dis 30:381, 1971.[25] The authors used skin markings and a plumbline on the thorax for lateral flexion.

reduction of lordosis between the 20- to 29-year-old group and the 40- to 49-year-old group in females.

In contrast to the preceding authors, the following studies reported no significant effects for gender on lumbar spine ROM. Loebl[22] found no significant gender differences between the 126 males and females aged 15 to 84 years for measurements of lumbar flexion and extension. Bookstein and associates[39] used a tape measure to measure the lumbar extension ROM in 75 elementary schoolchildren aged 6 to 11 years. The authors found no differences for age or gender, but they found a significant difference for age–gender interaction in the 6-year-old group. Girls aged 6 years had a mean range of extension of 4.1 centimeters, in contrast to the 6-year-old boys, who had a mean range of extension of 2.1 centimeters. Wong and colleagues[36] used an electrogoniometer and videofluoroscopy to assess the flexion–extension profile of the lumbar spine in different genders and age-groups. A total of 100 healthy volunteers (50 females and 50 males) aged 21 to 51 years and older participated in the study, but no statistically significant differences in the pattern of motion were found between the genders.

Race and Ethnicity

Trudelle-Jackson and colleagues[40] conducted a study of 917 women between the ages of 20 and 83 years. Normative values for lumbar extension and flexion were different for white and African American women and also differed between the following three age-groups: 20 to 39 years (n = 126), 40 to 59 years (n = 412), and older than 60 years (n = 228). An electronic inclinometer (BEP-VII) was used to take measurements in the fully extended and fully flexed positions to remove the influence of initial resting posture. Sixty degrees of lumbar extension for the 147 African American women was significantly greater than the lumbar extension value of 52 degrees for the 619 white women, but only a 2-degree difference was found between the two groups of women for flexion. The authors suggested that different criteria should be used to estimate impairment levels in women of different racial groups because the normative values for lumbar flexion and extension are different.

Occupation and Lifestyle

In the following brief section, one example of lifestyle effects on lumbar spine ROM is reviewed and two studies are reviewed regarding the effects of occupation.

Sjolie[41] compared low-back strength and low-back and hip mobility between a group of 38 adolescents living in a community without access to pedestrian roads and a group of 50 adolescents with excellent access to pedestrian roads. Low-back mobility was measured by means of the Modified Schober technique. The results showed that adolescents living in rural areas without easy access to pedestrian roads had less low-back extension and hamstring flexibility than did their counterparts in urban areas. The hypothesis that negative associations would exist between school bus use and physical performance was confirmed. The distance traveled by school bus was inversely associated with hamstring flexibility and other hip motions but not with low-back flexion. Walking or bicycling to leisure activities was positively associated with low-back strength, low-back extension ROM, and hip flexion and extension.

Freidrich and colleagues[42] conducted a comprehensive examination of spinal posture during stooped walking in 22 male sewer workers aged 24 to 49 years. Working in a stooped posture has been identified as one of the risk factors associated with spinal disorders. Five posture levels corresponding to standardized sewer heights ranging in decreasing size from 150 to 105 centimeters were taped by a video-based motion-analysis system. The results showed that the lumbar spine abruptly changed from the usual lordotic position in normal upright walking to a kyphotic position in mild, 150-centimeter headroom restriction. As ceiling height decreased, the neck progressively assumed a more extended lordotic position; the thoracic spine extended and flattened, becoming less kyphotic; and the lumbar spine became more kyphotic. As expected, the older workers showed decreased segmental mobility in the lumbar spine and an increase in cervical lordosis with decreasing ceiling height.

Lumbar disk degeneration (LDD) is associated with heavy physical loading in U.S. industries. The following study[43] used magnetic resonance imaging (MRI) to study the dose-related incidence of LDD in two groups of individuals: 393 fruit market workers with a mean age of 51.2 years who carry heavy loads, and 160 respiratory patients at a walk-in clinic with a mean age of 49.3 years. The participants were assigned to the following three groupings based on job histories of lifting: low lifting level (n = 185), intermediate lifting level (n = 184), and high lifting level (n = 184). Each individual disk from L1–L2 to L5–S1 was evaluated for disk hydration, annulus tears, disk height, narrowing, bulging, protrusion, degeneration, foramen narrowing, and nerve root compression. Disk bulging caused by carrying intermediate loads was observed at L2–L3 and L3–L4. Bulging caused by carrying high lifting loads and nerve root compression was observed at L4–L5 and L5–S1. Dehydration was most frequently observed at L4–L5 (69%) followed by L5–S1 (63.7%), and disk bulging was most commonly found at the L4–L5 level (61%). The results supported the hypothesis that mechanical loading may play a crucial role in disk pathogenesis and a dose-response relationship between cumulative lifting load and LDD.

Functional Range of Motion

Functional ranges of motion are essential for carrying out activities of daily living (ADLs), and knowledge of normative values is essential for providing guidelines for therapists and for motivating patients.

Bible and coinvestigators[44] used a noninvasive electrogoniometer and a torsiometer to measure ROM of the lumbar spine in 60 healthy volunteers (30 women and 30 men) aged 20 to 70 years, who were evenly distributed among four age-groups. The volunteers were asked to perform maximum lumbar ROM in all planes and also to perform a series of 15 ADLs in order to determine the functional ROM requirements required for these activities. The functional ROM required to complete all 15 ADLs ranged from 3 to 49 degrees (median: 9 degrees) of flexion–extension, 2 to 11 degrees (median: 6 degrees) of lateral flexion, and 2 to 7 degrees (median: 5 degrees) of rotation. Picking up a 2-pound circular weight from the floor either using a bending or squatting technique required the most ROM. However, squatting and picking up the weight required significantly less sagittal motion compared with bending at the waist while keeping the knees extended (42 versus 48 degrees).

Hsieh and Pringle[45] used a CA-6000 Spine Motion Analyzer to measure the amount of lumbar motion required for selected activities of daily living performed by 48 healthy subjects with a mean age of 26.5 years. Activities included stand to sit, sit to stand, putting on socks, and picking up an object from the floor. The individual's peak flexion angles for the activities were normalized to the subject's own peak flexion angle in erect standing. Stand to sit and sit to stand (Fig. 12.57) required approximately 56% to 66% of lumbar flexion. The mean was 34.6 degrees for sit to stand and 41.8 degrees for stand to sit. Putting on socks (Fig. 12.58) required 90% of lumbar flexion ROM (mean 56.4 degrees), and picking up an object from the floor (Fig. 12.59) required 95% of lumbar flexion (mean 60.4 degrees). In view of these findings, one can understand how limitations in lumbar ROM may affect an individual's ability to carry out dressing and other activities of daily living.

Levine and associates[46] conducted a study with 20 healthy women (mean age 23.4 years) from a university student population to determine changes in lumbar spine motion in standing, walking, and running on a treadmill at three different gradients. According to results obtained from the Vicon Motion Analysis System, total lumbar spine ROM was greater during running than during walking and greater walking downhill than walking uphill or on a level surface. However, the maximum amount of lumbar extension (anterior pelvic tilt) was found in standing at the three gradients.

In a study by Guoan and coinvestigators,[47] the authors used an imaging technique and an MRI to measure vertebral motion in eight healthy volunteers during unrestricted weight-bearing functional activities. Coupled motions were measured in addition to flexion–extension, left-right flexion, and left–right twisting. The results showed that the upper vertebrae L2–L3 (5.4 degrees) and L3–L4 (4.3 degrees) had significantly higher ranges of flexion than the lower vertebrae L4–L5 (1.9 degrees) during a flexion–extension motion.

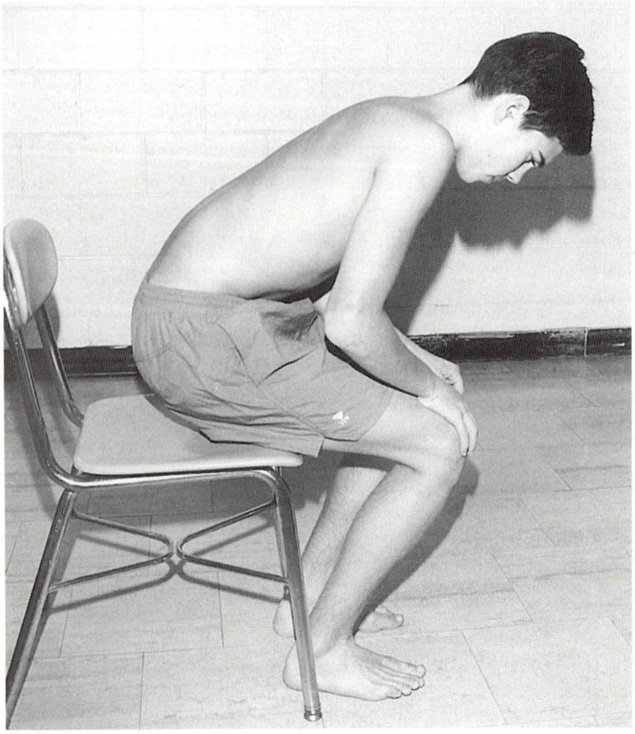

FIGURE 12.57 Sit to stand requires an average of 35 degrees of lumbar flexion.[45]

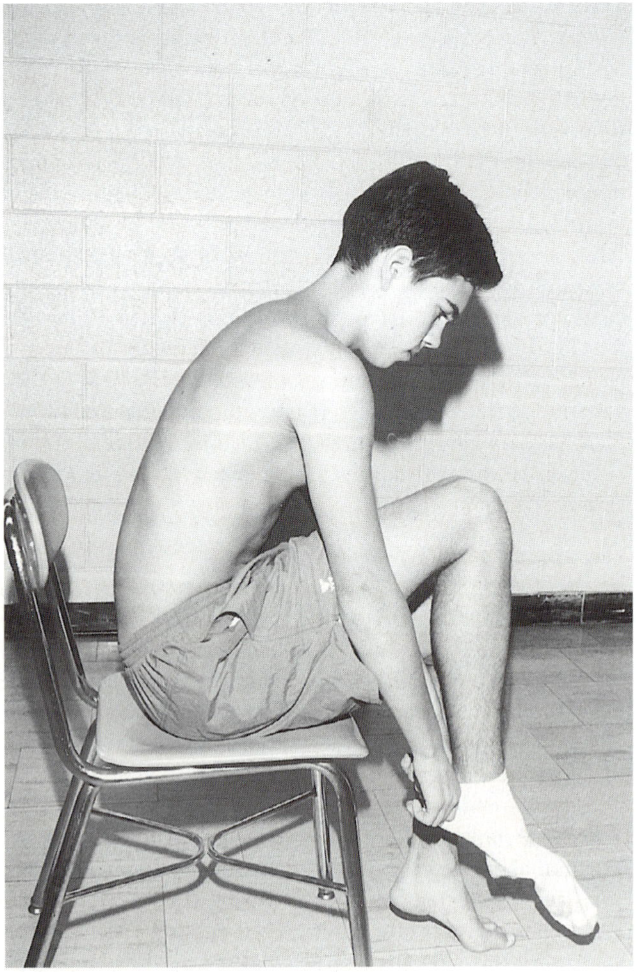

FIGURE 12.58 Putting on socks requires an average of 56 degrees of lumbar flexion.[45]

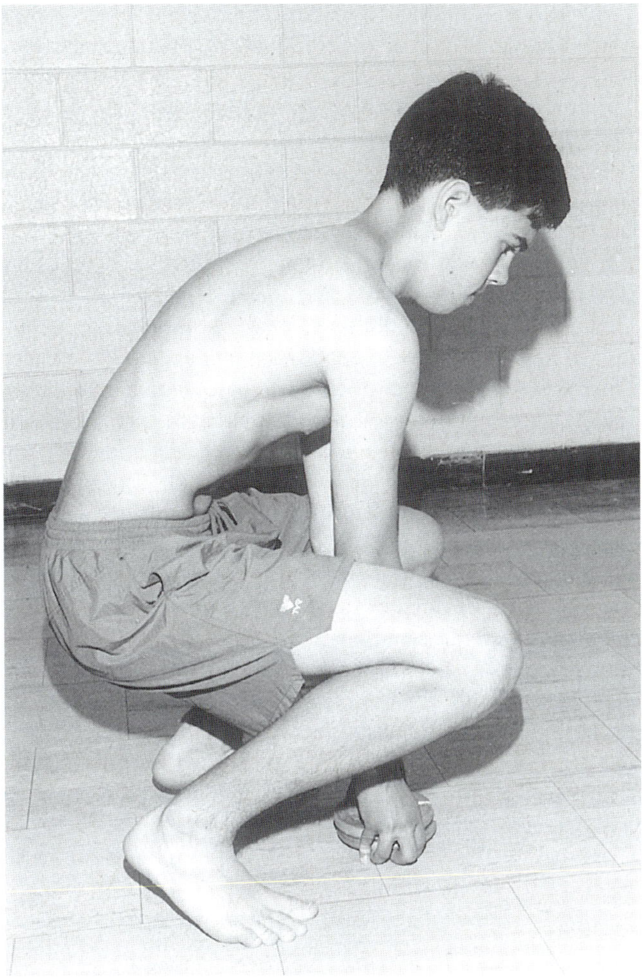

FIGURE 12.59 Picking up an object from the floor requires an average of 60 degrees of lumbar flexion.[45]

During lateral bending, L4–L5 had a higher but not significant range of left-to-right bending than both L2–L3 and L3–L4. In addition, the L4–L5 level had a significantly larger ROM in rotation than the L2–L3 level ($P < 0.05$).

Reliability and Validity

The following section on reliability and validity has been divided according to the instruments and methods used to obtain the measurements. However, some overlap occurs between the sections because several investigators have compared different methods and instruments within one study.

Many instruments have been used in attempts to measure the ROM of the thoracic spine. In a study by Johnson and colleagues,[48] 15 men and 30 women volunteers between the ages of 18 and 45 years performed five thoracic rotation ROM techniques. Three examiners used standard (20-centimeter) clear plastic goniometers to measure rotation in the following positions: seated with bar in front and with bar in back, half kneeling with bar in front and with bar in back, and the quadruped lumbar locked position. In the latter test position, the participant was placed in the quadruped position in which the upper extremity provided support on elbows and forearms. A bubble inclinometer was placed between the scapular spines at the T1–T2 level and rotation was performed by the participant placing an ipsilateral hand on the posterior aspect of the neck and rotating the thoracic spine while maintaining the quadruped position.

The lumbar-locked position of 40.8 degrees produced the smallest ROM value, whereas the largest amount of motion occurred in rotation in the half-kneeling position with the bar in front (60.6 degrees). All intratester and intertester ICC values were greater than 0.85 and all techniques had low standard error of measurement (SEMs less than 3 degrees and minimal detectable change [MDC] values less than 6 degrees) for measuring thoracic rotation in the seated, half kneeling, and lumbar locked position.

Some participants had difficulty maintaining balance in the half-kneeling position both with bar in front and bar in back. In fact, the presence of any condition that prevented the individual from kneeling would prevent testing in the half-kneeling position (see Table 12.5).

The following instruments have been used to measure thoracic kyphosis: digital clear plastic goniometers, inclinometers, the flexicurve kyphosis angle and flexicurve index, Debrunner

TABLE 12.5 Thoracic Spine: Intra- and Intertester Reliability of Measuring Rotation

Intratester (within day)	ICC	SEM	MDC	Intertester (within session)	ICC	SEM	MDC
Seated rotation (bar in back)	0.94	0.76	2.10	Seated rotation (bar in back)	0.85	2.03	5.61
Seated rotation (bar in front)	0.8	1.74	4.83	Seated rotation (bar in front)	0.87	1.72	4.77
Half-kneeling rotation (bar in back)	0.95	0.78	2.16	Half-kneeling rotation (bar in back)	0.92	1.26	3.49
Half-kneeling rotation (bar in front)	0.92	1.18	3.27	Half-kneeling rotation (bar in front)	0.94	1.03	2.84

ICC = Intraclass correlation coefficient; SEM = Standard error of measurement; MDC = Minimal detectable change.

Adapted from Johnson, KD, et al: Reliability of thoracic spine rotation range-of-motion measurements in healthy adults. J Athl Train 47(1):52, 2012.

kyphometer, SpinalMouse, tape measure, video camera, arcometer, and radiographs. Azadinia and colleagues[49] used the radiographic Cobb angle as a gold standard in a study of 105 patients with kyphosis. The digital inclinometer and flexicurve were also used to measure kyphosis. The digital inclinometer was reasonably valid for patients younger than 30 and older than 50 years, whereas the validity of the flexicurve in both age ranges was poor. The digital inclinometer had high intra- and interrater reliability in the same age-groups, whereas the flexicurve had only acceptable reliability for intrarater reliability and poor interrater reliability.

Greendale and colleagues[50] also used a modified Cobb angle as the criterion standard in 118 participants and employed the following measurement instruments: Debrunner kyphosis angle, the flexicurve index, and the flexicurve kyphosis angle. Contrary to the findings of Azadinia, results showed that all three measurement devices used in this study had strong and similar validity and reliability.

Barrett, McCreesh, and Lewis[1] measured thoracic kyphosis using two gravity-dependent inclinometers, the flexicurve index, and flexicurve angle. The feet of the inclinometers were placed over the spinous processes of T1–T2 and T12–L1. Intrarater reliability was excellent and very similar for all methods but the flexicurve index and the flexicurve angle had higher intrarater reliability than the inclinometer. However, for interrater reliability the double inclinometers showed excellent reliability, whereas the other two instruments showed only good reliability.

Similar instruments have been used in attempts to measure the ROM of the lumbar spine. The instrument that is unique to the lumbar spine is the BROM II. Littlewood and May[51] conducted a systematic review of 86 ROM studies to determine what low-tech measurement methods were valid for measuring lumbar spine ROM. Only four studies—those by Samo and colleagues,[52] Saur and colleagues,[53] Williams and colleagues,[17] and Tousignant and colleagues[54]—met the following criteria: English language only, validity evaluated by comparison with radiographs, adult subjects with nonspecific low-back pain, and measurement accuracy to enable judgment on validity. However, all failed to meet the criteria of blinding the examiners. Double inclinometers were used in three of the four studies, and the Modified-Modified Schober Test (MMST) was used in the other study. Littlewood and May[51] concluded that there was only limited supporting evidence for the validity of measuring total lumbar ROM with double inclinometers in comparison with radiographic analysis; there was conflicting evidence for the validity of measuring lumbar flexion ROM. In regard to the MMST, there was limited positive evidence for the lack of validity for measuring lumbar flexion ROM. The authors concluded that there is a need for scientific evidence on the validity of the measurement procedures.

MacDermid and colleagues[55] investigated the reliability and validity of a Tracker ME computerized dual inclinometer (CDI) compared with the MMST. Twenty individuals with back pain and 20 without back pain were selected through convenience sampling. Two examiners measured sagittal plane lumbar ROM for each individual. Two separate tests with the CDI and one test with the MMST were conducted. Intratrial reliability was high to very high for both the CDI (with ICCs of 0.85–0.96) and for the MMST (ICCs of 0.84–0.98). However, reliability was poor to moderate (ICCs of 0.16–0.59) when the CDI unit had to be repositioned either by the same examiner or a different one. Interrater reliability for the MMST was moderate to high (ICCs of 0.75–0.82) but concurrent validity showed that the correlation between the CDI and MMST was poor for lumbar flexion

In another review, Essendrop and colleagues[56] screened databases from 1980 to 1999 for reliability studies regarding the measurement of low-back ROM, strength, and endurance. Seventy-nine studies were located, six of which met the predetermined criteria for a quality study and focused on the measurement of low-back ROM. Noting the difficulty in making definite conclusions based on these limited studies, the authors reported that the tape measure was the most reliable instrument for flexion measurements. Reliable extension measurements were difficult to achieve with any of the reviewed instruments. The tape measure and Cybex EDI-320 goniometer were reliable for trunk lateral flexion when comparing groups but not individuals. Trunk rotation measurements were the most unreliable for all instruments including the double inclinometers, the Myrin single inclinometer, tape measure, and universal goniometer.

Reliability of the Inclinometer

The fifth edition of the AMA *Guides to the Evaluation of Permanent Impairment*[4] states that "measurement techniques using inclinometers are necessary to obtain reliable spinal mobility measurements." However, ROM is no longer suggested as a basis for defining impairment because of the variability of results and a lack of high quality evidence in the literature. Lumbar ROM has been removed from the sixth edition of the AMA Guide[5] as a reliable indicator of specific pathology or permanent functional status.

In a study by Williams and coworkers[17] that compared the measurements of the inclinometer with those of the tape measure, the authors found that the double inclinometer technique had questionable intertester reliability (Table 12.6). Reliability problems with the use of double inclinometers are often related to difficulty in identifying landmarks and in holding the inclinometers correctly. Other problems include a lack of sufficient practice to familiarize the examiner with the instruments.

Loebl[22] has stated that the only reliable technique for measuring lumbar spine motion is radiography. However, radiography is expensive and may pose a health risk to the subject; moreover, the validity of radiographic assessment of ROM is unreported. Loebl used an inclinometer to measure flexion and extension in nine subjects. He found that in five repeated active measurements, the ROM varied by 5 degrees in the most consistent subject and by 23 degrees in the most inconsistent subject. Variability decreased when

TABLE 12.6 Intratester and Intertester Reliability for Thoracolumbar and Lumbar ROM

Study	*n*	Sample	Method	Motions	Intratester ICC	Intertester ICC
Healthy Populations						
Madson et al[71]	40	Healthy adults 20–40 yr Mean age = 25.5	BROM*	Flexion	0.67	
				Extension	0.78	
				R lateral flexion	0.91	
				R rotation	0.88	
Kondratek et al[28]	15	Healthy children 5–11 yr	BROM II*	Flexion	0.53–0.71	
				Extension	0.82–0.94	
Petersen et al[77]	21	Healthy subjects 10–79 yr	OSI CA-6000†	Flexion	0.90	0.85
				Extension	0.96	0.96[+]
				R lateral flexion	0.89	0.85
				R rotation	0.95	0.90
Breum et al[70]	47	Healthy adults 18–38 yr, Mean age = 26	BROM	Flexion	0.91	0.77
				Extension	0.63	0.35
				R lateral flexion	0.89	0.89
				R rotation	0.57	
Patient Populations						
Nitschke et al[60]	61	Patients with back pain 20–65 yr	Universal goniometer	Flexion	0.92	0.84
				Extension	0.81	0.63
				R lateral flexion	0.76	0.62
			Dual inclinometers+	Flexion		
				Extension	0.90	0.52
				R lateral flexion	0.70	0.35
					0.90	0.18
Williams et al[17]	15	Children with low back pain	Dual inclinometers*	Flexion		0.60
				Extension		0.48
Kachingwe and Phillips[72]	91	Adults with low back pain Mean age = 28 yr	BROM* with 2 testers	Flexion	0.79, 0.84	0.74
				Extension	0.60, 0.74	0.55
				R lateral flexion	0.84, 0.85	0.79
				R rotation	0.68, 0.76	0.60
				L rotation	0.58, 0.69	0.64

ICC = Intraclass correlation coefficient; BROM = Back range of motion device; OSI CA-6000 = Spine Motion Analyzer; R = Right; L = Left.

*Lumbar ROM.

†Thoracolumbar ROM.

measurements were taken on an hourly basis rather than on a daily basis.

Mayer and associates[57] compared repeated measurements of lumbar ROM of 18 healthy subjects taken by 14 different examiners using three different instruments: a fluid-filled inclinometer, the kyphometer, and the electrical inclinometer. The three instruments were found to be equally reliable, but significant differences were found among examiners. Poor intertester reliability was the most significant source of variance. The authors identified sources of error as being caused by differences in instrument placement among examiners and inability to locate the necessary landmarks.

Saur and colleagues[53] used Pleurimeter V inclinometers to measure lumbar ROM in 54 patients with chronic low-back pain who were between 18 and 60 years of age. Measurements were taken with and without radiographic verification of the T12 and S1 landmarks used for positioning the inclinometers. Intertester reliability of the inclinometry technique for full cycle flexion–extension in a subgroup of 48 patients was high (Pearson correlation coefficient $r = 0.94$) and half cycle flexion was good ($r = 0.88$), but half cycle extension was poor ($r = 0.42$). The authors concluded that the Pleurimeter V was a reliable and valid method for measuring lumbar ROM and that with use of this instrument it was possible to differentiate lumbar spine movements from hip movements.

Chen and associates[58] investigated intertester and intratester reliability using three health professionals to measure lumbar ROM using a Pleurimeter V (double inclinometers), a carpenter's double inclinometer, and a computed single-sensor inclinometer. Intertester reliability was poor, with all ICCs less than 0.75; with a single exception, intratester reliability was less than 0.90. The authors determined that the largest source of measurement error was attributable to the examiners and associated factors and concluded that these three surface methods had only limited clinical usefulness.

Mayer and colleagues[59] used a Cybex EDI-320, a computed inclinometer with a single sensor, to measure lumbar ROM in 38 healthy individuals. Full cycle sagittal ROM was the most accurate measurement and extension was the least accurate. Clinical utility of lumbar sagittal plane ROM measurement appeared to be highly sensitive to the training of the test administrator in aspects of the process such as locating bony landmarks of T12 and S1 and maintaining inclinometer placement without rocking on the sacrum. Device error was negligible relative to the error associated with the test process itself. The authors found that practice was the most significant factor in eliminating the largest source of error when inexperienced examiners were used.

Nitschke and colleagues[60] used two examiners to compare the following measurement methods in a study involving 34 male and female subjects with chronic low-back pain: dual inclinometers for lumbar spine ROM (flexion, extension, and lateral flexion) and a plastic long-arm goniometer for thoracolumbar ROM (flexion, extension, lateral flexion, and rotation). Intertester reliability was poor for all measurements except for flexion taken with the long-arm goniometer (see Table 12.6). The dual inclinometer method had no systematic error, but there was a large random error for all measurements. The authors concluded that the standard error of measurement might be a better indicator of reliability than the ICC.

Salamh and Kolber[61] conducted a study to investigate the reliability, minimal detectable change, and concurrent validity of a gravity-based bubble inclinometer and an iPhone with an inclinometer application. Two investigators used both instruments to measure lumbar lordosis in 30 standing healthy participants. Good intrarater and interrater reliability was found for both the inclinometer (ICCs of .90 and 0.85, respectively) and for the iPhone application (with ICC values of 0.96 and 0.81, respectively). The minimum detectable change (MDC) indicated that a change of greater than or equal to 7 degrees and 6 degrees would be needed to exceed the threshold of error using the iPhone and inclinometer, respectively.

Validity of Inclinometers

Saur and colleagues[53] found that the correlation of radiographic ROM measurements with inclinometer ROM measurements demonstrated an almost linear correlation for flexion (r = 0.98) and total lumbar flexion–extension ROM (r = 0.97), but extension did not correlate as well (r = 0.75).

In contrast to the findings of Saur and colleagues,[53] poor criterion validity using inclinometers was reported by Samo and coworkers.[52] Samo compared radiographic measurements of lumbar ROM in 30 subjects with measurements taken with the following three instruments: a Pleurimeter V (double inclinometers), a carpenter's double inclinometer, and a computed single-sensor inclinometer. All ICCs between radiographs and each method were less than the 0.90 established by the authors as the criterion. Therefore, the authors judged that each method had poor validity.

MacDermid and colleagues[55] conducted a study to determine concurrent validity, test-retest, and inter- and intrarater reliability of lumbar flexion and extension measurements using the Tracker M.E., a computerized dual inclinometer (CDI), and the Modified-Modified Schober Test (MMST). The two measurement methods were tested on 40 individuals with a mean age of 26 (8) years. Half of the group had experienced low-back pain in the preceding month and the other half of the group had not had any back pain. Intratrial reliability was high to very high for both the CDI (ICCs = 0.85–0.96) and MMST (ICCs = 0.84–0.98). However, reliability was poor to moderate when the CDI unit had to be repositioned either by the same examiner (ICCs = 0.16–0.59) or by a different examiner. Interrater reliability for the MMST method was moderate to high (ICCs = 0.75–0.82), which was better than the correlation obtained by the CDI (ICCs = 0.45–0.52). Correlations between the CDI and MMST were poor for flexion (0.32) and poor to moderate for extension measurements (–0.42–0.51). The authors concluded that the MMST method was more reliable than the CDI. The Tracker M.E. dual inclinometer is considered better than a single inclinometer, but the concurrent validity and reliability of this system are yet to be proved.

Reliability of Universal Goniometers

Nitschke and colleagues[60] compared lumbar spine ROM measurements taken with the universal goniometer and double inclinometers in a study involving 34 males and females with low-back pain. The goniometer was used to measure all ranges of lumbar spine motion. Intertester reliability was poor for all measurements for both instruments except for flexion using the goniometer (see Table 12.6).

Fitzgerald and associates[12] used the universal goniometer to measure thoracolumbar lateral flexion and extension. Two testers measured half cycle motions in 17 volunteers who were physical therapy students. The intertester reliability was high for left lateral flexion (r = 0.91), good for extension (r = 0.88), and fair for right lateral flexion (r = 0.76).

Olson and Goehring[62] developed and tested an inexpensive method of measuring lower trunk rotation using a 14-inch plastic goniometer and a specific protocol in 41 participants who had a mean age of 23.3 years. Intrarater reliability ranged from 0.59 to 0.82 for right rotation and 0.76 to 0.82 for left rotation. Interreliability ranged from 0.62 to 0.83 for right rotation and from 0.75 to 0.77 for left rotation.

Validity of Universal Goniometers

A recent study was conducted by Wellmon and colleagues[63] to examine the concurrent validity and interrater reliability of the universal goniometer, inclinometer, and the following two goniometric mobile applications (apps): Goniometer

Records and Goniometer Pro. These apps were installed on the following smartphones: Apple iPhone 5, LG Android, and Samsung S111 Android. Three standardized angles that replicated the movement of a hinge joint in the human body were constructed to measure angular changes. The measurements were taken by three experienced physical therapist raters who used the three different devices. Interrater reliability for each of the smartphone apps, inclinometer, and UG were excellent (ICCs = 0.995–0.1000). Concurrent validity also was also excellent and the differences between instruments was low (−0.4–1.2 degrees). The error inherent in the measurement because of the smartphone, the installed apps, and examiner skill accounted for less than 2 degrees of measurement variability. Therefore, the authors concluded that the three smartphones with two installed apps were a viable substitute for a UG or inclinometer when measuring angular changes that typically occur during evaluation of ROM.

Nattrass and coworkers[64] compared measurements of the thoracolumbar spine taken with the universal goniometer and measurements of the lumbar spine taken with the Dualer Electronic Inclinometer with three measures of impairment. Thirty-four patients between 20 and 65 years of age with chronic low-back pain were the subjects for the study. The results showed that only flexion ROM measured with the goniometer demonstrated greater than 50% of the variance in common with one of the disability measures.

Reliability of the Modified-Modified Schober Test

Williams and coworkers[17] measured flexion and extension on 15 patient volunteers with a mean age of 36 years who had chronic low-back pain. The authors compared the MMST, which is also referred to as the simplified skin distraction method, with the double inclinometer method. Intratester Pearson correlation coefficients for the MMST were an r of 0.89 for tester 1, an r of 0.78 for tester 2, and an r of 0.83 for tester 3. Intertester Pearson correlation coefficients between the three physical therapist testers were an r of 0.72 for flexion and an r of 0.77 for extension with use of the MMST. The therapists underwent training in the use of standardized procedures for each method prior to testing. According to the testers, the MMST was easier and quicker to use than the double inclinometer method. The only disadvantage to using the MMST method is that norms have not been established for all age-groups.

Tousignant and associates[55] used the MMST to obtain lumbar flexion ROM measurements in 31 patients with low-back pain. The authors found excellent intratester reliability (ICC = 0.95) and very good intertester reliability (ICC = 0.91).

MacDermid and colleagues[55] investigated the reliability and validity of a Tracker M.E. computerized dual inclinometer (CDI), which they compared with the Modified-Modified Schober Test (MMST). Intratrial reliability was high to very high for both the CDI with (ICCs = 0.85–0.96) and for the MMST (ICCs = 0.84–0.98). Interrater reliability for the MMST was moderate to high (ICCs = 0.75–0.82) but concurrent validity showed that the correlation between the CDI and MMST was poor for lumbar flexion

Validity of the Modified-Modified Schober Test

The ease of finding landmarks for measuring lumbar flexion and extension with the MMST appears to make this method a better choice than the Schober and MST; however, more studies are needed to confirm its validity. Tousignant and associates[54] used the MMST to obtain lumbar flexion ROM measurements in 31 patients with low-back pain. The authors compared these measurements with measurements calculated on x-rays as the gold standard. The comparison showed that the MMST had moderate validity (r = 0.67; 95% confidence interval = 0.44–0.84). The minimum metrically detectable change of 1 centimeter was determined to be excellent in this group of patients, but because of the moderate validity finding, the authors suggest that further studies need to be performed to establish the test's validity.

Reliability of Prone Press-Up Test for Extension

Bandy and Reese[65] compared the reliability of the prone press-up to measure lumbar extension under two conditions: with and without a strap to control pelvic motion. Sixty-three unimpaired individuals with a mean age of 26 years participated as subjects in the study. Measurements of extension ROM were taken by both an experienced group and a student group using a tape measure. Intratester reliability was excellent for the experienced group in both the strapped (ICC = 0.91) and unstrapped (ICC = 0.90) conditions and good for the student group. Intertester reliability for both the strapped and unstrapped conditions was good (ICC = 0.87 and ICC = 0.85, respectively). Unfortunately, this test is not appropriate for the very young, many older adults, or anyone with upper-extremity weakness. The test is included in this book as a measure of thoracolumbar motion.

Reliability and Validity of the Fingertip-to-Floor Test for Forward Flexion

Perret and colleagues[9] included 32 patients with low-back pain with a mean age of 52 years in a reliability study. Intratester and intertester reliability were excellent (ICC = 0.99). Ten patients with low-back pain (mean age of 42 years) participated in the validity study. Two lateral radiographs were taken: one of the dorsal spine with the patients in the neutral standing position and one taken in full trunk flexion. Spearman's correlation coefficient for this validity test of trunk flexion was excellent (r = 0.96). Seventy-two patients with low-back pain participated in the responsiveness study. High values were found for responsiveness for the fingertip-to-floor method, which showed that the fingertip test has very good sensitivity to change.

Haywood and colleagues[66] also assessed reliability, validity, and responsiveness of the fingertip-to-floor forward flexion test in 77 patients with ankylosing spondylitis. The authors found both intratester and intertester reliability to be excellent, with ICCs between 0.94 and 0.99. The test was the most responsive to self-perceived changes in health at

6 months. Authors recommended this test for clinical practice and research.

Viitanen and associates[67] found that the fingertip-to-floor test had significant correlations with thoracolumbar changes seen on x-ray (calcifications of disc, ossification of ligaments, and changes in apophyseal joints).

Pile and associates[68] found that the sagittal plane fingertip-to-floor test had an excellent intertester reliability (ICC = 0.95) in a study in which three physical therapists, a rheumatologist, and a rheumatology registrar measured 10 patients twice.

Lindell and coworkers,[7] in a study of 50 subjects (30 patients with low-back or neck pain and 20 healthy participants), found intratester reliability to be excellent, with an ICC of 0.95 and SEM of 0.9 centimeters for both an experienced physiotherapist and a medically untrained research assistant. Intertester reliability was also excellent, with ICC values greater than 0.95 and SEM values ranging from 0.9 to 1.2 centimeters.

Gauvin, Riddle, and Rothstein[69] used a modified version of the fingertip-to-floor test by placing subjects on a stool and then measuring the distance from the tip of the subject's middle finger to the floor. Seventy-three patients with low-back pain participated in the study, and both intratester (ICC = 0.98) and intertester (ICC = 0.95) reliability were excellent. The modified version of the test is supposed to account for the fact that many people can easily reach the floor and beyond but the fingertip-to-floor test does not account for this fact.

Reliability of the Fingertip-to-Thigh Test for Lateral Flexion

Alaranta and associates,[16] in a study involving 508 white- and blue-collar workers between the ages of 35 and 54 years, found that the intertester reliability was high at an interval of 1 week for the fingertip-to-thigh method of assessing thoracolumbar lateral flexion. Intratester reliability at the interval of 1 year was remarkably good for the large time interval between tests (Table 12.7).

Jones and colleagues,[15] in a study of 119 children aged 11 to 16 years (30 children with low-back pain and 89 asymptomatic children), found excellent correlation coefficients for right and left lateral flexion in the group with low-back pain ($r = 0.93$ to 0.95) and in the asymptomatic group ($r = 0.99$). Limits of agreement, expressed as the mean difference between test and retest ±1.96 × SD of the difference between test and retest, were 0.16 millimeters ± 6.78 for right lateral flexion for the asymptomatic children but much larger for the symptomatic group (0.50 millimeters ± 16.93 millimeters). The authors concluded that there was very little systematic bias but all measures exhibited random error, which was larger in the symptomatic group (see Table 12.7).

Lindell and coworkers[7] conducted a study of 50 subjects (30 patients with low-back or neck pain, and 20 healthy subjects) who were tested by two examiners. The intratester reliability for the fingertip-to-thigh test for lateral bending was excellent for the experienced physiotherapist (ICC = 0.94–0.99, SEM = 0.5–1.0 centimeters) and fair for the medically untrained tester (ICC = 0.73–0.86, SEM = 1.4–1.6 centimeters). Intertester reliability was fair to excellent depending on the group and side tested, with ICCs ranging from 0.79 to 0.98 and SEMs ranging from 0.9 to 1.5 centimeters.

Reliability of Back Range of Motion Device

Reliability results are inconclusive, and it appears that additional research needs to be done on this method of measurement to warrant the expenditure involved in purchasing the

TABLE 12.7 Reliability of Thoracolumbar Lateral Flexion ROM: Tape Measure

Test / Author	Fingertip-to-Thigh Alaranta et al[16]		Fingertip-to-Thigh Lindell et al[7]		Fingertip-to-Thigh Jones et al[15]		Fingertip-to-Floor Haywood et al[66]		Fingertip-to-Floor Pile et al[68]
Sample	508 employed workers* 35–45 yr		20 healthy and 30 patients with back or neck pain 22–55 yr		89 healthy and 30 children with LBP 11–16 yr		Patients with AS 18–75 yr		Patients with AS† 28–73 yr
	n = 34	*n* = 93	*n* = 20	*n* = 30	*n* = 89	*n* = 30	*n* = 26	*n* = 51	*n* = 10
Motion	***Intra R***	***Inter R***	***Intra ICC***	***Inter ICC***	***Intra R***	***Intra R***	***Intra ICC***	***Inter ICC***	***Inter***
Right and left	0.81	0.91							
Right			0.99	0.93	0.99	0.93	0.98	0.98	0.83
Left			0.94	0.95	0.99	0.95	0.95	0.95	0.79

AS = Ankylosing spondylitis; ICC = Intraclass correlation coefficient; LBP = Low-back pain; *r* = Pearson product moment correlation coefficient; Intra = Intratester reliability; Inter = Intertester reliability.

* Some workers had back or neck pain and some had no pain.

back range of motion (BROM) device. The BROM II device is a revised and improved version of the original BROM. A research group investigating the reliability of the BROM II device agreed that the instrument had high reliability for measuring lumbar lateral flexion and low reliability for measuring extension. Breum, Wiberg, and Bolton[70] concluded that the BROM II device could measure flexion and rotation reliably, whereas Madson, Youdas, and Suman[71] determined that rotation but not flexion could be reliably measured (see Table 12.6). Potential sources of error identified by the authors included slippage of the device over the sacrum during flexion and extension and variations in the identification of landmarks from one measurement to another.

Kondratek and colleagues[28] used the BROM II to conduct one of the few studies on lumbar ROM in children. The subjects were 225 normally developing children aged 5 to 11 years. Two physical therapists who were experienced in working with children were trained in the use of the BROM II. Intrarater reliability on 15 children was good to excellent for one tester for all half-cycle motions except for flexion, which was unacceptable (ICC = 0.53). The intratester reliability for the second tester ranged from an ICC of 0.71 for flexion and an ICC of 0.76 for right lateral flexion to an ICC of 0.91 for right rotation.

Kachingwe and Phillips[72] employed two testers to use the BROM to measure lumbar motions in 91 healthy men and women with a mean age of 28 years. Intratester reliability for lateral flexion was good (ICC = 0.85–0.83), forward flexion was good to fair (ICC = 0.84–0.79), and extension and rotation were fair to poor (ICC = 0.76–0.58). Intertester reliability was fair to poor for all lumbar motions and for pelvic inclination (ICC = 0.76–0.58).

Reliability of Motion Analysis Systems

A number of researchers have investigated the reliability of motion-analysis systems, including the CA-6000 Spine Motion Analyzer and the FASTRAK. Two research groups found that intratester reliability for measuring lumbar flexion was very high with use of the CA-6000.[27,45] In one of the studies, both intratester and intertester reliability ranged from good to high for lumbar forward flexion and extension, but intratester and intertester reliability were poor for rotation.[27]

Steffan and colleagues[73] used the FASTRAK system to measure segmental motion in forward lumbar flexion by tracking sensors attached to Kirschner wires that had been inserted into the spinous processes of L3 and L4 in 16 healthy men. Segmental forward flexion showed large intersubject variation.

Van Herp and associates[31] used the Polhemus Navigation Sciences 3 Space System to measure ROM in 100 healthy subjects (50 male and 50 female subjects) ranging in age from 20 to 77 years of age. Recorded ranges of motion including flexion, extension, and lateral flexion and rotation showed a level of agreement with x-ray data, indicating good concurrent validity.

The following two studies[74,75] are examples of the experimentation with wearable motion sensors such as accelerometers, gyroscopes, and magnetic sensors, and they are evidence of the continuing search for measurement systems that are less expensive and complex than three-dimensional motion-analysis systems.

Consumuller and colleagues[74] introduced a new instrument called Eponics SPINE, which employs advanced strain gauge measurement technology based on two sensor strips (the Spine DMS system). The latter system allows for the noninvasive assessment of lumbar and thoracolumbar motion for periods of up to 24 hours. Built-in accelerometers allow additional detection of orientation of the upper body to Earth's gravitational field. This new spine evaluation system is lightweight and portable and maximum flexion, extension, and lordosis angles showed good agreement with the x-ray and Spinal Mouse data.

Alghtani and colleagues[75] tested the reliability of a novel motion-analysis device for measuring spinal motion and describing relative motion of the different segments of the thoracolumbar spine. To measure range of motion, sensors were placed on the spinous processes of T1, T4, T8, T12, L3, and S1. Intraclass correlation coefficients were high, ranging from 0.88 to 0.99 for all motions and regions of the spine.

In another study, Bedeker and colleagues[76] used a mobile device goniometer (iPod mobile device) to measure flexion range of motion of the lumbar spine. The spinous processes of T12 to S1 were marked and the results showed that intrarater reliability was excellent ($r = 0.920$) and interrater reliability ICC was good ($r = 8.12$).

Summary

The sampling of research studies reviewed in this chapter reflects the considerable amount of effort that has been directed toward finding reliable and valid methods for measuring spinal motion that the average therapist can afford. Each method reviewed has advantages and disadvantages, and clinicians should select a method that appears to be appropriate for their particular clinical situation.

REFERENCES

1. Barrett, E, McCreesh, KM, and Lewis, J: Intrarater and interrater reliability of the flexicurve and manual inclinometer for the measurement of thoracic kyphosis. Rehabil Res Pract 12, 2013.
2. Cyriax, JH, and Cyriax, P: Illustrated Manual of Orthopaedic Medicine. Butterworths, London, 1983
3. Bogduk, N: Clinical Anatomy of the Lumbar Spine and Sacrum, ed 3. Churchill Livingstone, New York, 1997.
4. American Medical Association: Guides to the Evaluation of Permanent Impairment, ed 5. AMA, Chicago, 2000.
5. American Medical Association: Guides to the Evaluation of Permanent Impairment, ed 6. AMA, Chicago, 2008.
6. Quack, C, et al: Do MRI findings correlate with mobility tests? An explorative analysis of the test validity with regard to structure. Eur Spine J 16:803, 2007.
7. Lindell, O, Eriksson, L, and Strender, L-E: The reliability of a 10-test package for patients with prolonged back and neck pain: Could an examiner without formal medical education be used without loss of quality? A methodological study. BMC Musculoskelet Disord 8:31, 2007.
8. Artun, E, et al: Screening of the spine in adolescents: Inter and intra-rater reliability and measurement error of commonly used clinical tests. BMC Musculoskelet Disord 15:37, 2014.
9. Perret, C, et al: Validity, reliability, and responsiveness of the fingertip-to-floor test. Arch Phys Med Rehabil 82:1566, 2001.
10. Gerhardt, J, Cocchiarella, L, and Lea, R: The Practical Guide to Range of Motion Assessment. American Medical Association, Chicago, 2002.
11. American Academy of Orthopaedic Surgeons: Joint Motion: Method of Measuring and Recording. AAOS Chicago, 1993.
12. Fitzgerald, GK, et al: Objective assessment with establishment of normal values for lumbar spine range of motion. Phys Ther 63:1776, 1983.
13. Sahrmann, SA: Diagnosis and Treatment of Movement Impairment Syndromes. Mosby, St. Louis, 2002.
14. Mellin, GP: Accuracy of measuring lateral flexion of the spine with a tape measure. Clin Biomech 1:85, 1986.
15. Jones, MA, et al: Measurement error associated with spinal mobility measures in children with and without low-back pain. Acta Paediatr 91:1339, 2002.
16. Alaranta, H, et al: Flexibility of the spine: Normative values of goniometric and tape measurements. Scand J Rehabil Med 26:147, 1994.
17. Williams, R, et al: Reliability of the modified-modified Schober and double inclinometer methods for measuring lumbar flexion and extension. Phys Ther 73:26, 1993.
18. Van Adrichem, JAM, and van der Korst, JK: Assessment of the flexibility of the lumbar spine: A pilot study in children and adolescents. Scand J Rheumatol 2:87, 1973.
19. Greene, WB, and Heckman, JD (eds): The Clinical Measurement of Joint Motion. American Academy of Orthopaedic Surgeons, Rosemont, IL, 1994.
20. Macrae, IF, and Wright, V: Measurement of back movement. Ann Rheum Dis 28:584,1969.
21. Neumann, DA: Kinesiology of the Musculoskeletal System: Foundations for Rehabilitation. Mosby, St. Louis, 2010.
22. Loebl, WY: Measurement of spinal posture and range of spinal movement. Ann Phys Med 9:103, 1967.
23. Ng, JK, et al: Range of motion and lordosis of the lumbar spine: Reliability of measurement and normative values. Spine 26:53, 2001.
24. Sullivan, MS, Dickinson, CE, and Troup, JDG: The influence of age and gender on lumbar spine range of motion. A study of 1126 healthy subjects. Spine 19:682, 1994.
25. Moll, JMH, and Wright, V: Normal range of spinal mobility: An objective clinical study. Ann Rheum Dis 30:381, 1971.
26. Gracovetsky, S, et al: A database for estimating normal spinal motion derived from non-invasive measurements. Spine 20:1036, 1995.
27. McGregor, AH, McCarthy, D, and Hughes, SP: Motion characteristics of the lumbar spine in the normal population. Spine 20:2421, 1995.
28. Kondratek, M, et al: Normative values for active lumbar range of motion in children. Pediatr Phys Ther 19:236, 2007.
29. Troke, M, et al: A normative database of lumbar ranges of motion. Man Ther 10:198, 2005.
30. Troke, M, et al: A new comprehensive normative database of lumbar spine ranges of motion. Clin Rehabil 15:371, 2001.
31. Van Herp, G, et al: Three dimensional lumbar spine kinematics: A study of range of movement in 100 healthy subjects aged 20 to 60+ years. Rheumatology 39:1337, 2000.
32. Dreischarf, M, et al: Age-related loss of lumbar lordosis and mobility: A study of 323 asymptomatic volunteers. PLoS One 9(12):e116, 2014.
33. Lee, ES, et al. The effect of age on sagittal plane profile of the lumbar spine according to standing, supine, and various sitting positions. J Orthop Surg Res 9:11, 2014.
34. Saidu, IA, et al: Lumbar spinal mobility changes among adults with increasing age. J Midlife Health 2(2):365, 2011.
35. Bible, JE, et al: Quantifying the effects of degeneration and other patient factors on lumbar segmental range of motion using multivariate analysis. Spine 15:33(16):1793, 2008.
36. Wong, KWN, et al: The flexion-extension profile of lumbar spine in 100 healthy volunteers. Spine 29:1636, 2004.
37. Battie, MC, Levalalti, E, and Videman, T: Heritability of lumbar flexibility and the role of disc degeneration and body weight. J Appl Physiol 104(2):379, 2008.
38. Intolo, P, et al: The effect of age on lumbar range of motion: A systematic review. Man Ther 14:596, 2009.
39. Bookstein, NA, et al: Lumbar extension range of motion in elementary school children [abstract]. Phys Ther 72:S35, 1992.
40. Trudelle-Jackson, E, et al. Lumbar spine flexion and extension extremes of motion in women of different age and racial groups. Spine 35(16):1539, 2010.
41. Sjolie, AN: Access to pedestrian roads, daily activities and physical performance of adolescents. Spine 25:1965, 2000.
42. Freidrich, M, et al: Spinal posture during stooped walking under vertical space constraints. Spine 25:1118, 2000.
43. Hung,Y-J, et al: The dose-response relationship between cumulative lifting-load and lumbar disk degeneration based upon magnetic resonance imaging findings. Phys Ther 94:1582, 2014.
44. Bible, JE, et al: Normal functional range of motion of the lumbar spine during 15 activities of daily living. J Spinal Disord Tech 23(2):106, 2010.
45. Hsieh, CY, and Pringle, RK: Range of motion of the lumbar spine required for four activities of daily living. J Manipulative Physiol Ther 17:353, 1994.
46. Levine, D, et al: Sagittal lumbar spine position during standing, walking and running at various gradients. J Athl Train 42:29, 2007.
47. Guoan, L, et al: Segmental in vivo-vertebral motion during functional human lumbar spine activities. Eur Spine J, 18(7):1013, 2009.
48. Johnson, KD, et al: Reliability of thoracic spine rotation range-of-motion measurements in healthy adults. J Athl Train 47(1):52, 2012.
49. Azadinia, F, et al: The validity and reliability of noninvasive methods for measuring kyphosis. J Spinal Disord Tech 27(6):E212, 2014.
50. Greendale, GA, et al. The reliability and validity of three non-radiological measures of thoracic kyphosis and their relations to the standing radiological Cobb angle. Osteoporosis 22(6):1897, 2011.
51. Littlewood, C, and May, S: Measurement of range of movement in the lumbar spine: What methods are valid? A systematic review. Physiotherapy 93:201, 2007.
52. Samo, DG, et al: Validity of three lumbar sagittal motion measurement methods: Surface inclinometers compared with radiographs. J Occup Environ Med 39:209, 1997.
53. Saur, PMM, et al: Lumbar range of motion: Reliability and validity of the inclinometer technique in the clinical measurement of trunk flexibility. Spine 21:1332, 1996.
54. Tousignant, M, et al: The Modified-Modified Schober test for range of motion assessment of lumbar flexion in patients with low back pain: A study of criterion validity, intra- and interrater reliability and minimum metrically detectable change. Disabil Rehabil 27:553, 2005.
55. MacDermid, JC, et al: The reliability and validity of the computerized double inclinometer in measuring lumbar mobility. Modified-Modified Schober Test 8:358, 2014.
56. Essendrop, M, et al: Measures of low back function: A review of reproducibility studies. Clin Biomech 17:235, 2002.
57. Mayer, RS, et al: Variance in the measurement of sagittal lumbar range of motion among examiners, subjects, and instruments. Spine 20:1489, 1995.
58. Chen, SP, et al: Reliability of the lumbar sagittal motion measurement methods: Surface inclinometers. J Occup Environ Med 39:217, 1997.
59. Mayer, TG, et al: Spinal range of motion: Accuracy and sources of error with inclinometric measurement. Spine 22:1976, 1997.
60. Nitschke, JE, et al: Reliability of the American Medical Association Guides' Model for Measuring Spinal Range of Motion: Its implication for whole-person impairment ratings. Spine 24:262, 1999.
61. Salamh, PA, and Kolber, M: The reliability, minimal detectable change and concurrent validity of a gravity-based bubble inclinometer and

iPhone application for measuring standing lumbar lordosis. Physiother Theory Pract 30(1):62, 2014.
62. Olson, KA, and Goehring, MT: Intra and interrater reliability of a goniometric lower trunk rotation measurement. J Back Musculoskelet Rehabil 22:157, 2009.
63. Wellmon, GH, et al: Validity and reliability of two goniometric mobile apps: Device application and examiner factors. J Sport Rehabil 5:6, 2015.
64. Nattrass, CL, et al: Lumbar spine range of motion as a measure of physical and functional impairment: An investigation of validity [abstract]. Clin Rehabil 13:211, 1999
65. Bandy, WD, and Reese, NB: Strapped versus unstrapped technique of the prone press-up for measurement of lumbar extension using a tape measure: Differences in magnitude and reliability of measurements. Arch Phys Med Rehabil 85:99, 2004.
66. Haywood, KL, et al: Spinal mobility in ankylosing spondylitis: Reliability, validity and responsiveness. Rheumatology 43:750, 2004.
67. Viitanen, JV, et al: Clinical assessment of spinal mobility measurements in ankylosing spondylitis: A compact set for follow-up and trials? Clin Rheumatol 19:131, 2000.
68. Pile, KD, et al: Clinical assessment of ankylosing spondylitis: A study of observer variation in spinal measurements. Br J Rheumatol 30:29, 1991.
69. Gauvin, MG, Riddle, DL, and Rothstein, JM: Reliability of clinical measurements of forward bending using the modified fingertip-to-floor method. Phys Ther 70:443, 2000.
70. Breum, J, Wiberg, J, and Bolton, JE: Reliability and concurrent validity of the BROM II for measuring lumbar mobility. J Manipulative Physiol Ther 18:497, 1995.
71. Madson, TJ, Youdas, JW, and Suman, VJ: Reproducibility of lumbar spine range of motion measurements using the back range of motion device. J Orthop Sports Phys Ther 29:470, 1999.
72. Kachingwe, AF, and Phillips, BJ: Inter and intrarater reliability of a back range of motion instrument. Arch Phys Med Rehabil 86:2347, 2005.
73. Steffan, T, et al: A new technique for measuring lumbar segmental motion in vivo: Method, accuracy and preliminary results. Spine 22:156, 1997.
74. Consumuller, T, et al: Comparative evaluation of a novel measure to assess lumbar spine posture and range of motion. Eur Spine J 21(11):2170, 2012.
75. Alghtani, RS, et al: JM: Reliability of an accelerometer-based device for quantifying multiregional spinal range of motion. J Manipulative Physiol Ther 38(4):275, 2015.
76. Bedeker, N, et al: Inter and intra reliability of mobile device goniometer for measuring lumbar spine flexion range of motion. J Back Musculoskelet Rehabil, 27(2):161, 2014.

CHAPTER 13

The Temporomandibular Joint

Cynthia C. Norkin, PT, EdD

Structure and Function

Temporomandibular Joint

The temporomandibular joint (TMJ) is the articulation between the mandible, the articular disc, and the temporal bone of the skull (Fig. 13.1A, B). The disc divides the joint into two distinct parts, which are referred to as the upper and lower joints. The larger upper joint is formed by the convex articular eminence, concave mandibular fossa of the temporal bone, and the superior surface of the disc. The lower joint consists of the convex surface of the mandibular condyle and the concave inferior surface of the disc.[1–3] The articular disc helps the convex mandible conform to the convex articular surface of the temporal bone,[2] adds stability to the joint, and helps guide the mandibular condyle during motion.[4]

The TMJ capsule is described as being thin and loose above the disc but taut below the disc in the lower joint. Short capsular fibers surround the joint and extend between the mandibular condyle and the articular disc and between the disc and the temporal eminence.[3] Longer capsular fibers extend from the temporal bone to the mandible.

The primary ligament associated with the TMJ is the temporomandibular ligament, which stabilizes the lateral side of joint capsule. The stylomandibular and the sphenomandibular ligaments located medial to the joint capsule (Fig. 13.2) are considered accessory ligaments.[5,6] The primary muscles associated with the TMJ are the medial and lateral pterygoids, temporalis, and masseter (Fig. 13.3), as well as the digastric, stylohyoid, mylohyoid, and geniohyoid.

Osteokinematics

The upper joint is an amphiarthrodial gliding joint, and the lower joint is a hinge joint. The TMJ as a whole allows motions in three planes around three axes. All of the motions except mouth closing begin from the resting position of the joint in which the teeth are slightly separated (freeway space).[3,6] The amount of freeway space, which usually varies from 2 to 4 millimeters, allows free anterior, posterior, and lateral movement of the mandible.

The functional motions permitted are mandibular depression (mouth opening), mandibular elevation (mouth closing), protrusion (anterior translation; Fig.13.4), and retrusion (posterior translation; Fig. 13.5), and right and left lateral excursion or laterotrusion (lateral deviation; Fig. 13.6A, B).

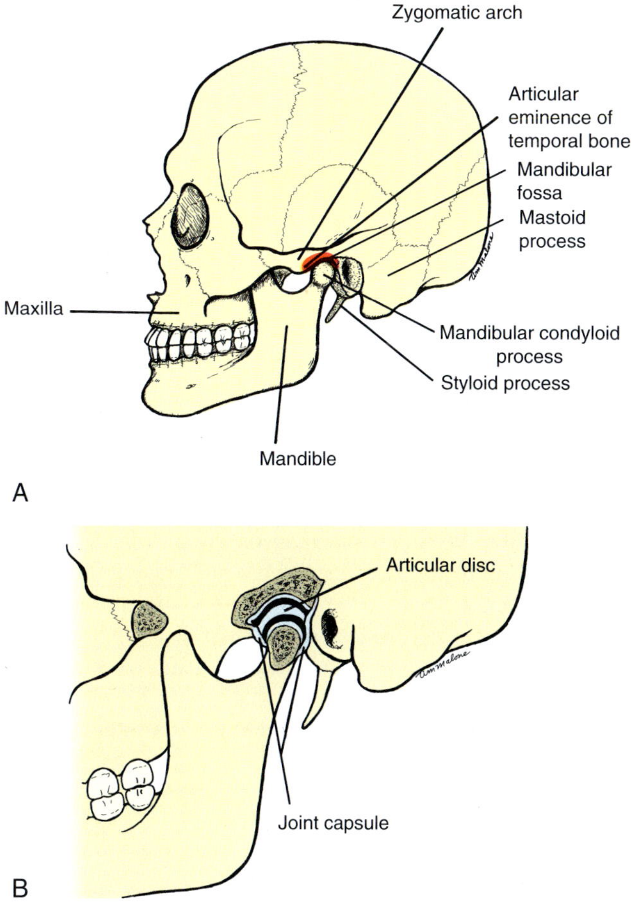

FIGURE 13.1 (A) Lateral view of the skull showing the temporomandibular joint (TMJ) and surrounding structures. (B) A lateral view of the TMJ showing the articular disc and a portion of the joint capsule.

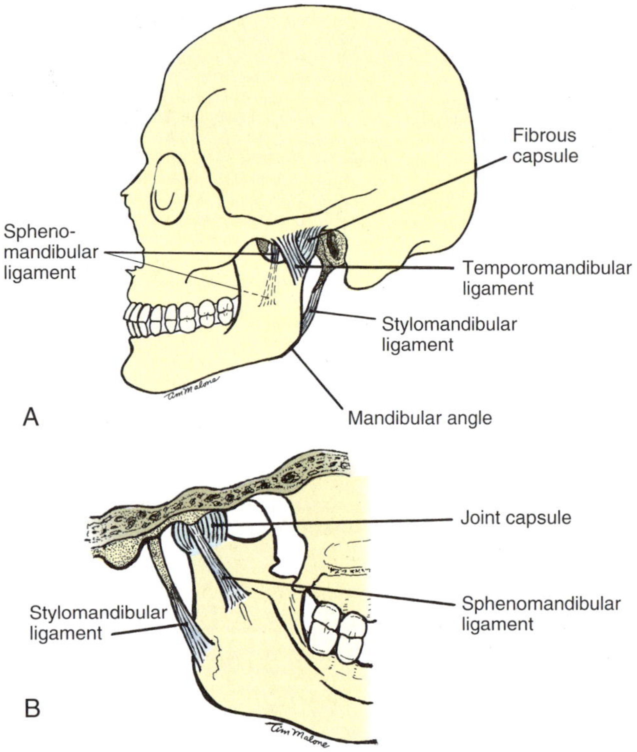

FIGURE 13.2 (A) A lateral view of the temporomandibular joint showing the oblique fibers of the temporomandibular ligament and the stylomandibular and sphenomandibular ligaments. (B) A medial view of the temporomandibular joint showing the medial portion of the joint capsule and the stylomandibular and sphenomandibular ligaments.

Maximal contact of the teeth in mouth closing is called centric occlusion.

Reinforcement of the TMJ is provided primarily by the temporomandibular ligament, which limits mouth opening, retrusion, and lateral excursion. The functions of the stylomandibular and sphenomandibular ligaments are somewhat controversial, but these ligaments appear to help suspend the mandible from the cranium.[4] According to Magee,[7] the ligaments keep the condyle, disc, and temporal bone in close approximation. These ligaments also may prevent excessive protrusion, but their exact function has not been verified.

The inferior head of the lateral pterygoid muscles and the digastric muscles produce mandibular depression (mouth opening),[1,3–7] whereas the mylohyoid and geniohyoid muscles assist in the motion, especially against resistance.[3,7] Mandibular elevation (mouth closing) is produced by bilateral contractions of the temporalis, masseter, and medial pterygoid muscles (see Fig. 13.3).[1,3–7] Mandibular protrusion is a result of bilateral action of the masseter,[1,7] medial,[1,3,7] and lateral[3–8] pterygoid muscles, which may be assisted by the mylohyoid, stylohyoid, and digastric muscles.[7] Retrusion is brought about by bilateral action of the posterior fibers of the temporalis muscles[1,3–7]; by the digastric,[1,3–7] middle, and deep fibers of the masseter[3,7]; and by the stylohyoid, mylohyoid,[1,7] and geniohyoid[1,3,7] muscles. Mandibular lateral excursion is produced

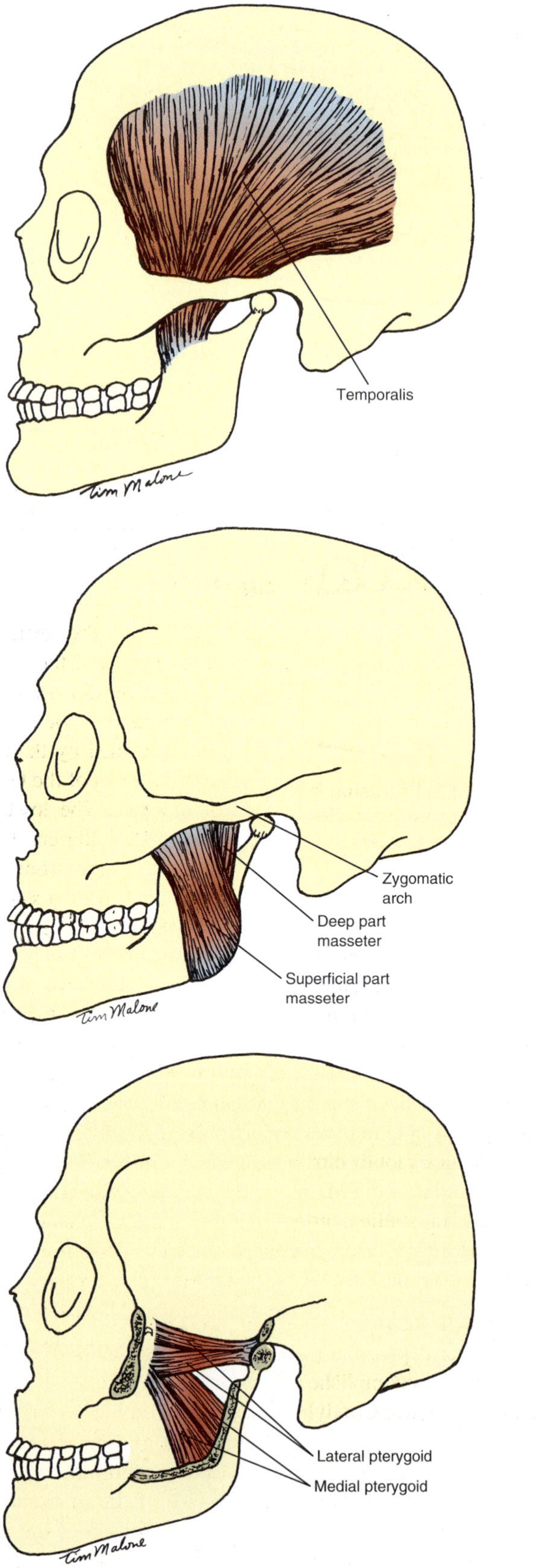

FIGURE 13.3 The temporal and masseter muscles along with the pterygoid muscles are considered the primary muscles of mastication.

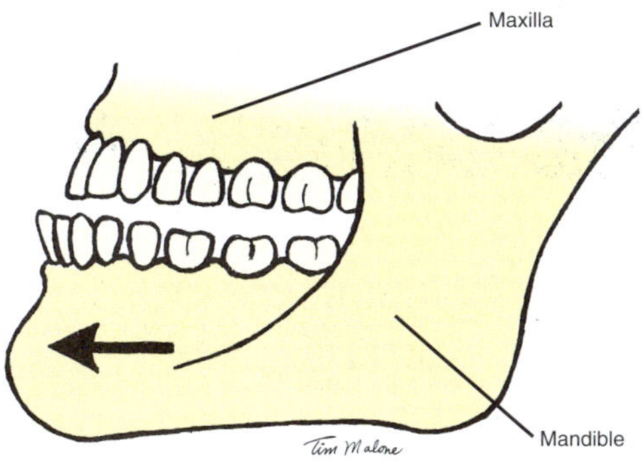

FIGURE 13.4 Protrusion is an anterior motion of the mandible in relation to the maxilla.

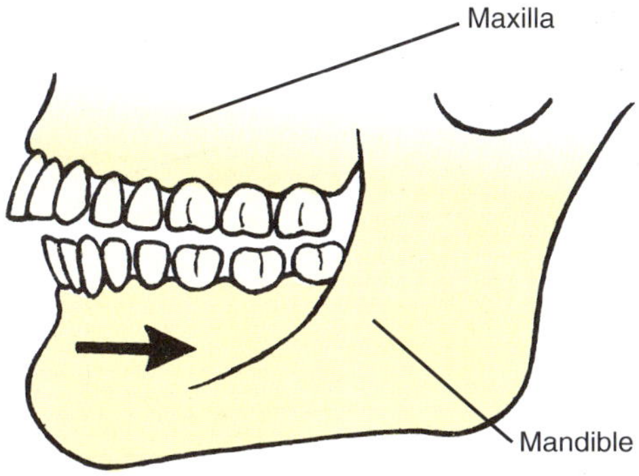

FIGURE 13.5 Retrusion is a posterior motion of the mandible in relation to the maxilla.

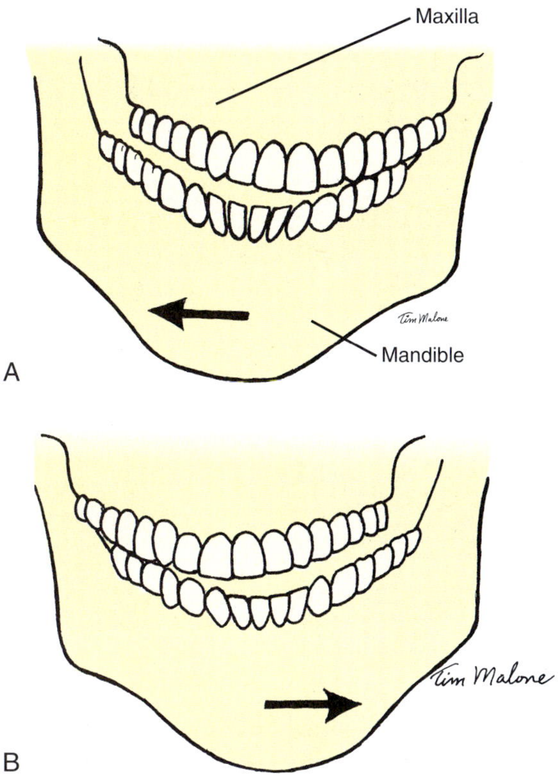

FIGURE 13.6 Lateral excursion is a lateral motion of the mandible to either side. (A) Right lateral excursion. (B) Left lateral excursion.

by a unilateral contraction of the medial and lateral pterygoid muscles,[1–7] which produce contralateral motion, whereas a unilateral contraction of the temporalis muscle causes lateral motion to the same side.

Cervical spine muscles may be activated in conjunction with TMJ muscles because of the close functional relationship that exists between the head and the neck.[1,4–11] Extension of the head and neck has been found to occur simultaneously with mouth opening, whereas flexion of the head and neck accompanies mouth closing. These coordinated and parallel movements at the TMJ and cervical spine joints have been observed in studies, and researchers suggest that preprogrammed neural commands may simultaneously activate both jaw and neck muscles.[9–11]

Arthrokinematics

Mandibular depression (mouth opening) occurs in the sagittal plane and is accomplished by rotation and sliding of the mandibular condyles. Condylar rotation is combined with anterior and inferior sliding of the condyles on the inferior surface of the discs, which also slide anteriorly (translate) along the temporal articular eminences. Mandibular elevation (mouth closing) is accomplished by rotation of the mandibular condyles on the discs and sliding of the discs with the condyles posteriorly and superiorly on the temporal articular eminences.

In protrusion, the bilateral condyles and discs translate together anteriorly and inferiorly along the temporal articular eminences. The movement takes place at the upper joint, and no rotation occurs during this motion. In lateral excursion, one mandibular condyle and disc slide inferiorly, anteriorly, and medially along the articular eminence. The other mandibular condyle rotates about a vertical axis and slides medially within the mandibular fossa. For example, in left lateral excursion, the left condyle spins and the right condyle slides anteriorly.

Capsular Pattern

In the capsular pattern, mandibular depression is limited.[7]

RANGE OF MOTION TESTING PROCEDURES: Temporomandibular Joint

Landmarks for Testing Procedures

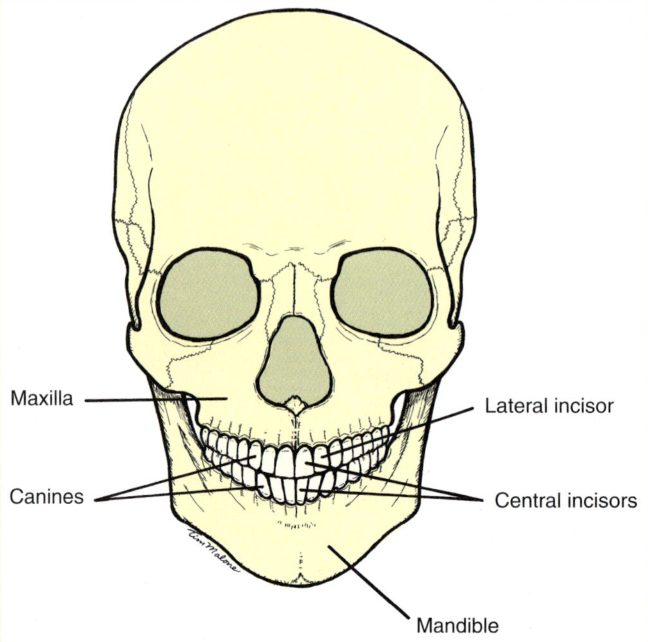

FIGURE 13.7 The adult has between 28 and 32 permanent teeth, including 8 incisors, 4 canines, 8 premolars, and 8 to 12 molars. The central incisors serve as landmarks for ruler placement to measure motion at the TMJ.

DEPRESSION OF THE MANDIBLE (MOUTH OPENING)

Motion occurs in the sagittal plane around a medial–lateral axis. Functionally the mandible is able to depress approximately 35 to 50 millimeters so that the individual's three fingers or two knuckles can be placed between the upper and lower central incisor teeth, although an opening of only 25 to 35 millimeters is needed for normal activities (Fig. 13.8). A slightly more restricted normal range of adult values (40 to 50 millimeters) was arrived at by consensus judgment at a 1995 Permanent Impairment Conference by representatives of major societies and academies whose members treat TMJ disorders.[12] Similar normative mean values for adult mouth opening varied from a low of 41 millimeters to a high of 58.6 millimeters. These values are presented in Table 13.1 in the Research Findings Section.

The Research Diagnostic Criteria for Temporomandibular Disorders (RDC/TMD) recommends that the examiner observe pain-free active mouth opening and describe fully any deviations of the mandible that take place during the motion.[13] The observation of active mouth opening should be followed with measurements of maximal active mouth opening and passive mouth opening.

Testing Position

Place the individual sitting, with the cervical spine in 0 degrees of flexion, extension, lateral flexion, and rotation.

Stabilization

Stabilize the posterior aspect of the head and neck to prevent flexion, extension, lateral flexion, and rotation of the cervical spine.

Testing Motions

Active Pain-Free Mouth Opening

Ask the individual to open the mouth slowly and as far as possible without pain. Observe the motion for any lateral excursion of the mandible. In normal active movement, no lateral mandibular motion occurs during mandibular depression (Fig. 13.9). If lateral excursion does occur, it may take the form of either a C-shaped or an S-shaped curve. With a C-shaped curve, the lateral excursion is to one side (Fig. 13.10) and should be noted on the recording form. With an S-shaped curve, the lateral excursion occurs first to one side and then to the opposite side[7]; the deviation should be described on the recording form (Fig. 13.11).

Active Mouth Opening

Ask the individual to make an effort to open the mouth as wide as possible even if pain is present.

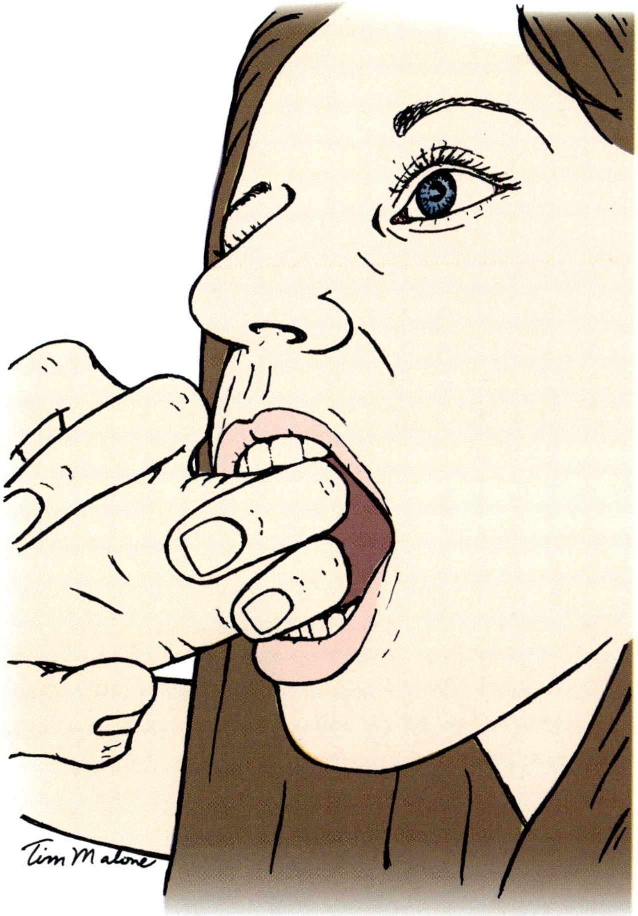

FIGURE 13.8 Normal mouth opening should be sufficient to allow two knuckles or three fingers to be placed between the upper and lower central incisor teeth.

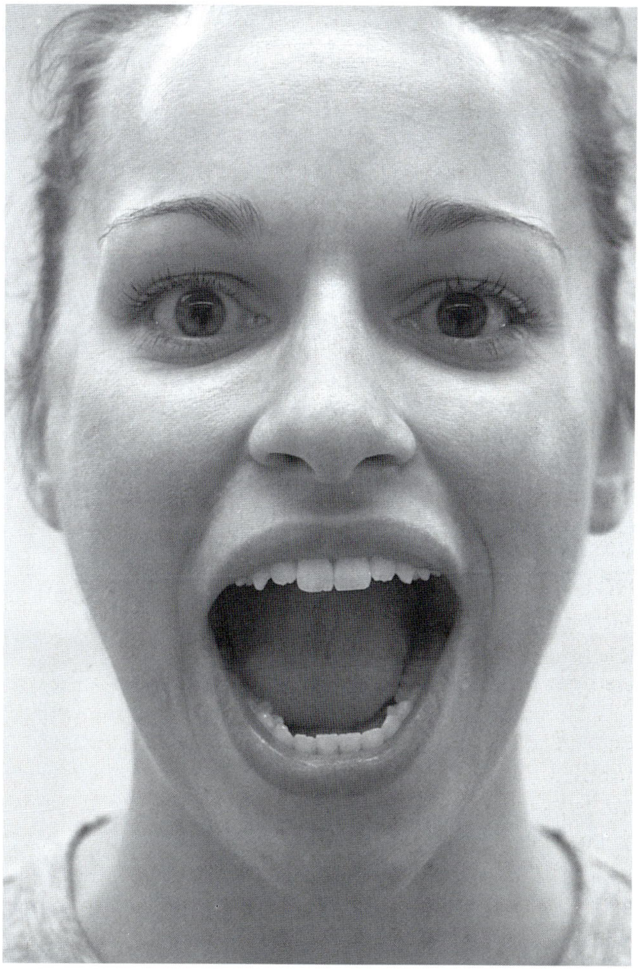

FIGURE 13.9 Normal maximal active mouth opening.

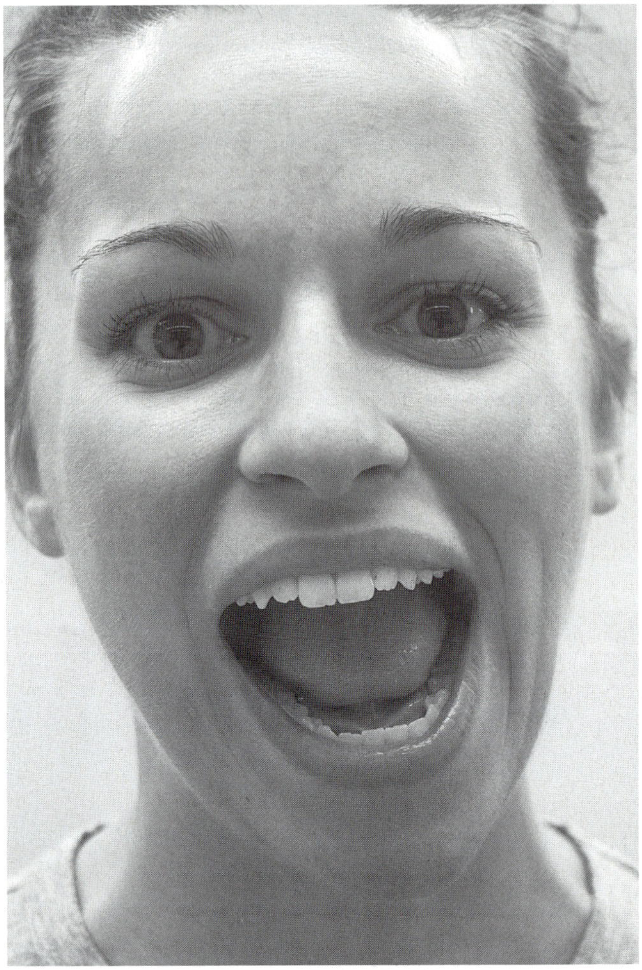

FIGURE 13.10 Abnormal mouth opening with lateral deviation to the left.

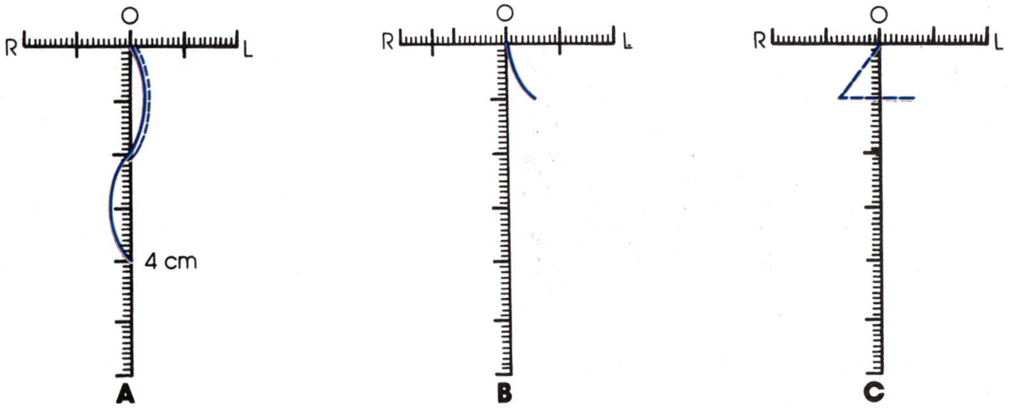

FIGURE 13.11 Examples of recording temporomandibular motions. (A) Lateral deviation R and L on opening, maximal opening is 4 centimeters; lateral excursions are equal and 1 centimeter in each direction; protrusion on functional opening (*dashed line*). (B) Opening limited to 1 centimeter; deviation to the left on opening; lateral excursion greater to the R than to L. (C) Protrusion is 1 centimeter; lateral deviation to R on protrusion (indicates weak pterygoid on opposite side). Adapted from Magee, DJ: Orthopedic Physical Assessment, ed 4. WB Saunders, Philadelphia, 2002:195; with permission.

Testing Motions

Passive Mouth Opening

Grasp the mandible so that it fits between the thumb and the index finger, and pull the mandible inferiorly (Fig. 13.12). The individual may assist with the motion by opening the mouth as far as possible. The end of the motion occurs when resistance is felt and attempts to produce additional motion cause the head to nod forward (cervical flexion).

Normal End-Feel

The end-feel is firm owing to stretching of the joint capsule; retrodiscal tissue; the temporomandibular ligament; and the masseter, temporalis, and medial pterygoid muscles.[6,7]

Measurement Method

Use a millimeter ruler to measure the vertical distance between the edge of the upper central incisor and the corresponding edge of the lower central incisor. The correct ruler placement is shown in Figure 13.13.

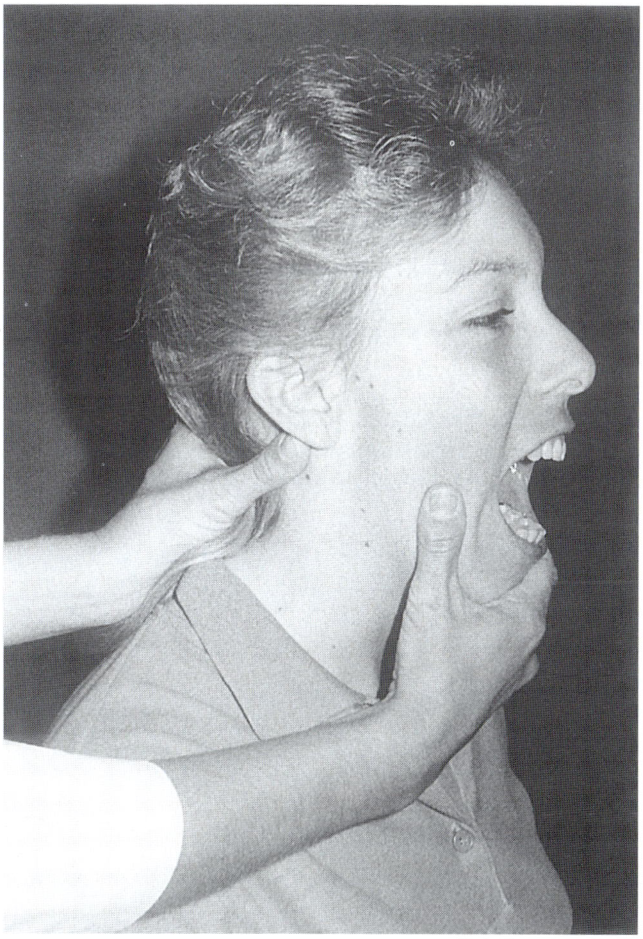

FIGURE 13.12 At the end of passive mandibular depression (mouth opening), one of the examiner's hands maintains the end of the range of motion by pulling the jaw inferiorly. The examiner's other hand holds the back of the individual's head to prevent cervical motion.

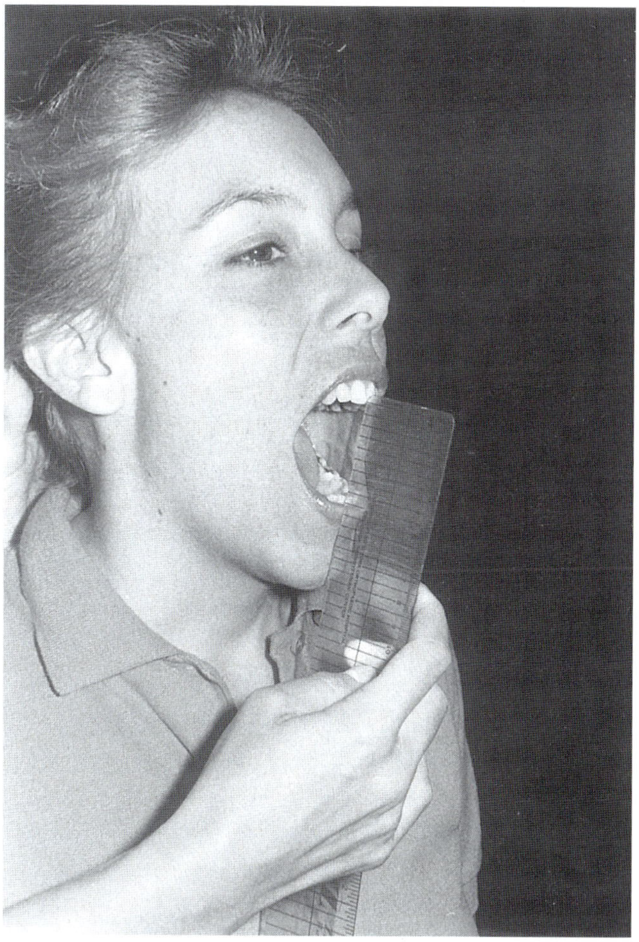

FIGURE 13.13 Use a millimeter ruler to measure the vertical distance between the edge of a lower central incisor and the edge of the opposing upper central incisor to measure mouth opening.

OVERBITE

Overbite, which is the amount that the upper teeth extend over the lower teeth when the mouth is closed, is usually added to the mouth opening measurements. This addition provides a more accurate measurement of mouth opening ROM, especially in persons with a large overbite. Most normal values published from research studies add the amount of overbite to mouth-opening values as recommended by the RDC/TMD criteria.

Measurement Method

When the individual's mouth is closed, use a nontoxic marking pencil to make a horizontal line on the lower central incisors at the bottom edge of the overlapping upper central incisors[14] (Fig. 13.14). After the line is drawn and the person's mouth is opened, measure the amount of overbite between the horizontal line and upper edge of the mandibular central incisors (Fig. 13.15).

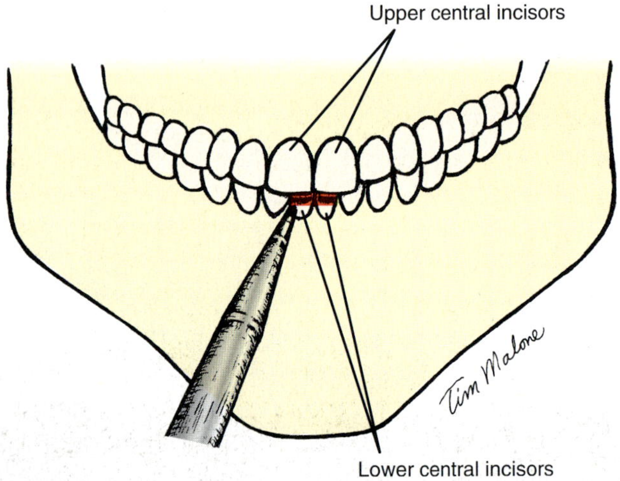

FIGURE 13.14 To measure the amount of overbite, use a nontoxic marking pencil to draw a horizontal line across the lower central incisors where the upper central incisors overlap when the mouth is closed.

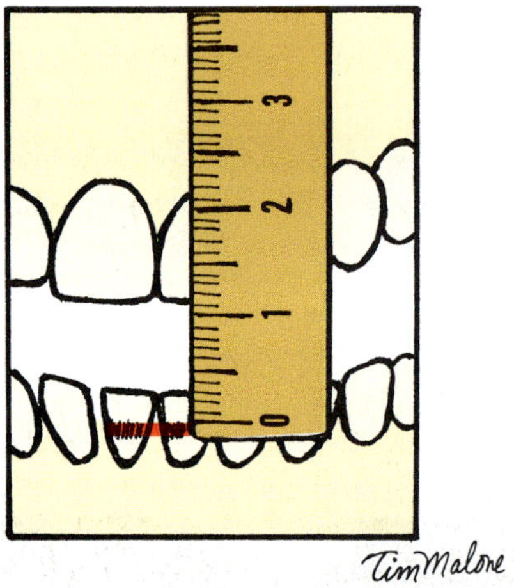

FIGURE 13.15 Ask the individual to open the mouth slightly so that it is possible to measure the amount of overbite as the distance from the horizontal line drawn on the lower central incisors to the top edge of the lower incisors.

PROTRUSION OF THE MANDIBLE

Protrusion of the mandible is a translatory motion that occurs in the transverse plane. Normally, the lower central incisor teeth are able to protrude 6 to 9 millimeters beyond the upper central incisor teeth. However, the normal ROM for adults ranged from 3 millimeters in one study[7] to 10 millimeters in another.[6] See Table 13.2 in the Research Findings section for additional normal values and the effects of age and gender on ROM.

Testing Position

Place the individual sitting, with the cervical spine in 0 degrees of flexion, extension, lateral flexion, and rotation. The TMJ is opened slightly.

Stabilization

Stabilize the posterior aspect of the head and neck to prevent flexion, extension, lateral flexion, and rotation of the cervical spine.

Testing Motions

Active Protrusion

Have the individual push the lower jaw as far forward as possible without moving the head forward.

Passive Protrusion

Grasp the mandible between the thumb and the fingers from underneath the chin. The individual may assist with the movement by pushing the chin anteriorly as far as possible. The end of the motion occurs when resistance is felt and attempts at additional motion cause anterior motion of the head (Fig. 13.16).

Normal End-Feel

The end-feel is firm owing to stretching of the joint capsule; stylomandibular and sphenomandibular ligaments; and the temporalis, masseter, digastric, stylohyoid, mylohyoid, and geniohyoid muscles.[3,7]

Measurement Method

Measure the distance between the lower central incisor and the upper central incisor teeth with a tape measure or ruler (Fig. 13.17). Alternatively, two vertical lines drawn on the upper and lower canines or lateral incisors may be used as the landmarks for measurement.[14]

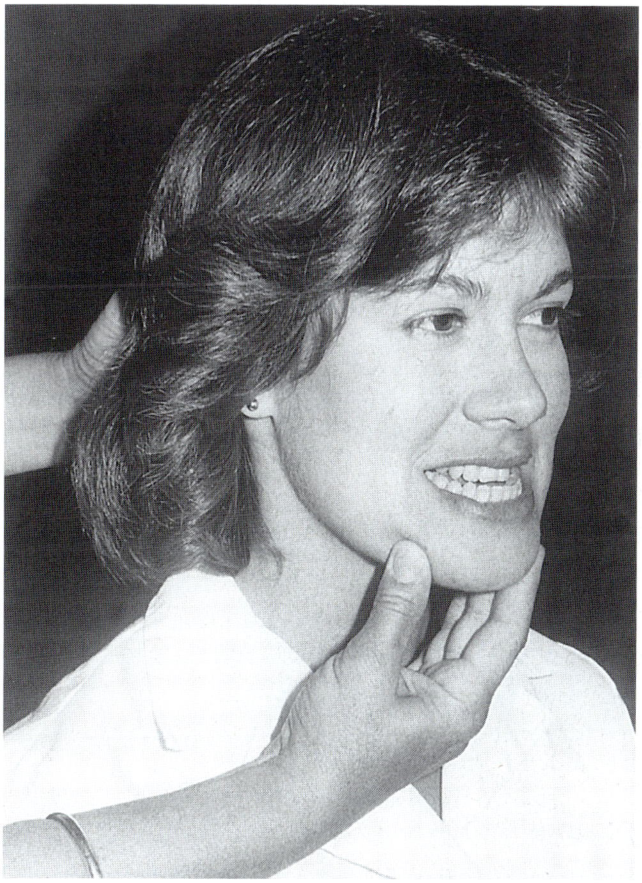

FIGURE 13.16 At the end of passive mandibular protrusion range of motion, the examiner uses one hand to stabilize the posterior aspect of the individual's head while her other hand moves the mandible into protrusion.

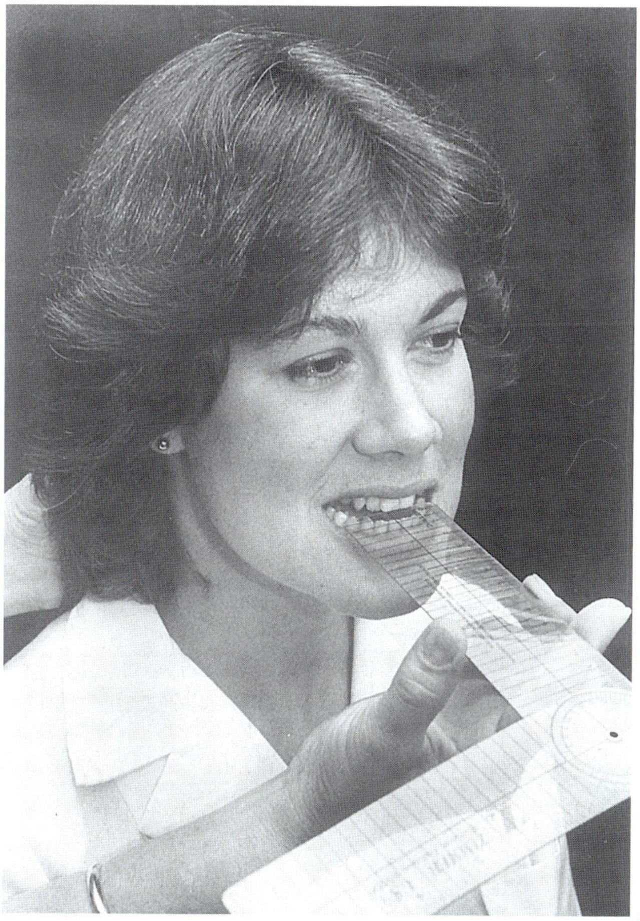

FIGURE 13.17 At the end of mandibular protrusion range of motion, the examiner uses the end of a plastic goniometer to measure the distance between the individual's upper and lower central incisors. The individual maintains the end of range position.

LATERAL EXCURSION OF THE MANDIBLE

This translatory motion occurs in the transverse plane. The amount of lateral movement to the right and left sides is not usually symmetrical, and there is some evidence that movement to the left is greater than to the right.[15] The normal ROM for adults is between 10 and 12 millimeters, as shown in one study,[2] but may range from 10 to 15 millimeters, as shown in another.[7] According to the consensus judgment of the Permanent Impairment Conference,[12] the normal ROM is between 8 and 12 millimeters. See Table 13.2 in the Research Findings section for additional normal values and the effects of age and gender on ROM.

Testing Position

Place the individual sitting, with the cervical spine in 0 degrees of flexion, extension, lateral flexion, and rotation. The TMJ is opened slightly so that the upper and lower teeth are not touching prior to the start of the motion.

Stabilization

Stabilize the posterior aspect of the head and neck to prevent flexion, extension, lateral flexion, and rotation of the cervical spine.

Testing Motions

Active Lateral Excursion

Have the individual slide the lower jaw as far to the right as possible. Have the individual move the lower jaw as far to the left as possible.

Passive Lateral Excursion

Grasp the mandible between the fingers and the thumb and move it to the side. The end of the motion occurs when resistance is felt and attempts to produce additional motion cause lateral cervical flexion (be careful to avoid depression, elevation, and protrusion and retrusion during the movement; Fig. 13.18).

Normal End-Feel

The normal end-feel is firm owing to stretching of the joint capsule; the temporomandibular ligaments; and the temporalis and medial and lateral pterygoid muscles.

Measurement Method

Measure the lateral distance between the center of the lower incisors and the center of the upper central incisors with a millimeter ruler (Fig. 13.19). The distance that the mandible has moved laterally in relation to the maxilla is evident by comparing the position of the upper and lower central incisors in Figures 13.19 and 13.20.

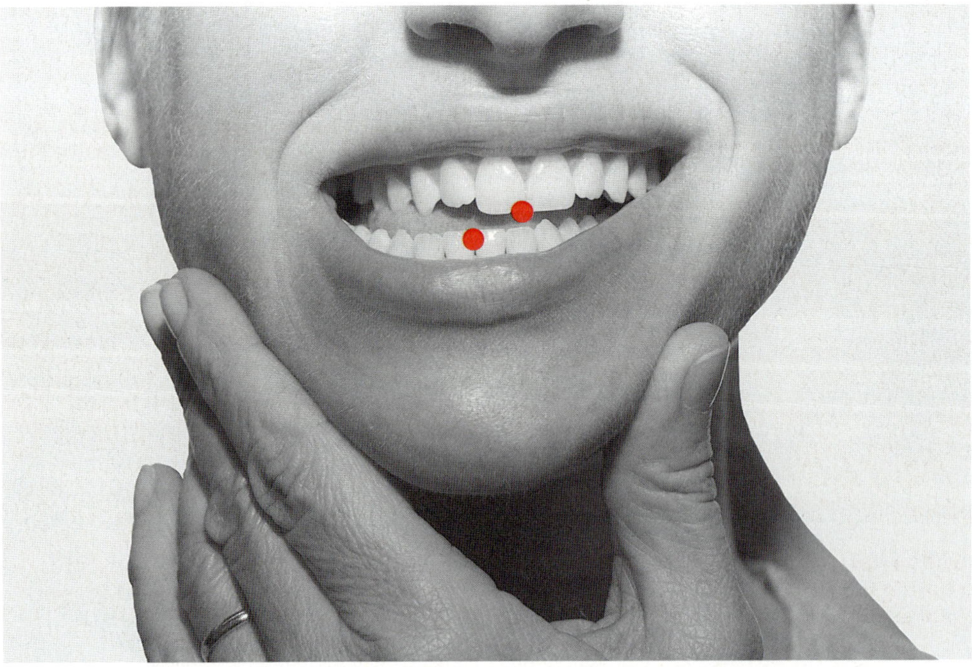

FIGURE 13.18 At the end of passive mandibular lateral excursion range of motion, the examiner uses one hand to prevent cervical motion and the other hand to maintain a lateral pull on the mandible.

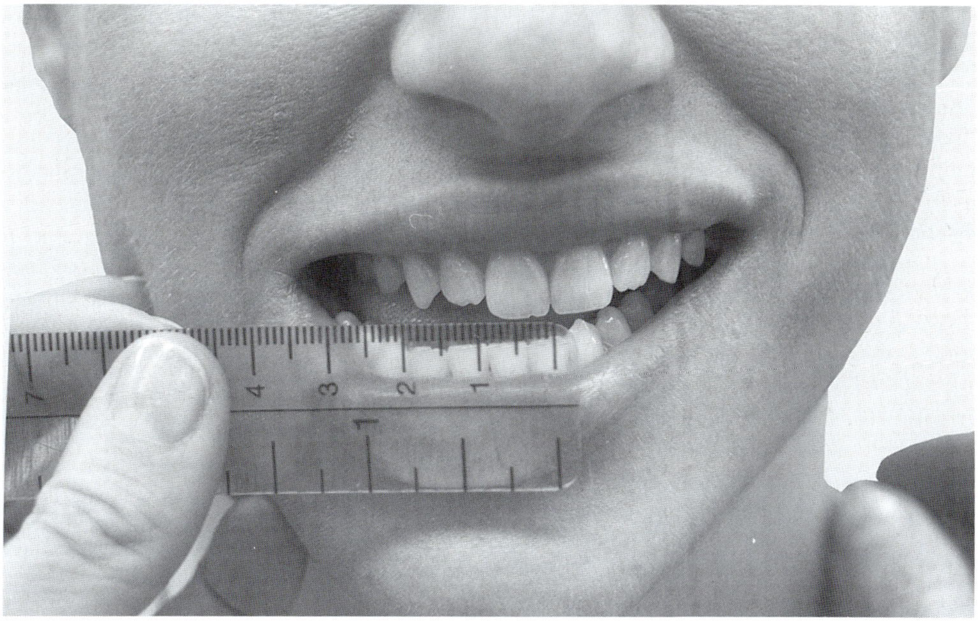

FIGURE 13.19 The examiner uses a millimeter ruler to measure the lateral distance between the center of the two upper incisors and the center of the two low incisors. Align the ruler with the upper incisors first because these teeth have not moved during the motion.

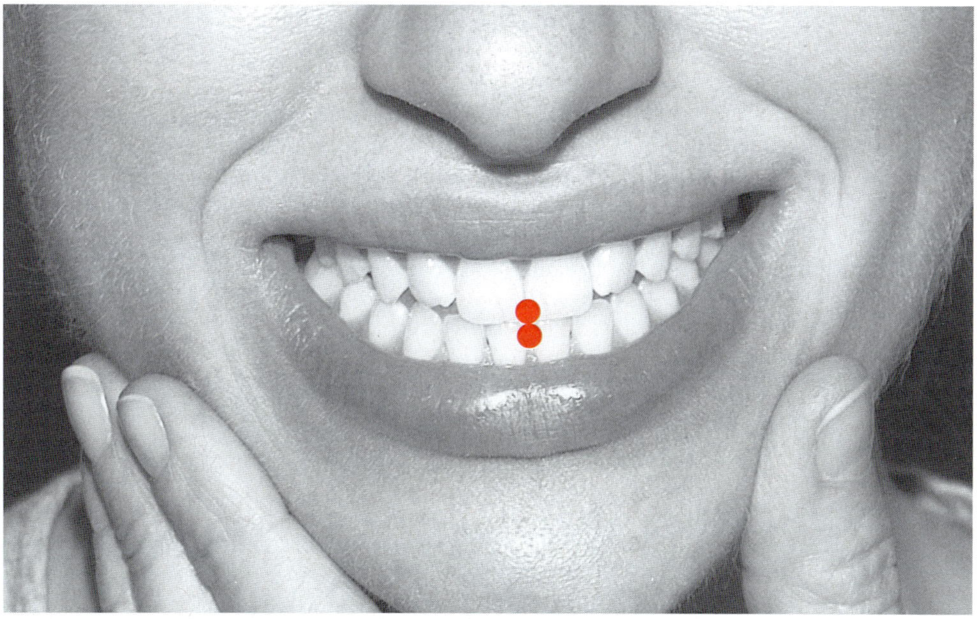

FIGURE 13.20 Note the difference between the alignment of the lower and upper central incisors in the neutral position compared with alignment of these incisors at the end of lateral excursion as shown in Figures 3.18 and 3.19.

Research Findings

The search for normative ROM values for TMJ joint motions is ongoing and includes various age-groups of males and females in different populations and ethnic groups. A sampling of these studies is included in this section and in the sections that follow on the effects of age and gender on TMJ ROM.

In one of the few studies conducted to determine reference values for children, Cortese, Oliver, and Biondi[16] found that the normal range of mouth opening in boys and girls with a mean age of 4.6 years was 38.6 millimeters. For children in the study with a mean age of 6.9 years, the ROM was found to be 42.0 millimeters. Hirsch and colleagues,[17] in a study involving children and adolescents 10 to 17 years old, found that the mean ROM for mouth opening was 50.6 millimeters.

Normal values for maximum active mouth opening ROM are shown in Table 13.1. Normal mean values for the ROM in protrusion and lateral excursive motions are presented from four sources in Table 13.2.

Effects of Age, Gender, and Other Factors

Age

Temporomandibular joint ROM in children tends to show an increase in ROM as age increases between the ages of 3 and 17 years.[16,17] Similar to other areas of the body, the ROM in adults tends to decrease rather than increase as age increases from 16 or 17 years onward. As with other areas of the body, some TMJ motions appear to be affected by age more than other TMJ motions in both adults and children.

Cortese, Oliver, and Biondi[16] determined ROM values in a sample of 212 boys and girls aged 3 to 11 years. The ROM in mouth opening and lateral excursion was found to be smaller in young children (3 to 4 years) compared with slightly older children (11 years), but no change in protrusion ROM was observed.

Machedo, Medeiros, and de Felicio[18] used digital calipers to measure the range of mandibular motion in 240 Brazilian children in three different age-groups (6 to 8 years, 8 to 10 years, and 10.1 to 12 years). Mean values for the entire sample were 44.5 millimeters for maximum mandibular opening; 7.7 millimeters for lateral excursion to the right; 7.0 millimeters for lateral excursion to the left; and 7.5 millimeters for protrusion. A gradual increase in the range of mandibular movements occurred with significant differences mainly between 6 and 8 years and 10.1 and 12 years. No differences were found between genders.

In a population-based study involving 1,011 German male and female children and adolescents between 10 and 17 years, Hirsch and colleagues[17] also found an increase in the ROM of some motions as age increased. A significant difference occurred between maximum active mouth opening in the 10- to 13-year-old group compared with the 14- to 17-year-old group, with the older adolescent group having a greater range of mouth opening. The authors determined that maximal unassisted mouth opening increased by 0.4 millimeters per year of age. Lateral excursion and protrusion also were influenced by age, with lateral excursion increasing 0.1 millimeters per year of age, whereas protrusion decreased 0.1 millimeter per year of age.

Gallagher and coworkers[22] conducted a population-based study of mouth opening in 1,513 Irish adults aged 16 to 99 years. In this study, maximum mouth opening showed a decrease in ROM from 45 millimeters in the 16- to 24-year-old group of males to 41 millimeters in the 65- to 99-year-old group of males. In fact, active ROM in all TMJ motions except for retrusion decreased with increasing age in the 100 subjects in the study. However, as noted, the loss of ROM was only 4 millimeters.

TABLE 13.1 Maximum Active Mouth Opening ROM in Subjects Aged 10 to 99 Years: Normal Linear Distance in Millimeters*

Author	Hirsch et al[17]	Marklund and Wänman[19]	Goulet et al[20]	Celic et al[21]	Gallagher et al[22]		Turp et al[15]	
	Males and females, German	Males and females, Swedish	Males and females	Males, Croatian	Males and females, Irish		Males and females, German	
	10–17 yr	18–48 yr	Mean age 29 yr	19–28 yr	16–99 yr		Mean age 26.1 yr	
					Males	Females	Males	Females
Sample	*n* = 1011	*n* = 371	*n* = 36	*n* = 60	*n* = 657	*n* = 856	*n* = 58	*n* = 83
	Mean (SD)	**Mean (SD)**	**Mean (SD)**	**Mean (SD)**	**Mean**	**Mean**	**Mean (SD)**	**Mean (SD)**
ROM	50.6 (6.4)	55.3 (6.1)	52.6 (6.3)	50.8 (5.0)	43	41	58.6 (7.1)	54.6 (7.9)

SD = Standard deviation.

*All measurements were obtained with a millimeter ruler, and all measurements include the amount of overbite except for measurements taken by Gallagher et al.

TABLE 13.2 Mandibular Protrusion and Lateral Excursion Range of Motion: Normal Linear Distance in Millimeters*

Author	Hirsch et al[17]	Celic et al[21]	Walker et al[14]	Turp et al[15]	
Sample	486 males and 525 females 10–17 yr *n* = 1011	Males and females 19–28 yr *n* = 60	3 males and 12 females 21–61 yr *n* = 15	Males and females Mean age = 26.1 yr *n* = 141 Male female	
Motion	***Mean (SD)***	***Mean (SD)***	***Mean (SD)***	***Mean (SD)***	***Mean (SD)***
Protrusion	8.2 (2.5)	7.9 (2.5)	7.1 (2.3)	—	
Left lateral excursion	10.6 (2.3)	10.1 (3.0)	8.6 (2.1)	12.1 (2.3)	11.5 (2.4)
Right lateral excursion	10.2 (2.2)	10.0 (2.8)	9.2 (2.6)	11.0 (2.6)	10.9 (2.1)

SD = Standard deviation.

* All measurements were obtained with a millimeter ruler.

In contrast to the preceding studies, Hassel, Rammelsberg, and Schmitter,[23] in a comparison of ROM between a group of 44 young adults aged 18 to 45 years and a group of 43 elderly patients aged 68 to 96 years, found that mouth-opening ROM did not decrease from the youngest to the oldest groups. However, the ROM in protrusion and lateral excursion followed the normal pattern and decreased from the youngest to the oldest group.

Gender

A definite gender difference appears to be present in adults aged 16 to 99 years, with males having larger ROM in mouth opening than females.[24,25] Studies also have found that male adults have a larger ROM in lateral excursion than females.[15] Furthermore, Hirsch and colleagues[17] detected a gender effect in 10- to 17-year-olds, with males having a significantly larger (1.8 millimeters) ROM in maximum active mouth opening than females. However, according to Cortese, Oliver, and Biondi,[16] the gender effect on mouth opening does not appear to be present in young children 3 to 11 years of age.

Gallagher and coworkers,[22] in a study of mouth opening in 1,513 Irish males and females, determined that the 657 males aged 16 to 99 years had greater maximum active mouth-opening ROM compared with the 856 females in the study. Lewis, Buschang, and Throckmorton[25] found that the healthy 26-year-old males in their study had significantly greater mouth-opening ROM (mean = 52.1 millimeters) than females (mean = 46.0 millimeters).

Mandibular Length

The ROM in mouth opening appears to be related to the length of the mandible. Dijkstra and colleagues,[26] in a study of mouth opening in 13 females and 15 males, found that the linear distance between the upper and the lower incisors during mandibular depression was significantly influenced by mandibular length. In a subsequent study, Dijkstra and associates[27] investigated the relationship between incisor distances, mandibular length, and angle of mouth opening in 91 healthy subjects (59 women and 32 men) ranging from 13 to 56 years of age (mean 27.2 years). Mouth opening was influenced by both mandibular length and angle of mouth opening. Therefore, it is possible that subjects with the same mouth-opening distance may differ from one another in regard to TMJ mobility. Lewis, Buschang, and Throckmorton[25] found that mandibular length accounted for some of the gender differences in mouth opening and for most of the gender differences in condylar translation in mouth opening.

To adjust for mandibular length, Miller and coworkers[28] developed a "mouth-opening index," called the temporomandibular opening index (TOI), which was determined by using the following formula: TOI = (PO – MVO/PO + MVO) × 100, in which PO is passive opening, and MVO refers to maximal voluntary opening. In a subsequent study, Miller and associates[29] compared the TOI in patients with a temporomandibular disorder (TMD) with the TOI in a control group of individuals without TMDs. Based on the results of the study, the authors concluded that the TOI appeared to be independent of age, gender, and mandibular length. Moipolai, Karic, and Miller,[30] in a study of 42 asymptomatic individuals, used analysis of covariance to assess the association between the TOI and age, gender, ramus length, and gonial angle. No relationship between the variables and the TOI was found. In a more recent study, Miller, Karic, and Myers[31] found that the TOI was able to distinguish between two groups of patients with myogenous TMD, a finding that should make the TOI valuable as a diagnostic tool.

Head and Neck Positions and Motions

Head and neck positions and motions are closely linked with mouth opening and closing movements. Also, the ROM of mouth opening is affected by the static position of the head and neck, so examiners need to be aware of the individual's head and neck position during measurements of the TMJ. According to Zafar,[9,10] there is a functional linkage between the temporomandibular and craniocervical regions, with head and neck extension movements being an integral part of natural active mouth opening and head and neck flexion being an integral part of mouth closing.

Higbie and associates[32] investigated the effects of static head positions (forward, neutral, and retracted) on mouth opening in 20 healthy males and 20 healthy females between 18 and 54 years of age. Mouth-opening ROM measured with a millimeter ruler was significantly different among the three positions. Mouth opening was greatest (mean = 44.5 millimeters, standard deviation [SD] = 5.3) in the forward head position, which includes extension of the upper cervical region; it was less in the neutral head position (mean = 41.5 millimeters, SD = 4.8); and it was least (mean = 36.2 millimeters, SD = 4.5) in the retracted head position, which includes cervical flexion. Day-to-day reliability was found to vary from a Pearson correlation coefficient r value of 0.90 to 0.97, depending on head position, and the standard error of measurement (SEM) ranged from 0.77 to 1.69 millimeters, also depending on head position. As a result of the findings, the authors concluded that the head position should be controlled when mouth-opening measurements are taken. However, the authors found that an error of 1 to 2 millimeters occurred regardless of the position in which the head was placed.

Temporomandibular Disorders

The structure of the TMJs and the fact that these joints get so much use predispose these joints, associated ligaments, and musculature to injury, mechanical problems, and degenerative changes. For example, the articular disc may become entrapped, deformed, or torn; the capsule may become thickened; the ligaments may become shortened or lengthened; and the muscles may become inflamed, contracted, and hypertrophied. These problems may give rise to a variety of symptoms and signs that are included in the temporomandibular disorders (TMD) classification.

According to the American Dental Association, TMD refers to a group of disorders characterized by TMJ pain, TMJ sounds during mandibular motion, and restriction of mandibular motion in both mouth opening and in lateral and protrusive motion.[33] Additional symptoms include muscular pain and deviation of mandibular movement during opening, which is defined as displacement of the mandible at least 2 millimeters to the right or left of the middle. Although TMD is often found in adults, the signs and symptoms of TMDs are found in up to 87% of children and a higher frequency of TMD appears to occur in females in puberty; a reduction in prevalence rates occurs after menopause. The latter finding suggests that female hormones may play a role in the disorder.

Other signs and symptoms include facial pain; muscular pain[34]; tenderness in the region of the TMJ, either unilaterally or bilaterally; headaches; and stiffness of the neck. Also, TMDs appear to be more prevalent in females of all ages after puberty, although the actual percentage of women affected varies among investigators.[34]

Possible reasons for a gender preference have been attributed to a number of factors including, among others, greater stress levels in women, hormonal influences, and habits of adolescent girls that are extremely harmful to the temporomandibular joints (e.g., intensive gum chewing, continuous arm leaning, ice crushing, nail biting, biting foreign objects, jaw play, clenching, and bruxism).[35–39]

In a 2012 study of 424 6- to 8-year-old boys and girls by Vierola and colleagues at the University of Eastern Finland,[40] the authors found that 226 children (53%) had experienced pain in the lower limbs and head during the past 3 months. Pain was most prevalent in the lower limbs (35%) and head (32%). No gender differences were found.

Karibe and investigators[41] examined 160 young patients who were divided into the following three groups (6–12 years), (13–15 years) and (16–18 years). No significant gender differences were found except for headache and neck pain in group three. Pain intensity and tightness in the jaw/face, headache and neck pain as well as ADL difficulty in prolonged jaw opening, eating soft or hard food, and sleeping differed among the three groups with late adolescents having higher pain intensity in the facial region and greater difficulty in ADLs.

A retrospective chart review of TMJ magnetic resonance imaging was conducted by Su and colleagues[42] to determine disc and bone changes in former patients. The authors found that disc changes were more prevalent in adolescents, whereas bone changes were more prevalent in the elderly patients. Anterior disc displacement was the most common finding and was most prevalent in adolescents.

Between September 2011 and December 2011, Bagis and investigators physically examined 243 consecutive patients (171 females and 72 males, mean age 41) and had the patients complete a questionnaire regarding limited mouth opening.[43] The most common symptom in both genders was pain in the temporal muscle followed by pain during mouth opening (89%). Temporomandibular joint pain in the masseter muscle, clicking and grinding, and antidepressant use were more frequent in females than in males. Increased age and missing teeth had significant adverse effects on prevalence of temporomandibular disorders.

A number of studies have investigated TMJ disorders in populations of children, adolescents, and elderly individuals.[17,20,21,31,34–39,44–46] Celic and colleagues[21] investigated the range of mandibular movements in a young male population of 180 patients with TMD disorders and 60 control subjects. A significant difference was found in maximal active mouth opening and active lateral excursion and protrusion between the controls and patients with TMD. Studies in the review by de Sena[34] reported prevalence in signs and symptoms varying from 3% to 53% for TMJ tenderness, from 5% to 81% for muscular tenderness, from 8% to 48% for joint sounds, and from 2% to 63% for restricted mouth opening. According to these authors, TMD needs to be better evaluated in the population because if diagnosed late, it may progress to a state of irreversible destruction of the intracapsular structures of the TMJ and perhaps cause abnormal craniofascial growth and mandibular dysfunction in adulthood.[34]

Cooper and Kleinberg[47] reviewed the records of 4,528 men, women, and children patients between the ages of 11 and

70 years and found that the prevalence of TMDs was highest between the ages of 21 and 50 years. The authors also found a gender difference in that 77% of the patients were females.

In a study of 114 males and 194 female university students with a mean age of 23 years, Marklund and Wänman[19] found that the persistence of signs and symptoms over the period of a year was higher in female students (77%). However, the 1-year incidence of TMJ signs and symptoms (12%) was not significantly different between men and women.

A great deal of the recent literature has been devoted to temporomandibular dysfunction in various populations worldwide. Schmid-Schwap and colleagues,[48] in a study of 404 females with a mean age of 41 (range of 12 to 96 years) and 98 males with a mean age of 41 (range of 16 to 78 years), found that the females showed significantly higher pain intensity and a significantly lower degree of mouth opening than did the males. Also, palpation of the masticatory muscles and the TMJ revealed that the females had significantly higher tenderness than did the males. In addition, the females had a different age distribution of TMD in that they had peaks of prevalence in the age-group below 25 years and in the group aged from 55 to 60 years, whereas the males had a more even age distribution.

Goncalves and coworkers[49] found that out of a total of 230 inhabitants aged 15 to 65 years, 39% reported at least one symptom of TMD. Pain was noted by 25% of the population and sounds in the TMJ were the most common symptom, followed by TMJ pain and masticating muscle pain.

In a systematic review of the literature performed to determine the diagnostic accuracy of clinical tests used for the identification of temporomandibular joint disorders, Reneker and coinvestigators found that only three studies out of seven were of high quality.[50] All seven studies used tests such as joint sounds or joint movements but no studies investigated TMD versus a non-TMD condition. The authors concluded that owing to the lack of clear findings in the articles that would lead to a diagnosis of TMD, there was insufficient evidence to support or reject the tests being used.

Reliability and Validity

As is the case in other areas of the body, some TMJ motions appear to be more reliably measured than other motions in both asymptomatic and symptomatic subjects. Mouth opening (active and passive) measured with a millimeter ruler as the vertical distance between the upper and lower central incisors has consistently demonstrated good to excellent reliability (see Table 13.3).[14,20,53] Measurements of protrusion have also shown good reliability, but lateral excursion has consistently shown poor to good reliability.[25,48,50–53]

Walker, Bohannon, and Cameron[14] determined that all six TMJ motions measured with a millimeter ruler were reliable. Two testers took measurements at three sessions, each of which was separated by a week. The 30 subjects who were measured included 15 patients with a TMD (13 females and 2 males with a mean age of 35.2 years) and 15 subjects without a TMD (12 females and 3 males with a mean age of 42.9 years). The intratester reliability intraclass correlation coefficients (ICCs) for tester 1 ranged from 0.82 to 0.99, and the intratester reliability for tester 2 ranged from 0.70 to 0.90. However, only mouth-opening measurements had construct validity and were useful for discriminating between subjects with and without TMDs. The technical error of measurement (difference between measurements that would have to be exceeded if the measurements were to be truly different) was 2.5 millimeters for the mouth-opening measurement in subjects without a TMD.

Higbie and associates[32] also found that ROM measurements of mouth opening were highly reliable with the use of a millimeter ruler. Two examiners measured 20 males and 20 females with a mean age of 32.9 years. Intratester, intertester, and test-retest reliability ICCs ranged from

TABLE 13.3 Intertester Reliability of Mandibular Measurements Using a Millimeter Ruler

Author	Goulet et al[20]	Walker et al[14]	Walker et al[14]	John et al[53]
Testers Sample	5 experienced 10 males and 62 females; 36 patients with TMD and 36 without TMD Mean age 29 yr *n* = 72	2 experienced 2 male and 13 female patients with TMD 20–52 yr *n* = 15	2 experienced 3 males and 12 females without TMD 21–61 yr *n* = 15	4 experienced 11 patients with TMD and 25 without TMD 17–71 yr *n* = 36
Motion	***ICC***	***ICC***	***ICC***	***ICC***
Mouth opening	0.87	0.99	0.98	0.93
Right lateral excursion	0.59	0.96	0.90	0.73
Left lateral excursion	0.68	0.94	0.95	0.79
Protrusion	—	0.98	0.95	0.91

ICC = Intraclass correlation coefficient; TMD = Temporomandibular disorder.

0.90 to 0.97, depending on head position. Standard error of measurement values indicated that an error of 1 to 2 millimeters existed for the measurement technique used in the study.

Kropmans and colleagues[51] found similar high reliability in a study of mouth opening involving 5 male and 20 female patients with painfully restricted TMJs. Intratester, intertester, and test-retest reliability varied between 0.90 and 0.96. However, in contrast to the findings of Walker, Bohannon, and Cameron[14] and those of Higbie and associates,[32] the authors found that the smallest detectable difference of maximal mouth opening in this group of subjects varied from 9 to 6 millimeters. Based on these results, a clinician would have to measure at least 9 millimeters of improvement in maximal mouth opening in this group of patients to say that improvement had occurred.

Reliability appears to be improved when examiners participate in a calibration training program in which examiners are calibrated to a standardized set of examination procedures and criteria, as described by the RDC/TMD.[52,53] Lobbezoo and colleagues[54] found that calibration training resulted in good to excellent interexaminer reliability of both active and passive mouth-opening measurements and protrusion ROM. Only lateral excursion ROM measurements had fair interexaminer reliability.

In a study by Leher and colleagues,[55] no significant difference was found in the reliability of ROM measurements between inexperienced dental students and experienced practitioners who had participated in a calibration program. The authors concluded that calibration training was more important than experience. However, both groups had unacceptable reliability scores for lateral excursive motions. Lausten, Glaros, and Williams[56] compared novice and expert examiners' ability to measure TMJ ROM following calibration training. The novices were able to measure maximum active mouth-opening ROM with a high degree of reliability, but, similar to Leher's results, neither group was able to measure lateral excursive motions reliably.

Baltran-Alocreu and colleagues[57] conducted a study of 50 asymptomatic adults designed to determine the inter- and intrarater reliability of mandibular ROM measurements taken with the individual positioned in a neutral supine craniocervical position. Two raters measured maximum mouth opening, protrusion, and lateral excursion using a craniomandibular scale (described as a thin plastic device) that allows assessment of the mandibular motions of lateral excursion and protrusion in two phases. Results showed that intratester reliability was excellent for maximum mouth opening and protrusion (ICC = 0.99–0.93) and moderate for both lateral excursion measurements (ICC = 0.77–0.62). Interrater reliability for maximal mouth opening and protrusion were excellent (ICC range = 0.96–0.92); however, lateral excursion ICC values were in the moderate range (ICC = 0.71–0.51). The SEM for mouth opening ranged from 0.74 to 0.82 millimeters and protrusion SEM ranged from 0.29 to 0.49 millimeters. The authors suggest that studies be conducted using the craniocervical position with individuals who have been diagnosed with temporomandibular disorders.

REFERENCES

1. Hoover, D, and Ritzline, P: The Temporomandibular Joint. In Levangie, PK, and Norkin, CC: Joint Structure and Function: A Comprehensive Analysis, ed 5. FA Davis, Philadelphia, 2011.
2. Iglarsh, ZA, and Synder-Mackler, L: The Temporomandibular Joint and the Cervical Spine. In Richardson, JK, and Iglarsh, ZA (eds): Clinical Orthopaedic Physical Therapy. WB Saunders, Philadelphia, 1994.
3. Williams, PL: Gray's Anatomy, ed 38. Churchill Livingstone, New York, 1995.
4. Neumann, DA: Kinesiology of the Musculoskeletal System: Foundations for Physical Rehabilitation, ed 2, Mosby, Inc., St. Louis, 2010.
5. Otis, CA: Kinesiology: The Mechanics and Pathomechanics of Human Movement. Lippincott Williams & Wilkins, Philadelphia, 2004.
6. Harrison, AL: The Temporomandibular Joint. In Malone, TR, McPoil, T, and Nitz, AJ (eds): Orthopedic and Sports Physical Therapy, ed 3. CV Mosby, St. Louis, 1997.
7. Magee, DJ: Orthopedic Physical Assessment, ed 4. WB Saunders, Philadelphia, 2002.
8. Cailliet, R: Soft Tissue Pain and Disability, ed 3. FA Davis, Philadelphia, 1996.
9. Zafar, H, Nordh, E, and Eriksson, PO: Temporal coordination between mandibular and head-neck movements during jaw opening-closing tasks in man. Arch Oral Biol 45:675, 2000.
10. Zafar, H: Integrated jaw and neck function in man. Studies of mandibular and head-neck movements during jaw opening-closing tasks. Swed Dent J 143(Suppl):1, 2000.
11. Eriksson, PO, et al: Co-ordinated mandibular and head-neck movements during rhythmic jaw activities in man. J Dent Res 79:1378, 2000.
12. Phillips, DJ, et al: Guide to evaluation of permanent impairment of the temporomandibular joint. Cranio 15(2):170, 1996.
13. Dworkin, SF, and Le Resche, L: Research diagnostic criteria for temporomandibular disorders. J Craniomandib Disord 6:301, 1992.
14. Walker, N, Bohannon, RW, and Cameron, D: Discriminant validity of temporomandibular joint range of motion measurements obtained with a ruler. J Orthop Sports Phys Ther 30:484, 2000.
15. Turp, JC, Alpaslan, C, and Gerds, T: Is there a greater mandibular movement capacity towards the left? Verification of an observation from 1921. J Oral Rehabil 32:242, 2005.
16. Cortese, SG, Oliver, LM, and Biondi, AM: Determination of mandibular movements in children without temporomandibular disorders. J Craniomandibular Pract 25:200, 2007.
17. Hirsch, C, et al: Mandibular jaw movement capacity in 10–17-yr-old children and adolescents: Normative values and the influence of gender, age, and temporomandibular disorders. Eur J Oral Sci 114:465, 2006.
18. Machedo, BCZ, Medeiros, APM, de Felicio, CM: Limites de movimentos mandibulares cm criancas [Mandibular movement in children]. Pro Fono 21(3):189, 2009.
19. Marklund, S, and Wänman, A: Incidence and prevalence of temporomandibular joint pain and dysfunction: A one-year prospective study of university students. Acta Odontol Scand 65:119, 2007.
20. Goulet, J-P, et al: The reproducibility of muscle and joint tenderness detection methods and maximum mandibular movement measurement for the temporomandibular system. J Orofacial Pain 12:17, 1998.
21. Celic, R, et al: Measurement of mandibular movement in patients with temporomandibular disorders and in asymptomatic subjects. Coll Antropol 2(Suppl):43, 2003.
22. Gallagher, C, et al: The normal range of mouth opening in an Irish population. J Oral Rehabil 31:110, 2004.
23. Hassel, AJ, Rammelsberg, P, and Schmitter, M: Inter-examiner reliability in the clinical examination of temporomandibular disorders: Influence of age. Community Dent Oral Epidemiol 34:41, 2006.
24. Thurnwald, PA: The effect of age and gender on normal temporomandibular joint motion. Physiother Theory Pract 7:209, 1991.
25. Lewis, RP, Buschang, PH, and Throckmorton, GS: Sex differences in mandibular movements during opening and closing. Am J Orthod Dentofacial Orthop 120:294, 2001.
26. Dijkstra, PU, et al: Temporomandibular joint mobility assessment: A comparison between four methods. J Oral Rehabil 22:439, 1995.
27. Dijkstra, PU, et al: Influence of mandibular length on mouth opening. J Oral Rehabil 26:117, 1999.
28. Miller, VJ, et al: A mouth opening index for patients with temporomandibular disorders. J Oral Rehabil 26:534, 1999.
29. Miller, VJ, et al: The temporomandibular opening index (TOI) in patients with closed lock and a control group with no temporomandibular disorders (TMD): An initial study. J Oral Rehabil 27:815, 2000.
30. Moipolai, P, Karic, VV, and Miller, VJ: The effect of gonial angle, ramus length, age and gender on temporomandibular opening index. J Oral Rehabil 30:1195, 2003.
31. Miller, VJ, Karic, VV, and Myers, SL: Differences in initial symptom scores between myogenous TMD patients with high and low TOI scores. J Craniomandibular Pract 24:25, 2006.
32. Higbie, EJ, et al: Effect of head position on vertical mandibular opening. J Orthop Sports Phys Ther 29:127, 1999.
33. Esposito, CJ, Panucci, PJ, and Farman, AG: Associations in 425 patients having temporomandibular disorders. J Kentucky Med Assoc 98:213, 2001.
34. De Sena, MF, et al. Prevalence of temporomandibular dysfunction in children and adolescents. Rev Paul Pediatr 31(4):1538, 2013.
35. Gavish, A, et al: Oral habits and their association with signs and symptoms of temporomandibular disorders in adolescent girls. J Oral Rehabil 27:22, 2000.
36. Winocur, E, et al: Oral habits among adolescent girls and their association with symptoms of temporomandibular disorders. J Oral Rehabil 28:624, 2001.
37. Rauhala, K, et al: Facial pain and temporomandibular disorders: An epidemiological study of the northern Finland 1966 birth cohort. J Craniomandibular Pract 18:40, 2000.
38. Kutilla, M, et al: TMD treatment need in relation to age, gender, stress and diagnostic subgroup. J Orofac Pain 12:67, 1998.
39. Warren, MP, and Fried, JL: Temporomandibular disorders and hormones in women. Cells Tissues Organs 169:187, 2000.
40. Vierola, A, et al: Clinical signs of temporomandibular disorders and various pain conditions among children 6–8 years of age: The PANIC study. J Orofac Pain 26(1):17, 2012.
41. Karibe, H, et al: Comparison of subjective symptoms of TMD's in young patients by age and gender. 1 Cranio 30(2):14, 2012.
42. Su, N, et al: TMJ changes in adolescent TMD patients seen on MRI in a clinical setting. N Y State Dent J 81(3):27, 2015.
43. Bagis, B, et al: Gender differences in prevalence of signs and symptoms of temporomandibular disorders: A retrospective study of 243 consecutive patients. Int J Med Sci 9(7):539, 2012.
44. Sonmez, H, et al: Prevalence of temporomandibular dysfunction in Turkish children with mixed and permanent dentition. J Oral Rehabil 28:280, 2001.
45. Alamoudi, N, et al: Temporomandibular disorders among school children. J Clin Pediatr Dent 22:323, 1998.
46. Nilsson, IM: Reliability, validity, incidence and impact of temporomandibular pain disorders in adolescents. Swed Dent J 183(Suppl):7, 2007.
47. Cooper, BC, and Kleinberg, I: Examination of a large patient population for the presence of symptoms and signs of temporomandibular disorders. J Craniomandibular Pract 25:115, 2007.
48. Schmid-Schwap, M, et al: Sex-specific differences in patients with temporomandibular disorders. J Orofac Pain 27(1):42, 2013.
49. Goncalves, DA, et al: Symptoms of temporomandibular disorders in the population: An epidemiological study. J Orofac Pain 24(3):270, 2010.
50. Reneker, J, et al: Diagnostic accuracy of clinical tests and signs of temporomandibular joint disorders: A systematic review of the literature. J Orthop Sports Phys Ther 41(6):408, 2011.
51. Kropmans, T, et al: Smallest detectable difference of maximal mouth opening in patients with painfully restricted temporomandibular joint function. Eur J Oral Sci 108:9, 2000.
52. List, T, et al: Recalibration improves inter-examiner reliability of TMD examination. Acta Odontol Scand 64:146, 2006.
53. John, MT, and Zwignenberg, AJ: Interobserver variables in assessment of signs of TMD. Int J Prosthodontics 14:265, 2001.
54. Lobbezoo, F, et al: Use of the research diagnostic criteria for temporomandibular disorders for multinational research: Translation efforts and reliability assessments in the Netherlands. J Orofac Pain 19:301, 2005.
55. Leher, A, et al: Is there a difference in the reliable measurement of temporomandibular disorder signs between experienced and inexperienced examiners? J Orofac Pain 19:58, 2005.
56. Lausten, LL, Glaros, AC, and Williams, K: Inter-examiner reliability of physical assessment methods for assessing temporomandibular disorders. Gen Dent 52:509, 2004.
57. Baltran-Alocreu, H, et al: Intra-rater and inter-rater reliability of mandibular range of motion measures considering a neutral craniocervical position. J Phys Ther Sci 26(6):915, 2014.

APPENDIX A

NORMATIVE RANGE OF MOTION VALUES

TABLE A.1 Shoulder, Elbow, Forearm, and Wrist Motion: Mean Values in Degrees

Author	Wanatabe et al*[1]	Boone and Azen[2]	Green and Wolf[3]	Walker et al[4]	Macedo and Magee[5]	AAOS[6]	AMA[7]
	0–2 yr *n* = 45	1–54 yr *n* = 109 M	18–55 yr *n* = 20 (10 M, 10 F)	65–85 yr *n* = 60 (30 M, 30 F)	18–59 yr *n* = 90 F		
Motion							
Shoulder Complex							
Flexion	172–180	167	156	165	188	180	≥180
Extension	78–89	62	—	44	70	60	≥50
Abduction	177–187	184	168	165	188	180	≥170
Medial rotation	72–90	69	49	62	94	70	≥80
Lateral rotation	118–134	104	84	81	108	90	≥60
Elbow and Forearm							
Flexion	148–158	143	145	143	149	150	≥140
Extension	—	1	0	4†	2	0	≥0
Pronation	90–96	76	84	71	92	80	≥80
Supination	81–93	82	77	74	96	80	≥80
Wrist							
Flexion	88–96	76	73	64	93	80	≥60
Extension	82–89	75	65	63	86	70	≥60
Radial deviation	—	22	25	19	18	20	≥20
Ulnar deviation	—	36	39	26	41	30	≥30

AAOS = American Academy of Orthopaedic Surgeons; AMA = American Medical Association; M = Males; F = Females.

All values obtained with a universal goniometer.

* Values in this column represent a range of means.

† Value refers to extension limitation.

TABLE A.2 Glenohumeral Motion: Mean Values in Degrees

Author	Ellenbecker et al[8]	Ellenbecker et al[8]	Boon and Smith[9]	Macedo and Magee[5]	Lannan et al[10]
	11–17 yr *n* = 113 M	11–17 yr *n* = 90 F	12–18 yr *n* = 50 (18 M, 32 F)	18–59 yr *n* = 90 F	21–40 yr *n* = 60 (20 M, 40 F)
Motion					
Glenohumeral					
Flexion	—	—	—	41	106
Extension	—	—	—	27	20
Abduction	—	—	—	85	129
Medial rotation	51	56	63	64	49
Lateral rotation	103	105	108	94	94

M = Males; F = Females.

Values obtained with a universal goniometer.

TABLE A.3 Finger Motions: Mean Values in Degrees

Author	Skarilova and Plevkova*[11]	Mallon et al‡[12]	Smahel and Klimova*[13,14]	Hume et al†[15]	AAOS[6]	AMA[7]
	20–25 yr *n* = 200 (100 M, 100 F)	18–35 yr *n* = 120 (60 M, 60 F)	18–28 yr *n* = 101 (52 M, 49 F)	26–28 yr *n* = 35 M		
Motion						
Finger MCP						
Flexion	91	95	92	100	90	≥90
Extension	26	20	25	—	45	≥20
Finger PIP						
Flexion	108	105	111	105	100	≥100
Extension	—	7	—	0	0	≥0
Finger DIP						
Flexion	85	68	81	85	90	≥70
Extension	—	8	—	0	0	≥0

MCP = Metacarpophalangeal; PIP = Proximal interphalangeal; DIP = Distal interphalangeal; AAOS = American Academy of Orthopaedic Surgeons; AMA = American Medical Association; F = Females; M = Males.

* Values obtained with a metallic slide goniometer on dorsal aspect.

† Values obtained with a computerized Greenleaf goniometer.

‡ Values obtained with a goniometer applied to the dorsal aspect.

TABLE A.4 Thumb Motions: Mean Values in Degrees

Author	Skarilova and Plevkova*[11] 20–25 yr n = 200 (100 M, 100 F)	Skarilova and Plevkova*[11] 20–25 yr n = 200 (100 M, 100 F)	Jenkins et al†[16] 16–72 yr n = 119 (50 M, 69 F)	DeSmet et al‡[17] 16–83 yr n = 101 (43 M, 58 F)	AAOS[6]	AMA[7]
Motion	**Active**	**Passive**	**Active**			
Thumb CMC						
Abduction	—	—	—	—	70	—
Flexion	—	—	—	—	15	—
Extension	—	—	—	—	20, 80	≥35§
Thumb MCP						
Flexion	57	67	59	54	50	≥60
Extension	14	23	—	—	0	≥0
Thumb IP						
Flexion	79	86	67	80	80	≥80
Extension	23	35	—	—	20	≥10

CMC = Carpometacarpal; MCP = Metacarpophalangeal; IP = Interphalangeal; AAOS = American Academy of Orthopaedic Surgeons; AMA = American Medical Association; M = Males; F = Females.

* Values obtained with a metallic slide goniometer on dorsal aspect.

† Values obtained with a universal goniometer on lateral aspect.

‡ Values obtained with a digital goniometer on dorsal aspect.

§ Range of motion value of 35 degrees is the difference between the minimal angle (15 degrees) of separation between first and second metacarpals and the maximal angle (50 degrees) of separation in what was referred to as radial abduction.

TABLE A.5 Hip and Knee Motions: Mean Values in Degrees

Author	Waugh et al[18] 6–65 hr n = 40	Drews et al[19] 12 hr–6 days n = 54 (26 M, 28 F)	Schwarze and Denton[20] 1–3 days n = 1,000 (473 (M, 527 F)	Wanatabe et al[1] 4 weeks n = 62	Phelps et al[21] 9 mo n = 25 M and F	Boone and Azen[2] 1–54 yr n = 109 M	Roach and Miles[22] 25–74 yr n = 1,683 (821 M, 862 F)	AAOS[6]	AMA[7]
Motion									
Hip									
Flexion	—	—	—	138	—	122	121	120	≥100
Extension	46*	28*†	20*	12*	10*	10	19	20	<10*
Abduction	—	55‡	78‡	51	—	46	42		>25
Adduction	—	6‡	15‡	—	—	27	—		>15
Medial rotation	—	80‡	58	24	52	47	32	45	>20
Lateral rotation	—	114‡	80	66	47	47	32	45	>30
Knee									
Flexion	—	—	150	—	—	142	132	135	≥110
Extension	15*	20*	15*	—	—	—	—	10	<5*

AAOS = American Academy of Orthopaedic Surgeons; AMA = American Medical Association; M = Males; F = Females.

* Values refer to extension limitations.

† Tested with subjects in side-lying position

‡ Tested with subjects in supine position

TABLE A.6 Ankle and Foot Motions: Mean Values in Degrees

Author	Waugh et al[18]	Wanatabe et al[1]	Boone and Azen[2]	McPoil and Cornwall[25]	Mecagni et al[24]	AAOS[6]	AMA[7]
	6–65 hr *n* = 40 (18 M, 22 F)	4–8 mo *n* = 54	1–54 yr *n* = 109 M	26.1 yr *n* = 27 (9 M, 18 F)	64–87 yr *n* = 34 F		
Motion							
Ankle							
Dorsiflexion	59	51	13	16	11	20	>10
Plantar flexion	26	60	56	—	64	50	>20
Inversion	—	—	37	19 (Subtalar)	26	35	>20 (Subtalar)
Eversion	—	—	21	12 (Subtalar)	17	15	>10 (Subtalar)
First MTP							
Flexion	—	—	—	—	—	45	—
Extension	—	—	—	86	—	70	>30

AAOS = American Academy of Orthopaedic Surgeons; AMA = American Medical Association; M = Males; F = Females.
All range of motion values in the table obtained with a universal goniometer.

TABLE A.7 Cervical Spine Motions: Mean Values in Degrees and Centimeters

Author	Youdas et al*[26]						Lantz et al†[27]		Hsieh and Young‡[28]	Balogun et al§[29]		AAOS[6]	AMA[30]
	11–19 yr *n* = 40 (20M, 20F)		30–39 yr *n* = 41 (20 M, 21 F)		70–79 yr *n* = 40 (20 M, 20 F)		20–39 yr *n* = 63		14–31 yr *n* = 34 (27 M, 7 F)	18–26 yr *n* = 21 (15 M, 6 F)			
Motion	**M**	**F**	**M**	**F**	**M**	**F**	**Active**	**Passive**					
Cervical Spine													
Flexion	64	—	47	—	39	—	60	74	1.0 cm	4.3 cm	32	45	50
Extension	86	84	68	78	54	55	56	53	22 cm	19 cm	64	45	60
Right lateral flexion	45	49	43	47	26	28	43	48	11 cm	13 cm	41	45	45
Right rotation	74	75	67	72	50	53	72	79	12 cm	11 cm	64	60	80

AAOS = American Academy of Orthopaedic Surgeons; AMA = American Medical Association; F = Female; M = Male.

* Values in degrees were obtained for active range of motion using the cervical range of motion (CROM) instrument.

† Values in degrees were obtained for active and passive range of motion with use of the OSI CA-6000 Spinal Motion Analyzer.

‡ Values in centimeters were obtained with a tape measure.

§ Values in centimeters obtained with a tape measure appear in the last column, whereas values in degrees obtained with a Myrin gravity-referenced goniometer appear in the second column.

TABLE A.8 Thoracic and Lumbar Spine Motions: Mean Values in Degrees and Centimeters

Author	Haley et al*[30]	Moll and Wright*[32]	Van Adrichem and van der Korst†[32]		Breum et al‡[34]		McGregor et al§[35]		Fitzgerald et al¶[36]	AAOS[6]	AMA[30]
	5–9 yr *n* = 282 (140 M, 142 F)	15–75 yr *n* = 237 (119 M, 118 F)	15–18 yr *n* = 66 (34 M, 32 F)		18–38 yr *n* = 47 (27 M, 20 F)		50–59 yr *n* = 41 (21 M, 20 F)		20–82 yr *n* = 172 (168 M, 4 F)		
Motion			**M**	**F**	**M**	**F**	**M**	**F**			
Thoracolumbar Motions											
Flexion	6–7 cm	5–7 cm	7 cm	6 cm	56	54	55	60	—	80	60
Extension	—	—	—	—	22	21	21	18	16–41	25	25
Right lateral flexion	—	—	—	—	33	31	30	30	18–38	35	25
Right rotation	—	—	—	—	8	8	26	26	—	45	30

AAOS = American Academy of Orthopaedic Surgeons; AMA = American Medical Association; F = Female; M = Male.

* Lumbar values obtained with use of the Modified Schober Test.

† Lumbar values obtained using the Modified-Modified Schober (simplified skin distraction) Test.

‡ Lumbar values in the first column were obtained with the BROM II. Lumbar values in the second column were obtained with double inclinometers.

§ Lumbar values obtained with the OSI CA-6000.

¶ Range of motion (ROM) values for thoracolumbar extension and lateral flexion were obtained with a universal goniometer. Lower values are for those aged 70–79 years and higher values are for those aged 20–29 years.

NB: The AAOS values for thoracolumbar motions were obtained with a universal goniometer. The AMA values were obtained with use of the two-inclinometer method for lumbar motions of flexion, extension, and lateral flexion. The AMA value for rotation is for the thoracic spine.

TABLE A.9 Temporomandibular Motions: Mean Values in Millimeters

Author	Walker et al*[37]	Hirsch et al*[38]		Thurnwald†[39]			
	21–61 yr *n* = 15 (3 M, 12 F)	10–17 yr *n* = 1,011 (486 M, 525 F)		17–25 yr *n* = 50 (25 M, 25 F)		50–65 yr *n* = 50 (25 M, 25 F)	
Motion		**M**	**F**	**M**	**F**	**M**	**F**
Temporomandibular Joint Motions							
Opening	43	51	51	61	55	58	51
Left lateral excursion	9	11	10	9	8	8	6
Right lateral excursion	9	10	10	10	9	7	9
Protrusion	7	8	8	5	5	5	4

* Values were obtained for active range of motion (ROM) with an 11-cm plastic ruler marked in millimeters.

† Values were obtained for active ROM with Vernier callipers as the measuring instrument.

REFERENCES

1. Wanatabe, H, et al: The range of joint motion of the extremities in healthy Japanese people: The differences according to age. (Cited in Walker, JM: Musculoskeletal development: A review. Phys Ther 71:878, 1991.)
2. Boone, DC, and Azen, SP: Normal range of motion of joints in male subjects. J Bone Joint Surg 61:756, 1979.
3. Greene, BL, and Wolf, SL: Upper extremity joint movement: Comparison of two measurement devices. Arch Phys Med Rehabil 70:288, 1989.
4. Walker, JM, et al: Active mobility of the extremities in older subjects. Phys Ther 4:919, 1984.
5. Macedo, LG, and Magee, DJ: Effects of age on passive range of motion of selected peripheral joints in healthy adult females. Physiother Theory Pract 25:145, 2009.
6. American Academy of Orthopaedic Surgeons: Joint Motion: Method of Measuring and Recording. AAOS, Chicago, 1965.
7. Rondinelli, RD (ed): Guides to the Evaluation of Permanent Impairment, ed 6. American Medical Association, Chicago 2008.
8. Ellenbecker, TS, et al: Glenohumeral joint internal and external rotation range of motion in elite junior tennis players. J Orthop Sports Phys Ther 24:336, 1996.
9. Boon, AJ, and Smith, J: Manual scapular stabilization: Its effect on shoulder rotational range of motion. Arch Phys Med Rehabil 81:978, 2000.
10. Lannan, D, Lehman, T, and Toland, M: Establishment of normative data for the range of motion of the glenohumeral joint [master's thesis]. Lowell, University of Massachusetts, 1996.
11. Skarilova, B, and Plevkova, A: Ranges of joint motion of the adult hand. Acta Chir Plast 38:67, 1996.
12. Mallon, WJ, Brown, HR, and Nunley, JA: Digital ranges of motion: Normal values in young adults. J Hand Surg 16:882, 1991.
13. Smahel, Z, and Klimova, A: The influence of age and exercise on the mobility of hand joints 1: Metacarpophalangeal joint of the three-phalangeal fingers. Acta Chir Plast 46:81, 2004.
14. Smahel, Z, and Klimova, A: The influence of age and exercise on the mobility of hand joints 2: Interphalangeal joints of the three-phalangeal fingers. Acta Chir Plast 46:122, 2004.
15. Hume, M, et al: Functional range of motion of the joints of the hand. J Hand Surg 15:240, 1990.
16. Jenkins, M, et al: Thumb joint motion: What is normal? J Hand Surg 23:796, 1998.
17. DeSmett, L, et al: Metacarpophalangeal and interphalangeal flexion of the thumb: Influence of sex and age, relation to ligamentous injury. Acta Orthop Belg 59:37, 1993.
18. Waugh, KG, et al: Measurement of selected hip, knee and ankle joint motions in newborns. Phys Ther 63:1616, 1983.
19. Drews, JE, Vraciu, JK, and Pellino, G: Range of motion of the lower extremities of newborns. Phys Occup Ther Pediatr 4:49, 1884.
20. Schwarze, DJ, and Denton, JR: Normal values of neonatal limbs: An evaluation of 1000 neonates. J Pediatr Orthop 13:758, 1993.
21. Phelps, E, Smith, LJ, and Hallum, A: Normal ranges of hip motion of infants between 9 and 24 months of age. Dev Med Child Neurol 27:785, 1985.
22. Roach, KE, and Miles, TP: Normal hip and knee active range of motion: The relationship of age. Phys Ther 71:656, 1991.
23. Greene, WB, and Heckman, JD (eds): The Clinical Measurement of Joint Motion. American Academy of Orthopaedic Surgeons, Rosemont, IL, 1994.
24. Mecagni, C, et al: Balance and ankle range of motion in community dwelling women aged 64-87 years: A correlational study. Phys Ther 80:1004, 2000.
25. McPoil, TG, and Cornwall, MW: The relationship between static lower extremity measurements and rearfoot motion during walking. Phys Ther 24:309, 1996.
26. Youdas, J, et al: Normal range of motion of the cervical spine: An initial goniometric study. Phys Ther 72:770, 1992.
27. Lantz, CA, Chen, J, and Buch, D: Clinical validity and stability of active and passive cervical range of motion with regard to total and uniplanar motion. Spine 24:1082, 1999.
28. Hsieh, C-Y, and Yeung, BW: Active neck motion measurements with a tape measure. J Orthop Sports Phys Ther 8:88, 1986.
29. Balogun, JA, et al: Inter-and intratester reliability of measuring neck motions with tape measure and Myrin Gravity-Reference Goniometer. J Orthop Sports Phys Ther 9:248, 1989.
30. Cocchiarella, L, and Andersson, GBJ (eds): American Medical Association: Guides to the Evaluation of Permanent Impairment, ed 5. American Medical Association, Chicago 2001.
31. Haley, SM, Tada, WL, and Carmichael, EM: Spinal mobility in young children. Phys Ther 66:1697, 1986.
32. Moll, JMH, and Wright, V: Normal range of spinal mobility: An objective clinical study. Ann Rheum Dis 30:381, 1971.
33. van Adrichem, JAM, and van der Korst, JK: Assessment of flexibility of the lumbar spine. A pilot study in children and adolescents. Scand J Rheumatol 2:87, 1973.
34. Breum, J, Wiberg, J, and Bolton, JE: Reliability and concurrent validity of the BROM II for measuring lumbar mobility. J Manipulative Physiol Ther 18:497, 1995.
35. Mcgregor, AH, MacCarthy, ID, and Hughes, SP: Motion characteristics of the lumbar spine in the normal population. Spine 20:2421, 1995.
36. Fitzgerald, GK, et al: Objective assessment with establishment of normal values for lumbar spine range of motion. Phys Ther 63:1776, 1983.
37. Walker, N, Bohannon, RW, and Cameron, D: Validity of temporomandibular joint range of motion measurements obtained with a ruler. J Orthop Sports Phys Ther 30:484, 2000.
38. Hirsch, C, et al: Mandibular jaw movement capacity in 10–17-yr-old children and adolescents: Normative values and the influence of gender, age, and temporomandibular disorders. Eur J Oral Sci 114:465, 2006.
39. Thurnwald, PA: The effect of age and gender on normal temporomandibular joint movement. Physiother Theory Pract 7:209, 1991.

APPENDIX B

SUMMARY GUIDES FOR MEASURING RANGE OF MOTION

Chapter 4: The Shoulder

Summary Guide for Measuring Shoulder Range of Motion With a Goniometer

Motion	Testing Position	Stabilization	Fulcrum	Proximal Arm Landmarks	Distal Arm Landmarks
Glenohumeral (GH) flexion	Supine, knees flexed; elbow in extension and forearm in neutral with palm facing body; do not abduct the shoulder	Scapula to prevent posterior tilt, upward rotation and elevation	Greater tubercle	Midaxillary line of thorax	Lateral midline of humerus
Shoulder complex flexion	Same as GH flexion	Thorax to prevent extension of spine	Same as GH flexion	Same as GH flexion	Same as GH flexion
GH extension	Prone, face turned away from shoulder being tested; elbow in slight flexion and forearm in neutral with palm facing body; do not abduct the shoulder	Scapula to prevent elevation and anterior tilt	Greater tubercle	Midaxillary line of thorax	Lateral midline of humerus using lateral epicondyle for reference
Shoulder complex extension	Same as GH extension	Thorax to prevent forward flexion of spine	Same as GH extension	Same as GH extension	Same as GH extension
GH abduction	Supine, with shoulder laterally rotated and elbow extended	Scapula to prevent upward rotation and elevation	Anterior aspect of acromion process	Parallel to anterior midline of sternum	Anterior midline of humerus; medial epicondyle may be helpful
Shoulder complex abduction	Same as GH abduction	Thorax to prevent lateral flexion of spine	Same as GH abduction	Same as GH abduction	Same as GH abduction

(table continues on page 544)

Summary Guide for Measuring Shoulder Range of Motion With a Goniometer (continued)

Motion	Testing Position	Stabilization	Fulcrum	Proximal Arm Landmarks	Distal Arm Landmarks
Glenohumeral (GH) medial rotation	Supine, shoulder in 90° abduction and elbow in 90° flexion; palm faces caudally; towel roll under distal humerus to level	Scapula to prevent anterior tilt or protraction	Olecranon process	Perpendicular or parallel to the floor	Lateral midline of ulna using olecranon and ulnar styloid for reference
Shoulder complex medial rotation	Same as GH medial rotation	Distal humerus to maintain 90° of shoulder abduction and 90° of elbow flexion; body weight stabilizes trunk	Same as GH medial rotation	Same as GH medial rotation	Same as GH medial rotation
GH lateral rotation	Same as GH medial rotation	Scapula to prevent posterior tilt or retraction	Same as GH medial rotation	Same as GH medial rotation	Same as GH medial rotation
Shoulder complex lateral rotation	Same as GH medial rotation	Distal humerus to maintain 90° of shoulder abduction and 90° of elbow flexion; body weight and plinth stabilize trunk	Same as GH medial rotation	Same as GH medial rotation	Same as GH medial rotation

GH = Glenohumeral.

Chapter 5: The Elbow and Forearm

Summary Guide for Measuring Elbow and Forearm Range of Motion With a Goniometer

Motion	Testing Position	Stabilization	Fulcrum	Proximal Arm Landmarks	Distal Arm Landmarks
Flexion	Supine, shoulder in neutral; towel roll under distal humerus, forearm in full supination	Humerus to prevent flexion of shoulder	Lateral epicondyle of humerus	Lateral midline of humerus, center of acromial process	Lateral midline of radius, radial head and styloid process
Extension	Same as flexion	Humerus to prevent shoulder extension; pad assists	Same as flexion	Same as flexion	Same as flexion
Pronation	Sitting, shoulder in neutral so arm is next to trunk; elbow in 90° flexion and forearm supported; start with thumb pointing toward ceiling	Distal end of humerus to prevent medial rotation and abduction of shoulder	Lateral and proximal to ulnar styloid process	Parallel to anterior midline of humerus	Dorsal surface of forearm just proximal to styloid processes
Supination	Same as pronation	Distal end of humerus to prevent lateral rotation and adduction of shoulder	Medial and proximal to ulnar styloid process	Parallel to anterior midline of humerus	Ventral surface of forearm just proximal to styloid processes

Chapter 6: The Wrist

Summary Guide for Measuring Wrist Range of Motion With a Universal Goniometer					
Motion	**Testing Position**	**Stabilization**	**Fulcrum**	**Proximal Arm Landmarks**	**Distal Arm Landmarks**
Flexion	Sitting, shoulder, in 90° abduction, elbow in 90° flexion, and forearm in neutral so palm facing the ground; forearm is resting on a supporting surface while the wrist and hand are off; wrist in 0° of radial and ulnar deviation; fingers are relaxed	Radius and ulna to prevent motion of the elbow and forearm	Lateral aspect of wrist over triquetrum	Lateral midline of ulna, using olecranon and ulnar styloid process for reference	Lateral midline of fifth metacarpal
Extension	Same as flexion	Same as flexion	Same as flexion	Same as flexion	Same as flexion
Radial deviation	Sitting, shoulder in 90° abduction, elbow in 90° flexion, and forearm in neutral so palm facing the ground; forearm and hand are resting on supporting surface; wrist in 0° of flexion and extension	Radius and ulna to prevent elbow flexion and motion of the forearm	Dorsal aspect of wrist over the capitate	Dorsal midline of forearm, using lateral epicondyle of humerus as landmark	Dorsal midline of third metacarpal
Ulnar deviation	Same as radial deviation	Radius and ulna to prevent elbow extension and motion of the forearm	Same as radial deviation	Same as radial deviation	Same as radial deviation

Chapter 7: The Hand

Summary Guide for Measuring Hand Range of Motion With a Universal Goniometer					
Motion	**Testing Position**	**Stabilization**	**Fulcrum**	**Proximal Arm Landmarks**	**Distal Arm Landmarks**
Fingers					
Finger MCP flexion	Sitting, forearm and hand on a supporting surface; forearm in 0° supination and pronation; wrist in neutral; MCP joint in 0° abduction and adduction; PIP and DIP joints relaxed	Metacarpal to prevent wrist motion	Dorsal aspect of MCP joint	Dorsal midline of metacarpal	Dorsal midline of proximal phalanx
MCP extension	Same as MCP flexion	Same as MCP flexion	Same as MCP flexion	Same as MCP flexion	Same as MCP flexion
MCP abduction	Sitting, forearm and hand on a supporting surface; forearm in full pronation so palm is facing the floor; wrist in neutral; MCP joint in 0° flexion and extension; PIP and DIP joints extended	Metacarpal to prevent wrist motion	Dorsal aspect of MCP joint	Dorsal midline of metacarpal	Dorsal midline of proximal phalanx
MCP adduction	Same as MCP abduction	Same as MCP abduction	Same as MCP abduction	Same as MCP abduction	Same as MCP abduction

(table continues on page 546)

Summary Guide for Measuring Hand Range of Motion With a Universal Goniometer (continued)

Motion	Testing Position	Stabilization	Fulcrum	Proximal Arm Landmarks	Distal Arm Landmarks
Fingers					
PIP flexion	Sitting, forearm and hand on a supporting surface; forearm in 0° pronation and supination; wrist and MCP joints in neutral	Proximal phalanx to prevent MCP joint motion	Dorsal aspect of PIP joint	Dorsal midline of proximal phalanx	Dorsal midline of middle phalanx
PIP extension	Same as PIP flexion	Same as PIP flexion	Same as PIP flexion	Same as PIP flexion	Same as PIP flexion
DIP flexion	Sitting, forearm and hand on a supporting surface; forearm in 0° pronation and supination; wrist, MCP and PIP joints in neutral	Middle phalanx to prevent PIP joint motion	Dorsal aspect of DIP joint	Dorsal midline of middle phalanx	Dorsal midline of distal phalanx
DIP extension	Same as DIP flexion	Same as DIP flexion	Same as DIP flexion	Same as DIP flexion	Same as DIP flexion
Thumb					
CMC flexion	Sitting, forearm and hand on a supporting surface; forearm in full supination so palm faces ceiling; wrist in neutral; start with thumb in contact with the lateral aspect of the second metacarpal so thumb is in the plane of the hand; MCP and IP joints relaxed	Carpals, distal radius, and ulna to prevent wrist motion	Palmar aspect of first CMC joint	Ventral midline of the radius using radial head and styloid process for reference	Palmar midline of first metacarpal. ROM is difference between angular measurements in starting position and ending position
Alternative CMC flexion	Same as CMC flexion	Same as CMC flexion	Palmar aspect of first CMC joint	Palmar aspect of trapezium and pisiform	Palmar midline of first metacarpal. ROM is difference between angular measurements in starting position and ending position
CMC extension (radial abduction)	Same as CMC flexion	Same as CMC flexion	Same as CMC flexion	Same as CMC flexion	Same as CMC flexion
Alternative CMC extension	Same as CMC flexion	Same as CMC flexion	Same as alternative CMC flexion	Same as alternative CMC flexion	Same as alternative CMC flexion
CMC abduction (palmar abduction)	Sitting, forearm and hand on a supporting surface; forearm and wrist in neutral; start with thumb in contact with the lateral aspect of the second metacarpal, then move perpendicular to plane of the hand; MCP and IP joints in 0° flexion and extension	Carpals and second metacarpal to prevent wrist motion	Junction of midlines of first and second metacarpals—usually lateral aspect of scaphoid or radial styloid process	Lateral midline of second metacarpal	Dorsal midline of first metacarpal
CMC adduction	Same as CMC abduction	Same as CMC abduction	Same as CMC abduction	Same as CMC abduction	Same as CMC abduction

Summary Guide for Measuring Hand Range of Motion With a Universal Goniometer (continued)

Motion	Testing Position	Stabilization	Fulcrum	Proximal Arm Landmarks	Distal Arm Landmarks
Thumb					
MCP flexion	Sitting, forearm and hand on a supporting surface; forearm in full supination so palm is facing ceiling; wrist, CMC, and IP joints in neutral	First metacarpal to prevent wrist motion and CMC flexion	Dorsal aspect of first MCP joint	Dorsal midline of first metacarpal	Dorsal midline of first proximal phalanx
MCP extension	Same as MCP flexion	First metacarpal to prevent wrist motion and CMC extension	Same as MCP flexion	Same as MCP flexion	Same as MCP flexion
IP flexion	Sitting, forearm and hand on a supporting surface; forearm in full supination so palm is facing ceiling; wrist, CMC, and MCP joints in neutral	First proximal phalanx to prevent MCP flexion	Dorsal aspect of first IP joint	Dorsal midline of first proximal phalanx	Dorsal midline of first distal phalanx
IP extension	Same as PIP flexion	First proximal phalanx to prevent MCP extension	Same as IP flexion	Same as IP flexion	Same as IP flexion

MCP = Metacarpophalangeal; PIP = Proximal interphalangeal; DIP = Distal interphalangeal; CMC = Carpometacarpal; IP = Interphalangeal.

Chapter 8: The Hip

Summary Guide for Measuring Hip Range of Motion With a Goniometer

Motion	Testing Position	Stabilization	Fulcrum	Proximal Arm Landmarks	Distal Arm Landmarks
Flexion	Supine, hip in 0° abduction, adduction, and rotation; knees flexed	Pelvis (PSIS) to prevent posterior tilt	Greater trochanter	Lateral midline of pelvis	Lateral epicondyle
Extension	Prone, hip in 0° abduction, adduction, and rotation; knee extended	Pelvis (ASIS) to prevent anterior tilt	Same as flexion	Same as flexion	Same as flexion
Abduction	Supine, hip in 0° flexion, extension, and rotation; knee extended	Pelvis (iliac crest) to prevent lateral tilt (rise)	ASIS	Line from ASIS to ASIS	Anterior midline of femur and patella
Adduction	Supine, hip in 0° flexion, extension, and rotation; knee extended. Abduct the contralateral hip	Pelvis (iliac crest) to prevent lateral tilt (drop)	Same as abduction	Same as abduction	Same as abduction
Medial rotation	Sitting, hip in 90° flexion and 0° abduction; towel roll under distal femur to keep thigh horizontal	Pelvis (iliac crest) to prevent lateral tilt (rise)	Anterior aspect of patella	Perpendicular to floor	Anterior midline of tibia, midway between malleoli
Lateral rotation	Same as medial rotation; contralateral knee flexion to complete ROM	Pelvis (iliac crest) to prevent lateral tilt (drop)	Same as medial rotation	Same as medial rotation	Same as medial rotation

PSIS = Posterior superior iliac spine; ASIS = Anterior superior iliac spine.

Chapter 9: The Knee

Summary Guide for Measurement of Knee ROM With a Universal Goniometer

Motion	Testing Position	Stabilization	Fulcrum	Proximal Arm Landmarks	Distal Arm Landmarks
Flexion	Supine, starting with hip and knee in extension; towel roll under ankle	Allow hip to flex during the motion, but stabilize femur to prevent rotation, abduction, or adduction	Lateral epicondyle of femur	Lateral midline of femur using lateral epicondyle and greater trochanter for reference	Lateral midline of the fibula using the lateral malleolus and fibular head for reference
Extension	Supine, same as starting position for flexion	Stabilize femur to maintain a neutral hip position; do not allow hip to flex	Same as flexion	Same as flexion	Same as flexion

Chapter 10: The Ankle and Foot

Summary Guide for Measuring Ankle, Foot, and Toe Range of Motion With a Universal Goniometer

Motion	Testing Position	Stabilization	Fulcrum	Proximal Arm Landmarks	Distal Arm Landmarks
Ankle					
Ankle dorsiflexion	*Non-weight-bearing:* Sitting with hip and knee flexed 90°; foot in 0° inversion and eversion *Weight-bearing:* Standing on firm surface with hip in neutral rotation; foot in 0° inversion and eversion	Tibia and fibula to prevent hip and knee motion Calcaneus to keep heel in contact with standing surface while knee flexes and moves forward	Lateral malleolus	Lateral midline of fibula using head of fibula for reference	Parallel to lateral midline of fifth metatarsal
Ankle plantarflexion	Same as non-weight-bearing ankle dorsiflexion	Same as non-weight-bearing ankle dorsiflexion	Same as ankle dorsiflexion	Same as ankle dorsiflexion	Same as ankle dorsiflexion
Foot					
Tarsal inversion	Sitting with hip and knee flexed 90°; hip in neutral rotation and abduction	Tibia and fibula to prevent knee extension and hip lateral rotation and abduction	Anterior aspect of ankle midway between malleoli	Anterior midline of lower leg using tibial tuberosity as reference	Anterior midline of second metatarsal
Tarsal eversion	Same as tarsal inversion	Tibia and fibula to prevent knee flexion and hip medial rotation and adduction	Same as tarsal inversion	Same as tarsal inversion	Same as tarsal inversion

Summary Guide for Measuring Ankle, Foot, and Toe Range of Motion With a Universal Goniometer (continued)

Motion	Testing Position	Stabilization	Fulcrum	Proximal Arm Landmarks	Distal Arm Landmarks
Foot					
Subtalar (rearfoot) inversion	Prone with foot over edge of plinth; hip and knee in neutral	Tibia and fibula to prevent lateral hip and knee rotation and hip adduction	Posterior aspect of ankle midway between malleoli	Posterior midline of lower leg	Posterior midline of calcaneus
Subtalar (rearfoot) eversion	Same as subtalar inversion	Tibia and fibula to prevent medial hip and knee rotation and hip abduction	Same as subtalar inversion	Same as subtalar inversion	Same as subtalar inversion
Transverse tarsal (midtarsal) inversion	Sitting with hip and knee flexed 90°; hip in neutral rotation and abduction	Talus and calcaneus to prevent inversion	Anterior aspect of ankle slightly distal to point midway between malleoli	Anterior midline of lower leg using tibial tuberosity as reference	Anterior midline of second metatarsal
Transverse tarsal (midtarsal) eversion	Same as transverse tarsal inversion	Talus and calcaneus to prevent eversion	Same as transverse tarsal inversion	Same as transverse tarsal inversion	Same as transverse tarsal inversion
Toes					
MTP flexion	Supine or sitting with ankle in neutral; MCP joint in 0° abduction and adduction	Metatarsal to prevent plantarflexion of ankle and inversion or eversion of foot	Dorsal aspect of MCP joint	Dorsal midline of metatarsal	Dorsal midline of proximal phalanx
MTP extension	Same as MTP flexion	Metatarsal to prevent dorsiflexion of ankle and inversion or eversion of foot	Same as MTP flexion	Same as MTP flexion	Same as MTP flexion
MTP abduction	Same as MTP flexion	Metatarsal to prevent inversion or eversion of foot	Dorsal aspect of MTP joint	Dorsal midline of metatarsal	Dorsal midline of proximal phalanx
MTP adduction	Same as MTP abduction	Same as MTP abduction	Same as MTP abduction	Same as MTP abduction	Same as MTP abduction
IP flexion	Supine or sitting with ankle, foot, and MCP joint in neutral	Phalanx proximal to joint being tested to prevent ankle, foot, and MTP joint motion	Dorsal aspect of joint being tested	Dorsal midline of phalanx proximal to joint being tested	Dorsal midline of phalanx distal to joint being measured
IP extension	Same as IP flexion	Same as IP flexion	Same as IP flexion	Same as IP flexion	Same as IP flexion

MTP = Metatarsophalangeal; IP = Interphalangeal.

Chapter 11: The Cervical Spine

Summary Guide for Measuring Cervical Spine Range of Motion With a Universal Goniometer

Motion	Testing Position	Stabilization	Fulcrum	Proximal Arm Landmarks	Distal Arm Landmarks
Flexion	Sitting with lumbar spine supported by back of a chair	Shoulder girdle and chest to prevent forward flexion of thoracic spine	External auditory meatus	Either perpendicular or parallel to the ground	Align with base of nares
Extension	Same as flexion	Shoulder girdle and chest to prevent extension of the thoracic spine; a strap across the chest may be used	Same as flexion	Same as flexion	Same as flexion
Lateral flexion	Same as flexion	Shoulder girdle and chest to prevent lateral flexion of thoracic and lumbar spine	Spinous process of C7 vertebra	Perpendicular to the floor over spinous processes of thoracic vertebrae	Align with dorsal midline of head using the occipital protuberance as a reference
Rotation	Same as flexion	Shoulder girdle and chest to prevent thoracic and lumbar spine rotation; a strap across the chest may be used	Center of cranial aspect of the head	Parallel to imaginary line between the right and left acromial processes	Align arm with tip of the nose

Chapter 12: The Thoracic and Lumbar Spine

Summary Guide for Measuring Thoracolumbar Range of Motion With a Tape Measure

Motion	Testing Position	Stabilization	Tape Alignment	Testing Motion	ROM Measurement
Thoracolumbar flexion	Standing upright with feet shoulder width apart, arms relaxed at side, and spine in neutral	Pelvis to prevent anterior tilt	Mark spinous processes of T1 and S2 vertebrae (between PSIS); measure and record distance between T1 and S2	Have individual bend forward slowly, keeping arms relaxed and knees extended; measure and record distance between T1 and S2	Difference between starting and ending distances is the ROM
Thoracolumbar extension	Standing upright with feet shoulder width apart, knees extended, and spine in neutral	Pelvis to prevent posterior tilting		Have individual extend spine backward as far as possible measure and red distance between T1 and S2	

Summary Guide for Measuring Thoracolumbar Range of Motion With a Tape Measure (continued)

Motion	Testing Position	Stabilization	Tape Alignment	Testing Motion	ROM Measurement
Thoracolumbar lateral flexion	Standing with back against wall, feet shoulder width apart, knees extended, and arms relaxed at sides of body	Pelvis to prevent lateral tilting	Mark the individual's thigh at the level of the tip of the individual's middle finger	Have individual bend sideways, keeping both feet on the floor; place a second mark on the individual's thigh at the new position of the tip of the middle finger	Distance between the first and second marks on the thigh is the ROM

ROM = Range of motion; PSIS = Posterior superior iliac spine.

Summary Guide for Measuring Lumbar Range of Motion With Single Inclinometer

Motion	Testing Position	Testing Motion	Retest Motion	ROM Measurement
Lumbar flexion	Standing upright with feet shoulder width apart and knees extended; zero inclinometer on T12 vertebra; inclinometer is in sagittal plane	Have individual bend forward as far as possible while examiner maintains inclinometer on T12; record measurement at the end of the motion	Have individual stand upright and zero inclinometer on S2 (between PSIS). Individual then bends forward again while the examiner maintains inclinometer on S2; record measurement at the end of the motion	Subtract the S2 measurement (hip motion) from the T12 measurement to obtain lumbar flexion ROM
Lumbar extension	Same as flexion	Have individual bend backward as far as possible while examiner maintains inclinometer on T12; record measurement at the end of the motion	Have individual stand upright and zero the inclinometer at S2. Have individual bend backward again as examiner maintains inclinometer on S2; record measurement at the end of motion	Subtract S2 (hip motion) measurement from T12 measurement to obtain lumbar extension ROM
Lateral flexion	Standing upright with feet shoulder width apart; zero inclinometer over T12; inclinometer is in frontal plane	Have individual bend to the side as far as possible without raising heel from the floor while examiner maintains inclinometer on T12; record measurement at end of the motion	Have individual return to upright standing position and zero inclinometer on S2. Have individual bend sideways again while examiner maintains inclinometer at S2; record measurement at the end of the motion	Subtract S2 (hip motion) from the T12 measurement to obtain lateral flexion ROM

ROM = Range of motion.

Chapter 13: The Temporomandibular Joint

Summary Guide for Measuring Temporomandibular Joint Range of Motion With a Tape Measure or Ruler				
Motion	**Testing Position**	**Stabilization**	**Testing Motion**	**ROM Measurement**
Mouth opening	Sitting with cervical spine in neutral	Posterior aspect of head and neck to prevent motion of the cervical spine	Open mouth with no lateral mandibular motion	Measure vertical distance between edge of the upper central incisor and edge of the corresponding lower central incisor with a millimeter ruler
Mandibular protrusion	Sitting with cervical spine in neutral and TMJ slightly open	Posterior aspect of head and neck to prevent motion of the cervical spine	Extend lower jaw forward as far as possible without moving head forward	Measure distance between lower central incisor and upper central incisor with a ruler
Lateral excursion of mandible	Sitting with cervical spine in neutral and TMJ slightly open	Posterior aspect of head and neck to prevent motion of the cervical spine	Slide mandible as far as possible to the right and then to the left	Measure lateral distance between the center of the lower incisor and the center of the upper incisors with a ruler

TMJ = Temporomandibular joint.

APPENDIX C

JOINT MEASUREMENTS BY BODY POSITION

Joint/Body Region	Position			
	Prone	*Supine*	*Sitting*	*Standing*
Shoulder	Extension	Flexion Abduction Medial rotation Lateral rotation		
Elbow		Flexion		
Forearm			Pronation Supination	
Wrist			All motions	
Hand			All motions	
Hip	Extension Lateral rotation* Medial rotation*	Flexion Abduction Adduction	Medial rotation Lateral rotation	
Knee		Flexion		
Ankle and foot	Subtalar inversion Subtalar eversion	Dorsiflexion Plantar flexion Inversion Eversion Midtarsal inversion Midtarsal eversion	Dorsiflexion Plantar flexion Inversion Eversion Midtarsal inversion Midtarsal eversion	
Toes		All motions	All motions	
Cervical spine		Rotation†	Flexion Extension Lateral flexion Rotation	
Thoracolumbar spine			Rotation	Flexion Extension Lateral flexion Rotation†‡
Temporomandibular joint			All motions	

* Alternative position.

† Measurement position using single inclinometer.

‡ Measurement position using double inclinometer.

APPENDIX D

NUMERICAL RECORDING FORMS

- Range of Motion—Upper Extremity
- Range of Motion—Hand
- Range of Motion—Lower Extremity
- Range of Motion—Temporomandibular Joint and Spine
- Muscle Length

Range of Motion—Upper Extremity

Patient's Name: ______________________________ Date of Birth ____________

Left				Right		
			Date			
			Examiner's Initials			
			Shoulder Complex			
			Flexion			
			Extension			
			Abduction			
			Medial Rotation			
			Lateral Rotation			
			Comments:			
			Glenohumeral			
			Flexion			
			Extension			
			Abduction			
			Medial Rotation			
			Lateral Rotation			
			Comments:			
			Elbow and Forearm			
			Flexion			
			Supination			
			Pronation			
			Comments:			
			Wrist			
			Flexion			
			Extension			
			Ulnar Deviation			
			Radial Deviation			
			Comments:			

Range of Motion—Hand

Patient's Name: ______________________ Date of Birth ____________

Left				Right		
			Date			
			Examiner's Initials			
			Thumb			
			CMC Flexion			
			CMC Extension			
			CMC Abduction			
			CMC Opposition			
			MCP Flexion			
			IP Flexion			
			Index Finger			
			MCP Flexion			
			MCP Extension			
			MCP Abduction			
			PIP Flexion			
			DIP Flexion			
			Middle Finger			
			MCP Flexion			
			MCP Extension			
			MCP Radial Abduction			
			MCP Ulnar Abduction			
			PIP Flexion			
			DIP Flexion			
			Ring Finger			
			MCP Flexion			
			MCP Extension			
			MCP Abduction			
			PIP Flexion			
			DIP Flexion			
			Little Finger			
			MCP Flexion			
			MCP Extension			
			MCP Abduction			
			PIP Flexion			
			DIP Flexion			
			Comments:			

Range of Motion—Lower Extremity						
Patient's Name: ______				Date of Birth ______		
Left				Right		
			Date			
			Examiner's Initials			
			Hip			
			Flexion			
			Extension			
			Abduction			
			Adduction			
			Medial Rotation			
			Lateral Rotation			
			Knee			
			Flexion			
			Ankle & Foot			
			Dorsiflexion			
			Plantarflexion			
			Tarsal Inversion			
			Tarsal Eversion			
			Subtalar Inversion			
			Subtalar Eversion			
			Midtarsal Inversion			
			Midtarsal Eversion			
			Great Toe			
			MTP Flexion			
			MTP Extension			
			MTP Abduction			
			IP Flexion			
			Toe ____			
			MTP Flexion			
			MTP Extension			
			MTP Abduction			
			PIP Flexion			
			DIP Flexion			
			Comments:			

Range of Motion—Temporomandibular Joint and Spine

Patient's Name: ______________________________ Date of Birth ____________

Left				Right		
			Date			
			Examiner's Initials			
			Temporomandibular Joint			
			Depression (opening)			
			Overbite			
			Protrusion			
			Lateral Excursion			
			Comments:			
			Cervical Spine			
			Flexion			
			Extension			
			Lateral Flexion			
			Rotation			
			Comments:			
			Thoracolumbar Spine			
			Flexion			
			Extension			
			Lateral Flexion			
			Rotation			
			Comments:			
			Lumbar Spine			
			Flexion			
			Extension			
			Lateral Flexion			
			Comments:			

Muscle Length

Patient's Name: ____________________ Date of Birth ____________

Left				Right		
			Date			
			Examiner's Initials			
			Upper Extremity			
			Biceps Brachii			
			Triceps Brachii			
			Flexor Digitorum Profundus and Superficialis			
			Extensor Digitorum, Indicis, and Digiti Minimi			
			Lumbricals, Palmar and Dorsal Interossei			
			Comments:			
			Lower Extremity			
			Hip Flexors—Thomas Test			
			Rectus Femoris—Ely Test			
			Hamstrings—SLR			
			Hamstrings—Distal Hamstring Length Test			
			Tensor Fascia Lata—Ober Test			
			Tensor Fascia Lata—Modified Ober Test			
			Gastrocnemius—Non-weight-bearing			
			Gastrocnemius—Weight-bearing			
			Comments:			

Index

Page numbers followed by "f" denote figures, "t" denote tables, and "b" denote boxes.

D

E

H

I

J

K

L

T

U

V

W

Z